SURGERY

Official Publication

SOCIETY OF UNIVERSITY SURGEONS

SOCIETY FOR VASCULAR SURGERY

Editors in Chief

Editorial Board

Editors Emeritus

Volume 75

January—June, 1974

THE C. V. MOSBY COMPANY
St. Louis

VOLUME 75

Printed in the United States of America

Volume 75 *Number* 1

SURGERY

CONTENTS, JANUARY, 1974

ORIGINAL COMMUNICATIONS

page 1 **Protective effect of glycogen and glucose on the anoxic arrested heart.** Robert L. Hewitt, M.D., David M. Lolley, M.D., George A. Adrouny, Ph.D., *and* Theodore Drapnas, M.D., *New Orleans, La.*

11 **Cardiorespiratory effects of hypertonic glucose in the critically ill patient.** Frank Pindyk, M.D., Michael R. Drucker, M.D., Robert S. Brown, M.D., *and* William C. Shoemaker, M.D., *New York, N. Y.*

20 **Strangulated obturator hernia.** Stephen W. Gray, Ph.D., John E. Skandalakis, M.D., Ph.D., F.A.C.S., Raul E. Soria, M.D., *and* Joseph S. Rowe, Jr., M.D., *Atlanta, Ga.*

28 **Stress at vascular anastomosis in relation to host artery: Synthetic graft diameter,** C. E. Kinley, M. D., F.R.C.S.(C), P. E. Paasche, B.Sc., A. S., MacDonald, M.D., F.R.C.S.(C), *and* A. E. Marble, M.Eng., P.Eng., *Halifax, Nova Scotia, Canada*

continued on page 7

Vol. 75, No. 1, January, 1974. SURGERY is published monthly by the C. V. Mosby Company, 11830 Westline Industrial Drive, St. Louis, Mo. 63141.

Annual subscription rates.

	U. S.	*Canada, Mexico*	*Other countries*
Institutional*	$29.00	$32.00	$32.75
Personal†	$21.00	$24.00	$24.75
Student, intern, resident†	$14.70	$17.70	$18.45

Single copies are $3.50 postpaid. Remittances should be made by check, draft, post office or express money order, payable to this Journal.

*Institutional (multiple-reader) subscriptions are available to public and private libraries, schools, hospitals, and clinics; city, county, state, provincial, and national government bureaus and departments; and all commercial and private institutions and organizations.

†Personal subscriptions and all student-rate subscriptions must be in the names of, billed to, and paid by individuals.

Subscriptions may begin at any time.

Second class postage paid at St. Louis, Mo. Printed in the U. S. A.

Our line expands to meet your needs

New
PARKE-DAVIS
ReadiFlex®
THIGH-HIGH STYLE
Hospital Elastic Stockings

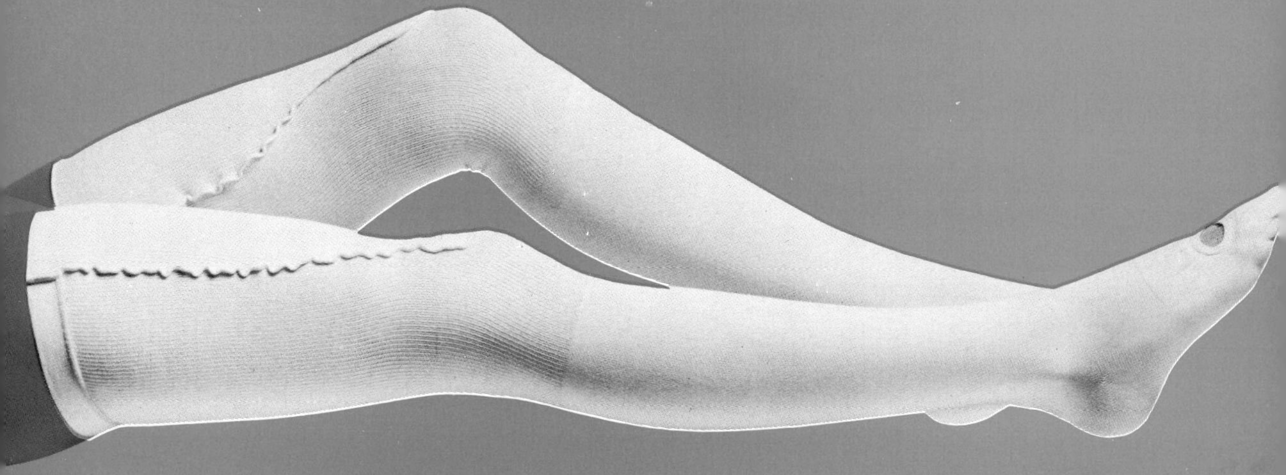

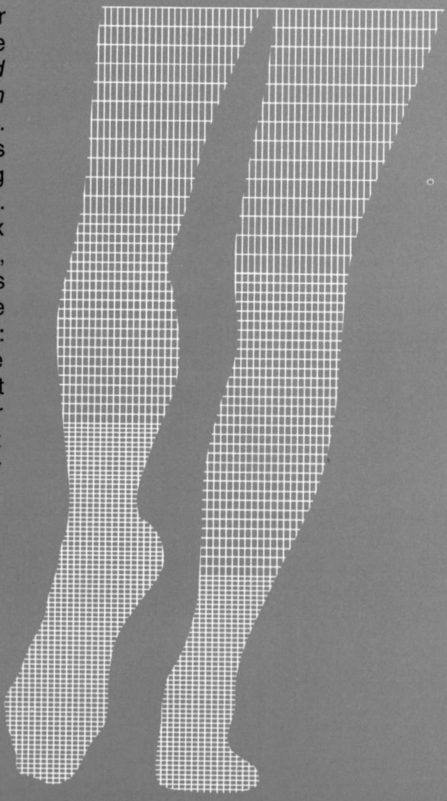

Now you can offer your patients the big advantage of ReadiFlex *controlled graduated compression* from ankles to thighs. Dependable control is woven into the stocking and stays in.

When you specify ReadiFlex Hospital Elastic Stockings, you select products designed to provide these important advantages:

- comfortable fit for the patient
- will not bind or overly constrict
- easy to fit and apply
- closed-toe styling with convenient viewing port
- also available in knee length—open or closed toe—and in new light-weight closed toe
- color coded for proper size identification
- may be machine washed and dried
- Spandex content means excellent life when cared for as directed.

Available through surgical supply dealers. Write for name of your nearest dealer.

Medical-Surgical Products Division
PARKE, DAVIS & COMPANY,
Detroit, Michigan 48232

PD-JA-0967-1-MS (5-73)

CONTENTS *continued*

page 31 **Surgical correction of advanced fibromuscular dysplasia of the renal arteries.** Folkert O. Belzer, M.D., Oscar Salvatierra, M.D., Dorothee Perloff, M.D., *and* Henry Grausz, M.D., *San Francisco, Calif.*

38 **Rewriting and the by-line: Is the author the writer?** Lois DeBakey, Ph.D., *Houston, Texas*

49 **The transplanted parathyroid gland: Evaluation of cryopreservation and other environmental factors which affect its function.** Samuel A. Wells, Jr., M.D., *and* Christine Christiansen, B.S., *Bethesda, Md.*

56 **Colon perforation associated with steroid therapy.** Sylvester Sterioff, M.D., Mark B. Orringer, M.D., *and* John L. Cameron, M.D., *Baltimore, Md.*

59 **Nomarski differential-interference contrast microscopy: Application in dermal wound healing studies.** T. N. Salthouse, F.I.M.L.T., F.R.P.S., *Somerville, N. J.*

64 **Reticuloendothelial dysfunction and endotoxemia following portal vein occlusion.** Isik Olcay, M.D., Akio Kitahama, M.D., Robert H. Miller, M.D., Theodore Drapanas, M.D., Rafael A. Trejo, M.D., Ph.D., *and* N. R. Di Luzio, Ph.D., *New Orleans, La.*

71 **Comparative efficacy of hypo-, iso-, and hypertonic sodium solutions in experimental burn shock.** Charles L. Fox, Jr., M.D., *and* John W. Stanford, M.S., *New York, N. Y.*

80 **Anatomic control of vertebral arteriovenous fistulas.** Thomas W. Kornmesser, M.D., *and* John J. Bergan, M.D., *Chicago, Ill.*

87 **Deglutition after resection of oral, laryngeal, and pharyngeal cancers.** Raymond C. Doberneck, M.D., Ph.D., *and* John E. Antoine, M.D., *Albuquerque, N. M.*

91 **Vascular pressure-flow relationships in denervated and reimplanted lungs of dogs.** Otto A. Wagner, M.D., L. Henry Edmunds, Jr., M.D., *Philadelphia, Pa., and* David C. Heilbron, Ph.D., *San Francisco, Calif.*

101 **Direct measurement of vagal release of gastrin.** Horst D. Becker, M.D., David D. Reeder, M.D., *and* James C. Thompson, M.D., *Galveston, Texas.*

107 **Juvenile gastrointestinal polyposis in a female infant: Report of a case and review of the literature of a recently recognized syndrome.** Charles R. Sachatello, M.D., *Lexington, Ky.,* Il Song Hahn, M.D., *and* Charles B. Carrington, M.D., *New Haven, Conn.*

continued on page 9

The extra margin of safety.

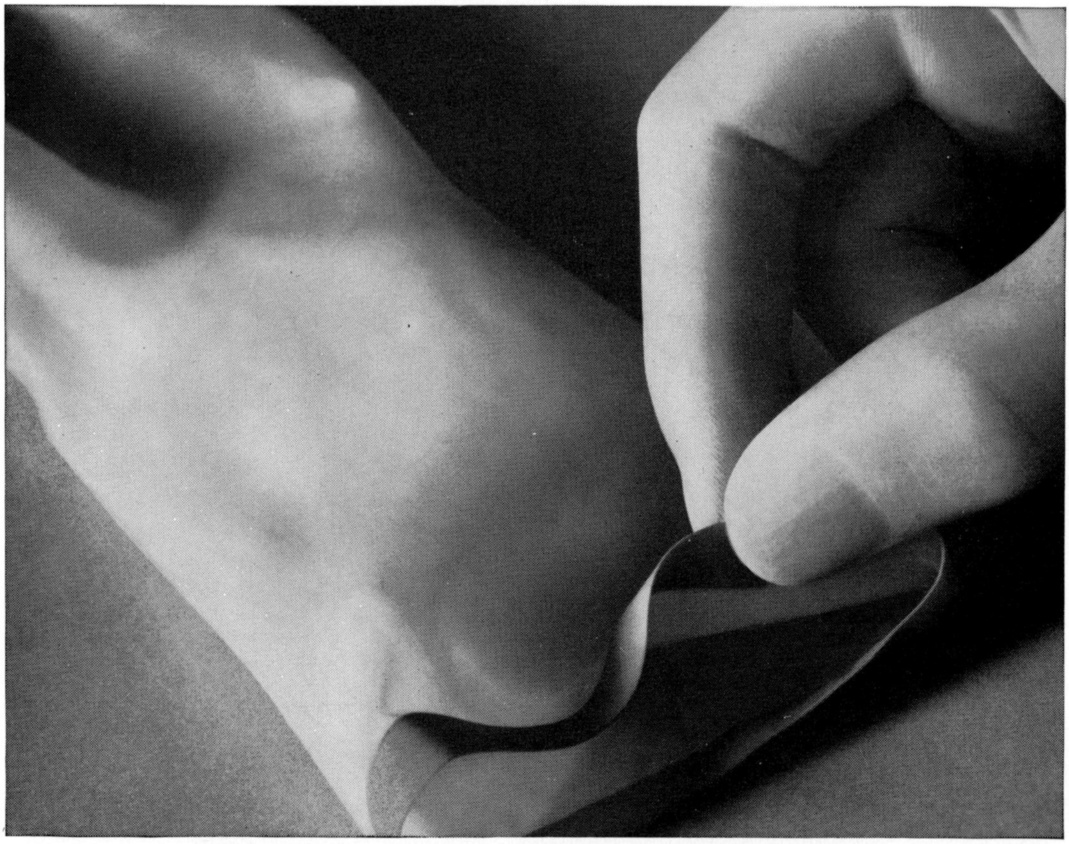

The Pioneer Rollpruf Band.

Right from the beginning, Rollpruf Sheers' flat-banded cuff gives you the edge in safety. It's color coded for mistake-proof sizing. It won't tear during gloving, because the band doubles cuff reinforcement. And Rollpruf's cuff *can't* roll down during surgery.

But we didn't stop there. We put an extra margin of safety all the way through Rollpruf Sheers. Precise production control eliminates weak spots . . . and each glove is thoroughly inspected at the factory. Look to Rollpruf Sheers . . . for the extra margin of safety that goes from cuff to fingertips. THE PIONEER RUBBER COMPANY, 387 Tiffin Road, Willard, Ohio.

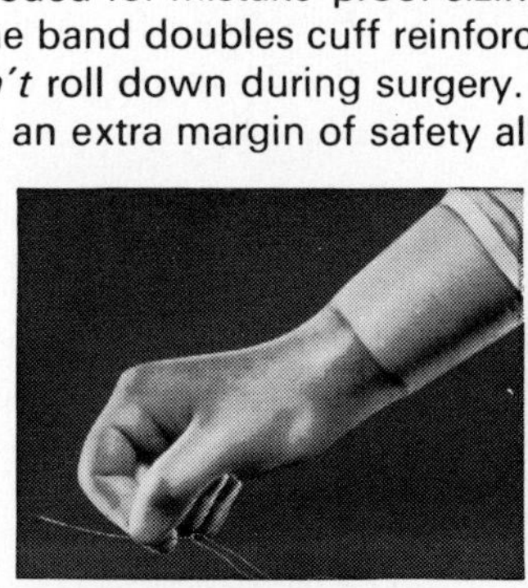

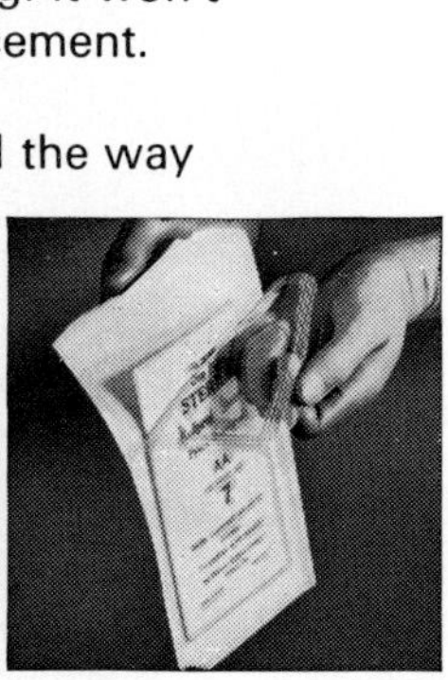

ROLLPRUF® SHEERS®

CONTENTS *continued*

CLINICAL REVIEWS

page 114 **Postoperative deep vein thrombosis and pulmonary embolism: A selective review and personal viewpoint.** John Joakim Skillman, M.D., *Bethesda, Md.*

123 **The mechanism of infection in patients with diabetes mellitus: A review of leukocyte malfunction.** Howard D. Robertson, First Lieutenant, USAF (MC), *and* Hiram C. Polk, Jr., M.D., F.A.C.S., *Louisville, Ky.*

BRIEF CLINICAL REPORTS

129 **A simplified method of ureteroileotomy in renal homotransplantation.** Thomas L. Marchioro, M.D., *and* James A. Tremann, M.D., *Seattle, Wash.*

132 **Successful management of mycotic aortic aneurysm: Report of a case.** Paul A. Cooke, M.B., B.Ch., *Johannesburg, Republic of South Africa, and* William K. Ehrenfeld, M.D., *San Francisco, Calif.*

137 **Routine venography in placement of the Mobin-Uddin vena cava filter: Dual filter placement in a patient with an accessory vena filter (cardinal vein).** Mark M. Kartchner, M.D., *and* A. J. Bogosian, *Tucson, Ariz.*

140 **Fate of a nylon vascular prosthesis for aortic replacement: 14 year follow-up study.** Peter B. Yaw, M.D., T. W. Grisell, M.D., W. M. Wahle, M.D., H. B Shumacker, M.D., *and* John L. Glover, M.D., *Indianapolis, Ind.*

EDITORIALS

145 **Hypertonic glucose and improved critical organ performance.** Richard H. Egdahl, M.D., *Boston, Mass.*

148 **Surgical anatomy.** John E. Skandalakis, M.D., Ph.D., F.A.C.S., Joseph S. Rowe, Jr., M.D., *and* Stephen W. Gray, Ph.D., *Atlanta, Ga.*

150 **Undergraduate medical education in Great Britain.** Gordon W. Philpott, M.D., *St. Louis, Mo.*

LETTERS TO THE EDITORS

153 **Arteriovenous shunting after sympathectomy.** Buck A. Rhodes, Ph.D., Vincent Lopez-Majano, M.D., Ph.D., *and* Henry N. Wagner, Jr., M.D., *Baltimore, Md.*

154 **Reply.** John P. Delaney, M.D., *and* Jon Scarpino, M.D., *Minneapolis, Minn.*

Volume 75 *Number* 2

SURGERY

CONTENTS, FEBRUARY, 1974

ORIGINAL COMMUNICATIONS

page 155 **A comparison of intraoperative tests of completeness of vagal section.** G. Grassi, M.D., *and* C. Orecchia, M.D., *Rome, Italy*

161 **Liver arterialization with portacaval shunt in the cirrhotic rat.** Y. Lecompte, M.D., D. Franco, M.D., E. D. Martin, M.D., *and* H. Bismuth, M.D., *Villejuif, France*

169 **Halsted and American surgery.** Edward F. X. Hughes, M.D., M.P.H., *New York, N. Y.*

178 **Nonpulsatile vs. pulsatile canine kidney perfusion.** R. Grundmann, M.D., H. Pitschi, F. Berr, *and* H. Pichlmaier, M.D., *Munich, Germany*

185 **Microvascular anastomosis: A device for holding stay sutures and a new vascular clamp.** R. D. Acland, F.R.C.S., *Bearsden, Glasgow, Scotland*

continued on page 7

Vol. 75, No. 2, February, 1974. SURGERY is published monthly by The C. V. Mosby Company, 11830 Westline Industrial Drive, St. Louis, Mo. 63141.

Annual subscription rates.

	U. S.	*Canada, Mexico*	*Other countries*
Institutional*	$29.00	$32.00	$32.75
Personal†	$21.00	$24.00	$24.75
Student, intern, resident†	$14.70	$17.70	$18.45

Single copies are $3.50 postpaid. Remittances should be made by check, draft, post office or express money order, payable to this Journal.

*Institutional (multiple-reader) subscriptions are available to public and private libraries, schools, hospitals, and clinics; city, county, state, provincial, and national government bureaus and departments; and all commercial and private institutions and organizations.
†Personal subscriptions and all student-rate subscriptions must be in the names of, billed to, and paid by individuals. All student-rate requests must indicate training status and name of institution.

Subscriptions may begin at any time.

Second class postage paid at St. Louis, Mo. Printed in the U. S. A.

CONTENTS *continued*

page 188 **Treatment and prevention of acute hepatic encephalopathy by intravenous levodopa.** O. Abramsky, M.D., *and* Z. Goldschmidt, M.D., *Jerusalem, Israel*

194 **Intravenous infusion of hydrochloric acid for treatment of severe metabolic alkalosis.** George M. Abouna, M.D., F.R.C.S., Philip R. Veazey, M.D., *and* Daniel B. Terry, Jr., M.D., *Augusta, Ga.*

203 **Elevation in host splenic and in allograft parenchymal and capsular histidine decarboxylase activity and weights following renal allografting in rats.** Thomas C. Moore, M.D., *Torrance, Calif.,* Michael C. Sinclair, M.D., *and* Carlos A. E. Lemmi, M.A., *Los Angeles, Calif.*

213 **Successful reversal of lethal carbon monoxide intoxication by total body asanguineous hypothermic perfusion.** Juan C. Agostini, M.D., Ruben G. Ramirez, M.D., Solomon N. Albert, M.D., Leo R. Goldbaum, Ph.D., *and* Karel B. Absolon, M.D., Ph.D., *Washington, D. C.*

220 **Effect of adenosine triphosphate–magnesium chloride administration in shock.** Irshad H. Chaudry, Ph.D., Mohammed M. Sayeed, Ph.D., *and* Arthur E. Baue, M.D., *St. Louis, Mo.*

228 **Experiences in the management of surgically correctable biliary atresia.** Eitoku Arima, M.D., Eric W. Fonkalsrud, M.D., *and* Robert C. Neerhout, M.D., *Los Angeles, Calif.*

233 **Identification of vagal structures at the esophageal hiatus.** John E. Skandalakis, M.D., Ph.D., F.A.C.S., Joseph S. Rowe, Jr., M.D., Stephen W. Gray, Ph.D., *and* John A. Androulakis, M.D., *Atlanta, Ga.*

238 **"Smooth loop" arteriovenous fistulas for hemodialysis.** Allastair M. Karmody, M.B., Ch.M., F.R.C.S.(Eng. and Edin.), *and* Neil Lempert, M.D., F.A.C.S., *Albany, N. Y.*

243 **Investigations of the enterobiliary metabolism of lecithin.** Ronald K. Tompkins, M.D., *and* William King, III, A.B., *Los Angeles, Calif.*

253 **Factors affecting survival from acute subdural hematoma.** T. Richards, M.D., *and* J. Hoff, M.D., *San Francisco, Calif.*

259 **The academic surgeon and the emergency department.** Robert B. Rutherford, M.D., F.A.C.S., *Denver, Colo.*

266 **Relative secretion of cholesterol-4-^{14}C in the bile and upper and lower small intestinal washings of the bile fistula rabbit.** Henry Buchwald, M.D., Ph.D., Roger L. Gebhard, M.D., *and* Richard L. Varco, M.D., Ph.D., *Minneapolis, Minn.*

continued on page 9

CONTENTS *continued*

CLINICAL REVIEW

page 274 **Problems associated with the massive transfusion of stored blood.** John A. Collins, M.D., *St. Louis, Mo.*

BRIEF CLINICAL REPORTS

296 **Starch pleuritis: A postthoracotomy syndrome possibly caused by surgical glove powder.** Andrew L. Warshaw, M.D., *and* Lawrence J. Mills, M.D., *Boston, Mass.*

299 **A simplified correction of subclavian steal syndrome.** Harry H. LeVeen, M.D., Vincent A. Piccone, Jr., M.D., Carlos Diaz, M.D., George Christoudias, M.D., Walter Slade, M.D., *and* Iris Norstrand, M.D., *Brooklyn, N. Y.*

305 **A simple and inexpensive tunneler for use in peripheral vascular surgery.** Robert M. Blumenberg, M.D., *and* Michael L. Gelfand, M.D., *Schenectady, N. Y.*

EDITORIALS

308 **How to be an adequate vagotomist.** John Alexander-Williams, *Birmingham, England*

312 **Diminished surgical infection by systemic antibiotic administration in potentially contaminated operations.** Hiram C. Polk, Jr., M.D., *Louisville, Ky.*

315 **The role of paramedical personnel in organ procurement.** Folkert O. Belzer, M.D., *San Francisco, Calif.*

LETTERS TO THE EDITORS

317 **Pulse contour vs. dye-dilution methods.** E. L. Bradley, III, M.D., *Atlanta, Ga.*

318 **Length of residency.** Paul A. Carlson, M.D., *Fresno, Calif.*

...all indicate

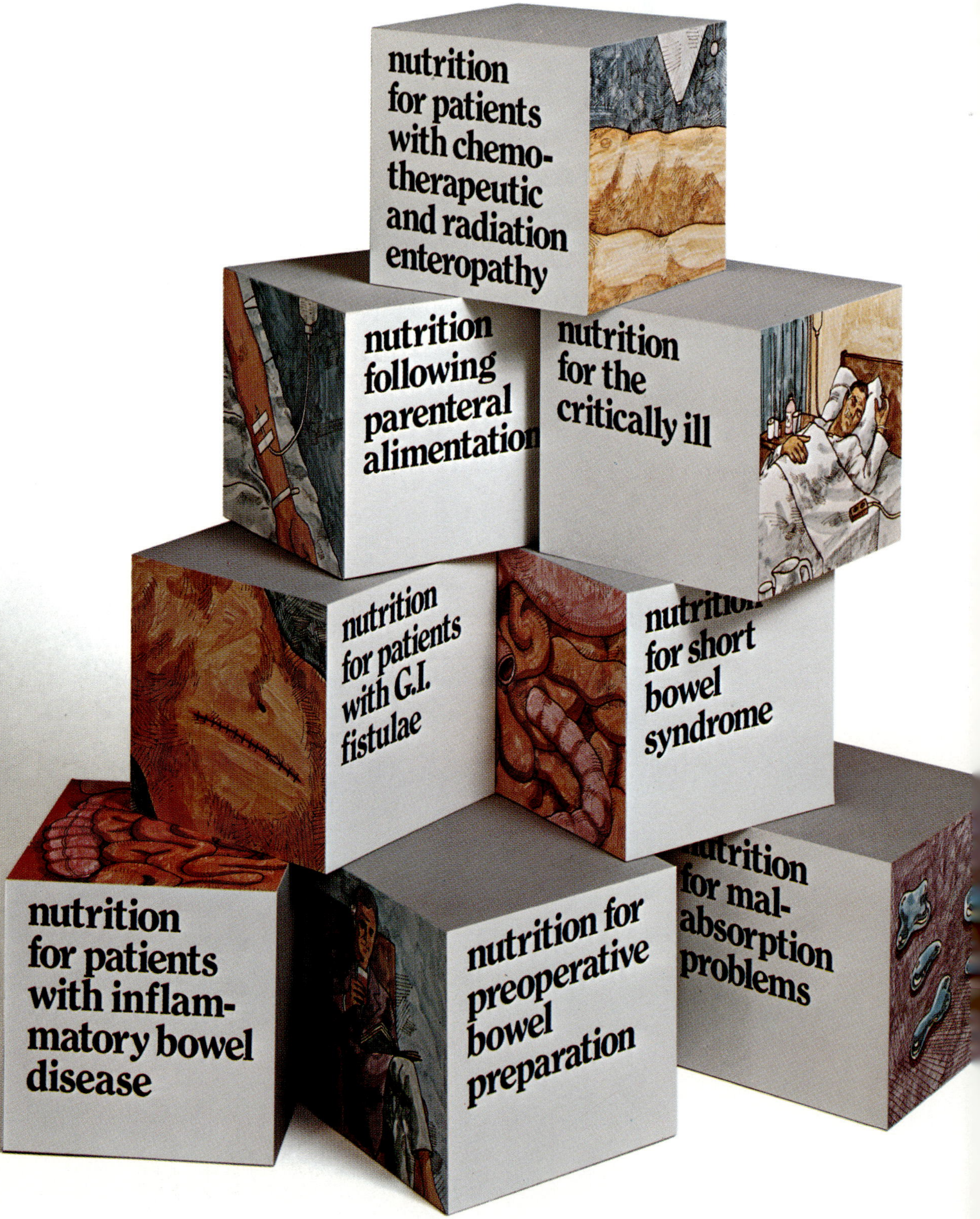

Volume 75 *Number* 3

SURGERY

CONTENTS, MARCH, 1974

ORIGINAL COMMUNICATIONS

page 319 **Surgical preparation, perfusion techniques, and cryoprotectants used in successful freezing of the kidney.** A. Eira Rebelo, M.D., Edmund F. Graham, Ph.D., Bo G. Crabo, D.V.M., Ph.D., Richard C. Lillehei, M.D., Ph.D., *and* Ronald H. Dietzman, M.D., Ph.D., *Minneapolis, Minn.*

332 **Surgery in the twenty-first century.** J. Englebert Dunphy, M.D., F.A.C.S., *San Francisco, Calif.*

338 **Transcholecystic extraction of residual calculi in common bile duct.** Rodolfo M. Mazzariello, M.D., *Buenos Aires, Argentina*

348 **Experimental lobar pneumonia in canine lung grafts.** Peter Schick, M.D., John R. Benfield, M.D., Bernard Gondos, M.D., Betty Hayakawa, M.A., Edwin Shors, B.S., Koichiro Shimada, M.D., *and* Michael Peter, M.D., *Torrance and Los Angeles, Calif.*

continued on page 7

Vol. 75, No. 3, March, 1974. SURGERY is published monthly by The C. V. Mosby Company, 11830 Westline Industrial Drive, St. Louis, Mo. 63141.

Annual subscription rates.

	U. S.	*Canada, Mexico*	*Other countries*
Institutional*	$29.00	$32.00	$32.75
Personal†	$21.00	$24.00	$24.75
Student, intern, resident†	$14.70	$17.70	$18.45

Single copies are $3.50 postpaid. Remittances should be made by check, draft, post office or express money order, payable to this Journal.

*Institutional (multiple-reader) subscriptions are available to public and private libraries, schools, hospitals, and clinics; city, county, state, provincial, and national government bureaus and departments; and all commercial and private institutions and organizations.

†Personal subscriptions and all student-rate subscriptions must be in the names of, billed to, and paid by individuals. All student-rate requests must indicate training status and name of institution.

Subscriptions may begin at any time.

Second class postage paid at St. Louis, Mo. Printed in the U. S. A.

CONTENTS *continued*

page 357 **Accelerated rejection of 36 immediate posttransplant functioning machine-preserved human cadaveric kidneys.** Thomas C. Moore, M.D., Thomas V. Berne, M.D., *and* Thomas S. English, *Los Angeles, Calif.*

368 **Prolonged survival of canine orthotopic small intestinal allografts preserved for 24 hours by hypothermic bloodless perfusion.** Luis H. Toledo-Pereyra, M.D., Richard L. Simmons, M.D., *and* John S. Najarian, M.D., *Minneapolis, Minn.*

377 **Exposure of the tibial-peroneal arteries by a single lateral approach.** Herbert Dardik, M.D., Irving Dardik, M.D., *and* Frank J. Veith, M.D., *Bronx, N. Y.*

383 **Nonoperative closure of atrial septal defects.** Terry D. King, M.D., *and* Noel L. Mills, M.D., *New Orleans, La.*

389 **Transplantation and reimplantation in the arts.** Bianca Tosatti, Ph.D. (Literature), *Genoa, Italy*

398 **Xenon-133 radiospirometry in electrophrenic respiration: Diaphragm pacing.** Glenn S. Forbes, M.D., W. W. L. Glenn, M.D., *and* R. C. Lange, Ph.D., *New Haven, Conn.*

408 **Hemodynamics of the terminal vascular bed in canine hemorrhagic shock.** Arnost Fronek, M.D., Ph.D., *and* Thomas Witzel, M.Sc., *La Jolla, Calif.*

416 **Method for maintaining the neonate's intraoperative core temperature.** Walton K. T. Shim, M.D., F.A.C.S., F.A.A.P., *and* Peter Halford, M.D., *Honolulu, Hawaii*

421 **Estimation of functional reserve of normal and regenerating dog livers.** Layton F. Rikkers, M.D., *and* Frank G. Moody, M.D., *Salt Lake City, Utah*

430 **Parabiotic inhibition of murine sarcoma growth.** Robert P. Feraci, M.D., *and* Lionel Schour, M.D., F.A.C.S., *Bethesda, Md.*

436 **Hernia presentation of cancer in the groin.** Glenn W. Geelhoed, M.D., Roger C. Millar, M.D., *and* Alfred S. Ketcham, M.D., *Bethesda, Md.*

442 **Hemodynamics of coronary circulation during ventricular fibrillation.** C. L. Sarin, M.D., Ch.M., F.R.C.S., *and* W. O. Nickel, M.D., F.A.C.S., *Detroit, Mich.*

continued on page 9

CONTENTS *continued*

page 447 **Alternatives for vascular access for hemodialysis: Experience with autogenous saphenous vein autografts and bovine heterografts.** M. Haimov, M.D., L. Burrows, M.D., A. Baez, M.D., M. Neff, M.D., *and* R. Slifkin, M.D., *New York, N. Y.*

453 **Hemodynamic effects of femoral venous occlusion in the subhuman primate.** Creighton B. Wright, M.D., Major, MC, USA, *and* Robert W. Hobson, M.D., Lieutenant Colonel, MC, USA, *Washington, D. C.*

461 **The effects of gastric exclusion operations on pancreatic exocrine secretion.** John W. Thomas, M.D., M.S., *Lexington, Ky., and* Edward E. Mason, M.D., Ph.D., F.A.C.S., *Iowa City, Iowa*

BRIEF CLINICAL REPORT

471 **Ascending aorta–bilateral femoral artery bypass for the totally occluded infrarenal abdominal aorta.** Stephen L. Frantz, M.D., Martin J. Kaplitt, M.D., Arthur R. Beil, Jr., *and* Harry L. Stein, M.D., *Manhasset, N. Y.*

LETTERS TO THE EDITORS

476 **No need for autoclavable information.** Mark M. Ravitch, M.D., *Pittsburgh, Pa.*

476 **Reply.** M. Bert Myers, M.D., *New Orleans, La.*

Microbicidal power

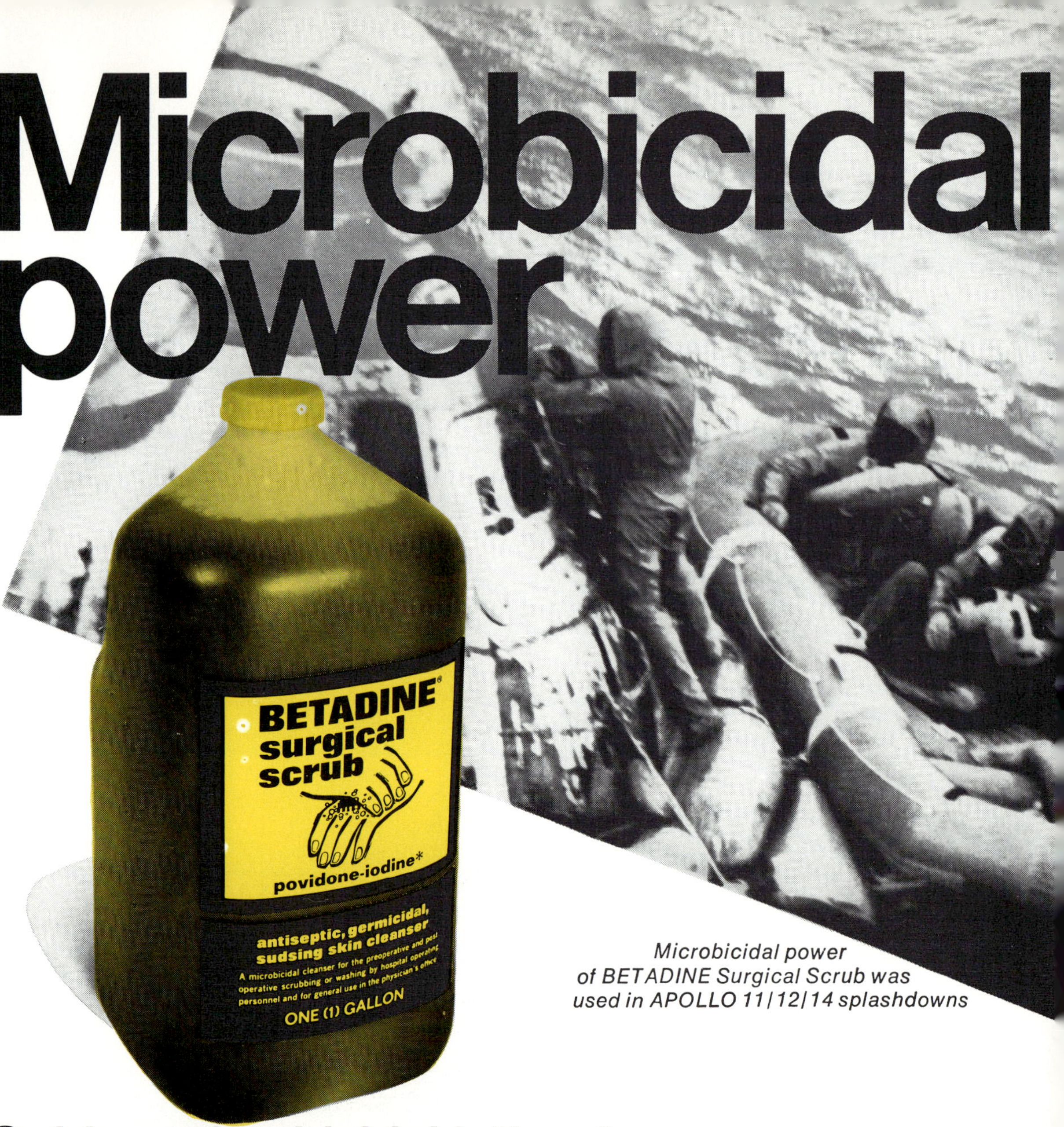

Microbicidal power of BETADINE Surgical Scrub was used in APOLLO 11/12/14 splashdowns

Golden microbicidal lather for optimal degerming of skin

Selected by NASA for decontamination procedures in Apollo 11/12/14 lunar missions splashdowns, BETADINE Surgical Scrub offers outstanding advantages for degerming the hands of the surgical team.

Some scrubs are merely bacteriostatic. **BETADINE Surgical Scrub is decisively microbicidal.**

Some scrubs inhibit mainly gram-positive bacteria. **BETADINE Surgical Scrub kills both gram-positive and gram-negative bacteria.**

Some scrubs have a limited antibacterial action. **BETADINE Surgical Scrub kills bacteria, fungi, viruses, protozoa, and yeasts.**

Some scrubs require repeated usage for several days before achieving their full antibacterial effect. **BETADINE Surgical Scrub is fully effective with each application.**

Use BETADINE Surgical Scrub for prompt, effective degerming action for operating personnel. BETADINE Surgical Scrub is virtually nonirritating. In the rare instance of local irritation or sensitivity, discontinue use in the individual. BETADINE Surgical Scrub does not stain the skin and natural fabrics. Bibliography available on request.

Purdue Frederick

Volume 75 Number 4

SURGERY

CONTENTS, APRIL, 1974

ORIGINAL COMMUNICATIONS

page 477 **Specific tissue and tumor responses of chimpanzees following immunization against human melanoma.** Maria O. Hornung, M.D., *and* Edward T. Krementz, M.D., *New Orleans, La.*

487 **The interaction of glucagon and glucose on cardiorespiratory variables in the critically ill patient.** Michael R. Drucker, M.D., Frank Pindyck, M.D., Robert S. Brown, M.D., David H. Elwyn, Ph.D., *and* William C. Shoemaker, M.D., *New York, N. Y.*

496 **Fatty acid absorption in jejunal autograft and allograft.** William P. Stamford, M.D., *and* Mark A. Hardy, M.D., *Bronx, N. Y.*

503 **Experimental cancer immunotherapy using a neuraminidase-treated non-viable frozen tumor vaccine.** Angelyn Rios *and* Richard L. Simmons, M.D., *Minneapolis, Minn.*

continued on page 5

Vol. 75, No. 4, April, 1974. SURGERY is published monthly by The C. V. Mosby Company, 11830 Westline Industrial Drive, St. Louis, Mo. 63141.

Annual subscription rates.

	U. S.	*Canada, Mexico*	*Other countries*
Institutional*	$29.00	$32.00	$32.75
Personal†	$21.00	$24.00	$24.75
Student, intern, resident†	$14.70	$17.70	$18.45

Single copies are $3.50 postpaid. Remittances should be made by check, draft, post office or express money order, payable to this Journal.

*Institutional (multiple-reader) subscriptions are available to public and private libraries, schools, hospitals, and clinics; city, county, state, provincial, and national government bureaus and departments; and all commercial and private institutions and organizations.
†Personal subscriptions and all student-rate subscriptions must be in the names of, billed to, and paid by individuals. All student-rate requests must indicate training status and name of institution.

Subscriptions may begin at any time.

Second class postage paid at St. Louis, Mo. Printed in the U. S. A.

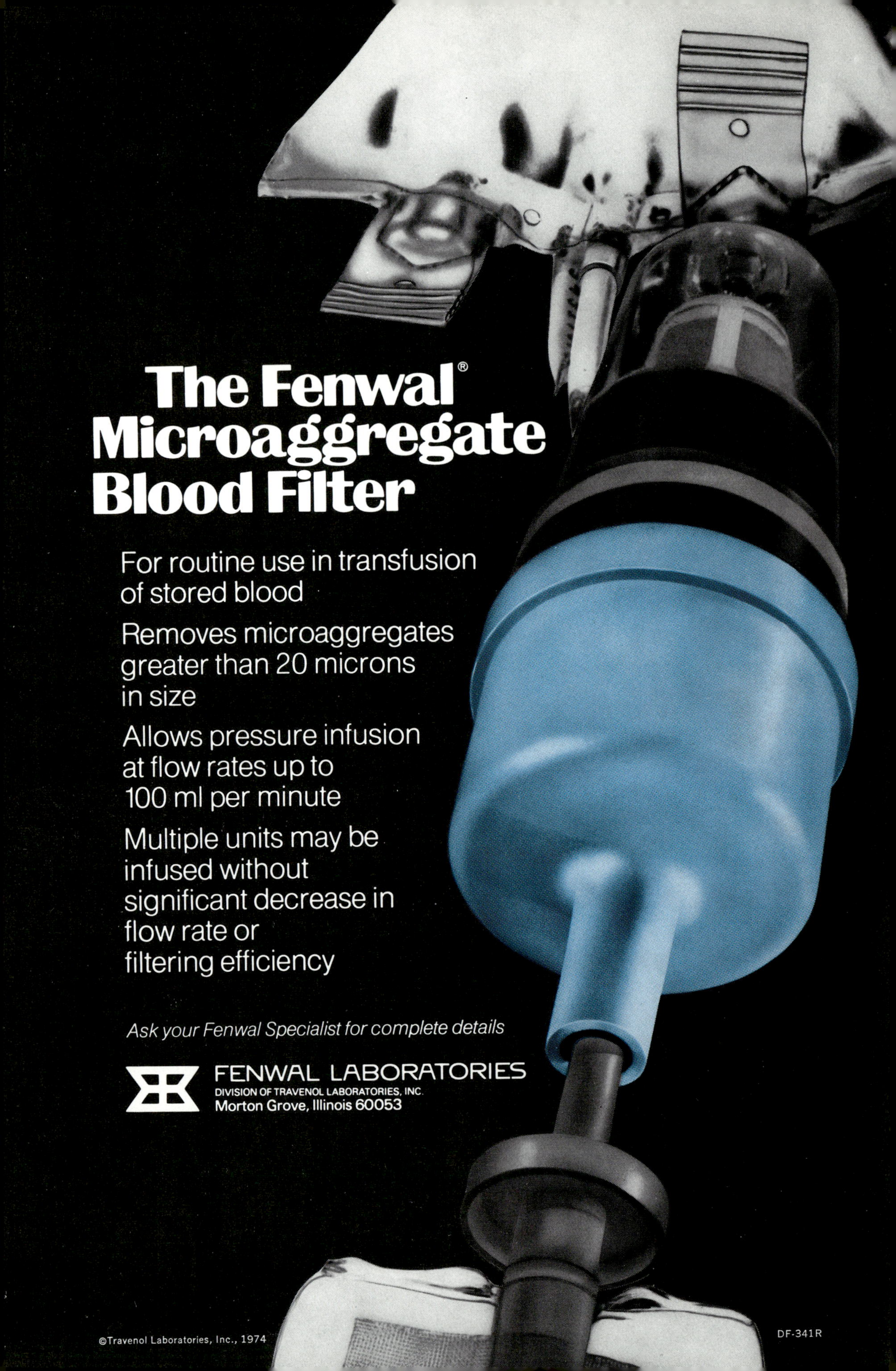
The Fenwal®
Microaggregate
Blood Filter
For routine use in transfusion of stored blood
Removes microaggregates greater than 20 microns in size
Allows pressure infusion at flow rates up to 100 ml per minute
Multiple units may be infused without significant decrease in flow rate or filtering efficiency
Ask your Fenwal Specialist for complete details
FENWAL LABORATORIES
DIVISION OF TRAVENOL LABORATORIES, INC.
Morton Grove, Illinois 60053
©Travenol Laboratories, Inc., 1974
DF-341R

page 508 **The adequacy of myocardial oxygen delivery in acute normovolemic anemia.** John Brazier, M.D., Norman Cooper, M.D., James V. Maloney, Jr., M.D., *and* Gerald Buckberg, M.D., *Los Angeles, Calif.*

517 **An experimental study of the antral gastrin mechanism.** S. R. Friesen, M.D., Ph.D., I. Crosby, M.D., M. D. Boggan, M.D., E. Fiallos, M.D., J. M. Lees, M.D., D. B. Cudnik, M.D., J. Underwood, III, M.D., M. S. Peckler, M.D., C. C. Craig, M.D., R. H. Friesen, M.D., R. E. Bolinger, M.D., *Kansas, City, Kan., and* J. E. McGuigan, M.D., *Gainesville, Fla.*

528 **Regional organ preservation program in the New England area.** Sang In Cho, M.D., Robert P. DerHagopian, M.D., Robert S. Krane, M.D., *and* Donald C. Nabseth, M.D., *Boston, Mass.*

535 **The prevention and treatment of the persistent perineal sinus.** William Silen, M.D., *and* Donald J. Glotzer, M.D., *Boston, Mass.*

543 **Delayed presentation of carotid intimal tear following blunt craniocervical trauma.** Michael M. Crissey, M.D., *and* Eugene F. Bernstein, M.D., *La Jolla, Calif.*

550 **Transvenous adrenal destruction: Clinical trials in patients with metastatic malignancy.** C. E. Zimmerman, M.D., H. Eisenberg, M.D., R. Spark, M.D., and C. B. Rosoff, M.D., *Boston, Mass.*

557 **Venoarterial bypass with a membrane oxygenator: Successful respiratory support in a woman following pulmonary hemorrhage secondary to renal failure.** E. Lawrence Hanson, M.D., Philip A. Drinker, Ph.D., Hillary F. Don, M.D., Stephen H. Van Devanter, M.D., Jacques Bonnet-Eymard, M.D., *and* Francis D. Moore, M.D., *Boston, Mass.*

566 **Ultrapore filter–induced thrombocytopenia.** Alfred S. Gervin, Major, MC, USA, Kenneth Mason, B.S., *Washington, D. C.,* Tom Limbird, B.S., and Donald Silver, M.D., *Durham, N. C.*

573 **Chronic salt-loading of donor and recipient in renal transplantation.** Sherman Jay Silber, M.D., *Melbourne, Australia*

578 **Hazards of surgical treatment due to microorganisms in the bile.** M. R. B. Keighley, D. M. Lister, S. I. Jacobs, *and* G. R. Giles, *Leeds, England*

continued on page 7

CONTENTS *continued*

page 584 **Venous drainage of the ischemic kidney.** Richard Brodman, M.D., William W. Pfaff, M.D., Birdwell Finlayson, M.D., *and* Raymond L. Hackett, M.D., *Gainesville, Fla.*

589 **The blood supply of experimental liver metastases. IV. Changes in vascularity with increasing tumor growth.** Norman B. Ackerman, M.D., Ph.D., *Kansas City, Mo.*

597 **Beta-islet cell tumors of the pancreas: Results of a study on 1,067 cases.** Paride Stefanini, M.D., Manlio Carboni, M.D., F.I.C.S., Neri Patrassi, M.D., F.I.C.S., *and* Antonio Basoli, M.D., *Rome, Italy*

BRIEF CLINICAL REPORTS

610 **The crossover femoropopliteal bypass.** M. Haimov, M.D., *New York, N. Y.*

613 **Inferior vena caval obstruction caused by expansion of an abdominal aortic aneurysm: Report of a case and review of the literature.** Richard L. Snider, M.D., John M. Porter, M.D., *and* Larry R. Eidemiller, M.D., *Portland, Ore.*

617 **Pinhole colonic perforation in breech-born infants.** A. Andersson, M.D., P.-A. Hofer, M.D., D. E. W. Holmlund, M.D., *and* H. Wendel, M.D., *Umeå, Sweden*

621 **Amyloidoma (a solitary nodule of the lung).** João Batista Marchesini, M.D., Albano de Almeida Chaves Luis, M.D., *and* Marco Aurelio Cravo, M.D., *Curitiba, Parana, Brazil*

EDITORIALS

626 **A single step.** George Zuidema, M.D., *Baltimore, Md.*

629 **Magnification and coronary artery surgery.** William W. L. Glenn, M.D., *New Haven, Conn.*

LETTERS TO THE EDITORS

630 **The young surgeon's dilemma.** Herbert Dardik, M.D., *Fort Lee, N. J.*

630 **Reply.** John A. Drews, M.D., *Torrance, Calif.*

Volume 75 *Number* 5

SURGERY

CONTENTS, MAY, 1974

ORIGINAL COMMUNICATIONS

page 631 **Morphology of the connective tissue grown in response to implanted silicone rubber: A light and electron microscopic study.** Pablo Hernández-Jáuregui, V.M.D., Carlos Esperanza-García, M.D., *and* Amador González-Angulo, M.D., *Mexico City, Mexico*

638 **The protection of the skin of fracture patients immobilized in plaster of Paris.** Cyril Boroda, M.B.B.S., M.R.C.S., *and* George L. Mouzas, M.D., F.I.C.S., *London, England*

643 **Inhibited platelet adhesion: A non-thrombogenic characteristic of a heparin-coated surface.** H. Lagergren, M.D., P. Olsson, M.D., *and* J. Swedenborg, M.D., *Stockholm, Sweden*

651 **A simplified kidney preservation system: Further development and results of extended perfusion.** I. R. Hardie, G. J. A. Clunie, Glenda Balderson, J. F. Leditschke, *and* I. J. Leslie, *Brisbane, Queensland, Australia*

660 **Thymidine incorporation in esophageal wounds of zinc-deficient rats.** R. A. MacMahon, M.S.(Colo.), F.R.C.S.(Edin.), F.R.A.C.S., L. J. Cussen, F.R.C.P.A., F. T. McDermott, F.R.C.S.(Eng.), F.R.A.C.S., *and* B. E. James, M.Sc., *Melbourne, Australia*

continued on page 7

Vol. 75, No. 5, May, 1974. SURGERY is published monthly by The C. V. Mosby Company, 11830 Westline Industrial Drive, St. Louis, Mo. 63141.

Annual subscription rates.

	U. S.	*Canada, Mexico*	*Other countries*
Institutional*	$29.00	$32.00	$32.75
Personal†	$21.00	$24.00	$24.75
Student, intern, resident†	$14.70	$17.70	$18.45

Single copies are $3.50 postpaid. Remittances should be made by check, draft, post office or express money order, payable to this Journal.

*Institutional (multiple-reader) subscriptions are available to public and private libraries, schools, hospitals, and clinics; city, county, state, provincial, and national government bureaus and departments; and all commercial and private institutions and organizations.
†Personal subscriptions and all student-rate subscriptions must be in the names of, billed to, and paid by individuals. All student-rate requests must indicate training status and name of institution.

Subscriptions may begin at any time.

Second class postage paid at St. Louis, Mo. Printed in the U. S. A.

CONTENTS *continued*

page 664 **Spontaneous perforation of the extrahepatic bile ducts and bile peritonitis in infancy.** John R. Lilly, M.D., William H. Weintraub, M.D., *and* R. Peter Altman, M.D., *Washington, D. C.*

674 **A simple esophageal bypass operation by the high gastric division.** Hiroshi Akiyama, M.D., *and* Mamoru Hiyama, M.D., *Tokyo, Japan*

682 **Surgical treatment of abdominal angina: Review of 25 patients.** George J. Reul, Jr., M.D., Don C. Wukasch, M.D., Frank M. Sandiford, M.D., Luigi Chiarillo, M.D., Grady L. Hallman, M.D., *and* Denton A. Cooley, M.D., *Houston, Texas*

690 **Congenital incomplete prepyloric diaphragm in infants and children.** Dimitris C. Keramidas, M.D., *Athens, Greece*

695 **Diagnosis, pathology, and treatment of Buerger's disease.** Shigehiko Shionoya, M.D., Ichiro Ban, M.D., Yukifumi Nakata, M.D., Junichi Matsubara, M.D., Kenzo Shinjo, M.D., Masafumi Hirai, M.D., Seiichi Kawai, M.D., Shoichi Suzuki, M.D., *and* Wen Hsiung Tsai, M.D., *Nagoya, Japan*

701 **Effect of atropine on basal and food-stimulated serum gastrin levels in man.** Horst D. Becker, M.D., David D. Reeder, M.D., *and* James C. Thompson, M.D., *Galveston, Texas*

705 **Ureterosigmoid conduit urinary diversion.** S. Martin Lindenauer, M.D., Joseph C. Cerny, M.D., *and* George W. Morley, M.D., *Ann Arbor, Mich.*

715 **Trends in the current management of primary hyperparathyroidism.** Roderick C. Haff, Lieutenant Colonel, USAF, MC, *and* Raymond G. Armstrong, Colonel, USAF, MC, *Lackland Air Force Base, Texas*

720 **Increased gastrin release following penetrating central nervous system injury.** John C. Bowen, M.D., *Houston, Texas,* William H. Fleming, M.D., *Atlanta, Ga., and* James C. Thompson, M.D., *Galveston, Texas*

725 **Correction of coagulation in the hemophilic dog by transplantation of lymphatic tissue.** Carl G. Groth, M.D., William E. Hathaway, M.D., Ake Gustafson, M.D., W. Peter Geis, M.D., Charles W. Putnam, M.D., Christer Bjorken, K. A. Porter, M.D., *London, England, and* Thomas E. Starzl, M.D., Ph.D., *Denver, Colo.*

734 **Microangiography of the renal vasculature following total renal artery occlusion.** Richard F. Brodman, M.D., Raymond L. Hackett, M.D., Birdwell Finlayson, M.D., Ph.D., *and* William W. Pfaff, M.D., *Gainesville, Fla.*

continued on page 9

CONTENTS *continued*

page 740 **Non-simultaneous bilateral breast carcinoma.** Sukawat Watanatittan, M.D., *and* M. D. Ram, M.D., M.S.(Surg.), F.R.C.S., F.A.C.S., *Cleveland, Ohio*

746 **Obturator intestinal obstruction following renal allotransplantation: Relief with hyperosmolar enemas.** Michael Berger, M.D., John S. Schuessler, M.D., Hugo F. Carvajal, M.D., William B. Lorentz, Jr., M.D., Luther B. Travis, M.D., *and* Kenneth R. T. Tyson, M.D., *Galveston, Texas*

750 **Factors altering pulmonary capillary perfusion.** Michael L. Schwartz, M. D., William R. C. Murphy, M.D., Demetre M. Nicoloff, M.D., *and* Edward W. Humphrey, MD., Ph.D., *Minneapolis, Minn.*

755 **The effect of endogenous secretin and cholecystokinin on pentagastrin-stimulated innervated and denervated gastric mucosa.** John A. Dorighi, M.D., Donald L. Kaminski, M.D., *and* Vallee L. Willman, M.D., *St. Louis, Mo.*

763 **Hypermetabolism in sepsis: Correlation with fever and tachycardia.** D. F. J. Halmagyi, M.D., D.Sc., J. Broell, M.S., F. E. Gump, M.D., *and* J. M. Kinney, M.D., *New York, N. Y.*

771 **Extraperitoneal endarterectomy for unilateral iliofemoral occlusive disease.** Toshio Inahara, M.D., *and* Jose D. Pineda, M.D., *Portland, Ore.*

776 **A broadening of vision: Observation on the practice of surgery in a university hospital in Great Britain.** Nicholas L. Tilney, M.D., *Boston, Mass.*

CLINICAL REVIEW

783 **Measurement of hepatic blood flow in man.** E. L. Bradley, III, M.D., *Atlanta, Ga.*

BRIEF CLINICAL REPORTS

790 **Lipoma, a cause of paralysis of deep radial (posterior interosseous) nerve: Report of a case and review of the literature.** Kwang-Tzen Wu, M.D., Francis R. Jordan, M.D., *and* Charles Eckert, M.D., *Albany, N. Y.*

796 **Interscapulothoracic amputation for the complications of breast cancer: A new approach.** Peter I. Pressman, M.D., *New York, N. Y.*

LETTERS TO THE EDITORS

802 **Scientists and medical writing.** William F. Hewitt, Ph.D., *Smyrna, N. Y.*

802 **Reply: Honesty in authorship.** Lois DeBakey, Ph.D., *Houston, Texas*

Volume 75 *Number* 6

SURGERY

CONTENTS, JUNE, 1974

SOCIETY OF UNIVERSITY SURGEONS

page 805 **Functional characteristics of surgically induced jejunal neomucosa.** H. Bradley Binnington, M.D., Hatton Sumner, M.D., Peggy Lesker, B.A., David A. Alpers, M.D., *and* Jessie L. Ternberg, M.D., *St. Louis, Mo.*

811 **Depletion of brain norepinephrine in acute hepatic coma.** John M. Dodsworth, M.B., F.R.C.S.E., J. Howard James, B.S., Michael C. Cummings, B.S., *and* Josef E. Fischer, M.D., *Boston, Mass.*

821 **Effect of small bowel bypass on gastric secretory function: Postintestinal exclusion hypersecretion, a phenomenon in search of a syndrome.** Henry Buchwald, M.D., Ph.D., John J. Coyle, M.D., *and* Richard L. Varco, M.D., Ph.D., *Minneapolis, Minn.*

continued on page 7

Vol. 75, No. 6, June, 1974. SURGERY is published monthly by The C. V. Mosby Company, 11830 Westline Industrial Drive, St. Louis, Mo. 63141.

Annual subscription rates.

	U. S.	*Canada, Mexico*	*Other countries*
Institutional*	$29.00	$32.00	$32.75
Personal†	$21.00	$24.00	$24.75
Student, intern, resident†	$14.70	$17.70	$18.45

Single copies are $3.50 postpaid. Remittances should be made by check, draft, post office or express money order, payable to this Journal.

*Institutional (multiple-reader) subscriptions are available to public and private libraries, schools, hospitals, and clinics; city, county, state, provincial, and national government bureaus and departments; and all commercial and private institutions and organizations.
†Personal subscriptions and all student-rate subscriptions must be in the names of, billed to, and paid by individuals. All student-rate requests must indicate training status and name of institution.

Subscriptions may begin at any time.

Second class postage paid at St. Louis, Mo. Printed in the U. S. A.

CONTENTS *continued*

page 829 **Transient kwashiorkor: A cause of fatty liver following small bowel bypass.** John J. White, M.D., C.M., Richard T. Moxley, III, M.D., Thomas Pozefsky, M.D., *and* Dean H. Lockwood, M.D., Baltimore, Md.

841 **Serum calcium, serum gastrin, and gastric acid secretion before and after parathyroidectomy for hyperparathyroidism.** John F. Stremple, M.D., F.A.C.S., *and* Charles G. Watson, M.D., F.A.C.S., *Pittsburgh, Pa.*

853 **Influence of vasopressin and topical bile salts on the gastric mucosal barrier of the subhuman primate.** W. P. Ritchie, Jr., M.D., Ph.D., *Washington, D. C., and Charlottesville, Va.*

861 **Physiologic factors in the selection of patients for superficial temporal artery–to–middle cerebral artery anastomosis.** George Austin, M.D., David Laffin, *and* William Hayward, *Loma Linda, Calif.*

869 **Altered action of parathyroid hormone by chlorpropamide.** Patricia J. Numann, M.D., *and* Arnold M. Moses, M.D., *Syracuse, N. Y.*

874 **Gas tensions in healing tissues of traumatized patients.** R. Bruce Heppenstall, M.D., Fred N. Littooy, M.D., Richard Fuchs, George F. Sheldon, M.D., *and* Thomas K. Hunt, M.D., *San Francisco, Calif.*

881 **Pulmonary changes due to hemorrhagic shock resuscitation with isotonic and hypertonic saline.** Robert L. Fulton, M.D., *Louisville, Ky., and* Ronald P. Fischer, M.D., Ph.D., *Albuquerque, N. M.*

892 **Topical lipid protection of burned subjects and their wounds.** Carl Jelenko, III, M.D., Mogan L. Wheeler, B.S., Ann P. Anderson, Dianne Callaway, B.S., *and* Robert A. Scott, Jr., *Augusta, Ga.*

continued on page 9

CONTENTS *continued*

page 900 **Total body potassium in surgical patients.** Harry M. Shizgal, M.D., Robert S. Kurtz, M.D., *and* C. Douglas Wood, M.D., *Montreal, Quebec, Canada*

908 **Are there educational advantages to a surgical clerkship in a university hospital?** Sidney Levitsky, M.D., Rene L. Nerenberg, M.A., C. Thomas Bombeck, M.D., *and* Lloyd M. Nyhus, M.D., *Chicago, Ill.*

915 **Objectives and methods in undergraduate surgical education.** Ralph G. DePalma, M.D., Robert J. Izant, M.D., Alf Jordan, M.D., William D. Holden, M.D., *Cleveland, Ohio, and* T. Joseph Sheehan, Ph.D., *Hartford, Conn.*

925 **Microcrystalline collagen as a topical hemostatic agent for vascular surgery.** William M. Abbott, M.D., *and* W. Gerald Austen, M.D., *Boston, Mass.*

934 **Emergency concepts in the control of surgical infections.** J. Wesley Alexander, M.D., Sc.D., *Cincinnati, Ohio*

Volume 75 *Number* 1

SURGERY

JANUARY, 1974

Original communications

Protective effect of glycogen and glucose on the anoxic arrested heart

Robert L. Hewitt, M.D., David M. Lolley, M.D., George A. Adrouny, Ph.D., *and* **Theodore Drapanas, M.D.,** *New Orleans, La.*

The possibility that enhancement of anaerobic metabolism during anoxic cardiac arrest would result in protection to the heart was investigated in dogs subjected to 30 minutes of anoxic arrest during cardiopulmonary bypass at 37° C. Energy substrate was provided by increasing cardiac glycogen levels and by perfusing the arrested heart with glucose solution. Cardiac glycogen was significantly elevated by restricting animals to a fat diet for three days, and the elevation in cardiac glycogen level was observed to result in increased glycogenolysis. Provision of energy substrate, either as glycogen or as glucose, during the anoxic period resulted in significant preservation of cardiac function as determined by cardiac output, left ventricular work, maximum rate of development of isometic tension of the left ventricle per unit of integrated isometric tension (dp/dt/ITT) and rate of development of isometric tension per unit of instantaneous pressure (dp/dt/IP). Potassium and insulin in combination with glucose also resulted in significant protection as determined by ability of the heart to be resuscitated following the anoxic interval. The results of this study support the concept that significant cardiac preservation during anoxic arrest may result from maintenance of energy generation through enhancement of anaerobic metabolism with available energy substrate.

From the Department of Surgery, Tulane University School of Medicine, New Orleans, La.

FAILURE OF the hypoxic heart to maintain contractility may be due to an insufficiency in the process of energy generation.[5] The possibility exists that a failure in energy production may precede irreversible structural changes during anoxic cardiac arrest and result in decreased cardiac contractility and function following restoration of coronary blood flow. Irreversible rigor of the heart that occasionally follows elective anoxic cardiac arrest has also been attributed to loss of myocardial energy stores leading to

Accepted for publication March 28, 1973.

adenosine triphosphate (ATP) depletion at a cellular level.[8] If these observations are correct, protection of the heart during anoxia might be expected by enhancing anaerobic metabolism through an increase in available energy substrate. Cardiac glycogen and exogenous glucose are known to be substrates for anaerobic metabolism during cardiac anoxia. Scheuer and Stezoski[14] demonstrated that increased myocardial glycogen stores in the isolated anoxic heart enhanced glycogenolysis and anerobic ATP production and resulted in preservation of function. Recently, a protective effect of increased myocardial glycogen upon cardiac function during anoxia was demonstrated in the intact working heart.[6] Glucose has also been found to improve anaerobic metabolism in the isolated heart,[11] and Austen and associates[2] demonstrated significant protection to the intact working heart with glucose loading prior to anoxic arrest as determined by ventricular function studies. The present study was designed to determine if utilization of stored glycogen and exogenous glucose during anoxic cardiac arrest might also have a protective effect upon subsequent cardiac function.

METHODS

Twenty-five dogs were studied during and immediately following cardiopulmonary bypass at 37° C. and ischemic cardiac arrest for 30 minutes. Cardiac function was measured prior to cardiopulmonary bypass and anoxic cardiac arrest and then exactly 20 minutes following restoration of coronary blood flow.

Five groups comparable in weight were studied as follows: Group I (22.9 ± 1.50 kilograms), was the control group in which the aorta was cross-clamped for 30 minutes and the right and left ventricles were vented. In Group II (21.9 ± 1.84 kilograms), the heart was perfused with isotonic saline through the aortic root during arrest; perfusion was accomplished with gravity flow through a No. 16 Jelco cannula placed into the aorta, and perfusion pressures ranged between 30 and 40 mm. Hg. In Group III (23.0 ± 1.71 kilograms), cardiac glycogen was increased by the administration of a diet consisting of butcher fat initiated three days prior to the experiment,[6] and the heart was perfused with isotonic saline. In Group IV (22.0 ± 1.50 kilograms), the heart was perfused with five percent dextrose in water, and in Group V (23.0 ± 1.02 kilograms), the heart was perfused with five percent dextrose in water containing regular insulin (100 U.) and KCl (20 mEq. per liter). Sodium bicarbonate (4 mEq. per liter) was added to give a pH of 7.76 ± 0.02. In Groups II, III, IV, and V approximately 1,000 ml. of perfusate at 28° C. was used during the 30 minutes of anoxia in each experiment. The left ventricular vent in all experiments was led to the oxygenator. The perfusate collected from the right ventricle was collected separately for subsequent measurement of electrolyte content in Groups II, III, IV, and V and for glucose content as well in Groups IV and V. The pulmonary artery was occluded at the time of aortic root infusion to achieve bloodless right ventricular drainage.

The animals were anesthetized with pentobarbital sodium (25 mg. per kilogram of body weight) and ventilated with oxygen (100 percent) through an endotracheal tube with the use of an automatic pressure-regulated respirator (Bird). Esophageal temperature was monitored and maintained at 37° C. Electrocardiogram was monitored with the use of standard leads. Following median sternotomy and administration of heparin intravenously (400 U. per kilogram of body weight), cannulas for venous return were placed into the superior vena cava and inferior vena cava through the right atrium, and arterial flow was directed into a femoral artery. The cardiopulmonary bypass included a Bentley Temptrol Oxygenator (Q-120), using a gas mixture of 95 percent O_2 and five percent CO_2, and a roller pump; the prime consisted of Ringer's lactate solution (30 ml. per kilogram of body weight) containing 1.5 mEq. of KCl per kilogram of body weight. The contents of the bypass circuit were returned to the animal upon

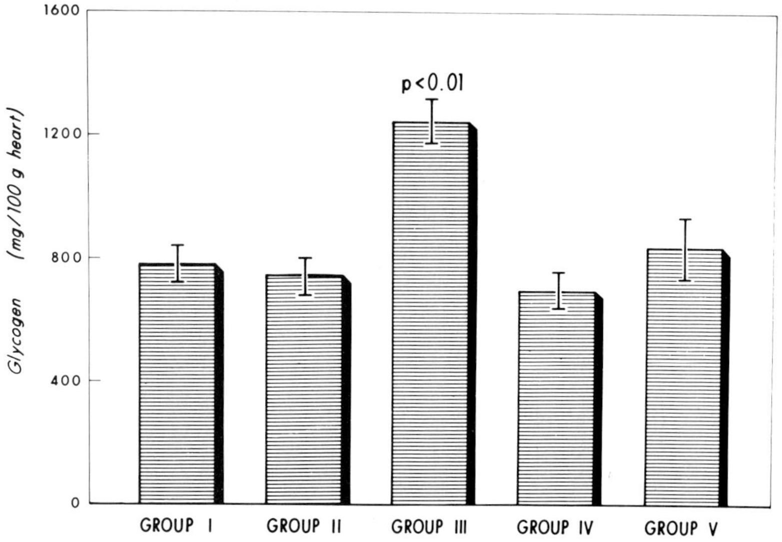

Fig. 1. Myocardial glycogen levels (mean values ± standard error).

completion of bypass. Mean aortic flow was determined by an electromagnetic flow probe around the ascending aorta and a sine-wave flowmeter (Statham, Model 4000). Right atrial, left atrial, and aortic pressures were monitored, and left ventricular pressure was recorded through a 25 cm. length of polyethylene tubing (internal diameter, 0.070 inch and outer diameter, 0.110 inch) placed into the ventricle and connected directly to a pressure transducer (Statham, Type P32AA). A Sanborn Recorder (Model 150) was used for recording of all pressures. Arterial blood was sampled and monitored for P_{O_2}, pH, and P_{CO_2} with the use of an Instrumentation Laboratories pH Gas Analyzer.

The dp/dt max (mm. per second) was calculated from the left ventricular pressure curve tangent during isometric contractions.[15] The index of contractility, dp/dt max/IIT (sec.$^{-2}$), was used as a measure of the quality of contractile elements and was calculated by obtaining the isometric integrated tension (IIT) by planometric integration of the isometric phase under the left ventricular pressure curve.[6, 15] The dp/dt max/IP (sec.$^{-1}$) was also used as a measure of contraction since this factor is essentially independent of external pressure changes.[6, 12]

Left ventricular work was determined by the following formula[13]:

$$\text{Stroke work (grammeters)} = \frac{\text{mean arterial pressure cm. } H_2O - \text{left atrial pressure cm. } H_2O \times \text{stroke volume}}{100}$$

Stroke volume was obtained from the aortic flow rate and the heart rate.

Through a small purse-string suture in the left ventricular apex, a full-thickness myocardial biopsy was taken using a dermal punch (5 mm.). The biopsy was immediately placed in dry ice and frozen. Cardiac glycogen was isolated from potassium hydroxide digests of muscle and assayed by the anthrone method.[1] A second biopsy was taken just prior to the termination of the ischemic interval.

Cardiac function was measured exactly 20 minutes following restoration of coronary blood flow and then was compared with function measured just prior to the initiation of cardiopulmonary bypass. Manual cardiac massage and electrical defibrillation were used as necessary for restoration of heart beat, but pharmacologic agents were not administered. All animals were removed from cardiopulmonary bypass within the 20 minute interval following restoration of coronary flow.

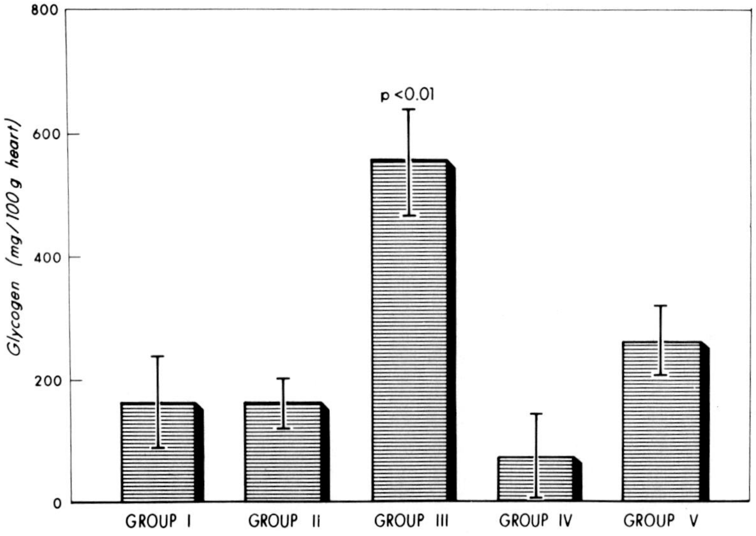

Fig. 2. Myocardial glycogen utilization during anoxia (mean values ± standard error).

The right ventricular effluent in Groups II, III, IV, and V was measured for Na^+ and K^+ with the use of a Coleman (Model No. 21) flame photometer, and for glucose in Groups IV and V with an orthotoluidine method. Right ventricular sump fluid was also assayed for lactic acid by using an enzymatic method (Sigma Kit No. 826-UV).

RESULTS

The results of cardiac glycogen measurements are shown in Fig. 1. Myocardial glycogen was significantly elevated ($p < 0.01$) in Group III, 1,244 ± 74 mg. per 100 Gm. heart muscle as compared to other groups (I: 779 ± 62; II: 745 ± 60; IV: 698 ± 60; and V: 844 ± 100 mg. per 100 Gm.). Glycogen utilization during anoxia for Group III was 555 ± 87 mg. per 100 Gm. heart muscle, significantly greater ($p < 0.01$) than for the other groups which did not differ significantly from each other (Fig. 2). To define further a correlation between glycogen level and glycogen utilized during the anoxic interval, the two groups perfused with saline (Groups II and III) were inspected, and glycogen utilized was plotted against glycogen levels. To avoid a possible spurious correlation, the mean of the initial and second glycogen levels for each animal in Groups II and III was used rather than the initial glycogen level. A correlation coefficient of 0.645 was found ($p < 0.05$) (Fig. 3).

Glucose utilization was observed in Group IV and in Group V as evidenced by decreases in glucose concentration in the right ventricular effluent to 2,159 ± 457 mg. percent and to 2,695 ± 850 mg. percent as compared to that of the perfusate (5,000 mg. percent). Myocardial potassium loss as measured in the right ventricular effluent for Groups II, III, and IV was 2.33 ± 0.64, 1.40 ± 0.24, and 1.07 ± 0.40 mEq. per 100 Gm. of heart muscle, respectively, although these differences were not statistically different from each other (Fig. 4). In Group V, a decrease in potassium concentration of the perfusate indicated that potassium was gained rather than lost by the myocardium. Sodium levels of the right ventricular effluent were determined for the two groups perfused with isotonic saline, Groups II and III, and were significantly decreased in each group (107 ± 15 mEq. per liter and 78 ± 15 mEq. per liter, respectively) from perfusate level (155 mEq. per liter) ($p < 0.01$), but these values were not significantly different from each other.

Among Groups II, III, IV, and V, no significant differences in lactic acid concentration or pH were observed in the right

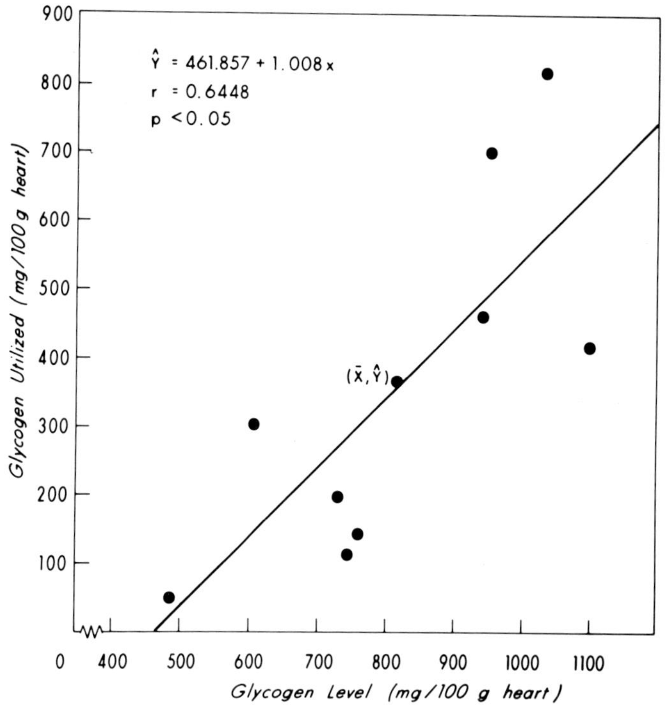

Fig. 3. Correlation of glycogen utilized and glycogen level (mean of initial level and second level) for saline perfused groups (II and III).

ventricular effluent. Lactic acid as determined from the right ventricular effluent for Groups II, III, IV, and V was: 212 ± 52, 145 ± 51, 273 ± 104, and 100 ± 17 mg. per 100 Gm. heart, respectively; and pH of the effluent was 7.18 ± 0.07, 7.01 ± 0.12, 6.95 ± 0.11, and 7.12 ± 0.12 for the Groups II, III, IV, and V, respectively.

Left ventricular temperatures monitored during the experiments declined slowly in all groups during the 30 minutes of anoxic arrest, and upon completion of the 30 minute period were as low as 32° C. to 34° C. in Group I and as low as 28° C. to 32° C. in Groups II, III, IV, and V. No attempt was made to warm the heart during the anoxic period.

Cardiac function was measured exactly 20 minutes following restoration of coronary flow and compared to control measurements. Manual cardiac massage and electrical defibrillation were used as required for restoration of heart contractions, but pharmacologic agents were not administered. Cardiac output after arrest and expressed as percent of original value was observed to be significantly better for Groups III, IV, and V as compared to Group I as measured 20 minutes after restoration of coronary flow (Fig. 5). Left ventricular work was depressed in Groups I, II, III, and IV following ischemic arrest, and was significantly better in Group IV and Group V as compared to Group I (Fig. 6). Maximum dp/dt/IP and maximum dp/dt/IIT determined 20 minutes after restoration of coronary flow and expressed as percent of original level prior to bypass and cardiac arrest were also significantly better for Group III, Group IV, and Group V as compared with Group I (Fig. 7). The time in minutes from restoration of coronary flow until normal sinus rhythm as measured by electrocardiogram is demonstrated in Table I. A significant difference in performance was observed in Group V as evidenced by a shorter period for recovery of normal rhythm than observed in other groups. Also as demonstrated in Table II, as a significantly fewer number of electroshocks were required for

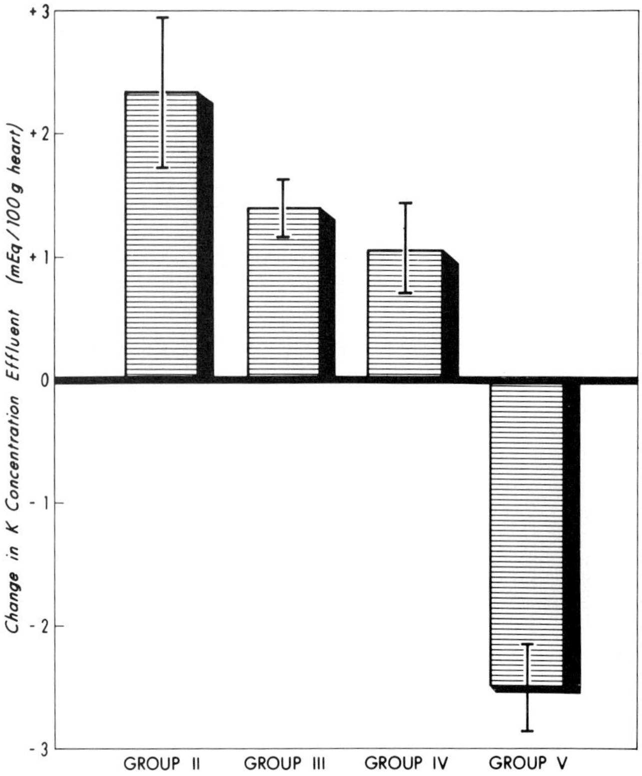

Fig. 4. Myocardial potassium loss as determined from right ventricular effluent (mean values ± standard error).

Table I. *Minutes resuscitation time until normal sinus rhythm*

Group	*Mean*	*S.E.M.*
I	13.5	2.16
II	12.6	2.79
III	11.2	2.22
IV	10.6	1.17
V	6.3	0.71*

*$p < 0.05$.

Table II. *Number of electroshocks for defibrillation*

Group	*Mean*	*S.E.M.*
I	8.5	2.9
II	13.4	3.17
III	7.8	2.03
IV	4.8	1.56
V	2.67	1.36*

*$p < 0.01$.

defibrillation in Group V as compared to other groups.

DISCUSSION

Results of the present study confirm that carbohydrate substrate either as stored myocardial glycogen or as exogenous glucose affords a degree of protection to the anoxic arrested heart as measured by subsequent cardiac function. Cardiac output, left ventricular work, and contractile function as determined by maximum dp/dt/IP and maximum dp/dt/IIT were significantly better 20 minutes following restoration of coronary flow in the group with increased myocardial glycogen (III) and in the two groups with glucose perfusion (IV and V) than in the control group (I). Significantly less time for recovery to a normal sinus rhythm following restoration of coronary flow and significantly less difficulty in defibrillation were observed when potassium and insulin were added to the glucose solution perfusate (Group V) as compared to control animals. The shorter period for cardiac resuscitation and the decreased use of electrical defibrillation in

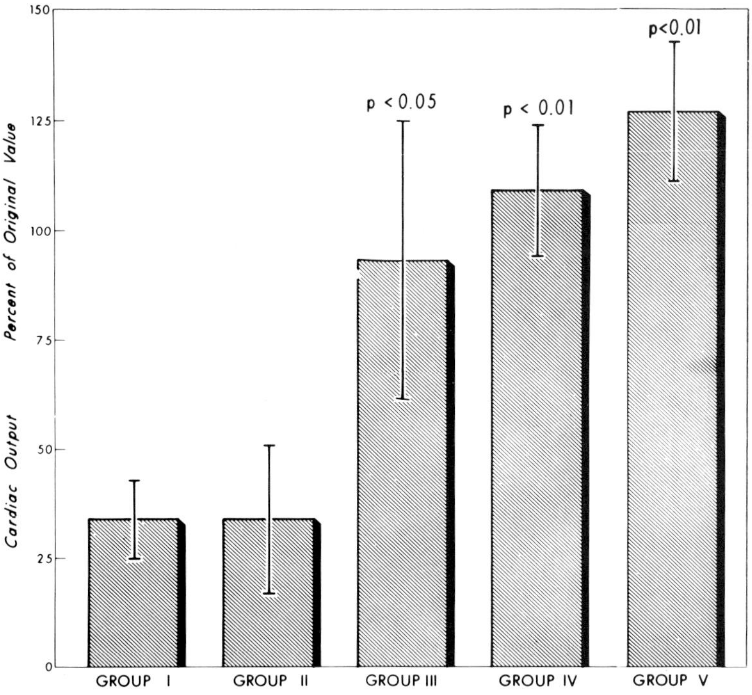

Fig. 5. Cardiac output as measured 20 minutes after restoration of coronary flow and expressed as percent of original value.

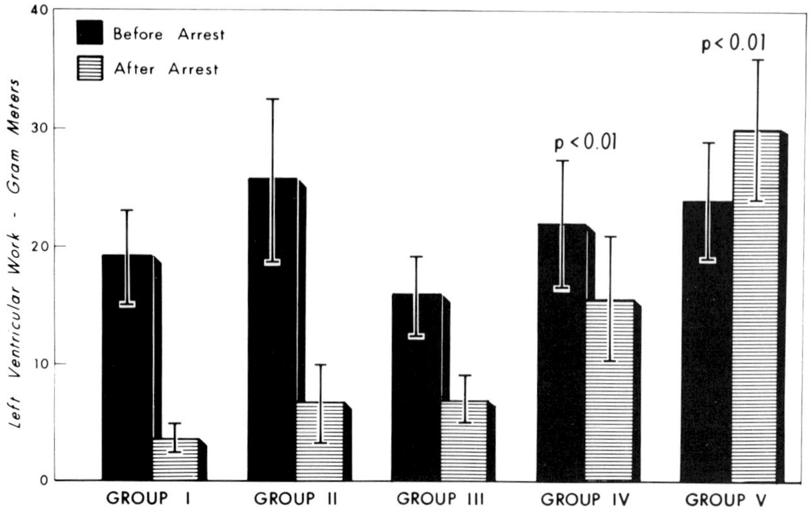

Fig. 6. Left ventricular work in grammeters (mean values ± standard error).

Group V must also be considered as possible factors in that group's having the best overall cardiac performance following arrest as compared to other groups. The benefit of the addition of potassium and insulin to the glucose perfusate as determined by cardiac function following arrest corroborates work of other investigators.[3, 11] The transport of glucose and potassium across the cell membrane and possibly other salutory effects appear to result from the availability of insulin and potassium in combination with glucose during cardiac anoxia.

Cardiac function in all groups was possibly

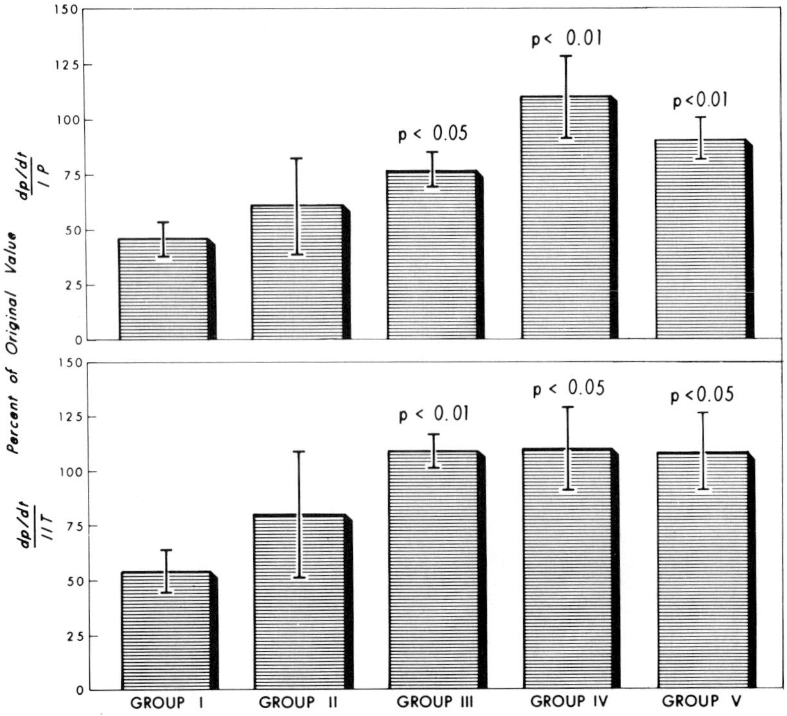

Fig. 7. The dp/dt max/IP (sec.$^{-1}$) and dp/dt max/IIT (sec.$^{-2}$) (mean values ± standard error).

afforded a degree of protection by the relatively low cardiac temperatures attained during anoxic arrest. This decline in temperature was achieved slowly during the anoxic period and was not significantly different among the groups perfused (II, III, IV, and V). Although not statistically different, the observed differences in temperature between Group I and the perfused groups should be considered in evaluating the results of function.

The accumulation of lactic acid and other acid metabolites has been observed to be a limiting factor in glycogenolysis.[4] Unpublished data from our laboratory have indicated that isolated glycogen-rich hearts (1,400 to 1,950 mg. per 100 Gm. heart) did not use glycogen at an increased rate over hearts with normal glycogen unless perfusion of the coronary vascular system with isotonic saline was performed as described in the present experiments. Noteworthy was the observation that the cardiac performance of Group II, saline perfusion, was not significantly different from the control group (I). Lactate recovery in the perfusion effluent was not significantly different for the groups perfused (II, III, IV, and V) and did not appear to reflect levels of glycogenolysis or glucose uptake. This observation is consistent with that of other investigators[7] and may be related to accumulation of other intermediate products in the Embden-Myerhof pathway or to a lag between intracellular and extracellular lactate levels secondary to slow diffusion rates.

Inability of the hypoxic heart to develop contractile force may be related to alterations in energy utilization for maintenance of ionic gradient and excitation-contraction coupling, both of which are ATP-dependent processes.[5] A shift in the composition of Na^+ and K^+ has been observed to occur before a defect in ability of the sarcotubular system to bind calcium become apparent. One possible mechanism in loss of potassium from the heart during isolated heart perfusion is paralysis of the membrane ATPase system, which is dependent upon high-energy phosphate regeneration.[10] The possibility that an

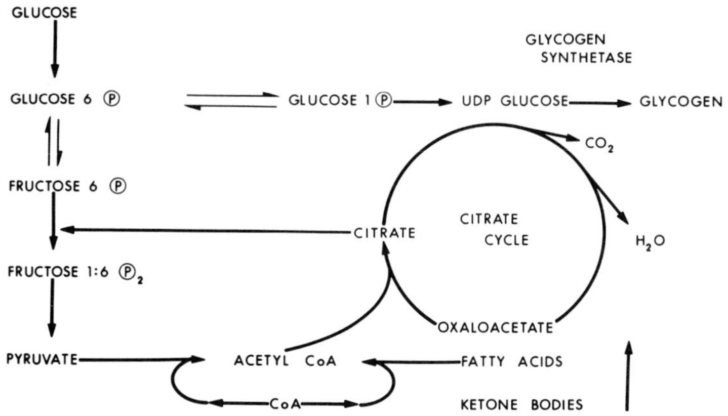

Fig. 8. Control of glucose metabolism in muscle by fatty acid metabolism. Increased acetyl CoA results in increased citrate level, which, through feedback inhibition, decreases phosphofructokinase activity, and leads to an increase in glucose-6-phosphate and ultimately glycogen. The increase in glucose-6-phosphate also promotes glycogen deposition by activating glycogen synthetase. (Adapted from Williams, R. H.: Textbook of endocrinology, Philadelphia, 1968, W. B. Saunders Company, p. 647.)

increase in anaerobic metabolism alone would protect the ATPase system and membrane transfer of Na^+ and K^+ is an attractive concept. Indeed, in the present experiments, Groups III (glycogen) and IV (glucose) did demonstrate a lesser myocardial loss of K^+ as measured in the perfusion effluent than did Group II (isotonic saline), but these differences were not statistically significant. Potassium loss was anticipated from perfusion of the heart with the noncolloid, K^+-free solution as well as a result of anoxic tissue injury. The addition of potassium and insulin to the glucose perfusate (Group V) resulted in an apparent increase in myocardial potassium. The significant decrease in sodium concentration in the perfusion effluent from Groups II and III (saline perfusion groups) indicates the probability of Na^+ gain by the myocardium during the anoxic perfusion.

The administration of a diet consisting exclusively of fat for three to five days has been observed to be a reliable method of increasing myocardial glycogen levels.[6, 9] The mechanism is believed to be related to an increase in fatty acids resulting in an increase in acetyl CoA through the Randle cycle and ultimately through an increase in citrate level (Fig. 8).[1, 16] An increase in the acetyl CoA to CoA ratio leads to an increase in the concentration of citrate, which favors the inhibition of phosphofructokinase. The result is a decrease in glycolysis and a buildup of glucose-6-phosphate, which is converted to glycogen. The increase in glucose-6-phosphate also promotes glycogen deposition by activating glycogen synthetase. The increased utilization of glycogen during anoxia resulting from increased glycogen content has been observed consistently and is believed to be related to a mass action effect of the increased stored glycogen or to the possibility that elevated glycogen stores represent a more labile fraction than normal glycogen stores.[6]

REFERENCES

1. Adrouny, G. A.: Differential patterns of glycogen metabolism in cardiac and skeletal muscles, Am. J. Physiol. **217:** 686, 1969.
2. Austen, W. G., Greenberg, J. J., and Piccinini, J. C.: Myocardial function and contractile force affected by glucose loading the heart during anoxia, SURGERY **57:** 839, 1965.
3. Calva, E., Mujica, A. B., and Sodi-Pallares, D.: Oxidative phosphorylation in cardiac infarct. Effect of glycose-KCl-insulin solution, Am. J. Physiol. **209:** 371, 1965.
4. Conn, H. L., Jr., Wood, J. C., and Morales, G. S.: Rate of change in myocardial glycogen and lactic acid following arrest of coronary circulation, Circ. Res. **7:** 721, 1959.
5. Dhalla, N. S., Yates, J. C., Walz, D. A., McDonald, V. A., and Olson, R. E.: Correlation between changes in the endogenous energy stores and myocardial function due to

hypoxia in the isolated perfused rat heart, Can. J. Physiol. Pharmacol. **50:** 334, 1972.

6. Hewitt, R. L., Lolley, D. M., Adrouny, G. A., and Drapanas, T.: Protective effect of myocardial glycogen on cardiac function during anoxia, SURGERY **73:** 444, 1973.
7. Huckabee, W. E.: Relationship of pyruvate and lactate during anaerobic metabolism. V. Coronary adequacy, Am. J. Physiol. **200:** 1169, 1961.
8. Katz, A. M., and Michihiko, T.: The "stone heart": A challenge to the biochemist, Am. J. Cardiol. **29:** 578, 1972.
9. Lolley, D. M., and Hewitt, R. L.: Protective effect of glycogen and glucose on the anoxic arrested heart during cardiopulmonary bypass, Surg. Forum **23:** 145, 1972.
10. Martin, D. R., Scott, D. F., Downes, G. L., and Belzer, F. O.: Primary cause of unsuccessful liver and heart preservation: Cold sensitivity of the ATPase system, Ann. Surg. **175:** 111, 1972.
11. Morgan, H. E., Randle, P. J., and Regan, D. M.: Regulation of glucose uptake by muscle. III. The effects of insulin, anoxia, salicylate and 2:4-dinitrophenol on membrane transport and intracellular phosphorylation of glucose in the isolated rat heart, Biochem. J. **73:** 573, 1959.
12. Nejad, N. S., Klein, M. D., Mirsky, I., and Lown, B.: Assessment of myocardial contractility from ventricular pressure recordings, Cardiovasc. Res. **5:** 15, 1971.
13. Sarnoff, S. J., and Berglund, E.: Ventricular function. I. Starling's Law of the heart studies by means of simultaneous right and left ventricular function curves in the dog, Circulation **9:** 706, 1954.
14. Scheuer, J., and Stezoski, S. W.: Protective role of increased myocardial glycogen stores in cardiac anoxia in the rat, Circ. Res. **27:** 835, 1970.
15. Siegel, J. H., and Sonnenblick, E. H.: Isometric time-tension relationships as an index of myocardial contractility, Circ. Res. **12:** 597, 1963.
16. Williams, R. H.: Textbook of endocrinology, Philadelphia, 1968, W. B. Saunders Company, p. 647.

Cardiorespiratory effects of hypertonic glucose in the critically ill patient

Frank Pindyck, M.D., Michael R. Drucker, M.D., Robert S. Brown, M.D., *and* **William C. Shoemaker, M.D.,*** *New York, N. Y.*

To test the hypothesis that inadequate energy substrates may be important to nutritional and metabolic failure in critically ill patients, we measured hemodynamic and oxygen transport effects of glucose (1 Gm. per kilogram of body weight) given intravenously over a 30 minute period in a series of severely stressed patients. The responses of patients who had been maintained on the standard clinical fluid regimen of five percent glucose were compared with those given 2,000 calories per day by intravenous administration of hypertonic glucose. The glucose load produced a marked improvement in hemodynamic and oxygen transport variables in the patient group maintained on five percent glucose; patients whose caloric needs were maintained with 50 percent glucose did not show significant changes. The findings suggest that insufficient nutrition may contribute to cardiorespiratory deterioration in the acutely ill patient and that these physiologic variables are improved by administration of adequate energy substrates in the form of hypertonic glucose.

From the Department of Surgery, Mount Sinai School of Medicine of the City University of New York

RECENT investigations have suggested that oxidative metabolism in the acutely ill patient is considerably different from the nonstressed individual. The hemodynamic and oxygen transport alterations that occur during shock and postoperative states provoke far reaching changes in body metabolism.

Poor tissue perfusion and inadequate oxygen delivery have been observed during many forms of acute illness; the resultant hypoxia has led investigators to explore associated metabolic changes. Under normal conditions, the peripheral and cardiac muscles utilize a variety of substrates. Fatty acids provide a major contribution to energy production in the fully oxygenated myocardium, but when the oxygenation of the cardiac muscle is limited, there is decreased oxidative phosphorylation and increased anaerobic glycolysis.[15] As fatty acids cannot supply energy anaerobically, glucose becomes the major source of energy. This suggests that glucose administration may be a useful therapy for the hypoxemia of critical illness.

The armamentarium for acute illness includes many different types of intravenous fluids for maintenance and replacement. Since few of these have a glucose concentration in excess of five percent, the available calories are inadequate relative to the metabolic needs of the severely stressed patient.

Supported in part by United States Army Contract No. DADA-17-69-C-9089 and United States Public Health Service Grant No. GM 01707.

Accepted for publication Oct. 21, 1973.

*Current address (1973-1974): William C. Shoemaker, M.D., 100 E. Valencia Mesa Dr., Fullerton, Calif. 92635.

Table I. *Clinical data of the series*

Patient	*Age (yr.)*	*Sex*	*Diagnosis*	*Surgery*	*Outcome*	*Group*
F. L.	79	M	Aortic aneurysm, pneumonia, debility	None	Died	1
I. I.	76	M	Stab wound, left ventricle	Thoracotomy	Survived	2
J. R.	91	M	Ruptured aortic aneurysm	Aortofemoral bypass	Died	2
B. F.	47	M	Cardiogenic shock	None	Died	1
A. K.	80	M	Massive upper gastrointestinal bleeder	Gastrotomy, ligation of arterial bleeding point	Survived	1, 2*
H. S.	58	M	Auto accident, spinal cord transection, ruptured spleen	Splenectomy	Died after complications, 30 days after injury	2
H. L.	79	M	Auto accident, multiple fractures	None	Survived	1
J. S.	78	M	Ruptured aortic aneurysm	Aortofemoral bypass	Died	1
H. G.	46	M	Stab wounds, right ventricular, and laceration of liver	Thoracotomy, laparotomy	Survived	2
J. S.	56	M	Cancer of esophagus	Esophagogastrectomy	Survived	1, 2
D. W.	70	M	Intestinal obstruction, septic shock	Laparotomy and lysis of adhesions	Died	1, 2
P. M.	90	M	Septic shock secondary to urosepsis	None	Died	1, 2
D. H.	80	M	Cancer of colon with obstruction, debility, dehydration	Transverse colostomy	Survived	2
E. R.	68	F	Massive pulmonary embolism	None	Survived	1, 2

*The patients of Groups 1 and 2 were studied as Group 1 having received only five percent dextrose; then after 24 to 48 hours of hyperalimentation, they were restudied as group 2 patients.

Under ordinary circumstances of elective surgical procedures in healthy persons, attention to the metabolic consequences of trauma and illness is usually not important to patient survival. But in chronic wasting diseases, severe accidental trauma and extensive surgical procedures, inadequate nutrition may significantly limit survival.

Hyperglycemia in response to shock has been known since it was observed by Claude Bernard[3] in 1877. More recently, hyperglycemia was seen in Vietnam casualities and in myocardial infarction patients.[4, 12] Catechol amine release with resultant increased hepatic glycogenolysis has been suggested as the cause of the observed hyperglycemia[21]; since hyperglycemia was prevented by adrenal medullectomy prior to the hypovolemic shock, it was concluded that hyperglycemia was produced by adrenal medullary catechol amine release.[8] Subsequently, Walker and associates[24] and Hume[11] demonstrated markedly increased rates of catechol release from the adrenal gland with the onset of hemorrhage. These and other hepatic physiologic responses may be reproduced by exogenous administration of epinephrine.[17] But the stimulation of gluconeogenesis and the inhibition of peripheral glucose uptake by steroids as well as the inhibition of pancreatic release of insulin observed with high circulating catechol amine levels are possible contributory factors to hyperglycemia.[14] When stress or hemorrhage was prolonged, hypoglycemia occurred as hepatic glycogen stores became depleted.[10, 20] Allison[1] observed increased survival of severely burned patients following the intravenous administration of large doses of glucose and insulin in combination with standard burn therapy.

In the present report, we studied the cardiorespiratory effects of large doses of exogenous glucose given to a group of severely stressed surgical patients. Our hypothesis is that the severely ill patient requires oxidative substrates as well as oxygen and that the effectiveness of a given therapy may be estimated by changes in hemodynamic and oxygen transport patterns which reflect the over-all state of tissue perfusion.

MATERIALS AND METHODS

Clinical material. Nineteen studies were performed on fourteen patients with severe accidental or surgical trauma. Table I lists the pertinent clinical data. The patients' ages ranged from 47 to 90 years. Etiologic factors responsible for their acute illness included hemorrhage, dehydration and debility, sepsis, accidental and operative trauma, alone or in combination. All patients survived the study period. However, six died in a continued state of shock after the study; one died later in his hospitalization of complications following the acute illness, and seven survived and left the hospital apparently well. The patients were subdivided into two groups in an effort to evaluate cardiorespiratory responses to the glucose administration. Group I patients were those patients maintained on the standard regimen of five percent glucose infusions prior to the study period. Group II patients received at least 2,000 calories per day as 50 percent glucose intravenously prior to the study period.

Protocol. After three to six control measurements, glucose, in the dose of 1 Gm. per kilogram of body weight, was administered intravenously over a 30 minute period. Cardiopulmonary measurements were observed at 15, 30, 45, 60, 90, and 120 minutes following the beginning of the infusion. To differentiate the hemodilution effect of glucose from its metabolic action, an equal dose of mannitol (1 Gm. per kilogram of body weight) was given in an equal volume of water during a subsequent period; cardiorespiratory variables were measured in a comparable manner. Mannitol was used as a control because it is structurally similar to glucose and has similar osmotic effects, but it is not metabolized by the body.

Methods. The patients were studied by previously described methods[5, 18] Briefly, catheters were placed into the radial artery and superior vena cava percutaneously or via cutdown. A flow-directed Swan-Ganz catheter was placed into the pulmonary artery by way of a brachial vein cutdown or percutaneous puncture. Central venous pressure, arterial pressures, and pulmonary artery and precapillary wedge pressures were recorded with Statham pressure transducers and recorded on an Offner multiple channel recorder. The position of the Swan-Ganz catheter was determined by pressure tracings as the tip was advanced.

Cardiac output was estimated by the indicator dilution technique with indocyanine green. Arterial and mixed venous blood (from the pulmonary artery catheter) were obtained anaerobically at the time of the cardiac output measurements. The P_{O_2}, P_{CO_2}, and pH were measured at 37° C. by an Instrumentation Laboratories (IL) blood gas analyzer with micro-blood pH assembly. Direct measurement of arterial and mixed venous O_2 saturations and hemoglobin concentrations were also recorded by an IL-70 co-oximeter. Systemic vascular resistance, pulmonary vascular resistance, and stroke volume as well as left and right ventricular stroke work were calculated according to standard formulas. For comparative purposes, all measurements involving flow were divided by the surface area and expressed as indexed values. Oxygen extraction was expressed as ratio of the (A-V) O_2 content difference to the arterial O_2 content. Oxygen availability was calculated as the product of cardiac index and arterial oxygen content. Oxygen consumption was calculated as the product of cardiac index and the (A-V) O_2 content difference. Previously, O_2 consumption was measured concomitantly by this method and with the direct Fick measurements. The results of simultaneous measurements by these two independent methods agree within an experiment error of ten percent.[18]

RESULTS

Hemodynamic responses. Cardiorespiratory data before and after glucose infusion (1 Gm. per kilogram of body weight) in Group I and II patients are presented in Table II. The time courses of the hemodynamic re-

Table II. *Cardiorespiratory variables before and after administration of glucose or mannitol*

	Group I		
	Control	Post glucose	P value†
Mean arterial pressure (mm. Hg)	78 ± 5*	87 ± 6	0.05
Cardiac index (1 · min.$^{-1}$ · M.$^{-2}$)	3.8 ± 0.5	5.8 ± 0.9	0.05
Heart rate (beats/min.)	96 ± 6	100 ± 7	N.S.
Stroke volume (ml. · M.$^{-2}$)	40 ± 5	58 ± 8	0.05
Left stroke work (Gm. · M. · M.$^{-2}$)	43 ± 6	68 ± 4	0.05
Right stroke work (Gm. · M. · M.$^{-2}$)	12 ± 1	20 ± 2	N.S.
Systemic vascular resistance (dyne · sec. · cm.$^{-5}$ · M.$^{-2}$)	1,826 ± 261	1,268 ± 185	0.05
Pulmonary vascular resistance (dyne · sec. · cm.$^{-5}$ · M.$^{-2}$)	341 ± 83	225 ± 57	N.S.
Central venous pressure (cm. H_2O)	5.6 ± 2	7.9 ± 2	N.S.
Precapillary wedge pressure (cm. H_2O)	5 ± 2.5	9 ± 1.8	0.05
Oxygen extraction	26 ± 2	28 ± 3	N.S.
Oxygen availability (ml. · min.$^{-1}$ · M.$^{-2}$)	517 ± 66	697 ± 70	0.05
Oxygen consumption (ml. · min.$^{-1}$ · M.$^{-2}$)	128 ± 15	190 ± 33	0.05

*Mean ± Standard Error.

†N.S. = Not significant.

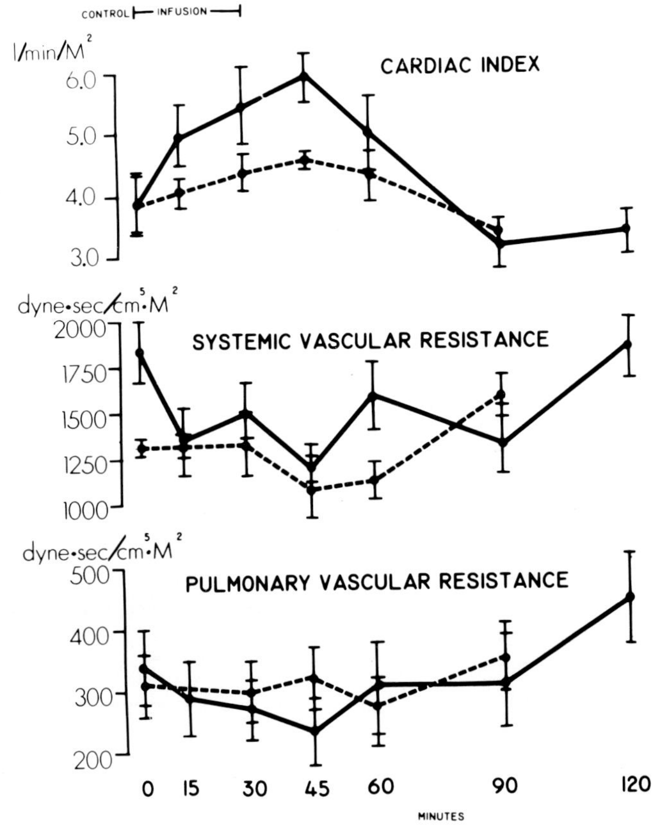

Fig. 1. Changes in cardiorespiratory variables after glucose. Serial changes in cardiac index and systemic and pulmonary vascular resistance before, during, and after administration of hypertonic glucose (1 Gm. per kilogram) over a 30 minute period. Note: Group I patients (solid lines), who had previously been maintained on five percent glucose, had greater responses to the glucose load. Dots connected by solid (Group I) or dashed (Group II) lines indicate mean values; vertical bars represent standard errors.

Group II			*Mannitol series*		
Control	*Post glucose*	*P value†*	*Control*	*Post mannitol*	*P value†*
71 ± 1	77 ± 6	N.S.	94 ± 18	95 ± 17	N.S.
4.2 ± 0.2	4.8 ± 0.1	N.S.	3.8 ± 0.6	4.0 ± 0.6	N.S.
878 ± 3	82 ± 3	N.S.	97 ± 6	95 ± 7	N.S.
54 ± 3	61 ± 2	N.S.	43 ± 13	45 ± 12	N.S.
53 ± 4	56 ± 4	N.S.	53 ± 12	55 ± 11	N.S.
16 ± 3	18 ± 2	N.S.	13 ± 2	16 ± 2	N.S.
1,307 ± 90	1,014 ± 75	N.S.	1,941 ± 390	1,725 ± 334	N.S.
311 ± 59	252 ± 72	N.S.	456 ± 54	368 ± 120	N.S.
5.6 ± 4	6.3 ± 3	N.S.	6.8 ± 4	12 ± 4	N.S.
7.7 ± 1	12 ± 1	0.05	8 ± 2.5	14 ± 3.6	0.05
25 ± 2	23 ± 2	N.S.	33 ± 1	33 ± 2	N.S.
546 ± 50	570 ± 45	N.S.	620 ± 68	627 ± 35	N.S.
134 ± 11	117 ± 12	N.S.	159 ± 7	130 ± 30	N.S.

sponses to glucose by the two groups are illustrated in Figs. 1 and 2. Responses in Groups I and II began shortly after the infusion and reached their maximum values at 37 and 43 minutes, respectively, after the beginning of the infusion. Increased cardiac index, stroke volume, and stroke work following the glucose infusion were associated with reduced systemic (peripheral) vascular and pulmonary vascular resistances in both groups, but Group I patients had greater responses. Significant change in precapillary wedge pressure was noted in both groups, but no significant heart rate or central venous pressure changes were noted in either group.

Myocardial performance, as illustrated by the Starling myocardial function curves, greatly improved in Group I patients but was not significantly changed in Group II patients (Fig. 3).

The hemodynamic responses of the mannitol infusion are summarized in Table II. There were relatively slight increases in central venous pressure and precapillary wedge pressure which reached maximal values at the end of the infusion. This is in keeping with the plasma expanding properties of an osmotically active substance. However, the improvements in hemodynamics were less than that observed after the glucose infusion in Group I patients. Except for the increase in precapillary wedge pressures, the changes were not statistically significant in mannitol and Group II. Fig. 4 compares the response to mannitol with that of 50 percent glucose in a representative patient; the marked response to hypertonic glucose and the absence of an appreciable left ventricular stroke work response to mannitol were seen in each of the patients studied.

Blood gas, pH, and oxygen metabolism. Oxygen transport data of Groups I and II are summarized in Table II and illustrated in Fig. 5. Arterial and venous Po_2 contents closely paralleled each other in both groups, but Group II patients had higher arterial Po_2 values after the glucose infusion. However, the increase in Po_2 was not reflected in an increase in actual peripheral oxygen exchange. No significant changes after glucose administration were recorded in Pco_2 or pH measurements.

Oxygen availability in Group I, rose markedly and reached a maximal value at the time of the maximal hemodynamic response; it did not change significantly in Group II. Small changes in oxygen extraction ratios were noted in both groups, but they were not significant. Changes in oxygen consumption rates in Group I patients were pronounced and significant; they increased an average of 63 ± 23 ml. per minute per

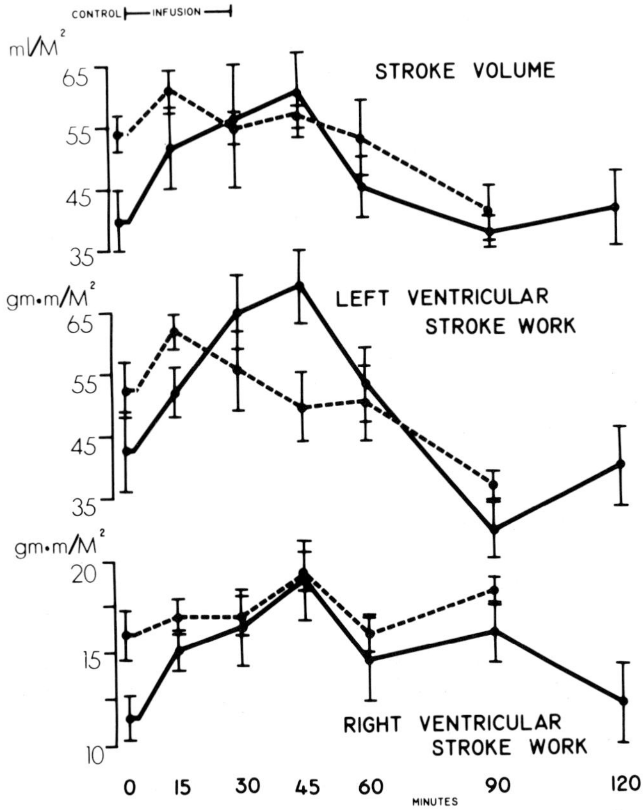

Fig. 2. Changes in cardiorespiratory variables after glucose. Serial changes in stroke volume and left and right ventricular work before, during, and after hypertonic glucose administration. Note: Group I patients had greater responses. Solid line represents Group I and dashed line represents Group II.

square meter at the point of their maxima. The oxygen consumption of Group II patients did not change significantly.

Responses of oxygen metabolism during the mannitol infusion were similar to those of patients in Group II. Oxygen consumption decreased slightly, but the decrease was not significant. There were no significant changes in pH, P_{CO_2}, P_{O_2}, oxygen extraction, and oxygen saturation after mannitol administration.

DISCUSSION

The present study provides evidence that during acute illness, increased amounts of glucose can produce significant hemodynamic and oxygen transport improvement. The observed differences in response to equal volumes of glucose and mannitol suggests that the improvement is not related to volume expansion but rather to the apparent utilization of glucose as an energy substrate for tissue metabolism. Though energy needs during illness presently are not precisely quantifiable, increased requirements during many forms of serious illness are suggested by increased body temperature and increased oxygen consumption rates.[18, 22] In our two groups of patients, the beneficial effects of added glucose were more pronounced in those patients maintained on 5 percent glucose infusions (Group I) than those maintained on 50 percent glucose therapy (Group II). This observation reinforces the concept that during stress, available energy sources may be insufficient to meet the metabolic needs of the patient.

Controversy has developed concerning glucose metabolism during acute illness. Basically, two major lines of speculation have

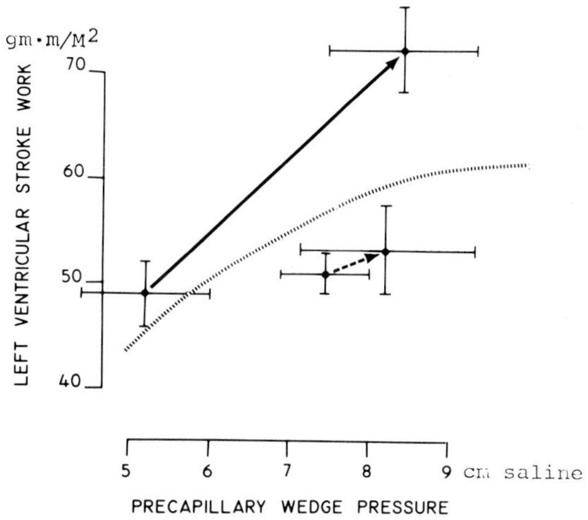

Fig. 3. Left ventricular stroke work values plotted against their corresponding precapillary wedge pressures in the control period and at the time of the maximal response (indicated by the arrow). Note the greater improvement in myocardial performance in the Group I patients. Dotted line represents data of a series of normal volunteer subjects given a volume load to define a segment of the normal Starling function curve. Solid line represents Group I and dashed line represents Group II.

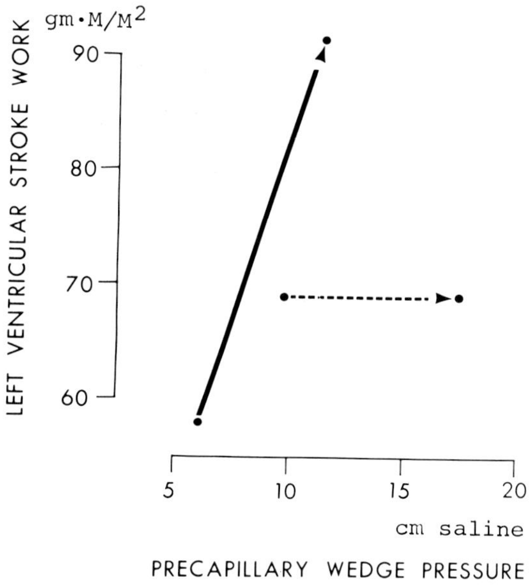

Fig. 4. Data of a representative depleted patient (No. 284) given hypertonic glucose (solid line) and then given mannitol (dashed line). Note the marked stroke work response to glucose and the lack of response to mannitol.

evolved. The first relates to insufficiently available energy substrates which are needed to supply the increased metabolic needs of the critically ill patient. Proponents of this view site the work of Field and Cori,[9] who showed that glucose loading progressively increased glucose utilization under aerobic conditions; saturation of the transport system occurred at serum glucose levels of 1,000 mg. percent. Morgan and associates[13] have shown in the perfused rat heart that the saturation levels are even higher under anaerobic conditions and that hypoxia increased glucose transport across the cell membrane and stimulated glucose phosphorylation. Drucker and DeKiewitt[6] in experiments on the rat diaphragm showed depletion of energy substrate stores and uptake of glucose by the diaphragm during prolonged shock.

The second line of speculation relates to the inefficient utilization of the available substrate. Proponents of this view cite the work of a number of investigators[2, 16, 22] who have shown a lack of insulin response to endogenous and exogenous glucose in a variety of critically ill patients. Further support stems from the discovery of possible defective intracellular mechanisms that have recently been shown to be operative during critical illness. ATP (adenosine triphosphate) and cyclic AMP (adenosine 3,'5-monophosphate), necessary for the actions of many hormones which are present in greater abundance in stress, have been shown to be depleted during experimental hemorrhagic shock and to remain depleted even after reinfusion of the shed blood.[16]

Our data lends support to the first of these contents, namely, that insufficient energy substrates may be responsible in large part for the metabolic deterioration of critically ill patients. The Group I patients would not have had improvement in hemodynamic variables and oxygen consumption rates, if inefficient glucose utilization were the major problem. However, both contentions may, to some extent, be operative during critical illness. The problem has been the inability to estimate metabolic failure in quantitative

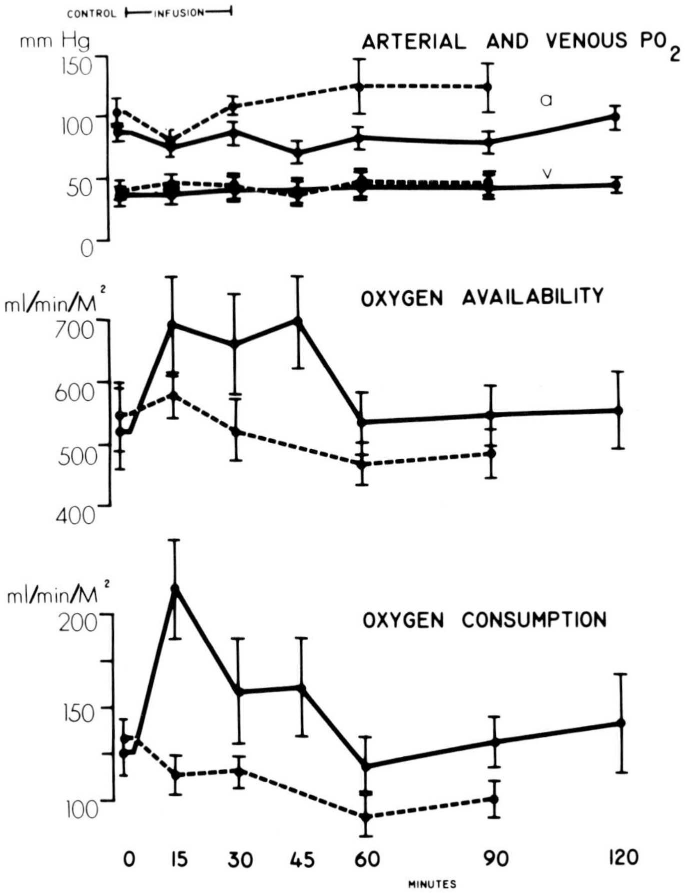

Fig. 5. Changes in cardiorespiratory variables after glucose administration. Serial changes in arterial and mixed venous Po_2, oxygen availability, and oxygen consumption before, during, and after hypertonic glucose administration. Note the marked increase in oxygen availability and consumption in the Group I patients, suggesting that these patients had been depleted of oxidative substrates and that this energy depletion had limited cardiorespiratory function.

terms and to relate it to the shock syndromes as a whole. Previous work from this laboratory has shown that cardiorespiratory alterations of shock patients vary in time.[19] Specific patterns seen early in shock are not present later on, and patterns seen terminally or preterminally are not the same as in the acute early stage. The metabolic response of the critically ill patient may be approached in a similar manner. Inadequate oxygen delivery and poor perfusion are seen at different times during acute illness. Hypoxemia may trigger increased anaerobic glycolysis which may require increased amounts of carbohydrate to maintain cellular function. In a previous report,[7] we showed this to be the case with respect to the hemodynamic effects of glucagon. Lack of oxidative substrates, increased metabolic needs, or both may lead to hypoxia and acidosis with inefficient utilization of the available substrates; i.e., insufficient supply may lead to inefficient utilization and compound the deficit.

REFERENCES

1. Allison, S. P.: Discussion of paper by Carey et al.,[3] Ann. Surg. **172:** 349, 1970.
2. Allison, S. P., Hinton, P., and Chamberlain, M. J.: Intravenous glucose tolerance, insulin and free fatty acid levels in burned patients, Lancet **2:** 1113, 1968.
3. Bernard, C.: Leçons sur le diabète et la glycogenese animale, Paris,1877, Vaillière.

4. Carey, L. C., Lowery, B. D., and Cloutier, C. T.: Blood sugar and insulin response of humans in shock, Ann. Surg. **172:** 342, 1970.
5. Carey, J. S., Brown, R. S., Mohr, P. A., and Shoemaker, W. C.: Cardiovascular function in shock due to hemorrhage, trauma and sepsis, Circulation **35:** 327, 1967.
6. Drucker, W. R., and Dekiewiet, J. C.: Glucose uptake in diaphragms from rats myocardial subjected to hemorrhage shock, Am. J. Physiol. **206:** 317, 1964.
7. Drucker, M., Pindyck, F., Brown, R. S., et al.: Enhancement of hemodynamic responses of glucagon following parenteral hypertonic glucose, Surg. Forum **23:** 58, 1972.
8. Engel, F. L., Winston, M. G., and Long, C. N. H.: Biochemical studies on shock: Metabolism of amino acid and carbohydrate during hemorrhagic shock in rat, J. Exp. Med. **77:** 397, 1943.
9. Field, R. A., and Cori, C. F.: The relationship between glucose load and utilization in normal and diabetic rats, *in* Cox, C. F., Foglia, V. G., Lelon, L. F., and Ochoa, S., editors: Perspectives in biology, Amsterdam, 1963, Elsevier Publishing Company.
10. Henneman, D. H., and Shoemaker, W. C.: Effect of glucagon and epinephrine on regional metabolism of glucose, pyruvate, lactate, and citrate in normal conscious dogs, Endocrinology **68:** 889, 1961.
11. Hume, D.: Some neurohumoral and endocrine aspects of shock, *in* Seeley, S. F., and Weisiger, J. R., editors: Recent progress and present problems in the field of shock, Fed. Proc. **20** (Suppl. 9): 87, 1961.
12. Mackensie, G. J., Taylor, S. H., Flenley, D. C., McDonald, A. H., Staunton, H. P., and Donald, K. W.: Circulatory and respiratory studies in myocardial infarction and circulatory shock, Lancet **2:** 825, 1964.
13. Morgan, H. E., Randle, P. J., and Reagan, D. M.: Regulation of glucose uptake by muscle. The effect of insulin, anoxia, salicylate, and 2:4 dinotrophenol on membrane transport and intracellular phosphorylation of glucose in the isolated rat heart, Biochem. J. **73:** 573, 1959.
14. Park, D., Graber, A. L., and Kuzaya, J.: The effect of epinephrine on immunoreactive insulin levels in man, J. Clin. Invest. **45:** 228, 1966.
15. Scheuer, J.: Myocardial metabolism in cardiac hypoxia, Am. J. Cardiol. **19:** 385, 1967.
16. Rutenberg, A. M., Bell, M. L., Butcher, R. W., et al.: Adenosine 3′,5′-monophosphate levels in hemorrhagic shock, Ann. Surg. **174:** 461, 1971.
17. Shoemaker, W. C.: Action of epinephrine and other hormones associated with the stress response of potassium movements, Rev. Surg. **25:** 9, 1968.
18. Shoemaker, W. C.: Cardiorespiratory patterns in complicated and uncomplicated septic shock, Ann. Surg. **174:** 119, 1971.
19. Shoemaker, W. C.: Cardiorespiratory patterns of surviving and nonsurviving postoperative patients, Surg. Gynecol. Obstet. **134:** 810, 1972.
20. Shoemaker, W. C., and Elwyn, D. H.: Liver: Functional interactions within the intact animal, Ann. Rev. Physiol. **31:** 327, 1969.
21. Stoner, H. B., and Threlfall, C. J.: Biochemical response to injury, Oxford, 1960, Blackwell Scientific Publications.
22. Taylor, S. H., Saxton, C., Majid, P. A., et al.: Insulin secretion following myocardial infarction: With particular respect to pathogenics of cardiogenic shock, Lancet **2:** 1373, 1969.
23. Tilstone, W. J., and Cuthbertson, D. P.: Protein component of the disturbance of energy metabolism in trauma, *in* Porter, R., and Knight, J., editors: Energy metabolism in trauma, London, 1970, J. & A. Churchill, Ltd.
24. Walker, W. F., Zileli, M. S., Reutter, F. W., Shoemaker, W. C., Friend, D., and Moore, F. D.: Adrenal medullary secretion in hemorrhagic shock, Am. J. Physiol. **197:** 773, 1959.

Strangulated obturator hernia

Stephen W. Gray, Ph.D., John E. Skandalakis, M.D., Ph.D., F.A.C.S., Raul E. Soria, M.D., *and* **Joseph S. Rowe, Jr., M.D.,** *Atlanta, Ga.*

A fatal case of strangulated obturator hernia is presented and 49 additional cases from the literature since 1946 are reviewed. Obturator hernia is uncommon in women and rare in men. Two thirds of reported cases occur in the seventh and eighth decades of life. The ileum is the organ most frequently found in the hernial sac. A history of previous attacks, spontaneously relieved, is common. Pain on the inner surface of the thigh extending to the knee (Howship-Romberg Sign) was present in over half of the patients. In no case was obturator hernia diagnosed in the absence of this sign. Presence of the sign did not always lead to correct diagnosis. The abdominal approach is the only one recommended in view of the low rate of correct diagnosis as well as the strong possibility that resection of the incarcerated bowel may be necessary. The sac should be ligated and large defects should be closed routinely to prevent recurrence.

From the Department of Surgery and the Department of Pathology, The Piedmont Hospital, and the Department of Anatomy, Emory Medical School, Atlanta, Ga.

Any crevice in the pelvic wall, however smoothly it is covered by peritoneum, is the potential site of a hernial sac. If such a sac forms, a loop of intestine or other pelvic organ will enter it, enlarge the sac, produce first obstruction and finally strangulation.

Among such openings, the obturator canal becomes a hernia site only occasionally. In addition to being uncommon, an obturator hernia forms no visible swelling until it becomes very large.

Perhaps the earliest report of an obturator hernia was that of Pierre Roland Arnaud de Ronsil, who presented two cases to the Royal Academy of Sciences of Paris about 1724.[14] The existence of so unusual a hernia without external manifestation was not accepted and seems not to have been published. In 1743, de Garengeot reported a case and collected six others. G. Arnaud de Ronsil, the son of the discoverer, first successfully reduced an obturator hernia.[24]

Although its reality was soon admitted, recognition of obturator hernia before operation is still the exception rather than the rule. Up to 1946, preoperative diagnosis was made correctly in 23 percent of reported cases.[24] Since 1946, diagnostic accuracy has increased to only 31.3 percent.

We were prompted to review the recently reported cases of this unusual lesion following the preoperative death of a patient from an undiagnosed obturator hernia. In many of the cases, including our own, correct diagnosis prior to surgery appears to be almost as rare as it was a century ago.

CASE REPORT

A 79-year-old woman was admitted to the hospital with complaint of intermittent, nonpenetrat-

Accepted for publication April 13, 1973.

ing, upper abdominal pain for three or four years. She frequently obtained relief by vomiting. The vomitus was usually green without obvious blood or odor. Stools were normal.

History revealed a weight loss of about 37 pounds over the last five years. At admission, the patient weighed 80 pounds. She smoked one package of cigarettes daily and coughed considerably. There were no cardiovascular complaints; the results of genitourinary and neuromuscular examinations were negative. There was no history of surgery or trauma.

On examination, the emaciated woman looked chronically ill, but she was mentally alert, intelligent, and cooperative. The skin was parchment-like and showed loss of subcutaneous tissue. The extremities were thin. The abdomen was scaphoid and no abnormal organs, masses, or pulsations were observed. Bowel peristalsis was thought to be slightly hyperactive on auscultation. The pelvic examination was not contributory. Proctosigmoidoscopy revealed normal mucosa to about 15 cm.

Results of tests at admission were as follows: WBC, 8,500 (71 percent neutrophils, 24 percent lymphocytes, and 5 percent monocytes); hemoglobin, 17.5 Gm.; hematocrit, 50 percent; stool guaiac, trace positive; blood urea nitrogen, 30 mg.; total bilirubin and serum amylase levels were normal. Abdominal x-ray was suggestive of partial small bowel obstruction with mild dilatation of the jejunum.

In the hospital, the vomiting persisted in spite of strong antiemetic drugs. The abdominal pain became more severe; the patient became markedly dehydrated; she vomited, aspirated, went into cardiac arrest, and died seven days after her admission.

Necropsy revealed generalized peritonitis with a positive culture of *E. coli* and *Candidae albicans*. There was a strangulated left Richter's obturator hernia of the jejunum 23 cm. distal to the ligament of Treitz. A perforation (0.5 × 0.8 cm.) was surrounded by necrosis and inflammatory cells.

ANATOMICAL CONSIDERATIONS

The obturator region. The obturator or adductor region is in the medial, upper third of the thigh, between the extensor and flexor muscle groups. Within this region lies the obturator canal and the origin of the adductor muscles from the obturator membrane and the margins of the obturator foramen.

The region, as defined by Anson and McVay,[4] is bounded medially by the pubic arch, the perineum, and the gracilis muscle, laterally by the hip joint and the shaft of the femur, superiorly by the horizontal ramus of the pubis, and inferiorly by the insertion of the adductor magnus on the adductor tubercle of the femur.

The obturator foramen. The obturator foramen, the largest foramen in the body, is formed by rami of the ischium and pubis. It lies on the anterolateral pelvic wall, inferior to the acetabulum. All but a small area of this huge foramen is closed by the obturator membrane, the fibers of which are continuous with the periosteum of the enclosing bones and with the tendinous attachments of the internal and external obturator muscles.

Developmentally, the foramen and its membrane represent an area of potential bone formation that never proceeds to completion. In this sense, the obturator foramen is a lacuna, and the obturator canal is the true foramen.

The obturator canal and its contents. The obturator canal is a tunnel 2 to 3 cm. long which begins in the pelvis at the defect in the obturator membrane and passes obliquely downward to end outside the pelvis in the obturator region of the thigh. It is bounded superiorly and laterally by the wall of the obturator groove of the pubic bone, inferiorly by the free edge of the obturator membrane and the internal and external obturator muscles. Through this canal pass the obturator nerve, artery, and vein. The relations of these structures to each other and to other structures within the pelvis may be seen in Figs. 1 and 2.

FORMATION OF THE OBTURATOR HERNIA

First stage (prehernial). Preperitoneal connective tissue and fat enter the pelvic orifice of the obturator canal (Fig. 3, *B*). Such "pilot tags," without dimpling of the peritoneum, are not rare. Anson and colleagues[3] found six examples among 360 body halves dissected. Singer and associates[20] found nine such tags among 14 female bodies and seven among 30 male bodies dissected. The frequency of pilot tags in cadavers and the rarity of actual obturator hernia in patients

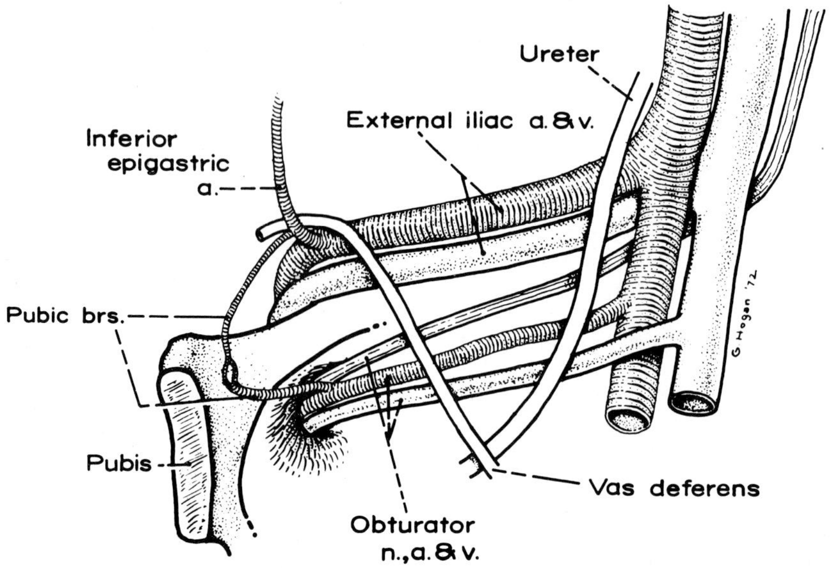

Fig. 1. The medial wall of the male pelvis showing the structures traversing the obturator canal and their relation to the ureter, ductus deferens, and iliac vessels.

suggests that few cases progress beyond the asymptomatic prehernial stage.

Second stage. The second stage (Fig. 3, *C*) begins with the appearance of a dimple in the peritoneum over the internal opening of the obturator canal and progresses to the formation of a peritoneal sac which may remain empty. The sac may follow the anterior or the posterior division of the obturator nerve (Fig. 4).

Third stage. The third stage begins with the onset of symptoms produced by entrance of an organ, usually the ileum, into the sac (Fig. 3, *D*). At first the herniation is transitory and reduces spontaneously. Later in the third stage, the herniated knuckle of ileum may fail to reduce spontaneously. If only a portion of the ileal circumference is incarcerated (Richter's hernia), the obstruction may be partial or complete. If an entire loop enters the sac, the obstruction will be complete (Fig. 3, *E*). Adhesions are not common, and the hernia usually can be reduced by traction. Necrosis of the incarcerated loop, however, may result in preoperative perforation or tearing during forcible reduction.

REVIEW OF THE LITERATURE

Incidence. In its anterior position, obturator hernia is close to the much more common inguinal and femoral hernias; in frequency it belongs to a group of rare hernias of the pelvic wall. Little is known of its incidence. Rogers[15] states that there were 12 cases of obturator hernia among 3,000 mechanical intestinal obstructions treated over 22 years at the Los Angeles County General Hospital.

Watson[24] found 442 cases of obturator hernia in the literature up to 1946. We have collected and analyzed 49 cases, in addition to one of our own, reported in the English language literature since 1946.

Sex, age, and side affected. Only seven of 49 cases occurred in males (Table I). The sex ratio is thus 1:6. Singer and colleagues[20] believe that the more vertical direction of the axis of the obturator canal in the male reduces the predisposition to hernia. The patients reported since 1945 are older than than those reported earlier. The modal group (36.7 percent) was in the eighth decade of life; in the earlier study, the modal age fell in the seventh decade. In the present series,

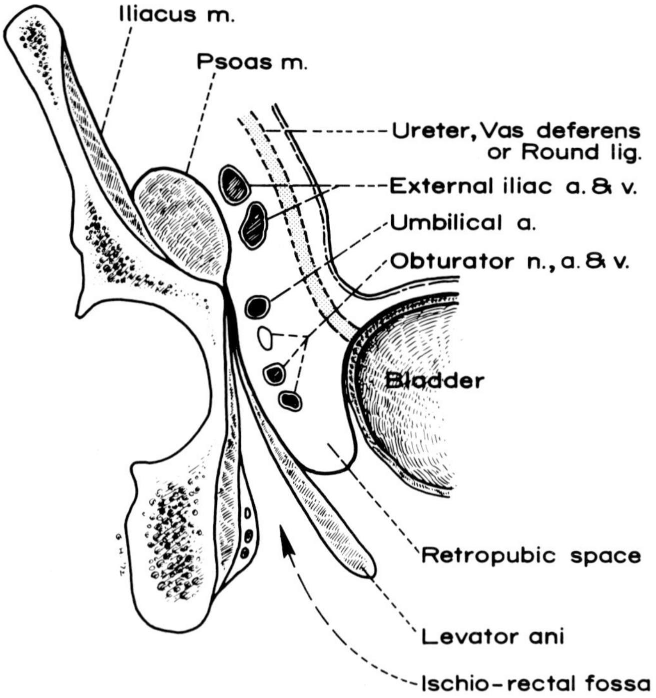

Fig. 2. Diagrammatic coronal section of the lateral wall of the pelvis showing the relations of the obturator nerve and vessels to other structures of the pelvis.

males appear to be affected earlier in life than females.

The right and left sides are about equally affected in male patients, but in female patients the right obturator foramen is involved three times as often as is the left (Table II). Among patients described as emaciated or among those who had undergone a marked weight loss, the ratio of left- to right-sided lesions is 1:1.3. Among those not so described, the ratio is 1:3.5. Thus, the left side appears to be more susceptible to hernia in thin patients than in those of normal habitus.

Contents of the sac. The hernial sac contained small bowel in most cases. A few other structures were occasionally found (Table III).

Symptoms and signs of obturator hernia. Symptoms of obturator hernia are acute, becoming progressively more severe, and are relieved only by reduction of the hernia (Table IV). Seventeen patients had a history of previous attacks, each relieved spontaneously

Table I. *Sex and age at operation*

Age (yr.)	*Male*	*Female*	*Total*
30–39	1	1	2
40–49	—	1	1
50–59	—	4	4
60–69	5	10	15
70–79	1	17	18
80–89	—	8	8
90–99	—	1	1
Total	7	42	49

until the last one. The longest such history was eight years. Two patients with empty peritoneal sacs found during elective surgery were asymptomatic.

Obstruction. Signs and symptoms of partial or complete intestinal obstruction were the presenting complaint in 43 of the 50 cases. Abdominal pain and vomiting were almost universally present; abdominal distention, tenderness and constipation were mentioned in less than half of the reports.

Hip-knee pain. More than half the pa-

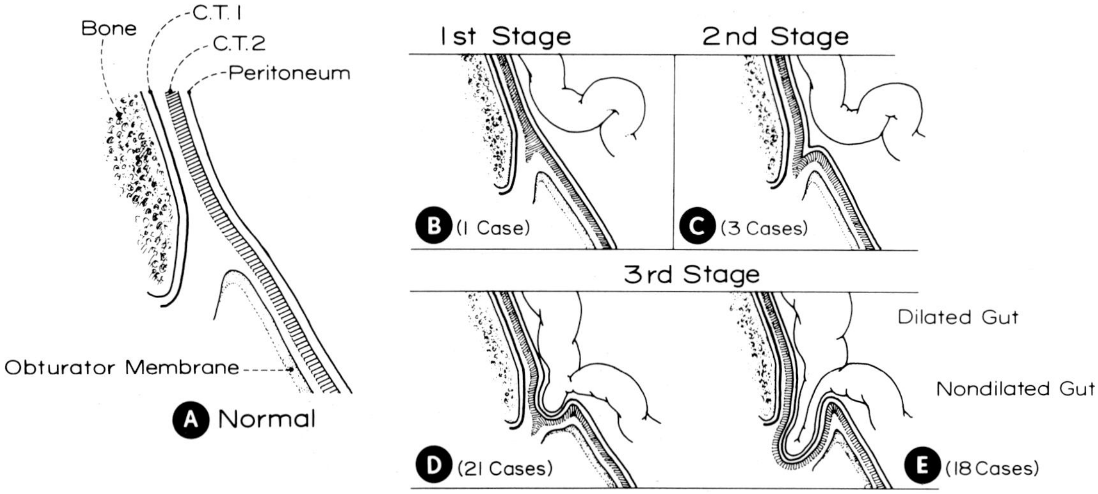

Fig. 3. The genesis of obturator hernia. *A,* Section through the obturator canal, pubic bone (above), and obturator membrane (below) form the boundaries. *B,* First stage: "pilot tag" of preperitoneal connective tissue in obturator canal. *C,* Second stage: peritoneal invagination beginning. *D,* Third stage: partial incarceration (Richter's) of an ileal loop. *E,* Third stage: complete herniation of ileal loop. C.T. 1 is the periosteal layer; C.T. 2 is the preperitoneal connective tissue.

Table II. *Sex and side affected**

Side	*Male*	*Female*	*Total*
Right	3	30	33
Left	4	11	15
Unknown	—	1	1
Total	7	42	49

*$Chi^2 = 4.497$; $P < 0.05$.

Table III. *Contents of obturator hernia sac*

Contents	*No.*
Ileum	29*
"Small intestine"	13*
Jejunum	2*
Appendix	2
Sigmoid epiploicae	1
Omentum	(1)*
Uterine tube	(1)*
None	2
Pilot tag only, no sac	1
Total	50

*Of the 44 hernias of the ileum, "small intestine," and jejunum, 20 were of the Richter type.

Table IV. *Signs and symptoms accompanying obturator hernia*

Sign or symptom	*No. of cases*
Obstruction	43 (+5 equivocal)
Howship-Romberg sign	27 (+4 equivocal)
Emaciation or weight loss	21
History of previous attacks	17
Palpable mass	9
Obstruction only	6

tients experienced pain extending down the inner surface of the thigh to the knee and sometimes lower, occasionally radiating to the hip joint. Flexion of the thigh usually relieves this pain; extension, adduction, or medial rotation exacerbates it. This is the Howship-Romberg sign. The pain results from compression by the hernia of the obturator nerve where it passes through the canal, especially affecting the cutaneous branch of the anterior division. The nerve contains motor as well as sensory fibers, and adductor weakness could probably be shown if pain from the sensory fibers did not mask it. Both sensory loss and motor weakness has been demonstrated following section of the obturator nerve.

The sign is not constant; many patients do not experience the pain. Its presence, however, is an indication of pressure on the obturator nerve. If the presence of a tumor of one of the pelvic organs is ruled out, the pressure can only be attributed to herniation into the obturator canal. The physician tak-

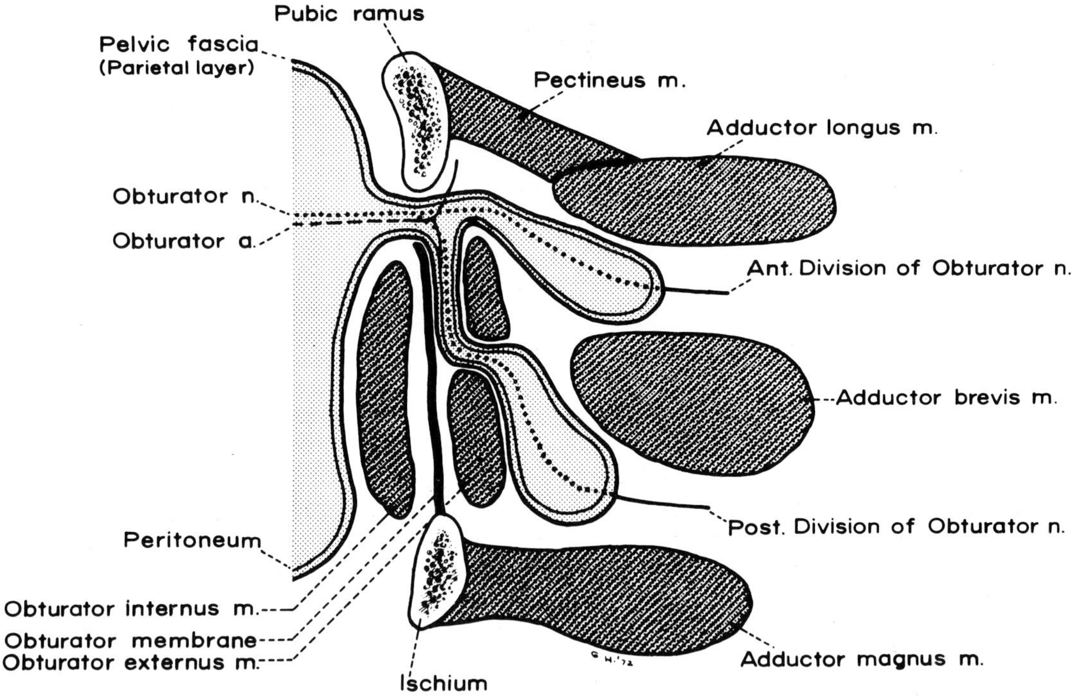

Fig. 4. Diagrammatic sagittal section of the upper thigh showing the potential pathways of obturator hernias. The hernial sac may follow either the anterior or posterior division of the obturator nerve.

ing the history must not overlook the significance of the medial thigh pain in elderly patients with numerous rheumatic pains of long standing.

Palpable mass. A hernial mass is palpable in only a few patients. The optimum position for palpation is with the patient supine and the thigh flexed, adducted and rotated outward. Rectal and vaginal palpation may aid in locating the mass. Tenderness or pain over the tumor will suggest strangulation of the hernia.

Diagnosis. The diagnosis of complete or partial intestinal obstruction was obvious in almost all of the cases. The nature of the obstruction was, however, often in doubt.

Obturator hernia was correctly diagnosed before operation in 15 of the 48 symptomatic patients (31.3 percent). In these 15 cases, the Howship-Romberg sign was the only factor consistently present. In another 12 cases, the presence of the sign failed to lead to a correct diagnosis, but in no case was obturator hernia diagnosed in absence of the sign.

The existence of a palpable mass or the history of previous attacks contributed to correct diagnosis only when they were accompanied by the Howship-Romberg sign. Although right-sided hernias are more frequent, this did not appear to influence diagnosis.

TREATMENT

An ileal loop, herniated into the obturator canal, may reduce spontaneously, ending a short episode of pain and partial obstruction. If it becomes stangulated, surgical intervention will be necessary. Treated early, the healthy intestinal loop may require only reduction. If surgery is delayed, gangrene will begin and the strangulated loop must be resected with anastomosis of the healthy intestine. Still longer delay will result in rupture of the strangulated loop and the onset of peritonitis.

The approach. The abdominal approach is the preferred method of treatment. Shackelford[19] suggests four advantages to this

Table V. *Summary of treatment of obturator hernia*

	No repair of defect	*Defect closed only*	*Sac excised only*	*Sac excised and defect closed*
Reduction only	4	13	3	3
Reduction and resection with anastomosis	9	9	2	3
Spontaneous reduction before operation	—	—	—	1
No operation	1	—	—	—
Potential hernia only	—	2	—	—
Total	14	24	5	7

approach. (1) It establishes the diagnosis. (2) It is the best way to expose the obturator ring. (3) It is the least dangerous to obturator vessels. (4) It permits intestinal resection where necessary.

The first advantage becomes important when the surgeon remembers that in the present series, 33 cases (66.0 percent) were not diagnosed as obturator hernia. The fourth advantage gains significance by the fact that in 23 patients (46.0 percent), resection of a portion of the intestine was necessary.

Two other surgical approaches have been advocated: (1) the Cheatle-Henry retropubic approach,[21] and (2) the inguinal approach.[19]

These approaches avoid entering the peritoneal cavity. Both give good results if it can be certain that (1) the patient's obstruction is actually caused by an obturator hernia and (2) that the incarcerated structures will not require resection. As these are the least predictable aspects of the lesion, the surgeon who uses these approaches will often be forced to make a second incision and approach the site of the obstruction through the abdominal wall. He should be prepared for this possibility before starting to operate.

Repair of the defect. As in other hernias, after the contents of the sac are reduced, the sac itself should be inverted, ligated, and the redundant portion excised. The stump, sutured to the margins of the obturator opening, will close the defect. More effective closure of the defect may be obtained by the use of a flap of autogenous fascia, prepared ox fascia, tantalum mesh, or a Teflon patch. Rogers[14, 15] has summarized the use of these and other materials for closing the obturator defect.

Among the 49 patients operated upon, no repair of the defect was mentioned in 13 (26.5 percent) (Table V). This deviation from the usual principles of hernia repair occurs because of the advanced age and acute illness of the patients afflicted with obturator hernia. In spite of this high percentage of unclosed defects, recurrence of the hernia was reported in only one patient.[16] Shackelford[19] stated that ten percent of such obturator hernias have recurred "in the past"; he gives no figures.

Mortality. Six of the 50 patients (12 percent) died, five after operation (ten percent) and one before. The average ages of those dying and those surviving the operation were 78.7 and 68.3 years, respectively. Four of the patients died of acute cardiovascular disease; two of these also had infection of their wounds. One patient who had undergone operation died from peritonitis following resection of the intestine. One patient, whose case is presented here, died of peritonitis from a ruptured jejunum before surgery could be performed.

REFERENCES

1. Adams, H. D., and Smith, D. C.: Obturator hernia; report of successful operative case, J. A. M. A. **137:** 948, 1948.
2. Ang, H. B.: Obturator hernia, Aust. N. Z. J. Surg. **40:** 86, 1970.
3. Anson, B. J., McCormick, L. J., and Cleveland, H. C.: Anatomy of hernial regions: Obturator hernia and general considerations, Surg. Gynecol. Obstet. **90:** 31, 1950.
4. Anson, B. J., and McVay, C. B.: Surgical

anatomy, Philadelphia, 1971, W. B. Saunders Company, vol. 2, p. 1123.
5. Ch'iu, H.-H.: Strangulated obturator hernia: Report of a case, Chin. Med. J. **75:** 328, 1957.
6. Craig, R. D. P.: Strangulated obturator hernia: A report of 4 cases, Br. J. Surg. **49:** 426, 1962.
7. Desmond, A. M., and Hutter, F.: Strangulated obturator hernia, Br. J. Surg. **35:** 318, 1948.
8. Gilfillan, R. R.: Obturator hernia, Can. J. Surg. **1:** 366, 1958.
9. Harper, J. R., and Holt, J. H.: Obturator hernia, Am. J. Surg. **92:** 562, 1956.
10. Joseph, W. L., Kipen, C. S., and Longmire, W. P., Jr.: Obturator hernia as a cause of acute intestinal obstruction, Am. J. Surg. **115:** 301, 1968.
11. Kwong, K. H., and Ong, G. B.: Obturator hernia, Br. J. Surg. **53:** 23, 1966.
12. Pender, B. W. T.: Recurrent obstruction of obturator hernia, Br. Med. J. **2:** 1038, 1950.
13. Pernworth, P.: Obturator hernia: Report of operation for irreducible incarceration, Am. J. Surg. **71:** 539, 1946.
14. Rogers, F. A.: Strangulated obturator hernia, Surgery **48:** 394, 1960.
15. Rogers, F. A.: Strangulated obturator hernia, *in* Nyhus, L. M., and Harkins, H. N., editors: Hernia, Philadelphia, 1964, J. B. Lippincott Company.
16. Rose, T. F.: Obturator hernia: Some difficulties in pre-operative diagnosis illustrated by two cases with unusual features, Med. J. Aust. **1:** 13, 1954.
17. Rothman, M.: The repair of obturator hernia with peritoneal graft, N. Y. J. Med. **51:** 1186, 1951.
18. Rowe, E. B., and Bynum, G. A.: Obturator hernia, Am. J. Surg. **18:** 770, 1952.
19. Shackleford, R. T.: Surgery of the alimentary tract, Philadelphia, 1955, W. B. Saunders Company, pp. 2369-2377.
20. Singer, R., Leary, P. M., and Hofmeyer, N. G.: Obturator hernia, S. Afr. Med. J. **29:** 73, 1955.
21. Soothill, E. F.: Obturator hernia, Guys Hosp. Rep. **103:** 43, 1954.
22. Throckmorton, T. D.: Repair of obturator hernia with a tantalum gauze implant, Surgery **27:** 888, 1950.
23. Waterfall, M. C.: Recovery from strangulated obturator hernia, Br. Med. J. **1:** 585, 1950.
24. Watson, L. F.: Hernia, ed. 3, St. Louis, Mo., 1948, The C. V. Mosby Company, pp. 457-475.
25. Yanover, R. R., Podolsky, W. G., and Marks, C. R.: Obturator hernia, N. Y. J. Med. **50:** 2317, 1950.

Stress at vascular anastomosis in relation to host artery: Synthetic graft diameter

C. E. Kinley, M.D., F.R.C.S.(C), P. E. Paasche, B.Sc., A. S. MacDonald, M.D., F.R.C.S.(C), *and* A. E. Marble, M.Eng., P.Eng., *Halifax, Nova Scotia, Canada*

Shear stress at host artery: Synthetic graft anastomoses was calculated from measurements made on Dacron prostheses placed in the abdominal aorta of dogs. Results indicate that the minimum stress at the anastomoses occurs when the graft-to-host artery radius ratio is approximately 1.4 cm. A comparison of stress magnitudes indicates that for any ratio between 1.0 and 1.6, the stress at the anastomoses is less than one-thirtieth of the yield stress for No. 6-0 suture, suggesting that failure is not due to suture rupture but to suture tearing through the arterial wall.

From the Department of Surgery, Faculty of Medicine, Dalhousie University, Halifax, Nova Scotia, Canada.

In a previous paper,[3] our group has shown that prosthetic vascular grafts are essentially nondistensible, whereas, the host artery has a diameter change of 10% over the cardiac cycle of pressures.[3] Follow-up studies[4] have shown that the prosthetic graft becomes more rigid as time passes, whereas host artery distensibility remains constant. This observation of large distensibility difference prompted us to investigate the magnitudes of the stresses existing at the anastomoses of the graft:host artery. Fig. 1 shows such an anastomoses, as well as the three stresses acting on the suture line. Fig. 1 indicates that both the axial stress and the shear stress are acting parallel to the suture. A mathematical model which relates these stresses to the intravascular pressure, and the physical properties of the vessel wall was derived by our group.[7] This model indicated that because of the large distensibility difference, the shear stress in the arterial wall just distal to the anastomoses is significantly larger than that found in the normal healthy artery. The model predicted that the minimum shear stress occurred at a graft-host artery radius of approximately 1.4 cm. Previous studies of the optimum ratio of graft-to-host artery radius has been based on blood flow.[5, 8] From these studies, Szilagi and associates[8] concluded that the ratio should be less than 1.6 in order to insure laminar flow and greater than 1.4 in order to accommodate the taper of the artery. In order to obtain some verification of the above ratio, our group has carried out dog experiments in which measurements were made in order to calculate shear stresses at anastomoses.

Supported from Canadian Heart Foundation (Grant No. 1200-365-018).

Accepted for publication July 18, 1973.

METHODS

Experiments were performed on five healthy mongrel dogs, ranging in weight from 18 to 22 kilograms. The dogs were anesthetized with pentobarbital sodium, (30 mg. per kilogram of body weight) and intubated. A laparotomy was performed to expose the abdominal aorta and a 4 to 5 cm. segment of this artery was replaced by a Dacron prosthesis. This prosthesis was selected so that the graft-host artery radius ratio at normal diastolic pressure (i.e., 80 mm. Hg) was in the range of 1.0 to 1.5. The graft was anastomosed end to end with the use of simple, continuous No. 4-0 Ethiflex. The abdominal incision was closed, and the dogs were allowed normal activity for a period of time which allowed the prosthesis to be enveloped by fibrous tissue. The animals were again anesthetized and a laparotomy carried out to expose the anastomoses for measurements. The lateral intravascular pressure was measured at the anastomotic site by using a No. 7 Fr. catheter* coupled to a Hewlett Packard transducer and a recorder (Hewlett Packard Model No. 7858A). The strain was measured on the host artery 1 mm. distal to the anastomoses with the use of a mercury in Silastic strain gauge coupled to a wheatstone bridge and the abovementioned recorder. A diagram of the measurement apparatus is shown in Fig. 2. Strain was continuously recorded for an intravascular pressure range of 100 to 200 mm. Hg. The higher pressures were induced by administration of 0.4 c.c. of epinephrine.

RESULTS

The strain measurements obtained from the five-dog experiments were converted to stress by first calculating the modulus of elasticity from the strain and pressure data by using equations given by Paasche and associates.[7] The shear stress data were plotted for a pressure range of 100 to 200 mm. Hg as shown in Fig. 3 for five ratios of graft:host artery radius. Each line on the graft shows the change in shear stress with pressure for a given graft-to-artery radius ratio. The reader will note that as the ratio increases from 1.05 to 1.45, the shear stress changes from a positive value of 10 × 10⁴ to a negative value of –2 × 10⁴ dynes/cm.². This change in shear stress from positive to negative can be explained as a change in the direction of the shear stress vector. In the mathematical model, the shear stress was taken as positive when directed radially inward toward the center of the artery. For the higher ratios, the shear stress has an outward direction for lower pressures, which causes the shear stress to be negative. When the pressure increases to 200 mm. Hg, the direction of the stress vector changes, and a

*U.S. Catheter & Instrument Corp., Glens Falls, N. Y.

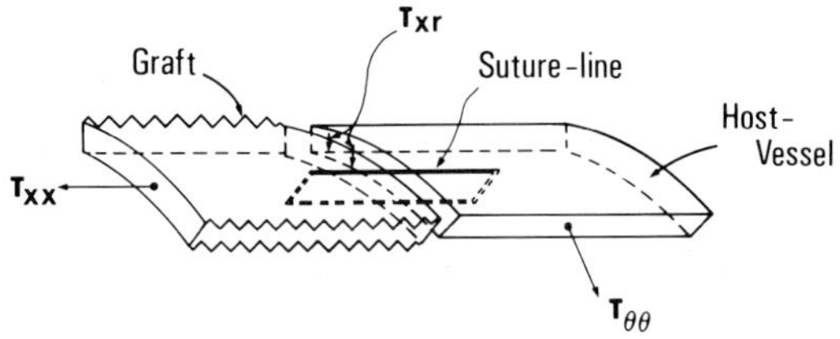

Fig. 1. Graft:host vessel anastomoses showing stresses acting on the suture line. The stresses are: T_{xx} (axial stress), $T_{\theta\theta}$ (hoop stress), and T_{xr} (shear stress).

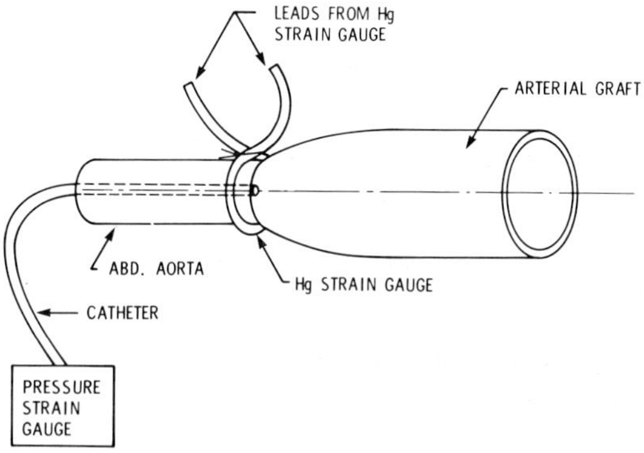

Fig. 2. Measurement apparatus used for acquisition of intravascular pressure and strain data near the anastomoses.

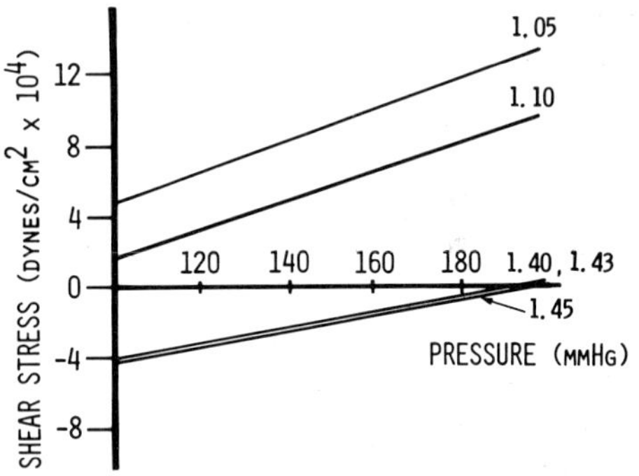

Fig. 3. Shear stress versus intravascular pressure for five graft: host artery radius ratios.

positive shear stress is developed. For the lower ratios, the inward direction of the shear stress is maintained for all pressures.

DISCUSSION

These experimental results seem to confirm the theorectical model's prediction that the minimum anastomotic shear stress occurs at a graft:host artery ratio of 1.4. However, the shear stresses determined are in the order of one-thirtieth of the tensile breaking stress of the suture materials used in this study. This suggests that disruption of suture lines in vascular prosthesis is not due to suture line shearing, but to the tearing of the artery by the suture. This is a result of excess shear stress caused by the marked contrast in graft: host artery distensibility. Work by others[2, 6] has shown that a truly nonabsorbable suture is required for permanent security of synthetic vascular grafts. Silk is not suitable, because the silk fibers fragment and are removed by mononuclear phagocytes, as was demonstrated by Cutler and Dunphy.[1] Three possible solutions to this problem are: (1) an investigation in order to determine the best pattern for suturing grafts to host-arteries; (2) the use of the ratio of 1.4; and finally, (3) the design of grafts which simulate the elastic properties of host arteries.

REFERENCES

1. Cutler, E. C., and Dunphy, J. E.: The use of silk in infected wounds, N. Engl. J. Med. **224:** 101, 1941.
2. Gardner T. J., Brawley, R. K., and Gott, V. L.: Anastomotic false aneurysm, SURGERY **72:** 474, 1972.
3. Gozna, E. R., Marble, A. E., Shaw, A. J., and Winter, D. A.: Distension and geometric taper of the thoracic aortic, Can. J. Surg. **15:** 113, 1972.
4. Gozna, E. R., Marble, A. E., Mason, W. F., and Winter, D. A.: The necessity for elastic properties in synthetic arterial Grafts, Can. J. Surg. In press.
5. Malan, E., Noseda, G., and Longo, T.: Approach to fluid dynamic problems in reconstructive vascular surgery, SURGERY **66:** 994, 1969.
6. Moore, W. S., and Hall, A. D.: Late suture failure in the pathogenesis of anastomotic false aneurysms. Ann. Surg. **172:** 1064, 1970.
7. Paasche, P. E., Kinley, C. E., Dolan, F. G., Gozna, E. R., and Marble, A. E.: Consideration of suture line stresses in the selection of synthetic grafts for implantation, J. Biomechanics **6:** 253, 1973.
8. Szilagi, D. E., Whitcomb, J. G., Schenker, W., and Waibel, P.: The laws of fluid flow and arterial grafting, SURGERY **47:** 55, 1960.

Surgical correction of advanced fibromuscular dysplasia of the renal arteries

Folkert O. Belzer, M.D., Oscar Salvatierra, M.D., Dorothee Perloff, M.D., *and* Henry Grausz, M.D., *San Francisco, Calif.*

A new technique for the treatment of advanced renal artery stenosis is presented. Complete correction of bilateral disease and normalization of blood pressure were obtained without antihypertensive medications in two patients. In the first patient, the levels of renal vein renins were normal before operation, became significant after unilateral correction, and were low after bilateral correction of renal artery stenosis. In the second patient, unilateral correction of renal artery stenosis and contralateral nephrectomy also resulted in normal renin levels after surgery. The role and significance of renin values in bilateral disease are discussed. The cases presented here are the first reported cases of clinical renal vascular reconstruction performed with the use of extracorporeal hypothermic continuous perfusion and are also the first cases of successful correction of bilateral lesions as well as that of a single kidney using in vitro reconstruction. This extracorporeal microsurgical technique should allow some previously inoperable patients to be considered for surgical correction.

From the Departments of Surgery and Medicine, University of California School of Medicine, San Francisco, Calif.

PATIENTS WITH hypertension associated with fibromuscular dysplasia and extensive arterial involvement often cannot be treated by conventional renal vascular surgery because surgical correction of renal artery stenosis is usually impossible if the disease extends into the branch arteries. If the disease in the branch arteries is minimal, dilatation, as suggested by Frye and associates[3] and others,[6] might be possible. However, this method is not applicable if the disease is extensive.

A new surgical technique will be described which makes it possible to correct previously inoperable lesions. The method was recently used in two patients with hypertension and bilateral fibromuscular disease involving primary branches of the renal artery. The procedure is described and the problems involved in the evaluation of bilateral renal artery stenosis by renin determination will be discussed.

REPORT OF CASES

Case 1. A 38-year-old white woman was admitted to the University of California Hospital, San Francisco, on Feb. 27, 1972, for evaluation of severe hypertension that had been difficult to manage by antihypertensive medication.

In February, 1970, the patient was found to have increased blood pressure in the range of 280/180 mm. Hg. An intravenous pyelogram showed that the left kidney measured 15 cm. and the right kidney measured 13 cm. The contrast medium appeared in greater concentration on the right side. The excretion of I^{131} Hippuran was

This work was supported in part by Grant No. AM-11290-06 from the National Institutes of Health.

Accepted for publication July 18, 1973.

Reprint requests: Folkert O. Belzer, M.D., Department of Surgery, University of California, San Francisco, Third and Parnassus Avenues, San Francisco, Calif. 94143.

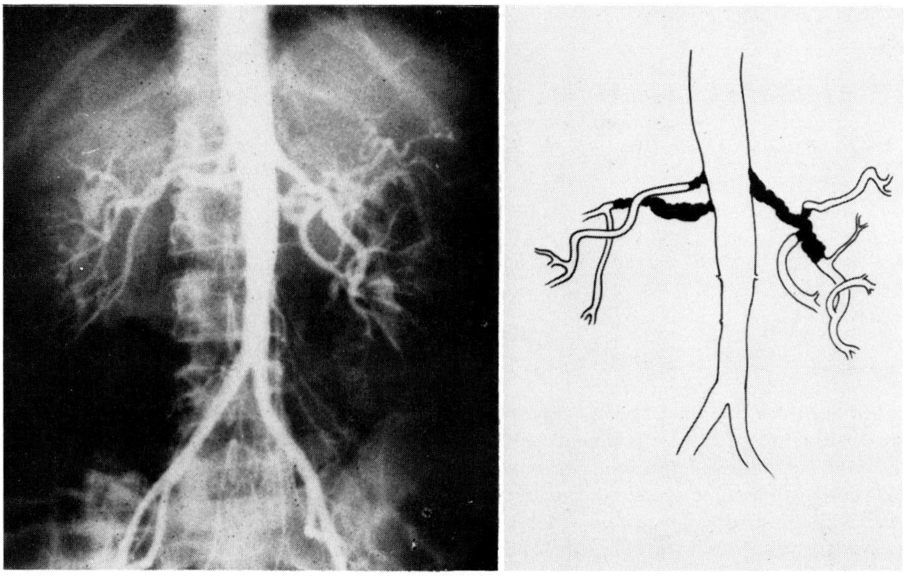

Fig. 1. Case 1. Preoperative arteriogram (*left*) and schematic drawing (*right*). Extent of fibromuscular hyperplasia of the renal arteries is shown in black.

Table I. *Renin determinations (ng./ml./3 hr.)*

	Right renal vein	*Left renal vein*	*Inferior vena cava*
Case 1			
Before left autotrans-plantation	8.7	11.4	7.2
After left trans-plantation	8.6	5.5	6.2
After bilateral transplantation	1.86	1.67	2.15
Case 2			
Before operation	40.0	19.2	19.2
After operation	—	—	5.0

symmetrical. Renal angiography showed that the left renal artery was severely affected by fibromuscular dysplasia extending beyond the first branching of the renal artery (Fig. 1). The right renal artery was duplicated and the smaller upper artery was narrowed at its origin. The lower pole artery in its midportion showed a localized dissection into the wall with severe narrowing (Fig. 1). The levels of urinary VMA (vanillylmandelic acid), serum electrolytes, serum creatinine, and serum calcium were all within normal limits.

The lesions were considered inoperable, and the patient was followed in the Hypertension Clinic and was treated with the following antihypertensive medications daily: Hydrodiuril, 100 mg.; Aldomet, 2 Gm.; Apresoline, 75 mg.; Guanethidine, 30 mg.; and Librium, 75 mg. In July, 1970, the patient was hospitalized because of substernal chest pain. Serial electrocardiograms showed subendocardial infarction and left ventricular hypertrophy. The patient made an uncomplicated recovery and on Jan. 24, 1972, a second renal angiogram again showed that the bilateral fibromuscular dysplasia unchanged from the earlier study. Renin measurements in renal venous blood are shown in Table I. During the three-year period following initial diagnosis of hypertension, the patient was considered on several occasions for surgical repair of the renal vascular lesions, but each time it was concluded that her lesions were inoperable.

On Feb. 27, 1972, the patient was hospitalized for extracorporeal microvascular repair of her left kidney followed by autotransplantation because of incapacitating symptoms of headache, weakness, repeated episodes of epistaxis and uncontrolled hypertension. Her preoperative blood pressure was 240/120 mm. Hg in the supine position, 180/110 mm. Hg while sitting, and 110/90 mm. Hg while standing. The fundi had marked arteriolar tortuosity and AV nicking. There was no evidence of hemorrhages, exudates, or papilledema. The chest was clear to percussion and auscultation. The heart beat was regular. The point of maximal impulse was 2 cm. to the left of the midclavicular line. A loud S_1 was present in the apex. A paradoxical split of S2 was heard at the base. No murmurs were heard. The abdomen was soft without organomegaly. A high-pitched bruit was heard

Table II. *Blood pressures and medication*

	Average office blood pressure (mm. Hg)	Portometer readings: Average systolic (mm. Hg)	Portometer readings: Average diastolic (mm. Hg)	Portometer readings: Average pulse	Medications
Case 1					
Before	240/140	180	124	94	None
Before	137/117	142	108	96	Guanethidine (30 mg.) Aldomet (2 Gm.) Apresoline (100 mg.) Hydrodiuril (100 mg.) Librium (75 mg.)
After left autotransplant	170/110	120	95	84	Aldomet (1 Gm.) Inderal (200 mg.) Valium (40 mg.)
After bilateral autotransplant	140/80	108	72	78	None
Case 2					
Before operation	220/120				Guanethidine (75 mg.) Hydrodiuril (100 mg.) Aldomet (2 Gm.) Hydralazine (300 mg.)
After operation	130/90				None

over the midepigastrium. The levels of serum electrolytes and the results of sequential multiple analyzer (with 12 different vital determinations) (SMA-12) and a complete blood count were within normal limits. Serum creatinine was 0.6 mg. percent and BUN (blood urea nitrogen) was 6.0 mg. percent. Creatinine clearance was 106 ml. per minute and the results of urinalysis were normal.

On Feb. 28, 1972, left nephrectomy was performed through a transabdominal approach. The kidney was placed on a specially constructed platform installed on the renal preservation unit. Arterial reconstruction was performed under continuous hypothermic pulsatile perfusion with the use of type-specific homologous cryoprecipitated plasma. The left hypogastric artery was used to replace the diseased segment of left renal artery. Segmental branches were reanastomosed with interrupted sutures of No. 6-0 and No. 7-0 silk. After repair, the kidney was implanted into the left iliac fossa with anastomoses of the renal vein end to side to the common iliac vein and the hypogastric artery end to side to the common iliac artery. The ureter was implanted into the bladder by a standard ureteroneocystostomy technique.

A renal arteriogram one week after implantation showed all anastomoses to be patent without obstruction. However, the distal renal artery, which had appeared to be normal preoperatively, had undergone some aneurysmal dilatation. This was thought to be due to localized disease of the distal renal artery which had been protected because of its proximal obstruction but had undergone dilatation after the obstruction had been relieved. The patient was observed for six months. A renal arteriogram showed that the aneurysmal dilatation had remained constant or perhaps had slightly decreased. Her blood pressure fell initially but returned to hypertensive levels four weeks after surgery. Control with antihypertensive medication was less difficult (Table II).

On Sept. 7, 1972, reconstruction of the right renal artery was performed by the same technique. Fig. 2 shows the classic signs of severe fibromuscular hyperplasia in the right renal artery. The postoperative course was normal, and the patient was discharged on the eighth postoperative day. A renal arteriogram now showed good anatomical repair without obstruction (Fig. 3).

Six months after a second operation, the patient is entirely asymptomatic and normotensive without antihypertensive medications. Blood pressure readings taken in the office by portometer before, between, and after surgical procedures are shown in Table II. (It should be mentioned that portometer readings are usually lower than blood pressures taken in the office.[11]) Renin values, before, between, and after the second surgical procedure are shown in Table I.

The patient's renal function continues to be excellent. The serum creatinine is 0.8 mg. percent, the BUN is 17 mg. percent, and creatinine clearance is 120 c.c. per minute.

Case 2. A 43-year-old white woman was admitted to the University of California Hospital, San Francisco, on March 7, 1973, for evaluation of severe hypertension. In 1968, the patient was

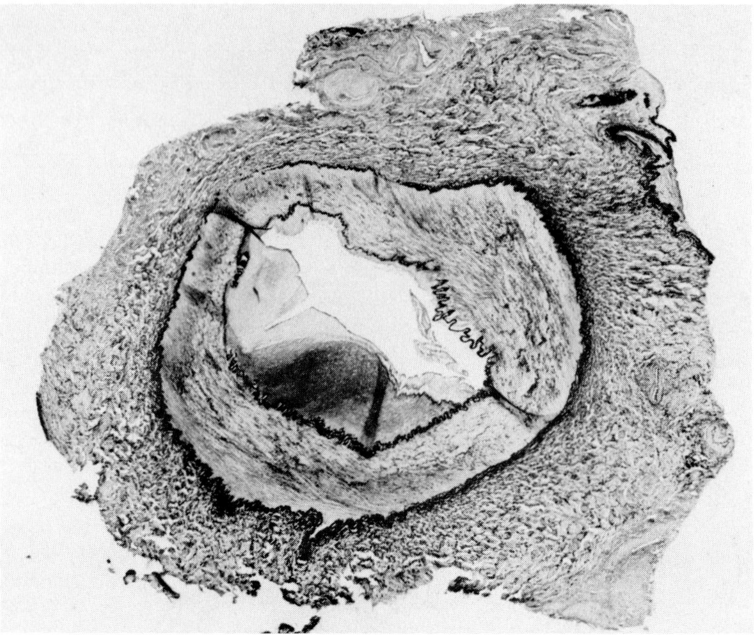

Fig. 2. Case 1. Cross-section of right main renal artery distal to area of dissection, showing severe fibromuscular hyperplasia. (van Giesen's stain; original magnification ×40.)

first found to be hypertensive, although she had been normotensive on previous examinations by the same physician. In 1971, she had been hospitalized by her physician for further studies. At that time, arteriography showed a small right kidney with extensive fibromuscular dysplasia of the left renal artery and three small arteries supplying the right contracted kidney.

In August, 1971, she underwent a left renal artery, saphenous vein bypass graft. The graft thrombosed shortly after surgery and she was admitted to the University of California Hospital. She had generalized cardiomegaly, electrocardiographic evidence of left ventricular hypertrophy, hypokalemia, proteinuria, and a serum creatinine level in the range of 2.1 to 2.9 mg. percent with a clearance of 31 ml. per minute. Angiography was again performed. The lesion of the left renal artery was thought to be inoperable, and it was decided that adequate medical control of hypertension should be attempted.

During the next year, the patient's hypertension was difficult to control and she was again admitted to the University of California Hospital in August, 1972, for further attempts to control blood pressure.

In February of 1973, the patient was seen in the emergency room for acute pulmonary edema and was subsequently readmitted to the hospital because of inadequate control of hypertension. Her blood pressure was 220/125 mm. Hg in the left arm in the supine position, 165/110 mm. Hg in the sitting position, and 165/105 mm. Hg while standing. Her heart was enlarged almost to the anterior axillary line with a 2+ left ventricular heave. The fundi showed Grade II changes but there were no hemorrhages, exudates, or papilledema.

Laboratory findings on admission included: hematocrit, 34 percent; blood urea nitrogen, 53 mg. percent; serum creatinine, 2.5 mg. percent; and creatinine clearance, 24 ml. per minute. Split function studies showed that the right kidney contributed 20 percent of the renal function. Blood pressures and medications are shown in Table II.

Another arteriogram was performed (Fig. 3). A selective left renal arteriogram showed severe involvement of the left main renal artery, an aneurysm of the upper branch artery, and severe constriction in the main renal artery branch distal to the first bifurcation (Fig. 4). Renin values are shown in Table I.

On March 21, 1973, left nephrectomy was performed through a transabdominal approach. The kidney was placed on isolated perfusion, and the reconstruction was performed under continuous pulsatile perfusion. The hypogastric arteries were severely involved by arteriosclerotic disease. In order to obtain a suitable arterial bifurcation graft, splenectomy was performed and the splenic artery was used. Interrupted sutures of No. 6-0 and No. 7-0 silk were used for anastomosis of segmental branches to the splenic artery branches.

After repair, the proximal end of the hypo-

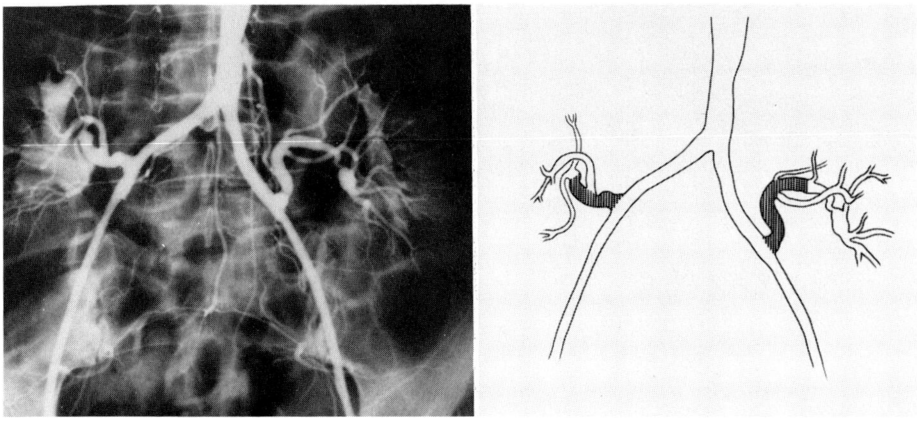

Fig. 3. Case 1. Postoperative arteriogram (*left*) and schematic drawing (*right*). Shaded area represents interposed hypogastric arteries.

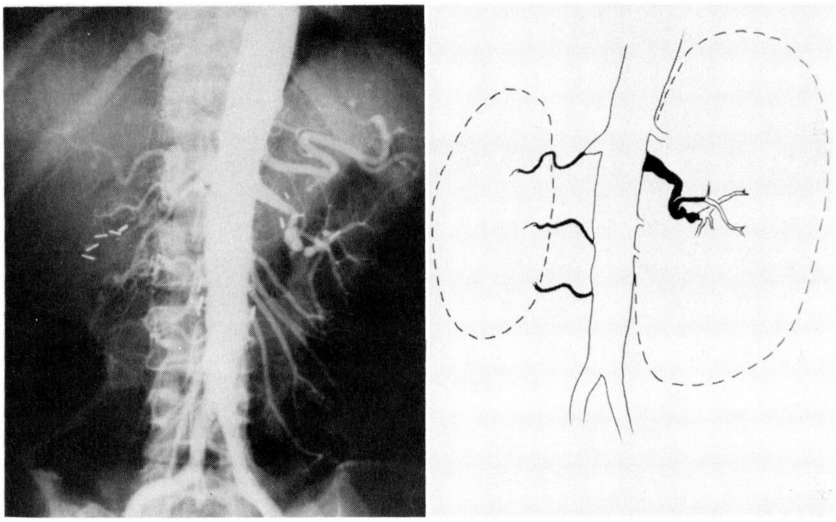

Fig. 4. Case 2. Preoperative arteriogram (*left*) and schematic drawing (*right*). Note splenic artery with bifurcation which was used for reconstruction.

gastric artery was endarterectomized, and the kidney was implanted into the left iliac fossa with end-to-side anastomosis of the renal vein to the common iliac vein and end-to-end anastomosis of the hypogastric artery to the splenic artery. The ureter was implanted into the bladder by standard ureteroneocystostomy technique (Fig. 5).

The patient did well after operation, and her blood pressure immediately returned to normal. The serum creatinine level rose to 3.5 mg. percent, and creatinine clearance dropped to 16 ml. per minute. When she was discharged on the eighth postoperative day, serum creatinine was 3.2 mg. percent and creatinine clearance was 22 ml. per minute.

A renal arteriogram eight days after implantation showed all anastomoses to be patent without obstruction (Fig. 6). Four weeks postoperatively the patient is normotensive without any hypotensive medications. Renal function studies four weeks postoperatively showed that her creatinine was 2.4 mg. percent, BUN was 32 mg. percent, and creatinine clearance was 30 ml. per minute.

DISCUSSION

As shown in Table I, the first patient's initial renal vein renin concentrations were within normal limits. The renin concentration ratio became significant on the right after correction of the left renal artery stenosis, when the criterion of 1½-fold increase on the affected side with suppression

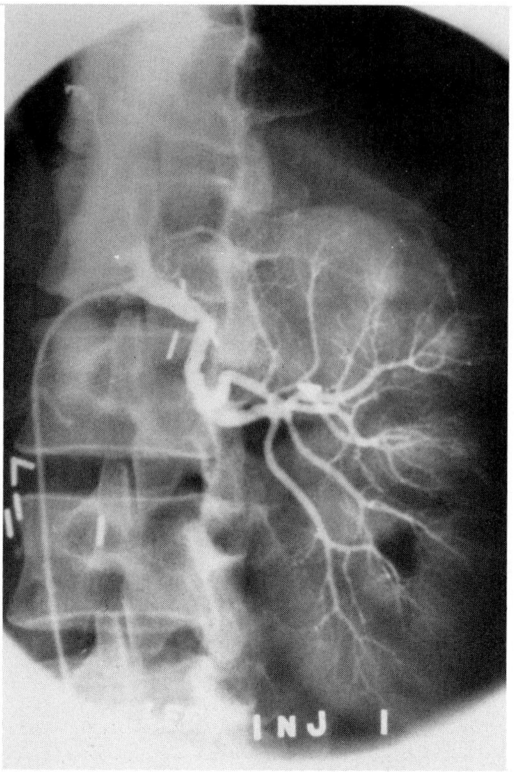

Fig. 5. Case 2. Selective arteriogram of left kidney.

on the unaffected side was used.[10] After both reconstruction procedures, the patient was normotensive without antihypertensive medication and the concentrations of the renal vein renins were extremely low. This suggests that although initial renin values were normal, the patient had significant renal vascular occlusion of the right renal artery which caused hypertension. The renin values in Case 2 (shown in Table I) suggest that hypertension was primarily due to occlusion of the right renal artery. However, reconstruction of the left kidney was performed because of the severe, progressive, obstructive nature of the left renal artery lesion and increasing azotemia. The fact that renal function has improved four weeks after surgery, although she had lost 20 percent of her functioning renal tissue, seems to have verified this decision.

The significance of renin values in bilateral renal disease is not fully understood.[5] Although we have presented only two cases, our data suggest that the criteria used in unilateral disease may not be entirely applicable to patients with bilateral renal artery stenosis. Criteria for renal vein renin concentrations in patients with bilateral disease have not been established.

The technique of in vitro renal vascular reconstruction, both in animals and man, was first reported by Mori and associates.[9] The technique of reconstruction with the use of extracorporeal hypothermic continuous perfusion was first described by us in laboratory animals in 1970.[1] This technique has several advantages over in vitro reconstruction with the use of only hypothermia, as described by other authors.[4, 7-9]

First, dissection of the extrarenal vascular tree is simplified because the vessels are distended; transection of minute vessels is immediately detected and can be readily controlled at that time. Second, the technique permits ample time for the procedure as this method has proved to be successful for preservation of human kidneys for as long as 70 hours. Meticulous attention to vascular reconstruction can thus be performed. At the end of the reconstruction, perfusion pressure can be temporarily set at normal systolic pressure and vascular leaks can be identified and controlled, thus alleviating the problems of excessive blood loss after reimplantation. Continuous perfusion in combination with standard donor nephrectomy technique prevents the occurrence of postoperative "tubular necrosis." Avoidance of this complication is essential since "tubular necrosis" is associated with marked reduction in renal blood flow.[2] Decreased renal blood flow in combination with multiple small vessel anastomoses would favor thrombosis at the anastomotic sites, and maintenance of normal renal blood flow after reimplantation is essential.

In both of the cases presented here, the ureter was divided, and after reconstruction, it was reimplanted into the bladder by a standard ureteroneocystomy technique. This avoids redundancy of the ureter after reimplantation into the iliac fossa, and we have found ureteral complications after transplantation to be very low. As an alternative, the

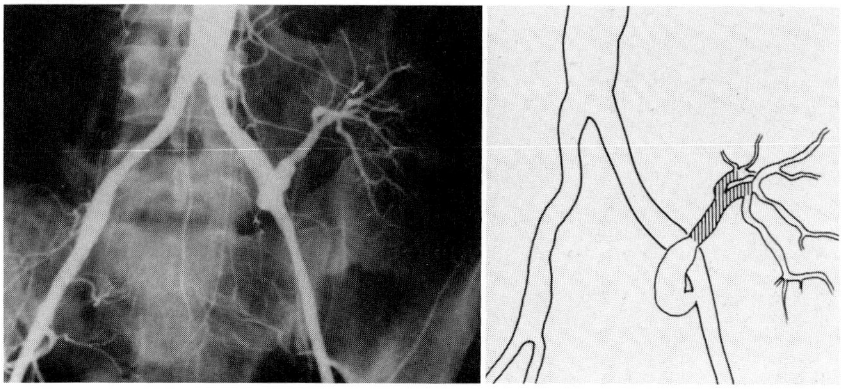

Fig. 6. Case 2. Postoperative arteriogram (*left*) and schematic drawing (*right*). Shaded area represents interposed splenic artery.

dissecting platform can be placed over the patient's abdomen and the ureter can then be left intact. If this procedure is used, an atraumatic clamp or sling should be placed around the ureter so that back-bleeding from the ureteral vessels into the perfusion reservoir will not occur.

The technique we have described permits corrective surgery of previously inoperable fibromuscular dysplasia or hyperplasia of the renal arteries extending beyond the segmental branches. This technique can be used in all patients with bilateral disease and in selected patients with unilateral disease.

The authors wish to thank Mr. Robert Hoffman and Mr. Kenneth Steiper for their excellent technical assistance.

REFERENCES

1. Belzer, F. O., Keaveny, T. V., Reed, T. W., and Pryor, J. P.: A new method of renal artery reconstruction, SURGERY **68:** 619, 1970.
2. Biber, T. U. L., Mylle, M., Baines, A. D., and Gottschalk, C. W.: A study by micropuncture and microdissection of acute renal damage in rats, Am. J. Med. **44:** 664, 1968.
3. Fry, W. J., Brink, B. E., and Thompson, N. W.: New techniques in the treatment of extensive fibromuscular disease involving the renal arteries, SURGERY **68:** 959, 1970.
4. Gelin, L. E., Claes, G., Gustafsson, G., and Strom, B.: Total bloodlessness for extracorporeal organ repair, Rev. Surg. **28:** 305, 1971.
5. Judson, W. E., and Helmer, O. M.: Diagnostic values of renin activity in renal venous plasma in renovascular hypertension, Hypertension **13:** 79, 1965.
6. Lamis, P. A., Stanton, P. E., Wilson, J. P., and Letton, A. H.: Fibromuscular disease of the segmental renal arteries, Arch. Surg. **106:** 109, 1973.
7. Lawson, R. K., Hodges, C. V., Pitre, T. M.: Nephrectomy, microvascular repair and autotransplantation. Surg. Forum **23:** 539, 1972.
8. Lim, R. C., Eastman, A. B., and Blaisdell, F. W.: Renal autotransplantation. Adjunct to repair of renal vascular lesions, Arch. Surg. **105:** 847, 1972.
9. Mori, S., Awane, Y., and Ueno, A.: Ex situ repair of renal artery for renovascular hypertension, Arch. Surg. **94:** 370, 1967.
10. Pawsey, C. G. K., Vandongen, R., and Gordon, R. D.: Renal venous renin ratio in the diagnosis of renovascular hypertension: Measurement during active secretion of renin, Med. J. Aust. **1:** 121, 1971.
11. Werdegar, D., Sokolow, M., and Perloff, D.: Portable recordings of blood pressure: A new approach to assessments of the severity and prognosis of hypertension, Trans. Assoc. Life Ins. Med. Dir. Am. **51:** 93, 1967.

Rewriting and the by-line: Is the author the writer?

Lois DeBakey, Ph.D.,* *Houston, Texas*

When a manuscript requires major revision to be acceptable for publication, the editor should return it to the author rather than rewrite the paper himself. Should an editor, or anyone else, rewrite an author's paper without changing the authorship, the by-line will no longer identify the actual author. Such a practice not only discourages scientists and physicians from improving their literary skills, but also involves functional risks, has undesirable ethical and aesthetic implications, and imposes an added economic burden on publishers of journals. The editor's insistence that authors revise their own manuscripts to meet high literary standards will suppress the submission of substandard or immature manuscripts and will ultimately elevate the caliber of scientific publications.

From Baylor College of Medicine, Houston, Texas, and Tulane University School of Medicine, New Orleans, La.

"I AM UNABLE to recognize the galley proof I received as the article I submitted to you for publication. Not only have you taken excessive liberties with my style, but you have also markedly altered my meaning so that the paper no longer conveys my thoughts. When you informed me that my paper had been accepted, you stated that its publication was 'subject to minor editorial changes.' If you do not wish to publish my article essentially as I wrote it, please return it to me immediately."

This fictional, but not improbable, communication from an irate author to a journal editor raises an interesting question: When an editor receives a manuscript whose content he considers scientifically sound but whose general literary form he disapproves of, should the editor rewrite it himself or return it to the author for the revamping deemed necessary for publication? Or, phrased in another way: To what extent is it appropriate for an editor of a scientific journal to emend a manuscript before publication? My position is that the published version of a scientific manuscript, as a scholarly product, should represent primarily the ratiocinative and literary efforts of the person(s) listed in the by-line and only incidentally those of an editor or others.

The key word in the question posed is "rewrite," the definition of which will vary from one editor to another. The point at which revision becomes extensive enough to be considered rewriting is not easy to identify. We can, however, eliminate as irrelevant to the present discussion nonsubstantive changes that merely make the manuscript conform to the policies of the journal about mechanical matters, such as abbreviations, citation of references, and the like. We can similarly eliminate an occasional grammatical change such as might be needed to clarify ambiguity or remedy awkward or faulty syntax. One other qualification: we are not here considering worthy manuscripts by foreign authors with a serious language prob-

Accepted for publication July 24, 1973.

*Professor of Scientific Communications, Baylor College of Medicine, Houston, Texas, and Lecturer, Tulane University School of Medicine, New Orleans, La.

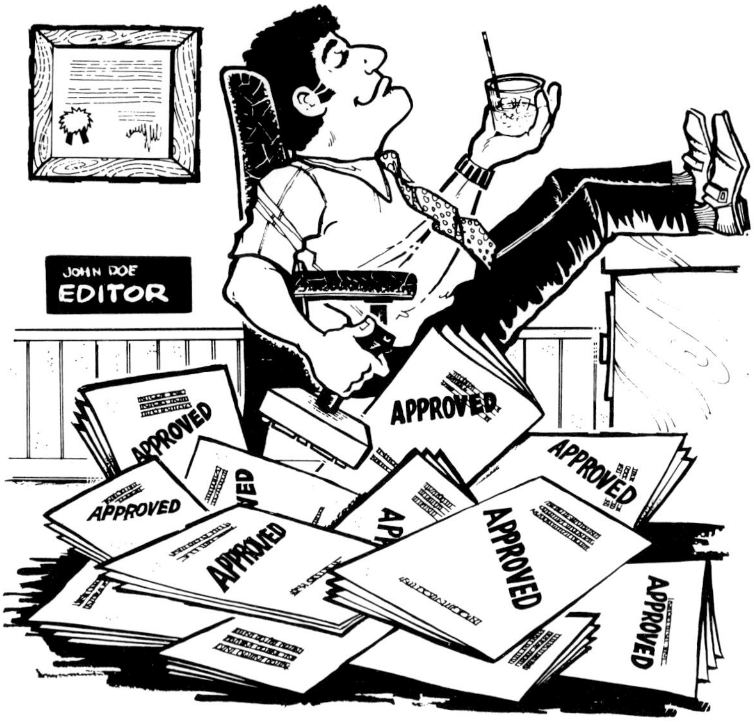

Fig. 1. The uncritical editor.

lem. What we are concerned with is major reorganization, excision, or recasting—perhaps even reconstruction of tables and graphs—changes which may indeed present the report in more lucid, logical, and readable form, but which may also distort meaning drastically, depending on how the changes are made.

The extent to which an editor of a scientific journal emends a manuscript before publication will vary according to the editor's views of his functions and responsibilities (Figs. 1 and 2). (For simplicity, "editor" in this discussion will be used to refer to the journal editor and his staff, including copy editors.) Some editors consider their primary responsibility to be the selection of scientifically valid and important material and a lesser function to be the maintenance of high literary standards. To protect the scientific integrity of their journals and the credulity of their readers, they will reject manuscripts which they think contain unwarranted hypotheses, illogical arguments, or invalid data, but they are usually less exacting about the quality of the prose. Other editors see their roles as encompassing both scientific and literary responsibilities and therefore evaluate not only content, but form and language as well. Such editors consider it more important to save the reader's time and effort than to gratify the ego of the author. They are less likely, therefore, to ignore disorderly sequence, illogical locutions, confused syntax, verbosity, or faulty diction.

Even among those who agree that the editor of a scientific journal has a responsibility to maintain general literary standards suitable to a scholarly publication, opinions differ about how he should meet this responsibility. Should he reject outright any manuscript that does not meet such standards? Or, should he accept a scientifically sound but crudely written manuscript on the condition that the author improve its literary quality? Or, should he and his staff undertake to rewrite a manuscript whose content he considers worthy but whose literary quality he considers unsatisfactory?

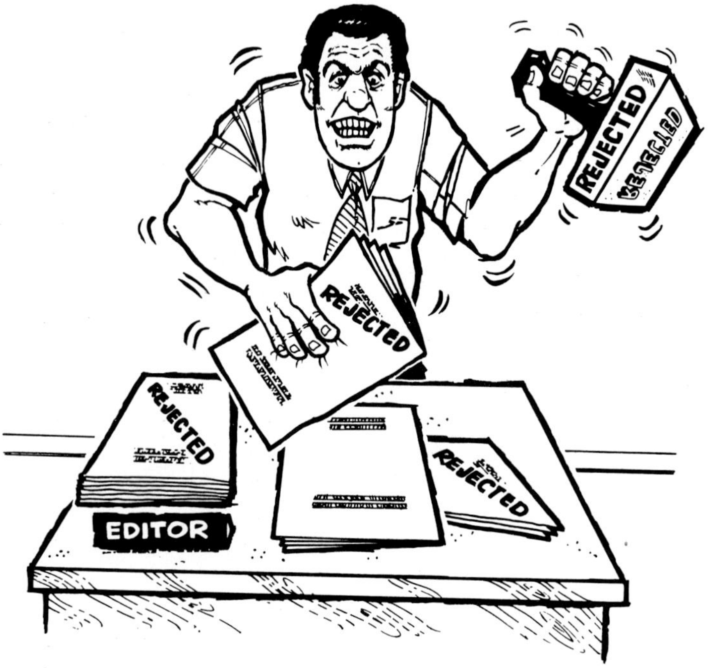

Fig. 2. The hypercritical editor.

WHOSE RESPONSIBILITY IS THE MANUSCRIPT?

Despite the view by some scientists of the report as a necessary but uninspiring chore after completion of the exciting research, the report is an integral part of the research project, since it is the permanent record of the performance and the means by which the researcher communicates to others any advance in knowledge resulting from his study. The preparation of the report is therefore the responsibility of the investigator; certainly no one should understand better than he the significance and implications of the results of the study. Such a report in a professional journal, moreover, is assumed to represent scholarship, and not the efforts of an auctorial surrogate. Allowing a ghostwriter to write or rewrite the report is therefore a form of deception that has a number of serious implications, some of which will be discussed later.

Anyone who produces a worthy piece of research should be able to prepare a clear, orderly account of that research. If he cannot, he should learn to do so, for he has not completed the project until he produces such a report. I make that statement with the conviction that anyone capable of productive research can learn, by the application of certain basic principles of good exposition, to write an accurate, lucid, and comprehensible, if not masterful, scientific report.[3] I am also convinced that clear writing requires clear thinking, and I strongly suspect that murky writing is preceded by murky thinking. With extensive practice in analyzing and rewriting under supervision, an author can discipline himself to think through his ideas thoroughly and clearly and then to seek the precise language that will convey those thoughts efficiently.[1, 2]

Extensive rewriting has some of the same educational, ethical, functional, aesthetic, and economic implications as ghostwriting, and I would like to explore a few of these implications in the succeeding paragraphs.

Educational considerations. Few journal editors consider it their responsibility to educate authors in effective self-expression, except, perhaps, by example. But even if we concede that the editor has such a responsibility, will his rewriting of substandard articles serve this purpose? I think not. That course is self-defeating, for writing well is a skill that is acquired through practice. As long as the editor does the revising or rewriting, the author will never recognize or learn to apply the principles of reason and exposition required to make a scientific article cogent, valid, and readable. Rather extensive experience has convinced me that only the rare author profits from major reorganization, revision, or rewriting of his article by an editor. Authors' responses to editorial changes are of two general types. Occasionally, an overly sensitive author will object strenuously—and emotionally—to any editorial changes, on the grounds that his "style" has been altered, even though the changes may be grammatical and functional rather than rhetorical. Most authors, however, will read the revised version and, unless they happen to detect any distortions in meaning, will accept it without profiting educationally from any editorial improvements. Some do not even read galley proofs critically; after an article has been published, someone may call an editorial blunder to the author's attention, but, of course, it is then too late to rectify the error.

Even when an author conscientiously reviews editorial revisions, he may not grasp the expository principles underlying the changes, although he may instinctively recognize that the revised version is an improvement over his original copy. Without an understanding of these principles, he will probably continue to commit the same literary infractions or infelicities as before. The most an author generally learns from an editor's changes are certain word preferences of the journal, such as *necropsy* for *autopsy* or *roentgenogram* for *x-ray,* or certain mechanical stylistic preferences, such as English rather than Latin plurals or closed rather than open punctuation. Rarely will an author be able to improve the organization and development of his next presentation on the basis of an editor's reordering and recasting of a paper. Personal conferences are generally needed to effect such improvement, and sporadic correspondence-course lessons by an occasional editor are therefore largely fruitless.

Nor is every scientific journal editor qualified to provide instruction in scientific writing. Many editors are selected for these posts because of their eminence in their fields of specialization, not because of any special training or aptitude in scientific writing or editing, and they are therefore hesitant to criticize the language, literary structure, or statistical supplements in manuscripts. Copy editors in redacting offices do not always have a background in logic or scientific exposition, but more often have degrees in English literature, which does not necessarily provide adequate training in grammar and composition and never in tabular and graphic construction. Unless a manuscript editor is properly qualified in scientific writing, his or her changes may be capricious, inane, or even mutilating.[8] The author who is guided by such changes may be misled.

Although it is not his duty to do so, the manuscript reviewer is generous who takes the time and effort to make detailed suggestions to authors for the improvement of their manuscripts, and authors who study such suggestions can gain valuable pointers about scientific exposition. On the other hand, the editor who accepts one poorly prepared paper after another, trying himself to rehabilitate it before publication, is sanctioning substandard writing and discouraging self-improvement on the part of authors. Only when editors establish high literary standards for all scientific journals will authors recognize the need to acquire greater literary proficiency than current scientific journals reflect.

Will the editor risk the loss of valuable scientific material by insisting on high literary as well as scientific standards for manuscripts? Not if his journal is highly esteemed. Authors want their manuscripts published in prestigious journals, and if the editor stipulates that literary improvement is a condition for publication or even reconsideration, most authors will try to meet those standards rather than submit their manu-

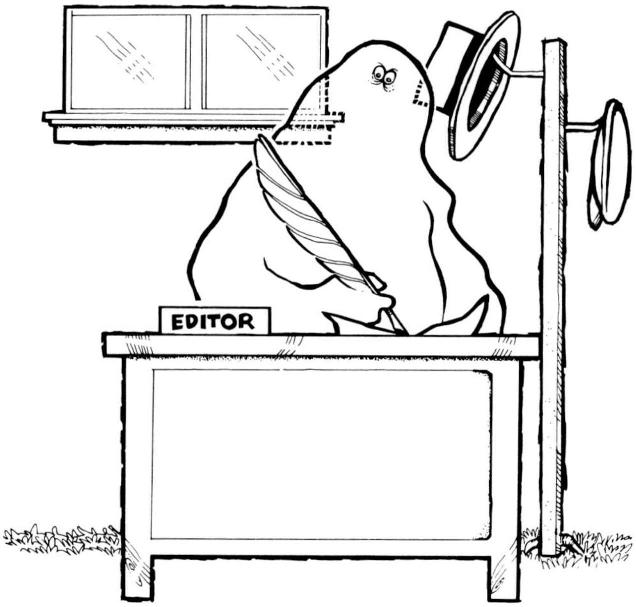

Fig. 3. The ghostwriter-editor.

scripts to a mediocre journal. The editor of a respected journal, moreover, is generally faced with an excess rather than a paucity of material and can therefore afford to be selective.

Ethical considerations. When an editor rewrites an article, the published version no longer represents exclusively the intellectual efforts of the original author. The editor, in effect, becomes a spectral scribe (Fig. 3), having recast the article to fit his notions of the most appropriate structure and language. In the process, he may have altered the content, intentionally or inadvertently. Although we have come to expect ghostwriting in the fields of politics, entertainment, and even religion, phantom authors have no place in education or medical science, where intellectual integrity is requisite. The fact that academic promotion, election to elite organizations, and other professional advancement and accolades are based to a considerable extent on professional writings makes authenticity of authorship important. Editors who solicit articles from a particular "author" because of the lucidity and general literary competence of his previous publications are victims of deception if the "author's" articles were ghostwritten. Similarly deluded is the committee that bestows an award for outstanding contributions to scientific communication on someone whose bibliography has been ghostwritten (Fig. 4). If a person will pose as the author of a piece written by another, how much confidence can be placed in the veracity of the report itself?

Functional considerations. Are there functional risks in rewriting? Yes. The editor may unwittingly impose his personal concepts, convictions, or biases on an article that he rewrites, or he may introduce inaccuracies. Moreover, it may be difficult to judge the scientific validity of an article that is so poorly composed as to require rewriting before publication. Extensive reordering of a report by an editor may lead to misinterpretation of the author's data and thus to unwarranted conclusions.

A paper that requires major overhauling, including reorganization, may reflect basic defects in substance. Just as clear exposition is closely linked to clear thinking, so shoddy prose may be related to an ill-defined thesis, errors in experimental design, or faulty collection and analysis of data. When major

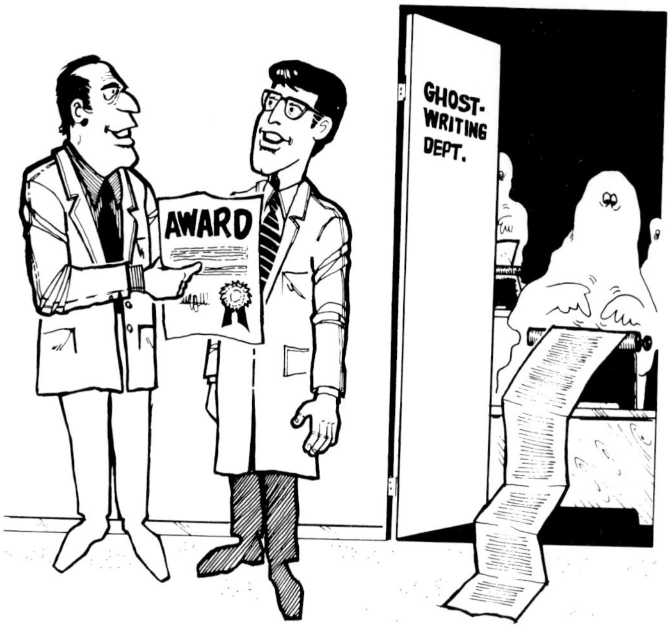

Fig. 4. The auctorial impostor.

reorganization of content provides a more logical sequence of ideas or when reconstruction of tables and graphs leads to new or different implications of the data, one may reasonably assume that the author's original thought processes were faulty or that he has not learned to coordinate rational thought with lucid language. In either case, the editor should not gloss over the deficiency. He is, after all, in an excellent position to promote orderly thinking by requiring orderly writing.

Some may argue that it is the content, not the form, of a report that matters and that, moreover, few scientific readers can distinguish good from poor exposition. But can form and content be wholly separated? Certainly, an assumption that most readers are undiscriminating should not be used to justify literary mediocrity in the material an editor accepts for publication. Furthermore, even the relatively insensitive reader judges an idea partly (even though perhaps subconsciously) by its mode of expression. He is likely to read from beginning to end an article that contains useful data presented in an appealing, easily interpretable form, but he will probably skip the one written in such cumbersome prose that he must exert inordinate mental effort to understand it.

Aesthetic considerations. The editor who rewrites a manuscript inevitably imposes his personal literary character on it. If he uses the blue pencil liberally on all articles, the entire journal will assume a stereotype that will bore the reader. Such a practice discourages stylistic individuality among authors, many of whom are already convinced that if their articles are to be accepted, they must not deviate from the bromidic style of many contemporary scientific journals. As a result, each generation of writers perpetuates the drab, desiccated, distended prose of the preceding generation. In language particularly, most of us are unwitting mimics, and the aphorism is largely true that we write what we read. Almost all scientific reports today are of a piece, cast in the same predictable mold. The rigidity of their structure and phraseology is reminiscent of a government form, whose blanks the author merely fills in with different data. Small wonder that the reader's eyes may follow a whole paragraph or even a whole page of print without a single idea being absorbed.

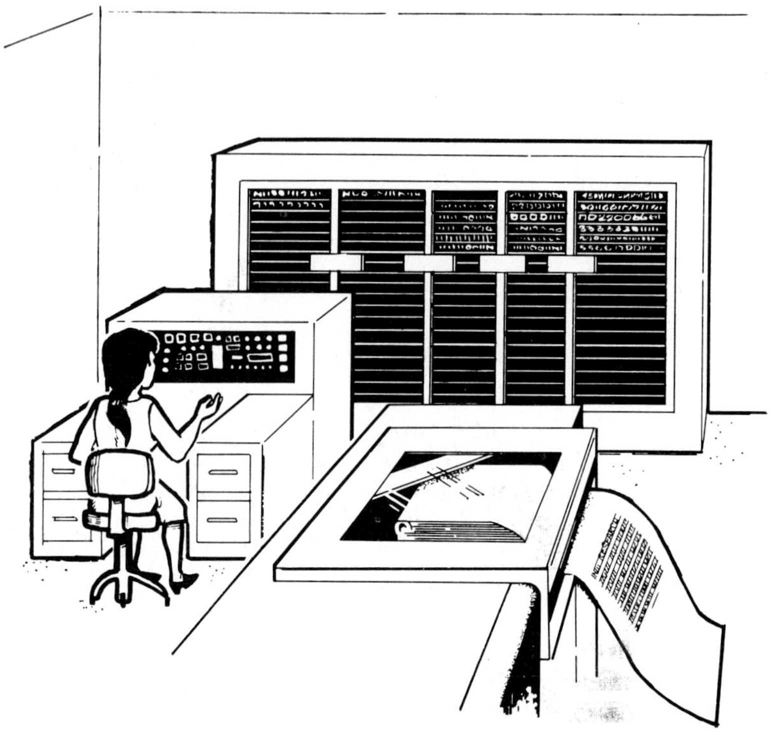

Fig. 5. The computer-author.

The frozen forms and clichés abounding in that kind of impotent prose are so familiar to the reader that they fail to engage his attention or activate his mind. Instead, his thoughts surrender to the omnipresent distractions waiting impatiently to intrude on every active mind.

I see no reason why a scientific report cannot be clear, accurate, and communicative while at the same time pleasing to read. Authors should be encouraged to experiment with new combinations of words to achieve some originality. I am not advocating rhetorical flourishes or artifice, but rather a more appealing and more individual style than the prolonged, ossified exposition now in vogue. Certainly, few reports reflect the excitement of scientific research; they read rather like the dead cellulose on which they are printed, as though produced not by a human being, but by an inanimate object, perhaps a rigidly programmed computer (Fig. 5).

Economic considerations. Not insignificant today, when publishing costs continue to mount steadily, is the additional expense incident to extensive revision by the editorial staff of a journal. From an economic standpoint, it seems impractical for a journal editor or his assistants to rewrite articles submitted for publication.

SURVEY OF JOURNAL EDITORS

In a casual survey which I made of selected journal editors, few indicated that they had done major reorganizing, elucidating, or condensing of manuscripts. One who had done so pointed up an interesting risk associated with the practice: the author liked the editor's rewritten version so well that he submitted it to another journal for publication. A more serious risk for an author is for the editor, on rewriting an article, to discover some flaw, not previously evident, in the scientific validity of the author's central thesis. Such a discovery would naturally mean rejection. Almost all editors agreed that rewriting by editors had no noticeable beneficial effect on subsequent articles by the same authors.

One editor stated that he and his staff have to rewrite most manuscripts to make them attractive enough for subscribers to read articles through completely. Even though the articles published in this journal are thus essentially *written by the editor* or one of his associates, the by-line contains the name of the original author, because, as the editor reasons, the reader is attracted by an authority's name. Curiously, this practice implies that "author" can no longer be equated with "writer."

In another case, an editor was impressed by the large size of a series of cases reported in a manuscript, but, on examining the author's analysis of the data, was dubious of the methods used and the results obtained. When he re-analyzed the data, he arrived at a conclusion that was diametrically opposed to that which the author had reached. He then rewrote the article, using his own analysis and conclusions, and published it under the original author's name. The authenticity of the authorship in this case could be legitimately challenged, it seems to me, since both content and form had been drastically changed.

The New England Journal of Medicine recently published two versions of a manuscript, one by the authors and another by a science writer.[6] The accompanying editorial, however, seemed to me to vitiate the experiment. According to Franz Ingelfinger,[7] the editor:

> The transformation, it turns out, is far from easy. In the first place . . . [the science writer] was asked . . . to avoid the use of additional information. . . . Secondly, the section on methods—a section that in the *Journal* is as a matter of course already presented in an abbreviated and simplified form—does not lend itself to rewriting. Thirdly, the science writer can hardly be expected to present a crystal-clear logic culminating in some readily understood and essentially simple conclusion when the nature of the subject investigated and the findings themselves are so complex as to preclude the formulation of any sharply defined concepts.[7]

Putting aside any judgment that the rewritten version may be no improvement over

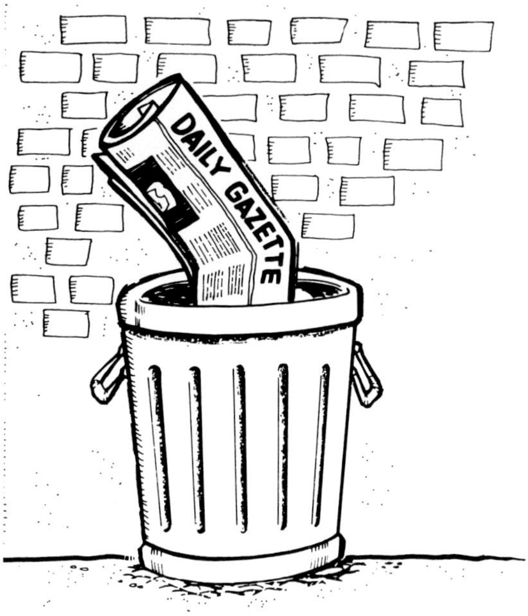

Fig. 6. The disposable daily.

the authors' original text or that it contains grammatical or rhetorical flaws, let us consider the implicit suggestion that the style of a popular journalist may be more "readable" than that of a scientist-author. Material written by science writers is published in newspapers, magazines, and other media which are generally discarded as soon as items of interest are read. It is reasonable, then, that the journalist should use the vernacular, including slang, colloquialisms, fad words, and other ephemeral diction for his perishable product (Fig. 6). The journalism student is, in fact, encouraged to exploit these linguistic devices to give his writing "flavor." The scientific article, on the other hand, is a permanent document and becomes a part of the scientific archives, to be consulted by future generations of scientists and clinicians (Fig. 7). Is it not logical to expect its language to be more stable and durable?

The purposes and audiences of the two genres, moreover, are decidedly different and call for different presentations. The newspaper reader is generally interested only in the results of scientific research as they affect him; he has neither the educational background nor the interest to delve deeply into the methods used or the theoretical

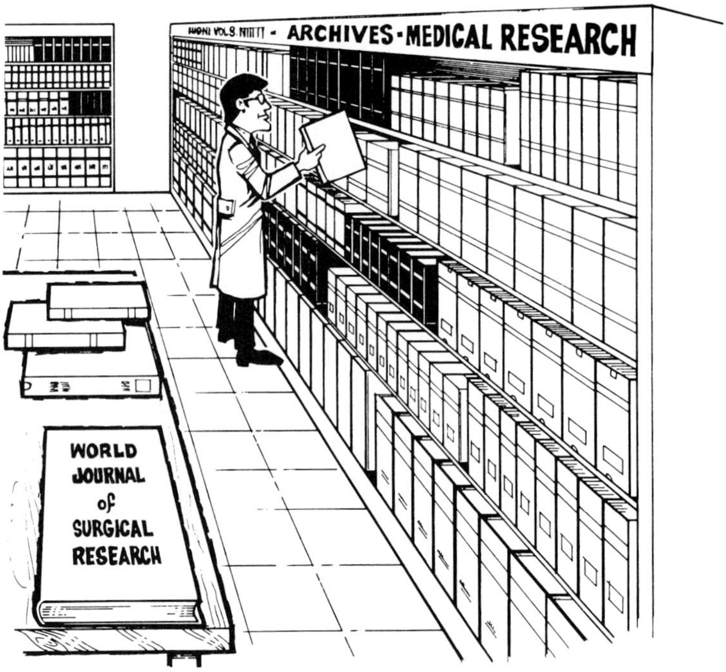

Fig. 7. The permanent publication.

basis of the experiments. Science writing, by nature, is more selective, superficial, and sensational than scientific writing, and the abstraction so imposed is more likely to result in distortion (Fig. 8). Unfortunately, the lay reader's first impression is usually lasting. To the reader of scientific journals, unlike the lay reader of popular publications, the method and the theoretical concepts and implications are all-important. The scholarly article, moreover, is usually read thoughtfully and analytically rather than hastily and superficially.

The discussion in a scientific report is an extremely important section, in which the scientist indicates the significance and implications of his experimental observations. These can best be presented by the person who has, himself, made the observations and analyzed the data rather than by someone entirely removed from the study and untrained in the discipline involved or in the scientific method. An eyewitness account is obviously more authentic than a secondhand report, since every time an account of an event is retold, additional chance is introduced for personal coloring, misinterpretation, or frank error. The problems in citation introduced by including in the bylines of scientific articles the phrase "as told to ——————" reinforce my objection to the whole idea.

Propriety and communicability of language are governed in part by the purpose of the message and by the audience to which it is directed. This is not to say that scientific writing need be unreadable; it certainly need not be.[3-5] But a far more rational and effective solution to the present sad state of scientific publications is to teach the scientific author how to improve his own communicative skills rather than have popular journalists or ghostwriters employed to do the author's job for him. If a science writer can learn to write readable prose, then certainly the scientist, with his higher education, should also be able to acquire that skill. Should the author abdicate his scholarship to a "ghost," we can expect accuracy, precision, and documentation in scientific reporting to suffer accordingly.

An editor who alters manuscripts drastically may (although not necessarily) produce a journal that is more readable and compre-

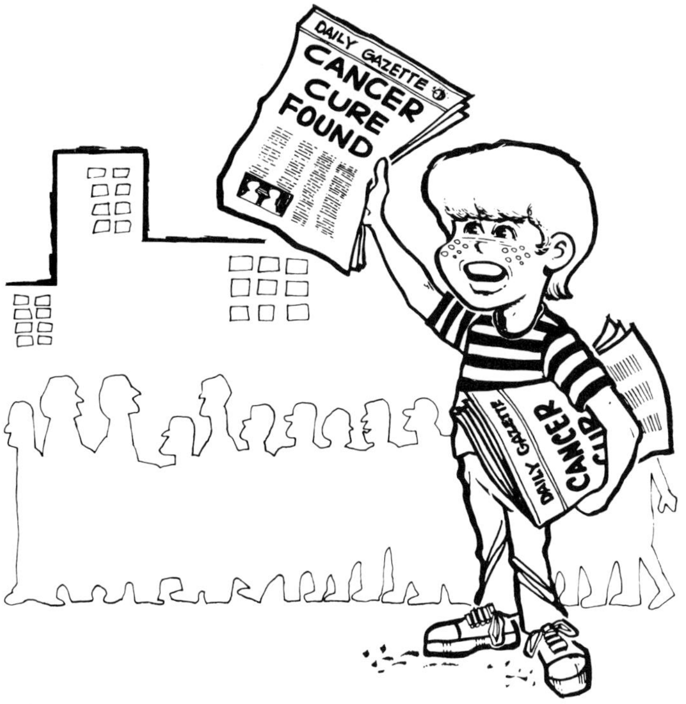

Fig. 8. The free press.

hensible than it would otherwise be. The reader, then, profits, but how does this practice affect authors and the quality of journals? I have heard authors say, "Why worry about the grammar? The editor will fix that." With such an attitude, the rewriting of manuscripts by editors may only lead to submission of more and more drivel, from which authors will expect editors to recover (or produce) important information and recast it into acceptable form. Because all editors do not have the time or staff to edit manuscripts heavily, many articles are published in less than exemplary form.

CONCLUSION

When a manuscript that appears to have some scientific merit requires drastic change to make it acceptable for publication, the editor would do well to return it to the author for rehabilitation. Such vast changes may be needed to remedy disarrayed parts, statistical errors, ambiguous or confusing statements, frequent grammatical infractions, pervasive verbiage, or other serious flaws. When the author's summary or abstract is noninformative or when his references are erroneous or deficient, the editor should require the author to rectify these himself. On the other hand, the editor may properly abbreviate or clarify a faulty title; remove an occasional rhetorical, grammatical, or mechanical flaw; or make other such minor improvements in a manuscript. Needless to say, the editor should not make changes simply to satisfy his own whims or personal idiosyncrasies regarding diction or style.

A published article is primarily the responsibility of the person who created it and only secondarily the responsibility of the editor, through whose hands it passes on the way to publication. Presumably the author is writing because he has worthwhile information to communicate, and it is reasonable to expect such an informed person to know how to convey that information intelligibly. If he does not, the editor should encourage him to cure the literary disorder, rather than to expect, or accept, symptomatic treatment indefinitely. By insisting that authors submit manuscripts that can be published without major revision, the editor will discourage submission of substandard manuscripts and will help suppress hasty, premature, or immature publications. And by refusing to rewrite an author's manuscript, the editor will not be a party to a spurious by-line.

REFERENCES

1. DeBakey, L.: Instruction in scientific communications, J. Med. Educ. **40:** 928, 1965.
2. DeBakey, L.: Competent medical exposition: The need and the attainment, Bull. Am. Coll. Surg. **52:** 85, 1967.
3. DeBakey, L.: Releasing literary inhibitions in scientific reporting, Can. Med. Assoc. J. **99:** 360, 1968.
4. DeBakey, L.: Every careless word that men utter. I. The English language, Anesth. Analg. **49:** 567, 1970.
5. DeBakey, L.: Every careless word that men utter. II. The language of science, Anesth. Analg. **49:** 827, 1970.
6. Gutterman, J. U., Rossen, R. D., Butler, W. T., McCredie, K. B., Bodey, G. P., Sr., Freireich, E. J., and Hersh, E. M.: Immunoglobulin on tumor cells and tumor-induced lymphocyte blastogenesis in human acute leukemia, N. Engl. J. Med. **288:** 169, 1973.
7. Ingelfinger, F. J.: Twin bill on tumor immunity, N. Engl. J. Med. **288:** 211, 1973.
8. Morgan, W. K. C.: Verbal blemishes seen as virtues (letter to the editor), N. Engl. J. Med. **287:** 941, 1972.

The transplanted parathyroid gland: Evaluation of cryopreservation and other environmental factors which affect its function

Samuel A. Wells, Jr., M.D.,* *and* **Christine Christiansen, B.S.,** *Bethesda, Md.*

Pairs of fresh syngeneic parathyroid grafts restored the serum calcium to normal within 20 days after implantation into hypocalcemic inbred Fischer rats. Likewise, syngeneic parathyroid glands when maintained in Waymouth's tissue culture medium for 12 hours at room temperature or dried for three hours at room temperature functioned identically as fresh parathyroid glands when implanted into hypocalcemic hosts. When gradually frozen in ten percent dimethyl sulfoxide, ten percent syngeneic rat serum, and 80 percent Waymouth's tissue culture medium, parathyroid glands functioned normally after preservation at 196° C. for nine months and in some cases for one year. Histologic evaluation of functioning transplanted parathyroid tissue revealed that the grafts appeared indistinguishable from fresh normal parathyroid tissue.

From the Tumor Immunology Section, Surgery Branch, National Cancer Institute, National Institutes of Health, Bethesda, Md.

IT HAS recently been shown in our laboratory that canine parathyroid glands when diced into small pieces and implanted intramuscularly function normally as autografts[8] and as allografts if the host is immunosuppressed.[9]

In the present study, parathyroid glands were frozen for periods of 3, 6, 9, or 12 months, and their functional capacity and histological appearance were evaluated after transplantation into syngeneic hypoparathyroid hosts. Also assessed was the effect of drying and prolonged lack of blood supply on parathyroid graft function.

Rats were used in these experiments because of the large number of animals needed for statistical analysis and because of this rodent's ability to tolerate the aparathyroid state asymptomatically.

Accepted for publication July 30, 1973.

*Present address: Department of Surgery, Duke University Medical Center, Durham, N. C. 27710.

MATERIALS AND METHODS

Rats. Highly inbred Fischer rats weighing 180 to 200 grams were obtained from the National Institutes of Health breeding colony and used throughout the experiment.

Diet. Rats were maintained on a standard NIH (National Institutes of Health) laboratory pellet diet except for occasional periods (see below) when they were placed on a low calcium diet.* All rats received water and food ad libitum.

Serum calcium. The rats were bled at varying intervals from the retro-orbital plexus, and the serum was separated and stored in siliconized tubes with plastic tops. Serum calcium was determined by the method of Kessler and Wolfman[3] (normal range 8.5 to 10.9 mg. per 100 ml.).

Histology. Removed parathyroid grafts were fixed in ten percent formalin and subse-

*Nutritional Biochemicals Company, Cleveland, Ohio.

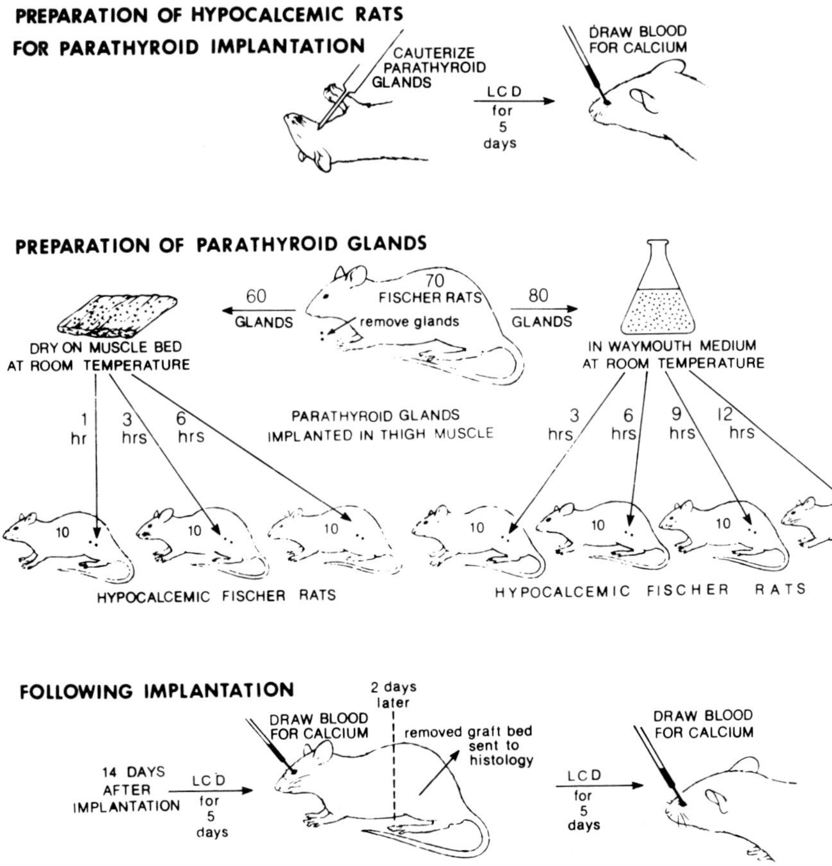

Fig. 1. The course of Experiment 1 (the effect of drying and/or lack of blood supply on parathyroid graft function).

quently sectioned and stained with hematoxylin and eosin.

Hypocalcemic rats. Fischer rats were anesthetized with pentobarbital intraperitoneally (50 mg. per kilogram), and their necks were shaved and cleaned with alcohol. The thyroid gland was exposed, and each of the two parathyroid glands and a circumferential rim of thyroid tissue were ablated with the electrocautery. The neck was closed and the animals were placed on a low calcium diet for five days at which time serum calcium was measured (Fig. 1). Only hypocalcemic (serum calcium below 6.0 mg. per 100 ml.) animals were used for subsequent grafting experiments.

Statistical analysis of data. Comparisons of results between groups of animals were analyzed by the paired t test and by the two sample t test.

Experiment 1. Effect of drying and/or lack of blood supply on parathyroid graft function. Seventy Fischer rats were anesthetized and under aseptic conditions both parathyroid glands were removed from each rat giving a total of 140 glands. Sixty parathyroid glands were placed on a muscle bed to dry at room temperature. One hour later, 20 of the 60 glands were implanted (two glands per animal) into the flank muscles of 10 hypocalcemic Fischer rats. At three hours and six hours, the other two groups of 20 parathyroid glands were similarly implanted into hypocalcemic recipients (Fig. 1).

The remaining 80 of the original 140 parathyroid glands were placed in Waymouth's tissue culture medium at room temperature. At 3, 6, 9, and 12 hours thereafter groups of 20 parathyroid glands were removed from the medium, and pairs were implanted intra-

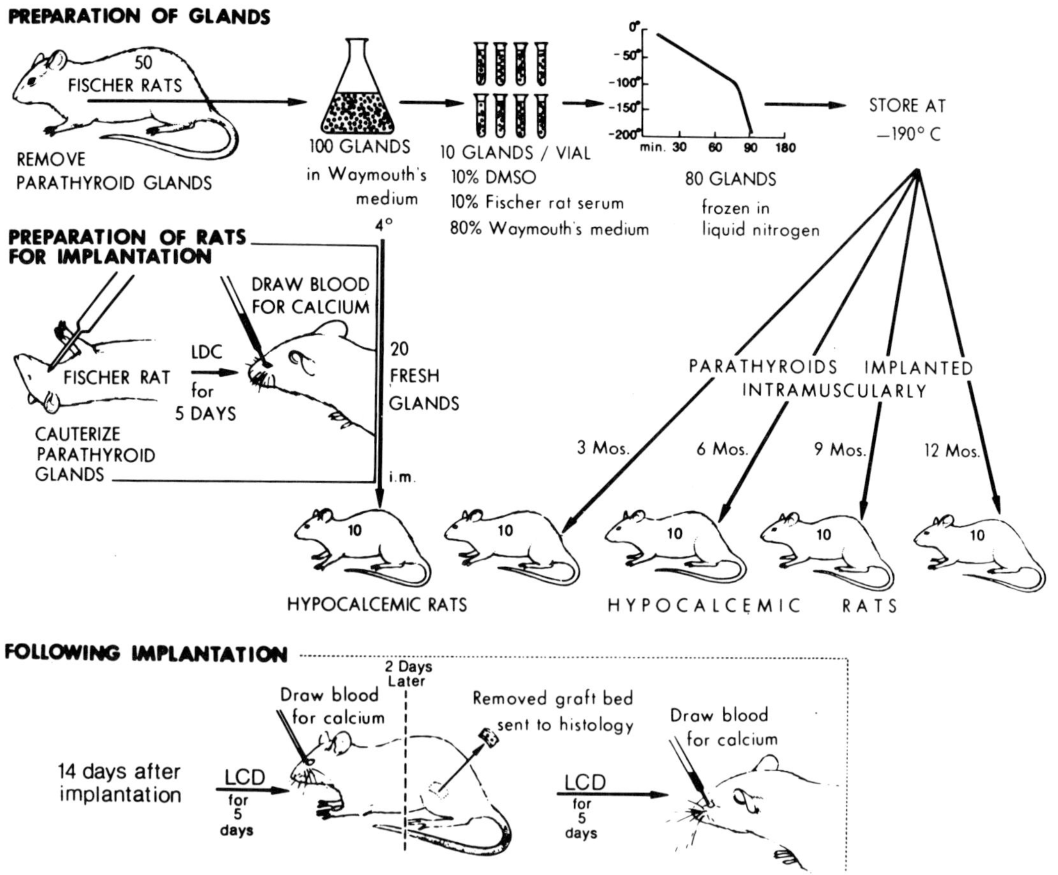

Fig. 2. The course of Experiment 2 (the assessment of parathyroid gland function after cryopreservation for 3, 6, 9, and 12 months).

muscularly into ten hypocalcemic animals.

After two weeks, the 70 recipient Fischer rats were placed on a low calcium diet for five days, the serum calcium concentration was determined, and two days later the parathyroid grafts were excised for histological evaluation. The rats were again placed on a low calcium diet for five days and the serum calcium was measured.

Experiment 2. The assessment of parathyroid gland function after cryopreservation for 3, 6, 9, and 12 months. The course of this experiment is outlined in Fig. 2. Fifty inbred Fischer rats were anesthetized and their parathyroid glands were removed and immediately placed into Waymouth's medium at 4° C. Ten pairs of these 100 fresh parathyroid glands were immediately implanted intramuscularly into the flanks of ten hypocalcemic Fischer rats. One would expect optimal function of these freshly transplanted parathyroid glands, and these ten animals serve as the control group for the transplanted animals in both parts of Experiment 1 as well as in the present experiment. The remaining 80 parathyroid glands were equally divided into groups of ten and immediately placed into eight chilled vials containing 10 percent dimethyl sulfoxide (DMSO), ten percent syngeneic rat serum, and 80 percent Waymouth's medium. The filled volume of the 3 ml. vials was about 1.5 ml. The vials were then placed in a Linde BF-4 freezing chamber* and cooled at a rate of 1° C. per minute to –80° C. The vials were then frozen at a rapid rate to –200° C. and immediately

*Union Carbide Corporation, Linde Division, Cryogenic Products Department, New York, N. Y.

Table I. *Effect of exposure at room temperature with or without drying on parathyroid graft function (serum Ca^{++} values in milligrams per 100 ml. ± S.E.M.)*

Status of parathyroid graft	Serum Ca^{++} of rats: Before graft	With graft	After graft removed	No. of grafted rats with normal Ca^{++}/ No. of grafted rats
Fresh	4.4 ± 0.7	9.9 ± 1.0*	5.3 ± 0.8	8/9
Dry, 1 hr.	5.2 ± 0.5	9.6 ± 1.1*	5.6 ± 1.0	8/9
Dry, 3 hr.	5.6 ± 1.2	9.9 ± 0.5*	5.9 ± 0.7	10/10
Dry, 6 hr.	5.6 ± 0.8	6.9 ± 2.9†	4.2 ± 0.4	4/9
Waymouth's, 3 hr.	5.5 ± 0.4	10.5 ± 0.4*	5.3 ± 0.5	10/10
Waymouth's, 6 hr.	5.5 ± 0.3	10.9 ± 0.8*	5.1 ± 0.5	10/10
Waymouth's, 9 hr.	5.3 ± 0.5	10.9 ± 0.3*	5.4 ± 0.3	9/9
Waymouth's, 12 hr.	5.7 ± 0.5	9.5 ± 1.5*	5.4 ± 0.5	7/10

*Serum Ca^{++} of rats with graft differs significantly ($p < 0.001$) from serum Ca^{++} of rats before grafting and serum Ca^{++} after graft was removed.

†Serum Ca^{++} of rats with graft does not differ statistically from serum Ca^{++} of rats before grafting.

placed into a liquid nitrogen freezer where they were maintained at −196° C. At 3, 6, 9, and 12 months, two of the eight vials were removed from the liquid nitrogen freezer and immediately thawed by shaking in a 37° C. waterbath. The 20 thawed glands were then washed three times with Waymouth's medium at 4° C. and immediately implanted into ten hypocalcemic Fischer rats. After each group of animals had received the transplants, they were observed for 14 days and then placed on a low calcium diet for five days. Serum calcium was then determined, and two days later the intramuscular parathyroid graft was removed. Serum calcium was again evaluated after the animals had been on a low calcium diet for five days.

RESULTS

Rat parathyroid glands dried at room temperature for one and three hours elevated the mean serum calcium concentration of hypocalcemic rats to the normal range by 20 days following implantation. The success rates in the two groups were 90 percent and 100 percent, respectively (Table I). When the parathyroid grafts were removed, the serum calcium dropped markedly to the pregrafting level. The removed parathyroid grafts appeared normal histologically.

Of the nine rats transplanted with parathyroid glands dried at room temperature for six hours, four had a normal serum calcium concentration by 20 days. The mean serum calcium concentration of the whole group, however, was not significantly different from that before grafting. There was an excellent correlation between parathyroid graft function and histological appearance.

Each group of rat parathyroid glands maintained in Waymouth's medium at room temperature for 3, 6, 9, and 12 hours was able to restore the mean serum calcium concentration to the normal range within three weeks after implantation into hypocalcemic syngeneic recipients (Table I). The success rate was 100 percent in the first three groups and 70 percent in the 12 hour group. Within five days after the parathyroid grafts had been removed from the rats in each of these four groups, the serum calcium concentration had fallen to the pretransplantation level. Histologically, the removed parathyroid grafts appeared normal (Fig. 3*A*).

In all groups of rats except those grafted with parathyroid glands dried at room temperature for six hours, the mean serum calcium concentration was elevated to the normal range within three weeks after grafting and was found to be significantly higher ($p < 0.001$) than the serum calcium concentration both before grafting and after the grafts had been removed (Table I).

Hypocalcemic rats transplanted with pairs of syngeneic parathyroid glands which had been frozen for 3, 6, or 9 months had mean serum calcium levels which were within the normal range 20 days after grafting. Following removal of the parathyroid grafts, which appeared histologically normal (Fig. 3*B*), the

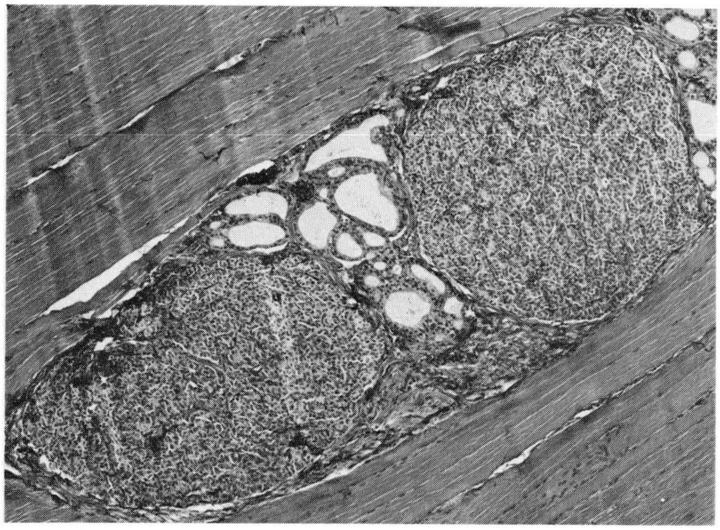

Fig. 3*A*. Parathyroid gland transplanted for three weeks after being incubated in Waymouth's tissue culture medium at room temperature for 12 hours. Parathyroid architecture is normal. Note thyroid follicles adjacent to parathyroid implants. (Hematoxylin and eosin; ×88.)

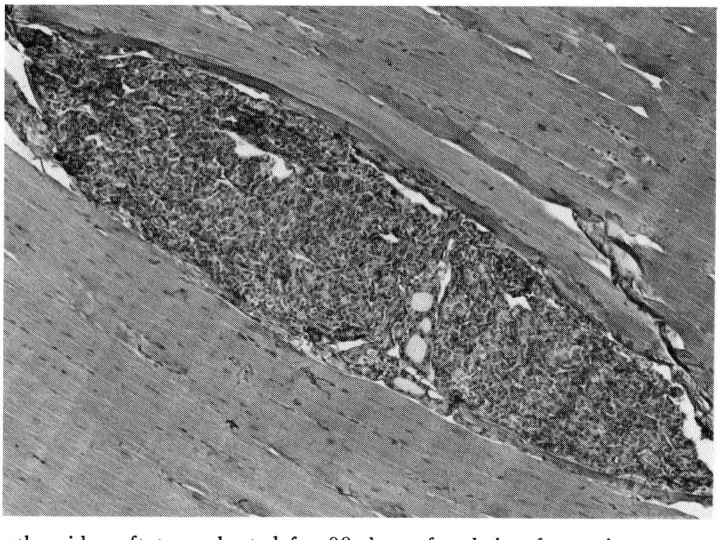

Fig. 3*B*. Parathyroid graft transplanted for 20 days after being frozen in ten percent dimethyl sulfoxide, ten percent rat serum, and 80 percent Waymouth's tissue culture medium at −196° C. for nine months. Parathyroid architecture is normal. Small thyroid follicles are present. (Hematoxylin and eosin; ×72.)

mean serum calcium concentration fell to pregrafting hypocalcemic levels. Of the grafts, 80 to 90 percent were successful in these three groups (Table II). Nine of the 11 hypocalcemic animals transplanted with parathyroid glands which had been frozen for one year had no change in the serum calcium concentration at 20 and 28 days following grafting, and destroyed glandular architecture was noted histologically. There were two animals in the group, however, which had normal serum calcium levels 20 days after grafting, and their parathyroid grafts appeared normal histologically.

The mean serum calcium concentration of the groups of animals grafted with parathy-

Table II. *Function of parathyroid glands after freezing in DMSO and serum for 3, 6, 9, or 12 months (serum Ca^{++} values in milligrams per 100 ml. ± S.E.M.)*

Status of parathyroid graft	*Serum Ca^{++} of rats*			*No. of grafted rats with normal Ca^{++}/No. of grafted rats*
	Before graft	*With graft*	*After graft removed*	
Fresh	4.4 ± 0.7	9.9 ± 1.0*	5.3 ± 0.8	8/9
Frozen 3 mo.	3.6 ± 0.4	9.8 ± 0.9*	5.8 ± 0.6	8/9
Frozen 6 mo.	5.6 ± 0.5	9.2 ± 1.4*	5.8 ± 0.7	10/12
Frozen 9 mo.	5.7 ± 0.4	8.9 ± 1.2*	5.2 ± 0.8	8/10
Frozen 12 mo.	5.4 ± 0.5	5.8 ± 2.0†	6.0 ± 2.2‡	2/11

*Serum Ca^{++} of rats with graft differs significantly ($p < 0.001$) from serum Ca^{++} of rats before grafting and serum Ca^{++} after graft was removed.

†Serum Ca^{++} of rats with parathyroid graft not significantly different from serum Ca^{++} of rats before grafting or serum Ca^{++} after graft removed.

‡Serum Ca^{++} of rats 28 days after implantation. Serum Ca^{++} concentration was not determined in this group after the grafts were removed.

roid glands frozen for 3, 6, and 9 months differed significantly ($p < 0.001$) both from the mean serum calcium concentration before grafting and that after the grafts had been removed.

DISCUSSION

Since Shaffner and associates[6] first demonstrated that fowl spermatozoa could be successfully stored at –76° C., numerous other investigators have viably frozen single cell suspensions of mammalian tissues for prolonged periods.

In 1957, Parkes[4] demonstrated that rat ovaries, frozen at –190° C. in 15 percent glycerol-saline for one year, maintained normal function following implantation. He also showed that a serum-glycerol mixture led to a more stable preservation of the frozen ovaries than did freezing in glycerol-saline alone. Recently, Bartlett and Reade[1] demonstrated that mouse tooth germs could be frozen in DMSO in a viable state for three months. Following implantation into syngeneic hosts, the developing teeth produced normal dental hard and soft tissue elements.

In 1950, Blumenthal and Walsh[2] noted that parathyroid autotransplants frozen at –70° for 24 hours appeared histologically normal 13 days after grafting. Russell and associates[5] in 1961 demonstrated that rat parathyroid glands could be viably frozen in 15 percent glycerol at –196° C. In one hypocalcemic animal, the serum calcium was restored to normal by a parathyroid autotransplant frozen for four months. More recently, Sonoda and co-workers[7] have shown that canine parathyroid autografts are capable of functioning after preservation in 15 percent DMSO for seven days.

Our data demonstrate that rat parathyroid glands dried at room temperature for up to three hours are capable of functioning normally following syngeneic transplantation. Drying for six hours had a deleterious effect, however, and the majority of transplanted glands failed to function. If the parathyroid glands were maintained in tissue culture medium at room temperature, their viability was prolonged and the large majority of grafted glands functioned normally even after incubation at room temperature for twelve hours.

Almost all of the parathyroid glands which were frozen in ten percent dimethyl sulfoxide and syngeneic rat serum and stored at –196° C. for as long as nine months functioned well and after excision appeared normal histologically. Even at one year, some glands maintained viability as evidenced by their ability to elevate the serum calcium to normal in hypocalcemic rats.

The successful preservation of rat parathyroid glands is in all likelihood due to their very small size, which allows for rapid permeability of the dimethyl sulfoxide and a relatively equal rate of freezing throughout the gland. Preliminary studies in our laboratory have shown that larger parathyroid glands such as those in dog and man require dicing into very small pieces prior to freezing and implantation to maximize viability.

We gratefully acknowledge the help of Dr. William M. O'Fallon, Associate Professor of Community Health Sciences, for help in statistical analysis data.

REFERENCES

1. Bartlett, P. F., and Reade, P. C.: Cryopreservation of developing teeth, Cryobiology **9:** 205, 1972.
2. Blumenthal, H. T., and Walsh, L. B.: Survival of guinea pig thyroid and parathyroid autotransplants previously subjected to extremely low temperatures, Proc. Soc. Exp. Biol. Med. **73:** 62, 1950.
3. Kessler, G., and Wolfman, M.: An automated procedure for the simultaneous determination of calcium and phosphorus, Clin. Chem. **10:** 686, 1964.
4. Parkes, A. S.: Viability of ovarian tissue after freezing, Proc. Roy. Soc. Lond. [Biol.] **147:** 520, 1957.
5. Russell, P. S., Wood, M. L., and Gittes, R. F.: Preservation of living tissue in the frozen state: A study using parathyroid tissue, J. Surg. Res. **1:** 23, 1961.
6. Shaffner, C. S., Henderson, E. W., and Carol, C. G.: The viability of spermatozoa after vitrification and dehydration at low temperatures, Nature **164:** 666, 1941.
7. Sonoda, T., Ohkawa, T., Takeuchi, M., et al.: Successful parathyroid preservation: Experimental study, SURGERY **64:** 791, 1968.
8. Wells, S. A., Burdick, J. F., Ketcham, A. S., et al.: Transplantation of the parathyroid glands in dogs: Biochemical, histological, and radioimmunoassay proof of function, Transplantation **15:** 179, 1973.
9. Wells, S. A., Burdick, J. F., Christiansen, C. L., et al.: Long-term survival of dogs transplanted with parathyroid glands as autografts and as allografts in immunosuppressed hosts, Trans. Proc. **5:** 769, 1973.

Colon perforations associated with steroid therapy

Sylvester Sterioff, M.D., Mark B. Orringer, M.D., *and* **John L. Cameron, M.D.,**
Baltimore, Md.

Ten patients on systemic steroid therapy for a variety of diseases developed acute colon perforation secondary to diverticulitis or vasculitis. In eight patients, there was delay in diagnosis. Fever, abdominal pain, and tenderness were frequently present. Abdominal guarding and leukocytosis are inconstant findings. The prognosis is grave if free perforation exists. Recommendations for clinical recognition and management are proposed.

From The Department of Surgery, The Johns Hopkins University School of Medicine, Baltimore, Md.

SYSTEMIC corticosteroid therapy is followed in a significant number of patients by serious intra-abdominal pathology. In some instances, such as peptic ulcer disease, the pathology is thought to be secondary to steroid administration. Pancreatitis, also, has been implicated as a complication of systemic steroid treatment. Other intra-abdominal catastrophies, such as acute colon perforation, have not been recognized as frequently, nor have they been thought directly caused by the steroid therapy. Recently, ten patients on steroid therapy with acute colon perforations have been seen at The John Hopkins Medical Institutions. This report describes our clinical experience with these patients and makes recommendations for their clinical management.

CLINICAL MATERIAL

Ten patients on systemic steroid therapy have been recognized as having acute colon perforations in the past two years. Seven were female and three male; the average age was 46 years. All patients were on oral prednisone for a variety of underlying illnesses. The dose ranged from 10 to 80 mg. per day with a mean of 20 mg. per day. The duration of medication ranged from five days to six years with a mean of ten months. The underlying diseases and their frequency were: disseminated lupus erythematosis (DLE) (four); postrenal transplant (three); postbone-marrow transplant for acute monocytic leukemia (one); emphysema and bronchial asthma (one); and rheumatoid arthritis (one). In addition to prednisone, most patients were on other medications for treatment of their underlying disorders; however, there was no other single drug common to all.

In eight patients there was some delay in the diagnosis of the colon perforation. Fever and abdominal tenderness were present in almost all patients. Leukocytosis and rebound tenderness were often absent (Table I). In only two patients was an unequivocal diagnosis made of a perforated viscus by the con-

Accepted for publication Aug. 13, 1973.

Reprint requests: Sylvester Sterioff, M.D., Dept. of Surgery, Baltimore City Hospitals, 4940 Eastern Ave., Baltimore, Md. 21224.

Table I. *Clinical signs in ten patients*

Signs	*No.*
Abdominal tenderness	8/10
Abdominal guarding or rebound	1/10
Bowel sounds absent or decreased	6/10
Fever (over 100° F.)	8/10
Leukocytosis (> 10,000 per min.[3])	4/10

Table II. *Surgical therapy*

Surgical procedures	*No.*
Proximal colostomy and drainage	4
Exteriorization	2
Drainage alone	2
Resection (elective)	1
None (autopsy)	1

sulting surgeon on initial physical examination. The diagnosis was eventually made by x-ray evidence of free intraperitoneal air, by barium enema, and in one case at autopsy. Eight patients had perforated diverticula, all in the rectosigmoid. Two patients with DLE had a vasculitis involving the transverse colon with necrosis, ulceration, and perforation.

Standard surgical approaches were made with either exteriorization of the perforation, proximal colostomy and drainage, or simply drainage of an abscess (Table II). Only three of the ten patients survived. All three survivors had walled off the perforation prior to presentation and a well-defined abscess was demonstrated by barium enema. All six patients with free intraperitoneal perforation died, as did one patient with a diverticular abscess. The immediate causes of death were: sepsis (four); pulmonary complications (two); and stress bleeding (one).

COMMENTS

Clinical evidence of intra-abdominal catastrophies may be obscured in patients whose inflammatory response is depressed by steroid therapy. In this series, there was a delay in recognition of colon perforation in eight of the ten patients. Although the presence of fever and abdominal tenderness was commonplace, the suspicion of serious intra-abdominal pathology was frequently allayed by the absence of leukocytosis and involuntary guarding or rebound tenderness. These inconsistent clinical signs in a patient with a precarious underlying condition lead to some procrastination and falsely hopeful observation.

An inability to localize the perforation adequately seems to be present in these patients. This has also been noted by Cantor and Shorb.[1] Penn and associates[8] reported two renal transplant patients with perforated sigmoid diverticulitis, both of whom died, and noted that Monaco also had two transplant patients with a similar fate.[8] In an unreported series, De Bakey had three patients with perforated diverticulitis in his first ten patients with cardiac transplants.[8] Misra and co-workers[7] observed six renal transplant patients, all with kidneys from cadaver sources and presumably on systemic steroids, with perforated sigmoid diverticulitis. Four of the six patients died as a result of the diverticulitis.

The effect of steroids on the colon has not been established. As first suggested by ReMine,[10] steroids may inhibit the normal inflammatory response and the antifibroblastic activity may predispose to perforation. Our observations and the references noted here imply that frequent lack of containment of the inflammatory process is commonplace with single perforated diverticula. Another conclusion could be that inflammation of diverticula occurs frequently, however, with normal responses, the process is contained.

The occurrence of perforation of any area of the gastrointestinal tract associated with all collagen vascular disease, has been well documented, whether treated with steroids or not.[2, 5] Of the four DLE patients reported here, two had vasculitis, whereas two had diverticular complications.

The relatively young age of the patients reported with diverticulitis is noteworthy. Five of the patients were under 50 years and two of these were under 40 years. Eusebio and Eisenberg[3] have pointed out that two to four percent of patients admitted for diverticular disease are under the age of 40 years. There is generally a low level of awareness of this possibility and in 64 young patients the admission diagnosis was made correctly in only eight. Although it is attractive to imply that the apparently increased number of young people in our report who developed diverticular complications indicates a causal effect of the steroid administration, the number of patients is obviously too small for such a conclusion.

From this limited observation, we cannot establish an increased incidence of diverticular disease in a steroid-treated population; we can show an increased mortality rate from the complication. The increasing recognition of the problem[4, 7, 10, 11] may indicate a real increase in incidence, and the occurrence of colon perforation with steroid therapy may prove to be a causal association.

As mentioned, the diagnosis was made frequently by x-ray evidence, including barium enema, without the serious complication of barium peritonitis. The infrequent occurrence of free flow of barium into the peritoneal cavity has recently been documented,[6] and with good communciation between clinician and fluoroscopist, there should even be less chance. Contrast enema with a water-soluble contrast material (Gastrografin) is a safe alternative.

RECOMMENDATIONS

Clinical recognition will be aided by remembering that in any steroid-treated patient with fever and abdominal symptoms, the colon should be suspect. Reliance on the usual physical findings, such as abdominal guarding, rebound tenderness, or leukocytosis will lead to delay in diagnosis. X-ray evidence of free intraperitoneal air or early contrast enema for confirmation of colonic disease are the most reliable diagnostic aids. The prognosis is considerably better if a walled-off abscess is demonstrated.

Proximal diversion by means of a colostomy, and extraperitoneal drainage of the abscess cavity followed by elective resection when the inflammatory process is quiescent, is recommended therapy. For free perforation of a vasculitis lesion or a diverticulum, exteriorization and resection of the involved area, leaving a colostomy and a distal mucous fistula is advocated. If the area of perforation cannot be mobilized, the perforation should be plicated and a proximal colostomy constructed. Appropriate systemic antibiotic agents for colonic flora have been used in all instances.

REFERENCES

1. Canter, J. W., and Shorb, P. E.: Acute perforation of colonic diverticula associated with prolonged adrenocortico-steroid therapy, Am. J. Surg. **121:** 46, 1971.
2. Couris, C. D., Block, M. A., and Rube, C. E.: Gastrointestinal complications of collagen disease, Arch. Surg. **89:** 695, 1964.
3. Eusebio, E. B., and Eisenberg, M. M.: Natural history of diverticular disease of the colon in young patients, Am. J. Surg. **125:** 308, 1973.
4. Fein, B. T.: Perforation and inflammation of diverticula of the colon secondary to long-term adrenocortico-steroid therapy for bronchial asthma and pulmonary emphysema, South. Med. J. **54:** 355, 1961.
5. Finkbiner, R. B., and Decker, J. P.: Ulceration and perforation of the intestine due to necrotizing arteriolitis, N. Engl. J. Med. **268:** 14, 1963.
6. Gardner, H., and Miller, R. E.: Barium peritonitis, Am. J. Surg. **125:** 350, 1973.
7. Misra, M. K., Pinkus, G. S., Birtch, A. G., and Wilson, R. E.: Major colonic diseases complicating renal transplantation, SURGERY **73:** 942, 1973.
8. Penn, I., Brettschneider, L., Simpson, K., Martin, A., and Starzl, T. E.: Major colonic problems in human homotransplant recipients, Arch. Surg. **100:** 61, 1970.
9. Renshaw, T. S., and Phelps, D. B.: Perforation of colonic diverticula, J. Bone Joint Surg. **54A:** 1070, 1972.
10. ReMine, W.: Discussion of Paper by Sautter and Ziffren,[11] Arch. Surg. **79:** 354, 1959.
11. Sautter, R. D., and Ziffren, S. E.: Adrenocortical steroid therapy resulting in unusual gastrointestinal complications, Arch. Surg. **79:** 346, 1959.

Nomarski differential-interference contrast microscopy: Application in dermal wound healing studies

T. N. Salthouse, F.I.M.L.T., F.R.P.S., *Somerville, N. J.*

A combination of Masson's collagen stain and Nomarski differential-interference contrast microscopy was applied to sections of guinea pig dermal wounds. Appreciation of collagen fiber orientation and wound architecture was greatly enhanced in comparison to standard transmission microscope optics. This was accomplished by the specific staining of the connective tissue elements and the "shadow cast" optical relief effect of the interference contrast system. It was considered to be more generally useful than scanning electron microscopy.

From the Histology-Histochemistry Section, Ethicon Research Foundation, Somerville, N. J.

Since its introduction, the Nomarski differential-interference contrast (DIC) system of optical miçroscopy has been applied to the study of a variety of biological specimens.[1, 5-7] Generally, unstained material is examined as in phase contrast microscopy. Recently the examination of stained sections by this system was suggested by Geissinger and Duitschaever,[6] and stained sections from dermal wound healing sites were employed in our study.

It is unnecessary to describe in detail the optical principles of this sysem. A clear exposition of the principles and equipment properties has been given by Allen and associates.[1] By the application of this system, phase objects are seen as though "shadow-cast." DIC is a function of the gradient in phase difference across the object with a related azimuth effect. Because of the "optical relief" effect, additional detail in stained sections can be observed. We have noted that this effect can greatly assist in the observation of connective tissue orientation in sections treated by collagen-staining procedures. Our appreciation of collagen fiber ingrowth in healing wounds was considerably enhanced by the application of DIC.

Scanning electron microscopy has been applied and found to be valuable by Forrester and associates[4] for examining collagen fibril orientation in sutured and taped wounds. However, we believe that additional information of wound tissue architecture can be gained by a combination of selective connective tissue staining and differential-interference contrast optics.

Wolman and Gillman[9] have recently applied the polarizing microscope to the study of collagen in dermal wound healing, and they have reported differences in birefringence with age of collagen.

Hunt,[8] in a recent editorial comment, considered that new and powerful tools were being ignored in wound healing research. The Nomarski differential-interference contrast system could be such a tool. The optical equipment for DIC microscopy is relatively inexpensive and can be applied by anyone with an average knowledge of optical mi-

Accepted for publication Aug. 22, 1973.

croscopy. Our own experience with this system is descibed and some photomicrographs are presented which may suggest applications to others working in this general area of research.

MATERIALS AND METHODS

Ten female guinea pigs were divided into five groups of two animals each for this histologic study. These were part of a larger study of wound strength and lathyrism which will be reported separately. A 3 cm. incision was made through the dermis and panniculus in the middorsal region. The wounds were closed by three interrupted No. 4-0 Ethilon sutures, 1 cm. apart and 0.3 cm. from the wound edge. Two animals each were killed at five, ten, fifteen, and twenty days after wounding. Two animals were killed without wounding for control sections of dermis.

The wound area with surrounding dermis and panniculus was excised and placed in Bouin's fixative for 18 hours and then treated in 70 percent ethanol for 24 hours. The tissue was embedded in paraffin by normal histologic procedues.[2] Sections across the wound and between the sutures were cut serially at a thickness of 5 μ. One section was stained by hematoxylin and eosin, one by Masson's trichrome connective tissue procedure, and the third section was subjected to van Gieson's procedure.[2] A fourth section was cut at a thickness of 15 μ and mounted on ⅜ diameter copper studs for subsequent examination by scanning electron microscopy. After removal of the wax with xylene and ethanol, the studs with attached sections were treated in buffered (pH 5.4) alpha-amylase solution, as suggested by Finlay and co-workers.[3] After having been washed and dried, the sections were coated with gold-palladium in vacuo and examined in a Joel scanning electron microscope.

The stained sections were examined by normal transmitted light and with Zeiss-Nomarski differential-interference contrast equipment,[1] consisting of interference contrast condenser, interference contrast slides (Wollaston prism), and polarizing filter. Planachromat 16 and 40 objectives were adjusted to give a "shadow casting" effect but no change in the original stain coloration. The unstained sections were examined by DIC alone.

RESULTS AND DISCUSSION

In general, our appreciation of collagen fiber orientation in both normal dermis and in healing wounds was greatly enhanced by application of DIC (Figs. 1 through 6). The combination of Masson's connective tissue staining and examination or photomicrography with Nomarski optics yielded more information of wound morphology than normal light microscopy alone.

The parallel orientation of fibroblasts and newly formed collagen in the area of the incisions was clearly demonstrated by this combination applied to stained sections of five-day wounds (Fig. 1). The further development of collagen in this same area is seen at ten days in Fig. 3. Differences in the appearance of older and newly synthesized collagen fibers are clearly visible (Fig. 3, 10 day wound, compared with Fig. 5, 20 day wound).

Other combinations such as van Gieson's picrofuchsin with DIC (Fig. 6) or hematoxylin and eosin staining with DIC did not permit the differentiation of collagen and fibroblasts that was observed with the Masson-DIC combination. DIC with unstained sections was of little value.

Scanning electron micrographs (Fig. 7) did not, in our judgment, provide as useful differential morphologic information as the staining-DIC combination. Furthermore, specimen preparation and examination is considerably more time-consuming, and the possibility of artifactual change by enzyme treatment is present. With scanning electron microscopy, specific identification of collagen is not possible, whereas with the Masson trichrome–DIC technique, the collagen fibers can be readily identified.

Our purpose in advocating the application of Nomarski differential contrast microscopy is the belief that it can assist other scientists working in the field of wound healing morphology.

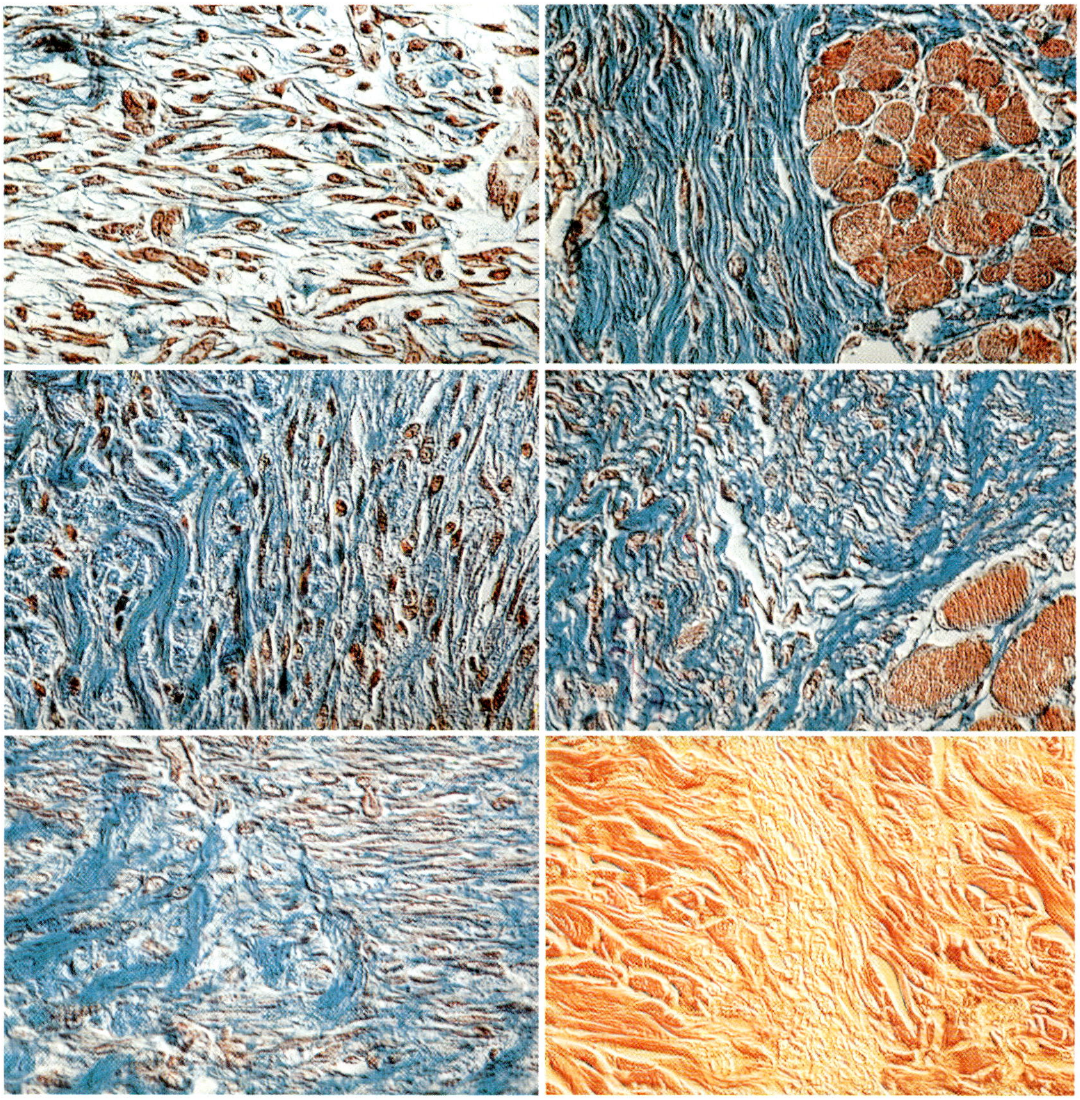

2

4

6

Figs. 1 through 6. In Figs. 1 through 5, stained by a Masson trichrome procedure, collagen is stained blue-green and muscle and nuclei are stained brick red. In Fig. 6, stained by the van Gieson method, collagen is stained orange and the other elements are stained yellow. It will be seen that the effect of applying the optics of differential-interference contrast (DIC) to the stained slides is to delineate tissue structure by a "shadow casting." This optical relief aids the observation of both fiber orientation and separation.

Fig. 1. Linear arrangement of fibroblast (red) and young collagen (blue-green) at incision line of five-day wound. Note "shadow cast" appearance of cells and collagen. (Masson trichrome with DIC. ×300.)

Fig. 2. The orientation of the dermal collagen and panniculus muscle fibers is well demonstrated by the Masson trichrome–DIC combination. Normal guinea pig dermis. (×300.)

Fig. 3. Wound area *(right)* and older original collagen *(left)* in ten-day wound demonstrated. (Masson trichrome–DIC. ×300.)

Fig. 4. Twenty-day wound. Arrangement of collagen fibers in incisional gap of panniculus muscle. (Masson trichrome–DIC. ×300.)

Fig. 5. Comparative difference in fibroblast orientation in wound area and original dermis is well delineated by Masson trichrome–DIC application in 20-day wound. (×300.)

Fig. 6. Van Gieson picrofuchsin–DIC combination. Although collagen fibers are demonstrated by "optical relief," differentiation of detail is not so apparent as with the Masson trichrome–DIC combination from the area of the incision of a ten-day wound. (×300.)

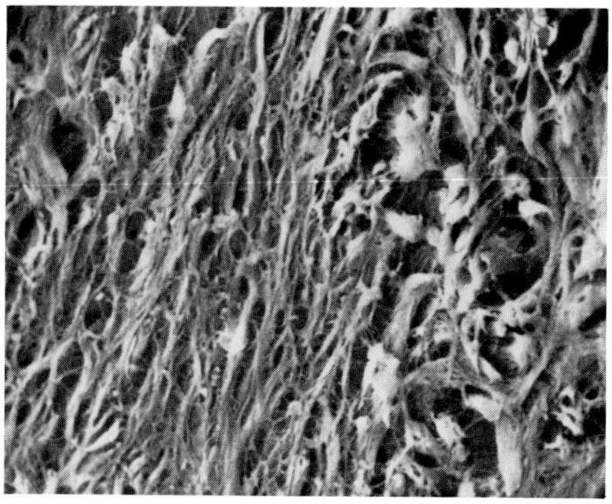

Fig. 7. Wound area section at ten days. The area is similar to that in Fig. 3. It was prepared for scanning electron microscopy by the procedure of Finlay and associates.[3] Orientation of collagen fibers with some interlocking elements. (×500.)

Mr. P. J. Lehn and Mrs. B. F. Matalga were responsible for organizing these studies.

REFERENCES

1. Allen, R. D., David, G. B., and Nomarski, G.: The Zeiss-Nomarski differential-interference equipment for transmitted-light microscopy, Z. Wiss. Mikrosk. **69:** 193, 1969.
2. Disbrey, B. D., and Rack, J. H.: Histological laboratory methods, Edinburgh, 1970, E. & S. Livingstone, Ltd.
3. Finlay, J. B., Hunter, A. A., and Stevens, F. S.: Preparation of human skin for high-resolution scanning electron microscopy using phosphate-buffered crude bacterial α-amylase, J. Microsc. **93:** 73, 1971.
4. Forrester, J. C., Zederfeldt, B. H., Hayes, T. L., and Hunt, T. K.: Tape-closed and sutured wounds: A comparison by tensiometry and scanning electron microscopy, Br. J. Surg. **57:** 729, 1970.
5. Geissinger, H. D., and Bond, E. F.: Nomarski differential-interference contrast microscopy and scanning electron microscopy of tissue sections and fibroblast cell culture monolayers, Mikroskopie **27:** 32, 1971.
6. Geissinger, H. D., and Duitschaever, C. L.: Nomarski differential-contrast microscopy in transillumination: Its use on unstained or stained sections, smears, and wet mounts, or on fluorochromed sections cell-culture monolayers, J. Microsc. **94:** 107, 1971.
7. Geissinger, H. D., Sontegard, R., and Reschauer, G. A.: Qualitative and quantitative Nomarski differential-interference contrast-fluorescence microscopy on cell culture monolayers, Mikroskopie **27:** 129, 1971.
8. Hunt, T. K.: Standards for wound healing research, SURGERY **73:** 153, 1973.
9. Wolman, M., and Gillman, T.: A polarized light study of collagen in dermal wound healing, Br. J. Exp. Pathol. **53:** 85, 1972.

Reticuloendothelial dysfunction and endotoxemia following portal vein occlusion

Isik Olcay, M.D., Akio Kitahama, M.D., Robert H. Miller, M.D., Theodore Drapanas, M.D., Rafael A. Trejo, M.D., Ph.D., *and* **N. R. Di Luzio, Ph.D.,** *New Orleans, La.*

Acute temporary ligation of the portal vein (PV) produces death in various animal species. The influence of PV occlusion (PVO) on reticuloendothelial (RE) function and endotoxemia was studied in both conventional and germ-free rats. Although endotoxin was not detected in portal or systemic blood samples prior to PVO, endotoxin was invariably present in the portal circulation five minutes after PVO. Portal endotoxin concentration continued to increase throughout the 30 minute occlusive interval. Systemic endotoxemia was detected late during the occlusion episode. Following the restoration of portal flow, systemic endotoxin levels initially increased and were subsequently reduced six hours later. Systemic endotoxemia was invariably associated with portal endotoxemia. In contrast to the findings in conventional rats, endotoxin was not detected in portal vein or systemic samples of gnotobiotic animals during PVO. Phagocytic activity, measured six hours after PVO, was significantly depressed in both the conventional and germ-free animals, denoting that RE depression following ischemic insult to the liver was not due to endotoxemia. The demonstration of the development of systemic as well as portal endotoxemia following gut vascular stasis in association with RE dysfunction may well contribute to the pathophysiology of PVO injury.

From the Departments of Surgery and Physiology, Tulane University School of Medicine, New Orleans, La.

ACUTE LIGATION of the portal vein (PV) has been demonstrated to be fatal in a variety of animals.[3, 12, 16] The mechanism by which this insult leads to a high degree of mortality in cows,[3] cats, and dogs,[12, 16] is unknown. Several theories have been advanced to explain lethality following ligation of the portal vein. Lautenbach,[17] as well as Netter,[18] proposed that an undesignated toxin produced in the gut caused death. Elman and Cole[12] concluded that death was not caused by elaboration of a toxin from the gastrointestinal tract but was due to pooling of splanchnic blood resulting in hypovolemic shock. Boyce and associates[6] proposed that in addition to splanchnic pooling, a neurogenic component also contributed to the development of death following portal occlusion.

Recently, Fine and colleagues[13, 14] and Wiznitzer and colleagues[26] advanced the thesis that failure of the reticuloendothelial system (RES) to neutralize endotoxins released from gram-negative bacteria of the gut contributes to the shock syndrome and

Supported, in part, by the American Heart Association, the Louisiana Heart Association, and National Institutes of Health Grant No. AM-13935.

Accepted for publication Aug. 22, 1973.

Address correspondence to: N. R. Di Luzio, Ph.D., Department of Physiology, Tulane University School of Medicine, 1430 Tulane Ave., New Orleans, La. 70112.

lethality. Fine and associates[13] also maintained that shock is a type of trauma which impairs the RES; the degree of which is related to the intensity and duration of the shock episode.

In light of Fine's experiments implicating endotoxin in a variety of shock models, studies were undertaken to evaluate RE function and the occurrence of endotoxemia following portal vein occlusion (PVO). Upon finding that PVO resulted in phagocytic impairment and portal as well as systemic endotoxemia in conventional rats, additional experiments in germ-free animals were undertaken to ascertain the contribution of gastroingestin-derived endotoxins to RES depression.

MATERIALS AND METHODS

Male Charles River rats were used as conventional animals. Germ-free rats of both sexes were obtained from the Tulane Medical Center's germ-free colony. A total of 191 rats, weighing between 250 and 400 grams, were divided into six groups as follows: I, conventional, nonoperated (24); II, conventional, sham operated (64); III, conventional, portal vein occluded (69); IV, germ free, nonoperated (14); V, germ free, sham operated (10); and VI, germ free, portal vein occluded (10).

All rats were anesthetized with sodium pentobarbital (Nembutal), intraperitoneally, with a dose of 4 mg. per 100 Gm. of body weight; all the surgical manipulations were done under sterile conditions. The abdomen was opened with a midline incision and the PV was isolated. PVO was accomplished by placing a small vascular clamp on the PV for 30 minutes.

In control and experimental animals, heparinized blood samples for plasma endotoxin determinations were taken from the PV proximal to the occlusion site and from the heart at five and twenty-nine minutes during the PVO period, as well as five minutes, thirty minutes, and six hours after releasing the vascular clamp. Because of the volume of blood required for endotoxin analyses, different rats were used at each time interval with at least eight animals being sampled. Plasma endotoxin levels were determined in duplicate by the Limulus lysate test.[20, 21] Twofold serial dilutions of plasma were performed for the quantitation of endotoxins. *E. coli* endotoxin (Difco Laboratories) was employed as a standard, and the test was sensitive to 0.005 μg of endotoxin.

Phagocytic activity of the RES was evaluated six hours after the sham operation or the restoration of portal blood flow by using the gelatinized ^{131}I-RE test lipid emulsion as previously described.[11] The lipid emulsion was injected intravenously in 68 control and experimental animals in a dose of 50 mg. per 100 Gm. of body weight in the dorsal vein of the penis. Blood samples were obtained at 1, 3, 5, 7, and 9 minutes for determination of blood radioactivity. The localization of the lipid emulsion in lung, spleen, and liver was measured ten minutes after injection. The intravascular half-time was determined, and the extrapolated zero time concentration was employed in the determination of circulating blood volume.

The mortality rate in the sham-operated and in the portal vein–occluded groups was determined at 72 hours following release of the PVO.

Statistical significance was ascertained according to Student's t test with the level of significance established at 95 percent.

RESULTS

PVO for 30 minutes in conventional, i.e., non–germ-free, rats was associated with a 25 percent mortality rate, usually within the first 12 hours following occlusion. No deaths were observed in the sham-operated group at the end of the 72 hour period. Additional studies indicated that 15, 20, or 25 minutes of PVO did not induce any deaths. In contrast, a 60 minute period of ligation induced 100 percent mortality rate. In germ-free rats, mortality studies were not conducted due to technical reasons.

None of the conventional rats showed endotoxin in either portal or systemic blood prior to PVO (Fig. 1). Endotoxin was, however, detected in the portal blood after five

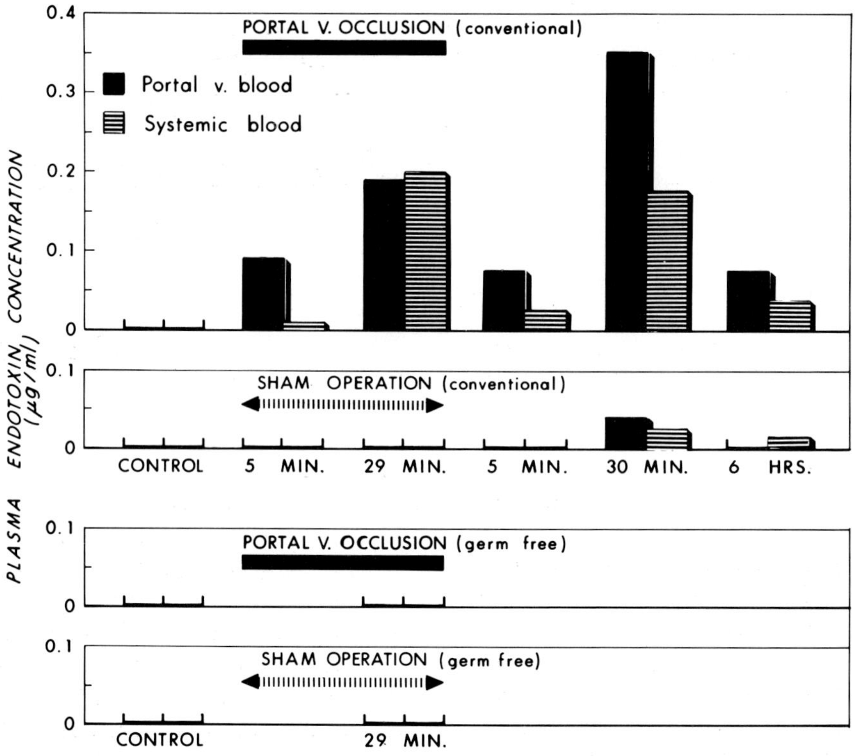

Fig. 1. Mean plasma endotoxin concentrations as measured by the Limulus test in portal (■) and systemic (▤) samples of conventional and germ-free rats. Endotoxin determinations were performed prior to, during, or subsequent to PVO or sham procedures in both conventional and germ-free rats.

minutes of occlusion in seven of eight (87.5 percent) of the conventional rats. The mean plasma endotoxin concentration was 0.09 µg per milliliter with a range of 0.05 to 0.20 µg per milliliter. In contrast to the high incidence of portal vein endotoxemia at the five-minute occlusive period, in only one of eight (12.5 percent) of the rats was endotoxin evident in the systemic circulation. In this animal, an endotoxin concentration of 0.05 µg per milliliter was found. Twenty-nine minutes into the occlusion episode, six of ten (60 percent) animals had endotoxin in the PV and five of ten (50 percent) had systemic endotoxemia. The mean endotoxin concentration of 0.2 µg per milliliter was comparable in both portal and systemic blood at this period. The endotoxin concentration in portal plasma ranged from 0.2 to 0.8 µg per milliliter, while the systemic plasma ranged from 0.05 to 0.8 µg per milliliter.

Five minutes after restoration of the splanchnic circulation, endotoxin was present in the portal blood of nine of 16 (56.3 percent) animals and in the systemic blood in three of 15 (20 percent) animals. The mean value in the portal samples was 0.08 µg per milliliter (range: 0.05 to 0.40 µg per milliliter) while that in the systemic samples was 0.02 µg per milliliter. The concentration of endotoxin in systemic blood was 0.05, 0.1, and 0.1 µg per milliliter in the three endotoxin-positive animals. Thirty minutes after release of the clamp, the mean endotoxin concentration was 0.36 µg per milliliter in the portal blood (range: 0.2 to 0.8 µg per milliliter) and 0.18 µg per milliliter in the systemic blood (range: 0.1 to 0.4 µg per milliliter) with endotoxin being present in eight or nine (89 percent) of the animals in the PV and in an identical number of animals in the systemic circulation.

Six hours after termination of the occlusion, two of nine (22 percent) of the con-

Table I. *Effect of occlusion of the portal vein on the intravascular removal rate and organ distribution of the gelatinized* ^{131}*I-RE test lipid emulsion**

Group	Intravascular t/2 (min.)	Organ distribution Liver (% ID/TO)	Lung (% ID/TO)	Spleen (% ID/TO)
Non-operated	16.9 ± 1.5	46.2 ± 2.7	1.0 ± 0.05	3.2 ± 0.2
Sham operated	13.4 ± 0.6	42.8 ± 3.4	1.2 ± 0.07	3.6 ± 0.4
Portal vein occluded	37.6 ± 4.6	29.5 ± 3.0	1.6 ± 0.1	2.6 ± 0.3

*Rats were injected intravenously with the lipid emulsion (50 mg. per 100 Gm.) six hours after the release of the portal occlusion. Tissue distribution of the emulsion was measured ten minutes after injection. The distribution data are expressed as percent of injected dose (% ID) per total organ (TO). Intravascular clearance data are derived from 16 to 17 rats per group while the tissue localization data are compiled from eight to nine rats per group. Values are expressed as means ± standard error.

ventional rats had endotoxin concentrations in portal blood of 0.2 and 0.4 μg per milliliter. Endotoxin was present in peripheral blood of only one rat at a concentration of 0.4 μg per milliliter, which was identical to the portal concentration.

In sham-operated conventional rats, endotoxin was not detected in either the portal or the systemic plasma until thirty minutes after the termination of the sham procedures. Three of eleven (27 percent) had endotoxin in the portal plasma, with values of 0.1, 0.2, and 0.2 μg per milliliter. The mean endotoxin concentration of eleven rats was 0.04 μg per milliliter. Two of the three rats which had portal vein endotoxemia had systemic endotoxin concentrations of 0.2 μg per milliliter. Endotoxin was not present in the portal blood six hours following the sham operation. One of nine (11.1 percent) of the sham-operated did have a systemic endotoxin concentration of 0.2 μg per milliliter. These findings may reflect bacterial and/or endotoxin contamination.

In agreement with the observation of the absence of endotoxin in portal or systemic circulation of normal rats prior to occlusion, endotoxins were not detected in the portal or systemic plasma of germ-free animals. In contrast to the findings in the normal group of portal vein and systemic endotoxemia during the occlusion period, endotoxin was not detected in portal or systemic plasma of any of the germ-free animals.

In conventional animals, PVO significantly impaired phagocytic activity of the RES (Table I). The intravascular clearance rate (t/2) of the lipid emulsion was significantly ($p < 0.001$) depressed in the portal vein–occluded group. No impairment in clearance was observed in the sham-operated group. The hepatic uptake of the lipid emulsion in the portal vein–occluded group was diminished significantly ($p < 0.02$) when compared to either the sham-operated or non-operated group. In contrast to the depressed particle uptake by liver, uptake by spleen or lung of the lipid emulsion was normal. The changes in organ distribution of the lipid emulsion were not the result of alterations in incubating blood volume since comparable blood volumes were found in the control and experimental groups. In all groups, the predominant organ of localization of the lipid emulsion was liver with lung and spleen accounting for a relatively minor fraction of the removed lipid.

In germ-free rats, the uptake of the lipid emulsion by liver was also significantly decreased ($p < 0.02$) in the portal vein–occluded group when compared to the non-operated control group (Table II). The uptake was decreased 36 percent relative to the sham-operated controls. This value is, however, not statistically significantly different. The uptake of the lipid emulsion by spleen in the germ-free rats, which approximates three percent of the injected dose, was not significantly impaired in the portal vein–occluded group. Likewise, lung uptake by the group which underwent 30 minutes of occlusion was essentially unaltered.

Table II. *Influence of occlusion of the portal vein on the organ distribution of the gelatinized ^{131}I-RE test lipid emulsion in germ-free rats**

Group	Organ distribution† Liver (% ID/TO)	Lung (% ID/TO)	Spleen (% ID/TO)
Non-operated	32.9 ± 5.2	0.9 ± 0.1	3.1 ± 0.3
Sham operated	25.7 ± 4.9	1.6 ± 0.5	1.9 ± 0.6
Portal vein occluded	16.2 ± 1.8	1.4 ± 0.2	2.3 ± 0.5

*Values derived from 5-9 rats per group are expressed as means ± standard error.

†Distribution data are expressed as percent of injected dose (% ID) per total organ (TO).

DISCUSSION

The present study indicates that temporary PVO in the rat results in a high number of deaths as previously described in such animal species as the cow, cat, and dog.[3, 12, 16] The nature of the unique susceptibility of these various animal species to PVO has not been established.

Another model of intestinal ischemic insult associated with a high percentage of deaths is superior mesenteric artery occlusion (SMAO). Since endotoxemia[8, 25] and RES depression[1, 4, 5] have been demonstrated to occur following SMAO, our studies were conducted to relate the possible occurrence of endotoxema and RES depression in the shock episode following PVO. In essential agreement with the findings in SMAO shock, endotoxemia was present in both the portal and systemic circulation of conventional rats after temporary PVO. The endotoxemia of the experimental group, i.e., occluded, was significantly higher and occurred with greater frequency than that of the sham-operated animals.

In contrast to the findings of endotoxemia in conventional animals following PVO, endotoxin was not demonstrable in any of the blood samples of germ-free animals. These findings support the reports of other investigators[10, 15, 22, 23] that endotoxins originate from the gram-negative flora of the gut. The conclusions of these investigators were based upon the employment of nonabsorbable antibiotic agents rather than the use of germ-free animals.

The pathway by which endotoxin from the gut enters into the systemic circulation has been considered by Cuevas and Fine.[10] These investigators postulated that the peritoneal surface plays the most important role in the absorption of endotoxin since they were unable to demonstrate endotoxin in the PV of rabbits following SMAO. Battersby and associates[3] demonstrated the presence of gram-negative, coliform bacteria in both the portal as well as the systemic blood following occlusion of the PV in the calf. These investigators also observed the presence of the same gram-negative organism in the serosanguinous transudate present in the peritoneal cavity following the occlusive interval. In our study, systemic endotoxemia found during the PVO period indicates that in the rat there must be at least one additional pathway, such as the lymphatic channels, by which the endotoxin can reach the systemic circulation. However, in contrast to the observations of Cuevas and Fine[9] of the absence of endotoxins in the PV in the SMAO model, endotoxins appeared in the portal blood immediately following PVO.

It was noted that all animals which had systemic endotoxemia had endotoxin present in the portal sample. There were no rats in which a negative test for endotoxin in portal blood was accompanied with a positive test for endotoxin in the systemic sample. Therefore, in this model, the PV is an important route for endotoxin transfer from the gut to the systemic circulation. It remains to be established whether the differences in presence or absence of endotoxins in the PV as denoted by Cuevas and Fine[10] reflect the animal species employed or the nature of the shock model.

In normal animals, prior to any experimental operative procedure, neither the PV nor the systemic circulation had detectable levels of endotoxin. This finding is in essential agreement with the observation of Tamakuma and associates[25] of undetectable endotoxin levels in normal rabbits.

Since Kupffer cells are the major site of removal of endotoxin,[7] the increasing plasma endotoxin concentration from the 5 to 30 minute period following release of the clamp suggests that the ischemic cells inadequately removed endotoxins present in the pooled splanchnic blood. Indeed, Greene and colleagues[15] have reported that the incidence of endotoxemia varies with the size of the endotoxin pool in the gut. Additionally, they demonstrated that failure of RE cells of the liver to extract endotoxins results in generalized endotoxemia.

The marked drop in systemic endotoxin concentrations seen in the five-minute postocclusion sample may be explained on the basis that the liver, the major site of the RES, has been excluded from the circulation during the occlusion process by two mechanisms. First, the clamp on the PV prevents blood from reaching the liver from the gut. Second, it has been demonstrated in a variety of animals that during the period of PVO, there is a marked decrease in the systemic blood pressure.[3, 12, 16] With the resulting hypotension, there would be reduced perfusion of the liver by way of the hepatic artery which would further reduce the liver's ability to remove and possibly detoxify endotoxins. Upon removal of the clamp on the PV, systemic blood pressure returns to normal,[3] at which time the liver would then receive blood from the portal vein and hepatic artery. Thus, the liver, although somewhat impaired by the ischemic insult, would be initially able to remove some of the endotoxin present in the portal as well as the systemic blood, thereby reducing the endotoxin concentration. Additionally, the possibility exists that the liver may act as a reservoir during the immediate postocclusion period.

Since certain endotoxins have the ability to impair RES function,[2, 24] the exposure of the liver to high titers of endotoxin during the period immediately following removal of the occlusion may result in RES depression leading to a marked elevation of the systemic endotoxin levels such as that observed in the 30 minute sample.

Although several studies have been performed on animals following PVO,[3, 12, 16, 19] the status of RE function has not been ascertained. Thirty minutes of PVO produced significant RE depression in the conventional rats. The intravascular clearance rate of the lipid emulsion in the operated conventional rats was significantly prolonged. Depression in phagocytosis was due exclusively to Kupffer cell dysfunction. The uptake of the lipid emulsion by the liver of the portal vein–occluded germ-free rats was also significantly depressed when compared to nonoperated control germ-free animals.

The role of substances other than endotoxins in the mediation of RE depression has been postulated by several investigations. Blattberg and Levy[4] and again Blattberg and colleagues[5] proposed that a circulating RE depressing substance was found in the ischemic dog intestine and that RE depression occurs with or without the presence of a gram-negative flora in the gut. Altura and Hershey[1] showed that intestinal ischemia induced by SMAO produces RE depression. The degree of depression in RE function correlated with the magnitude of the ischemic insult. In the present study, RE depression and endotoxemia were produced following PVO in the conventional animals. Significant RE depression also occurred following PVO in gnotobiotic rats, although endotoxemia was not present. Our studies therefore demonstrate that endotoxins are not the cause of RE depression.

The present findings denote that in addition to venous pooling and resulting hypotension which characterizes PVO, an added insult to the host occurs in the form of portal and systemic endotoxemia as well as RE depression. These composite events may well be contributory to the pathophysiology of acute temporary PVO.

REFERENCES

1. Altura, B. M., and Hershey, S. G.: Acute intestinal ischemia shock and reticuloendothelial system function, J. Reticuloendothel. Soc. **10:** 361, 1971.
2. Arredondo, M. I., and Kampschmidt, R.: Effect of endotoxins on phagocytic activity of the reticuloendothelial system of the rat, Proc. Soc. Exp. Biol. Med. **112:** 78, 1963.
3. Battersby, C., Balderson, G., Sinch, J., and Burnett, W.: Acute occlusion of the portal vein in the calf, J. Surg. Res. **11:** 95, 1971.
4. Blattberg, B., and Levy, M. N.: Reticuloendothelial depression with superior mesenteric artery occlusion, Am. J. Physiol. **204:** 899, 1963.
5. Blattberg, B., Levy, M. N., and Strong, I.: Effect of a reticuloendothelial-depressing substance on survival from shock, J. Reticuloendothel. Soc. **3:** 65, 1966.
6. Boyce, F. F., Lambert, R., and McFetridge, E. M.: Occlusion of the portal vein: An experimental study with its clinical application, J. Lab. Clin. Med. **20:** 935, 1935.
7. Braude, A. I., Carey, F. J., and Zalesky, M.: Studies with radioactive endotoxin. II. Correlation of physiologic effects with distribution of radioactivity in rabbits injected with lethal doses of *E. coli* endotoxin labelled with radioactive sodium chromate, J. Clin. Invest. **34:** 858, 1955.
8. Cuevas, P., and Fine, J.: Demonstration of a lethal endotoxemia in experimental occlusion of the superior mesenteric artery, Surg. Gynecol. Obstet. **133:** 81, 1971.
9. Cuevas, P., and Fine, J.: Route of absorption of endotoxin from the intestine in nonseptic shock, J. Reticuloendothel. Soc. **11:** 535, 1972.
10. Cuevas, P., and Fine, J.: Production of fatal endotoxic shock by vasoactive substances, Gastroenterology **64:** 285, 1973.
11. Di Luzio, N. R., Pisano, J. C., and Saba, T. M.: Evaluation of the mechanism of glucan-induced stimulation of the reticuloendothelial system, J. Reticuloendothel. Soc. **7:** 731, 1970.
12. Elman, R., and Cole, W. H.: Hemorrhage and shock as causes of death following acute portal obstruction, Arch. Surg. **28:** 1166, 1934.
13. Fine, J., Frank, E. D., Ravin, H. A., Rutenberg, S. H., and Schweinberg, F. B.: The bacterial factor in traumatic shock, N. Engl. J. Med. **260:** 214, 1959.
14. Fine, J., Rutenberg, S., and Schweinberg, F. B.: The role of the reticuloendothelial system in hemorrhagic shock, J. Exp. Med. **110:** 547, 1959.
15. Greene, R., Wiznitzer, T., Rutenberg, S., Frank, E., and Fine, J.: Hepatic clearance of endotoxin absorbed from the intestine, Proc. Soc. Exp. Biol. Med. **108:** 261, 1961.
16. Johnston, F. R. C.: Acute ligation of the portal vein, SURGERY **41:** 958, 1957.
17. Lautenbach, B. F.: On a new function of the liver, M. Times and Reg. **7:** 387, 1876-77.
18. Netter: Des poisons chimiques qui apparaisent dans les matières organiques en voie dedécomposition et des maladies qu'ils peuvent provoquer, Arch. Gen. de Méd. **2:** 447, 1884.
19. Onnis, M., Shumacker, H. B., Jr., and Bounous, G.: Response to occlusion of the portal vein, Arch. Surg. **85:** 897, 1962.
20. Reinhold, R. B., and Fine, J.: A technique for quantitative measurement of endotoxin in human plasma, Proc. Soc. Exp. Biol. Med. **137:** 334, 1971.
21. Rojas-Corona, R. R., Skarnes, R., Tamakuma, S., and Fine, J.: The Limulus coagulation test for endotoxin. A comparison with other assay methods, Proc. Soc. Exp. Biol. Med. **132:** 599, 1969.
22. Schweinberg, F. B., and Fine, J.: Evidence for a lethal endotoxemia as the fundamental feature of irreversibility in three types of traumatic shock, J. Exp. Med. **112:** 793, 1960.
23. Schweinburg, F. B., Shapiro, P. B., Frank, E. D., and Fine, J.: Host resistance in hemorrhagic shock. IX. Demonstration of circulating lethal toxin in hemorrhagic shock, Proc. Soc. Exp. Biol. Med. **95:** 646, 1957.
24. Serafin, D., Stone, H. H., Kolb, L. D., Martin, J. D., Jr.: Alterations in reticuloendothelial functions as produced by the administration of bacterial toxins, Am. Surg. **34:** 714, 1968.
25. Tamakuma, S., Rojas-Corona, R., Cuevas, P., and Fine, J.: Demonstration of a lethal endotoxemia of intestinal origin in refractory non-septic shock, Ann. Surg. **173:** 219, 1971.
26. Wiznitzer, T., Better, N., Rachlin, W., Atkins, N., Frank, E. D., and Fine, J.: *In vivo* detoxification of endotoxin by the reticuloendothelial system, J. Exp. Med. **112:** 1157, 1960.

Comparative efficacy of hypo-, iso-, and hypertonic sodium solutions in experimental burn shock

Charles L. Fox, Jr., M.D., *and* **John W. Stanford, M.S.,** *New York, N. Y.*

This study was designed to ascertain the most effective electrolyte solution for resuscitation after potentially fatal thermal injury. Solutions containing from 75 to 300 mEq. per liter of sodium with various concentrations of chloride were administered in graduated dosages to mice subjected to a standardized scald. Their effectiveness was evaluated by comparison of the 24 hour mortality rates and also the changes in body weight, urine, and plasma electrolytes. Several solutions were effective; the optimal intake was approximately 22.5 mEq. of sodium per kilogram. This was most efficiently given in a solution containing 225 mEq. of sodium and 160 mEq. of chloride per liter. Greater survival resulted where the Na:Cl ratio more closely approximated that in plasma. Hypotonic solutions such as are generally used in patients were less effective at all dosage levels.

From the Department of Surgery, Columbia University College of Physicians and Surgeons, New York, N. Y.

THE FLUID therapy of burns has changed in the past four decades. The demonstration that colloid does not enhance the efficacy of electrolyte solutions in restoring cardiac output[37] affirms clinical reports[1, 7, 13, 14, 21, 23, 32] of resuscitation of patients without plasma or blood. These emphasize the essentiality of the sodium and water intakes.

Following burns or surgical trauma, ADH (antidiuretic hormone) is increased[31] with retention of excess water even in patients who recover.[20] The increase in aldosterone after trauma and in various edema states can be suppressed by a high intake of sodium as was demonstrated in the nephrotic syndrome prior to the advent of steroids.[17, 18, 33, 41] After experimental thermal trauma, alkaline sodium salt solutions induced considerably more excretion of sodium, potassium, and water than other agents.[14]

Inasmuch as more sodium than water is translocated to burned tissues (which lose potassium), the over-all shift is *hypertonic* in terms of sodium.[12, 14-16, 22, 40, 41] Thus, hypertonic solutions might facilitate sodium replacement, reduce the total water intake, expedite excretion of potassium released from traumatized cells, and equal the net tissue gain in sodium and water. Hypertonic sodium chloride solutions have been used,[2, 5, 23, 26] but the likelihood of increasing the acidosis by using only sodium chloride was not considered.[34, 35, 43] As early as 1918, Cannon measured the acidosis in man after injury and successfully utilized hypertonic alkaline solutions.[18] Burn patients are now being resuscitated with hypertonic alkaline solutions with less edema and less gain in weight.[3, 27, 28]

In clinical practice, six different regimens

This study was aided in part by The John A. Hartford Foundation, Inc., and Research Grant No. GM-18275-02 from the National Institutes of Health.

Accepted for publication Sept. 4, 1973.

Presented in part at the 1972 meeting of the American Burn Association.

Table I. *Composition of solutions used (milliequivalents per liter)*

Na	Cl	HCO₃*	K	Mg	Ca
300	100	200	0	0	0
300	170	130	0	0	0
225	100	135	5	2	3
225	160	75	5	2	3
225	225	0	0	0	0
154	154	0	0	0	0
150	100	58	5	3	0
140	98	50	5	3	0
130	126	18	14	5	0
130	109	28	4	0	3
100	75	30	4	1	0
75	56	23	3	1	0

*HCO_3 obtained by metabolism of acetate and d,l-lactate.

Table II. *Comparison of solutions with sodium intakes near 22.5 mEq. per kilogram*

Solution (mEq./L.)		Dose		Mortality at 24 hr. (percent)	No. of mice
Na	Cl	Sodium (mEq./Kg.)	Volume (ml./Kg.)		
300	170	22.5	75	0	20
300	100	22.5	75	4	112
225	225	22.5	100	7	30
225	160	22.5	100	3	60
225	100	22.5	100	5	180
150	150	22.5	150	13	30
150	100	22.5	150	9	120
140	100	21.0	150	0	20
130	109	26.0	200	8	40
130	109	19.5	150	5	40
100	75	22.5	225	10	80
75	56	22.5	300	19	47
Controls		None		78	310

are described by six authors in *Contemporary Burn Management.*[36] Inasmuch as variations in the patients and their burns make comparisons difficult, utilizing a standardized thermal injury might facilitate evaluation of solutions with varying sodium and chloride concentrations by gauging survival, urine output, weight changes, and other indices.

MATERIALS AND METHODS

Female albino mice from a closed colony (Hemlock Farms) weighing 22 to 24 grams, were used. Food and water were given ad libitum up to the beginning of the experiments and withheld for 24 hours subsequently. For burn trauma, unshaven mice were anesthetized with ether and then immersed to the axilla in water as described by Rosenthal and Tabor.[40] The temperatures of 72 or 73° C. for six or seven seconds were selected to obtain 80 percent mortality rate in 24 hours in untreated mice. Groups of ten mice were kept in metal cages with a bedding of woodchips in a room air-conditioned at 25° C. For metabolic experiments, a slightly less severe scald at 70° C. was used so that urine could be collected without mortality from pooled groups of five treated mice kept in stainless steel metabolism cages.

Fluid therapy was administered intraperitoneally via a No. 26 gauge needle two hours after the burn was inflicted; volumes over 225 ml. per kilogram were given in divided doses two and five hours post burn. In each experiment, the scalded animals were divided randomly into groups of 20 to provide one control group and five therapy groups. This schedule limited the number of animals that could be handled in each experiment and hence, each fluid was tested

Table III. *Comparison of solutions with sodium intakes near 15 mEq. per kilogram*

Solution (mEq./L.)		Dose		Mortality at 24 hr. (percent)	No. of mice
Na	Cl	Sodium (mEq./Kg.)	Volume (ml./Kg.)		
300	252	15.0	50	6	16
300	170	15.0	50	8	40
300	100	15.0	50	18	60
260	218	15.0	58	10	20
225	189	15.0	67	6	16
225	160	15.0	67	15	20
150	126	15.0	100	19	16
150	100	15.0	100	6	70
130	109	15.0	115	3	36
130	126	11.0	100	5	20
130	109	13.0	100	13	60
100	75	15.0	150	14	70
75	56	15.0	200	20	30

Table IV. *Comparison of solutions with minimal sodium intakes of 11.25 to 3.8 mEq. per kilogram*

Solution (mEq./L.)		Dose		Mortality at 24 hr. (percent)	No. of mice
Na	Cl	Sodium (mEq./Kg.)	Volume (ml./Kg.)		
300	100	9.0	30	57	30
300	170	7.5	25	30	20
225	100	11.25	50	8	61
225	160	9.0	40	5	20
225	160	7.5	33	15	20
150	100	11.25	75	18	80
150	100	7.5	50	27	70
130	109	7.5	58	10	40
100	75	10.0	100	33	30
100	75	5.0	50	35	40
75	56	7.5	100	20	30
75	56	3.8	50	30	40

three to five times in different experiments; over 3,000 mice were used.

The sodium concentration of the solutions ranged from 75 to 300 mEq. per liter with various sodium to chloride ratios as shown in Table I. Hypertonic solutions containing only 100 mEq. per liter of chloride and others with sodium to chloride ratios closer to that of plasma were tested. The volume of fluid administered ranged from 37.5 to 346 ml. per kilogram of body weight.

RESULTS OF FLUID THERAPY TRIALS

Tables II through V show the mortality results with four levels of sodium input and in untreated controls. It should be noted that at a fixed sodium input, the volume of solution administered decreased as the sodium concentration of the solution was increased.

Maximum survival occurred with a sodium intake of 22 to 24 mEq. per kilogram of body weight (Table II) obtained from appropriate volumes of solutions varying from 100 to 300 mEq. per liter of sodium. For statistical comparison with other sodium intakes it was necessary to exclude the solutions containing only sodium chloride and the 75 mEq. per liter sodium solution in order to pass the chi-square test for homogeneity ($P > 0.05$). This appeared justifiable in the case of the sodium chloride solutions since their composition (Na = Cl) differs markedly from the other solutions. In the

Table V. *Comparison of solutions with maximal sodium intakes of 30 to 45 mEq. per kilogram*

Solution (mEq./L.)		Dose		Mortality at 24 hr. (percent)	No. of mice
Na	Cl	Sodium (mEq./Kg.)	Volume (ml./Kg.)		
300	170	45.0	150	20	20
300	170	30.0	100	0	20
300	100	30.0	100	17	60
225	160	45.0	200	15	20
225	160	33.75	150	10	20
225	100	33.75	150	16	50
150	100	45.0	300	5	20
150	100	30.0	200	0	20
130	109	45.0	346	0	20
130	109	39.0	300	5	20
100	75	30.0	300	22	32

Table VI. *Na/Cl ratio and efficacy of sodium solutions*

Solutions (mEq./L.)		Dose		Mortality at 24 hr. (percent)	No. of animals
Na	Cl	Sodium (mEq./Kg.)	Volume (ml./Kg.)		
150	150	22.5	150	13	30
150	100	22.5	150	9	120
225	225	22.5	100	7	30
225	160	22.5	100	3	60
225	100	22.5	100	5	180
300	170	22.5	75	0	20
300	100	22.5	75	4	112
225	160	9.0	40	5	20
225	100	11.25	50	8	61
300	170	30.0	100	0	20
300	100	30.0	100	17	60
300	170	15.0	50	8	40
300	100	15.0	50	18	60

case of the 75 mEq. per liter sodium solution, the high mortality rate suggested that this solution exceeded the limits of physiologically acceptable tonicity and volume.

When the sodium intake was reduced (Table III) to 15 mEq. per kilogram ($P > 0.5$ in the chi-square test for consistency), the mortality values were significantly increased over those in Table II with 22.5 mEq. per kilogram of sodium ($P < 0.005$).

Further reduction in sodium intake to 11.25 or below (Table IV) was followed by further increase in mortality rate.

In Table V are shown the results with the maximal sodium intakes of 30 to 45 mEq. per kilogram. These results pass the chi-square test for consistency ($P > 0.05$) when the data for the isotonic solutions (containing 130 or 150 mEq. per liter of sodium) are omitted. The difference in mortality rate between the isotonic solutions and the others is highly significant ($P < 0.005$). The mortality rate with these isotonic solutions used in substantially greater volume is similar to the mortality rate observed with the smaller volumes used in Table II. In contrast, the mortality rates of the nonisotonic groups in Table V are significantly greater than the values analyzed in Table II ($P < 0.005$).

The ratio of sodium to chloride appears important as shown in Table VI. In all experiments, the hypertonic solutions containing 160 or 170 mEq. per liter of chloride

Table VII. *Comparative efficacy of various sodium solutions in terms of volume of fluid administered*

Sodium solution (mEq./L.)		Amount of fluid administered (ml.)/Kg. body weight									
		300		200		150		100		50	
Na	Cl	Mortality (%)*	Na† (mEq.)	Mortality (%)*	Na† (mEq.)	Mortality (%)*	Na† (mEq.)	Mortality (%)*	Na† (mEq.)	Mortality (%)*	Na† (mEq.)
300	170	–	–	–	–	20	45	0	30	8‡	15
225	160	–	–	–	–	10	34	**3**	**23**	8‡	11
150	100	5	45	0	30	**9**	**23**	6	15	27	8
130	109	5	39	**8**	**26**	5	20	13	13	10	7
100	75	22	30	**10**	**20**	14	15	33	10	35	5
75	56	**19§**	**23**	20	15	–	–	20	8	30	4

*Percent of treated mice that died in 24 hours: 78 percent of 310 untreated mice died in 24 hours.

†Intake of sodium in milliequivalents per kilogram of body weight.

‡These solutions in this dosage were more effective ($P < 0.005$).

§Solution intake values in boldface type demonstrate those which delivered optimum sodium intake.

(Na:Cl ratios like plasma) yielded lower mortality rates than did the hypertonic solutions with higher Na:Cl ratios (2:1) or the solutions containing only Na = Cl. Although these differences are not statistically significant, their consistent tendency is noteworthy especially since the rodent is known to handle NaCl more easily than man.

Inasmuch as the dosage of fluids is usually expressed as milliliters of fluid per kilogram of body weight rather than in terms of milliequivalents of sodium per kilogram, the therapy experiments have been thus summarized in Table VII. The over-all results suggest that excess sodium with too little water or excess water with too little sodium are deleterious. With the lowest fluid intake (50 ml. per kilogram), the hypertonic solutions were significantly more effective ($P < 0.005$). The optimal sodium intake of approximately 22.5 mEq. per kilogram is shown in italics. The hypertonic fluids were effective in minimal volumes, but the other solutions were required in substantially larger volumes.

CHANGES IN ELECTROLYTES, URINE VOLUME, HEMATOCRIT AND BODY WEIGHT AFTER FLUID THERAPY

In attempting to discern optimal fluid therapy, the metabolic studies summarized in Tables VIIIA and VIIIB provide additional information. With the optimal sodium intake of 22.5 mEq. per kilogram, the volume of urine increased as the volume of the administered solution increased. The large volume of urine after the hypotonic fluid would represent 3 to 4 L. in 24 hours in an adult human and comprised one third of the fluid administered compared to only one sixth of that administered with hypertonic solutions. As the sodium concentration of the administered fluid was increased, the concentration of sodium in the urine increased also; nevertheless, 85 percent or more of that administered was retained. After the burn at the higher temperature (the more severe injury), the concentration of sodium in the urine was lower than after the less severe burn, suggesting greater retention of sodium with more severe thermal trauma. The percentage of sodium retained exceeded the percentage of water retained. The water excess is most obvious after the hypotonic fluid therapy in which twice as much water is excreted as after other intakes.

The urine potassium and urea concentrations are elevated similarily in proportion to the sodium concentration of the fluid administered and the smaller urine volumes. The excess potassium excretions were approximately 20 percent of the sodium administered; this indicates the portion of administered sodium exchanged with intracellular potassium.[14, 16, 40] The urea nitrogen and potassium excretions, which may be taken as

Table VIIIA. *Urinary excretion and weight loss after hypo-, iso-, and hypertonic fluid therapy**

	Hypotonic	Isotonic	Hypertonic	
Solution used				
Sodium (mEq./L.)	100	150	225	300
Dose† ml./100 Gm.)	22.5	15.0	10.0	7.5
Body weight loss (Gm./100 Gm.)	1.4	0.3	4.5	4.6
Urine concentration				
Volume* (ml./100 Gm.)	4.2	1.1	1.5	1.2
Sodium (mEq./L.)	19	80	85	140
Chloride (mEq./L.)	43	95	54	67
Potassium (mEq./L.)	103	277	287	364
Urea nitrogen (Gm./L.)	12	22	50	47

*Type of burn: Scald 7 seconds at 73° C. Average of five experiments with five mice per group.
†Values adjusted to 100 Gm. of mouse weight; sodium intake 22.5 mEq. per killigram.

Table VIIIB. *Urinary excretion and weight loss after hypo-, iso-, and hypertonic fluid therapy**

	Hypotonic	Isotonic	Hypertonic	
Solutions used				
Sodium (mEq./L.)	100	150	225	300
Dose (ml./100 Gm.)	22.5	15.0	10.0	7.5
Body weight loss† (Gm./100 Gm.)	2.9	0.3	5.2	7.9
Urine concentration				
Volume† (ml./100 Gm.)	7.5	3.3	1.6	1.3
Percent of intake	35	22	16	17
Sodium (mEq./L.)	49	111	192	239
Chloride (mEq./L.)	65	103	65	63
Potassium (mEq./L.)	74	142	316	307
Urea nitrogen (Gm./L.)	11	30	35	36

*Type of burn: Scald 7 seconds at 70° C. Average of five experiments with five mice per group.
†Adjusted to 100 Gm. of mouse weight; sodium intake 22.5 mEq. per kilogram.

Table IX. *Plasma volume and electrolytes after various Na solutions**

Fluid sodium (mEq./L.)	Hematocrit (%)	Plasma values: Protein (Gm. %)	Na (mEq./L.)	Cl (mEq./L.)	HCO_3 (mEq./L.)
None	74	5.7	134	101	23
100	59	3.6	136	104	22
150	62	3.8	146	106	30
225	59	4.0	156	116	30
300	62	4.1	162	118	34
Normal	46	6.0	150	110	30

*Mice received 22.5 mEq. per kilogram of sodium intraperitoneally. Values are average of five mice per group taken at six hours post burn.

indicative of tissue breakdown and renal function, were approximately similar.

The changes in body weight are compared to the untreated controls, which exhibited negative water balance and lost weight. Among treated animals, the maximum weight loss occurred after the hypertonic fluid; the minimum occurred after isotonic fluid therapy, with maximal retention of Na and Cl.

The effects of the fluid therapy on the hematocrit and plasma electrolyte values are shown in Table II. These changes and the rise in hematocrit were transient; by 18 hours, nearly normal values were observed.

DISCUSSION

Previous investigators[1, 7, 13, 14, 23, 26, 28, 32, 36, 40] found that maximal survival after extensive thermal trauma was attained by administration of 15 to 18 percent of body weight of an isotonic sodium salt solution. This delivers 22.5 to 24 mEq. per kilogram of sodium: the optimum intake found in our studies with solutions ranging from 100 to 300 mEq. per liter of sodium.

After thermal injury, the therapeutic goal is to restore circulatory, pulmonary and renal function. The influx of sodium into the burned regions, which exceeds their gain in water, reduces the total "available" sodium. In man, experimental sodium loss resulted in severe circulatory and renal dysfunction.[25] In animals similar events occur,[6, 9, 10] together with a marked fall in O_2 consumption, glucose utilization, cardiac output, and respiratory control efficiency after sodium removal produced with minimal changes in body water and potassium.[19] Severe burns are further complicated by metabolic acidosis[34, 35] which depresses renal function[43] and is responsive to alkali therapy.[14, 18, 34, 35] Because of these dangerous physiological consequences, "lost" sodium needs to be replaced with appropriate anions.

The basic question is how to compensate for the effects of thermal injury and avoid excess of water or sodium. Isotonic solutions were utilized initially.[1, 7, 13, 23, 32] As shown in Table V, hypertonic or hypotonic solutions were deleterious in large volumes, but isotonic balanced solutions were required in large volumes to attain minimal mortality rate. Markley and associates[24] found that volumes of 400 ml. per kilogram were effective, and patients receiving similar volumes have become edematous but survived.

Following the observations that evaporative water loss is increased in burned patients,[30, 39] large supplements of electrolyte free water were added to resuscitation regimens. Thus the Evans and Bigger,[11] Cope and Moore,[4a] Brooke Army,[36] and Birmingham[8, 21] formulas have become hypotonic with sodium lowered to 100 mEq. per liter or below. Further evaluation[1, 3, 4, 28] has shown that free water replacement is not required until *after* resuscitation.

Colloid solutions are added to improve the circulatory dynamics, but capillaries damaged by thermal injury are unable to retain plasma proteins within the circulatory system. Hence, Rhoads and associates[38] advised delaying plasma administration until after 48 hours. Pruitt and Mason[37] have observed that colloid therapy did *not* augment plasma volume but that both colloid and electrolyte solutions equally raised cardiac output to supranormal levels in the first 24 hours and now advocate omitting colloids from the Brooke Army formula.[36]

In contrast to the above formulas which result in substantial weight gain and edema, resuscitation with hypertonic alkaline solutions (and no colloid) is accomplished with less fluid intake, less gain in weight, less edema, and with urine output averaging 30 ml. per hour.[3, 27, 28] Subsequently, Monafo treated over 100 patients with a solution containing 250 mEq. per liter of sodium and 150 mEq. per liter of chloride and observed similar advantages with less hypernatremia.

The results of the present study are in agreement with those reported by Markley and associates.[24] With hypertonic solutions the required sodium intake was achieved with the relatively low volume of 75 to 100 ml. per kilogram and less weight gain occurred. With isotonic solutions, the volume was increased to the range of 150 to 300 ml. per kilogram, and the largest gains in body weight were observed. The hypotonic solutions required the largest fluid intake of 225 to 300 ml. per kilogram, and the 75 mEq. per liter solution resulted in considerably higher mortality rate. Patients treated with the regimens currently in use receive hypotonic mixtures that require maximal fluid volumes to attain the optimal sodium intake. The disadvantages of these frequently used hypotonic solutions are clearly discernible.

The 225Na-160Cl solution offers the advantages of resuscitation with less fluid intake and early onset of adequate urine and sodium excretion. The upper limit of sodium intake (22 to 24 mEq. per kilogram) should be observed carefully. Clinical trials are needed to confirm this efficacy and decrease in edema.

Its additional usefulness for both hemorrhagic and traumatic shock is under study in view of the reports of the value of other hypertonic solutions in hemorrhagic shock.[2, 29]

ADDENDUM

Since this paper was submitted, similar results in dogs subjected to thermal trauma have just been published by Moylan, J. A., Jr., Reckler, J. M., and Mason, A. D., Jr.: Resuscitation with hypertonic lactate saline in thermal injury, Am. J. Surg. 125: 580, 1973. Although the mortality rate was not observed, their evaluation of efficacy of resuscitation based on cardiac output showed that "the efficacy of resuscitation as evaluated by the selected indexes was roughly equal with the Brooke formula, half-Brooke formula, and hypertonic lactate [Na 300, Cl 100, Monafo[27]] saline solution." They conclude that inasmuch as hypertonic saline resuscitation produced natriuresis and no gain in weight this solution may be as advantageous clinically in patients with limited cardiopulmonary reserve.

The authors express their thanks to Professors J. W. Fertig, A. A. O. Varma, and Mrs. M. H. Park in the Department of Public Health for their invaluable assistance with the statistical evaluations.

REFERENCES

1. Baxter, C. R., and Shires, T.: Physiological response to crystalloid resuscitation of severe burns, Ann. N. Y. Acad. Sci. **150:** 874, 1968.
2. Brookes, D. K., Williams W. G., Manley, R. W., and Whiteman, P.: Osmolar and electrolyte changes in hemorrhagic shock. Hypertonic solutions in the prevention of tissue damage, Lancet **1:** 521, 1963.
3. Caldwell, F. T., Casali, R. E., Flanigan, W. J., and Bowser, B.: What constitutes the proper solution for resuscitation of the severely burned patient? Am. J. Surg. **122:** 655, 1971.
4. Casali, R. E., Caldwell, F. T., et al.: Critical factors in resuscitation of the severely burned rat: The relative merit of volume, tonicity, sodium load, and concentration of the solution used, Ann. Surg. **175:** 138, 1972.

4a. Cope, O., and Moore, F. D.: The redistribution of body water and the fluid therapy of the burned patient, Ann. Surg. **126:** 1010, 1947.

5. Danowski, T. A., Winkler, A. W., and Elkinton, J. R.: The treatment of shock due to salt depletion; comparison of the hemodynamic effects of isotonic saline; of hypertonic saline and of isotonic glucose solutions, J. Clin. Invest. **25:** 130, 1946.
6. Darrow, D. C., and Yannett, H.: The changes in the distribution of body water accompanying increase and decrease in extracellular electrolyte, J. Clin. Invest. **14:** 266, 1935.
7. Davidson, E. C.: Sodium chloride metabolism in cutaneous burns and its possible significance for a rational therapy, Arch. Surg. **13:** 262, 1926.
8. Davies, J. W. L.: Plasma therapy, Mod. Treat. **4:** 1236, 1967.
9. Dillon, J.: A bioassay of treatment of hemorrhagic shock, Arch. Surg. **93:** 537, 1966.
10. Elkinton, J. R., Danowski, T. S., and Winkler, A. W. Hemodynamic changes in salt depletion and in dehydration, J. Clin. Invest. **25:** 120, 1946.
11. Evans, E. I., and Bigger, I. A.: Rationale of whole blood therapy in severe burns: Clinical study, Ann. Surg. **122:** 693, 1945.
12. Flear, C. T. G., Pickering, J., and McNeill, I. F.: Observations on water and electrolyte changes in skeletal muscle during major surgery, J. Surg. Res. **9:** 369, 1969.
13. Fox, C. L., Jr.: Oral sodium lactate in the treatment of burn shock, J. A. M. A. **124:** 207, 1944.
14. Fox, C. L., Jr.: The role of alkaline sodium salt solutions in the treatment of severe burns, Ann. N. Y. Acad. Sci. **150:** 823, 1968.
15. Fox, C. L., Jr., and Keston, A. S.: The mechanism of shock from burns and trauma traced with radiosodium. Surg. Gynecol. Obstet. **80:** 561, 1945.
16. Fox, C. L., Jr., and Baer, H.: The redistribution of potassium, sodium and water in burns and trauma and its relation to the phenomena of shock, Am. J. Physiol. **151:** 155, 1947.
17. Fox, C. L., Jr., and McCune, D. J.: Electrolyte changes in nephrosis—Occurrence of diuresis following administration of sodium and potassium salts, Am. J. Med. Sci. **216:** 1, 1948.
18. Fox, C. L., Jr.: Physiological basis for balanced electrolyte solutions in surgery, *in* Fox, C. L., Jr., and Nahas, G. G., editors: Body fluid replacement in the surgical patient, New York, 1970, Grune & Stratton, Inc., p. 256.
19. Fulton, R. L., and Ridolpho, P.: Physiologic effects of acute sodium depletion, Ann. Surg. **173:** 344, 1970.
20. Gump, F. E., Kinney, J. M., Iles, M., and Long, C. C.: Duration and significance of large fluid loads administered for circulatory support, J. Trauma **10:** 431, 1970.
21. Jackson, D., and Cason, J. S.: Treatment of burn shock with oral hypotonic saline-bicarbonate solution, *in* Research in Burns, Trans-

actions of Second International Congress, Edinburgh, 1965, E. & S. Livingston, Ltd. p. 61.
22. Leape, L. L.: Initial changes in burns: Tissue changes in burned and unburned skin of rhesus monkeys, J. Trauma **10:** 488, 1970.
23. Markley, K., Bocanegra, M., Bazan, A., Temple, R., Chiappori, M., Morales, G., and Carrion, A.: Clinical evaluation of saline solution therapy in burn shock, J. A. M. A. **161:** 1465, 1956.
24. Markley, K., Smallman, E., and Millican, R. C.: The efficacy and tonicity of iso-, hypo- and hypertonic sodium solutions in the treatment of burn shock in mice, Surgery **57:** 698, 1965.
25. McCance, R. A.: Experimental sodium chloride deficiency in man, Proc. R. Soc. Lond. (Biol.) **119:** 245, 1935.
26. McCarthy, M. D., and Newlin, N.: Range of efficacy of sodium chloride solutions in treating severe thermal injury in the rat, J. Lab. Clin. Med. **41:** 416, 1953.
27. Monafo, W. W.: The treatment of burn shock by the intravenous and oral administration of hypertonic lactated saline solution, J. Trauma **10:** 575, 1970.
28. Monafo, W. W.: The Treatment of burns: Principles and practice, St. Louis, 1971, Warren H. Green, Inc., p. 83.
29. Monafo, W. W.: Bioassay of murine hemorrhagic shock. II. The relationship of sodium, osmolal, anionic, and water loads to survival, J. Trauma **11:** 940, 1971.
30. Moncrief, J. A., and Mason, A. D., Jr.: Evaporative water loss in the burned patient, J. Trauma **4:** 180, 1964.
31. Moran, W. H., Jr., and Zimmermann, B.: Mechanisms of antidiuretic hormone (ADH) control of importance to the surgical patient, Surgery **62:** 639, 1967.
32. Moyer, C. A., Margraf, H. W., and Monafo, W. W.: Burn shock and extravascular sodium deficiency—treatment with Ringer's solution with lactate, Arch. Surg. **90:** 799, 1965.
33. Osman, A. A.: Guy's Hosp. Rep. **76:** 412, 1926; **77:** 386, 1927.
34. Peaston, M. J. T.: Metabolic acidosis in burns. Brit. Med. J. **1:** 809, 1968.
35. Peaston, M. J. T.: Use of electrolytes in severe burns, *in* Fox, C. L., Jr., and Nahas, G. G., editors: Body fluid replacement in the surgical patient, New York, 1970, Grune & Stratton, Inc. p. 229.
36. Polk, H. C., and Stone, H. H., editors: Contemporary burn management, Boston, 1971, Little, Brown and Company.
37. Pruitt, B. A., and Mason, A. D., Jr.: Hemodynamic studies of burned patients during resuscitation, *in* Research in burns, Transactions of Third International Congress, Prague, 1970, p. 83.
38. Rhoads, J. E., Wolff, W. A., and Lee, W. E.: The use of adrenal cortical extract in the treatment of traumatic shock of burns, Ann. Surg. **113:** 955, 1941.
39. Roe, C. E. and Kinney, J. M.: Water and heat exchange in third-degree burns, Surgery **56:** 212, 1964.
40. Rosenthal, S. M., and Tabor, H.: Electrolyte changes and chemotherapy in experimental burn and traumatic shock and hemorrhage, Arch. Surg. **51:** 244, 1945.
41. Schlutz, F. W., and Collier, J. L.: Treatment of nephrosis in the young child, J. A. M. A. **109:** 1959, 1937.
42. Winfield, J. M., Fox, C. L., Jr., and Mersheimer, W. L.: Etiologic factors in postoperative salt retention and its prevention, Ann. Surg. **134:** 626, 1951.
43. Zimmerman, W. E.: Acidosis in severe burns, Ann. N. Y. Acad. Sci. **150:** 584, 1968.

Anatomic control of vertebral arteriovenous fistulas

Thomas W. Kornmesser, M.D., *and* **John J. Bergan, M.D.,** *Chicago, Ill.*

Occurrence of the vertebral arteriovenous fistula is uncommon. When it does occur, significant morbidity may result. Numerous variations of staged procedures, both direct and indirect, have been utilized for cure. A straightforward, direct one-stage surgical approach is presented. This primarily involves eversion of the sternocleidomastoid muscle after its division at the mastoid process, thus giving access to the intertransverse process portion of the vertebral artery. Sound anatomic and surgical principles are applied to this otherwise troublesome problem. Two patients are presented who have been successfully treated with this approach.

From the Department of Surgery, Northwestern University Medical School, Chicago, Ill.

ARTERIOVENOUS fistulas of the vertebral artery are relatively uncommon. When they occur, usually due to penetrating trauma, they present a surgical dilemma because of a general unfamiliarity of surgeons with the possible accessibility of the lesion. The condition may be acutely life-threatening, not only because of external blood loss but also because of internal retropharyngeal bleeding with consequent upper respiratory obstruction. Also, artery-to-vein shunting may cause acute midbrain ischemia as a vertebral steal phenomenon occurs.

The purpose of this report is to indicate an anatomic approach that can be utilized to control vertebral arteriovenous fistulas directly, so that immediate surgical care can be applied at the time of injury.

Control of the arteriovenous fistula can be performed in a straightforward, one-stage operation by using minor modifications of standard cervical incisions familiar to most experienced surgeons. Need for knowledge of such an approach is indicated by the numerous variations of staged operations which have been used in the past.[1, 6, 12, 19, 28, 30-32, 35] Also, the method to be described obviates need for indirect methods recently advocated.[3, 4, 6, 17, 22]

SURGICAL APPROACH

It is generally thought that the main portion of the vertebral artery is in a relatively inaccessible area of the neck in the transverse foramina of the cervical vertebrae. Actually, this portion is easily approached when muscle masses of the sternocleidomastoid and splenius capitis are reflected laterally to obtain proximal and distal control of the vertebral artery. The first portion of the vertebral artery is exposed easily through a low collar incision (Fig. 1). This division of the vessel runs from the subclavian artery to the lowest foramina in the transverse process of the sixth cervical vertebra. The upper portion of the artery becomes available for surgical control where it leaves the transverse foramina

Supported in part by a grant-in-aid from the Chicago Heart Association and the Northwestern University Vascular Research Fund.

Accepted for publication Sept. 14, 1973.

of the atlas and before it enters the axis.

Arteriovenous (AV) fistulas are particularly common in the intertransverse portion of the vessel. This is because the numerous veins surrounding the artery travel as a plexus and do not become a single vein until low in the neck near the transverse process of the sixth cervical vertebra. The adventitia of the veins is intimately associated with periosteum of the intervertebral foramina. Thus, these vessels are fixed throughout their course.

With these considerations in mind, the patient is placed on the operating table in supine position with the head turned to the side opposite the lesion. His neck is hyperextended and a 6 cm. transverse supraclavicular incision is centered over the clavicular head of the sternocleidomastoid muscle. The object of this first portion of the operation is to ligate the proximal portion of the vertebral artery to interrupt arterial flow to the fistula from below. The clavicular head of the sternocleidomastoid muscle is transected and disection is carried deeply, reflecting the scalene fat pad and sectioning the scalenus anticus muscle while avoiding the phrenic nerve. The thyrocervical trunk is identified and divided as it may contribute to the AV fistula. The vertebral artery is medial to the thyrocervical artery and it is identified, ligated, and divided. To conclude this first portion of the operation, the wound is closed in layers without drainage.

A second incision is made along the anterior border of the sternocleidomastoid muscle, beginning at the mastoid process and curving inferiorly, as a standard anterior sternocleidomastoid cervical incision. The object of this portion of the operation is to control the vertebral artery near the base of the skull, thus interrupting the arterial stream as it feeds the fistula from above (Fig. 2). The upper portion of the incision is curved posteriorly over the mastoid process. This allows the sternocleidomastoid muscle to be everted, which is accomplished by dividing fibers that insert into the mastoid process itself. The fibers of the splenius capitis muscle are also sectioned. The entire

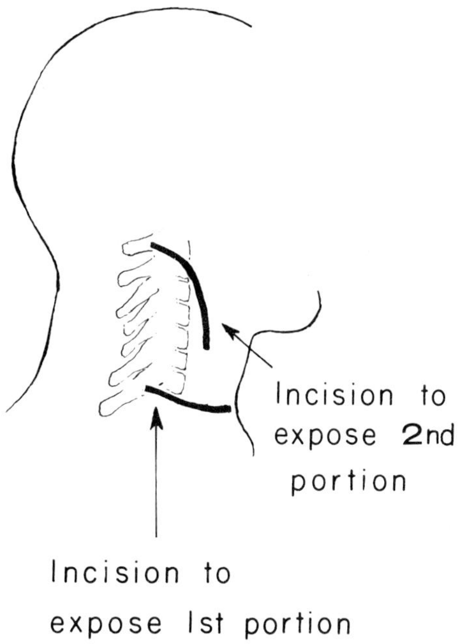

Fig. 1. A one-stage, two-incisional approach simplifies surgical cure of vertebral AV fistulas. The two incisions are diagrammed here.

portion of the sternocleidomastoid muscle within the incision is everted. Once this is done, the transverse process of the atlas is easily palpated. It is longer than that of the axis and lies 1 to 2 cm. anterior to the mastoid tip. The spinal accessory nerve is identified and protected. It enters the everted sternomastoid 4 to 5 cm. below the mastoid process. The jugular vein is avoided by keeping this part of the disection posterior to the transverse processes of the vertebrae. With this, the vertebral artery is found passing between the atlas and the axis. It is covered by thick prevertebral fascia, the origin of the levator scapulae and, some fibers of intertransverse muscle. As these are divided, the anterior ramus of the second cervical nerve is seen. It swells forth as overlying fascia is cut. The vertebral artery curving out between the atlas and the axis is identified at this point in the operation. It is now encircled and ligated. Once the second portion of the vertebral artery is ligated, attention can be turned to the transverse processes between the levels of the second and the sixth cervical vertebrae. The longus coli and

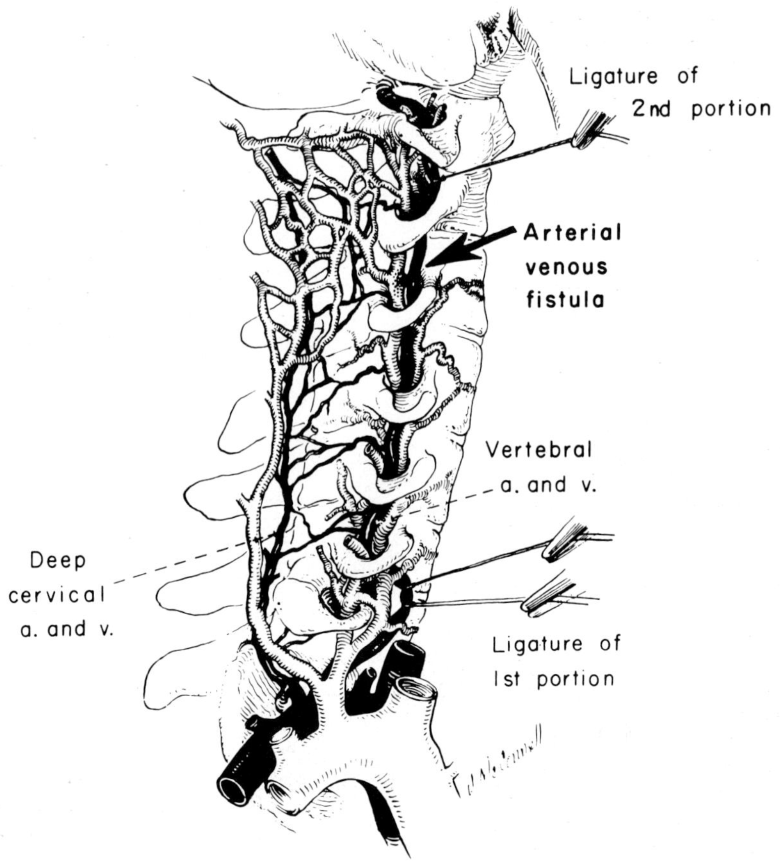

Fig. 2. Anatomically, there are two portions of the vertebral artery which present themselves for ligation. These are shown in this drawing.

longus capitis muscles are detached from the transverse processes of the cervical vertebrae. The transverse processes are then opened with a rongeur (Fig. 3). This exposes the vertebral artery and its surrounding plexus of veins.

The entire vertebral artery can be removed from its bony canal, thus ensuring that the arteriovenous fistula is cured. Bleeding points are controlled with bone wax at this time. Hypotensive anesthesia is a useful adjunct if experienced personnel are available for its administration.[18]

ILLUSTRATIVE CASE REPORTS

Case 1. A 43-year-old black woman sustained a knife wound to the right neck one year prior to admission. External blood loss was profuse, transfusions were given, and she was hospitalized for one week at that time. After the injury, she experienced a roaring noise in the right ear as well as periodic light-headedness and syncope.

Physical examination revealed a loud continuous bruit and thrill over the right posterior neck. The findings of neurological examination were normal. Angiography showed a large AV fistula of the right vertebral artery (Fig. 4).

Proximal and distal vertebral artery ligation with obliteration of the fistula at the level of the second and third cervical vertebrae was performed as described above. Postoperative angiography showed the fistula to be absent. The patient was asymptomatic without cervical bruit during a two-year follow-up period to 1973.

Comment. This case illustrates failure of diagnosis of the vertebral AV fistula at the time of injury, subsequent evidence of the vertebral steal phenomenon causing midbrain ischemia and syncope, and later surgical correction with a simple anatomic approach according to plan. A direct approach to the fistula during the initial hospitalization could have prevented later morbidity. Diagnosis of the fistula could have been made from the history of external blood loss and detection of the loud bruit.

Case 2. A 31-year-old white female underwent an anterior interbody fusion of the fourth and fifth cervical vertebrae. During the procedure an unusual amount of bleeding was reported. She was discharged but later readmitted with progressive weakness of the left arm and difficulty in swallowing.

Physical examination revealed decreased strength of the left deltoid and a decrease of the left triceps reflex. There was a fullness in the left anterior cervical triangle and a palpable thrill was present. A loud bruit was heard over the left side of the neck.

Upon admission, an esophagram demonstrated a large retropharyngeal mass. Brachial angiography demonstrated a leaking false aneurysm and an associated AV fistula of the left vertebral artery and vein (Fig. 5). The patient developed sudden upper respiratory obstruction and a tracheostomy was performed. The first portion of the left vertebral artery was ligated at this time through a separate incision. A decrease in the bruit and neck swelling resulted.

Within ten days, paratracheal bleeding developed from the inferior thyroid artery. The wound of the anterior fusion was found to be intact at this time. At definitive exploration, the second portion of the vertebral artery was ligated between the levels of the first and second cervical vertebrae, and the fistula was obliterated at the level of the third and fourth cervical vertebrae. Postoperatively, there was no cervical bruit, arm strength returned and the patient has remained asymptomatic during a two-year follow-up period to 1973.

Comment. This case illustrates the progressive nature of the AV fistula and subsequent development of a false aneurysm. Internal expansion of the false aneurysm leads to tracheal and esophageal compression, necessitating urgent treatment. Definitive one-stage repair of the anomaly cannot be undertaken without need to resort to tracheostomy, as was done in this case. However, elective correction of the fistula with a planned anatomic approach could have obviated the emergency tracheostomy with its attendant morbidity.

DISCUSSION

Matas[25] described the first traumatic vertebral arteriovenous fistula in 1893. Since that time, 79 have been reported.[1-8, 11-22, 24-35] The second portion of the artery has been the most common site of involvement due to the venous complexity described above. The left side has been more commonly involved than the right.

Interestingly, the most common cause of vertebral AV fistulas since 1960 has been percutaneous angiography. Both vertebral artery punctures done deliberately and accidental punctures produced during carotid angiography have been implicated. Prior to this time, penetrating wounds of the neck were the most common cause of this lesion. It is noteworthy that the anterior cervical interbody fusion has not previously been reported as a cause.[10] Cloward's[9, 10] personal experience with over 1,000 cases does not include a single vertebral artery injury. Though six arterial injuries are known to him, none of these resulted in a vertebral AV fistula. In direct inquiry, we were able to find other arterial injuries occurring during the Cloward procedure, but in no instance had a vertebral AV fistula resulted.[9]

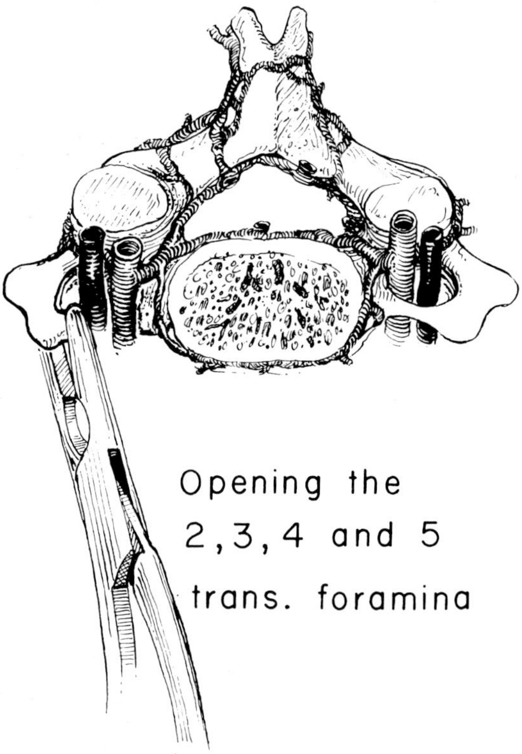

Fig. 3. Removal of the fingernail-thick bone over the transverse foramena allows removal of the vertebral artery and radical cure of the fistula.

A review of the surgical literature attending vertebral AV fistulas is anecdotal but not informative. Many surgical procedures have been advocated but no single best technique has emerged. In general, successful operations tend to be reported, and these have in

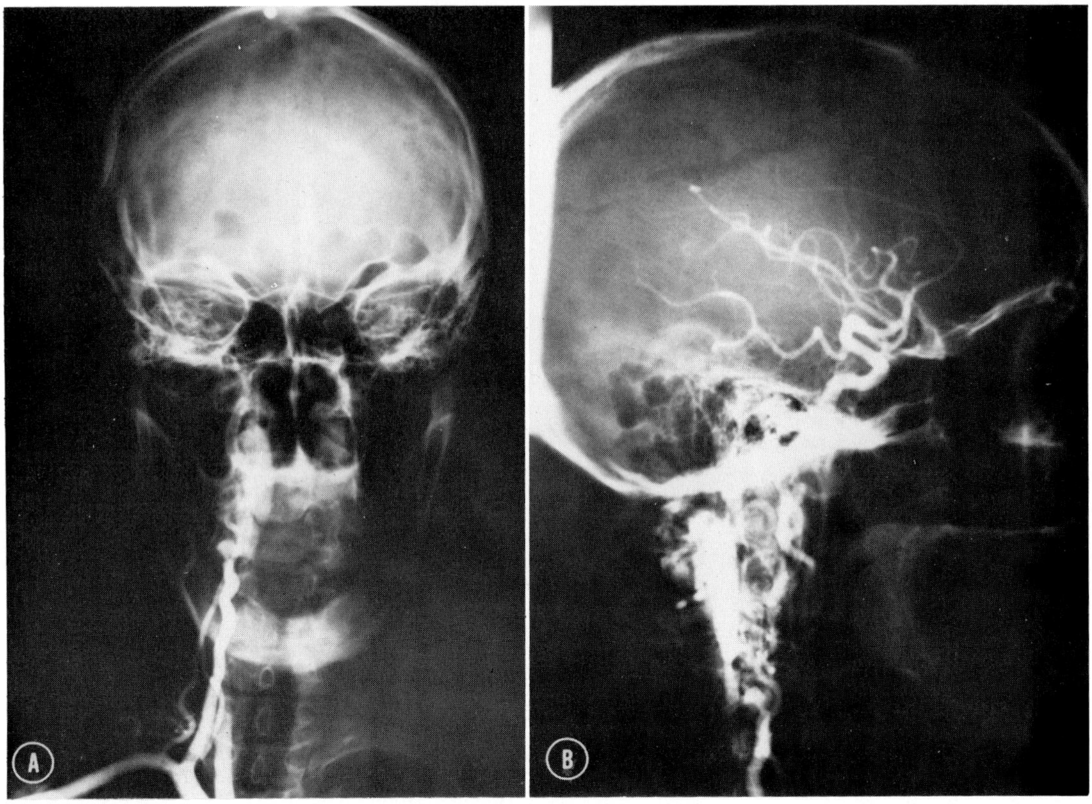

Fig. 4. The anteroposterior and lateral seriograms shown here clearly delineate the right vertebral AV fistula located at the level of the third cervical vertebra.

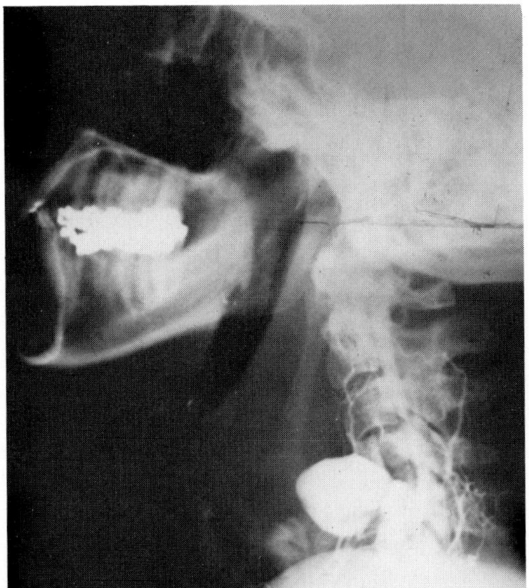

Fig. 5. The lateral arteriogram shown here demonstrated the AV fistula of the vertebral artery, its associated ruptured false aneurysm, and contrast media within the retropharyngeal hematoma.

common the principle of some form of distal and proximal control of the vessel. Direct attack upon the fistula itself has been very effective and in some cases dramatic. Planned staged approaches and unplanned staged attempts are recorded.

The most recent technique advocated in correction of vertebral AV fistulas was the use of an interarterial Fogarty balloon catheter placed at the fistula site under radiographic control. This technique, although used successfully in three patients, illustrated the need for simplified direct surgical approach rather than indirect techniques.[4]

In commenting on this subject, Lorrimer[23] said, "Experience with such injuries, however, has resulted in a prolonged, difficult and bloody operative procedure. It is surgically impossible to expose the artery distally to prevent back-bleeding with the patient in the supine position, the usual position for neck exploration or injury." This comment underscores the need for greater understanding of the anatomy of vertebral AV fistulas and the realization that a direct, planned anatomic approach is logical and feasible without need to resort to bloody surgical procedures.

Finally, it should be noted that AV fistulas caused by percutaneous vertebral arteriography usually close spontaneously and do not require surgical treatment. These remain the exceptions in recorded surgical experience.

REFERENCES

1. Aronson, N. I.: Traumatic arteriovenous fistula of the vertebral vessels. Angiographic demonstration and a rationale for treatment, Neurology **11:** 817, 1961.
2. Bergquist, E.: Bilateral arteriovenous fistula, Br. J. Radiol. **44:** 519, 1971.
3. Bergstrom, K., and Lodin, H.: Arteriovenous fistula as a complication of cerebral angiography. Report of three cases, Br. J. Radiol. **39:** 263, 1966.
4. Binkley, F. M., and Wylie, E. J.: A new technique for obliteration of cerebrovascular arteriovenous fistulae, Arch. Surg. **106:** 524, 1973.
5. Bjork, V. O.: Iatrogenic vertebral arteriovenous fistula, Thorax **21:** 367, 1966.
6. Chou, S. N., and French, L. A.: Arteriovenous fistula of the vertebral vessels in the neck. J. Neurosurg. **22:** 77, 1965.
7. Chou, S. N., Stoey, J. L., Seljeskog, E. A., and French, L. A.: Further experience with arteriovenous fistulas of the vertebral artery in the neck, SURGERY **62:** 779, 1967.
8. Cloete, G. N. P., Nel, L. J., and Van Wyk, F. A. K.: Arteriovenous fistula of the vertebral vessels in the neck, S. Afr. Med. J. **42:** 253, 1968.
9. Cloward, R. B.: Complications of anterior cervical disc operation and their treatment, SURGERY **69:** 175, 1971.
10. Cloward, R. B.: Personal communication.
11. Dutton, J., and Isherwood, I.: Iatrogenic vertebral A-V fistula, Neurochirurgia (Stuttg.) **13:** 49, 1970.
12. Elkin, D. C., and Harris, M. H.: Arteriovenous aneurysms of the vertebral vessels, Ann. Surg. **124:** 934, 1946.
13. Elkin, D. C., and Shumacker, H. B., Jr.: Arterial aneurysms and arteriovenous fistulas: General considerations in surgery in W.W. II vascular surgery, Office of the Surgeon General, Department of the Army, Washington, D. C., 1955.
14. Feath, W. H., and Dueker, H. W.: Arteriovenous vascular malformation of the cervical portion of the vertebral artery, Neurology **11:** 492, 1916.
15. Garland, H., Lamb, J. T., and Pearce, J.: Iatrogenic vertebral arteriovenous fistula, Br. Med. J. **1:** 429-430, 1965.
16. Gooddy, W., and Schecther, M. M.: Spontaneous arteriovenous fistula of the vertebral artery, Br. J. Radiol. **33:** 709, 1960.
17. Heifetz, C. J.: Traumatic aneurysm of the first portion of the left vertebral artery: Case report, Ann. Surg. **122:** 102, 1945.
18. Henry, A. K.: Extensive exposure, Edinburgh, 1966, E. & S. Livingstone, Ltd.
19. Jefferson, J., Bailey, R. A., and Kerr, A.: Suboccipital arteriovenous aneurysms of the vertebral artery, J. Bone Joint Surg. **38B:** 114, 1956.
20. Leape, L. L., and Palacios, E.: Acute traumatic vertebral arteriovenous fistula, Ann. Surg. **174:** 908, 1971.
21. Lester, J.: Arteriovenous fistula after percutaneous vertebral angiography, Acta Radiol. (Diagn.) (Stockh.) **5:** 337, 1966.
22. Linde, L. H., Fonkalsrud, E. W., Wilson, G. H., and Batzdorf, U.: Traumatic vertebral A-V fistula in a child, J. A. M. A. **213:** 1465, 1970.
23. Lorimer, W. S., Jr.: In discussion of Binkley, F. M. and Wylie, E. J.: A new technique for obliteration of cerebrovascular arteriovenous fistulae, Arch. Surg. **106:** 524, 1973.
24. McDowell, H. A., Jr.: Post arteriographic A-V fistula of the cervical vertebral artery, South. Med. J. **64:** 119, 1971.
25. Matas, R.: Traumatisms and traumatic aneurysms of the vertebral artery and their surgical treatment, with the report of a cured case, Ann. Surg. **18:** 477, 1893.
26. Morelli, R.: An angiographic complication of vertebral arteriovenous fistula, J. Neurol. Neurosurg., Psychiatry **30:** 264, 1967.
27. Newton, T. H., and Durrock, J.: Vertebral arteriovenous fistula complicating vertebral angiography. Acta Radiol. (Diagn.) (Stockh.) **5:** 428, 1966.
28. Ogilvie, W. H.: Extracranial aneurysms of the vertebral artery, Guys Hosp. Rep. **90:** 178, 1941.
29. Olson, R. W., Baker, H. L., Jr., and Svien, H. J.: Arteriovenous fistula: A complication of vertebral angiography, J. Neurosurg. **20:** 73, 1963.
30. Sher, M. H., Meyer, N. I., Lenhardt, H. F., and Trunimer, M. J.: Arteriovenous fistula involving the vertebral artery: Report of three cases, Ann. Surg. **163:** 408, 1966.
31. Shumacher, H. B., Jr.: Arteriovenous fistulas of the cervical portion of the vertebral vessels, Surg. Gynecol. & Obstet. **83:** 625, 1946.
32. Shumacher, H. B., Jr., Campbell, R. L., and Heimburger, R. F.: Operative treatment of

vertebral arteriovenous fistulas, J. Trauma **6:** 3, 1966.
33. Tsuji, H. K., Redington, J. J., and Kay, J. H.: Vertebral arteriovenous fistula, J. Thorac. Cardiovasc. Surg. **55:** 746, 1968.
34. Verbiest, H.: Extracranial and cervical arteriovenous aneurysms of the carotid and vertebral arteries, Johns Hopkins Med. J. **122:** 350, 1968.
35. Zilkha, A., and Schecter, M. M.: Arteriovenous fistulas of the major vessels of the neck, Acta Radiol. (Diagn.) (Stockh.) **9:** 560, 1969.

Deglutition after resection of oral, laryngeal, and pharyngeal cancers

Raymond C. Doberneck, M.D., Ph.D., *and* **John E. Antoine, M.D.,** *Albuquerque, N. M.*

Fifteen patients were studied by cineradiography after oral, laryngeal and hypopharyngeal resection. Moderate to severe impairment of mobility of tongue, pharynx, and epiglottis was observed in 12 patients but such impairment failed to correlate with clinical dysphagia. Five patients who had partial glossectomy were the only patients who had significant clinical dysphagia. The implications of these findings are discussed.

From the Departments of Surgery and Radiology, University of New Mexico School of Medicine and the Veterans Administration Hospital, Albuquerque, N. M.

DYSPHAGIA IS occasionally a perplexing problem after oral and pharyngeal resection.[5] Although such dysphagia improves in time, the problem often is incompletely resolved. Unfortunately, new techniques of reconstruction do not appear to have overcome the problem. The mechanism of such dysphagia is unclear and may relate to the structures resected or the impairment of mobility of residual structures. The present report attempts to delineate the abnormalities of swallowing following oral, pharyngeal, and laryngeal resections for cancer by utilizing cineradiography of the oral cavity, pharynx, and hypopharynx. Having delineated such abnormalities, their mechanism may become apparent.

MATERIAL AND METHOD

Fifteen patients who had resection of malignant tumors of the mouth, jaw, larynx, and pharnyx were studied by cineradiography with exposures at 15 to 30 frames per second. The patients swallowed thin liquid barium while in a sitting position and were studied between two and four weeks after operation. Swallowing as seen on the cine filmstrips was then analyzed by grading the component motions on a scale of zero

Supported in part by the Milheim Foundation for Cancer Research.

Accepted for publication Sept. 14, 1973.

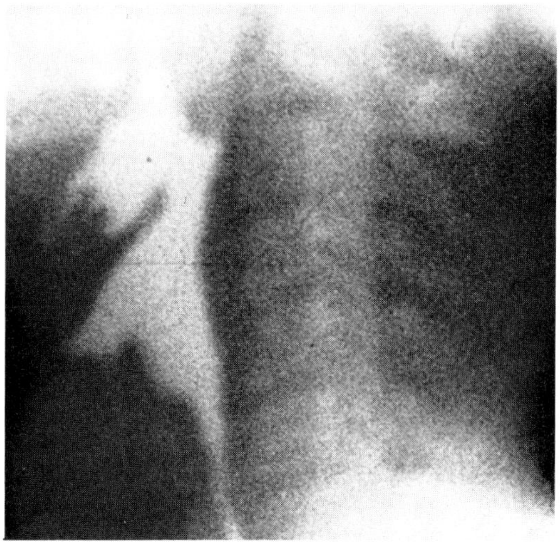

Fig. 1A. Frame from cineradiograph of patient swallowing after tongue-jaw-neck resection. Note erect epiglottis which fails to cover and protect glottis.

Table I. *Operations performed, impairment of deglutition, and dysphagia**

Patient No.	Operations performed	Tongue: Posterior	Tongue: Superior	Nasal Regurgitation	Aspiration
1	Total laryngectomy and neck dissection	1	1	0	0
2	Total laryngectomy and neck dissection	1	3	0	0
3	Total laryngectomy and neck dissection	0	0	0	0
4	Total laryngectomy and neck dissection	2	3	0	0
5	Hemiglossectomy, segmental mandibulectomy, and neck dissection	1	3	1	1
6	Hemiglossectomy, marginal mandibulectomy, and neck dissection	0	1	0	1
7	Hemiglossectomy, segmental mandibulectomy, and neck dissection	0	0	1	1
8	Hemiglossectomy, marginal mandibulectomy, and neck dissection	1	1	1	1
9	Hemiglossectomy, hemimandibulectomy, and neck dissection	1	1	0	3
10	Hemiglossectomy and neck dissection	3	3	2	2
11	Excision of tonsilar fossa and pillars, segmental mandibulectomy, and neck dissection	0	0	0	0
12	Hemiglossectomy and neck dissection	0	0	0	2
13	Hemimandibulectomy	0	0	0	0
14	Supraglottic laryngectomy and neck dissection	0	0	0	1
15	Excision of posterior hypopharynx	0	0	0	0

*0 = normal; 1 = mild impairment; 2 = moderate impairment; 3 = marked impairment.

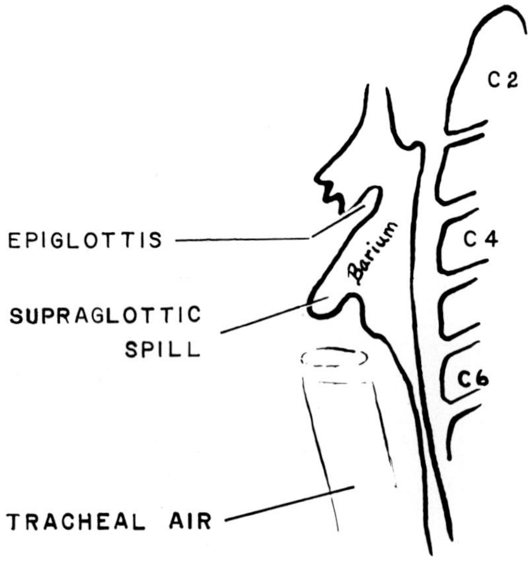

Fig. 1B. Line drawing of cineradiograph shown in Fig. 1*A*.

to three. The motions analyzed were those described by Bosma[1] and are recorded in Table I. A grade of zero indicated normal motion and a grade of three, absent motion. Grades of one and two indicated mild and moderate degrees of impairment, respectively, of a particular motion. The grades assigned each component motion were added together to give the total for each patient. As the basis for comparison and grading, cine film strips of patients with normal swallowing and most of the fifteen patients prior to operations were also studied. No patient had abnormal swallowing prior to operation.

The grading system was also applied to the degree of clinical dysphagia experienced by the patient after operation. A grade of zero indicated little or no dysphagia of brief duration. A grade of three indicated severe and prolonged dysphagia, while grades of one and two indicated mild and moderate degrees, respectively, of dysphagia of moderate duration.

RESULTS

The operations done, the grades assigned to each motion of swallowing after opera-

Grading of components of deglutition										
Pharynx, larynx and hyoid		*Epiglottis*		*Pharyngeal*	*Cricopharyngeus*	*Tongue,*	*Epiglottis,*	*Larynx and hyoid,*		
Anterior	*Superior*	*Posterior*	*Inferior*	*peristalsis*	*opening*	*anterior*	*superior*	*inferior*	*Total*	*Clinical dysphagia*
3	1	—	—	0	0	1	—	—	7	0
3	1	—	—	0	0	1	—	—	9	0
0	3	—	—	0	0	0	—	—	3	0
2	2	—	—	0	0	2	—	—	11	0
0	0	0	3	0	0	1	3	0	13	0
0	0	0	3	0	0	1	3	0	9	2
1	0	0	3	0	?	0	3	0	9	2
1	1	1	3	0	0	1	3	0	14	1
3	3	3	3	3	3	1	3	3	27	2
3	2	3	3	2	3	3	2	3	34	0
1	1	0	0	0	0	0	0	1	3	2
1	1	3	3	3	1	0	3	1	18	2
0	0	0	0	0	0	0	0	0	0	0
0	0	—	—	0	0	0	—	0	1	0
?	?	0	0	0	0	0	0	?	0	1

tion, the total of such grades, and the degrees of clinical dysphagia for all patients after operation are shown in Table I. None of six patients who had laryngeal or pharyngeal resections experienced more than minimal dysphagia, in spite of moderate degrees of impairment of motion of the tongue and pharynx. The total of the grades assigned to the motions of swallowing of such patients ranged from zero to eleven (average, 5.2). Four of six patients who had tongue-jaw-neck resections experienced marked dysphagia while the other two had mild or no dysphagia. The total of the grades assigned to the motions of swallowing of the patients with marked dysphagia ranged from 3 to 27 (average, 12.5) while such totals assigned to those with mild or no dysphagia were 13 and 14. One of two patients who had tongue-neck resections had marked dysphagia and the other had no dysphagia. The total of the grades assigned the motions of swallowing of the patient with marked dysphagia was 18, and of the patient with no dysphagia was 34. The patient who had mandibulectomy only had no dysphagia, and the total of the grades assigned to the motions of swallowing was zero.

COMMENT

The results of the present study show that marked alteration of the component motions of swallowing may occur after oral, pharyngeal, and hypopharyngeal resection. The alteration most frequently observed is impaired mobility of the epiglottis which correlates well with radiographic aspiration. In several patients the epiglottis remains erect and fails to cover and protect the glottis from the bolus of liquid barium (Fig. 1). Neither aspiration nor impaired mobility of the epiglottis correlate with clinical dysphagia. The second most frequently observed alteration is impairment of laryngopharyngeal mobility, and the third, is impairment of lingual mobility. Impairment of neither laryngopharyngeal nor lingual mobility correlates well with clinical dysphagia. Seven of eight patients who had lingual resection had varying degrees of impairment of residual structures but only five patients had marked clinical dysphagia. On the other hand, four of six patients who had laryngeal or hypopharyngeal resection had varying degrees of impairment of mobility, but none had even minimal clinical dysphagia. Thus, the loss of a structure appears to be more important than impairment of mobility of the residual structures. In this study, the tongue appears to be the critical structure.

Other factors not quantitated in the present study appear to be important in the production of clinical dysphagia. Motivation of the patient, as previously concluded by Conley,[2-4] appears to be of paramount importance. Sympathetic encouragement of the patient by his surgeon is therefore of vital importance to a prompt and successful convalescence.

REFERENCES

1. Bosma, J. F.: Deglutition: Pharyngeal Stage, Physiol. Rev. **37:** 275, 1957.
2. Conley, J. J.: Swallowing dysfunctions associated with radical surgery of the head and neck, Arch. Surg. **80:** 602, 1960.
3. Conley, J. J.: The crippled oral cavity, Plast. Reconstr. Surg. **30:** 469, 1962.
4. Conley, J. J., and Seaman, W.: Function in the crippled laryngopharynx, Ann. Otol. Rhinol. Laryngol. **72:** 441, 1963.
5. Shedd, D. P., Scatliff, J. A., and Kirchner, J. A.: A cineradiographic study of postresectional alterations in oropharyngeal physiology, Surg. Gynecol. Obstet. **110:** 69, 1960.

Vascular pressure-flow relationships in denervated and reimplanted lungs of dogs

Otto A. Wagner, M.D.,* L. Henry Edmunds, Jr., M.D., *Philadelphia, Pa., and,*
David C. Heilbron, Ph.D., *San Francisco, Calif.*

We studied vascular pressure-flow relationships, alveolar-arterial oxygen differences, and lung weights in normal, denervated, and reimplanted left lung of dogs two to three days after operation and in reimplanted left lungs six to eight weeks after operation. Pulmonary arterial blood flow to the left lung was measured with an electromagnetic flow probe and was altered by inflation or deflation of a balloon occluder around the right pulmonary artery and by infusion of dextran or withdrawal of blood. Pulmonary vascular pressure-flow regression slopes and intercepts varied between dogs within groups. Mean regression slopes of groups of normal, denervated, and reimplanted lungs studied six to eight weeks after operation did not differ significantly ($P > 0.06$) from each other, but all differed significantly ($P < 0.06$) from the mean regression slope of reimplanted lungs studied two to three days after operation. Although increases in lung weight and alveolar-arterial oxygen differences were greatest in dogs two to three days after excision and reimplantation of the lung, the magnitudes of these changes in individual dogs did not correlate with pressure-flow regression slopes.

From the Department of Surgery, the Office of Information Systems–Computer Center, and the Cardiovascular Research Institute, University of California, San Francisco, Calif.

VASCULAR RESISTANCE of the reimplanted canine lung increases temporarily after operation,[23, 26] but returns to normal within six weeks.[27] In the absence of anastomotic imperfections, this temporary increase in vascular resistance at resting blood flows is probably due to increased extravascular water[31] and postoperative atelectasis. Little is known about the vascular resistance of the reimplanted lung at greater than resting blood flows. Experimental evidence indicates that edema, peribronchial, perivascular, and alveolar hemorrhage develop acutely in many dogs if the entire cardiac output is forced through the reimplanted lung.[1, 6, 16, 26] Although several workers have measured pulmonary arterial pressure before and after occlusion of the pulmonary artery opposite the reimplanted lung, these limited data are contradictory.[8, 24, 25] Careful measurements of vascular pressure-flow relationships in reimplanted lungs have not been made, yet knowledge of these relationships is relevant to potential candidates for lung allografts who have moderate or severe pulmonary hypertension. In the present experiments, we studied vascular pressure-flow

This study was supported by National Institutes of Health Grants HL-11358 and HL-06285 from the National Heart and Lung Institute.

Accepted for publication Sept. 27, 1973.

Address all correspondence to: L. Henry Edmunds, Jr., M.D., Department of Surgery, University of Pennsylvania, 3400 Spruce Street, Philadelphia, Pennsylvania 19104.

*Present address: Otto A. Wagner, M.D., First Surgical Unit, University of Vienna, Alser Strasse 4, A-1090 Wien, Austria.

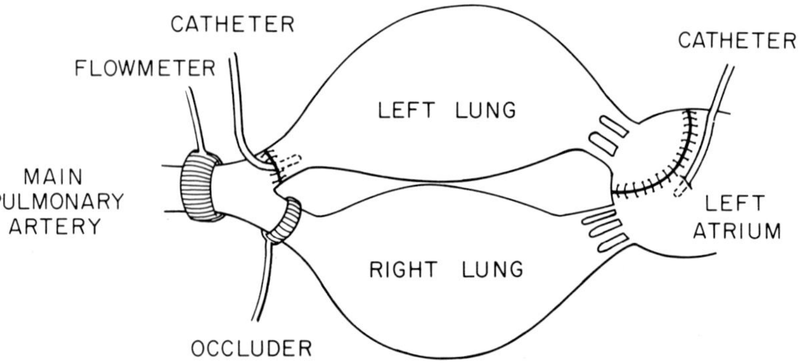

Fig. 1. Diagram of the positions of the flow probe, balloon occluder, and left atrial and left pulmonary arterial catheters in pressure-flow studies on 21 dogs. The tip of the pulmonary arterial catheter was always placed downstream to the arterial anastomosis (Groups 3 and 4).

relationships, alveolar-arterial oxygen differences, and lung weights in denervated lungs and in reimplanted lungs two to three days and six to eight weeks after operation.

METHODS

Twenty-four healthy mongrel dogs weighing 19.1 ± 1.9 S.D. kilograms were anesthetized with sodium pentobarbital (30 mg. per kilogram, given intravenously) and a left thoracotomy was performed. These animals were divided into four groups. In nine dogs (Group 1), which served as the control group, an electromagnetic flow probe* was placed around the main pulmonary artery, a balloon occluder† was placed around the right pulmonary artery, and catheters (0.050 inch, internal diameter; 0.090 inch, outer diameter) were inserted into the left atrium and left pulmonary artery (Fig. 1). Catheters were filled with heparin and capped, and the ends of all devices were passed through the chest wall and placed in a subcutaneous pocket.

In five dogs (Group 2), the left lung was denervated by excision of the left vagus nerve, sympathetic chain (TI-6), and stellate and caudal cervical ganglia after the flow probe, occluder, and catheters had been inserted. In ten dogs, the left lung was excised and reimplanted with the use of the intra-atrial wire technique[19] to ensure that the atrial anastomosis did not constrict the orifices of the pulmonary veins.[1, 8, 16, 19, 24, 25, 27, 29] In seven of these dogs (Group 3) a flow probe, balloon occluder, and catheters were inserted at the same operation. In three animals (Group 4), these devices were inserted at a second operation through the right chest six to eight weeks later. After all operations the chest was closed, with one drainage catheter left in place. All animals received penicillin (600,000 U., given intramuscularly), and streptomycin (0.75 Gm., given intramuscularly) for five days or until death. After insertion of flow probes and catheters, all dogs received digoxin (0.25 mg., given intramuscularly) daily.

Pulmonary vascular pressure-flow relationships were studied two to three days after implantation of the flow probe and catheters in all dogs. A chest roentgenogram was obtained 0.5 to 16 hours before the study. Dogs were anesthetized with sodium pentobarbital (20 to 30 mg. per kilogram, intravenously), placed supine, intubated, and permitted to breathe 100 percent oxygen spontaneously at 3 cm. H_2O end tidal pressure. The flow probe, occluder, and catheter endings were exteriorized, and a central venous catheter was inserted into the left jugular vein. Pressure catheters were connected to calibrated transducers.* The zero reference was a point two-thirds the depth of the chest above the table top. Phasic and

*Series 5000, Biotronex Labs, Inc., Silver Springs, Md.
†Model No. VO-4B, Rhodes Laboratories, Hartford, Conn.

*Model No. P23BB, Statham Instruments, Oxnard, Calif.

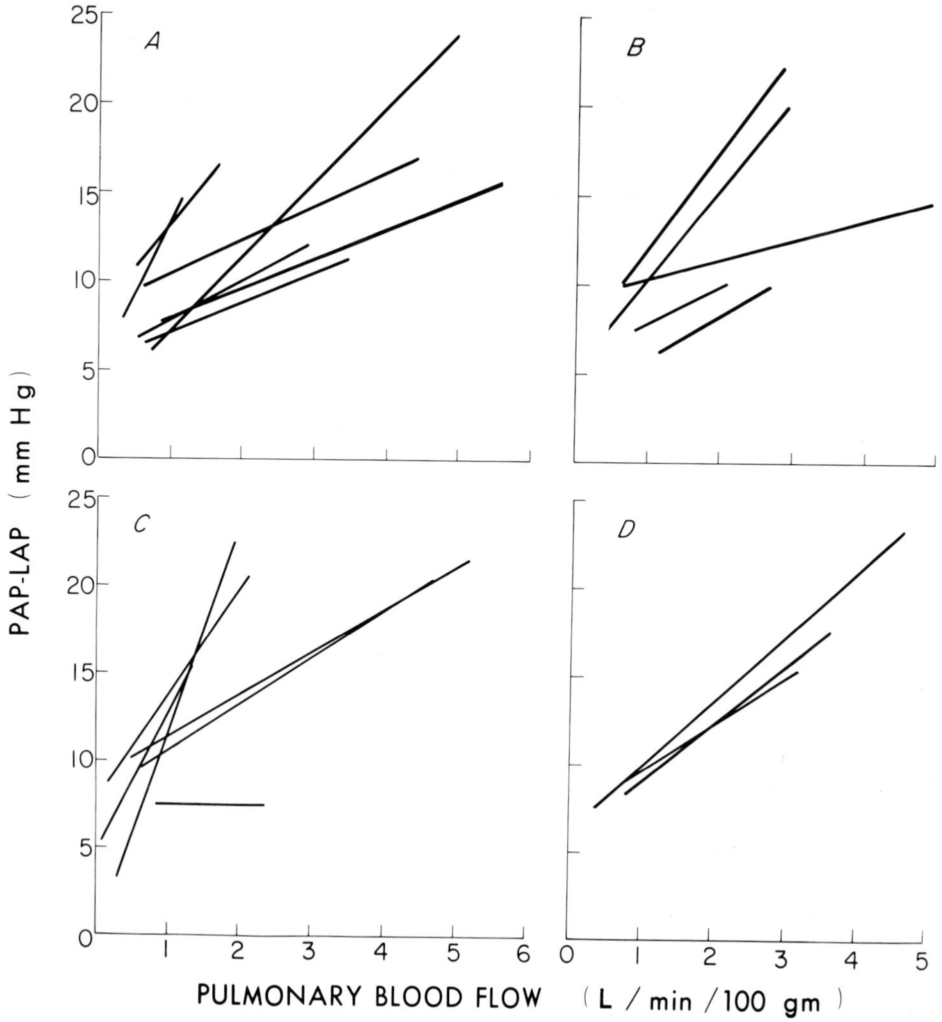

Fig. 2. Pressure-flow regression lines of the left lung of each dog within each group. *A,* Group 1: control; *B,* Group 2: denervated; *C,* Group 3: reimplanted 2 to 3 days; *D,* Group 4: reimplanted 6 to 8 weeks.

integrated blood flow were recorded from a flowmeter.* Pulmonary blood flow at end diastole was used as the zero reference. Each flow probe was calibrated by roller pump on four separate occasions during the study at hematocrits of 20 and 40.

The percentage of cardiac output that perfused the left lung was determined on three occasions by intravenous injection of different batches of radionuclide-labeled microspheres† (15,000 to 25,000 spheres, 15 μ ± 5 S.D. μ in diameter).[9] Microspheres were injected before and after inflation of the balloon occluder on the right pulmonary artery and after the balloon occluder was released. Blood flow to the left lung was increased by inflation of the balloon occluder and by rapid infusion of 6 percent dextran 70 in normal saline.[18] After each change in left pulmonary blood flow, two to five minutes elapsed before pressure and flow recordings were obtained. When left atrial pressure reached 7 to 17 mm. Hg, blood was withdrawn through a jugular venous catheter in 100 to 150 ml. increments by a roller

*Model No. BL-610, Biotronex Labs, Inc., Silver Springs, Md.

†Minnesota Mining and Manufacturing Company, St. Paul, Minn.

Table I

Group	No. of pressure-flow observations	Pulmonary blood flow (L./100 Gm. min.)		Range of mean pressure (mm. Hg)	
		Minimum	Maximum	Left atrium	Pulmonary artery
1	14	0.904	4.407	-4 / 4	7 /20
	23	0.922	4.345	1 / 7	11 /23.5
	30	0.556	1.602	-1 / 6.5	8 /22
	16	0.461	2.860	-1 / 2.5	4 /21.5
	15	0.682	3.402	0.5/12.5	5.5/22
	15	0.360	1.092	-4 / 3	4 /14.5
	16	0.768	4.668	-3.5/10	7 /32.5
	Total 129				
2	20	0.672	4.862	-3 /16	7 /27
	13	1.185	2.617	-0.5/ 6	6 /15
	24	0.842	1.987	1 / 7.5	9 /16
	29	0.569	2.774	2.5/13	11 /35
	30	0.457	2.479	1 /10	8 /28
	Total 116				
3	16	0.855	2.306	6 /14	11 /22
	15	0.631	4.623	-2 /12.5	9.5/29.5
	13	0.323	1.869	-1.5/ 9	6 /29
	32	0.522	4.738	0.5/17	8 /38
	15	0.111	1.299	-1 / 4.5	5.5/17.5
	23	0.191	2.039	-0.5/17	7.5/35
	Total 114				
4	49	0.806	3.572	-1.5/17	8 /35
	23	0.804	3.121	-1 / 9.5	9 /24
	32	0.373	4.558	1 /17	7 /38
	Total 104				

*With occluder inflated.

†Actual weight minus predicted weight divided by predicted weight multiplied by 100.

‡Average slope for group weighted for numbers of observations.

§Mean and standard deviation of the mean.

pump, and similar pressure and flow measurements were made. When cardiac output decreased below levels measured before dextran infusion, the balloon occluder was released and the third injection of microspheres was made.

Arterial pH, P_{CO_2}, and P_{O_2} were measured* before and after inflation of the occluder and after dextran infusion (maximal pulmonary blood flow) and after phlebotomy before the occluder was released. When necessary, sodium bicarbonate was infused, and the animal was manually ventilated to maintain arterial pH between 7.30 and 7.42 and Pa_{CO_2} below 50 mm. Hg. Alveolar oxygen tension was calculated from barometric pressure, arterial P_{CO_2}, and water vapor pressure.

After pressure-flow studies, all dogs were killed by bleeding. The positions of the catheters (downstream to the left pulmonary arterial anastomosis), balloon occluder, and flow probe were confirmed. Because of extensive atelectasis[26] or thrombosis around the left pulmonary arterial catheter,[23] two dogs in Group 1 and one dog in Group 3 were excluded from further study. The lungs of the remaining 21 dogs were excised, dissected into lobes, and weighed.* Each lobe was minced, put into plastic vials, and counted in a well-scintillation counter for one minute.[9] The percentage of cardiac output that reached each lobe at the time the microspheres were injected was calculated from the counts of each isotope.

The "predicted" weight of the left lung was calculated by multiplying the measured weight of the right lung by 0.7123.[15] The

*Radiometer, Inc., Cleveland, Ohio.

*Model No. P 120, Mettler Instrument Corp., Princeton, N. J.

Pressure-flow regression slope	Range hematocrit	Initial alveolar-arterial O_2 difference (mm. Hg)*	Change in alveolar-arterial O_2 difference (mm. Hg)*	Increase in left lung weight (%)†
1.687	33/40	171	+82	21.5
1.972	26/36	—	—	34.4
5.041	20/44	216	-30	33.9
2.245	43/48	243	-27	24.3
1.716	24/—	78	-40	9.9
8.560	28/40	185	-24	26.9
4.236	—/36	143	+37	11.5
3.637‡		173 ± 58§	-0.3	23.2 ± 9.8§
1.124	20/—	135	-40	36.6
2.481	28/39	306	+73	40.5
2.096	21/39	470	-41	27.6
5.543	15/33	293	-12	38.7
5.460	17/30	122	+1	5.2
3.341‡		265 ± 143§	-3.8	29.7 ± 14.6§
-0.006	15/29	251	+21	37.4
2.684	23/39	363	-60	58.4
12.123	18/—	282	+3	100.3
2.473	28/42	276	-44	74.2
7.978	25/31	40.3	+19	63.1
6.149	24/41	299	+234	120.1
5.234‡		312 ± 58§	28.8	75.6 ± 30.0§
3.406	20/36	143	+26	38.5
2.679	23/39	370	+2	59.6
3.739	23/36	146	+52	30.9
3.275‡		220 ± 130§	26.6	43.0 ± 14.9§

percentage increase in left lung weight was obtained by dividing the difference between the predicted and actual weights by the predicted weight. Actual blood flow to the left lung was calculated by multiplying flow measurements by the percentage of microspheres that reached the left lung. Left lung flows were corrected to flow per 100 Gm. of predicted weight per minute. Mean left atrial pressure was subtracted from mean pulmonary arterial pressure during end expiration to obtain the pressure difference across the lung during the time mean flow was recorded.

For each of the 21 left lungs, a least squares linear regression equation for pressure difference as a function of flow was calculated.[4] The pressure-flow relationship for each group of dogs was characterized by the mean of the individual regression slopes. For each pair of groups (six combinations), the hypothesis of equality of mean slopes was tested by a form of t test (see Appendix A). In this test, each difference in mean slopes was divided by an estimated standard deviation for that difference which was based on variances about regression for individual dogs. The significance levels of these six interrelated tests were assessed conservatively with the use of the Bonferroni inequality.[21]

RESULTS

Number of pressure-flow measurements, ranges of pulmonary blood flow, ranges of left atrial and pulmonary arterial pressures, pulmonary pressure-flow regression slopes, ranges of hematocrits, changes in alveolar-arterial oxygen differences, and the percentage increases in left lung weights have been tabulated for each dog (see Table I). At least 13 pressure-flow measurements were made in each dog. Some of the more im-

Table II. *Summary of group observations*

Group	No. of dogs	No. of pressure flow observations	Pressure-flow regression slopes: Group mean	Pressure-flow regression slopes: Group range	Change in alveolar-arterial Po_2 difference (mm. Hg)	Increase in left lung weight (%)*
1	7	129	3.637	1.687 - 8.560	-0.3	23.2 ± 9.8
2	5	116	3.341	1.124 - 5.543	-3.8	29.7 ± 14.6
3	6	114	5.234	-0.006 - 12.123	+28.8	75.6 ± 30
4	3	104	3.275	2.679 - 3.739	+26.6	43.0 ± 14.9

*Actual lung weight minus predicted lung weight × 100 divided by predicted lung weight. Values are means ± S.D.

portant data on each group are summarized in Table II and Fig. 2.

The inflated balloon occluder caused 91.2 to 100 percent of the cardiac output to pass into the left lung (calculated from microsphere injections). After injection of 15 μ microspheres, pulmonary arterial pressure and flow usually did not change; occasionally flow decreased for a few heart beats.

Regression slopes of pressure-flow relationships of the left lung of each dog within each group were plotted (Fig. 2). Within all groups except Group 4, slopes of pressure-flow relationships varied greatly (Fig. 2, Table II). The mean slope for left lungs of Group 3 dogs differed very significantly ($P < 0.006$)* from mean slopes for lungs of the dogs in Groups 2 and 4 and differed significantly ($P < 0.06$) from the mean slope for lungs in Group 1 animals. The mean slopes for Groups 1, 2, and 4 dogs did not differ significantly ($P > 0.06$) from one another.

Pulmonary vascular resistance, calculated as the difference between mean pulmonary arterial pressure and mean left atrial pressure (mm. Hg) divided by flow (liters per 100 Gm. minute), was plotted against flow for all observations within each group (Fig. 3). In all animals, pulmonary vascular resistance decreased as pulmonary blood flow increased.

When the balloon on the right pulmonary artery was inflated, alveolar-arterial oxygen differences were higher in the dogs in Groups 2 and 3 (mean 265 and 312, respectively) than in dogs in Groups 1 and 4 (mean 173 and 220, respectively). However, because of considerable variation between dogs, none of these means differed significantly ($P > 0.05$). Furthermore, no significant changes in mean alveolar-arterial oxygen differences occurred in any group during the experiments (Table II).

As expected, the greatest increase in lung weights occurred in dogs in Group 3 (Table II); however, there was no correlation between the increases in lung weight in this group and the pressure-flow regression slopes or the alveolar-arterial oxygen differences.

*Unorthodox critical probabilities arise because of the use of the Bonferroni inequality in conjunction with standard tables of the t distribution.

DISCUSSION

Pulmonary pressure-flow regression slopes and intercepts vary considerably between individuals in both men and dogs[13] and are affected by many factors including acidosis, hypoxia, hypercarbia, alveolar pressure, left atrial pressure, emboli, and vasoactive substances.[5, 13] These facts prompted the design of this study. We chose a closed-chest preparation and made many measurements over a considerable range of pulmonary blood flows in each animal. Although flowmeters are less accurate than calibrated pumps, we avoided extracorporeal perfusion because of associated platelet aggregate emboli,[6] and ill-defined neurohumoral changes. Necessarily, left atrial pressures varied, and the higher pressures, which reduce pulmonary vascular resistance[5, 22] were associated with higher flows. However, our preparation permitted a beating heart to perfuse the lungs during spontaneous respiration with a wide range of pulsatile blood flows. End expiratory lung volumes were approximately constant and known factors that alter pulmonary

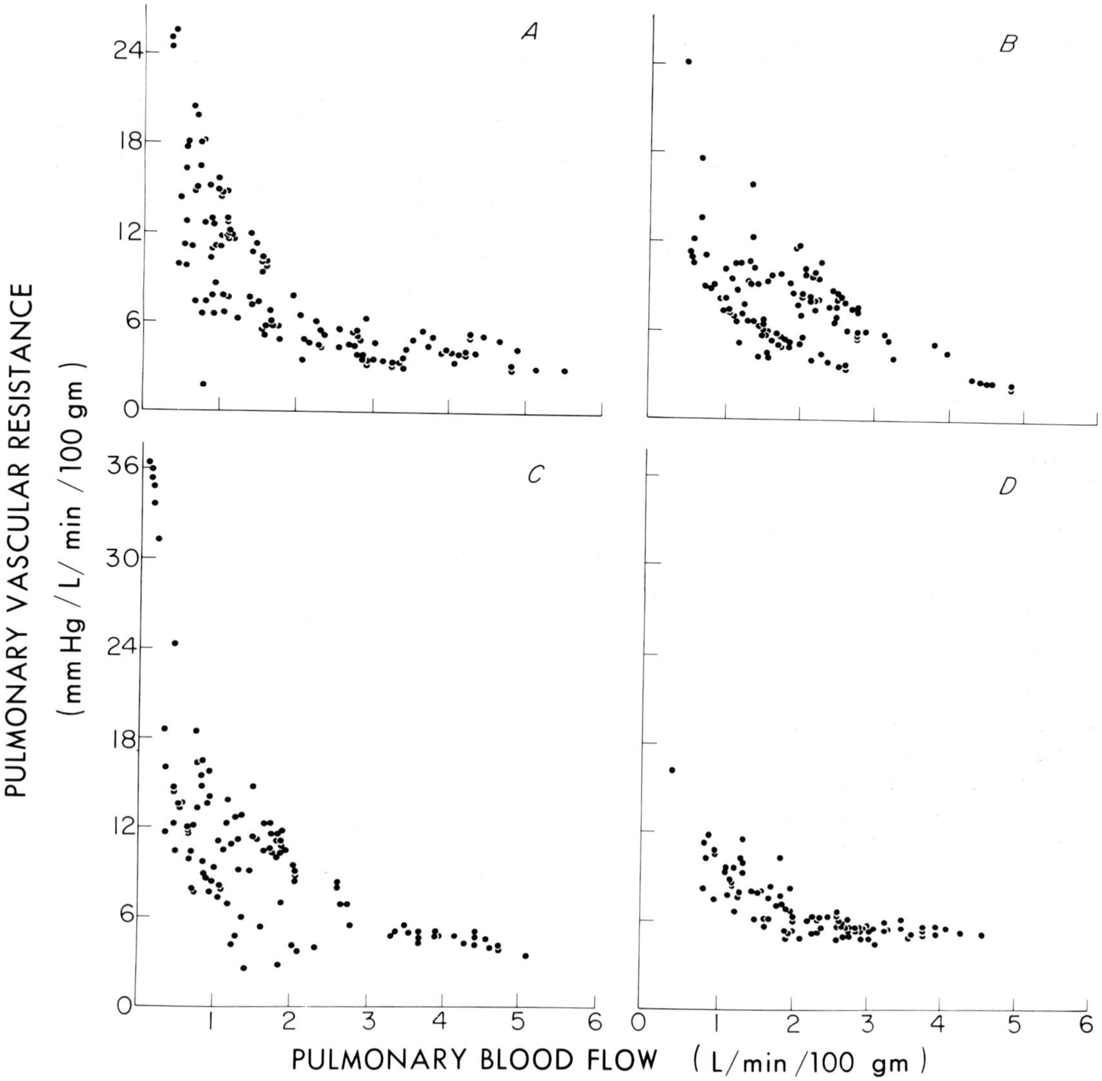

Fig. 3. Pulmonary vascular resistance (mean pulmonary arterial pressure minus mean left atrial pressure divided by flow) is plotted against simultaneous flow for the pooled data on the four groups of dogs. *A*, Group 1; *B*, Group 2; *C*, Group 3; *D*, Group 4.

pressure-flow relationships were controlled within narrow ranges. Furthermore, we corrected pulmonary blood flows for the size of the lung and used predicted left lung weights to avoid errors resulting from postoperative increases in lung fluids.

We studied our control group of dogs two to three days after thoracotomy, but the pulmonary arterial pressures at resting blood flows and the observed variations in pressure-flow regression slopes and intercepts were similar to those published by Rudolph and Auld[22] and by Fowler and Holmes.[14] These investigators used extracorporeal perfusion and open-chested dogs and did not correct flow measurements for the size of the lung; thus we cannot compare our data to theirs in detail. However, recent thoracotomy and postoperative miliary atelectasis (as indicated by the increased alveolar-arterial oxygen differences in the absence of atelectasis on chest roentgenograms), which were common to all of our dogs, did not appear to affect pulmonary vascular pressure-flow relationships.

Variation in pulmonary vascular pressure-flow relationships of individual dogs make comparisons between different studies and between different groups of dogs within the same study difficult. In order to make comparisons we chose to treat our groups of dogs as a fixed population rather than as a random sample of a larger population of dogs. As a result, the scope of inferences is limited to this fixed population. This simpler analysis avoided the heavy assumptions required for an extremely complex random slope analysis and, because of inequality of variance about regression between dogs, was more appropriate than the analogous t statistic with pooled variance estimate. The method of moments adjustment of the degrees of freedom reduced the sensitivity of the test, but it also reduced the chance of faulty inferences caused by inequality of variance.

Unilateral denervation of the lung did not alter pulmonary vascular pressure-flow regression slopes. Adrenergic and cholinergic nerves innervate large (greater than 30 μ) pulmonary vessels in the dog,[12] but the effect of sympathetic and parasympathetic stimulation on pulmonary vascular resistance remains controversial.[3, 17] Several workers have concluded that denervation of the lung causes increased pulmonary vascular resistance[1, 8, 16, 29]; however, we did not observe any difference in vascular pressure-flow relationships between the control and denervated groups of dogs. These data are consistent with the hypothesis that the pulmonary vasculature reacts passively to changes in blood flow.[13]

After excision and reimplantation of the lung, vascular pressure-flow regression slopes are temporarily increased, but within six to eight weeks the slopes are within the normal range. This temporary change coincides with other temporary changes in lung structure and function.[26] As we observed, lung weight and alveolar-arterial oxygen differences are increased after excision and reimplantation of the lung. In addition, ventilation and oxygen uptake is decreased,[7, 23] mucus transport is impaired,[10] and severed bronchial arteries and lymphatic vessels have not yet regenerated. Within two to six months, these and other temporary changes in lung structure and reductions in function are reversed,[7, 10, 20, 24, 26] and although afferent nerves have not regenerated,[11] the reimplanted lung without stenotic anastomoses has a normal gross and microscopic appearance[20, 26] and satisfactorily ventilates blood.

Some investigators have found an increase in the vascular resistance of reimplanted lungs one or more years after operation.[24, 29] Although no data for vascular pressure-flow regression slopes are available, Tisi and associates[24] measured vascular resistances of reimplanted lungs 2.5 to 4.0 years after operation before and after balloon occlusion of the opposite pulmonary artery. Vascular resistances were normal at resting blood flows, but with one exception were elevated when the opposite pulmonary artery was occluded. These investigators explained their findings on the fact that the reimplanted left lungs were smaller than normal; however, their data indicate that the ratio of left and right static lung volumes measured with neon were nearly identical to the volume ratios found by Frank in excised normal lungs of dogs.[15] In their animals, and in most other studies, the left atrial anastomosis was made in the conventional manner which places the suture line near the ostia of the left pulmonary veins and particularly near the left upper lobar vein.[2, 30] This anastomosis is not distensible, and at higher than resting blood flows may cause increased resistance. The intra-atrial wire technique avoids placement of the suture line near the ostia of the pulmonary veins. Since direct evidence of structural abnormalities of chronically reimplanted lungs is lacking[20, 26, 29] and since no known stimulus for a chronic process exists, we suspect that the observed deficiencies in the size and ventilatory function of the chronically reimplanted canine lung are directly related to the anastomoses, particularly the left atrial anastomosis.

APPENDIX A

For comparison of average slopes between groups let b_{ij} be the estimate of the true slope B_{ij} for animal j of Group i, s_{ij} be the estimated standard error of b_{ij} with m_{ij} degrees of freedom (the number of observations on that animal–2), and J_i the number of animals in Group i.

Comparisons between groups are based on t tests of equality of mean slopes for any two groups, where $\overline{b_i} = J_i^{-1} \Sigma_j b_{ij}$ estimates the true mean slope $\overline{B_i} = J_i^{-1} \Sigma_{ij} B_{ij}$ for Group i. Let 1, 2 be the indices of any two groups; then the (approximate) t statistic for the comparison is $d s_d^{-1}$ with n_d degrees of freedom, where $d = \overline{b}_1 - \overline{b}_2$, $s_d^2 = J_1^{-2} \Sigma_j s_{1j}^2 + J_2^{-2} \Sigma_j s_{2j}^2$, $n_d = s_d^4 [J_1^{-4} \Sigma_j (s_{1j}^4/m_{1j}) + J_2^{-4} \Sigma_j (s_{2j}^4/m_{2j})]^{-1}$.
The justifying assumptions are that each b_{ij} has a normal distribution with variance σ_{ij}^2 estimated by s_{ij}^2 and that the estimated variance of a difference d, s_d^2, is distributed as a multiple of a χ^2 variable with n_d degrees of freedom. The estimate of n_d is obtained by the method of moments. This statistic is a generalization of the t test with separate variance estimates[28] commonly used when groups to be compared are known to have different variances.

The authors are grateful for the contributions of B. Andersen, D. Berrigan, Y. Cain, B. Halliday, I. Hemassi, A. Martin, and S. Montgomery to this study.

REFERENCES

1. Allgood, R. J., Ebert, P. A., and Sabiston, D. C., Jr.: Immediate changes in pulmonary hemodynamics following lung autotransplantation, Ann. Surg. **167:** 352, 1968.
2. Benfield, J. R., and Coon, R.: The role of the left atrial anastomosis in pulmonary reimplantation, J. Thorac. Cardiovasc. Surg. **53:** 676-684, 1967.
3. Daly, I. de B., and Hebb, C.: Pulmonary vasomotor fibers in the cervical vagosympathetic nerve of the dog, Quart. J. Exp. Physiol. **37:** 19, 1952.
4. Draper, N., and Smith, H.: Applied regression analysis, New York, 1966, John Wiley & Sons, Inc., chap. 1.
5. Duke, H. N., and Lee, G. de J.: The regulation of blood flow through the lungs, Br. Med. Bull. **19:** 71, 1963.
6. Dutton, R. C., and Edmunds, L. H., Jr.: Measurement of emboli during extracorporeal perfusion, J. Thorac. Cardiovasc. Surg. **65:** 523, 1973.
7. Duvoisin, G. E., Fowler, W. S., Ellis, F. H., Jr., and Payne, W. S.: Causes of depressed pulmonary function following reimplantation of the canine lung, Chest **58:** 102, 1970.
8. Ebert, P. A., and Hudson, B. H.: Pulmonary hemodynamics following lung autotransplantation, J. Thorac. Cardiovasc. Surg. **62:** 188, 1971.
9. Edmunds, L. H., Jr., Gold, W. M., and Heymann, M. A.: Lobar distribution of pulmonary arterial blood flow in awake standing dogs, Am. J. Physiol. **219:** 1779, 1970.
10. Edmunds, L. H., Jr., Graf, P. D., Sagel, S. S., and Greenspan, R. H.: Radiographic observation of the clearance of tantalum and barium sulfate particles from airways, Invest. Radiol. **5:** 131, 1970.
11. Edmunds, L. H., Jr., Graf, P. D., and Nadel, J. A.: Reinnervation of the reimplanted canine lung. J. Appl. Physiol. **31:** 722, 1971.
12. Fillenz, M.: quoted by Hebb, C.: Motor innervation of the pulmonary blood vessels of mammals, *in* Fishman, A. P., and Hecht, H. H., editors: The pulmonary circulation and interstitial space, Chicago, Ill., 1969, University of Chicago Press, pp. 195-218.
13. Fowler, N. O.: The normal pulmonary arterial pressure-flow relationships during exercise, Am. J. Med. **47:** 1, 1969.
14. Fowler, N. O., and Holmes, J. C.: Pulmonary arterial pressure at high pulmonary flow, J. Clin. Invest. **44:** 2040, 1965.
15. Frank, N. R.: A comparison of static volume-pressure relations of excised pulmonary lobes of dogs, J. Appl. Physiol. **18:** 274, 1963.
16. Fujimura, S., Parmley, W. W., Tomoda, H., Norman, J. R., and Matloff, J. M.: Hemodynamic alterations after staged and simultaneous bilateral lung autotransplantation, J. Thorac. Cardiovasc. Surg. **63:** 527, 1972.
17. Ingram, R. H., Szidon, J. P., Skalak, R., and Fishman, A. P.: Effects of sympathetic nerve stimulation on the pulmonary arterial tree of the isolated lobe perfused in situ, Circ. Res. **22:** 801, 1968.
18. Keros, J., Ecker, R. R., and Rapaport, E.: Ventricular function curves in the exercising dog, Circ. Res. **25:** 557, 1969.
19. Kottmeier, P. K., Cheng, C., Fitzgerald, J., Hockman, R., and Emmanuel, G. E.: Growth and function of the replanted lung in young dogs, J. Pediatr. Surg. **4:** 66, 1969.
20. Marshall, R., and Gunning, A. J.: The long-term physiologic effects of lung reimplantation in the dog, J. Surg. Res. **6:** 185, 1966.
21. Miller, R. G., Jr.: Simultaneous statistical inference, New York, 1966, McGraw-Hill Book Company, chap. 2, sect. 3.
22. Rudolph, A. M., and Auld, P. A. M.: Physical factors affecting normal and serotonin-constricted pulmonary vessels, Am. J. Physiol. **198:** 864, 1960.
23. Strieder, D. J., Barnes, B. A., Aronow, S., Russell, P. S., and Kazemi, H.: Xenon 133 study of ventilation and perfusion in normal and transplanted dog lungs, J. Appl. Physiol. **23:** 359, 1967.
24. Tisi, G. M., Trummer, M. J., Cuomo, A. J., Ashburn, W. L., and Moser, K. M.: Long-term autotransplanted canine lungs: base-line

ventilatory and hemodynamic function, J. Appl. Physiol. **32:** 113, 1972.

25. Veith, F. J., Dougherty, J., Boley, S. J., and Koerner, S.: Flow and resistance characteristics of normal and transplanted lungs, Eur. Surg. Res. **2:** 41, 1970.
26. Veith, F. J., and Blumenstock, D. A.: Current research review: Lung transplantation, J. Surg. Res. **1:** 33, 1971.
27. Wagner, O. A., Cowan, G. S. M., Jr., and Edmunds, L. H., Jr.: Lobar pulmonary arterial blood flow in reimplanted canine lungs, J. Thorac. Cardivosac. Surg. **65:** 171, 1973.
28. Welch, B. L.: The generalization of Student's problem when different population variances are involved. Biometrika **34:** 28, 1947.
29. Wildevuur, C. R. H., Heemstra, H., Tammeling, G. J., Hilvering, C., Bouma, H. G. D., ten Hoor, F., Scherpenisse, L. A., Kleine, J. W., Orie, N. G. M., and Homan van der Heide, J. N.: Long-term observation of the changes in pulmonary arterial pressure after reimplantation of the canine lung, J. Thorac. Cardiovasc. Surg. **56:**799, 1968.
30. Yanes, H. O., Rudy, L. W., and Edmunds, L. H., Jr.: Pulmonary arterial blood flow in reimplanted lungs of dogs, SURGERY **71:** 576, 1972.
31. Cowan, E. S. M., Jr., Edmunds, L. H., Jr., and Erdmann, A. J., III: Analysis of weight gain in reimplanted dog lungs, Surg. Forum **24:** 269, 1973.

Direct measurement of vagal release of gastrin

Horst D. Becker, M.D., David D. Reeder, M.D., *and* **James C. Thompson, M.D.,**
Galveston, Texas

The concentration of gastrin in the antral venous blood of dogs was measured by radioimmunoassay during direct electrical stimulation of the branches of the vagus to the gastric antrum. In addition, we have studied the effects on the vagal release of gastrin caused by changes in antral pH and changes in the duration and magnitude of electrical stimuli. The gastrin response to electrical vagal stimulation was almost immediate. Acidification of the antrum greatly diminished the gastrin response to electrical stimulation of the vagus (5 v.) but did not abolish it. The increase in antral venous gastrin after stimulation with higher voltage (10 v.) was inhibited only slightly by antral acidification. When the antral pH was changed to pH 7.0, the concentration of gastrin rose rapidly. Stimulation of the antral vagus for two minutes resulted in release of gastrin from the isolated antrum for at least 30 minutes. These studies directly confirm the vagal release of gastrin and provide some data for quantification of the amount released.

From the Department of Surgery, The University of Texas Medical Branch, Galveston, Texas

A CONTINUOUS interplay between the vagus and gastrin seems to be essential for optimal activation of the oxyntic glands during the secretory response to a meal. Previous studies have shown that vagal stimulation by insulin,[3] by sham feeding,[15] or by electrical impulses[17] caused a minute but definite acid response from a denervated fundic pouch in dogs. The response to sham feeding was potentiated by raising antral pH towards neutral.[15] The development of highly sensitive radioimmunoassay techniques for measuring serum gastrin concentrations has allowed direct determination of the circulating levels of gastrin.[2, 8] In the present study, we have measured the concentration of gastrin in antral venous blood during selective direct electrical stimulation of the branches of the vagus to the gastric antrum. In addition, we have studied the effects on the vagal release of gastrin caused by changes in antral pH and changes in the duration and magnitude of electrical stimuli.

MATERIALS AND METHODS

Nineteen adult mongrel dogs, weighing from 18 to 21 kilograms, were divided into four groups. Each dog was fasted for 24 hours and anesthetized with pentobarbital sodium. At laparotomy a clamp was put across the antrofundic junction of the stomach and the antral vein was cannulated to allow intermittent sampling of the entire venous outflow as previously described.[8]

The anterior and posterior branches of

Supported by Grant No. AM 15241 from the National Institutes of Health and by a grant from The John A. Hartford Foundation, Inc.

Accepted for publication Oct. 3, 1973.

Reprint requests: James C. Thompson, M.D., Department of Surgery, The University of Texas Medical Branch, Galveston, Texas 77550.

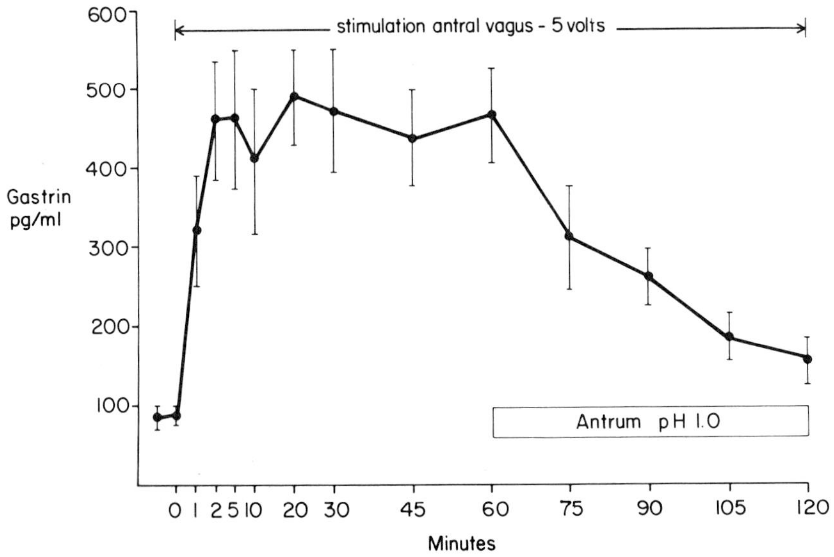

Fig. 1. Effect of continuous electrical stimulation of the antral vagus nerve on the concentration of gastrin in the antral venous outflow in five dogs. The isolated antrum was acidified during the final hour of the experiment. Narrow vertical bars in this and all subsequent figures indicate ± one SE.

the vagus were identified, dissected carefully from the surrounding tissues, and divided approximately 5 cm. proximal to the antral wall. A platinum electrode was placed on the distal portion of each nerve, approximately 1 cm. from the site of transection. Electrical impulses were delivered by a Grass stimulator (characteristics of stimulus: square wave impulses, 5 or 10 volts (v.), 1.0 milliamperes, 5 milliseconds, 20 impulses per second). A double-lumen catheter was placed into the antrum via a stab wound in the duodenum, and the pylorus was ligated around the catheter. The perfusates used in these studies were 0.9 percent NaCl, adjusted to pH 1.0 or pH 7.0 with either 0.1N HCl or 0.1N NaOH. The perfusates were allowed to flow into the antrum at the rate of 150 ml. per hour. At this rate, inflow pressure is less than 2 cm. H_2O. The antrum was drained by gravity through the other lumen of the tube, and antral distention was avoided. The pH of the secretions in the resting antrum and of the perfusates which drained from the antrum was determined with a glass pH electrode. Blood samples for gastrin radioimmunoassay were taken from the antral venous outflow in the basal state (time 0) and at intervals throughout the experiments.

Group I. In five dogs we tested the effect of vagal stimulation and antral acidification on the release of gastrin. After measurement of antral pH, the antral vagus received a 5 v. stimulus for 120 minutes. During the final 60 minutes of stimulation, the antrum was perfused with saline (pH 1.0).

Group II. In five dogs, the antrum was perfused first for 60 minutes with saline with a pH of 1.0, and then for 60 minutes with saline with a pH of 7.0. Electrical stimulation of the antral vagus (5 v.) was begun 30 minutes after initiation of the antral perfusion and was continued throughout the experiment.

Group III. In six dogs the antrum was perfused first for 45 minutes with saline with a pH of 1.0, then for 45 minutes with saline with a pH of 7.0, and finally for 60 minutes with saline with a pH of 1.0. The antral vagus was continually stimulated (10 v.) for 90 minutes, beginning 15 minutes after initiation of the study. After a 30 minute rest period, the antral vagus was stimulated again for ten minutes.

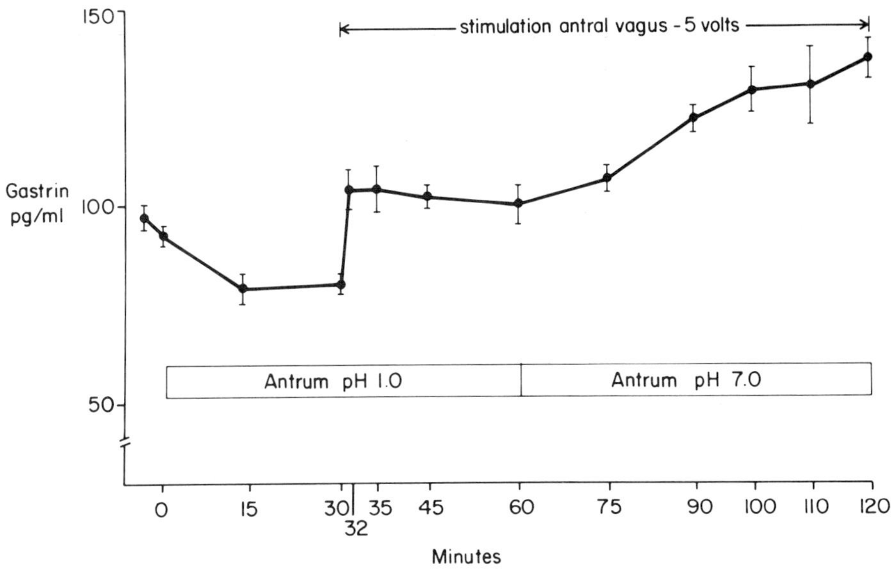

Fig. 2. Effect of antral acidification on basal and vagally stimulated gastrin concentrations in the antral venous outflow of five dogs. Periods of acidification and neutralization of the isolated antrum are shown.

Group IV. In order to test the duration of increased gastrin release after a brief period of vagal stimulation, the antral vagus was stimulated (5 v.) in three dogs for two minutes. Antral venous blood samples were collected for 60 minutes.

Radioimmunoassay of gastrin. Serum concentrations of gastrin were measured by radioimmunoassay.[8] Antigastrin antibodies were prepared in rabbits with synthetic human gastrin I (residues 2 to 17) conjugated to bovine serum albumin as immunogen. Synthetic human gastrin I is radioiodinated by means of the technique of Greenwood and Hunter.[6] The radioimmunoassay utilizes the double-antibody system described by Odell and associates.[14] Assays have a limit of sensitivity of about 10 picograms (pg.) per milliliter, and reproducibility of results is within ± 10 per cent.

Results are expressed as the mean of the observed gastrin concentration with the corresponding standard errors (± SE). Student's t test was used to determine statistical significance of the data. A p value of less than 0.05 was considered to indicate statistical significance.

RESULTS

Group I. Effect of 5 v. electrical stimulation of the antral vagus and antral acidification on gastrin release. The mean serum concentration of gastrin in two basal samples was 88 ± 9 pg. per milliliter (Fig. 1). The range of pH of the aspirated antral secretions was from 3.0 to 5.0. After one minute of electrical stimulation of the vagus, the gastrin levels had increased to 319 ± 78 pg. per milliliter. Peak gastrin levels of 488 ± 110 pg. per milliliter were observed 20 minutes after the initiation of the vagal stimulation. Antral perfusion with saline (pH 1.0) caused diminution in the antral venous gastrin concentration to 164 ± 22 pg. per milliliter after 60 minutes (time: 120 minutes).

Group II. Effect of prior antral acidification on gastrin release stimulated by 5 v. electrical current applied to the vagus. The mean basal concentration of serum gastrin in the antral venous blood was 95 ± 4 pg. per milliliter (Fig. 2). Acidification of the antrum by perfusion with saline (pH 1.0) caused a diminution of gastrin levels to 80 ± 4 pg. per milliliter ($p < 0.05$) after 30 minutes. Stimulation of the vagus in-

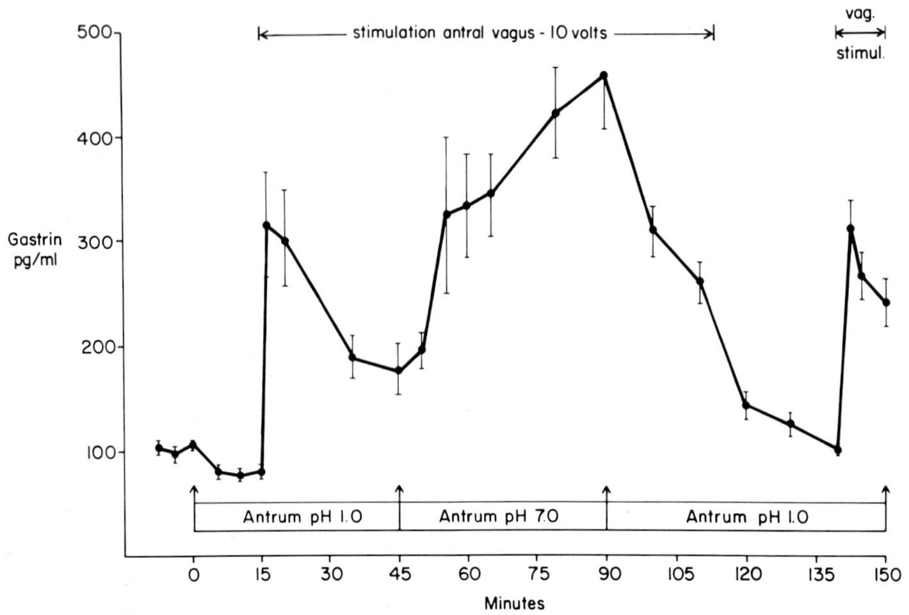

Fig. 3. Effect of antral acidification and neutralization on concentration of gastrin in the antral venous outflow during periods of electrical stimulation of the antral vagus nerve in six dogs.

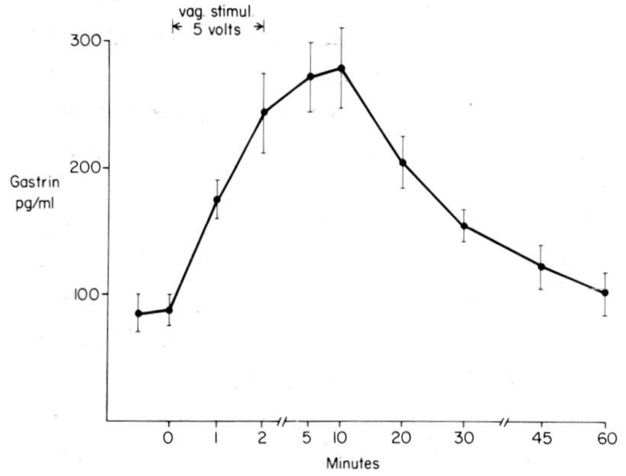

Fig. 4. Effect of a brief (two minutes) period of electrical stimulation of the antral vagus nerve on the duration of stimulated gastrin release as measured in the venous outflow of the isolated antrum in three dogs.

creased the gastrin concentration to 104 ± 8 pg. per milliliter ($p < 0.05$). When the pH of the antral perfusate was changed to pH 7.0, antral venous gastrin increased further to a peak of 137 ± 14 pg. per milliliter.

Group III. Effect of prior and subsequent antral acidification on gastrin release stimulated by 10 v. electrical current applied to the vagus. The mean basal gastrin concentration in antral venous serum was 102 ± 5 pg. per milliliter (Fig. 3). Acidification of the antrum decreased gastrin to 78 ± 5 pg. per milliliter ($p < 0.05$). Electrical stimulation (10 v.) of the antral vagus in the face of antral acidification increased the gastrin concentration in the antral venous outflow to 316 ± 53 pg. per milliliter after two minutes. During continuous vagal stimulation and perfusion of the antrum with saline, pH 1.0, gastrin decreased to 174 ± 21 pg. per milliliter. After the pH of the perfusate was changed to 7.0, gastrin increased to 459 ± 79 pg. per milliliter ($p < 0.02$). Acidification of the antrum resulted in an abrupt decrease to 256 ± 33 pg. per milliliter ($p < 0.01$). When the vagal stimulation was stopped, antral venous gastrin concentration fell to basal levels (104 ± 5 pg. per milliliter). When electrical vagal stimulation was begun again, the gastrin concentration rose to 312 ± 35 pg. per milliliter in two minutes ($p < 0.01$).

Group IV. Duration of gastrin secretion in response to brief (two minutes) vagal stimulation. The basal concentration of gastrin in antral vein serum was 86 ± 6 pg.

per milliliter (Fig. 4). One minute after initiation of stimulation of the antral vagus (5 v.), gastrin concentration increased to 175 ± 10 pg. per milliliter ($p < 0.01$). The maximal response (278 ± 26 pg. per milliliter) occurred at ten minutes (eight minutes after the stimulation was stopped). One hour after the brief vagal stimulation, antral venous gastrin had returned to near basal levels (103 ± 14 pg. per milliliter).

DISCUSSION

In 1942, Uvnäs[17] observed that electrical stimulation of the vagus in cats resulted in secretion of gastric acid. In cross-transfusion experiments, he showed that this secretion was apparently caused by a hormonal agent released after vagal stimulation, and he concluded that this hormonal agent could be gastrin. In the following years, doubts arose about the vagal release of gastrin because investigators could not demonstrate that sham feeding induced a secretory response from a Heidenhain pouch.[1, 12] Burstall and Schofield[3] and Pe Thein and Schofield,[15] using a perfusion technique for the determination of small amounts of acid secretion from a denervated fundic pouch, demonstrated a small but definite secretory response to sham feeding. This response was abolished by antrectomy or by antral acidification.

Several recent studies have focused on the role of the vagus in releasing gastrin. Jaffe and associates[9] showed an increase in the concentration of gastrin in the portal vein after insulin hypoglycemia in dogs. In man, the results of insulin hypoglycemia are still controversial. Hansky and associates[7] showed a significant increase of peripheral serum gastrin concentrations during insulin hypoglycemia in four duodenal ulcer patients. This response was potentiated by neutralization of the antrum. Ganguli and Elder[5] found significant increases in plasma gastrin concentration during insulin hypoglycemia in 10 of 13 patients. Other authors have been unable to confirm these findings.[2, 4] Stadil[16] found an increase in gastrin during induced hypoglycemia in duodenal ulcer patients, but truncal or selective gastric vagotomy did not reduce the gastrin response to vagal stimulation. These authors concluded that the release of gastrin by insulin is independent of vagal innervation of the stomach. Korman and colleagues,[10] however, have recently provided evidence that intact vagal innervation of the antrum is a requisite for the release of gastrin in response to insulin hypoglycemia.

In a recent study, Lanciault and coworkers[11] reported that electrical stimulation of the cervical vagi in dogs caused a rapid and significant rise in portal serum gastrin concentrations within 2.5 minutes of onset of stimulation. They suggested that innervation of the gastrin cells of the antral mucosa was direct and that the secretory granules are extruded rapidly after vagal stimulation.[11]

The present studies show that the release of gastrin in response to electrical stimulation of the antral vagus occurs almost immediately. Within only two minutes, maximal levels of gastrin were achieved. Acidification of the antrum diminished the gastrin response to vagal stimulation with 5 v. but did not abolish it. The immediate increase in antral venous concentrations of gastrin after vagal stimulation with 10 v. was only slightly inhibited by antral acidification, but this stimulated level of gastrin decreased rapidly during continuous acidification. When the antral pH was changed to 7.0, the gastrin concentration again rose rapidly.

Although it seems reasonable to us that the increase in antral venous gastrin concentration after selective stimulation of the antral branches of the vagus is reflected in an absolute increase in the amount of gastrin released, it is theoretically possible that a simultaneous diminution in blood flow from the antrum might result in a decrease in gastrin release.

Molina and colleagues[13] reported that after a single 15 minute period of electrical stimulation of the vagus nerve above the diaphragm, restimulation after four hours did not elicit further acid production. Infusion of gastrin, however, restored the gastric secretory response. They suggested that the antral gastrin release mechanism fatigued rapidly after electrical stimulation of the vagus. In our studies with dogs with isolated antra, a second electrical stimulus, applied directly to the antral branches of the vagus, elicited a similar release of gastrin. Since our experimental preparation was completely different from that of Molina and colleagues,[13] the results cannot be compared.

The persistence of elevated antral venous gastrin levels for nearly 60 minutes after a two-minute period of electrical stimulation of the vagus confirms the resilience of the gastrin cell to continued release and, presumably, to continued synthesis of gastrin.[8] These studies again illustrate the importance of feedback mechanisms of acid inhibition in the control of gastrin release.

REFERENCES

1. Babkin, B. P., and Schachter, M.: The chemical phase of gastric secretion and the surgery of the stomach, McGill Med. J. **13:** 127, 1944.
2. Berson, S. A., Walsh, J. H., and Yalow, R. S.: Radioimmunoassay of gastrin in human plasma and regulation of gastrin release, *in* Andersson, S., editor: Nobel Symposium XVI. Frontiers in gastrointestinal hormone research, Uppsala, Sweden, 1973, Almqvist and Wiksell, pp. 57-68.
3. Burstall, P. A., and Schofield, B.: Secretory effects of psychic stimulation and insulin hypoglycemia on Heidenhain gastric pouches in dogs, J. Physiol. **120:** 383, 1953.
4. Feurle, G., Ketterer, H., Becker, H. D., and Creutzfeldt, W.: Circadian serum gastrin concentrations in control persons and in patients with ulcer disease, Scand. J. Gastroenterol. **7:** 177, 1972.
5. Ganguli, P. C., and Elder, J. B.: Effect of insulin hypoglycemia on plasma gastrin concentration and gastric acid secretion in normal subjects, Gut **12:** 861, 1971.
6. Greenwood, F. C., and Hunter, W. M.: The preparation of ^{131}I-labeled human growth hormone of high specific radioactivity, Biochem. J. **89:** 114, 1963.
7. Hansky, J., Korman, M. G., Cowley, D. J., and Baron, J. H.: Serum gastrins in duodenal ulcer. Part II. Effect of insulin hypoglycemia, Gut **12:** 959, 1971.
8. Jackson, B. M., Reeder, D. D., and Thompson, J. C.: Dynamic characteristics of gastrin release, Am. J. Surg. **123:** 137, 1972.
9. Jaffe, B. M., McGuigan, J. E., and Newton, W. T.: Immunochemical measurement of the vagal release of gastrin, SURGERY **68:** 169, 1970.
10. Korman, M. G., Hansky, J., Coupland, G. A. E., and Cumberland, V. H.: Serum gastrin response to insulin hypoglycaemia: Studies after parietal cell vagotomy and after selective gastric vagotomy, Scand. J. Gastroenterol. **8:** 235, 1973.
11. Lanciault, G., Bonoma, C., Karreman, G., and Brooks, F. P.: Kinetics of gastrin release and degradation in response to electrical vagal stimulation in the dog, Proc. Soc. Exp. Biol. Med. **142:** 740, 1973.
12. Lin, R. K. S., and Moce, P.: Does vagal excitation liberate pyloric gastrin? Fed. Proc. **10:** 84, 1951.
13. Molina, J. E., Ritchie, W. P., Edlich, R. F., Tomiyama, Y., and Wangensteen, O. H.: Fatigue of the antral gastrin mechanism following electrical vagal stimulation, SURGERY **69:** 680, 1971.
14. Odell, W. D., Rayford, P. L., and Ross, G. T.: Simplified partially automated method for radioimmunoassay of human thyroid-stimulating, growth, luteinizing and follicle stimulating hormones, J. Lab. Clin. Med. **70:** 973, 1967.
15. Pe Thein, M., and Schofield, B.: Release of gastrin from the pyloric antrum following vagal stimulation by sham feeding in dogs, J. Physiol. **148:** 29, 1959.
16. Stadil, F.: Effect of vagotomy on gastrin release during insulin hypoglycemia in ulcer patients, Scand. J. Gastroenterol. **7:** 225, 1972.
17. Uvnäs, B.: The part played by the pyloric region in the cephalic phase of gastric secretion, Acta Physiol. Scand. **4:** 1, 1942.

Juvenile gastrointestinal polyposis in a female infant: Report of a case and review of the literature of a recently recognized syndrome

Charles R. Sachatello, M.D., *Lexington, Ky.,* **Il Song Hahn, M.D.,** *and*
Charles B. Carrington, M.D., *New Haven, Conn.*

A report of a female infant who died with extensive juvenile polyposis of the entire gastrointestinal tract is presented. The similarity of the clinical and pathological findings of this patient with several previously reported patients supports the contention that juvenile polyposis of infancy is a relatively distinct entity. This syndrome is characterized by gastrointestinal bleeding, diarrhea, rectal prolapse, and intussusception in infants and young children. It appears to be transmitted as a nonsex-linked recessive. Prognosis is directly related to the severity and extent of gastrointestinal involvement with juvenile polyps. Accurate pathologic interpretation of polypoid lesions is necessary to distinguish this syndrome from familial polyposis of the colon and Peutz Jeghers syndrome.

From the Department of Surgery, University of Kentucky Medical School, Lexington, Ky., and the Department of Pathology, Yale University School of Medicine, New Haven, Conn.

JUVENILE gastrointestinal polyposis has only recently been recognized to represent an entity distinct from the other more commonly known syndromes of gastrointestinal polypoid diseases, i.e., Peutz Jeghers syndrome and familial (adenomatous) polyposis coli.[3, 5, 13, 15]

This case report of a female infant who died more than a decade ago is presented because it helps clarify the often confusing spectrum of gastrointestinal polypoid diseases in infants and children.

CASE REPORT

At age two months, this white female infant had two bouts of pneumonia requiring hospitalization at Yale New Haven Hospital. She was found to have a grade 2/6 systolic murmur, cardiomegaly, hepatosplenomegaly, and she was diagnosed as having an interventricular septal defect.

Supported in part by the Jewel Fund for the Study of Intestinal Diseases.

Accepted for publication Oct. 9, 1973.

The infant was rehospitalized at age five months because of anemia and was found to have guaiac-positive stools. Flecks of bright red blood had been noted in the stool since one month of age. Sigmoidoscopy and air contrast studies demonstrated multiple polypoid defects in the large intestine.

Laparotomy revealed multiple polyps in both large and small intestine. Thirty-one polyps from the small intestine and 14 polyps from the large intestine were removed. An ileocecal intussusception caused by a large cecal polyp was reduced. A Meckel's diverticulum was noted and removed.

During the subsequent five months, the patient continued to manifest both guaiac-positive stools and numerous episodes of gastrointestinal bleeding requiring repeated transfusions. Rectal prolapse of multiple polyp–studded mucosa developed at age ten months, and six polyps were removed during sigmoidoscopy at this time.

At one year of age, the patient was noted to have peripheral edema. Total serum proteins were 4.7 Gm. percent with an albumin count of 1.8 Gm. percent. Repeat gastrointestinal series showed additional polyps in the small and large intestine.

A second laparotomy was performed at age 14 months. One large gastric polyp and innu-

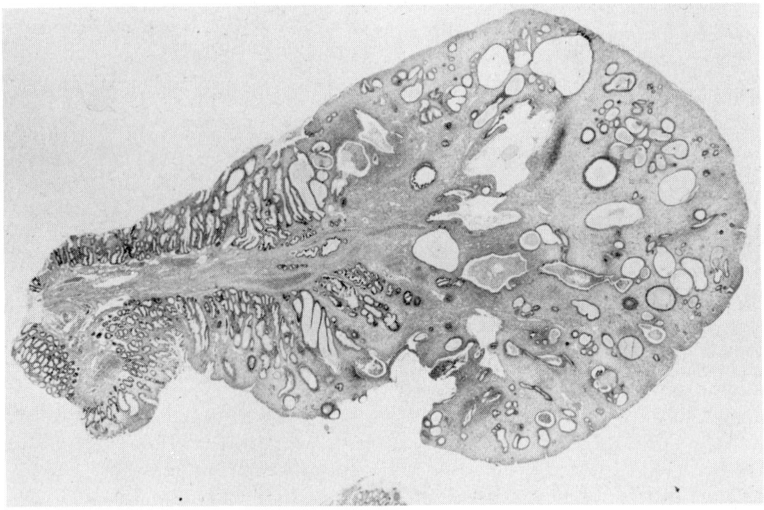

Fig. 1. This colonic polyp obtained from the segment of bowel resected at the age of 14 months is typical of the lesions in this patient. Note especially the smooth surface and the simple glands of various size. (Hematoxylin and eosin. Original magnification ×8.)

merable polyps in the small intestine were removed. The colon was described as filled and bulging with polyps and a subtotal colectomy was performed.

Recurrent bleeding, rectal prolapse, diarrhea, and inanition prompted readmission for the eighth time at age 22 months. Physical examination revealed a cachectic child with prominent abdominal distention and rectal prolapse. In addition, cardiomegaly, a loud systolic murmur, clubbing of her fingers, and hepatomegaly were noted. Laboratory data revealed anemia and hypoalbumenia (albumin, 1.9 Gm. percent). The child could not stand or walk, and she could sit only with support.

The patient was operated on for the third time, and multiple polyps were removed from the stomach, and the small and large bowel. She died in the immediate postoperative period.

PATHOLOGY

The polyps removed at each operation and those found at autopsy were available for study. The polyps ranged from 1 mm. to 3 cm. in size. The larger polyps tended to be predunculated while the smaller polyps were sessile. Small sessile polyps were apparent on the mucosal "stalks" of larger predunculated polyps. The surface epithelium was smooth and not lobulated as are ordinary adenomatous polyps. Mucosal ulcerations were noted on some polyps.

There were no unequivocal polyps in the stomach at autopsy, but the rugal folds were accentuated and some foci were thought to be undergoing polypoid transformation. The large gastric polyp removed at 14 months of age was similar to the intestinal polyps. The polyps were less numerous in the proximal small bowel and were scattered in normal mucosa. The specimens removed from the second and third operations (terminal ileum and colon) as well as the distal ileum and rectosigmoid colon noted at autopsy were virtually bulging because of the mass of polyps.

Microscopically, all the polyps were similar. The superficial epithelium of the polyp was composed of a single layer of goblet cells and colonic columnar epithelial cells with focal denudation, hemorrhage, and superficial ulcers. There was no granulomatous reaction.

The great bulk of the polypoid masses was comprised of innumerable and different sized glandular structures randomly scattered in a closely cellular stromal connective tissue (Figs. 1 and 2).

The glandular structures were lined by a single layer of goblet and columnar epithelial, cells compactly or loosely organized but without papillary formation. Some of the glands were cystically dilated with at-

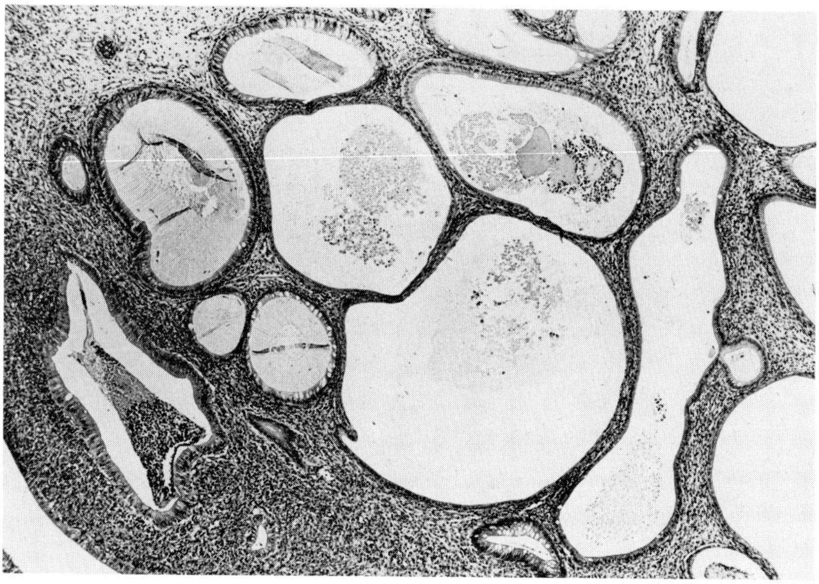

Fig. 2. In this view of another colonic polyp, the glandular epithelium is seen to consist of a single layer of columnar and goblet cells. There is no papillary hyperplasia. Some glands contain partly inspissated secretions, and in some dilated glands the epithelium is attenuated. (Hematoxylin and eosin. Original magnification ×70.)

tenuation of lining epithelium. The lumina of many of the glandular structures were filled with mucus, but some contained polymorphonuclear leukocytes.

The connective tissue framework was relatively acellular and was variably and randomly infiltrated by plasma cells, lymphocytes, and a few polymorphonuclear leukocytes.

At autopsy the oropharynx and esophagus were grossly and microscopically normal. The stomach, duodenum, and proximal jejunum demonstrated focal mucosal and submucosal hemorrhage, but otherwise the intervening mucosa was normal microscopically.

Extraintestinal autopsy findings included: fenestrated defect in membranous interventribular septum but without actual communication between ventricles; left ventricular cardiac hypertrophy; double pelvis of left kidney and double left ureter; and bifid uterus and vagina.

DISCUSSION

There is a striking similarity in this patient's clinical course and pathologic manifestations with those of several other infants now considered to have juvenile polyposis of infancy.[2-4, 6-9, 14]

A brief summary of several of these previously recorded cases follows.

Case 1.[7] A 10-month-old white male presented with a history of diarrhea since birth and was found to have prolapse of polypoid-studded rectal mucosa on initial examination. He was anemic, malnourished (7,500 grams) and "could not walk, crawl or sit up, and was scarcely able to hold up his head." He required repeated transfusions and treatment for rectal "prolapse of major proportion."

At 18 months of age the patient weighed 8,600 grams and was noted to have edema, clubbing of his fingers, and a chronic cough. Intestinal obstruction caused by an ileoileal intussusception required resection, and the infant died one day postoperatively.

Autopsy findings showed polypoid involvement from the cardia of the stomach to the anus.

Case 2.[6] A 4-month-old male presented with intermittent bloody stools, diarrhea, and constipation. Rectal prolapse of polypoid mucosa and abdominal distention were prominent on examination. Sigmoidoscopic removal of numerous polyps was performed on several occasions.

The infant died of intestinal obstruction at six months of age and was noted to have an infarcted ileoileal intussusception at autopsy. Polyps (approximately 170) were present in the fourth part of the duodenum, jejunum, and ileum.

Table I

Author and year	*Sex*	*"Diarrhea"*	*Rectal prolapse*	*Intussusception*
Ravitch[7] (1948)	Male	"From birth"	10 mo.	18 mo.
LeFevre and Jacques[6] (1951)	Male	Onset; 3 mo., bloody	4 mo.	6 mo.
Raymann (1969)	Male	9 mo., bloody	15 mo.	None
Arbeter and associates[2] (1970)	Male	6 wk.	—	7 mo.
Soper and Kent[14] (1971)	Male	3 mo., mucous	9 mo.	10 mo.
Ray and Heald[8] (1971)	Male	9 mo., bloody	2nd yr.	—
Present case	Female	5 mo., guaiac positive	9 mo.	5 mo.; incidental finding

Case 3.[14] A 9-month-old male with macrocephaly presented with rectal prolapse of polypoid-studded mucosa. Reduction required anesthesia.

At ten months, the patient developed an ileocolic intussusception requiring operative reduction. A second laparotomy was performed at one year of age, and 25 polyps were removed from the large and small intestine.

Persistent bloody diarrhea prompted a third laparotomy and colon resection at 18 months. The patient died postoperatively.

Autopsy examination revealed several gastric antral polyps, a few polyps in the duodenum and upper jujenum, and a larger number in the terminal ileum. Polyps were present in the colon with the rectum most involved.

Case 4.[8] A 10-month-old male presented with bloody diarrhea of one month's duration. A left colectomy was performed, and numerous polyps were noted in the specimen.

Rectal bleeding, prolapse, and anemia prompted a second exploratory operation at two years of age. Polyps were noted in the jejunum and ileum, and nine were removed. An abdominal colectomy with a cecorectal anastomosis was performed.

Upper gastrointestinal x-ray films demonstrated gastric, duodenal, jejunal, and ileal polyps at four years of age.

The patient has done well since and now (1973) is 18 years of age. Subsequent x-ray films have demonstrated that some polyps have grown while others have apparently sloughed.

Other possible cases. The seven patients summarized in Table I form the basis of this report. There are several other cases which may well be examples of this syndrome but which are lacking sufficient data for accurate classification:

Soper and Kent[14] cite a case report by Campanello[4] of a 5-month-old infant who died of a jejunal intussusception and who was found to have nearly 300 polyps in the jejunum and colon.

Veale and associates[15] cite a 15-month-old infant studied by I. M. P. Dawson. The patient died of recurrent gastrointestinal hemorrhage and had juvenile polyposis of the entire gastrointestinal tract discovered at autopsy.

Veale and associates[15] reported a female infant who presented at 18 months with rectal bleeding, rectal prolapse, and diarrhea. She had hydrocephalus, hypotonia, and clubbing of the fingers and toes. She had a protocolectomy and ileostomy, but she died at age three years and four months of inanition, polyposis, and hydrocephalus. It is not known whether this patient had gastric or intestinal polyps.

DIAGNOSIS

A composite clinical picture of an infant with juvenile polyposis would be the early

Operative treatment	*Status*	*Distribution of polyps*	*Other manifestation*
Resection of intussusception	Postoperative death	Cardia to anus, no skip areas	Clubbing; peripheral edema; motor retardation
Rectal fulguration	Died at 6 mo.	Jejunum; most numerous in ileum and colon	Duodenal ulcer
Subtotal colectomy ileorectal anastomosis at 16 mo.	Postoperative death	Entire small intestine; most polyps in ileum tract	Macrocephaly hypotonia; retarded motor development; xanthoma on upper lip; hyperlipidemia; 957 mg. %; clubbing; alopecia
Resection at 5 mo.; polypectomy at 7 mo.	Died at 16 mo.	Cardia to rectum	Bilateral hernia
Reduction of intussuception; multiple polypectomies lumus	Postoperative death at 18 mo.	Few in stomas duodenum and jejunum; most in ileum	Macrocephaly; retarded motor development
Colectomy—cecorectal anastomosis at age 2 yr.; repeated polypectomies at 14 years	Alive; known polyps at age 16 years	Stomach, and small and large intestine	None
Multiple polypectomies at 5 mo.; subtotal colectomy at age 14 mo.; colectomy at age 22 mo.	Postoperative death at 22 mo.	Stomach to anus; ileum and colon bulging with polyps	Meckel's diverticulum; peripheral edema; double renal and pelvis; uterus and vagina bifid

development of diarrhea, either bloody or mucoid, associated with anemia, failure to thrive, and an increased susceptibility to pneumonia. Rectal prolapse develops between eight and ten months of age and leads to significant morbidity. Either gastrointestinal bleeding or rectal prolapse would prompt barium contrast studies and the recognition of intestinal polypoid disease.

Sigmoidoscopy and biopsy would establish the diagnosis of multiple juvenile polyps. Laboratory data reveals anemia and hypoproteinemia and suggests protein-losing enteropathy. With the recognition that the infant did not have a premalignant form of intestinal polyposis and with the knowledge of the natural history of the disease, treatment would thereby be on a more rational basis.

The genetics of this syndrome are unclear. It appears to be a nonsex-linked recessive gene. The parents and siblings of the present patient are alive and well without gastrointestinal symptoms. There is no history of other cases of intestinal polyposis in any of the other families. The clinical course of each of these seven patients is summarized in Table I.

TREATMENT

Supportive treatment. Diarrhea should be treated vigorously with fluid replacement as well as specific antidiarrheal medication. Since the diarrhea may result from a low-grade infection of the polyps, a trial of broad-spectrum antibiotic agents would appear reasonable and worthwhile. Oral elemental diet preparations may be tried to see if decreasing roughage would lessen the tendency of juvenile polyps to become ulcerated and infected.

Supportive treatment must be both anticipatory and vigorous since each of these infants has suffered from severe recurrent anemia, diarrhea, malabsorption, malnutrition, and hypoproteinemia. Soper and Kent[14] suggest that prolonged intravenous hyperalimentation may be advantageous.

Operative treatment.

Rectal prolapse. As many rectal polyps as possible should be removed to reduce their tendency to act as the leading point of the prolapse. Since the polyps have no malignant potential, fulguration is appropriate. The scarring between the mucosa and submucosa resulting from repeated fulguration conceivably could reduce the tendency toward recurrent prolapse.

Intestinal polyps. The indications for operation are recurrent severe blood loss requiring transfusions, persistent diarrhea with weight loss, or signs of partial small bowel obstruction. The most severely involved areas of the gastrointestinal tract, usually the terminal ileum and colon, should be resected. Numerous enterotomies are indicated to remove isolated easily palpable polyps in the stomach and small bowel.

Careful barium contrast studies of the stomach and the small and large bowel should be available to help the surgeon plan his operative procedure. Although the distribution of the juvenile polyps is unpredictable, the polyps have been most numerous and largest in the terminal ileum and colon. Intussusception developed in each of the infants and led to emergency operations in three and death in three patients. Two patients in this series initially had a subtotal colectomy with some short-term benefit, only to require a repeat procedure because of extensive residual colon involvement.

Realistic appraisal of the intestinal pathology in several of these infants suggests that long-term survival may be possible in some but doubtful in others. The extent of initial involvement, the tendency of the juvenile polyps to recur, and their size will be the ultimate determinants. Factors that influence the degree of initial involvement are unknown, but it is quite likely that some of these patients begin to develop polyps in utero.

BEHAVIOR OF JUVENILE POLYPS AND RELATIONSHIP OF JUVENILE POLYPOSIS OF INFANCY TO OTHER FORMS OF JUVENILE POLYPOSIS

Although the polypoid lesions in each of these patients were classified as "adenomas," "adenomatous polyps," and "multiple polyps" initially, they appear now to be typical juvenile-type polyps.

Weller and McCall[16] consider juvenile polyps to represent hamartomas of connective tissue, and both tissue culture studies and electron microscopy support this view.[3, 10, 16] Alexander and associates[1] suggest an allergic etiology for some juvenile polyps. There is no evidence that juvenile polyps are either premalignant per se, or that they occur in individuals with an increased tendency to develop cancer elsewhere.

Although large series of children have been diagnosed as having one or more juvenile polyps, it is only recently that juvenile polyps have been recognized to occur in older patients, and to involve the entire gastrointestinal tract.[3, 5, 13]

It is uncertain at the present time whether juvenile polyposis is one disease with a spectrum of variable manifestations or whether there are several distinct entities of intestinal juvenile polyposis. Veale and associates[15] and Bussey[3] have collected records of more than thirty patients with multiple juvenile gastrointestinal polyps and consider this one syndrome with variable manifestations. Franklin and McSwain[5] reported five patients with multiple juvenile polyps.

Sachatello[12] prefers to classify the Juvenile Polyposis into three sub-groups: (1) juvenile polyposis of infancy; (2) juvenile polyposis coli; and (3) generalized juvenile gastrointestinal polyposis.

The reasons for this classification are as follows: (1) to emphasize that juvenile polyposis in infancy carries an unfavorable prognosis and is associated with recurrent gastrointestinal bleeding, rectal prolapse and intussusception; (2) to point out that the colon may be extensively involved with juvenile polyps (This distribution of polyps may lead to an erroneous diagnosis of familial, or adenomatous, polyposis coli and needlessly agressive treatment); (3) to indicate that some patients with generalized gastrointestinal polyposis have a distribution of polyps similar to that of Peutz-Jeghers syndrome (The former patients do not have melanin pigmentation).

The ultimate classification of the various forms of juvenile polyposis awaits detailed case reports describing the manifestations in other patients and eludication of the underlying developmental abnormalities.

SUMMARY

A case of extensive juvenile gastrointestinal polyposis in a female infant is reported. This patient is the first female to be recognized with this syndrome. Detailed study of her clinical course and intestinal pathology helps establish the natural history of a newly recognized entity, juvenile polyposis of infancy.

This syndrome is distinct from Peutz Jeghers syndrome and familial polyposis of the colon. It is characterized by gastrointestinal bleeding, diarrhea, recurrent rectal prolapse, inanition, and intussusception in infants.

Prognosis is directly related to the severity and extent of gastrointestinal involvement with juvenile polyps. Vigorous medical management and resection of the most severely involved areas of the gastrointestinal tract (usually ileum and colon) offer a reasonable possibility for long-term survival. Six of seven infants with extensive juvenile polyposis died before age two years.

REFERENCES

1. Alexander, R. H., Beckwith, J. B., Morgan, A., and Bill, A. H.: Juvenile polyps of the colon and their relationship to allergy, Am. J. Surg. **120:** 222, 1970.
2. Arbeter, A. M., Courtney, R. A., and Gaynor, A. F., Jr.: Diffuse gastrointestinal polyposis associated with chronic blood loss, hypoproteinemia and anasarca in an infant, J. Pediatr. **76:** 609, 1970.
3. Bussey, H. J. R.: Gastrointestinal polyposis, Gut **11:** 978, 1970.
4. Campanello, N.: Polyposi intestinale diffusa in un lattante, Rirasc. Med. **17:** 299, 1940.
5. Franklin, R., and McSwain, B.: Juvenile polyps of colon and rectum, Ann. Surg. **175:** 887, 1972.
6. LeFevre, H. W., Jr., and Jacques, T. F.: Multiple polyposis in an infant of four months, Am. J. Surg. **81:** 90, 1951.
7. Ravitch, M. M.: Polypoid adenomatosis of the entire gastrointestinal tract, Ann. Surg. **128:** 283, 1948.
8. Ray, J. E., and Heald, R. J.: Growing up with juvenile gastrointestinal polyposis, Dis. Colon Rectum **14:** 375, 1971.
9. Raymann, F. B.: Juvenile polyps with cachexia, Gastroenterology **57:** 431, 1969.
10. Romer, H., Cotte, C., and Essenfeld-Yahr, E.: Behavior of the rectal juvenile polyp in vitro, Gut **12:** 194, 1971.
11. Sachatello, C. R.: Familial polyposis of the colon, Cancer **28:** 581, 1971.
12. Sachatello, C. R.: Gastrointestinal polypoid diseases, J. Ky. Med. Assoc. **70:** 540, 1972.
13. Sachatello, C. R., Pickren, J. W., and Grace, J. T., Jr.: Generalized juvenile gastrointestinal polyposis, Gastroenterology **58:** 699, 1970.
14. Soper, R. T., and Kent, T. H.: Fatal juvenile polyposis in infancy, SURGERY **69:** 692, 1971.
15. Veale, A. M. O., McCall, I., Bussey, H. J. R., and Morson, B. C.: Juvenile polyposis coli, J. Med. Genet. **3:** 5, 1966.
16. Weller, R. O., and McCall, I.: Electron microscopic appearance of juvenile and Peutz Jeglers polyps, Gut **7:** 265, 1966.

Clinical reviews

Postoperative deep vein thrombosis and pulmonary embolism: A selective review and personal viewpoint

John Joakim Skillman, M.D., *Boston, Mass.*

Deep vein thrombosis (DVT) is a problem of far greater proportions than heretofore thought. The advent of the I^{125} fibrinogen scan in 1959 has added greatly to the knowledge of its natural history; and its use in routine screening has shown that DVT occurs in a large percentage of patients undergoing all types of surgical procedures. Pulmonary embolism is one of the commonest causes of death after operation; it is the greatest single cause of maternal deaths due to childbirth. Its late sequelae represent some of the commonest intractable problems in surgery. Presented in this review are noninvasive and invasive methods of establishing the diagnosis of DVT, the value of prophylactic physical and pharmacologic measures to prevent DVT, and the treatment of established DVT and pulmonary embolism.

From the Department of Surgery, Harvard Medical School and the Beth Israel Hospital, Boston, Mass.

THE MAGNITUDE of the problem of deep vein thrombosis (DVT) in injured patients was suggested by earlier reports such as the one by Sevitt and Gallagher[56] in 1959 who found that in an unselected series of fatally injured patients, 60 percent had DVT without pulmonary embolism and over 80 percent of elderly patients who died after a fractured femur had this complication. The advent of the I^{125} fibrinogen scan by Atkins and Hawkins[3] in 1965 has contributed greatly to our knowledge of the natural history of DVT, and with the adoption of this technique for routine screening, it has been shown that DVT occurs in 30 to 60 percent of patients undergoing general surgical operations,[13, 31] in 54 percent of patients undergoing orthopedic operations,[12] in 50 percent of patients having urological operations,[37, 44] and in 18 percent of patients having gynecological operations.[17] Pulmonary embolism is one of the commonest causes of death after operation.[31] Not only is pulmonary embolism a frequent occurrence in prostrating medical illness, but it is also the greatest single cause of maternal deaths due to childbirth.[26] Apart from the immediate risk to life, the late sequelae of swelling of the leg, varicose ulceration, and other trophic changes after DVT represent some of the commonest intractable problems in surgery.

In this selective review, I will consider

This work was supported by United States Public Health Service Grant No. HL 05422.

Accepted for publication July 19, 1973.

noninvasive and invasive methods of establishing the diagnosis of DVT, the value of prophylactic physical and pharmacologic measures to prevent DVT, and, finally, the treatment of established DVT and pulmonary embolism.

DIAGNOSIS OF DVT

Clinical examination. Clinical examination has been the mainstay of surgeons to make the diagnosis of DVT, and the signs of swelling of the ankle, leg, and thigh, tenderness of the calf and popliteal area, and a positive Homan's sign are well known. Unfortunately, many investigators have shown that if one relies solely on physical findings the diagnosis of DVT will be missed in about 50 percent of patients.[13] Because of the frequent failure of clinical examination to provide a positive diagnosis, an attempt has been made to find noninvasive methods to detect DVT, since ascending contrast phlebography cannot be clinically justified or routinely employed as a screening technique.

Noninvasive methods.

Impedance plethysmography. This technique has been employed by Mullick and sociates[43] to detect DVT; they originally reported only two of 79 patients in whom the results of venography disagreed with the impedance study. This technique is based on the assumption that if the venous system in the lower extremity is patent, the blood volume, and, therefore, the electrical impedence in the legs changes with respiration as venous returns waxes and wanes. In the presence of DVT, there should be little or no change in either limb blood volume or electrical impedance with respiration because of obstruction to venous blood flow and lack of transmission of the venous pulse. At our hospital, this technique has been used as a screening technique in 111 patients (410 examinations). Only 21 of the 111 patients were studied by both impedance plethysmography and venography, and false negative impedence studies occurred in more than one third of the 21 patients. Three patients who had positive impedance studies also had positive venograms and no instances of false positive impedance studies were found.[59] Others have found an over-all accuracy of only about 50 percent.[9] The reliability of the impedance technique to accurately detect DVT seems questionable to me when the test is negative. When the test is positive, its reliability appears to be greater than 90 percent.[9, 59] Patients who are unable to cooperate by holding still or taking a deep breath (approximately 20 percent of patients[59]) cannot be screened by this technique, a further limitation in its general applicability.

Ultrasonic velocity detection. This technique has been advocated to detect DVT by Strandness and Sumner[60] and also by Evans.[10] This method utilizes the Doppler principle. When ultrasound encounters moving particles in the blood, the frequency of the sound is shifted by an amount proportional to the velocity of flow. The backscattered frequencies and nonshifted signal from stationary tissues are detected by a receiving crystal and mixed to produce a beat signal which is amplified to drive a loudspeaker or provide an analogue output or both. Strandness and Sumner[60] reported that the ultrasonic technique accurately predicted DVT in 93 per cent of 53 patients who either had venography or operation for confirmation. They stated that considerable experience is needed to perform the technique well. Milne and co-workers[39] evaluated 75 general surgical patients by I^{125} scans, venography, and ultrasound, and they found that ultrasound gave a high incidence of false positive and false negative tests as compared to the I^{125} scans and venography. The ultrasound technique has the advantage of being able to detect DVT in the iliofemoral segment but shares with the impedance technique the disadvantage of not being able to detect accurately nonocclusive thrombi, especially in the soleal veins where flow may not be reduced.

I^{125} fibrinogen scanning. This technique has been used with increasing frequency, particularly by British investigators, especially Flanc and associates,[13, 14] Kakkar and co-workers,[30, 31] and Nicolaides[12, 31, 45] who have

had an extensive experience with this technique. The radioactive fibrinogen is incorporated into newly forming thrombi, and the activity is monitored by scanning over multiple positions in the leg and thigh with a portable scintillation counter. By using this technique, Kakkar and co-workers[30] found DVT in 30 percent of 132 consecutive postoperative patients. In 14 patients, venography showed that the thrombus was located only in the soleal or tibial veins, and spontaneous lysis of these thrombi occurred within 72 hours. In 26 patients, the thrombosis persisted for more than 72 hours, and four of these patients developed pulmonary embolism. Venography showed that nine of these 26 patients had thrombi which extended into the femoral or popliteal veins. Of the 40 patients with positive radioactive fibrinogen scans, 39 had positive phlebograms. The remaining 92 patients did not develop DVT, and none of these patients developed pulmonary embolism.

The radioactive fibrinogen technique has added greatly to our knowledge of the natural history of DVT. The test is not completely reliable in patients who have established DVT and in whom fibrinogen is not still being incorporated into clots.[36] It is also not reliable for the detection of iliac or pelvic vein thrombosis. This test has the advantage of being able to detect lysis of clots which are not clinically significant when serial studies are performed over five to seven days. It seems to me that the I^{125} fibrinogen scan is the single most sensitive, accurate, and useful noninvasive test to diagnose DVT. I think that the test should be used in all patients who have an increased tendency to develop postoperative DVT[31] and in whom some form of prophylactic anticoagulation is not employed. The radioactive fibrinogen technique has not yet become widespread in the United States, however, because of limited access to hepatitis-free labeled fibrinogen and because of the expense of trained personnel and monitoring equipment.

Invasive methods. All noninvasive techniques to establish the diagnosis of DVT must be compared with *ascending phlebography,* since this method is the most sensitive and complete and can also be applied for the iliofemoral venous segment. This method cannot be recommended as a routine screening procedure, however, because of time, labor, cost, and some risk to the patient. Occasional episodes of pain and tenderness strongly suggestive of dye-induced superficial phlebitis or even deep vein phlebitis have occurred in the leg after this examination, but no cases of pulmonary embolism following ascending contrast phlebography have thus far been seen in our own patient group. The present technique now in use at our hospital places the patient in the semi-upright position supporting his weight on the contralateral noninvolved foot.[50] Dye injection is made into the dorsal pedal vein and no tourniquet is used. Under fluoroscopic control, 75 to 125 ml. of contrast medium is injected over a 1½ to 3 minute period and serial films are taken in the anteroposterior and lateral positions. This specific technique regularly fills all the superficial and deep veins from foot to pelvis.

I believe that the use of ascending phlebography should be reserved for patients who have clinical signs and symptoms suggestive of DVT, in whom the alternative differential diagnoses of cellulitis, local calf hematoma following injury, or superficial phlebitis, conditions which do not require anticoagulation cannot easily be excluded. Noninvasive methods (impedance plethysmography or ultrasonic flow detection) may be useful adjuncts here, although if the results of these tests are negative, venography should be employed to settle the issue before embarking on a prolonged course of anticoagulation. The exceedingly low incidence of either false positive or false negative I^{125} fibrinogen scans makes venography unnecessary if a positive diagnosis has been established by this screening technique. In my opinion, patients with classical symptoms and physical findings of DVT do not require *any* additional diagnostic tests to justify the institution of a course of anticoagulant therapy.

VALUE OF PROPHYLACTIC MEASURES TO PREVENT DVT

Physical measures. The physical measures designed to reduce the incidence of postoperative DVT have been examined by two groups. Flanc and associates[14] studied the effect of an intensive program of prophylactic physical measures to prevent DVT in a consecutive group of 65 control patients admitted for elective surgery and a second group of 67 test patients who were instructed preoperatively by a physical therapist in active quadriceps exercises and in leg elevation with active plantar flexion exercises against a footboard and who also wore below-knee heavy-duty elastic stockings. The test group wore elastic stockings during operation and had exercises supervised six times daily in the postoperative period. Both groups were made to walk early. The diagnosis of DVT was based on the I^{125} fibrinogen scan. The incidence of DVT was 35 percent in the control group and 25 percent in the test group, an insignificant difference. However, when the patients were subdivided into those having major operations whose ages ranged between 61 and 80 years, the incidence of DVT was 61 percent in the control group and 24 percent in the test group, a significant difference ($p < 0.05$). In addition, the rate of spontaneous clot lysis was 5.9 days in the control group and 2.6 days in the test group, also a significant difference ($p < 0.01$). I strongly suspect that the intensive prophylactic measures used by Flanc and co-workers[14] would strain the resources of most hospitals, and yet, the result is a clear-cut benefit at least in the elderly group undergoing major operations.

Another nonrandomized study by Tsapogas and co-workers,[61] who also used I^{125} fibrinogen scans, showed that the use of below-knee elastic stockings, elevation of the foot of the bed 30 degrees, ambulation without sitting, and passive and active foot flexion exercises reduced the incidence of DVT from 14 percent in the control group to 4 percent in the test group. Statistical evaluation of the results of this study was not provided, but the authors concluded that these measures were strongly recommended. A randomized study by Rosengarten and co-workers,[52] who also employed I^{125} fibrinogen scans for diagnosis evaluated the effect of compression stockings in 50 patients over 40 years old undergoing elective operations. The incidence of DVT was 32 percent in *both* control and test groups.

It seems reasonable to conclude from these data that patients in the high-risk elderly group undergoing major surgery may be significantly protected from DVT by a combination of physical means, but one can only guess as to the individual merit of any one maneuver.

Drugs.

Warfarin. The efficacy of drugs which interfere with the development of red thrombi[8] in the prevention of DVT was initially based on autopsy evidence provided in the controlled clinical trial reported by Sevitt and Gallagher,[56] who used phenindione in 300 patients with fractured hips. Pulmonary embolism did not occur in any patients receiving anticoagulant agents, but this complication did develop in 18 percent of the control group, and fatal embolism occurred in ten percent. Clinically detectable DVT occurred in 29 percent of the control group, but only in three percent of the phenindione-treated patients. In another controlled study, Salzman and co-workers[53] found that clinically detectable thromboembolic complications were significantly reduced in patients with fracture of the hip when prophylactic warfarin was administered to keep the one-stage prothrombin time between 1.5 and 2.5 times control values.

Antiplatelet agents. Anatomic studies by Paterson[48] and by Sevitt[55] have identified platelet thrombi in valve cusps in established venous thrombosis. Adhesion of platelets to subendothelial connective tissue and aggregation of platelets are relatively unaffected by heparin and oral anticoagulants. These findings have led to the suggestion that agents which interfere with platelet function may be useful to prevent venous thromboembolism.

DEXTRAN. The value of dextran 40 to prevent venous thromboembolism has been established in patients having total hip replacement. Harris and co-workers[24] found that clinically detectable thromboembolic disease occurred in ten percent of 227 randomized patients treated with dextran 40 in comparison to 7.9 percent of patients receiving warfarin, an insignificant difference. A control group was not included in this study because of the already proved statistically higher 39 percent incidence of thromboembolic complications in a previously studied control group of patients who underwent vitallium mold arthroplasty of the hip[23] and who were not protected by prophylactic antithrombotic agents. Most other studies with dextran[2, 11, 27] have also shown protection. However, it is my view that the occasional side effects of hemodilution which may result in congestive heart failure, rare, but severe, allergic reactions, and renal failure, make this drug unacceptable as a standard form of prophylactic therapy for DVT.

DIPYRIDAMOLE AND ASPIRIN. Salzman and associates[54] examined the prophylactic effect of postoperative dipyridamole (400 mg. per day divided into four doses), aspirin (0.6 Gm. twice daily), dextran 40 (500 ml. of ten percent solution daily for 4 days and then every three days), and warfarin (in doses intended to achieve a prothrombin time of 1.5 to 2.0 times the control value) in 169 patients undergoing vitallium mold arthroplasty of the hip. Dipyridamole was dropped from the trial after 34 patients had been treated with this drug because 26 percent developed thromboembolic complications. The incidence of thromboembolism in the aspirin and dextran–treated groups was approximately the same as those patients receiving warfarin, and all three drugs gave significant protection in comparison to a 39 percent incidence of thromboembolism in a previously studied group of unprotected control patients. Another double-blind randomized study[51] published by the Medical Research Council in Britain which included 303 patients undergoing elective operations in whom the diagnosis of DVT was established by I^{125} fibrinogen scans indicated no protective effect of aspirin. On the basis of these studies, the use of dipyridamole and aspirin cannot be recommended as safe prophylactic antithrombotic measures.

Low dose subcutaneous heparin. A large number of controlled studies have now been published in which the use of low dose subcutaneous heparin (5,000 units of heparin given every twelve hours subcutaneously beginning preoperatively) to prevent DVT has been studied with the radioactive fibrinogen technique. The rationale for this therapy is based on the presence of a potent naturally occurring inhibitor to activated factor X in human plasma[63] and upon the observation that the activity of this inhibitor (antithrombin III) is enhanced by heparin.[64] These studies, principally by Nicolaides and associates, Kakkar and co-workers,[33, 34] Williams,[62] and Gordon-Smith and colleagues,[20] may be summarized by saying that the use of this form of heparin appears to give significant protection against the development of DVT in general surgical patients, but not in patients undergoing open prostatectomy,[62] operation for fracture of the hip,[34] or after myocardial infarction,[22] although a recent article by Gallus and co-workers[18] suggests that low dose subcutaneous heparin may protect against the development of DVT in this latter group. When the frequency of the dose of subcutaneous heparin is increased to every eight hours, the incidence of bleeding complications may be prohibitive, and the recent study by Gallus and co-workers[18] indicated that blood loss in the operative period is greater in heparin-treated patients. On the basis of this information, I believe it is reasonable to conclude that the use of subcutaneous low dose heparin (5,000 units, given subcutaneously every 12 hours) should be much more widely adopted as a prophylactic measure in general surgical patients.

Relative to the use of prophylactic measures certain questions arise:

Is there a high risk group? Kakkar and co-workers[31] studied this question by the I^{125}

fibrinogen technique in 203 consecutive patients over 40 years of age undergoing operations of large magnitude and concluded that: (1) Sixty-eight percent of patients with a previous history of DVT or pulmonary embolism developed DVT again ($p < 0.01$). Only 26 percent of those patients with no previous history developed DVT. Of six patients with a previous history of both DVT and pulmonary embolism, all six developed DVT again. (2) If varicose veins were present, DVT developed in 56 percent ($p < 0.01$). (3) Obese patients had a 48 percent incidence of DVT ($p < 0.01$). (4) DVT was significantly more common in patients in the 61 to 80 year age group (46 percent incidence of DVT, $p < 0.01$). (5) Patients with malignancy also had a higher incidence of DVT (41 percent, $p = 0.04$).

Therefore, a previous history of DVT or pulmonary embolism, presence of varicose veins, obesity, elderly age, and malignancy all predispose to DVT. Patients who demonstrate these predisposing factors should be placed on prophylactic low dose subcutaneous heparin or warfarin before operation. In the event that a contraindication to prophylactic anticoagulation exists, the I^{125} fibrinogen scan should be employed as a screening technique in this high-risk group of patients.

Where and when does DVT occur? Kakkar and co-workers[30] and Nicolaides and colleagues[45] have shown that DVT almost always starts in the tibial veins and soleal sinuses and then extends more proximally into the popliteal and femoral veins, although this technique does not sample the iliofemoral venous segment. However, Mavor and co-workers[36] have challenged the viewpoint that DVT resulting in pulmonary embolism usually starts in the calf veins, stating that about two thirds of all emboli arise from the iliofemoral segment. Mavor's conclusions were subsequently rebutted by Kakkar,[29] who pointed out that Mavor's criticisms were drawn from the use of I^{125} fibrinogen test under inappropriate circumstances, namely, the use of this test under situations of *established* DVT, since labeled fibrinogen may not be incorporated into a thrombus which is either stationary or dissolving.[28] Flanc and associates[13] and Kakkar and co-workers[31] have also shown that about half of the thrombi detected by the labeled fibrinogen technique develop *during the operation* itself.

What is the clinical significance of the diagnosis of DVT based on I^{125} fibrinogen scans? In patients who have raised counts persisting for more than 72 hours, Kakkar and colleagues[30] showed that about 35 percent will have extension of the clot into the popliteal and femoral veins, and when this occurs the chance of developing a pulmonary embolus are about 40 percent, whereas the risk of developing pulmonary embolism from thrombi that remain limited to the calf is extremely low. In other words, the chance of developing a pulmonary embolus when the I^{125} fibrinogen scan is positive is about 10 to 15 percent.[47]

TREATMENT OF ESTABLISHED DVT AND PULMONARY EMBOLISM

Intravenous heparin followed by administration of warfarin sodium (Coumadin) is the primary treatment for established DVT and pulmonary embolism in patients who do not have a major contraindication to anticoagulation therapy. It is not yet known with certainty what method of administration or dosage schedule of heparin is best. Heparin must be continued for approximately five days after the initiation of warfarin therapy even when the one-stage prothrombin time indicates therapeutic levels have been reached before this, since this test may be responsive to depression of clotting factors with a short half-life before clinical anticoagulation protection is reached. The major risk of this therapy is bleeding. It has recently been suggested that the activated partial thromboplastin time may be useful in monitoring heparin therapy,[18] although the precise relationship between the level of the partial thromboplastin time and the incidence of bleeding complications is not yet established.

Operative treatment. When therapy with anticoagulants for established DVT and pulmonary embolism is contraindicated or fails, some form of venous interruption is necessary.

Venous thrombectomy for iliofemoral DVT. This procedure was popular a number of years ago.[16, 21, 57] The major rationale for this treatment was the prevention of postphlebitic sequelae. Follow-up study of these patients showed that this treatment did not really prevent destruction of the venous valves, and postoperative venograms performed in patients who had thrombectomy demonstrated a high incidence of rethrombosis.[4, 16] It seems likely to me that venous thrombectomy is only indicated in the rare case of phlegmasia cerulea dolens when portions of the limb are threatened.[15, 19] Perhaps in these cases where extensive thrombosis predisposes the patient to gangrene, this procedure may have a role, although it is by no means clear even here.

Caval ligation. This is the preferred means of venous interruption for patients with DVT and pulmonary embolism. I believe this viewpoint is definitely justified for patients in whom the problem is multiple small emboli. When septic pulmonary emboli develop from a pelvic focus in women, caval ligation should be performed transabdominally just below the renal veins to prevent the development of a stagnant cul-de-sac, and the left ovarian vein should be ligated simultaneously. Various clips[1, 7, 38, 42] and plication[58] methods for inferior vena caval interruption have also been used successfully. The rationale for this partial interruption technique is that the clip or plication will not completely interrupt venous return and also that the postphlebitic sequelae might be decreased in comparison to patients who have caval ligation. Follow-up studies indicate that the vena cava frequently clots below the clip and pulmonary emboli from clots extending through the clips have been reported.[6] Nevertheless, these techniques have a role in seriously ill patients with congestive heart failure, since the immediate hemodynamic effects of caval ligation are minimized by their use.[25, 35]

Transvenous caval interruption with an umbrella filter. This procedure has been used extensively by Mobin-Uddin and colleagues.[41] It has the advantage of being able to perform the insertion under local anesthesia. Embolization of the filter, recurrent pulmonary embolization, malposition of the filter into the iliac or renal veins,[40] and perforation of the ureter[49] have been reported, however, and I do not believe that it is likely that this method will replace the more traditional types of caval interruption. Use of the umbrella filter should probably be restricted to patients who have severe congestive heart failure with refractory hypotension or to those patients who have recent myocardial infarction.[5]

Femoral vein interruption. This method appears to have a place in selected sick patients in whom phlebography (or fibrinogen scans) show clot confined to the calf. This procedure can be accomplished easily while the patient is under local anesthesia.

REFERENCES

1. Adams, J. T., and DeWeese, J. A.: Experimental and clinical evaluation of partial vein interruption in prevention of pulmonary emboli, SURGERY 57: 82, 1965.
2. Atik, M., Harkess, J. W., and Wickman, H.: Prevention of fatal pulmonary embolism, Surg. Gynecol. Obstet. **130:** 403, 1970.
3. Atkins, P., and Hawkins, L. A.: Detection of venous thrombosis in the legs, Lancet **2:** 1217, 1965.
4. Barner, H. B., Willman, V. L., Kaiser, G. C., and Hanlon, C. R.: Thrombectomy for ileofemoral venous thrombosis, J.A.M.A. **208:** 2442, 1969.
5. Crane, C.: The Mobin-Uddin inferior vena caval filter, Arch. Surg. **103:** 661, 1971.
6. DeMeester, T. R., Rutherford, R. B., Blazek, J. V., and Zuidema, G. D.: Plication of the inferior vena cava for thromboembolism, SURGERY **62:** 56, 1967.
7. DeWeese, M. S., and Hunter, D. C., Jr.: Vena cava filter for prevention of pulmonary embolism: Five-year clinical experience, Arch. Surg. **86:** 852, 1963.
8. Deykin, D.: Thrombogenesis, N. Engl. J. Med. **276:** 622, 1967.
9. Dmochowski, J. D., Adams, D. F., and Couch, N. P.: Impedance measurement in the

diagnosis of deep vein thrombosis, Arch. Surg. **104:** 170, 1972.
10. Evans, D. S.: The early diagnosis of deep-vein thrombosis by ultrasound, Br. J. Surg. **57:** 726, 1970.
11. Evarts, C. M., and Feil, E. J.: Prevention of thromboembolic disease after elective surgery of the hip, J. Bone Joint Surg. **53A:** 1271, 1971.
12. Field, E. S., Nicolaides, A. N., Kakkar, V. V., and Crellin, R. Q.: Deep vein thrombosis in patients with fractures of the femoral neck, Br. J. Surg. **59:** 377, 1972.
13. Flanc, C., Kakkar, V. V., and Clarke, M. B.: The detection of venous thrombosis of the legs using ^{125}I-labelled fibrinogen, Br. J. Surg. **55:** 742, 1968.
14. Flanc, C., Kakkar, V. V., and Clarke, M. B.: Postoperative deep-vein thrombosis—Effect of intensive prophylaxis, Lancet **1:** 477, 1969.
15. Fogarty, T. J., Cranley, J. J., Krause, R. J., Strasser, E. S., and Hafner, C. D.: Surgical management of phlegmasia cerulea dolens, Arch. Surg. **86:** 256, 1963.
16. Fogarty, T. J., Dennis, D., and Krippaehne, W. W.: Surgical management of ileofemoral venous thrombosis, Am. J. Surg. **112:** 211, 1966.
17. Friend, J. R., and Kakkar, V. V.: Deep vein thrombosis in obstetric and gynecological patients, *in* Kakkar, V. V., and Jouhar, A. J., editors: Thromboembolism: Diagnosis and treatment, Edinburgh, 1972, E. & S. Livingstone, Ltd., pp. 131-138.
18. Gallus, A. S., Hirsch, J., Tuttle, R. J., Trebilcock, R., O'Brien, S. E., Caroll, J. J., Minden, J. H., and Hudecki, S. M.: Small doses of heparin in prevention of venous thrombosis, N. Engl. J. Med. **288:** 545, 1973.
19. Galvin, C.: Phlegmasia cerulea dolens, Angiology **22:** 237, 1971.
20. Gordon-Smith, I. C., Grundy, D. J., LeQuesne, L. P., Newcombe, J. F., and Bramble, F. J.: Controlled trial of two regimens of subcutaneous heparin in prevention of postoperative deep-vein thrombosis, Lancet **1:** 1133, 1972.
21. Haller, J. A.: Thrombectomy for deep thrombophlebitis of the leg, N. Engl. J. Med. **267:** 65, 1962.
22. Handley, A. J.: Low-dose heparin after myocardial infarction, Lancet **2:** 623, 1972.
23. Harris, W. H., Salzman, E. W., and DeSanctis, R. W.: The prevention of thromboembolic disease by prophylactic anticoagulation—A controlled trial in elective hip surgery, J. Bone Joint Surg. **49A:** 81, 1967.
24. Harris, W. H., Salzman, E. W., DeSanctis, R. W., and Coutts, R. D.: Prevention of venous thromboembolism following total hip replacement—Warfarin versus Dextran 40, J.A.M.A. **220:** 1319, 1972.
25. Harsanyi, P. G., Rius-Garriga, J., and Moser, K. M.: Acute hemodynamic consequences of ligation of the inferior vena cava, J. Thorac. Cardiovasc. Surg. **57:** 442, 1969.
26. Jeffcoate, T. N. A., Miller, J., Roos, R. F., and Tindall, V. R.: Puerperal thromboembolism in relation to the inhibitor of lactation by oestrogen therapy, Br. Med. J. **4:** 19, 1968.
27. Johansson, S. R., Bygdernan, S., and Eliasson, R.: Effect of dextran on postoperative thrombosis, Acta Chir. Scand. Suppl. **387:** 80, 1968.
28. Kakkar, V. V.: The diagnosis of deep vein thrombosis using the ^{125}I fibrinogen test, Arch. Surg. **104:** 152, 1972.
29. Kakkar, V. V.: Letter to the editor, Lancet **1:** 909, 1972.
30. Kakkar, V. V., Howe, C. T., Flanc, C., and Clarke, M. B.: Natural history of postoperative deep-vein thrombosis, Lancet **2:** 230, 1969.
31. Kakkar, V. V., Howe, C. T., Nicolaides, A. N., Renney, J. T. G., and Clarke, M. B.: Deep vein thrombosis of the leg: Is there a high risk group? Am. J. Surg. **120:** 527, 1970.
32. Kakkar, V. V., Nicolaides, A. N., Renney, J. T. G., Friend, J. R., and Clarke, M. B.: ^{125}I-labelled fibrinogen test adapted for routine screening for deep vein thrombosis, Lancet **1:** 540, 1970.
33. Kakkar, V. V., Field, E. S., Nicolaides, A. N., Flute, P. T., Wessler, S., and Yin, E. T.: Low doses of heparin in prevention of deep vein thrombosis, Lancet **2:** 669, 1971.
34. Kakkar, V. V., Corrigan, T., Spindler, J., Fossard, D. P., Flute, P. T., and Crellin, R. Q.: Efficacy of low doses of heparin in prevention of deep vein thrombosis after major surgery, Lancet **2:** 101, 1972.
35. Little, J. M., and Goodman, A. H.: An experimental study of the hemodynamics of occlusion of the inferior vena cava, Surg., Gynecol. Obstet. **128:** 1, 1969.
36. Mavor, G. E., Mahaffy, R. G., Walker, M. G., Duthie, J. S., Dhall, D. P., Gaddie, J., and Reid, G. F.: Peripheral venous scanning with ^{125}I-tagged fibrinogen, Lancet **1:** 661, 1972.
37. Mayo, M. E., Halil, T., and Browse, N. L.: The incidence of deep vein thrombosis after prostatectomy, Br. J. Urol. **43:** 738, 1971.
38. Miles, R. M., Chapell, F., and Renner, O.: Partially occluding vena caval clip for prevention of pulmonary embolism, Am. Surg. **30:** 40, 1964.
39. Milne, R. M., Gunn, A. A., Griffiths, J. M.

T., and Ruckley, C. V.: Postoperative deep vein thrombosis—A comparison of diagnostic techniques, Lancet **2:** 445, 1971.
40. Mobin-Uddin, K., Trinkle, J. K., and Bryant, L. R.: Present status of the inferior vena cava umbrella filter, SURGERY **70:** 914, 1971.
41. Mobin-Uddin, K., Callard, G. M., Bolooki, H., Rubinson, R., Michie, D., and Jude, J. R.: Transvenous caval interruption with umbrella filter, N. Engl. J. Med. **286:** 55, 1972.
42. Moretz, W. H., Rhode, C. M., and Sheperd, M. H.: Prevention of pulmonary embolism by partial occlusion of the inferior vena cava, Am. Surg. **25:** 617, 1959.
43. Mullick, S. C., Wheeler, H. B., and Songster, G. P.: Diagnosis of deep venous thrombosis by measurement of electrical impedance, Am. J. Surg. **119:** 417, 1970.
44. Nicolaides, A. N., Field, E. S., Kakkar, V. V., Yates-Bell, A. J., Taylor, S., and Clarke, M. B.: Prostatectomy and deep-vein thrombosis, Br. J. Surg. **59:** 487, 1972.
45. Nicolaides, A. N., Kakkar, V. V., Field, E. S., and Fish, P.: Venous stasis and deep vein thrombosis, Br. J. Surg. **59:** 713, 1972.
46. Nicolaides, A. N., Dupont, P. A., DeSai, S., Lewis, J. D., Douglas, J. N., Dodsworth, H., Fourides, G., Luck, R. J., and Jamieson, C. W.: Small doses of subcutaneous sodium heparin in preventing deep venous thrombosis after major surgery, Lancet **2:** 890, 1972.
47. O'Brien, J. R., and Kakkar, V. V.: Peripheral venous scanning with ^{125}I-tagged fibrinogen, Lancet **1:** 909, 1972.
48. Paterson, J. C.: Pathology of venous thrombi, *in* Sherry, S., Brinkhous, K. M., Genton, E., et al., editors: Thrombosis, Washington, D. C., 1969, National Academy of Sciences, pp. 321-331.
49. Praiss, D. E., and Marmar, J. L.: Is the umbrella filter safe? (Letter to the Editor) N. Engl. J. Med. **286:** 1006, 1972.
50. Rabinov, K., and Paulin, S.: Roentgen diagnosis of venous thrombosis in the leg, Arch. Surg. **104:** 134, 1972.
51. Report of the Steering Committee of a trial sponsored by the Medical Research Council, Great Britain: Effect of aspirin on postoperative venous thrombosis, Lancet **2:** 441, 1972.
52. Rosengarten, D. S., Laird, J., Jeyasingh, K., and Martin, P.: The failure of compression stockings (Tubigrip) to prevent deep venous thrombosis after operation, Br. J. Surg. **57:** 296, 1970.
53. Salzman, E. W., Harris, W. H., and DeSanctis, R. W.: Anticoagulation for prevention of thromboembolism following fractures of the hip, N. Engl. J. Med. **275:** 122, 1966.
54. Salzman, E. W., Harris, W. H., and DeSanctis, R. W.: Reduction in venous thromboembolism by agents affecting platelet function, N. Engl. J. Med. **284:** 1287, 1971.
55. Sevitt, S.: Venous thrombosis in injured patients (with some observations on pathogenesis), *in* Sherry, S., Brinkhous, K. M., Gendon, E., et al., editors: Thrombosis, Washington, D. C., 1969, National Academy of Sciences, pp. 29-49.
56. Sevitt, S., and Gallagher, N. G.: Prevention of venous thrombosis and pulmonary embolism in injured patients: A trial of anticoagulant prophylaxis with phenindione in middle-aged and elderly patients with fractured necks of the femur, Lancet **2:** 981, 1959.
57. Smith, G. W.: Iliofemoral venous thrombectomy, Circulation **37:** 847, 1968.
58. Spencer, F. C., Quattlebaum, J. K., Quattlebaum, J. K., Jr., Sharp, E. H., and Jude, J. R.: Plication of inferior vena cava for pulmonary embolism: Report of 20 cases, Ann. Surg. **155:** 827, 1962.
59. Steer, M. L., Spotnitz, A. J., Cohen, S. I., Paulin, S., and Salzman, E. W.: Limitations of impedance phlebography for diagnosis of venous thrombosis, Arch. Surg. **106:** 44, 1973.
60. Strandness, D. E., and Sumner, D. S.: Ultrasonic velocity detector in the diagnosis of thrombophlebitis, Arch. Surg. **104:** 180, 1972.
61. Tsapogas, M. J., Miller, R., Peabody, R. A., and Eckert, C. L.: Detection of postoperative venous thrombosis and effectiveness of prophylactic measures, Arch. Surg. **101:** 149, 1970.
62. Williams, H. T.: Prevention of postoperative deep-vein thrombosis with perioperative subcutaneous heparin, Lancet **2:** 950, 1971.
63. Yin, E. T., and Wessler, S.: Heparin-accelerated inhibition of activated factor X by its natural plasma inhibitor, Biochim. Biophys. Acta **201:** 387, 1970.
64. Yin, E. T., Wessler, S., and Stoll, P.: Biological properties of the naturally occurring plasma inhibitor to activated factor X, J. Biol. Chem. **246:** 3703, 1971.

The mechanism of infection in patients with diabetes mellitus: A review of leukocyte malfunction

Howard D. Robertson, First Lieutenant, USAF (MC), *and*
Hiram C. Polk, Jr., M.D., F.A.C.S., *Louisville, Ky.*

Malfunction of the PMN (polymorphonuclear) leukocyte has been considered a potential cause of enhancement of bacterial infection in the diabetic individual. The cause of this malfunction remains unclear, but several factors have been implicated. In some experimental systems, hyperglycemia alone led to decreased phagocytosis, decreased diapedesis, and a decrease in intracellular killing of bacteria by the polymorphonuclear leukocyte. An intrinsic defect in the diabetic PMN with or without hyperglycemia is a possible cause of PMN malfunction. Ketoacidosis was necessary in another experimental model before leukocyte malfunction was noted. There are no significant differences in immunoglobulins A, G, and M on the surface of diabetic and normal PMN leukocytes, but antibodies to thyroid cytoplasm and gastric parietal cell cytoplasm are elevated significantly in diabetic patients. Metabolic pathways are altered in diabetic PMN, which may cause a malfunction in their ability to affect infectious organisms. These findings are all part of the answer to the mechanism of enhancement of infection in the diabetic patient. Careful review of these findings and the development of new experimental models will clarify this complex clinical and laboratory issue.

From the Department of Surgery and the Price Institute of Surgical Research, The University of Louisville School of Medicine, Louisville, Kentucky

Surgeons have long identified patients with diabetes mellitus as prone to infections which complicate operations and occasionally cause death. The cooperative study of the efficacy of ultraviolet light as an aid to reduction of surgical infections disclosed a statistically significant higher rate of infection among diabetic patients, but this difference disappeared when the infection rates were adjusted for differing age distributions between diabetic and nondiabetic patients.[16] Autopsy reports have shown that the average age at time of death in diabetic and nondiabetic patients is equal, but diabetic patients tend to have an increased incidence of coronary occlusion, peripheral vascular disease, infections of the extremeties, and acute pyelonephritis.[23] Although diabetic patients also have an increased incidence of urinary tract infections, diabetes has not been correlated with an increased risk of staphylococcal infections in operations on well-controlled diabetic patients.[8, 14, 29] Renal tuberculosis, osteomyelitis, mucormycosis, and vascular ulcers with secondary infection have an increased incidence in the diabetic patient.[11, 13] Although the question of incidence of various infections in the diabetic patient is very controversial, infection still is con-

Supported in part by grants from the Edelen Memorial Fund, Rodrigo Borges Fund, and the Lilly Research Foundation.

Accepted for publication Oct. 10, 1973.

The views and opinions expressed herein do not necessarily represent those of the Surgeon General, the Department of the Air Force, or the Department of Defense.

Table I. *Summary of effect of hyperglycemia and acidosis on leukocyte function*

Author(s)	Experimental model	Blood glucose (mg. %)	Observed effect on leukocyte
Ainsworth and Allison[1] (1970)	Rabbit ear chamber, glucose infusion, without ketoacidosis	876–3,640	Impaired sticking, decreased diapedesis
Bagdade and associates[3] (1970)	Poorly controlled diabetics without ketoacidosis	243–1,000	Decreased phagocytosis, decreased killing
Drachman and associates[9] (1966)	Chronic diabetic rats and stressed exudate system	300 every 3 wk.	Decreased phagocytosis
Bybee and Rogers[7] (1970)	Phagocytes from: Diabetic patients without acidosis	> 250	Normal activity
	Diabetic patients with acidosis	171–1,160	Decreased phagocytosis
Tan and associates[27, 28] (1971 and 1972)	Phagocytes from 31 nonketoacidotic diabetic patients	Not given, said to be unrelated	Nonketoacidotic diabetic 77.6* 18.7† Nondiabetic control 95.4* 3.1†
Brody and Merlie[6] (1970)	Phagocytes from known diabetic patients not receiving insulin	1 hr. glucose tolerance test 200	Decreased response to phytohemagglutinin
Ragab and associates[21] (1972)	Phagocytes from known diabetic patients taking insulin or chlorpropamide or diet	80–336	Normal response to phytohemagglutinin
Mowat and Baum[19] (1971)	Diabetic outpatient phagocytes	70–470	Decreased chemotaxis
	Normal outpatient phagocytes and glucose in vitro	300–900	Normal chemotaxis
Brayton and associates[4] (1970)	Leukocyte mobilization to a controlled abrasion of the forearm of various groups including:		
	Controlled diabetic patients	Not stated	Delayed leukocyte diapedesis
	Acidotic diabetic patients	Not stated	Delayed leukocyte diapedesis
	Uremic patients	Not stated	Normal leukocyte diapedesis
Briscoe and Allison[5] (1965)	Alloxan-treated rats	Not stated, but all animals had glucosuria	Normal phagocytosis, normal bacterial killing
Miller and Baker[18] (1972)	Juvenile diabetic PMN leukocytes	152–429	Normal phagocytosis Decreased chemotaxis

*Percent killed intracellular bacteria.

†Percent viable intracellular bacteria.

sidered more significant in the surgical candidate who has diabetes. The mechanism of action is not thoroughly understood. One important factor may well be the nonspecific host defense system. This paper reviews the role of malfunction of the polymorphonuclear (PMN) leukocytes in diabetes and related conditions.

LEUKOCYTE MALFUNCTION

Hyperglycemia has been shown to interfere with leukocyte function. Ainsworth and Allison,[1] using the ear chambers of rabbits, found impaired sticking of leukocytes to the endothelium of the vascular system; thus, a decrease in migration of leukocytes was observed when blood glucose levels were 800 to 3,600 mg. percent (Table I). Bagdade and associates[3] showed that decreased phagocytosis and killing of bacteria by phagocytes was directly related to high, fasting blood sugar levels. Drachman and colleagues[9] used a stressed phagocyte model in which leukocytes operated in a crowded exudate while ingesting pneumococci with antiphagocytic capsules. They found that leukocytes exposed to high concentrations of glucose in chronically diabetic rats had a diminished capacity for phagocytosis. In vivo impairment of phagocyte activity was also demonstrated and was alleged to be caused by the increased osmotic forces of hyperglycemia. The above experimental data tend to give credence to the importance of carefully controlled blood sugar levels in diabetic patients to prevent depression of host-immune mechanisms.

Evidence also exists that hyperglycemia does *not* affect leukocyte function. Tan and associates,[27, 28] while studying the phagocytosis of *S. aureus,* observed that 17 of 31 nonketoacidotic diabetic patients had impaired phagocytosis or an intracellular killing defect. The nondiabetic group had 95.4 percent killing of intracellular bacteria, and the total diabetic group had only 77.6 percent killing of intracellular bacteria. The nondiabetic subjects had 3.1 percent viable extracellular bacteria, and the diabetic group had 18.7 percent viable extracellular bacteria. These differences were not related to blood sugar levels nor were they corrected by normal serum. This evidence implies that the defect of the PMN leukocyte must be intrinsic and is not related to extrinsic environmental factors. Lymphocytes from the peripheral blood of 23 patients with well-controlled diabetes, studied by Ragab and colleagues,[21] were not significantly different from the lymphocytes of normal subjects in their response to phytohemagglutinin (PHA) and *Candida albicans* antigen. The fasting blood sugar value ranged from 80 to 336 mg. percent, with that of four individuals over 250 mg. percent. No relationship between blood sugar level and degree of response was noted. Brody and Merlie[6] found a decreased lymphocyte response to PHA in patients with a one-hour oral glucose tolerance test greater than 200 mg. percent, but again no correlation was made between glucose concentration and degree of response. Mowat and Baum[19] found no correlation between chemotaxis and fasting blood sugar levels. Delayed leukocyte diapedesis was found in both acidotic and nonacidotic diabetic patients, but similarly acidotic, nondiabetic patients having uremia alone showed normal leukocyte diapedesis.[4] Polymorphonuclear leukocytes of juvenile diabetic patients with blood glucose concentrations ranging from 152 to 429 mg. percent had normal phagocytosis but had a marked deficiency in chemotaxis. It was found that the PMN leukocytes were leukotactic-deficient and the sera from diabetic children was chemotatic-deficient.[18] Data from this group suggest that blood sugar concentrations in diabetic patients have no association with enhancement of infection as far as impaired phagocytosis or decreased leukocyte diapedesis can contribute to increased infection. These experiments indicate that rigid control of blood sugar levels is not needed to improve host resistance to infections.

Table II. *Bacteriuria in female diabetic and nondiabetic patients*

Source	*Diabetic (%)**	*Nondiabetic (%)**
Vejlsgaard[29]	18.8	7.9
Hansen[14]	18.5	3.7

*Percent with bacteriuria.

CLINICAL RELATIONSHIP TO BACTERIA AND DIABETES

Bacteriuria has been shown to occur in 18.8 percent of female diabetic patients and 7.9 percent of female nondiabetic patients by Vejlsgaard.[29] Hansen[14] found almost the same figures: 18.5 percent bacteriuria in diabetic female patients and 3.7 percent in nondiabetic female patients (Table II). Hansen stated there was no connection between a high glucose content in the urine specimen examined and bacteriuria.

In vitro growth studies show that gram-negative bacteria were inhibited by high levels of glucose while gram-positive bacteria thrived.[24] Among 214 patients, 81 percent of those with a blood glucose of less than 110 mg. percent developed gram-negative septicemia, and 82 percent with a blood glucose of greater than 120 mg. percent developed gram-positive septicemia.[24] These findings are pertinent in setting up experimental models as well as during the treatment of infections.

EFFECTS OF KETOACIDOSIS

Other authors have tried to relate leukocyte derangement to acidosis. The effects of

Table III. *Summary of the effect of various leukocyte and serum combinations on phagocytosis*

Source	*Leukocyte*	*Serum*		*Effect on phagocytosis*
Bybee and Rogers[7] and Henan and Delannay[15]	Nonketoacidotic diabetic	+ Normal or diabetic	=	Normal
	Normal	+ Normal or ketoacidotic	=	Normal
	Ketoacidotic diabetic	+ Normal or diabetic	=	Decreased
Bagdade and associates[3]	Keto- and nonketo-acidotic diabetic	+ Normal	=	Decreased
	Normal	+ Hyperglycemic diabetic	=	Decreased

alcohol and various diseases on leukocyte mobilization were studied, and a decreased leukocyte mobilization in diabetic patients was observed, suggesting an intrinsic abnormality in the PMN leukocyte, as the defect was not related to uremia or acidosis.[4] Ketoacidosis was necessary in experiments of Perillie and associates[20] and Bybee and Rogers[7] before decreased leukocyte phagocytosis was apparent (Table III). Bagdade and associates,[3] however, found decreased phagocytosis with either hyperglycemic diabetic serum or ketodiabetic and nonketodiabetic leukocytes. The experimental data presented by Bagdade and associates[3] give more evidence for serum and cell abnormalities in diabetic patients causing decreased phagocytosis, whereas Perillie and associates[20] and Bybee and Rogers[7] stress the importance of an intrinsic derangement of the ketodiabetic leukocyte as the cause of decreased phagocytosis. Alloxan-treated, nonketotic rats have not shown a decrease in leukocyte phagocytosis or killing power.[5] At two to four hours, leukocyte migration to controlled skin abrasions was less in diabetic patients than in nondiabetic patients, with those diabetic patients in an acidotic state having the fewest leukocytes at the skin abrasion after migration.[4]

IMMUNOLOGIC FACTORS

Yet another avenue of study into the problem of infection in diabetic patients is the immunologic aspect of the PMN leukocyte. Richardson[22] found no decrease in serum complement in diabetic patients. Irvine and associates,[17] however, discovered that antibodies to thyroid cytoplasm and gastric parietal cell cytoplasm were increased significantly in 1,054 diabetic patients as compared to 871 control subjects. No clear relationship between incidence of antibodies and duration of diabetes was found. They suggest a common genetic mechanism between autoimmunity and insulin-dependent diabetes. No significant differences of immunoglobulins A, G, or M (IgA, IgG, IgM) on the surface of PMN leukocytes in diabetic and nondiabetic patients have been found.[19]

METABOLIC FACTORS

Both polycythemia vera and chlorambucil-treated adenocarcinoma decreased the activity of leukocytes.[30] These cells as well as diabetic phagocytes tend to be hypermetabolic and have an increased oxygen uptake. Brody and Merlie[6] showed that most diabetic lymphocytes metabolized glucose through the direct oxidative pathway. A decreased incorporation of radioactive thymidine also was found. A quantitative relationship apparently exists between the amount of glucose passing through the hexose monophosphate pathway (which has as its function the generation of nicotinamide-adenine-dinucleotide phosphate [NADPH]) and the use of NADPH to reduce oxyribonucleotide to deoxyribonucleotide and thus induce synthesis of DNA. Perhaps the immunologic response of lymphocytes is mediated by DNA information produced from this metabolic pathway, and this information is abnormal in diabetic patients. Esmann[12] gives evidence that there is no difference between the leukocytes of diabetic and normal subjects with respect to NADPH production. However, NADPH thus produced may not enter the DNA-synthesizing process but be channeled to other pathways.[12]

Two metabolic defects of rabbit PMN leukocytes have been demonstrated.[15] One defect is modified intensity of metabolism—normal rabbit PMN leukocytes not in active phagocytosis in diabetic serum have decreased metabolism, decreased O_2 uptake, decreased lactic acid production, and decreased glucose uptake. There is also a defect involving an abnormal pathway—normal rabbit PMN leukocytes in active phagocytosis in diabetic serum take up abnormally high amounts of glucose, but only one part of the molecule is degraded while normal leukocytes in normal serum will degrade all the glucose.

Two other metabolic features should be noted here. Diabetic acidosis can be stimulated in the diabetic patient by gram-negative bacterial infection.[30] This, in turn, can cause hyperkalemia. Depletion of intracellular potassium causes an impairment of chemotaxis and thus increased infection.[31] Lactic acid tends to kill bacteria, but when ketones are added, the bacteria live longer.[10] One must ask whether the infection causes the diabetes to become uncontrolled or whether uncontrolled diabetes renders the diabetic patient more susceptible to infection. This question is particularly appropriate in light of Robson's[24] conclusion, as stated earlier, that gram-negative infections are inhibited by hyperglycemia but gram-positive infections are enhanced by hyperglycemia. Rocha and associates[25] have shown that plasma glucagon levels are raised in nondiabetic dogs with experimentally induced pneumococcal pneumonia. They have also found that alloxan-diabetic dogs with controlled insulin levels and artificially induced chronic hyperglucagonemia can cause hyperglycemia, polyuria, glycosuria, and urea excretion. Combining findings from these experiments with dogs and the observation that 22 nondiabetic patients hospitalized with bacterial infections had increased glucagon levels, Rocha and associates[25] conclude glucagon elevation may explain infection-induced deterioration observed in numerous diabetic patients.

Apparently two factors compromise this portion of the host defence system. Although controversial, one transferable serum factor may be hyperglycemia. There is also a cellular abnormality or biochemical alteration in the PMN leukocytes of the diabetic patient that impairs energy production required for both phagocytosis and bactericidal functions. These factors working separately or in combination have the potential to enhance infectious processes in the diabetic individual.

OTHER FACTORS

Other mechanisms involved in enhancing infectious processes in patients with diabetes mellitus are varied and largely speculative and proposed.[11] There may be a decreased host antibody production or interference with the bactericidal action of blood. Vascular insufficiency caused by lipid deposits in small vessels can lead to decreases in blood flow, granulocyte mobilization, diffusion of specific antibody, plasma factors, oxygen, and thus, increases in microaerophilic and anaerobic organisms. Nonspecific humoral factors such as lysozyme, properdin, betalysin, interferon, and pH must be explored in depth as their roles thus far are poorly defined.[2]

The authors express their appreciation for review of the manuscript and advice to Norton Waterman, M.D., and Martin Raff, M.D.

REFERENCES

1. Ainsworth, S. K., and Allison, F., Jr.: Studies on the pathogenesis of acute inflammation. IX. The influence of hyperosmolarity secondary to hyperglycemia upon the acute inflammatory response induced by thermal injury to ear chambers of rabbits, J. Clin. Invest. **49:** 433, 1970.
2. Alexander, J. W., and Good, R. A.: Immunobiology for surgeons, Philadelphia, 1970, W. B. Saunders Company, pp. 1-41.
3. Bagdade, J. D., Nielson, K. L., Root, R., and Bulger, R.: Host defense in diabetes mellitus: The feckless phagocyte during poor control

and ketoacidosis, Diabetes (Suppl. 1) **19:** 364, 1970.
4. Brayton, R. G., Stokes, P. E., Schwartz, M. S., et al: Effect of alcohol and various diseases on leukocyte mobilization, phagocytosis and intracellular bacterial killing, N. Engl. J. Med. **282:** 123, 1970.
5. Briscoe, H. F., and Allison, F., Jr.: Diabetes and host resistance. I. Effect of alloxan diabetes upon the phagocytic and bactericidal efficiency of rat leukocytes for Pneumococcus, J. Bact. **90:** 1537, 1965.
6. Brody, J. I., and Merlie, K.: Metabolic and biosynthetic features of lymphocytes from patients with diabetes mellitus: Similarities to lymphocytes in chronic lymphocytic leukemia, Br. J. Haemat. **19:** 193, 1970.
7. Bybee, J. D., and Rogers, D. E.: The phagocytic activity of polymorphonuclear leukocytes obtained from patients with diabetes mellitus, J. Lab. Clin. Med. **64:** 1, 1964.
8. Cohen, L. S., Fekety, F. R., and Cluff, L. E.: Studies of the epidemiology of staphylococcal infection, Ann. Surg. **159:** 321, 1964.
9. Drachman, R. H., Root, R. K., and Wood, W. B.: Studies on the effect of experimental nonketotic diabetes mellitus on antibacterial defense. I. Demonstration of a defect in phagocytosis, J. Exp. Med. **124:** 227, 1966.
10. Dubos, R.: Effect of ketone bodies and other metabolites on the survival and manipulation of staphylococci and tubercle bacilli, J. Exp. Med. **98:** 145, 1953.
11. Ellenburg, M., and Rifkin, H.: Diabetes mellitus: Theory and practice, New York, 1970, McGraw-Hill Book Co., Inc., pp. 734-743.
12. Esmann, V.: The metabolism of [1-^{14}C]-, [2-^{14}C]-, [3,4-^{14}C]-, and [6-^{14}C]- glucose in normal and diabetic polymorphonuclear leukocytes and during phagocytosis, Diabetologia **7:** 188, 1968.
13. Fajans, S. S., and Sussman, K. E., editors: Diabetes mellitus: Diagnosis and treatment, New York, 1971, American Diabetes Association, Inc., pp. 211-215.
14. Hansen, R. O.: Bacteriuria in diabetic and nondiabetic out-patients, Acta Med. Scand. **176:** 721, 1965.
15. Henan, M., and Delannay, A.: Experimental diabetes and anti-infection defenses in the organism. I. Metabolic modifications produced in vitro in the phagocytes of normal rabbits, at rest or active, by serum from diabetic rabbits, Ann. Inst. Pasteur (Paris) **115:** 908, 1968.
16. Howard, J. M., Chairman, *ad hoc* Committee: Postoperative wound infections: The influence of ultraviolet irradiation of operating room and of various factors, Ann. Surg. (Suppl.) 160, 1964.
17. Irvine, W. J., Clarke, B. F., Scarth, L., Cullen, D. R., and Duncan, L. J. P.: Thyroid and gastric autoimmunity in patients with diabetes mellitus, Lancet **2:** 165, 1970.
18. Miller, M. E., and Baker, L.: Leukocyte functions in juvenile diabetes mellitus: Humoral and cellular aspects, J. Pediatr. **81:** 980, 1971.
19. Mowat, A. G., and Baum, J.: Chemotaxis of polymorphonuclear leukocytes from patients with diabetes mellitus, N. Engl. J. Med. **284:** 621, 1971.
20. Perillie, P. E., Nolan, J. P., and Finch, S. C.: Studies of the resistance to infection in diabetes mellitus: Local exudative cellular response, J. Lab. Clin. Med. **59:** 1008, 1962.
21. Ragab, A. H., Hazlett, B., and Cowan, D. H.: Response of peripheral blood lymphocytes from patients with diabetes mellitus to phytohemagglutinin and candida albicans antigen, Diabetes **21:** 906, 1972.
22. Richardson, R.: Immunity in diabetes. IV. Measurement of phagocytic activity in diabetes mellitus, Am. J. Med. Sci. **204:** 29, 1942.
23. Robbins, S. L., and Tucker, A. W.: The cause of death in diabetes, N. Engl. J. Med. **231:** 865, 1944.
24. Robson, M. C.: A new look at diabetes mellitus and infection, Am. J. Surg. **120:** 681, 1970.
25. Rocha, D. M., Santeusanio, F., Faloona, G. R., and Unger, R. H.: Abnormal pancreatic alpha-cell function in bacterial infections, N. Engl. J. Med. **288:** 700, 1973.
26. Stockigt, J. R., and Taft, P.: The stimulation of diabetic acidosis by severe G-negative bacterial infection occurring in the diabetic, Med. J. Aust. **1:** 210, 1966.
27. Tan, J. S., Watanakunakorn, C., and Phair, J. P.: A modified assay of neutrophil function: Use of lysostaphin to differentiate defective phagocytosis from impaired intracellular killing, J. Lab. Clin. Med. **78:** 317, 1971.
28. Tan, J. S., Watanakunakorn, C., and Phair, J. P.: Host resistance in diabetes: Neutrophil dysfunction, J. Clin. Invest. **51:** 96a, 1972.
29. Vejlsgaard, R.: Studies on urinary infections in diabetes. I. Bacteriuria in patients with diabetes mellitus and in control subjects, Acta Med. Scand. **179:** 173, 1966.
30. Walters, M. I., Lessler, M. A., and Stevenson, T. D.: Oxidative metabolism of leukocytes from non-diabetic and diabetic patients, J. Lab. Clin. Med., **78:** 158, 1971.
31. Ward, P. A., and Becker, E. L.: Potassium reversible inhibtion of leukotaxis by ouabain, Life Sci. (Part 2) **9:** 355, 1970.

Brief clinical reports

A simplified method of ureteroileostomy in renal homotransplantation

Thomas L. Marchioro, M.D., *and* **James A. Tremann, M.D.,** *Seattle, Wash.*

The use of a new technique in renal homotransplantation, which combines the features of two procedures, has provided five patients with successful ureteroileostomies since March, 1970. The technique herein described reduces the amount of stasis, infection, and absorption of urinary constituents, and presents several advantages over the technique usually employed.

From the Department of Surgery, University of Washington School of Medicine, Seattle, Wash.

DISTAL URINARY tract obstruction is the underlying cause of renal failure in a small but definite number of patients. Transplantation in these patients has been performed with the use of a ureteroileostomy, as described by Kelly and associates[2] and Tunner and co-workers.[6] Both groups employ a technique such that urinary drainage is not dependent into the ileal conduit. This technique has been satisfactory, as evidenced by the later long-term follow-up report by Markland and colleagues.[3]

We believe the technique is unnecessarily cumbersome, however, and has certain disadvantages. By combining a technique originally reported by Starzl and associates[5] for the insertion of large adult homografts in small children, we have been able to provide dependent urinary drainage similar to that achieved with the standard ureteroileostomy for other purposes.

The ileal conduit is constructed at least two or three weeks prior to the proposed time of transplantation, or in the case of cadaveric recipients, at an indefinite interval prior to the obtaining of an appropriately matched kidney. The segment is kept quite short, as indicated in Fig. 1. This reduces the amount of stasis, infection, and absorption of urinary constituents.

At the time of transplantation, the kidney is placed according to the technique described by Starzl and colleagues[5] and illustrated in Fig. 1. The right colon is reflected off the posterior body wall, and the renal artery is anastomosed either to the terminal aorta or to the proximal right iliac artery. The renal vein is anastomosed end to side to the vena cava at the confluence of the two iliac veins. For practical purposes, the kidney now occupies the old renal fossa on the right.

The ureter is then implanted into the antimesenteric border of the ileal conduit. It may pass either in front of or behind the mesentery. A standard two-layered anastomosis, similar to that described by Bricker,[1] is used. In this position, the right colon, which now overlies the kidney, ureter, and ileal conduit, protects the ureter from entanglement with the small bowel, avoiding ureteric disruption and/or small bowel obstruction.

Accepted for publication July 18, 1973.

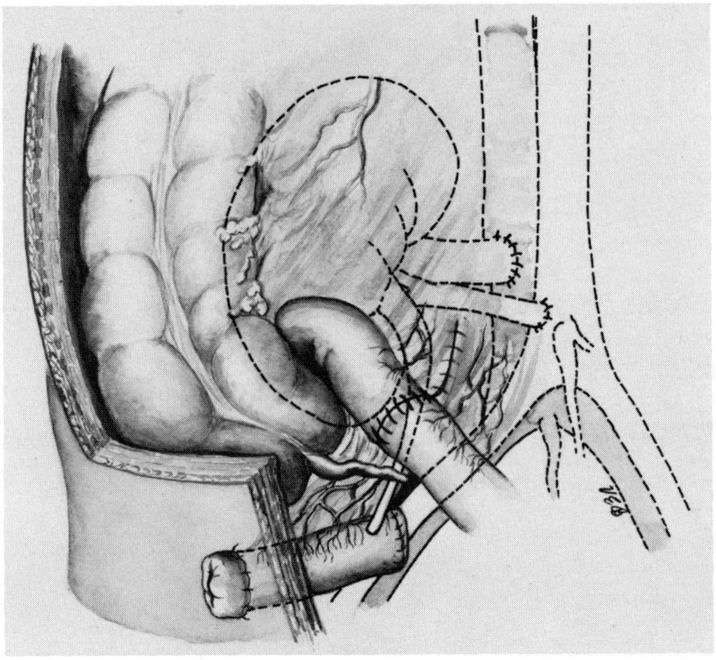

Fig. 1. For clarity, the cecum is shown lying cephalad of the ileal conduit. In actual practice, the conduit and ureter are covered by this structure, thus placing the kidney, ureter, and conduit retroperitoneally. (See text.)

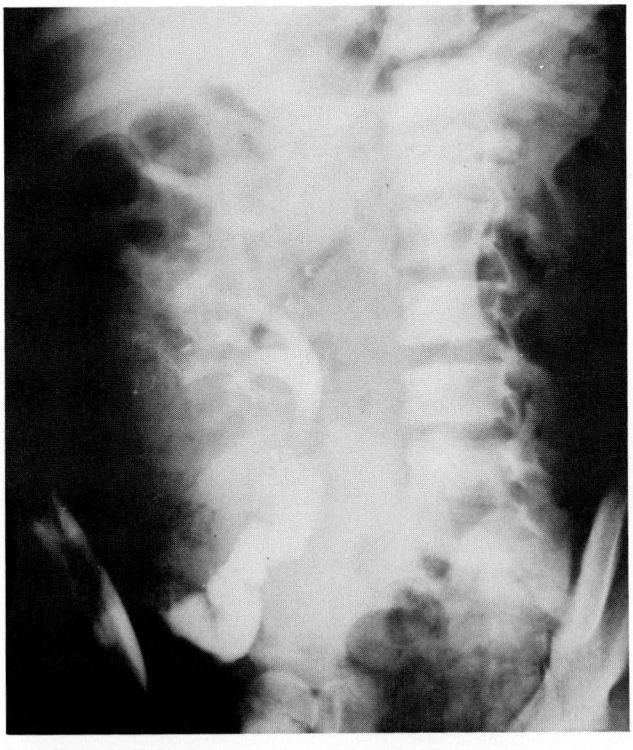

Fig. 2. Excretory urogram taken two months after transplantation of a related donor kidney into an ileal conduit by the technique illustrated in Fig. 1.

This technique has been used in five patients since March, 1970. In each case, the ureteric implant functioned well initially. Fig. 2 shows an excretory urogram demonstrating prompt drainage into the conduit. In this instance, the conduit was the first one constructed and was overly long. Subsequent conduits have been one-third to one-half as long as the one illustrated here.

In only one patient was there a serious complication of the technique. This patient developed a hernia 33 months after transplantation through the fascial opening of the ileal conduit. This caused slow deterioration of renal function until the hernia was corrected. She now has stable renal function with sterile urine three years after transplantation. In the remaining four patients, the ureteroileostomy functioned well until the time of death in two patients (one from coronary thrombosis 19 months after transplantation and another from peritonitis secondary to small bowel perforation at four months after operation) or rejection in two patients at three and 18 months.

We believe the technique to be at least as simple as that described by other authors with several distinct advantages. First, the kidney is placed above the ileal conduit and drainage is aided by gravity during most of the patient's waking hours. It has been shown by Schick and Tanagho[4] that ureteral peristalsis ceases if urine must be transported against gravity. Second, the conduit can be kept quite short, thus minimizing infection and reabsorption of urine by the ileal segment. Third, the ureter is entirely extraperitoneal, as is the conduit, because of the covering of the kidney and the ureter by the right colon. The only technical complication we encountered was not due to this innovation per se but was due to a hernia developing 33 months after transplantation, which could easily have happened with alternative techniques.

REFERENCES

1. Bricker, E. M.: Bladder substitution after pelvic evisceration, Surg. Clin. North Am. **30:** 1511, 1950.
2. Kelly, W. D., Merkel, F. K., and Markland, C.: Ileal urinary diversion in conjunction with renal homotransplantation, Lancet **1:** 222, 1966.
3. Markland, C., Kelly, W. D., Buselmeier, T., Kjellstrand, C., Simmons, R., and Najarian, J.: Renal transplantation into iliac urinary conduits, Transplant. Proc. **4:** 629, 1972.
4. Schick, E., and Tanagho, E. A.: The effect of gravity on ureteral peristalsis, J. Urol. **109:** 187, 1973.
5. Starzl, T. E., Marchioro, T. L., Morgan, W. W., and Waddell, W. R.: A technique for uses of adult renal homografts in children, Surg. Gynecol. Obstet. **119:** 106, 1964.
6. Tunner, W. S., Whitsell, J. C., Jr., Rubin, A., and Marshall, V. F.: Renal transplantation in children with damaged and repaired or replaced lower urinary tracts. Presented at the Fourth Annual Meeting of the Association for Academic Surgery, Denver, Colo., Nov. 19-20, 1970.

Successful management of mycotic aortic aneurysm: Report of a case

Paul A. Cooke, M.B., B.Ch.,* *Johannesburg, Republic of South Africa, and* **William K. Ehrenfeld, M.D.,** *San Francisco, Calif.*

Mycotic aneurysm of the abdominal aorta is a serious disorder that generally carries a grave prognosis. Few survivors have been reported. This report describes an operative approach that was successfully used in a patient with a mycotic abdominal aortic aneurysm. The diagnosis was made preoperatively and an axillofemoral graft was placed before the abdomen was entered, thus diminishing the chance for graft contamination. The infected aortic aneurysm was resected and blood supply to the viscera and lower extremities was not compromised.The importance of early surgery to avoid rupture and of distant bypassing to prevent presistent sepsis is emphasized. The gravity of these complications is discussed. This approach seems to be the most logical method in dealing with this problem. A review of the literature provides insight into some past diagnostic and therapeutic pitfalls.

From the Department of Surgery, University of California School of Medicine, San Francisco, Calif.

Mycotic aortic aneurysm carries a grave prognosis and few survivors have been reported. The most vexing problem in management is restoration of aortic continuity after resection of the infected aortic aneurysm. An axillofemoral bypass graft inserted before the abdomen is opened will prevent graft contamination and will provide blood supply to the pelvis and lower extremities.

CASE REPORT

A 52-year-old woman had a one-month history of epigastric pain, fever, and a weight loss of 14 pounds. Systemic lupus erythematosus had been diagnosed 22 years ago which was treated with prolonged courses of steroid therapy, but no treatment had been given for seven months prior to admission. Eight previous operations included a vagotomy and pyloroplasty, appendectomy, hysterectomy, cholecystectomy, three laparotomies for lysis of adhesions, and a cesarean section. She also had had several hospital admissions for recurrent pancreatitis.

On admission to the hospital, she had severe, persistent pain which radiated to the back and left flank. It was aggravated by movement, was not relieved by antacids, and was accompanied by nausea, vomiting, and general malaise.

She was dehydrated, cachectic, and obtunded. Body temperature was 38.5° C., pulse was 104 beats per minute, and blood pressure was 116/74 mm. Hg. She had a large visible epigastric pulsation and a palpable aneurysm which was remarkably tender. The peripheral arterial tree was otherwise free of clinically detectable disease. There was no evidence of subacute bacterial endocarditis or other cardiac disease.

Laboratory investigations provided the following data: hematocrit, 28.4; white blood count, 12.2; amylase, 232; erythrocyte sedimentation rate

Accepted for publication July 30, 1973.

Reprint requests: W. K. Ehrenfeld, M.D., Department of Surgery, University of California School of Medicine, San Francisco, Calif. 94143.

*Present address: Department of Surgery, University of the Witwatersrand, Johannesburgh, Republic of South Africa.

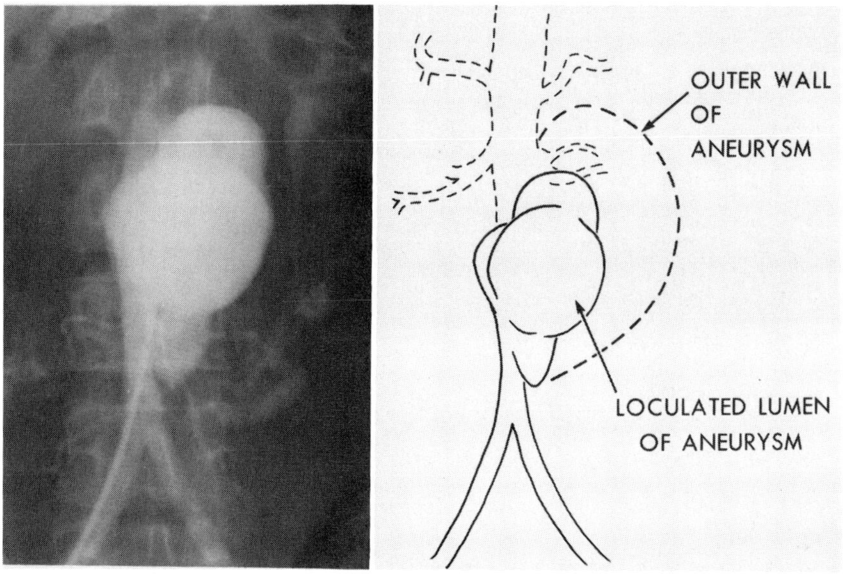

Fig. 1. Preoperative aortogram demonstrating a saccular loculated aneurysm arising from the abdominal aorta *(left)*. Schematic diagram *(right)* shows the findings at surgery in relation to the aortogram.

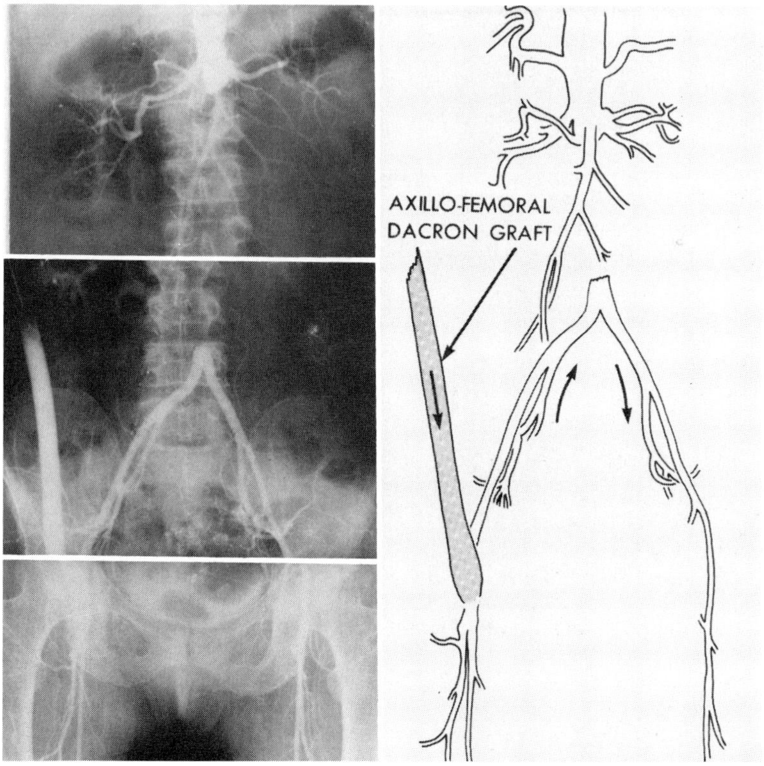

Fig. 2. Composite postoperative arteriogram *(left)* showing perfusion of the kidneys by the suprarenal aorta and of the pelvis and the lower limbs by the right axillofemoral graft. Schematic diagram *(right)* depicts the postoperative vascular status and direction of blood flow.

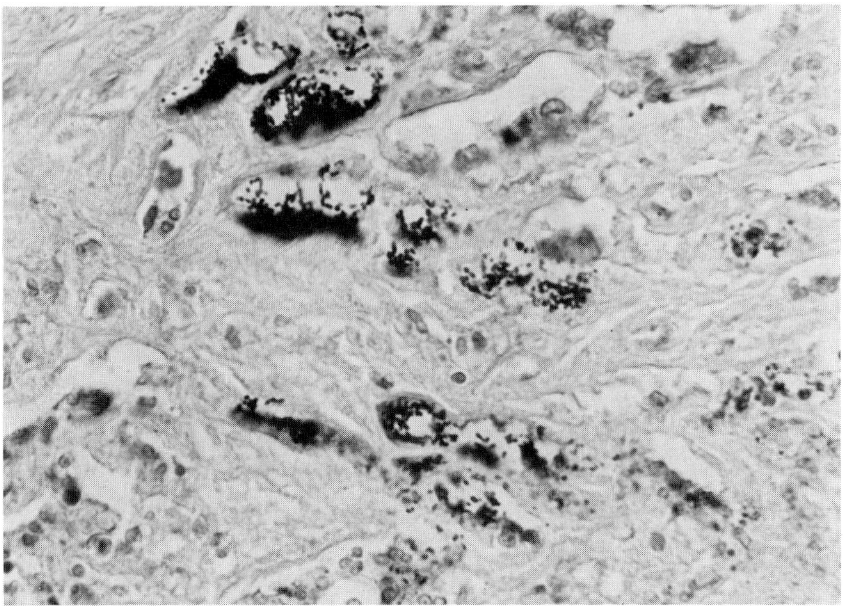

Fig. 3. Photomicrograph of a portion of the resected aneurysm wall showing degenerative atherosclerosis and plaques containing gram-positive cocci and macrophages with ingested cocci.

(ERS), 116 mm. per hour; albumin, 3.2 Gm. per 100 c.c.; gamma globulin, 2.7 Gm. per 100 c.c. A lupus erythematosus (LE) preparation was positive, and three consecutive blood cultures produced no growth. An intravenous pyelogram performed for microscopic hematuria was essentially normal, and an upper gastrointestinal series showed duodenal deformity consistent with a previous pyloroplasty. An abdominal aortogram demonstrated a saccular loculated aneurysm arising from the abdominal aorta (Fig. 1).

A mycotic aortic aneurysm was suspected, and operation was performed immediately. A right axillofemoral Dacron graft was inserted prior to laparotomy. A mass of adhesions was present in the abdomen, and a large inflammatory mass was densely adherent to a large broad-based saccular infrarenal aortic aneurysm. The aneurysm was evacuated and obliterated, and the infrarenal and distal aortic stumps were oversewn with wire sutures. An arterial clamp previously placed on the proximal right common femoral artery was removed after aortic occlusion, and blood flow to the pelvis and left leg was restored through the iliac arteries. The postoperative course was uneventful, and arteriograms demonstrated adequate perfusion of the kidneys by the suprarenal aorta and of the pelvis and lower limbs by the axillofemoral graft (Fig. 2). Microscopic examination of the aneurysm wall showed degenerative changes of atherosclerosis and plaques containing gram-positive cocci and macrophages with ingested cocci (Fig. 3).

DISCUSSION

Because of their obscure clinical manifestations, rapidly destructive nature, and frequency of rupture, cryptogenetic mycotic aneurysms are often not diagnosed until autopsy.[7, 9, 10, 12, 13, 28] Bennett and Cherry,[3] in a review of 34 reported cases of infected aortic aneurysms, found that the correct diagnosis was seldom made in time to permit surgical intervention and that rupture supervened in 79 percent of cases and was uniformly fatal. The insidious onset, prolonged febrile course, and vague symptomatology described by our patient are typical of "primary mycotic aneurysms," a term coined by Crane[14] in 1937 to denote lesions arising without an obvious primary intravascular source of infection or contiguous sepsis. In the patient reported here, pronounced systemic illness, toxic appearance, and the marked tenderness of the abdominal aneurysm led to the correct preoperative diagnosis. The unusual loculated, saccular configuration of the aneurysm in an otherwise normal-appearing vasculature further supported the diagnosis of mycotic aneurysm. Preadmission antibiotic therapy probably accounts for her negative blood cultures, although only 53 percent of the patients in Bennett's[2] collected series had positive blood cultures.

Once infection of an aortic aneurysm is suspected, immediate operation is imperative to avoid rupture and to remove the intravascular focus of infection. Intense antibiotic therapy alone is usually inadequate in controlling infection, and fatal rupture often occurs during antibiotic therapy.[3, 9, 15, 28]

We are aware of only two previously reported cases of successful resection and reconstruction. Sower and Whelan[29] claimed the first successfully treated case of a ruptured aorta due to *Salmonella choleraesuis* aortitis. They were concerned about introducing a large Dacron foreign body into an infected area but fortunately the outcome was favorable. Rob and Ngu[24] reported a patient who survived after infrarenal aortic ligation after a new mycotic aneurysm developed distal to a Dacron graft used to repalce an earlier mycotic aortic aneurysm. Although Robb[25] also reported the successful tangential resection of a mycotic aortic aneurysm, his patient had no evidence of infection at the time of surgery, three years after the successful antibiotic treatment of subacute bacterial endocarditis. His case represents the unusual situation in which infection has apparently been controlled by antibiotic agents prior to surgery.

Although spontaneous thrombosis and resolution has been noticed in small mycotic aneurysms,[1] rupture of infected aortic aneurysms may occur suddenly and earlier in their development than uninfected atherosclerotic aneurysms.[18] When these aneurysms ruptured, death was inevitable in spite of surgery.[3, 27, 30] Even complete antibiotic sterilization does not guarantee protection against continuing enlargement and subsequent rupture.[13, 19, 25]

Operative deaths[14, 31] are probably due to the patient's debilitated septic state at the time of surgery. Postoperative deaths, in ruptured and unruptured aneurysms, are attributable to persistent sepsis whether Dacron,[7, 17] Teflon,[18] or homograft prostheses[4] were used for the aortic reconstruction. Because direct aortic replacement frequently is unsuccessful in a contaminated area, the principle advocated by Shaw and Baue[26] of defunctioning and bypassing the infected segment has obvious application.

The axillofemoral graft, as described independently and almost simultaneously by Louw[20] and Blaisdell and Hall,[5] was devised mainly as an alternative to aortofemoral reconstruction in patients deemed unsuitable for major abdominal surgery. The axillofemoral graft has also proved to be of value in the treatment of infected intra-abdominal prosthetic grafts[5, 30] and to circumvent fistulas widely between bowel and plastic arterial prostheses.[16] The axillofemoral graft lends itself admirably to the management of mycotic aortic aneurysms, as is demonstrated by this case and one previously reported.[6] Six months after operation, our patient has no abdominal pain or evidence of systemic illness. She has good pedal pulses bilaterally. Because 50 percent of axillofemoral grafts have been reported to be occluded after 18 months,[23] we have considered later elective intra-abdominal graft placement in our patient. However, there is evidence that long-term patency is greater when a single graft is used to supply both lower extremities,[23] and prolonged success has been reported by Mannick and associates[22] and Louw.[21]

The operation was performed as an emergency in our patient to avoid rupture. Intense antibiotic therapy was begun preoperatively and the right axillofemoral graft was inserted with skin closure before the abdomen was opened in order to avoid contamination of the prosthesis. An arterial clamp was left in situ on the right common femoral artery through the groin incision to avoid aortoiliac competitive flow and possible intraoperative graft occlusion. The clamp was removed to restore flow to the left leg as soon as the terminal aorta was cross-clamped prior to proximal aortic resection. The patient's uneventful postoperative course attests to the feasibility of the procedure which we advocate as the treatment of choice for mycotic aortic aneurysm.

REFERENCES

1. Barker, W. F.: Mycotic aneurysms, Ann. Surg. **139:** 84, 1954.

2. Bennett, D. E.: Primary mycotic aneurysms of the aorta. Report of a case and review of the literature, Arch. Surg. **94:** 758, 1967.
3. Bennett, D. E., and Cherry, J. K.: Bacterial infection of aortic aneurysms. A clinico-pathological study, Am. J. Surg. **113:** 321, 1967.
4. Black, P. H., Kunz, L. J., and Swartz, M. N.: Salmonellosis—a review of some unusual aspects, N. Engl. J. Med. **262:** 811, 1960.
5. Blaisdell, F. W., and Hall, A. D.: Axillary-femoral artery bypass for lower extremity ischemia, SURGERY **54:** 563, 1963.
6. Bliss, B. P., and Barrett, G. S.: Axillo-femoral and axillo-profunda bypass grafts, Ann. R. Coll. Surg. Engl. **50:** 268, 1972.
7. Bosher, L. H., Jr., and Decker, A. M., Jr.: Experiences in vascular grafting for aortic and arterial aneurysms, Ann. Surg. **145:** 943, 1957.
8. Case records of the Massachusetts General Hospital: Clinico-Pathological Conference, Case 39291, N. Engl. J. Med. **249:** 110, 1953
9. Case records of the Massachusetts General Hospital: Clinico-Pathological Conference, Case 42511, N. Engl. J. Med. **255:** 1194, 1956.
10. Case records of the Massachusetts General Hospital: Clinico-Pathological Conference, Case 53-1961, N. Engl. J. Med. **265:** 189, 1961.
11. Case records of the Massachusetts General Hospital: Clinico-Pathological Conference, Case 8-1962, N. Engl. J. Med. **266:** 249, 1962.
12. Case records of the Massachusetts General Hospital: Clinico-Pathological Conference, Case 38-1971, N. Engl. J. Med. **285:** 739, 1971.
13. Cates, J. E., and Christie, R. V.: Subacute bacterial endocarditis: Review of 442 patients treated in 14 centers appointed by the Penicillin Trials Committee of the Medical Research Council, Q. J. Med. **20:** 93, 1951.
14. Crane, A. R.: Primary multilocular mycotic aneurysm of the aorta, Arch. Pathol. **24:** 634, 1937.
15. Currens, J. H., and Faulkner, J. M.: Gonococcal mycotic aneurysm of the aorta: Report of a case superimposed upon a syphilitic aorta, Ann. Intern. Med. **19:** 155, 1943.
16. Ehrenfeld, W. K., Lord, R. S. A., Stoney, R. J., and Wylie, E. J.: Subcutaneous arterial bypass grafts in the management of fistulae between the bowel and plastic arterial prostheses, Ann. Surg. **168:** 29, 1968.
17. Foster, J. H., and Vetto, R. M.: Aortic intra-aneurysmal abscess caused by a sigmoid-aortic fistula, Am. J. Surg. **104:** 850, 1962.
18. Hyde, R. D., and Davis, T. K. B.: Infection of an aortic aneurysm with *Salmonella choleraesuis,* Br. Med. J. **1:** 30, 1962.
19. Javett, S. M., and Kahn, E.: Rupture of a mycotic aneurysm of the thoracic aorta, Arch. Dis. Child. **27:** 294, 1952.
20. Louw, J. H.: Splenic-to-femoral and axillary-to-femoral bypass grafts in diffuse atherosclerotic occlusive disease, Lancet **1:** 1401, 1963.
21. Louw, J. H.: Axillary to femoral bypass graft for aorto-iliac occlusive disease, S. Afr. J. Surg. **8:** 15, 1970.
22. Mannick, J. A., Williams, L. E., and Nabseth, D. C.: The late results of axillofemoral grafts, SURGERY **68:** 1038, 1970.
23. Moore, W. S., Hall, A. D., and Blaisdell, F. W.: Late results of axillary-femoral bypass grafting, Am. J. Surg. **122:** 148, 1971.
24. Rob, C., and Ngu, V.: Mycotic aneurysms of undetermined etiology, Dtsch. Med. Wochenschr. **84:** 1157, 1960.
25. Robb, D.: Surgical treatment of mycotic aneurysm, SURGERY **52:** 847, 1962.
26. Shaw, R. S., and Baue, A. E.: Management of sepsis complicating arterial reconstructive surgery, SURGERY **53:** 75, 1963.
27. Smith, R. F., Szilagyi, D. E., and Colville, J. M.: Surgical treatment of mycotic aneurysms, Arch. Surg. **85:** 663, 1962.
28. Sommerville, R. L., Allen, E. V., and Edwards, J. E.: Bland and infected arteriosclerotic abdominal aortic aneurysms: A clinico-pathological study, Medicine **38:** 207, 1959.
29. Sower, N. D., and Whelan, T. J., Jr.: Suppurative arteritis due to Salmonella, SURGERY **52:** 851, 1962.
30. Urdaneta, L. F., Visudh-Arom, K., Delaney, J. P., and Castaneda, A. R.: Use of bilateral axillofemoral bypass prosthesis for the management of infected aortic bifurcation grafts: Report of a case with extended follow-up, SURGERY **65:** 753, 1969.
31. Zak, F. G., Strauss, L., and Sapura, I.: Rupture of diseased large arteries in the course of intrabacterial (Salmonella) infection, N. Engl. J. Med. **258:** 824, 1958.

Routine venography in placement of the Mobin-Uddin vena cava filter: Dual filter placement in a patient with an accessory vena cava (cardinal vein)

Mark M. Kartchner, M.D., *and* **A. J. Bogosian,** *Tucson, Ariz.*

One advantage of the routine use of venography during the placement of a Mobin-Uddin inferior vena cava umbrella is illustrated by the report of a patient with an accessory inferior vena cava (cardinal vein). The venography catheter also serves as a guide for the passage of the inferior vena cava umbrella. The authors believe routine catheter venography eliminates many of the complications associated with inferior vena cava filter placement.

IMPLANTATION of the Mobin-Uddin vena cava umbrella below the renal veins in the inferior vena cava has been developed as a means of preventing pulmonary emboli.[1-5] A number of major complications have arisen from its use.[6, 7] Studies are underway to further evaluate and correct these problems. It is our contention that the filter is a valuable adjunct in treatment of selected patients when placed correctly with the use of *routine* venography. Our current case study exemplifies one benefit from following such a protocol.

CASE STUDY

G. K. is a 59-year-old woman with a history of chronic intermittent pulmonary infections commencing in 1944. The patient was admitted to the hospital with a clinical and radiographic picture of pneumonia. After appropriate antibiotic treatment, the patient improved somewhat but was still slightly dyspneic. Bronchoscopic washings revealed no organisms and the evolving radiographic picture suggested the diagnosis of pulmonary embolism. Lung scan further delineated pulmonary perfusion defects consistent with pulmonary emboli. Because of the pulmonary findings, the decision was made to implant an inferior vena cava umbrella to prevent further pulmonary vascular insult. Preliminary venography under direct fluoroscopy demonstrated an absence of the left iliac vein which was consistent with total thrombotic occlusion. Further venographic examination of the renal veins demonstrated an extremely large tributary to the left renal vein, which drained the left iliac vein (Fig. 1). It was quite evident at this point that this was a residual cardinal vein (accessory vena cava). With the use of a venography catheter as a guide, separate umbrella filters were placed in the accessory vena cava, as well as the inferior vena cava (Figs. 2 and 3).

Accepted for publication Oct. 9, 1973.

METHOD

Routine venography prior to insertion of the inferior vena cava umbrella is accomplished with a straight arterial catheter under fluoroscopy. This is inserted through the internal jugular venotomy site used subsequently for passage of the filter intraducer. Dye injection under fluoroscopy is carried out at the level of the renal and inferior vena cava bifurcation. Routine venography is stressed for a number of reasons: (1) to assess the anatomy into which the filter will be placed, specifically the level of the renal veins and the bifurcation of the inferior vena

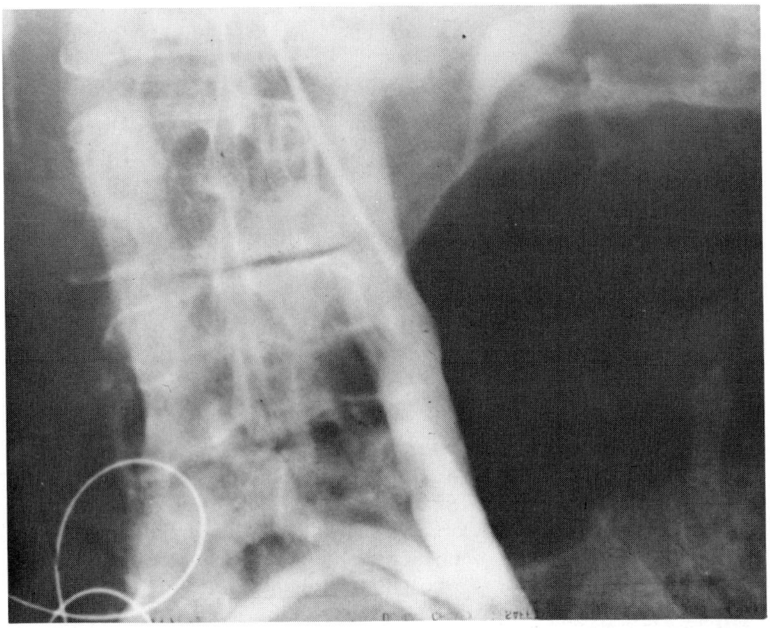

Fig. 1. Venographic demonstration of vena cava (*left*) and accessory vena cava (*right*).

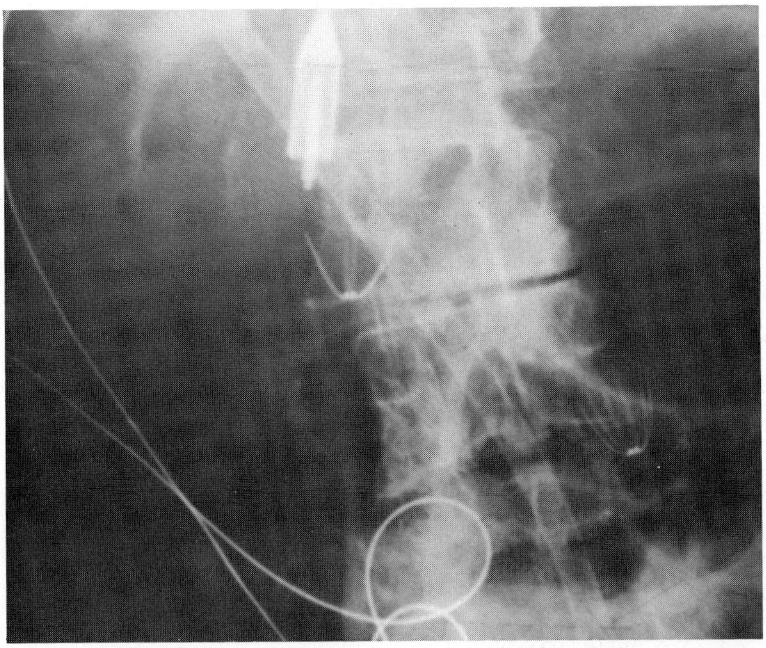

Fig. 2. Flat plate abdominal x-ray film of filters in place.

cava; (2) to demonstrate anatomical variants such as large collateral systems; (3) to size the inferior vena cava and avert filter placement in a mega cava, which has been reported as a cause of umbrella dislodgment and subsequent embolization; (4) to use the venography catheter as a guide to facilitate the passage of the filter intraducer through the right atrium, and avoiding the hepatic and renal veins. (The routine usage of venography has proven helpful in our current case as well as others where severe

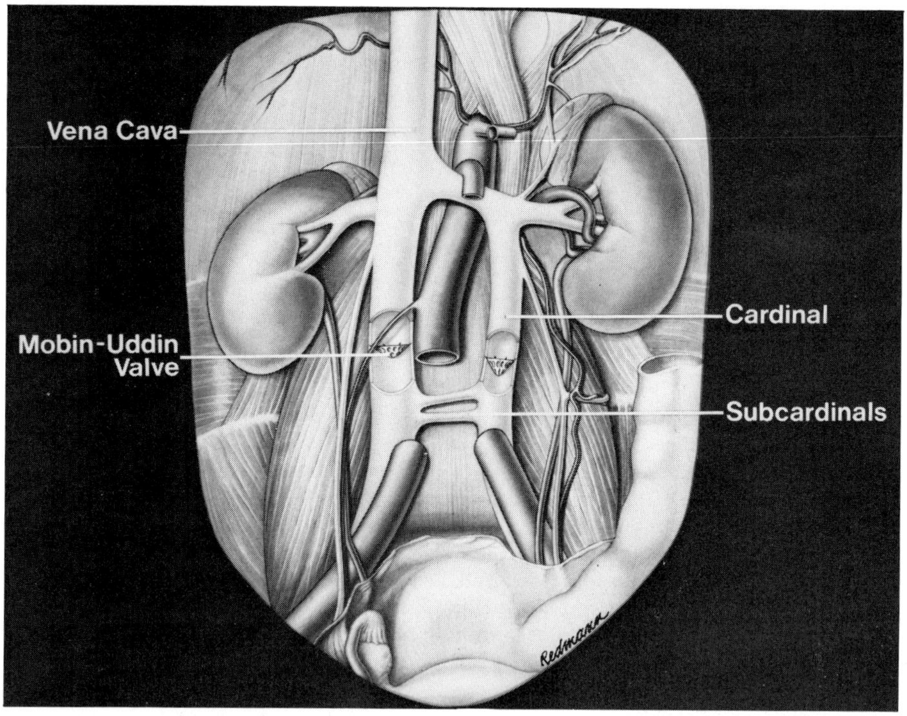

Fig. 3. Diagrammatic representation of anomalous anatomy with filters in place.

kyphoscoliosis or aberrant anatomy has interfered with umbrella filter placement.); (5) to document adequate seating of the umbrella filter after implantation.

DISCUSSION

With the assumption that major pulmonary embolism can be prevented by utilization of the Mobin-Uddin inferior vena cava umbrella,[2] it is desirable to ensure accurate placement and seating of this device. A number of complications including renal vein placement, iliac vein placement, malposition of the umbrella, and embolization have been reported. The routine use of catheter venography has allowed us to avoid many of the common complications and technical difficulties encountered in umbrella placement. Also recognition of anatomic variants by this technique permits their management, thereby alleviating the possibility of aberrant recurrent embolization.

REFERENCES

1. Beller, B. M., Talley, R. C., and Leslie, L. J.: Nonsurgical inferior vena cava obstruction for prevention of pulmonary emboli, J. A. M. A. **220:** 973, 1972.
2. Bergan, J. J., Crane, C., Mortez, W. H., Ochsner, A., Sautter, R. D., Sher, M. H., and Silver, D.: Forum: Preventing embolism: What method of canal interruption is preferred? Mod. Med. **41:** 93, 1973.
3. Lynch, J. D., Sketch, M. H., and Schultz, R. D.: Treatment of recurrent pulmonary embolism by intravenous interruption of the inferior vena cava, Nebr. Med. J. **57:** 354, 1972.
4. Mobin-Uddin, K., Smith, P. E., Martines, L. D., Lombardo, C. R., and Jude, J. R.: A vena cava filter for the prevention of pulmonary embolus, Surg. Forum **18:** 209, 1967.
5. Mobin-Uddin, K., McLean, R., and Jude, J. R.: A new catheter technique of interruption of inferior vena cava for prevention of pulmonary embolism, Am. Surg. **35:** 889, 1969.
6. Mobin-Uddin, K., Bolooki, H., and Jude, J. R.: Intravenous canal interruption for pulmonary embolism in cardiac disease, Circulation **41**(Suppl. 2): 153, 1970.
7. Mobin-Uddin, K., Trimble, J. K., and Bryant, L. R.: Present status of the inferior vena cava umbrella filter, SURGERY **70:** 914, 1971.
8. Nevin, W. S., and Beddingfield, G. W.: Case report: Migration of vena cava filter, J. A. M. A. **222:** 88, 1972.

Fate of a nylon vascular prosthesis for aortic replacement: 14 year follow-up study

Peter B. Yaw, M.D., T. W. Grisell, M.D., W. M. Wahle, M.D., H. B Shumacker, M.D., *and* John L. Glover, M.D., *Indianapolis, Ind.*

A 68-year-old woman underwent a second aortoiliac reconstruction procedure 14 years after placement of an Edwards-Tapp nylon graft. The only vestige of graft remaining was a mass of scar tissue on the anterior surface of the aorta, the iliac limbs having been completely absorbed. Tissue examination revealed fragments of fabric present intracellularly in phagocytes and also encased in fibrous tissue. A Dacron graft was inserted with a good result. Early research activities relating to development of suitable grafts are reviewed and some factors in the selection process are discussed. To our knowledge, this is the first report of an examination of a nylon graft implanted in human tissue for 14 years.

From the Departments of Surgery, Marion County General Hospital and Indiana University Medical Center, Indianapolis, Ind.

THE PIONEER work of Voorhees and associates[12] in 1952 showed the feasibility of using tubular cloth grafts as replacement of aortic segments in dogs with long-term patency. Many synthetic materials were subsequently tested experimentally, and in 1953 the first plastic aortic prostheses were placed by Shumacker and King[10] with the use of nylon and by Blakemore and Voorhees[3] with vinyon "N." Experimental evidence[6] quickly showed that nylon had a major disadvantage in that it rapidly lost tensile strength in tissues. Reported cases of degeneration of nylon grafts[8] are sparse, however, although a few cases of aneurysmal dilatation have been noted by one of us (H. B S.). A recent operative experience in which we observed some rather spectacular changes in a nylon cloth graft placed in the aortic position 14 years ago prompted this report.

Accepted for publication Oct. 10, 1973.

Reprint requests: Dr. P. B. Yaw, Department of Surgery, Marion County General Hospital, 960 Locke St., Indianapolis, Ind. 46202.

CASE REPORT

In 1958, a 54-year-old white woman underwent an aortic iliac graft operation because of severe intermittent claudication. The prosthesis used was an Edwards-Tapp nylon graft which was implanted end to side to the infrarenal aorta and end to side to the femoral arteries. The common iliac arteries were felt to be moderately altered by arteriosclerotic changes at this time, and the terminal aorta was severely involved with the same process. She recovered from the operation without difficulty but had no relief of her claudication. Although graft occlusion was suspected, angiography was not performed. Her claudication remained stable initially; but she developed mild angina pectoris, congestive heart failure, and symptoms suggestive of peptic ulcer disease in the ensuing years.

In 1972 she was hospitalized because of increasingly severe intermittent claudication in the right leg and mild pain at rest. Although neck and arm pulses were present and of normal intensity, there were no pulses in either groin or below that level. The aortic pulse seemed normal, and there was no evidence of an aneurysm. The blood pressure was 140/80.

Angiography by the axillary route revealed severe arteriosclerotic changes in the abdominal aorta and near-total obstruction of both iliac arteries. There was no filling of the old graft (Fig. 1). Later films revealed a right superficial femoral artery occlusion; but both popliteal systems were visualized. Another revascularization procedure seemed indicated.

At the time of operation, the only vestige of the aortic portion of the old graft was a nonpulsatile mass of scar tissue and atheromatous material on the anterior surface of the aorta (Fig. 2). The iliac limbs were absent, apparently having been completely absorbed. The iliac arteries were small (6 mm.) and still only moderately atherosclerotic. A knitted Dacron bifurcation graft was interpolated end to end to the aorta (at a higher level than previously) and end to side to both external iliac arteries. Although the patient required tracheostomy and ventilatory assistance in the postoperative period, she recovered satisfactorily and had an excellent result, as manifested by relief of claudication. Femoral pulses were strong bilaterally and pedal pulses were palpable, being stronger on the left side than the right.

Examination of the tissue removed from the aortic area revealed severe atheromatous changes and complete fragmentation of the nylon fabric. One could not, in fact, recognize any fabric in the gross specimen. In polarized light sections, there were microscopic fragments of fabric and thread within phagocytes and also embedded in fibrous tissue. Some of the fragments were obviously nylon, and some were probably from the silk suture used for the anastomosis (Figs. 3, 4, and 5).

About three months after the aortoiliac operation, the patient developed recurrent claudication and was found to have no pulse in the right groin. A femorofemoral tubular graft was placed crossing the midline above the pubis, with successful restoration of pulsatile flow. Follow-up examination at six months revealed an excellent pulse and no claudication.

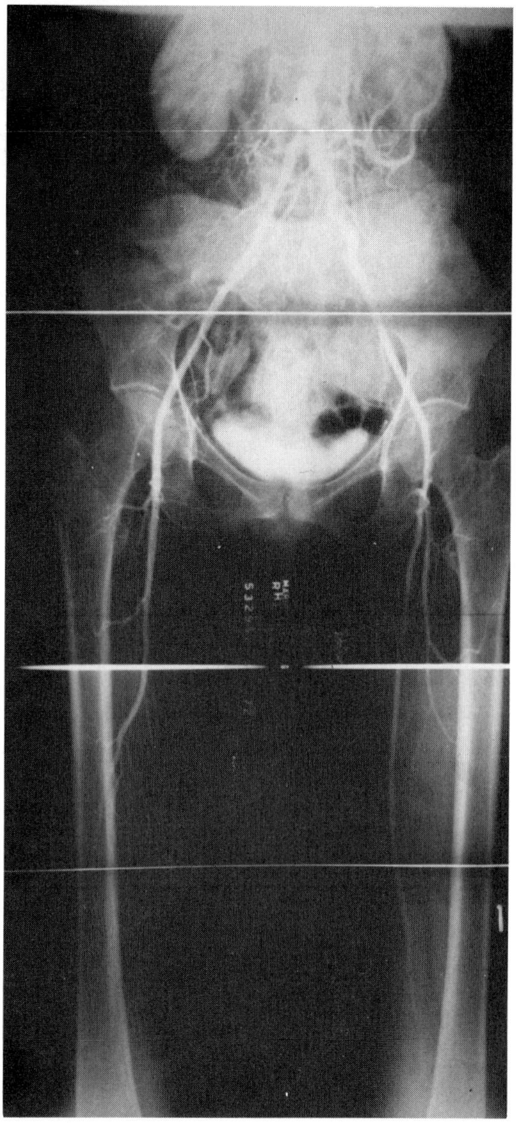

Fig. 1. Preoperative angiogram done 14 years after aortoiliac bypass. Note the high-grade obstruction at the aortic bifurcation and the right superficial femoral artery obstruction. There is no sign of the vascular prosthesis.

DISCUSSION

In the early 1950's, there was a great deal of effort to determine the best fabric for aortic and aortoiliac replacement. Aortic homografts had been used in many cases up to that time and give very adequate results, although late aneurysm formation occurred, as did calcification and occlusion. The major problems with homologous aorta, however, were supply, sterilization, storage, and availability of various sizes.

Early tissue acceptance of numerous fabrics was satisfactory,[1, 2, 5, 7, 9, 10] and the advantages of unlimited supply, various sizes, long shelf life, and ease of storage, and sterilization were obvious. The early fabric grafts did tend to fray at the cut ends and were more difficult to sew than the homografts. Also, they tended to kink rather than bend, causing occlusion in some cases. Early

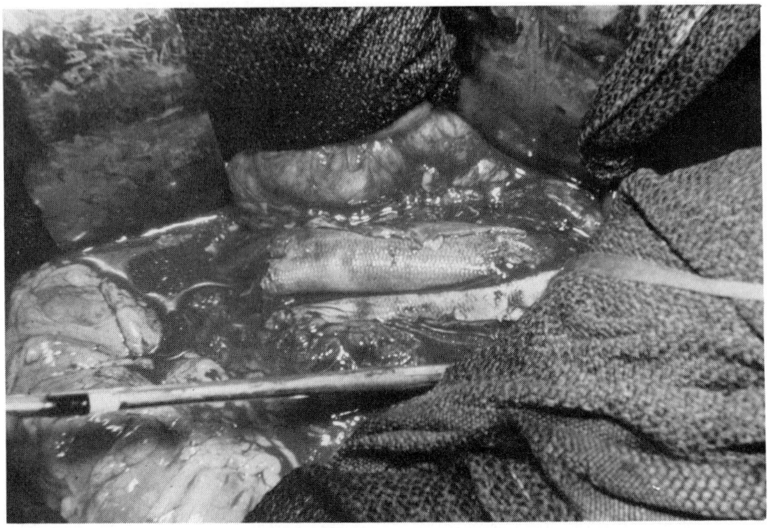

Fig. 2. Nylon aortic graft remnant in place. The weave pattern of the graft is obvious. The remnants of the two femoral limbs are seen in its inferior aspect. The patient's aorta lies just below the graft. Grossly, the specimen consisted entirely of atheromatous material without recognizable fabric. Microscopically, remnants of the nylon graft were seen (see Figs. 3, 4, and 5).

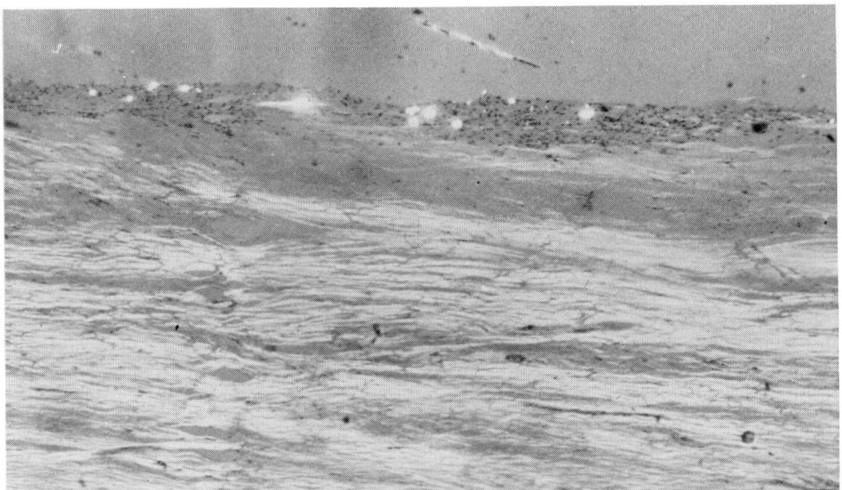

Fig. 3. Polarized photomicrograph showing birefringent mature collagen in the media and bright polarized spots of residual graft material on the intimal surface (top) and adventitis (bottom). (Hematoxylin and eosin stain. Original magnification, ×13.)

leakage through the fabric was another problem causing mild to moderate blood loss and some cases of exsanguination. Tightening the graft weave and crimping the fabric adequately handled these problems, however.

One of the first commercially available fabric grafts was the Edwards-Tapp braided nylon crimped graft. Shumacker and others used them with early good results. In 1957 Shumacker and associates[11] and later Barnett and Norman[2] and other investigators reported on the fate of nylon fabric grafts of

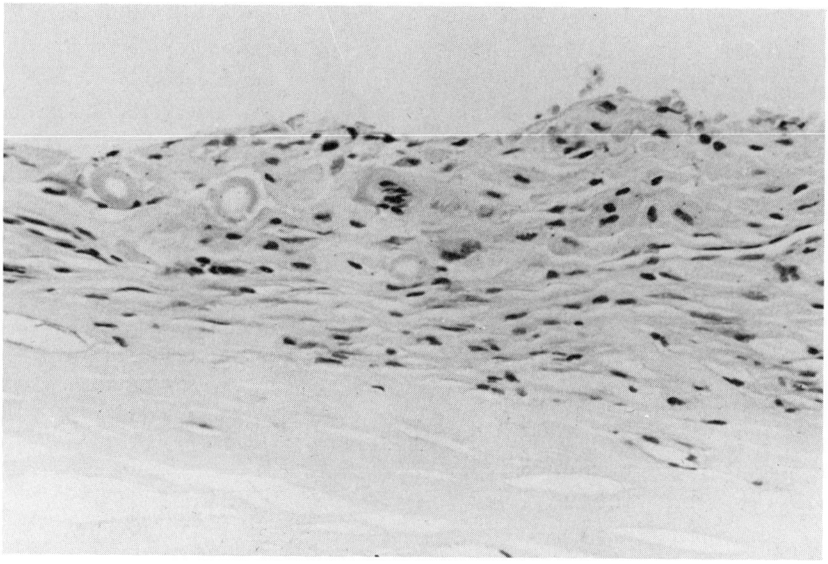

Fig. 4. View of intimal surface showing fibrosis, residual graft material (round amorphous material) and collagen fibers in the subintimal portion. (Hematoxylin and eosin stain. Original magnification, ×32.)

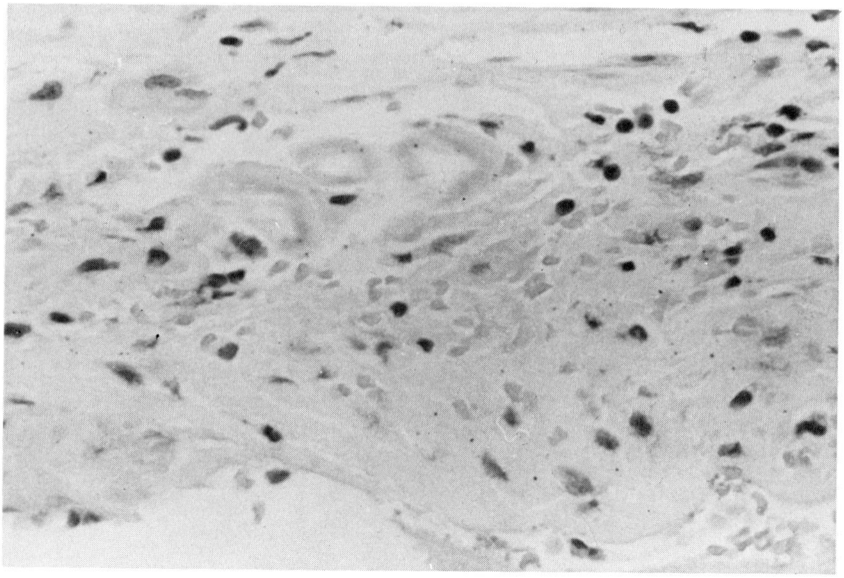

Fig. 5. High-power view of adventitial surface showing amorphous circular graft remnants in fibrous tissue. (Hematoxylin and eosin stain. Original magnification, ×120.)

various types in dogs and in humans for periods varying from one day up to two years in dogs and approximately two years in humans. They noted no graft fragmentation or aneurysm formation in their studies.

In 1956 in a report[4] to the Society for Vascular Surgery by a committee for the study of vascular prostheses, the conclusion was reached that many materials showed early acceptable results as vascular replacements, especially in the aortic and aorto-iliac positions where high pressure and rapid flow made thrombotic occlusion unlikely. Earlier investigators had noted that nylon lost from 75 to 80 percent of its original strength after six to eighteen months of implantation in tissue.[8] Although follow-up studies for as long as two years after placement of nylon grafts as aortic and aortoiliac replacements had shown no fragmentation or dilatation in dogs or humans, it was the feeling of the committee that Dacron and Teflon were the most satisfactory materials available at that time for the formation of vascular prostheses, since both materials retained their strength in tissues over long periods of time.[4] The committee stated that inertness, flexibility without kinking, strength, and ease of handling and suturing were properties that would be desirable in any successful aortic prosthesis. In 1960 Halpert and associates[6] reported the fate of abdominal aortic replacement homografts and prostheses including five nylon grafts. One of the nylon grafts in place for 43 months was found to be aneurysmal at reoperation for occlusion of one of the graft limbs. The other nylon grafts were in place for 37, 22, 12½, and 12 months, and they were intact at autopsy or at reoperation for another reason. They[6] recommended Dacron as the best prosthetic material available for aortic replacements. In the eight Dacron aortic replacements in their study that were in place from three to twenty-five months, there were no aneurysms formed.

Based on the experimental demonstration of loss of strength in tissue and the personal experience of various surgeons with aneurysmal formation, nylon fell into disuse after this time as a fabric for formation of vascular prostheses. The patient reported in this paper received one of the last nylon grafts (if not the last) used at Indiana University Medical Center and represents a 14 year follow-up study of this material in the aortoiliac position. We are unaware of any previous report of such a case, especially one showing complete fragmentation of the graft. Whether the early occlusion was related to the absorption is not known. It has been the policy of our surgical department since 1957 to follow all nylon aortic grafts closely, if possible, and replace them at the first sign of any degeneration.

This case does emphasize the danger of drawing early conclusions about the function and fate of materials implanted in tissue. It also demonstrates that successful reconstructive procedures can be accomplished despite failure of earlier attempts at bypass or replacement.

REFERENCES

1. Barnett, W. O.: Experimental nylon aortic substitutes, Arch. Surg. **76:** 1, 1958.
2. Barnett, W. O., and Norman, T. D.: A histologic study of the tissues surrounding experimental nylon aortic substitutes, Arch. Surg. **76:** 389, 1958.
3. Blakemore, A. H., and Voorhees, A. B.: The uses of tubes constructed from Vinyon "N" cloth in bridging arterial defects: Experimental and clinical, Ann. Surg. **140:** 324, 1954.
4. Creech, O., Jr., Deterling, R. A., Jr., Edwards, S., Julian, O. C., Linton, R., and Shumacker, H. B, Jr.: Vascular prostheses, Surgery **41:** 62, 1957.
5. Edwards, W. S., and Tapp, J. S.: Chemically treated nylon tubes as arterial grafts, Surgery **38:** 61, 1955.
6. Halpert, B., De Bakey, M. E., Jordan, G. L., and Henley, W. S.: The fate of homografts and prostheses of the human aorta, Surg. Gynecol. Obstet. **III:** 659, Dec. 1960.
7. Harris, E. J., Shumacker, H. B, Jr., Siderys, H., Moore, T. C., and Grice, P. E.: Pliable plastic aortic grafts, Arch. Surg. **71:** 449, 1955.
8. Harrison, J. H., and Adler, R. H.: Nylon as a vascular prosthesis in experimental animals with tensile strength studies, Surg. Gynecol. Obstet. **103:** 613, 1956.
9. Shumacker, H. B, Jr.: Plastic grafts for aortic substition in man, Arch. Surg. **75:** 413, 1957.
10. Shumacker, H. B, Jr., and King, M.: The use of pliable plastic tubes as aortic substitutes in man, Surg. Gynecol. Obstet. **99:** 287, 1954.
11. Shumacker, H. B, Jr., Kajikuri, H., Grice, P., Rodriguez, R., Riberi, A., Moore, T. C., and Siderys, H.: Comparative experimental study of aortic grafts, Surgery **41:** 943, 1957.
12. Voorhees, A. B., Jr., Jeretzki, A., III, and Blakemore, A. H.: The use of tubes constructed of vinyon "N" clot in bridging arterial defects, Ann. Surg. **135:** 332, 1952.

Editorials

Hypertonic glucose and improved critical organ performance

Richard H. Egdahl, M.D., *Boston, Mass.*

From the Department of Surgery, University Hospital, Boston University Medical Center, Boston, Mass.

TWO ARTICLES[2, 4] in this month's issue of SURGERY focus on the use of glucose as a substrate to improve critical organ performance under abnormal conditions.

Pindyck and co-workers[4] have demonstrated that pretreatment of critically ill patients with hypertonic glucose appears to increase the stores of substrate available for myocardial function. Hewitt and co-workers,[2] utilizing the anoxic arrested heart as a model, demonstrated a protective effect by increasing glycogen stores or administering glucose. This editorial constitutes a brief progress report on the current status of the use of hypertonic glucose in critically ill patients and suggests possible alternative metabolic approaches to the problem of cell energy needs under conditions dangerous to the organism.

The past few years have seen a series of papers from several different laboratories and clinical centers on the use of hypertonic glucose, either alone or with potassium and insulin added and under a variety of clinical circumstances. There are two basic purposes for which the hypertonic glucose has been administered. The first centers around the general nutrition of the patient and improvements in a variety of critical functions that occur with increase in effective caloric intake. This is the focus of the article by Pindyck and colleagues[4] and of papers by Hinton and co-workers[3] utilizing massive doses of glucose, potassium, and insulin (GKI) in severely burned patients. The other method of using glucose is illustrated by the paper by Hewitt and associates[4] in which specific organ function is improved by perfusing the individual organ with GKI and thereby increasing available substrate. The mechanism for increased myocardial function in the latter instance is thought to be increased utilization of glucose in anaerobic metabolism of the heart. In the case of systemic hypertonic glucose administration, it is probable that critical organs increase their stores of available substrate.

Although the utilization of hypertonic glucose offers intriguing possibilities, there are great dangers which accompany the use of large doses of insulin and potassium along with the glucose. On the one hand, if 50 percent glucose alone is given, the blood sugar may become extremely elevated and various complications may result. On the other hand, very large doses of insulin are necessary in order to keep the blood sugar near normal levels, and this provides the basis for possible dangerous or fatal hypoglycemic reactions. I have heard discussions about near fatal or fatal reactions from hypoglycemia in critically ill patients given hypertonic glucose and massive doses of insulin. For that reason, continued investiga-

Accepted for publication June 11, 1973.

tion of hypertonic glucose administration along with insulin should be carried out in only those institutions prepared to study most carefully their patients and derive data that can be used to decide whether the therapy clearly results in improved organ function and increased survival without excessive danger.

The most urgent study needed in this field is experimental evidence for *increased survival* with GKI, not just improvements in *isolated organ function*. Previous survival studies have yielded inconclusive results, although some reports suggest prolongation of survival time in shocked animals given GKI. Unless critical survival studies are carried out in appropriate experimental animals in different laboratories within the next few years, it is possible that this potentially valuable clinical therapy will find itself in the same therapeutic limbo that radical mastectomy is in for primary treatment of breast carcinoma. Failure of unbiased surgeons to set up appropriate clinical trials of various methods of primary treatment of breast cancer many years ago have put us in the position at the present time where it is difficult to make a truly informed decision as to the best initial therapy for that disease. Increasing numbers of studies showing favorable alterations in function of one organ or another with hypertonic glucose, without the basic buttressing of significant improvement in survival, may well lead to the utilization of GKI therapy in a variety of clinical circumstances without any real evidence that it is indeed over-all efficacious. Further difficulty centers around the widely differing dosages of glucose, insulin, and potassium which have been administered and the necessity to develop somewhat standard protocols for individuals who set out to confirm results of others. Finally, it is necessary to devise critical experiments to determine whether GKI acts exclusively on an increased caloric basis or if potassium and insulin provide an additional effect. Indeed, it has been suggested that effectiveness of the hyperalimentation regimen may be based upon beneficial endocrine effects, in addition to increased caloric intake.

There are other metabolic developments that may find future therapeutic application. It has been shown that both ATP (adenosine triphosphate) and cyclic AMP (adenosine 3′,5′-monophosphate) are decreased in liver and other organs in severe hemorrhagic shock. Preliminary results from Dr. Rutenburg's laboratory* indicate that administration of a cyclic AMP analogue to animals in shock results in significantly increased myocardial work capacity, decreased peripheral resistance, and increased survival rates. Further work along these lines is indicated in order to confirm and extend these findings. Administration of alpha-adrenergic blockers appears to restore the normal insulin response to the hyperglycemia of shock, and these findings suggest the possibility that the administration of alpha-adrenergic blockers may find a role in the metabolic treatment of shock. Blackburn and co-workers[1] have shown that if amino acids are substituted for glucose in intravenous solutions given to postoperative patients, a significant nitrogen-sparing effect occurs which may have beneficial effects on the patients' overall metabolic state.

We appear to be reaching the point where the major contribution of hyperalimentation to the metabolic treatment of critically ill patients may be supplemented by any of several fine tuning metabolic mechanisms involving specific substrates, chemicals, or pharmacological agents. If critical experiments are set up which show significantly increased survival in shocked animals given these new metabolic regimens, metabolic manipulations may find a secure place in the surgical armamentarium for treatment of critically ill patients. It does appear established that improved myocardial function and systemic hemodynamics result from increased carbohydrate substrate availability. What now remains to be demonstrated is whether experimental animal—and ultimate-

*Unpublished data.

ly patient survival—is increased by any of the new metabolic approaches.

REFERENCES

1. Blackburn, G. L., Flatt, J. P., Clowes, G. H. A., O'Donnell, T. F., and Hensle, T. E.: Protein sparing therapy during periods of starvation with sepsis or trauma, Ann. Surg. **177:** 588, 1973.
2. Hewitt, R. L., Lolley, D. M., Adrouny, G. A., and Drapanas, T.: Protective affect of glycogen and glucose on the anoxic arrested heart, Surgery **75:** 1, 1974.
3. Hinton, P., Littlejohn, S., Allison, S. P., and Lloyd, J.: Insulin and glucose to reduce catabolic response to injury in burned patients, Lancet **1:** 767, 1971.
4. Pindyck, F., Drucker, M. R., Brown, R. S., and Shoemaker, W. C.: Cardiorespiratory effects of hypertonic glucose in the critically ill patient, Surgery **75:** 11, 1974.

Surgical anatomy

John E. Skandalakis, M.D., Ph.D., F.A.C.S., Joseph S. Rowe, Jr., M.D., *and* **Stephen W. Gray, Ph.D.,** *Atlanta, Ga.*

. . . those surgeons who more and more have come to realize that a knowledge of anatomy in surgical procedures is the best safeguard to avoid surgical injuries."

Nicholas A. Michels[2]

From the Department of Surgical Education, Piedmont Hospital, and the Departments of Anatomy and Surgery, Emory University School of Medimine, Atlanta, Ga.

WE ARE DISTURBED to see surgical education devoting more and more attention to physiology and pathophysiology at the expense of surgical anatomy. Improvement in preoperative and postoperative care has drastically lowered the operative mortality rate in recent years, but the very terms tell us that the essence of surgery is the operation itself. The best of pre- and postoperative care will not make up for a bungled operation. Surgical anatomy is still the most important basis for surgery.

We are not blind to the contribution of physiology, pathophysiology, biochemistry, or cell biology. We are grateful for their progress and their help. We speak, not to condemn these sciences, but to defend anatomy, the "most unpopular science," and to hope that it will return to its proper emphasis in the medical curriculum.

If a patient does poorly two days after surgery, the surgeon can request another specialist to help him with problems of respiratory insufficiency or azotemia. Where will he get help when he can not find the recurrent laryngeal nerve or when he is confused by an anomalous biliary tree? Here, at the operation, he is alone—with only the knowledge he brought to the table with him.

One reason for the lack of emphasis on surgical anatomy is confusion between advances in the field of surgery and the knowledge required of each young surgeon. Many surgical anatomical problems have been worked out in the past, but each new surgeon must relearn for himself much information that has been left behind by the advancing wave of present surgical concern. It is not enough to produce surgeons who understand modern theories of gallstone formation (a subject of present interest) if he does not know how to recognize and manage an anomalous biliary tree (a subject of little present interest). Must the young surgeon be a second-rate physiologist before he becomes a first-rate anatomist?

Our concern is for greater interest in surgical anatomy, the field in which only the surgeon can be the authority, so that the young surgeon can do his daily work efficiently and accurately. With proper attention to surgical anatomy he can: (1) dissect swiftly along anatomical tissue planes; (2) correctly evaluate the technical literature; (3) be flexible enough to tailor his operation to the particular anatomy of each individual

Accepted for publication March 28, 1973.

patient; and (4) cope with unforeseen circumstances as they arise.

We are concerned with the teaching of anatomy by computers. We realize that our students and residents have too much to learn today, but "computer knowledge" based on words rather than on visualization will not be their Simon when their burden grows too heavy.

A much learned man, William Hunter,[1] stated "Were I to place a man of proper talents in the most direct road of becoming truly great in his profession, I would choose a good practical anatomist and put him into a large hospital to attend the sick and dissect the dead." For the student of surgery today, this statement of yesterday is still valid—very valid indeed.

REFERENCES

1. Hunter, W.: Two introductory lectures to his last course of anatomical lectures, etc., London, J. Johnson, 1784, Lecture 2.
2. Michels, N. A.: Blood supply and anatomy of the upper abdominal organ with a descriptive atlas, Philadelphia, 1955, J. B. Lippincott Company, p. 280.

Undergraduate medical education in Great Britain

Gordon W. Philpott, M.D.,* *St. Louis, Mo.*

From the Department of Surgery, Washington University School of Medicine, St. Louis, Mo.

FOR THE LAST decade, almost all institutions and social establishments have come under intense criticism throughout much of the Western world. In the United States, everything from God to country is fair game, and it is not surprising that Yale too should come under attack. Certainly, the educational system in general and undergraduate medical curricula in particular have been frequent targets. Although this criticism is somewhat more muted in Great Britain, it is becoming increasingly louder. Even though the British trainees seem considerably more cautious in verbalizing complaints than our own students, many of them are deeply concerned about the educational problems and are increasingly vocal in their criticisms. Furthermore, it is not just the youth who are seeking changes. The initial stimulus may have come from a militant minority, but it is no longer just a small band of dissident protestors, clamoring for change. Educators, administrators, students, and the public have banded together to demand solutions to the educational problems that have been building over the years.

One of the major problems is the vastness and ever-changing nature of medical and scientific knowledge that prevents even a superficial coverage for all students. With acceptance of this fact, and recognizing the greatly diverse roles and vocations that students will pursue, it has become quite obvious that medical curricula need more flexibility with the opportunity for individual student choice. In many of the undergraduate medical programs in Great Britain, the amount of elective time is increasing with a shortening of the required courses. Although this move toward a more flexible curriculum is not as prevalent as in the United States, it is a major change in some British schools.

As the student body enlarges and the formal curriculum becomes shorter and more flexible, it is even more imperative to identify what knowledge and skills are essential for *all* students, what are the best ways to teach them, and how to evaluate the results. These are extremely difficult and time-consuming areas that are all too often avoided by the medical faculty. It was reassuring to see that others are having as much trouble as we in fulfilling these goals. Although many of us are truly concerned about medical education, I think very few are willing or able to commit themselves fully to these tasks, and some are still dubious about the worth of doing so. As in this country, there were very few trained educators or behavioral scientists involved in the organization of medical curricula, particularly of the clinical years. Although there is still debate on the need to have some faculty with formal training in education in medical schools, I think most would agree that it can be helpful. Since it is difficult to find medical and surgical faculty willing to ex-

Accepted for publication July 12, 1973.

*James IV Surgical Traveler to England and Scotland for 1972.

tend the already long and arduous training period, one possible solution is to utilize willing faculty in existing medical education departments. This is being done in some of the British universities. For example, the Department of Medicine at the University of Glasgow has a Division of Medical Education that works closely with the Department of Education. At least one faculty member has a joint appointment with the two departments. This enthusiastic group of internists and educators are outlining essential material ("core curriculum") and examining different techniques for presenting it. One of the promising approaches that they are testing is the use of carefully prepared slide-taped lectures that are used in lieu of the standard lectures and that the student can go over at this leisure. This series of slide-tape material was prepared by experts on the faculty and is utilized in conjunction with a reduced number of tutorial sessions. This approach has been tried on a pilot basis for one or two sections of the "integrated" fourth year curriculum. Adequate evaluation of the results is admittedly difficult and subject to bias, but on the basis of comparative written and oral exams, the students using this approach improved at a much faster rate than did those taking the standard course. The original trial group of students was small (12) but has risen steadily (60 this year) and eventually may include the entire class.

The "integrated" clinical sciences courses in the fourth year of medical school seem to be quite similar to our pathophysiology courses with faculty from a number of different departments presenting lectures and tutorials in a multiple organ systems approach. Thus, for example, pathologists, internists, and surgeons take an active part in presenting the pathophysiology of a variety of organ systems such as the gastrointestinal tract, heart, or lungs. All of the medical schools I visited have apparently adopted this coordinated approach to the clinical sciences, and it seems to be successful in eliminating much of the repetition of material and in integrating the preclinical and clinical sciences in a meaningful way.

It was interesting to see that in Great Britain, just as in our country, the best teachers of the "classical areas" of pathophysiology and anatomy were often the clinicians. As the basic scientists have become more and more specialized into areas of cellular and subcellular biology, the task of "classical" human physiology and anatomy, which are so important to patient care, falls upon the clinician. In designing curricula, this changing pattern of available "talent" has to be taken into consideration. The trend for having surgeons and internists participate heavily in the preclinical years has apparently proved quite successful in England and Scotland as it has in the United States.

The patterns of medical care and the medical manpower needs of the society obviously have an important influence on undergraduate medical education. Well over half of all British medical students eventually become general practitioners under the National Health Service. This is in spite of the somewhat lower stated preference of students for becoming general practitioners (24 percent according to the Report of the Royal Commission on Medical Education, 1965-1968). Since the majority of faculty are specialists, contact with practitioners during medical school was, until recently, often minimal. Consequently, students frequently had inadequate views of the delivery of health care at the community level and of what the generalist was like. A number of institutions in Great Britain have now added Departments of General Practice with faculty that take an active part in undergraduate education. This should not only help the student become more familiar with the general practitioners and medical practice at the community level, but also, it should encourage a more critical, academic appraisal and study of the whole area of health-care delivery.

Last, I should like to make one final comment about all of the educational programs that I visited. It is blatantly clear that no revision of the curriculum, no matter how innovative, will ever take the place of an enthusiastic, interested, and available faculty. I was deeply impressed with the quality of dedicated teachers that I saw in every medical school and hospital. Everyone from the junior house officer to the chairmen of the departments seemed strongly motivated to teach. No matter what the other duties or pressures might be, the obligation to teach seems to be a tradition that is almost taken for granted in Great Britain. At no other time in my life, have I been more vividly reminded of the following comment by Sir William Osler: "The great possession of any university is its great names, not its wealth, nor the number of its schools, not the students who throng its halls, but the men who have trodden in its service, the thorny road through toil."

Letters to the editors

Arteriovenous shunting after sympathectomy

To the Editors:

The recent article by Delaney and Scarpino[2] contains several conclusions on which we would like to comment.

First, in their series of five control dogs, percent shunting in the hindlimb averaged 0.7 percent, with the highest value being 1.4 percent. Previous studies, including our own[1, 3-5] involving larger numbers of measurements, have revealed both a much higher average value and a wider variation in percent shunting in pentobarbital-anesthetized dogs. They explain this difference on the failure of previous investigators to control arterial blood gases. Like Delaney and Scarpino, we hypothesized that shunting was related to blood gases. When tested, however, this hypothesis was not supported by the experimental data. For example, we observed 37 percent shunting in a dog in which respiration was controlled and blood gases were monitored (pH: artery = 7.410, vein = 7.460; Pco_2: artery = 37, vein = 44; Po_2: artery = 107, vein = 66). In a series of 28 observations in eight dogs in which respiration was controlled and blood gases were monitored, correlation of blood gases and shunting were not observed. The details of these experiments will be reported shortly.[6] We suggest that general health of the animals, previous temperature adaption, and laboratory temperature at the time of the study probably influence shunting more than blood gases. For example, we observed that five of six dogs (Table I) increased hindlimb shunting of 15 -30 micra microspheres following local cooling (p = 0.97).

Second, Delaney and Scarpino[2] report that they have "demonstrated that acidosis is invariably associated with increased hindlimb AVA [arteriovenous anastomosis] flow but that very little shunting is found when arterial pH is in the 7.40 to 7.44 range." They do not refer to data on this critical point. We found 24.5 ± 15.8 percent shunting in a series of 22 measurements in eight different dogs in which arterial pH was within the 7.40 to 7.44 range (mean arterial pH = 7.418 ± 0.014).

Table I. *Effect of local cooling on shunting in the hindlimb of dog*

Experiment No.	*Percent shunting* — *Control leg*	*Percent shunting* — *Test leg 2 min. after icing*	*Percent shunting in test leg / Percent shunting in control leg*
1	1.3	3.4	2.02
2	2.4	12.6	5.25
3	4.5	8.8	1.96
4	0.0	0.0	1.00
5	7.2	17.3	2.40
6	4.7	8.0	1.70
Means ± S.D.	3.35 ± 2.62	8.35 ± 6.21	2.49 ± 1.47

Third, they show that shunting averaged around 20 percent in sympathectomized dogs compared to 3.3 percent or less in control or sham-operated dogs. In a series of ten dogs, we also found about 20 percent shunting in the sympathectomized hindlimb.[7] The measurements were made one week after unilateral sympathectomy. In each case, however, the control side showed an even higher percent shunting. Thus, we concluded that one week after sympathectomy, there was a reduction in AVA shunting in the pentobarbital-anesthetized dogs. This is opposite to the conclusion of Delaney and Scarpino.

We hope that further data will resolve these differences.

Buck A. Rhodes, Ph.D.
Vincent Lopez-Majano, M.D., Ph.D.
Henry N. Wagner, Jr., M.D.
Division of Nuclear Medicine
The Johns Hopkins School of Hygiene and Public Health
Baltimore, Md.

REFERENCES

1. Delaney, J. P.: Arteriovenous anastomotic blood flow in the mesenteric organs, Am. J. Physiol. **216:** 1556, 1969.

2. Delaney, J., and Scarpino, J.: Limb arteriovenous shunting following sympathetic denervation, SURGERY **73:** 202, 1973.
3. Lopez-Majano, V., Rhodes, B. A., and Wagner, H. N., Jr.: Arteriovenous shunting in extremities, J. Appl. Physiol. **27:** 782, 1969.
4. Piiper, J., and Schoedel, W.: Untersuchungen über die Durchblutung der arteri-venosen Anastomosen in der hinteren Extremität des Hundes mit Hilfe von Kugeln verschiedener grösse. Arch. Ges. Physiol. **258:** 489, 1954.
5. Spence, R. J., Rhodes, B. A., and Wagner, H. N., Jr.: Regulation of arteriovenous anastomotic and capillary blood flow in the dog leg, Am. J. Physiol. **222:** 326, 1972.
6. Rhodes, B. A., Lopez-Majano, V., and Wagner, H. N., Jr.: Dissociation of functional from anatomic shunting. To be published.
7. Valenta, J., Rhodes, B. A., and Rutherford, R. B.: Effect of lumbar sympathectomy on arteriovenous shunts of the lower extremity, an experimental study, Rozhl. Chir. **51:** 206, 1972.

Reply

To the Editors:

Drs. Wagner, Rhodes, Lopez-Majano and colleagues have been pioneers in the study of the physiology of arteriovenous shunting, and we admire their work. Many of their experiments parallel our own. Not only the paper discussed but other data, currently in press, differ from their observations. We have done numerous experiments in addition to those reported in which the control group invariably demonstrated a mean of less than five percent of limb flow traversing arteriovenous channels which exceeded 25 μ in diameter. Thus, the difference does not result from a paucity of experiments. The discrepancies are not readily explained. One possibility lies in a seemingly unimportant technical detail. The method described by Spence, Rhodes, and Wagner (Am. J. Physiol. **222:** 326, 1972) involves a rather extensive dissection of the femoral and external iliac arteries. Such dissection results in local periarterial denervation. Our technique involves percutaneous needle puncture of the femoral artery without otherwise disturbing the vessel. Possibly periarterial sympathetic denervation leads to a "control" state which in fact represents that of partial sympathectomy.

A second significant technical difference is their sequential injection of technetium-labeled albumin spheres while we employed Yterbium-labeled polystyrene spheres. Working with the albumin-labeled spheres we have found, as one might expect using soluble material, that there is an early and steady increase in thoracic radioactivity following injection into the femoral artery. The increase depends upon a rise in circulating technetium as well as accumulation of the technetium in the reticuloendothelial system, most notably the liver and spleen. Our conclusion was that to estimate arteriovenous shunting by means of technetium-labeled albumin spheres, one must evaluate the lung radioactivity within two or three minutes of injection. Repeated sequential injections would introduce variables impossible to quantitate. We doubt the validity of observations made in that manner and would suggest that use of inert plastic spheres allows for no circulation of the radioactive label and therefore more credible results.

With respect to local cooling we again differ. A paper currently in press (Proc. Soc. Exp. Biol. Med., 1973) describes a series of experiments in which systemic or local cooling or heating were carried out. Only systemic heating resulted in substantial enhancement of arteriovenous anastomotic blood flow. Here again a difference in technique is apparent. The duration of local cooling in our studies was between 30 and 60 minutes depending upon measurement of tissue temperatures. The Johns Hopkins experiments were carried out with two minutes of limb immersion in ice. The result would more likely be due to a neurogenic response than to tissue temperature changes.

The mechanisms controlling arteriovenous anastomotic blood flow remain incompletely defined but should gradually be resolved with improved methodology.

John P. Delaney, M.D.
Jon Scarpino, M.D.
Department of Surgery
University of Minnesota Medical School
Minneapolis, Minn. 55455.

Volume 75 Number 2

SURGERY

FEBRUARY, 1974

Original communications

A comparison of intraoperative tests of completeness of vagal section

G. Grassi, M.D., F.A.C.S., *and* C. Orecchia, M.D., *Rome, Italy*

The completeness of vagotomy was studied during operation in 769 patients by means of the Burge, Lee, and Grassi tests and checked three months postoperatively by Hollander's test. The tests were evaluated and their limitations discussed. Use of the Grassi test reduced the incidence of incomplete vagotomies from 10 to two percent. In 98 percent of these patients there was still no acid response in control studies made two years later. On the basis of these results, only total absence of an acid response to Hollander's test should be regarded as the index of completeness of a vagotomy; an acid response even if minimal is, in the author's opinion, attributable to incompleteness of the vagal denervation of the stomach.

From the San Giovanni Hospital, II Surgical Department (Prof. G. Grassi), Rome, Italy

If the results of vagotomy for duodenal ulcer are to be assessed fairly, it is imperative that the vagotomy be complete because it is impossible to calculate the percentage of success or failure of the surgical treatment adopted unless it is certain that vagal denervation of the stomach has been carried out completely.

In order to verify intraoperatively the completeness of vagal section, we have compared the electrostimulation test of Burge and Vane,[3, 4] the leuko-methylene blue test of Lee,[15] and the Congo red and pH test of Grassi.[7-12, 16-18] Follow-up studies with the Hollander test[13] were also performed in the immediate postoperative period and three months after operation.

It was the purpose of this study to compare the techniques by which the completeness of vagotomy could be assessed intraoperatively and to determine whether these results correlated with the postoperative assessment of vagal innervation to the stomach by the conventional Hollander tests.

Accepted for publication Jan. 25, 1973.

Reprint requests: Dr. Giuseppe Grassi, 7, Via Circo Massimo, 00153, Rome, Italy.

Table I

Vagotomy type	*No. performed*
Selective	1,026
Proximal selective	227
Selective anterior, truncal posterior	90
Truncal	60
Total	1,403

MATERIAL AND METHOD

Intraoperative tests for the completeness of the vagotomy were performed in 769 patients who were part of the series of 1,403 patients operated upon for duodenal ulcer in Surgical Division II of the San Giovanni Hospital in Rome from January, 1962, to December, 1971 (Table I).

In 150 of these patients (Table II) (123 selective vagotomies and 27 anterior selective and posterior truncular vagotomies) we performed Burge's test with the electrostimulator (which combines an electronic with a manometric element) according to the method described by its author, which may be briefly summarized as follows: Immediately after the vagotomy has been performed a rubber catheter with an inflatable balloon is introduced into the stomach and so placed that the balloon lies at the level of the lower esophagus and cardia. The balloon is inflated to a measured pressure of 150 mm. Hg, thus gently distending the esophagus, and a special forceps, with annular ends containing the electrodes, is applied around the cardia. The stomach is then clamped at the pylorus in the case of selective vagotomy, or at the junction of the fundus and antrum in the case of proximal selective vagotomy. Air is introduced into the stomach and the catheter is connected to the manometer. If vagotomy is incomplete, stimulation of the electrodes produces a motor response, manifested by a rise of manometric pressure; if section is complete, no response is obtained.

Three months after operation the completeness of the vagotomy was tested in 87 of these patients (Table III).

In 30 cases (20 selective vagotomies and 10 ultraselective—proximal selective—vagotomies) Lee's test was performed. This is a colorimetric method based on the fact that methylene blue, colorless when in contact with ascorbic acid in the absence of oxygen, in the presence of oxygen acquires a blue color which is more intense at the site of nerve fibers because of the oxidative processes occurring here.

To assess the value of this test, we divided the most easily identifiable branches of the vagus and then carried out the leuko-methylene blue test as described by its author. That is to say, a swab soaked in the liquid was applied to the cardial surface after selective vagotomy or to the lesser curvature as far as the antrum after proximal selective vagotomy. The methylene blue was then removed with a swab soaked in physiologic saline. As the nervous tissue remained bluer than the surrounding tissues we divided the relevant nerve branches, subsequently confirming the completeness of the denervation by performing Grassi's test. In addition, the resected fragments of tissue were examined histologically in order to define with precision what tissue elements were present.

In these patients, also, Hollander's test was done three months after operation.

We performed Grassi's intraoperative test in 619 patients, including the 30 in whom we had previously carried out Lee's test (Table II). This test is easy to perform and harmless to the patient. Its positivity or negativity is based on the secretory response observed during the operation by the method of measuring pH with a glass electrode or by a colorimetric method using as indicator a saturated solution of Congo red, which turns black in the presence of a pH lower than 3.5.

To carry out the test, an intravenous infusion of pentagastrin 0.6 mg. per kilogram per hour (or, if preferred, of histamine bichloridrate, 0.025 mg. per kilogram per hour), in 200 c.c. of physiologic saline is started as soon as the abdomen has been opened, in order to stimulate the acid-secreting cells of the gastric wall. When the vagotomy (truncular, selective, or ultrase-

Table II. *Intraoperative tests*

Vagotomy type	*Burge's test*	*Grassi*	*Total*
Selective	123	386*	509
Proximal select:ve	0	227†	227
Selective anterior, truncal posterior	27	4	31
Truncal	0	2	2
Total	150	619	769

*Twenty patients also had Lee's test.
†Ten patients also had Lee's test.

Table III

Vagotomy type	*No. checked with Hollander's test*			
	Burge No.	*Positive*	*Grassi No.*	*Positive*
Selective	73	4	195	3
Proximal selective	0	—	122	3
Selective anterior, truncal posterior	14	3	0	—
Truncal	0	—	0	—
Total	87	7 (8.0%)	317	6 (1.09%)

lective) is finished, we make an antral gastrotomy which can be used later for the construction of a pyloroplasty or, if the diameter of the pylorus is so satisfactory that we decide to omit this, can be sutured. Through the gastrotomy, we carefully cleanse the gastric wall of all secretions with the use of swabs and gauze strips—first soaked in distilled water and later dry.

Alternatively, pentagastrin or histamine in appropriate doses may be given by rapid intravenous injection at the conclusion of the denervation.

The index of completion of vagal section is attained when the pH (as measured by the pH electrode) in all parts of the gastric mucosa is between 5.5 and 7.0. If Congo red is used as the indicator, the absence of a black color despite continuing pharmacologic stimulation is the desired end point. If the glass electrode discloses any mucosal areas in which an acid pH persists even after further cleansing, or if the Congo red becomes black, we know that one or more vagal branches supplying these areas have not been divided; when these are cut the acidity will disappear.

It is important to point out that, to avoid errors of assessment in both Burge's and Grassi's tests, during the 48 hours preceding the operation, the patient must not be given atropine or any parasympatholytic drug which may block or reduce the transmission of the nerve impulse in Burge's test or the secretion of acid in Grassi's test.

Hollander's test was similarly performed in 317 of these patients (51.2 percent) three months after operation (Table III).

RESULTS

The use of Burge's electrostimulator in the course of the operation enabled an incomplete vagotomy to be avoided in 13 (9.3 percent) of 150 patients operated upon. In four of these patients the uncut branches belonged to the anterior vagus, in eight to the posterior vagus, and in one to both. In five it was necessary to repeat the test after revision of the vagotomy because a slight increase of intragastric pressure showed that a branch from the posterior vagus was still unsectioned.

Of the 150 patients operated upon, 87 (73 with selective vagotomies and 14 with anterior selective and posterior truncular vagotomies) were checked three months after operation by a Hollander test, the response to insulin being assessed according to the criteria of Hollander, Stempien,[19] and Bachrach,[1, 2] to assure the completeness of the vagotomy. In seven of these 87 patients (8 percent), four with selective vagotomies and three with anterior selective and posterior truncular vagotomies, the insulin response signified an incomplete vagotomy (Table III).

All of the 30 patients in whom Lee's test was performed during the operation were also checked by the Grassi test and this revealed uncut branches belonging to the anterior vagal branches to the fundus of the stomach; in four it belonged to the posterior vagus, corresponding to the fundus in two patients and to the antrofundal junction in two.

Grassi's test enabled vagotomy to be completed in 50 of 619 patients (eight percent). In 12 patients the uncut vagal branches came from the posterior trunk at the level of the fundus, in 10 from the anterior trunk, also at the fundal level, in 20 from both trunks at the antrofundal level, and in eight from the posterior trunk at the antrofundal level.

In 19 patients the test had to be repeated after revision of the vagotomy because of persisting areas of acidity, which disappeared after the small branches concerned had been divided.

Of the 619 patients operated upon, 317 (51.2 percent)—195 with selective and 122 with ultraselective vagotomies—were checked by means of Hollander's test three months after operation (Table III). The vagotomy was found to be incomplete in six patients (1.0 percent), three (1.5 percent) with selective vagotomies and three (2.5 percent) with ultraselective vagotomies. In the remaining 311 patients the insulin test showed no acid response (a flat curve).

DISCUSSION

The results obtained confirm the importance of intraoperative tests for completeness of a vagotomy. It must be pointed out, however, that while both Burge's and Grassi's test reduced the incidence of incomplete parasympathetic denervation to about eight and two percent, respectively, as compared with a value of 10 percent in patients in whom no intraoperative test is performed, Lee's test when checked by Grassi's test was found to lead to incompleteness of the vagotomy in 23 percent of cases. It must be further noted that Burge's test is an indirect one, its positivity or negativity depending on the presence or absence of a gastric motor reaction to electrostimulation. Since the relation between motility and secretory activity is not yet fully understood, and since the method reduces by only two percent the value for incompleteness found in patients not submitted to any intraoperative test, we may surmise that the reduction of incidence may be partly attributable to refinement of the technique and to the surgeon's increased experience, both of which reduce the probability of an incomplete gastric denervation being performed.

Furthermore, in ultraselective (proximal selective) vagotomy the clamp temporarily placed on the antrofundal junction makes it impossible to be sure that this ill-defined zone has been completely denervated. There may still be one or more uncut branches which, because they have ben compressed by the clamp, do not give a motor response but which may subsequently give a secretory response.

With regard to Lee's test, we believe that it may be helpful in some cases but that it cannot be considered a test of completeness of a vagotomy because connective tissue also stains to some extent, as was confirmed by the histologic examination in 22 percent of the cases, so that it cannot insure that all nerve branches have been sectioned.

Our best results to date have been obtained with Grassi's test, which is a direct method based on the abolition of the acid-secretory response to pentagastrin or histamine after vagototmy has been completed. It is equally valid in truncal, selective, and proximal vagotomy for it enables the vagal secretory branches supplying the acid-producing area to be identified with precision.

The results, especially those obtained in

the initial stage of our study, were perplexing, because we had not expected that the acid response to pentagastrin or histamine would be abolished by vagal section; but when, in order to verify the validity of the test, we applied it after carrying out anterior vagal denervation only, we observed that the whole of the anterior mucosal surface had a pH of 5.5 to 7.0 while pH values measured on the posterior surface were between 0.9 and 0.2. It was necessary, therefore, to exclude the possible interference of drugs or anesthetic agents capable of abolishing or reducing the acid response; the dose of the stimulant could not be regarded as insufficient, since it evoked a response from the gastric areas which remained innervated.

A tenable hypothesis is that after vagal denervation of the stomach there is a rise in the threshold of excitability to all stimuli of the parietal cells, so that stimula capable in normal conditions of evoking a secretory response become subliminal after vagotomy. This theory can be confirmed or refuted only by further experimental researches directed to that end.

Finally, we would emphasize the continued absence of *any* acid-secretory response in 305 of 311 patients (98 percent) who were negative at three months and who were rechecked by Hollander's test two years later. Except in six patients both the basal acid values and those after insulin stimulation showed no acid-secretory response (flat curves). These results lead us to conclude that it is arbitrary to fix numerical limits of positivity of Hollander's test, and that it should be counted as negative only in the *absence* of any acid response. This finding alone coincides with the purpose of vagotomy; to abolish the acid response of neurogenic origin. The presence of an acid response, even if it is within the limits accepted by most authors as indices of complete vagotomy, must, in our judgment and in the light of these results, be attributed to incomplete vagal denervation of the stomach. Whether or not this residual acidity is of a degree sufficient to cause recurrence is a question quite separate from that of fixing criteria for completeness of the vagal denervation for it is obvious that if a neurosecretory organ is denervated no secretory response at all can be mediated by the cut nerve fibers.

REFERENCES

1. Bachrach, W.: Laboratory criteria for completeness of vagotomy, Am. J. Dig. Dis. **7:** 1071, 1962.
2. Bachrach, W. H., and Bachrach, L. B.: Reevaluation of the Hollander test, Ann. N. Y. Acad. Sci. **46:** 915, 1967.
3. Burge, H., and Vane, J. R.: Method of testing for complete nerve section during vagotomy, Br. Med. J. **1:** 615, 1958.
4. Burge, H.: Vagotomy, London, 1964, Edward Arnold, Publisher.
5. Calleander, S. T., Rutief, F. P., and Witts, H. L. J.: The augmented histamine test with special reference to achloridrya, Gut **1:** 326, 1960.
6. Card, W. I., and Sircus, W.: *In* Jones, F. A., editor: Modern trends in gastroenterology, Series 2, London, 1964, Butterworth & Co., Ltd.
7. Grassi, G., and Orecchia, C.: Studio della secrezione gastrica nella malattia ulcerosa in fase operatoria, Chir. Gastroenterol. **3:** 69, 1969.
8. Grassi, G.: New test for complete nerve section during vagotomy, Br. J. Surg. **58:** 187, 1971.
9. Grassi, G., Orecchia, C., Cantarelli, I., Fivoli, E., and Sbuelz, B.: The results and comment on the intraoperative study of gastric secretion in peptic ulcer, Surgery in Italy **1:** 103, 1971.
10. Grassi, G., Orecchia, C., Sbuelz, B., and Cantarelli, I.: Variations in secretion during gastric resection for duodenal ulcer, Chir. Gastroenterol. **5:** 247, 1971.
11. Grassi, G., Orecchia, C., Sbuelz, B., Cantarelli, I., and Dell'Osso, A.: Completeness of vagotomy and gastric secretion stimulated by pentagastrin during operation for duodenal ulcer, Chir. Gastroenterol. **5:** 38, 1971.
12. Grassi, G., Orecchia, C., Cantarelli, I., and Sbuelz, G.: Intraoperative relation of gastric acidity and complete vagotomy, Surg. Gynecol. Obstet. **134:** 35, 1972.
13. Hollander, F.: Laboratory procedures in the study of vagotomy (with particular reference to the insulin test), Gastroenterology **11:** 419, 1948.
14. Jensen, H. E., Kragelund, E., and Amdrup, E.: Intraoperative studies of the stomach

(leucomethilene blue staining of the vagus, intragastric determinations of pH, and Congo red staining of the mucosa), Chir. Gastroenterol. **5:** 303, 1971.
15. Lee, M.: A selective staining to detect the vagus nerve in operation of vagotomy, Br. J. Surg. **56:** 10, 1960.
16. Orecchia, C., Sbuelz, B., Cantarelli, I., and Dell'Osso, A.: Sulle modalità tecniche del test di Grassi per la completa enervazione vagale gastrica, Chir. Gastroenterol. **4:** 417, 1970.
17. Orecchia, C., Sbuelz, B., and Grassi, G. B., Jr.: Our concept of vagotomy and results obtained (1245 cases), Chir. Gastroenterol. **5:** 2250, 1971.
18. Orecchia, C., and Sbuelz, B.: The present position of vagotomy (considerations of 1245 cases), Chir. Gastroenterol. **6:** 189, 1972.
19. Stempien, S. J.: Insulin gastric analysis: technique and interpretation, Am. J. Dig. Dis. **7:** 138, 1962.

Liver arterialization with portacaval shunt in the cirrhotic rat

Y. Lecompte, M.D., D. Franco, M.D., E. D. Martin, M.D., *and* H. Bismuth, M.D.,
Villejuif, France

Arterialization of the liver associated with portacaval shunt was performed in cirrhotic rats by creating an anastomosis between the right renal artery and the hepatic stump of the portal vein. This procedure prevented the onset of early postoperative liver failure which follows portacaval shunt alone. It appeared, however, to be harmful to the liver both structurally and functionally after a few weeks. This should be taken into account if arterialization is considered in cirrhotic patients.

From the Laboratoire de Chirurgie Expérimentale, INSERM U-17, and Unité de Chirurgie Hépato-biliaire, Hôpital Paul Brousse, Villejuif, France

THE INCIDENCE of liver failure in cirrhotic patients increases following portal systemic shunt, which seems to be accounted for by a decrease of hepatic blood flow (HBF).[17] Several new surgical methods have been proposed to reduce this unwanted effect of portacaval shunting (PCS), one of which being the arterialization of the hepatic stump of the portal vein following an end-to-side shunt.[1, 6, 13] Although this procedure may prevent postshunt decrease of HBF in animals with normal liver, its superiority in comparison to PCS alone with regard to postoperative liver function still remains to be shown in cirrhotic patients. It is too early yet to draw any definite conclusion from the recent clinical series[1, 13] in which arterialization was performed in cirrhotic patients. Comparative studies between arterialized and nonarterialized shunted patients need to be performed in order to know if arterialization is of any benefit. Furthermore, the effects of arterialization on the structure of the normal liver is damaging but these effects have not been studied in cirrhotic livers. This study was undertaken to investigate the consequences of arterialization on liver function and structure in cirrhotic rats and, in particular, to answer the following questions: (1) Does liver arterialization improve the postoperative course of shunted cirrhotic rats and (2) has it any damaging effect upon the liver?

MATERIAL AND METHODS

Hepatic cirrhosis was obtained in 29 male Charles River rats* by subcutaneous injection of carbon tetrachloride (0.1 ml. plus an equal volume of mineral oil per 100 Gm. of body weight) twice weekly for eight months. When shunted, the rats weighed from 300 to 400 Gm. During the postoperative study period, they were housed in individual cages, fed standard laboratory chow,† and had free

Supported by Research Grant No. 318 from UER Bicêtre, Université Paris-Sud.

Accepted for publication July 18, 1973.

Reprint requests: Y. Lecompte, M.D., Laboratoire de Chirurgie Expérimentale, Hôpital Paul Brousse, 14, av. P.V. Couturier, 94800 Villejuif, France.

*From Charles River, St Aubin les Elbeuf, France.
†From U.A.R., Villemoisson-sur-Orge, France.

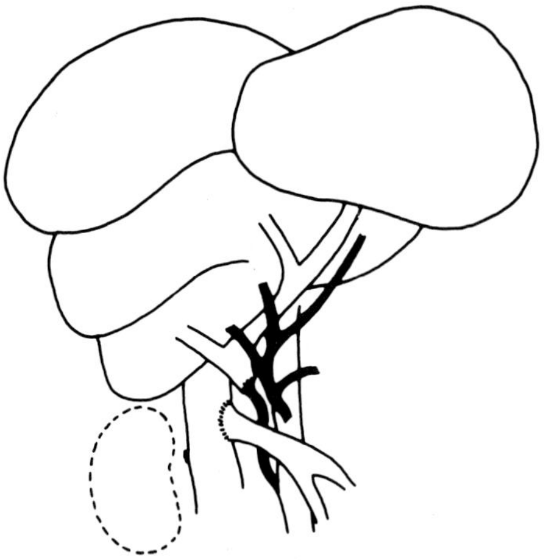

Fig. 1. Liver arterialization in the rat: The end-to-side portacaval shunt is associated with end-to-end anastomosis between the right renal artery and the hepatic end of the portal vein. The right kidney must be removed.

access to water. The cirrhotic rats were divided into two groups. Ten rats experienced only an end-to-side portacaval shunt, and they will be referred to as the PCS rats. Nineteen rats had PCS plus arterialization of the hepatic stump of the portal vein with the use of the right renal artery, and this group will be referred to as the ART rats. The PCS was constructed according to a previously described technique,[4] and the portal arterialization was performed according to a newly developed microsurgical technique (Fig. 1). After completion of the PCS, a right nephrectomy was performed. The right renal artery was then dissected free, and its distal end was passed beneath the vena cava from right to left. The renal artery was turned upward and anastomosed end to end to the hepatic stump of the portal vein with two No. 9-0 silk running sutures (Fig. 2). Since right nephrectomy was mandatory in arterialized rats, it was also performed in PCS rats. Administration of carbon tetrachloride was discontinued following surgery in all rats.

Portacaval anastomoses were patent in all animals. In the arterialized group, the patency of the renoportal anastomosis was tested, either by angiography (Fig. 3) during the study or by minium injection at the end of the study. In only one animal was the anastomosis not patent; this animal was therefore withdrawn from the study and is not included in the 29 rats mentioned above.

To determine postoperative hepatic function, serum transaminase (SGPT) levels, blood ammonia levels, and bromsulfalein plasma disappearance rate (BSP-PDR) were studied weekly for six weeks. Serum transaminases were, in addition, measured on the second and fourth postoperative days. Blood samples were taken by puncture of the retroorbital sinus while the animals were under light ether anesthesia. SGPT levels were measured by UV technique; the BSP-PDR was measured according to a modification of the technique described by Berthelot and associates.[3] Serum ammonia was measured with the use of the Hyland blood ammonia test.*

Liver sections were studied twice, once during the shunting and once postoperatively, either at the end of the study, six weeks after operation, or at the time of autopsy if an animal died during the course of the study. Liver sections were stained by trichrome for light microscopic examination.

RESULTS

Mortality rate. The mortality rate was high following both procedures. In the arterialized group, 11 animals (57 percent) died within the first 24 hours after operation, while three (33 percent) died in the shunted group. Five more arterialized rats died within the course of the study; two died on the fourteenth day and one each on the twenty-first, twenty-fifth, and twenty-eighth postoperative day. Three of these animals died from anesthesia while a blood sample was being taken. In the shunted group, two rats died on the thirteenth and thirty-eighth postoperative day.

Body weight. Animals in both groups lost weight during the study. This weight loss was slightly more pronounced in shunted rats by the end of the study (23 percent of

*Travenol Labs (California).

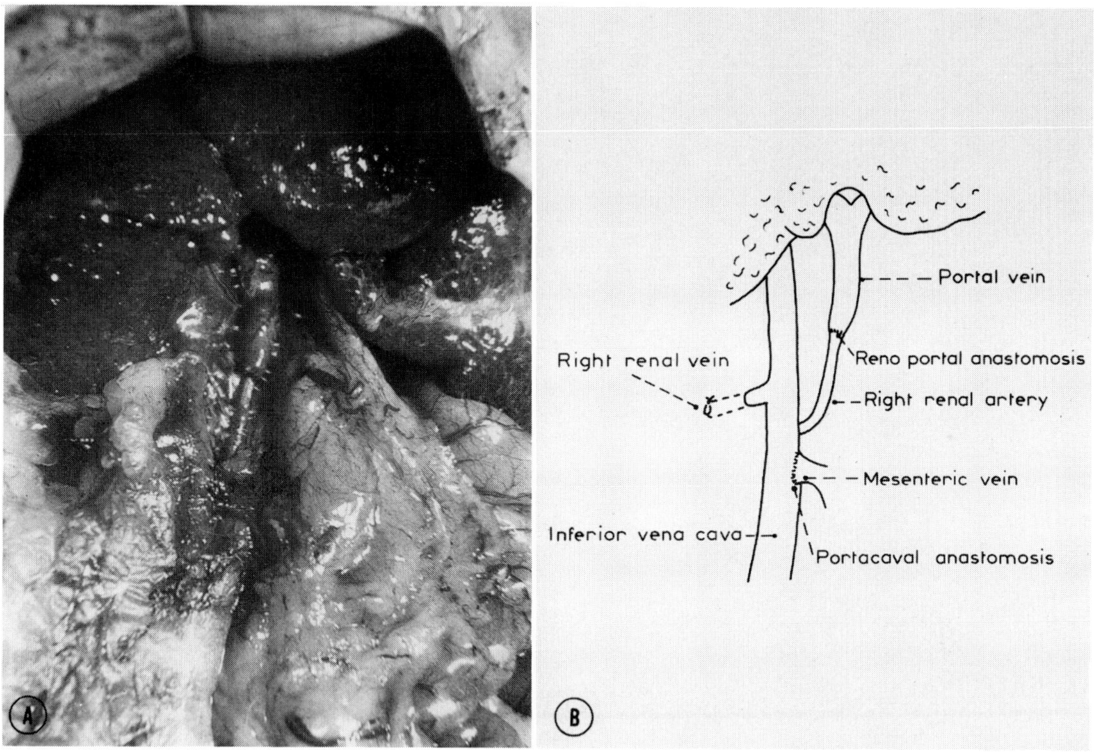

Fig. 2. Operative view of the procedure. *A*, Photograph and *B*, diagram.

Table I. *SGPT values (mIu. ml.$^{-1}$) following portacaval shunt and arterialization in cirrhotic rats*

(NS)
(p < 0.001)
(p < 0.001)

	Preoperative	*Postoperative*		
		Second day	*Fourth day*	*Seventh day*
Portacaval shunt	26 ± 12	313 ± 224	52 ± 15	23 ± 13
	NS	p < 0.001	p < 0.01	NS
Arterialization	29 ± 8	21 ± 17	17 ± 12	17 ± 5

preoperative body weight) than in the arterialized rats (14 percent of preoperative body weight), although the difference was not significant.

Serum transaminases (Table I). In PCS rats, SGPT increased significantly on the second postoperative day to 313 ± 224 mU. ml.$^{-1}$, ($p < 0.001$). Afterwards, it decreased slowly and returned to preoperative values within a week. In the arterialized group, SGPT remained at preoperative levels throughout the study. There was a significant difference between the two groups on the second ($p < 0.001$) and fourth ($p < 0.01$) postoperative days. There was no further difference between the two groups by the end of the study, that is, six weeks after operation.

BSP-PDR (Table II). In the PCS rats, there was a marked and significant decrease of BSP-PDR to 0.084 ± 0.006 on the seventh postoperative day as opposed to

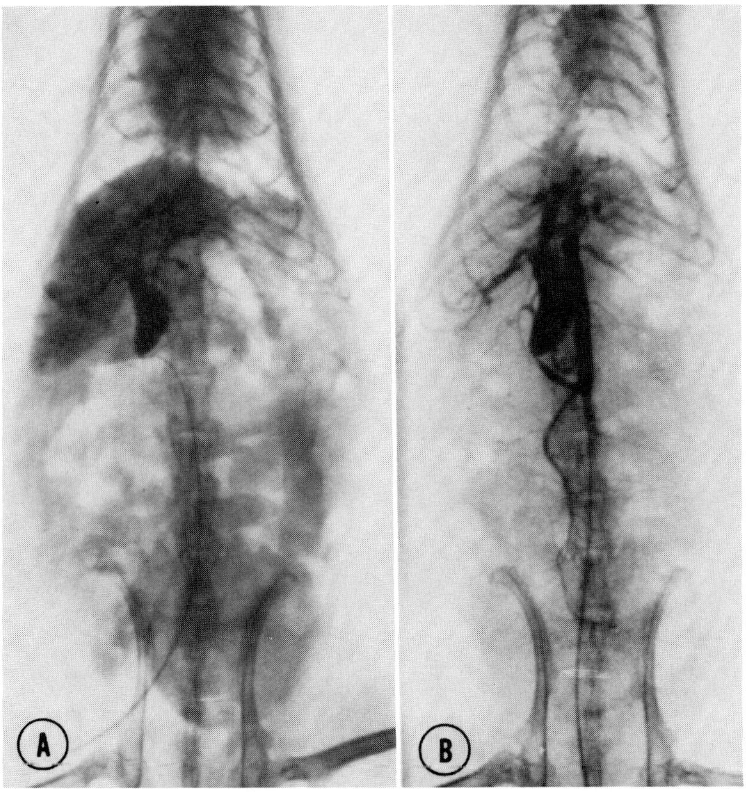

Fig. 3. Angiographic control. *A,* Selective angiography of the portal vein via the right renal artery. *B,* Aortogram showing the right renal artery and the portal vein. The hepatic artery is seen above the renal artery.

the preoperative value of 0.123 ± 0.023 ($p < 0.01$). Thereafter, the BSP-PDR levels remained significantly lower than preoperative levels. In the ART rats, decrease in the BSP-PDR was minimal at first; the seventh day postoperative levels did not differ significantly from the preoperative values. They then decreased slowly throughout the study and became significantly lower than preoperative values. The seventh postoperative day values were significantly different between the two groups ($p < 0.01$), but, thereafter, as the values of the arterialized group approached those of the control PCS group, no significant differences were noted.

Blood ammonia (Table III). In the PCS group, a sharp and significant rise in blood ammonia was observed on the seventh postoperative day and persisted for six weeks. In the ART group, the ammonia rise was slow and progressive, the difference between the two groups being significant on the seventh postoperative day ($p < 0.05$). Eventually, ammonia levels in the ART group reached the same levels as in the PCS group on the fourteenth postoperative day.

Pathological studies. All rats showed histological evidence of cirrhosis, including portal fibrosis, regeneration nodules, proliferation of biliary canaliculi within the portal tracts, and fatty degeneration of the hepatocytes (Fig. 4). In the PCS group, the hepatic structure remained identical even six weeks after shunting. In arterialized rats, striking histological changes were observed as early as two weeks following operation, and they were even more obvious by the end of the study at six weeks. These changes included a very important increase in portal fibrosis, spotty necrosis, and polymorphonuclear infiltration of the portal tracts (Fig. 5). There

Table II. *BSP-PDR expressed as the fractional clearance (k = 0.693/t½) following portacaval shunt and liver arterialization in cirrhotic rats*

	Preoperative	Postoperative: First week	Postoperative: Second week	Postoperative: Sixth week
Portacaval shunt	0.123 ± 0.023	0.084 ± 0.006	0.099 ± 0.023	0.095 ± 0.013
	NS	p < 0.01	NS	NS
Arterialization	0.128 ± 0.016	0.113 ± 0.018	0.109 ± 0.018	0.085 ± 0.010

Portacaval shunt, preoperative vs. sixth week: (p < 0.02); vs. second week: (p < 0.02); vs. first week: (p < 0.01)
Arterialization, preoperative vs. first week: (NS); vs. second week: (p < 0.02); vs. sixth week: (p < 0.001)

Table III. *Blood ammonia (μg. ml.⁻¹) following portacaval shunt and arterialization in cirrhotic rats*

	Preoperative	Postoperative: First week	Postoperative: Second week	Postoperative: Sixth week
Portacaval shunt	146 ± 92	328 ± 59	291 ± 88	292 ± 78
	NS	p < 0.05	NS	NS
Arterialization	98 ± 35	193 ± 56	283 ± 100	291 ± 39

Portacaval shunt, preoperative vs. sixth week: (p < 0.05); vs. second week: p < 0.01); vs. first week: (p < 0.02)
Arterialization, preoperative vs. first week: (p < 0.001); vs. second week: (p < 0.001); vs. sixth week: (p < 0.001)

was also a dilation of the intrahepatic portal branches with a thickening of their walls.

DISCUSSION

In the cirrhotic rat, portacaval shunting was the cause of an early postoperative liver function deterioration, as shown by a rise of the SGPT levels, a decrease of BSP-PDR, and an increase in blood ammonia. Arterialization of the hepatic end of the portal vein prevented these early changes. In arterialized animals, SGPT levels remained normal throughout the study and only minimal changes of BSP-PDR and blood ammonia were demonstrated during the early postoperative course. This correlates well with the findings of other experimental works on normal dogs in which blood ammonia clearance was higher in arterialized than in shunted animals.[10, 12]

The improvement of liver function following portal arterialization could be accounted for by an increased hepatic oxygen consumption or an increased hepatic blood supply. As for hepatic oxygen consumption, it has been shown by Bradley and associates[5]

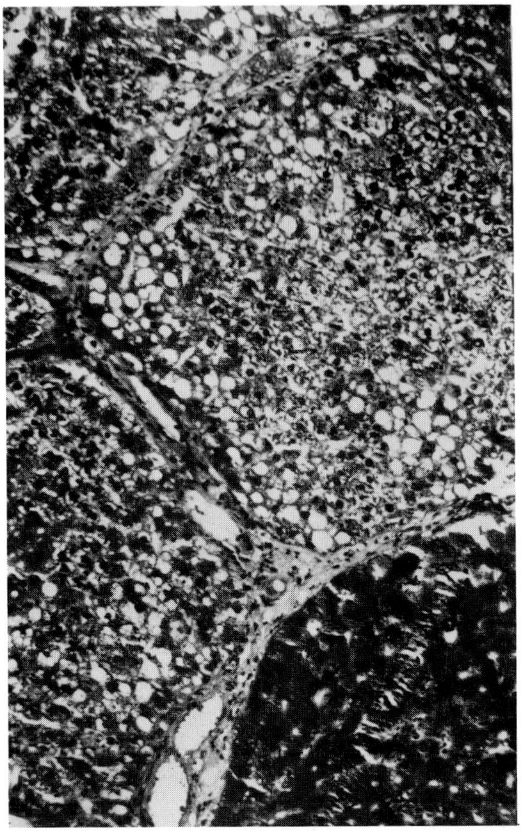

Fig. 4. Liver biopsy at six weeks following portacaval shunting in a cirrhotic rat. There is a well-developed fibrosis, a fatty degeneration of the hepatocytes, a slight infiltration of the portal spaces, and regeneration nodules.

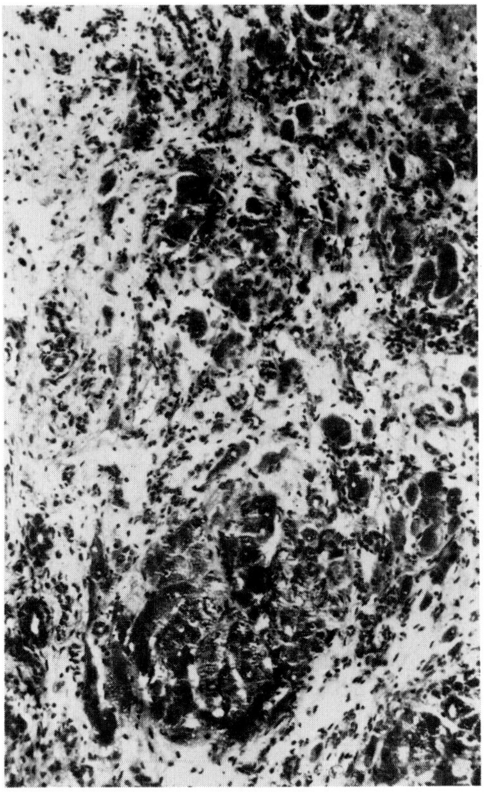

Fig. 5. Liver biopsy at six weeks after portacaval shunting and arterialization of the hepatic stump of the portal vein. Fibrosis is very dense, with many biliary canaliculi, there are only a few remaining hepatocytes, and there is marked infiltration by polymorphonuclear cells.

and by Basu and co-workers[9] that it was not affected by portacaval anastomosis in cirrhotic patients. In addition, there was no increase of hepatic oxygen consumption in the dogs arterialized by Fisher and associates[9] when compared to normal dogs. Thus, there is no evidence that an increase in oxygen uptake would be a main factor in improving the postoperative course of arterialized cirrhotic rats. On the other hand, it has been clearly demonstrated by Fisher and co-workers[9] and Tutassaura and Baird[16] that in normal dogs, HBF can be increased by adding arterialization to portacaval shunt. Although we did not measure HBF in the present work, it may be assumed that an increased HBF in the arterialized group accounted for the absence of early postoperative liver function deterioration observed in these animals.

Secondary late deterioration of liver function tests was evident in arterialized cirrhotic rats but not in shunted rats without arterialization. In the former group, the BSP-PDR slowly decreased and blood ammonia increased with time, while in the latter, it remained fairly stable. This was associated with dramatic changes in the structure of the arterialized livers, including an increase in the hallmarks of cirrhosis and occurrence of portal vasculitis. There is considerable disagreement in the literature concerning the effects of liver arterialization on liver structure. Rather and Cohn[14] and Zuidema and colleagues[18] have reported definite intrahepatic changes of portal vasculitis or even changes which resemble liver cirrhosis. An increase in the intrahepatic portal pressure was thought by Rather and Cohn[14] to be responsible for these structural changes. It has been reported by Fisher and associates[9] and by Schwartz and colleagues[15] that portal arterialization has minimal or no effect on hepatic structure in normal as well as in cirrhotic dogs. Fischer and co-workers[8] have even shown that liver regeneration may be enhanced by portal arterialization. It must be stressed, however, that in Fisher's experimental model,[7, 9] aortoportal anastomosis had become narrowed for a period of time and that there was a thrombosis of the main portal vein walls near its bifurcation; this may have decreased both arterioportal flow and intrahepatic portal pressure. Postanastomotic portal pressure was not recorded in our rats in order to avoid postoperative intra-abdominal bleeding; however, histological changes observed in this work resemble those seen after arterialization in dogs with normal livers. Secondary deterioration of liver function tests correlated well with the histology and may be due to these structural changes.

A decrease of HBF has been documented in most cirrhotic patients following portacaval shunting, and although it has never been actually proved, it is generally agreed that this may account for the high incidence of postoperative liver failure in these patients. It has been recently reported by Kessler and associates[11] that there was a particularly high risk of postshunt liver failure in patients whose intrahepatic portal pressure was markedly diminished following portal decompression. It is postulated that in these patients, the disappearance of portal blood was not compensated by a spontaneous increase in liver arterial blood flow. In such cases, arterialization would be of interest in overcoming the early postoperative risk of liver failure. However, it appears from the present work that long-term renoportal arterialization of the liver bears a high risk of liver damage in the cirrhotic rat. These damages may be due to the high rate flow and/or the high pressure created within the portal system by the arterioportal anastomosis. If this were to happen in man, it could lead to perform a low-rate flow arterioportal anastomosis or to consider arterialization as a temporary procedure.

We are gratefully indebted to B. Blondeau for her technical assistance and to M. B. Corlette, M.D., for revising the manuscript.

REFERENCES

1. Adamsons, R. J., Kinkhabwala, M., Moskowitz, H., Himmelfarb, E., Minkowitz, S., and Lerner, B.: Portacaval shunt with arterialization of the hepatic portion of the portal vein, Surg. Gynecol. Obstet. **135:** 529, 1972.
2. Basu, A. K., Chatterjee, C., and Mitra, S.: The importance of the haemodynamic changes in cases of cirrhosis of liver before and after porta-systemic shunt anastomosis, Br. J. Surg. **53:** 695, 1966.
3. Berthelot, P., Sicot, C., Desbuquois, B., Benhamou, J. P., and Rauvert, R.: Mesures simultanées des clearances de la bromesulfonephtaléine (BSP) et de l'or colloïdal radioactif Au^{198} chez le rat normal, Rev. Fr. Etud. Clin. Biol. **9:** 232, 1964.
4. Bismuth, H., Benhamou, J. P., and Lataste, J.: L'anastomose porto-cave expérimentale chez le rat normal. Technique et résultats préliminaires, Presse Med. **71:** 1859, 1963.
5. Bradley, S. E., Smythe, C. M., Fitzpatrick, H. F., and Blakemore, A. H.: The effect of portacaval shunt on estimated hepatic blood flow and oxygen uptake in cirrhosis, J. Clin. Invest. **32:** 526, 1953.
6. Burlui, D., Ratiu, O., Manesco, G., and Téju, G.: Artérialisation portale par la veine ombilicale reperméabilisée, Presse Med. **76:** 581, 1968.
7. Fisher, B., Russ, C., and Updegraff, H.: A suitable technique for total arterialization of the dog liver, SURGERY **35:** 879, 1954.
8. Fisher, B., Russ, C., Updegraff, H., and Fisher, E. R.: Effect of increased hepatic blood flow upon liver regeneration, Arch. Surg. **69:** 263, 1954.
9. Fisher, B., Russ, C., Fedor, E., Wilde, R., Engstrom, P., and Fisher, E. R.: Further experimental observations on animals with arterialized livers SURGERY **38:** 181, 1955.
10. Griffen, W. O., Bernstein, E. F., Nicoloff, D. M., Miller, E. O., Anderson, J. A., and Wangensteen, O. H.: The effect of liver arterialization upon ammonia clearance, Surg. Gynecol. Obstet. **115:** 704, 1962.

11. Kessler, R. E., Tice, D. A., and Zimmon, D. S.: Hemodynamic factors reflect prognosis after porta-caval shunt, Surg. Forum **23:** 334, 1972.
12. McCredie, J. A., Doggart, J. R., and Welbourn, R. B.: Total arterialization of the liver, Br. J. Surg. **45:** 83, 1957.
13. Maillard, J. N., Benhamou, J. P., and Rueff, B.: Total arterialization of the liver with portacaval shunt in the treatment of portal hypertension due to intrahepatic block, SURGERY, **67:** 883, 1970.
14. Rather, L. J., and Cohn, R.: Some effects upon the liver of complete arterialization of its blood supply. III. Acute vascular necrosis, SURGERY, **34:** 207, 1953.
15. Schwartz, S. I., Morton, J. H., and McGovern, G. R.: Experimental arterialization of the liver, SURGERY, **49:** 611, 1961.
16. Tutassaura, H., and Baird, R. J.: Hemodynamic observations following arterialization of the portal vein, Arch. Surg. **104:** 696, 1972.
17. Warren, W. D., Restrepo, J. E., Respess, J. C., and Muller, W. H.: The importance of hemodynamic studies in management of portal hypertension, Ann. Surg. **158:** 387, 1963.
18. Zuidema, G. D., Gaisford, W. D., Abell, M. R., Brody, T. M., Neill, S. A., and Child, C. G.: Segmental portal arterialization of canine liver, SURGERY **53:** 689, 1963.

Halsted and American surgery

Edward F. X. Hughes, M.D., M.P.H., *New York, N. Y.*

William Stewart Halsted demonstrated a consistent ability to achieve excellence in ever-changing settings—as athlete, student, private practitioner, innovative clinician, disciplined scientist, and pedagogue. His professional achievements and personal idiosyncrasies detail a fascinating American biography. Recent revelations confirm that his accomplishments as the first Professor of Surgery at Johns Hopkins were achieved against the backdrop of continuing drug addiction.

From the Department of Community Medicine, Mount Sinai School of Medicine, City University of New York, and the National Bureau of Economic Research, New York, N. Y.

IN AN American Mercury article of 1926, medical historian Fielding Garrison[11] stated that his recollection of Halsted was embodied in Sir Henry Taylor's line, "The world knows nothing of its greatest men." Then only four years after his death, Halsted was widely remembered as the first Professor of Surgery at Johns Hopkins, but the full details of his personal and professional accomplishments circulated only amid those who knew him intimately.

Gradually the publications of Cushing,[4, 5] MacCallum,[14] Fulton,[9] Crowe,[2] Penfield,[24] and Olch[22, 23] have shed light on the dramatic career of this accomplished surgeon and have set forth one of the most fascinating of American biographies.

Halsted's origins were far from humble. His great-grandfather had been a Revolutionary War physician in New Jersey and his grandfather was the founder of a prosperous dry goods firm in New York City. Under the latter's leadership the family grew wealthy and became socially prominent. Grandfather Halsted achieved some of his social prominence by helping to found Union Theological Seminary and by becoming a Governor of the New York Hospital where his grandson would later be a house physician.

Halsted's father, William, closely followed in his father's footsteps both in the family business and at the New York Hospital and, in addition, became a Trustee of the College of Physicians and Surgeons in New York. We can only wonder at what effect the strong medical associations of his three forebears had on Halsted's career, for he never discussed his motivation for medicine or the aspirations of his youth.

Halsted's early youth was uneventful. The position of his family entitled him to a private tutor until the age of ten. No record remains of his interaction with his tutor. The only incident of note during his ensuing stay in 1863 at a small New England boys' school was his attempt to run away. He was

Accepted for publication Aug. 22, 1973.

Reprint requests: Edward F. X. Hughes, M.D., Assistant Professor, Department of Community Medicine, Mount Sinai School of Medicine, Fifth Ave. and 100th St., New York, N. Y. 10029.

then 11 years old. After graduating from Andover in 1869, he was judged too immature to go to college. He secured private tutoring for a year and in 1870 he was allowed to enter Yale.

Here the future academician distinguished himself as a leader of men—on the playing field rather than in the classroom. After playing football brilliantly in the season of 1872, he was elected captain of the sport in his senior year and scored the winning goal in a game against Eaton. This was the highlight of his career at Yale. He also achieved moderate success as an actor, a baseball player, and a boxer. His academic career was, however, disappointing. He did show enough initiative, nonetheless, as a senior majoring in liberal arts, to buy a copy of Gray's *Anatomy* and a copy of Dalton's *Physiology* and to study them with interest. He also attended a few clinics at Yale Medical School. This information is contained in a later letter[15] and is the only record we have of his undergraduate science training and premedical preparation. In the letter, he states that he entered the College of Physicians and Surgeons in New York the next year. Of note, he makes no mention of his father's position on the school's Board of Trustees.

At the College of Physicians and Surgeons, Halsted transformed his life style completely. This ability to transform himself was to become a recurrent attribute. He applied himself to his work diligently, demonstrated an ability to think creatively, and amassed an excellent record. Having fortuitously read Dalton's *Physiology* while at Yale, he sought and achieved at "P. & S." the position of Dalton's first assistant in experiments on cerebral localization and gastric physiology. He profited immensely from this association as he did from summer pharmacy work and winter chemistry experiments. Besides attending regular classes, he participated in an evening tutorial session, called a "quiz," as was the custom of medical students of his day. These "quizzes" often comprised the most important part of a student's training as formal classes were often deemphasized by the faculty in favor of these profit-making side ventures.

The schedule of classes, quizzes, and extra work of the first two years exhausted Halsted. At the end of the second year, he felt that he could no longer memorize, and went to Block Island for a summer of reading and relaxation. He returned to New York in the fall in time for the Bellevue Hospital Internship examinations. Although only candidates who had completed the required three-year medical school course were expected to go on to internships, the examinations were open to all students.

It is now part of the Halsted legend that, fresh from Block Island, he placed fifth on the examination and became, without an M.D., an intern at Bellevue. Those of you who have recently taken internship examinations will enjoy Halsted's reflections on that day:

> As I have said I had little expectation of being admitted to Bellevue, for I was ineligible, not having a medical degree, nor had I taken the cram quiz. I recall contrasting my physical condition with that of the other fellows who presented themselves for the examination. Most of them were pale and nervous having remained in town all summer for the cram quizzes. Some of them told me that they had been bracing up on strychnine and quinine during the hot weather and I had a fine coat of tan and was in perfect health. I cannot recall being nervous for I was taking the examination as something of a lark, knowing I could try again in the spring.[16]

His internship year was an interesting one. He spent time on both medicine and surgery but it was surgery that attracted his special interest. Trauma cases composed a large part of the case load and, despite his busy schedule, he found time to work out original variations of Buck's traction for fractures of the neck of the femur. In time, these variations became standard procedures. He also measured hundreds of legs and demonstrated that the left was longer than the right. Through such innovative efforts, he grew close to many of the older physicians, who became his teachers and advisors.

His most valiant efforts, however, lay in attempting to introduce antiseptic surgery on to the Bellevue wards. It was 1877; Lister had just visited New York; there were only two surgeons in New York who followed his technique. It was so commonplace for surgeons to be opposed to it that Halsted was forever grateful to his chief-of-service for not having discouraged his efforts.

All his life, Halsted continued to concern himself with the dissemination and perfection of aseptic technique. As a staff man at Bellevue, only a few years later, he yelled at a senior surgeon for not washing his hands. This reprimand occasioned such opposition to the technique that Halsted had a tent erected in a vacant lot next to the hospital. Here he practiced antiseptic surgery unimpeded and achieved such startling results that his lead was followed throughout New York.

In the spring of his internship year, the young intern without an M.D. was invited to take the honors examination with his graduating classmates at "P. & S." He wrote for three and a half hours on arteries of the neck and won first prize, tantamount to graduating first in his class. He was granted an M.D. degree, became a house physician at the New York Hospital, and continued his interest in surgery. During his stay at New York Hospital, he claimed to have done the first two appendectomies in New York, preceding Fitz by six years. He also redesigned the temperature charts of the hospital and his modification came into common use.

Halsted soon started to attract the attention of his colleagues. His seniors were quick to see his potential and took pride in their friendship with him. Dr. William H. Welch, only two years his senior and destined to become the first Professor of Pathology at Johns Hopkins, was one of those who befriended Halsted. It was through the advice of Welch and others that Halsted sailed for Europe in the fall of 1880 for two years of intensive study of clinical surgery and basic science.

The tradition of eager young American physicians going to Europe to complete their education was well established by Halsted's time. American schools could not compete with the more aggressively scientific clinics of Europe and no American doctor could consider himself educated without a European experience. Many Americans deplored this state of affairs. In a speech to the medical faculty of the University of Pennsylvania 54 years earlier, Patrick Macaulay, a young physician only recently returned from study in Europe, stated, "The system of medical education in America is extremely defective. The defect is in our system and not our want of talent. A young gentleman enters a physician's office, he reads for 12 months, reports to some medical college and, after attendance at most of two courses of lectures, receives a degree. Unfortunate is the man who goes forth with a diploma in his pocket if his only opportunity of discerning or distinguishing the disease of mankind has been the lecture room."[3] Dr. Macaulay dreamed of a medical school tied to a university and to a hospital where the student would learn basic science and clinical medicine as a continuum. He set up practice in Baltimore and became a close friend of a rising merchant, Mr. Johns Hopkins. Out of this interaction came the medical environment of which Dr. Macaulay dreamed, an environment which was to contribute much to and derive much from the young surgeon who had just embarked for Europe.

The story of Halsted's days in Europe reads like a fairy tale for the medical historian. He toured the continent and, for periods of from one week to three months, studied at the clinics of Chiari, Zucherkandl, Billroth, Mynert, Woelfler, Mickulicz, and Volkmann. Here he found intellectual fervor that he had not experienced in America. Anatomy flourished, embryology was blossoming, and pathology and histology were booming. All clinics and lectures were open to the public, open debate and discussion was encouraged, and original investigation was prized. Antiseptic technique seemed suited to the German temperament and was practiced enthusiastically.

Here Halsted first learned to use silk. His study of the thyroid in Woelfler's laboratory led to his later work on goiter. In studying sections of breast carcinoma, he noted malignant cells in lymphatics and conceived his radical mastectomy. Through his study of anatomy he envisioned a surgical cure for inguinal hernia. The meticulousness and delicacy of German surgery had no equal in America and became engrained in his technique. The advantages of the arterial clamps used by the Germans staggered him, and he became an advocate of bloodless surgery.

He was so impressed by the European surgeons that many became his life-long friends and he became a frequent visitor to their clinics. The Germans, in turn, recognized his contributions by electing Halsted the first American member of the German Surgical Association.

With innumerable ideas and unbounded energy, Halsted landed in New York in 1880. It is not by accident that MacCallum subtitled his chapter on Halsted's New York days "Activity."[17] He was Assistant Surgeon at Roosevelt Hospital and tackled the job of organizing an Outpatient Department. He was also given the responsibility of introducing antiseptic technique and the privilege of operating on all patients that interested him. He began his series of radical mastectomies and herniorrhaphies, using silk in all procedures. In the Outpatient Department, he labored seven mornings a week with his three assistants and made significant contributions to the diagnosis of intracapsular fractures of the femur by leg measurements and to the treatment of gonococcal urethritis with bichloride of mercury. Also at Roosevelt Hospital, he collaborated on the use of plates and screws in humeral fractures.

At Chambers Street Hospital, he treated carbon monoxide inhalation by withdrawing arterial blood, shaking the defibrinated blood in the presence of air, and reinfusing it. Although these experiments were not properly controlled, they demonstrated the remarkability of the busy surgeon to think physiologically.

There was in Halsted a penchant for the dramatic. In 1881, he was called to his sister's bedside; she was felt to be terminal following a postpartum hemorrhage. When all attempts at hemostasis failed he thrust a syringe into his antecubital vein, transfused his blood into his sister, and watched her promptly recuperate.

It was only a year later that the 30-year-old surgeon was called to his mother's bedside. She was jaundiced, tender in the right upper quadrant of the abdomen, and chronically ill. All senior surgeons refused to operate but Halsted added two years to his mother's life by draining her pus-filled gallbladder. It was the first gallbladder operation he had ever done and is claimed to be only the third in America.

As if the above were not sufficient accomplishments for any man, Halsted assumed teaching responsibilities in a number of the city's medical schools and began an evening quiz for students. In no time at all, the young surgeon's quiz was the most popular. Students swarmed to learn at the feet of the charismatic, witty, and ruthlessly rigorous educator.

So it was that in the year 1884 Halsted was the fastest rising surgeon in New York. It was only natural that, upon reading in the Medical Record of October 11 of that year of the introduction of cocaine anesthesia of the cornea at the Heidelburg Ophthalmic Congress, Halsted and his associates should act. Within a few short weeks they were able to produce anesthesia in the distribution of the ulnar nerve by injecting each other's forearms. They demonstrated painless extraction of teeth and treated trigeminal neuralgia with the drug. Halsted went to Europe and demonstrated his findings to the skeptical Woelfler, who, Halsted humorously recalled in a letter to Osler, published the results without mentioning Halsted.

Little was known of the side-effects of cocaine and its users soon noted increased energy and a remarkable ability to resist fatigue. As 1885 stretched out, the deleterious effects of the drug became evident and Halsted and his three assistants realized that they were addicted.

The events that followed were critical for the career of the future professor and are among the most interesting in the history of American medicine. He attempted to keep on working but became erratic. In early 1886, he prepared a series of lectures for competition for the Professorship of Surgery at the College of Physicians and Surgeons, but they were never delivered. As he decompensated he approached his close friends, including Dr. Welch, now Professor of Pathology at Hopkins, and sought their advice. It was agreed that, under an assumed name, Halsted should enter the Butler Hospital in Providence, R. I., and undergo treatments for cure of his addiction. All was performed with utmost secrecy and only today is the controversy resolving as to how many times he went to the hospital, when he went, and how long he stayed. On Dec. 6, 1886, he was discharged and took up residence in the Baltimore home of Dr. Welch. He later returned in 1887 for a second stay of nine months, returning again to the home of Dr. Welch.[21, 22] Whipple claims that, on discharge, hospital records show he was completely free of addiction.[27*]

Halsted's assistants did not fare as well. Not one lived to overcome the habit. One of the most dramatic of all is the case of Dr. Halsted's talented first assistant, Dr. Richard Hall, who for reasons of health soon had to resign his newly appointed Professorship of Anatomy at P. & S. He moved to California and fought through "a long period of misery" to pull himself together to establish a successful private practice.[18]

The work of these unfortunate men is now recognized as the classic experiments in local anesthesia and the threshold of a major surgical advance. Though it is difficult to find documentation, Cushing said that Halsted was the first to perform spinal anesthesia.[5] Following his discharge, Halsted never used cocaine again in his practice—perhaps one of the rare unscientific prejudices in his career.

With residence in Dr. Welch's home came an invitation to work in his laboratory. Dr. Welch was then 36 years old and Halsted was 34. The relationship between these two men showed a devotion rare in medicine and was, at this most critical point in his life, crucial to Halsted's survival.

With Dr. Welch and the laboratory to help him, Halsted matured. The flashy surgeon of New York slowed down and in the relaxed pace of the laboratory reaped the harvest of ideas sown in Germany. This was the first laboratory of experimental pathology in America. Embryology, bacteriology, and histology were vigorously studied. His associates in that laboratory, William Councilman, Walter Reed, James Carrol, Simon Flexner, George Sternberg, and Franklin Mall are as significant in the development of American medicine as his earlier German friends were in their tradition.

The laboratory was education in action. Under Dr. Welch's able leadership, communication and collaboration were encouraged; mutual endeavor bred mutual edification. With Mall, Halsted performed his classic studies on intestinal surgery. In well-controlled, live animal experiments, with histologic follow-up, he demonstrated the strength of the submucosa over the serosa in retaining sutures. These studies revolutionized the field and, like his studies on anastomoses, became mainstays of abdominal surgery. With histologists, he studied wound healing and inflammation and showed that blood in the wound did not necessarily imply infection. With bacteriologists, he showed the etiologic role of necrotic tissue in infection and its relevance to peritonitis. He demonstrated the effectiveness of silk over catgut in hemostasis and continued its use in all procedures. All his work was carefully controlled and meticulous and he showed a freedom from haste rare among surgeons of that era. The traits that characterized his work soon characterized his personality. The extrovert surgeon of New York grew comtemplative, shy, and withdrawn; a second transformation remade William Stewart Halsted.

When the Johns Hopkins Hospital opened on May 7, 1889, Halsted's work on goiter was well under way. Macewen, Lister's successor at Glasgow, had refused the Professorship of Surgery and the position lay vacant. For

*Halsted also took a cruise to the Windward Islands during this period. Some claim Dr. William Welch accompanied him on this cruise but the evidence is conflicting.[2, 14, 27]

the period of one year Halsted was appointed Acting Surgeon to the Hospital and Surgeon-in-Chief to the Dispensary.

It is hypothesized that at this time there was still some question as to Halsted's cure and that this was responsible for his not being offered the professorship. Doubt was dissipated shortly thereafter when Osler wrote to President Gilman that "Halsted is doing remarkable work in surgery and I feel that his appointment to the University and Hospital would be quite safe."[6] (Later Osler was to have much more to say on this subject.)[24] In six months, Halsted was an Associate Professor; in nine months, Surgeon-in-Chief to the hospital; and in 1892, at the age of 39, Professor of Surgery.

The opening of the hospital gave him the patient load required to round out his work. Within three and a half years, he had operated on 86 inguinal hernias, 58 by his own method; and of those healing per primam, he had noted no recurrences. Prior to this series and Bassini's coincident work in Italy, a surgical cure of hernia was a rarity. His radical mastectomy series grew; in five years he had 50 cases with only six percent local recurrence and 21 percent regional recurrence. Kuster had had the best series prior to this with 56.6 percent recurrence. Halsted became the first to remove successfully an aneurysm of the subclavian artery and he carried out extensive clinical and physiologic experiments on the ligation of aneurysms of the abdominal aorta and common iliac vessels. He also made innovations in the surgery of the bile passages and demonstrated the role of bile regurgitation in the etiology of acute hemorrhagic pancreatitis. His hospital became a referral center for thyroid surgery and he dovetailed his experimental work with his clinical cases. He studied the postparathyroidectomy syndrome and attempted transplantation of this gland. From this work he evolved his concept of gland transplantation. He also maintained an active and diversified private practice.[22]

As his work broadened, Halsted became more withdrawn. Cushing complained that he was so shy he would ask a resident's permission to examine a patient. He often spent hours on such an examination. After removing a breast, he would repair to his laboratory alone, leaving the patient to his residents, and work over the specimen for hours. The once dynamic lecturer became a mumbler. Students sitting beyond the first row complained that they could hear only fragments of his laboriously detailed lectures. He pitched his approach, however, to the most gifted and, as the years went on, he became an abiding influence in their lives.

A flair for the dramatic still persisted in Halsted and, in the winter of 1889, when his unusually efficient scrub nurse was afflicted with dermatitis from an operating room solution, he addressed himself to the matter. One day in New York, he requested the Goodyear Rubber Company to make "a pair of very thin rubber gloves with gauntlets."[20] The gloves were the first of their kind to be introduced into an operating room and, as they relieved Miss Hampton's dermatitis, serendipity saw that their aseptic value was recognized. Miss Hampton did not have long to enjoy her gloves; she resigned in a few months to become Mrs. William Stewart Halsted.

The former Miss Hampton brought Halsted a retreat from the rigors of the academic life. She was the daughter of an old Southern planting family and soon, with her husband, purchased the family estate in the North Carolina mountains. Here Halsted summered. He developed a fondness for the growing of dahlias, for the care of horses, and for relaxation. He later noted that he had no live animal experiment follow-ups longer than nine months for he closed his laboratory each summer when he went to the mountains. He was fond of entertaining and found great joy in having his friends relax in this beautiful setting.

Halsted was also famous for his entertaining in Baltimore. He was an accomplished gourmet and overpowered his residents with nine-course dinners. He personally picked the terrapins for the stew, examined each coffee bean, and insisted on ironing the tablecloth while it lay on the table to insure the absence of wrinkles. This formal entertaining exacted a toll from Mrs. Halsted. She developed migraine, which worsened as her husband grew more meticulous, and eventually prohibited their entertaining in Baltimore.

Despite his idiosyncrasies Halsted enjoyed the unbridled respect of his colleagues and his protegés. In a letter to his fiancée, Cushing stated, "He is surely the best man in the country and I enjoy being his slave."[10] Slaves his residents were, but it is to Halsted's credit that he inspired in them the same love of knowledge which he possessed. The same vision and insight which characterized Halsted as surgeon and scientist distinguished him as educator. He was quick to praise and eager to encourage original thinking. He chose his men carefully, with an eye as much on their future potential as on their past accomplishments, and created an environment where they could grow as individuals. He incorporated his German and "Welch School" experiences into his own school and matured his men on that same blend of science and surgery he grew on. Seven professors of surgery grew in his school and disseminated Halsted's ideals across the country. Numerous departments of surgery across the country today boast of being founded by one of Halsted's residents and of following the basics of his program.

With his school secure, he turned his attention to the nation. He advocated university affiliation for medical schools and decried proprietary medical schools. Contrary to popular conception, he embraced the full-time system only late in life and then over Osler's objection.[22] His acceptance of the full-time salary system at Johns Hopkins is traditionally held as a crucial step in the spread of this plan, in which numerous universities followed Hopkins' example.

The scope of Halsted's ideals in education of surgeons is broad; but nowhere are his ideals better expressed than in his beautifully written Yale Medical Address of 1904 when he said, "We need a system and we shall have it, which will produce not only surgeons, but surgeons of the highest type, men who will stimulate the first youths of our country to study surgery and to devote their energies and their lives to raising the surgical science."[12] It is through the embodiment of these ideals in the training of the surgeon that Halsted rounded out his greatness.

Now, fifty years after Halsted's death in 1922, recent disclosures from Osler's long concealed work, *Inner History of the Johns Hopkins Hospital,* make the accomplishments of W. S. Halsted seem all the more remarkable.[24] This "secret history" was written in a locked book around 1893, four years after the opening of the Johns Hopkins Hospital, and was later updated. Osler originally left instructions that the contents of the history not be made public till the one hundredth anniversary of the Hospital. The work is now in the Osler Library of the McGill University and its contents regarding Halsted have recently been made public.[24]

In this record, Osler stated that when "we recommended Halsted as full surgeon to the hospital in 1890, I believed, and Welch did too, that he was no longer addicted to *morphia*" (emphasis added). About six months after the full position had been awarded, Osler noted Halsted having a severe chill and recorded that "this was the first intimation I had that he was still taking morphia." Over the years, Halsted grew very close to Osler and confided that "he had *never* been able to reduce the amount [of morphine] to less than three grains a day." Years later, Osler made a further entry in his secret history, stating, "subsequently (1898) he got the amount down to 1½ grains, and of late years (1912) [when Halsted was 60 years old] has possibly got on without it."

These remarkable revelations not only confirm the long-held suspicion that Halsted may have had a chronic drug problem but, for the first time, implicate morphine as the drug involved. The traditional view held that, if Halsted had a continuing drug problem, it involved cocaine. A re-examination of the evidence surrounding Halsted's first encounter with addiction continues to implicate cocaine as the drug to which he and his co-workers succumbed in their work in the Roosevelt Dispensary.[14, 23] Indeed, the syndrome of social disintegration that characterized Halsted's later New York period (as well as Hall's) is quite characteristic of cocaine abuse. Osler, however, relates that at the time of his recommendation of Halsted as full professor he felt he was free of morphine addiction.[24]

When and how did morphine enter the picture? Stout related that, while in New York, Halsted turned at one point to morphine and later to alcohol to counteract the agitation associated with cocaine.[23] The impression given by Stout, however, is that the utilization of morphine was a very transient event. Osler, at another point in his secret history, however, described Halsted's first two years in Baltimore living with Welch as a struggle "to recover from the cocaine and morphine habit which he had acquired in New York." It thus appears that Halsted began medicating himself with morphine in New York to ward off the effects of cocaine and that it was to this drug that he developed a long-term dependence. It also appears that he was able to give up cocaine through his stays in the Butler Hospital and with Dr. Welch. With morphine, however, he was to succeed in only concealing his continuing administration (and to succeed to a remarkable degree).

Prior to Halsted's work on the anesthetic properties of cocaine, the drug had been used at times to treat morphine addiction.[23, 25] In view of the widespread therapeutic use of alkaloid derivatives in Halsted's time, it is not unlikely that at one time or another morphine might have been employed to treat cocaine addiction.[26] Accordingly, it could be hypothesized that Halsted may have been treated with morphine while at Butler Hospital and there have developed his dependency. An examination of Halsted's medical records from Butler Hospital would settle this point but they have long since disappeared.[21] Osler's and Stout's testimony, however, combined with Whipple's description of the prehospitalization Windward Island trip as a "tragic experience," suggest that Halsted took his morphine habit with him to Butler Hospital.[23, 24, 27] A note of poignancy is added in this regard by MacCallum's stating, of Halsted's second visit to Butler, "There he sent for the manager and asked him to make sure he should have no money so that he could not buy any drug."[19]

On the basis of Osler's account, one can infer that Halsted's Baltimore period of maximum morphine intake lasted 10 to 12 years —until approximately 1898; his period of diminished intake lasted an additional 14 years, if not the entire 24 years remaining in his life. During his period of maximum dosage, Halsted was consuming almost 200 mg. of morphine a day. It was during this same period that Halsted not only accomplished much of his most important scientific work but also laid the groundwork for much of his later work. On this daily morphine dose, Osler noted "[Halsted] could do his work comfortably and maintain his excellent physical vigor."[24] At the time of this writing, a 200 mg. a day morphine habit is equivalent to a daily heroin habit on the streets of New York well in excess of $100.[1, 8] The magnitude of Halsted's triumphs during this period of high opiate intake provides an impressive backdrop to our present discussion of the efficacy of long-term chemotherapy for narcotics addiction.[7, 13]

I would like to thank Drs. Paul Russel, Henry Viets, James Feeney, Kurt Deuschle, William Shoemaker, and Robert Brown for their encouragement and advice through the writing of this paper, Dr. Peter Olch for his clarification of some historical ambiguities, and Drs. Vincent Dole and Bernard Bihari for clarification of the addiction problem.

REFERENCES

1. Bihari, B.: Personal communication, Morris Bernstein Institute, Beth Israel Medical Center, New York, N. Y.
2. Crowe, S. J.: Halsted of Johns Hopkins: The man and his men, Springfield, Ill., 1957, Charles C Thomas, Publisher.
3. Ibid.: p. 4.

4. Cushing, H.: The life of Sir William Osler, Oxford, 1925, Clarendon Press, 2 vols.
5. Cushing, H.: William Stewart Halsted, Science **56:** 461, 1922.
6. Op. cit.: **1:** 325.
7. Dole, V. P.: Methodone maintenance treatment for 25,000 heroin addicts, J. A. M. A. **215:** 1131, 1971.
8. Dole, V. P.: Personal communication. Rockefeller Institute, New York, N. Y.
9. Fulton, J. F.: Harvey Cushing: A biography, Springfield, Ill., Charles C Thomas, Publisher.
10. Ibid.: p. 139.
11. Garrison, F. A.: Halsted, Am. Mercury **28:** 396, 1926.
12. Halsted, W. S.: Surgical papers, Baltimore, 1924, Johns Hopkins Press, The training of surgeons **2:** 527.
13. Koran, L. M.: Heroin maintenance for heroin addicts: Issues and evidence, N. Engl. J. Med. **288:** 654, 1973.
14. MacCallum, W. G.: William Stewart Halsted—Surgeon. Baltimore, 1930, Johns Hopkins Press.
15. Ibid.: p. 11.
16. Ibid.: p. 16.
17. Ibid.: p. 29.
18. Ibid.: p. 52.
19. Ibid.: p. 57.
20. Ibid.: p. 81.
21. Olch, P. D.: Personal communication, History of Medicine Division, National Library of Medicine, NIH, Bethesda, Md.
22. Olch, P. D.: William S. Halsted and private practice: A re-examination, SURGERY **72:** 804, 1972.
23. Olch, P. D.: William S. Halsted's New York Period, 1874-1886, Bull. Hist. Med. **40:** 495, 1966.
24. Penfield, W.: Halsted of Johns Hopkins, J. A. M. A. **210:** 2214, 1969.
25. Terry, C. E., and Semple, M.: The opium problem, New York, 1928, The Bureau of Social Hygiene, Inc., p. 531.
26. Ibid.: p. 71.
27. Whipple, A. O.: Halsted's New York period, SURGERY **32:** 542, 1952.

Nonpulsatile vs. pulsatile canine kidney perfusion

R. Grundmann, M.D., H. Pitschi, F. Berr, *and* **H. Pichlmaier, M.D.,**
Munich, Germany

Dog kidneys were perfused in pairs. Pulsatile perfusion was used for one kidney of each pair and nonpulsatile perfusion for the other. All were transplanted after 48 hours' perfusion to the necks of recipient animals. Hypothermic human albumin was the perfusion fluid. In both groups there was no elevation of perfusion pressure, only slight enzyme release, small increase in kidney weight, and immediate posttransplantation function. There was no difference between P- and NP-perfused kidneys in PAH and inulin clearance, in urine electrolyte concentrations, or in osmolality. It is concluded that nonpulsatile and pulsatile perfusion yield equivalent results.

From Chirurgische Universitätsklinik München

SUCCESSFUL kidney transplantation requires reliable preservation. Preservation makes possible critical examination of the viability of the organ in vitro before implantation and allows time for selection of the most suitable recipient and for tissue typing.[9] The method applied most frequently is mechanical hypothermic perfusion of the kidney, in which it is continuously perfused under hypothermia (8° C.) with the use of cryoprecipitated plasma[2] or albumin[12] as the perfusion medium. One important point that is still under discussion is whether pulsatile perfusion of the organ, as originally applied by nearly all investigators,[1, 2, 23] is necessary or whether nonpulsatile perfusion yields equal results.[13] The latter has the advantage of being technically simpler and therefore more economical.

Recently we reported successful 72 hour canine kidney preservation by means of nonpulsatile perfusion in our own preservation system,[7, 10] which enabled us to conclude that equal length of preservation can be obtained with either pulsatile or nonpulsatile perfusion. The preservation period obtained, however, does not in itself determine the value of the method used. Rather, the immediate posttransplant function of the kidney, the ability to sustain life after simultaneous contralateral nephrectomy, and the state of preservation after perfusion (the degree of tubular damage) are all significant criteria.

For these reasons, one objective of the experiments described in this article was to examine the behavior (LDH release, kidney weight gain, and renal vascular resistance) of kidneys perfused by both pulsatile and nonpulsatile methods. Another objective was

This investigation was supported by the "Sonderforschungsbereich 37."

Accepted for publication Aug. 28, 1973.

Reprint requests: Dr. R. Gundmann, Chirurgische Klinik der Universitat München, 8 München 2, Nussbaumstr. 20, Munich, Germany.

 Vol. 75, No. 2, pp. 178-184

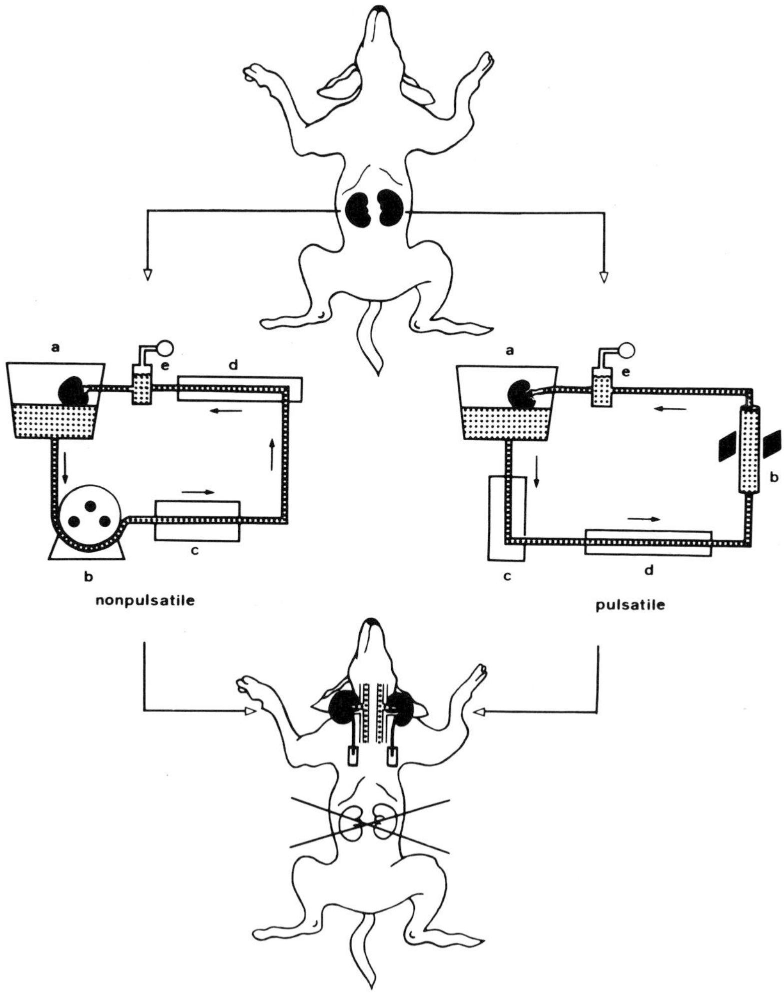

Fig. 1. Diagram of experimental arrangement. (*a*) Kidney chamber, (*b*) perfusion pump, (*c*) oxygenator, (*d*) heat exchanger, (*e*) bubble trap.

to examine the immediate posttransplant function of the kidneys. For that purpose, clearances of both PAH (para-aminohippuric acid) and inulin were verified in both P (pulsatile)- and NP (nonpulsatile)-perfused kidneys as a measure of secretion and filtration capacity. Furthermore, the urine osmolality and Na^+ and K^+ content were determined to evaluate concentration capacity.

The main difficulty in comparing various preservation methods lies in the fact that the results are influenced by different factors: (1) the structure of the preservation unit (quantity of evaporation; kinds of materials used), (2) the perfusate used (human albumin; cryoprecipitated plasma; electrolyte solution), (3) the perfusate volume, (4) the condition of the kidney prior to perfusion (warm and cold ischemia time; kidney diseases), and (5) operation techniques and anesthesia (condition of circulation; application of diuretics; infusion therapy; operation time, including performance of vascular anastomoses). It was therefore necessary to develop a model in which all experimental conditions were identical for P- and NP-perfused kidneys; only under such conditions can different results be attributed to the different types of pump.

MATERIALS AND METHODS

Through a midline incision bilateral nephrectomy was performed in 18 mongrel dogs weighing 20 to 25 kilograms. Anesthesia was introduced and maintained intravenously with pentobarbital sodium; a muscle relaxant was given; the animals' respiration was accomplished via intratracheal tube. Dogs with only one renal artery were used. The left kidney was removed first. The organ was flushed with 300 to 500 ml. of Ringer's lactate solution, at 4° C., containing 200 mg. of procaine and 5,000 U. of heparin sodium per liter, before being placed in the perfusion circuit.

Two different perfusion systems were used: each consisted of a kidney chamber, a heat exchanger, an oxygenator, a filter, a bubble trap, and a perfusion pump, but in one system there was a piston pump (pulsatile) and in the other a roller pump (nonpulsatile). In the NP-perfusion system the heat exchanger, filter, and oxygenator were placed behind the pump (between the pump and the kidney), whereas in the P-perfusion unit they were placed in front of the pump (between the pump and the kidney chamber) so that pulse amplitude would be as large as possible (Fig. 1). With the exception of the pumps, all parts of the two units were made of the same materials (the NP system has already been described).[7, 10]

Perfusion of either the left or the right kidney of the donor animal was alternated, either P or NP, and perfusion continued for 48 hours. The perfusion fluid used was human albumin, 800 ml. of which contained: human albumin 20 percent, 300 ml.; NaCl 0.9 percent, 500 ml.; dextrose 50 percent, 10 ml.; Mg_2SO_4 20 percent, 2 ml.; KCl 20 percent, 4 ml.; bicarbonate 4 percent, 7.5 ml.; penicillin, 1.5 Gm.; prednisolone, 100 mg.; insulin, 80 I.U. The final concentrations were: Na^+, 132 mEq. per liter; K^+, 12 mEq. per liter; dextrose, 600 mg. per 100 ml.; protein, 6 Gm. per 100 ml.; osmolality, 330 mOsm. per kilogram.

Room air was used for oxygenation, taken in by an air pump at a flow rate of 1 L. per minute through the oxygenator; additional O_2 or CO_2 was not needed. The temperature of the perfusate was approximately 7° C., the arterial oxygen tension was approximately 140 mm. Hg, and the pH ranged from 7.2 to 7.4. With pulsatile perfusion, the perfusion pressure was adjusted to 60/20 mm. Hg (37 mm. Hg mean pressure) at the beginning of preservation. With nonpulsatile perfusion, it ranged up to 30 mm. Hg. The perfusion pressure decreased in the first six hours and was then regulated to approximately 30 mm. Hg for pulsatile perfusion and 20 mm. Hg for nonpulsatile. In earlier experiments the lower pressure used in NP perfusion had proved particularly favorable.[10] During preservation the pH, LDH (lactic dehydrogenase), Na^+ and K^+ concentrations, and osmolality were measured regularly; pressure was registered continually by a pressure transducer; kidneys were weighed before and after perfusion. After 48 hours' preservation the kidneys were transplanted to the vessels on both sides of the neck of the recipient (allotransplantation)—renal vein to external jugular vein; renal artery to common carotid artery—and then bilateral nephrectomy was performed in the recipient. PAH and inulin were given intravenously to the recipient via an infusion pump and a serum PAH level of 2 mg. per 100 ml. and a serum inulin level of 25 mg. per 100 ml. were attained. After that, PAH and inulin clearances were determined simultaneously in both kidneys during the six hours after transplantation. The extraction ratio of PAH and inulin was calculated as follows:

$$\%\ \text{extraction} = \frac{a - v}{a} \times 100$$

where a is the arterial concentration and v is the renal vein concentration of PAH and inulin, respectively. Dextrose, protein, Na^+ and K^+ content, osmolality, and LDH and LAP concentration of the urine were measured. At the end of the experiment the kidneys were removed and histologically examined.

Table I. *Perfusion data*

Exp. No.	LDH concentration of perfusate: final value NP (mU./ml.)	LDH concentration of perfusate: final value P (mU./ml.)	Perfusion pressure: final value NP (mm. Hg)	Perfusion pressure: final value P (mm. Hg)	Flow rate during perfusion NP (ml./min.)	Flow rate during perfusion P (ml./min.)	Kidney weight (Gm.) NP Initial	Kidney weight (Gm.) NP Final	Kidney weight (Gm.) P Initial	Kidney weight (Gm.) P Final
1	372	372	18	29	120	112	105	120	111	117
2	181	277	20	30	64	96	62	66	62	68
3	315	286	20	28	82	98	76	81	76	82
4	105	115	20	29	80	95	76	86	76	78
5	267	220	21	29	68	98	79	88	83	102
6	75	75	17	28	64	82	98	106	96	102
7	220	191	19	26	88	86	68	74	66	72
8	162	200	18	28	72	80	68	68	66	66
9	239	191	17	27	82	88	58	64	56	63
10	120	124	18	31	90	108	97	98	98	100
11	143	138	18	28	102	120	96	96	82	83
12	410	229	22	35	98	128	74	86	82	96
13	124	105	18	27	72	95	74	81	77	77
14	277	305	18	30	84	108	88	94	86	92
15	143	134	16	28	76	100	78	88	83	97
16	210	172	18	30	68	104	75	86	75	88
17	115	124	20	37	72	144	62	72	58	76
18	95	86	18	33	76	128	72	78	70	80

RESULTS

In 18 experiments 36 kidneys were perfused—one pulsatile and one nonpulsatile in each pair.

Perfusion data. After an initial decrease the pressure remained almost constant in both P and NP perfusions. Elevation of renal vascular resistance was never observed. The enzyme release was small: the mean value of the LDH concentration after 48 hours' perfusion was 185 ± 83 mU. per milliliter with P perfusion and 198 ± 98 mU. per milliliter with NP. The kidney weight gain (a measure of edema formation during perfusion) amounted to 9.7 ± 8.6 percent of the initial value with P perfusion and 9.1 ± 5.1 percent with NP. Flow rates ranged to 1.37 ± 0.35 ml. per gram of kidney weight per minute with P perfusion (mean pressure 30 mm. Hg) and to 1.04 ± 0.18 ml. per gram of kidney weight per minute with NP perfusion (mean pressure 20 mm. Hg). The perfusion data of all kidneys are summarized in Table I.

Functional data. All kidneys produced urine immediately after establishment of circulation. Urinary samples were collected for six hours. PAH clearances ranged up to 40.7 ± 31.0 ml. per minute with P perfusion and 51.4 ± 39.2 ml. per minute with NP; inulin clearances ranged up to 7.2 ± 5.4 ml. per minute with P perfusion and 11.7 ± 6.2 ml. per minute with NP. Differences were not significant even when the glomerular filtration rate was stimulated by 40 mg. of furosemide (Fig. 2).

The urine concentrations of Na^+ and K^+ and the osmolality did not differ significantly (Table II) nor did the enzyme (LDH; LAP) concentrations of the urine. Histologic examination revealed no difference between results after P and NP perfusion.

In one experiment (No. 11) the kidneys became pink 15 minutes after transplantation and produced urine immediately; then they became dark and urine production ceased. Histologic examination demonstrated a hyperacute rejection of both kidneys. These two kidneys had been perfused with an albumin solution produced by another supplier. The sodium and protein contents of commercially available albumin solutions vary widely.

At the end of the clearance periods the

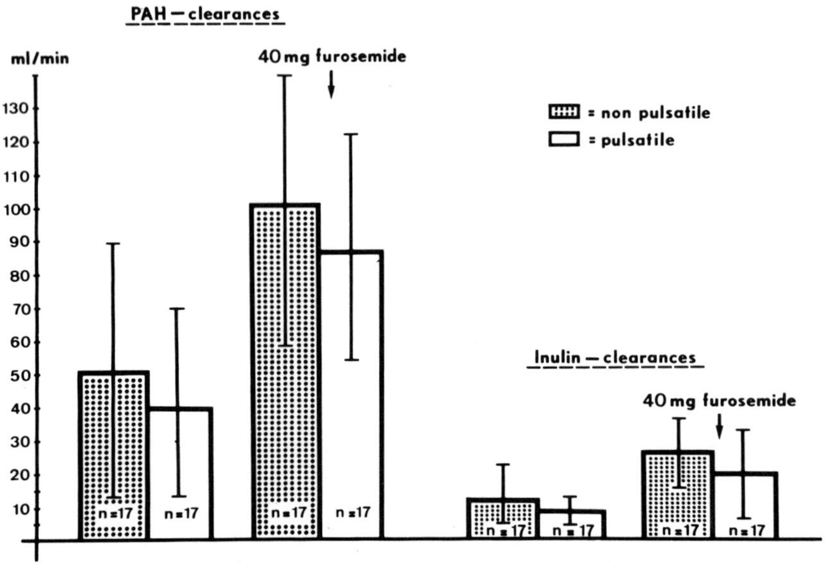

Fig. 2. PAH and inulin clearances after transplantation (mean values and standard deviation).

Table II. *Urine electrolytes and enzymes concentration 6 hours after transplantation (mean values and standard deviations)*

	Nonpulsatile perfusion (n = 17)*	Pulsatile perfusion (n = 17)*
Urine volume (ml./min.)	0.80 ± 0.39	0.58 ± 0.29
Sodium (mEq./L.)	75.25 ± 29.70	89.21 ± 32.69
Potassium (mEq./L.)	28.32 ± 8.35	26.46 ± 8.73
Osmolality (mOsm./Kg.)	304.42 ± 25.72	294.57 ± 21.50
LDH (mU./ml.)	127.0 ± 139.20	153.0 ± 172.80
LAP (mU./ml.)	22.88 ± 24.99	24.0 ± 21.83
Dextrose (mg./100 ml.)	36.97 ± 27.45	34.02 ± 48.10
Albumin (Gm./100 ml.)	0.53 ± 0.40	0.39 ± 0.37

*No significant difference between pulsatile and nonpulsatile perfusion.

PAH extraction ratio was 12.9 ± 8.4 percent with P perfusion and 15.4 ± 7.8 percent with NP; the inulin extraction ratio was 11.1 ± 10 percent with P perfusion and 11.4 ± 10 percent with NP. There were no significant differences.

DISCUSSION

Many investigators use pulsatile pumps in hypothermic mechanical kidney perfusion in order to avoid elevation of renal vascular resistance and kidney weight gain.[3] They feel that the pulsatile pump imitates physiologic conditions in vitro. In earlier experiments, however, we showed that successful 72 hour canine kidney preservation is possible with the use of hypothermic nonpulsatile perfusion. The results presented in this article further demonstrate that there is no difference in kidney function and preservation whether P or NP perfusion is used.

Reports in the literature regarding results of P and NP perfusion vary markedly. Ssentjurin[21] demonstrated that, at the same average pressure, flow rates are higher with NP than with P perfusion. Shephard and associates[20] stated the opposite. Hooker,[11] Gesell[5] and Many and associates[16] found reduced kidney function with NP perfusion but Goodyer and Glenn[6] did not confirm a reduction of glomerular filtration rate and of PAH and inulin clearance with NP perfusion. Nakayama and colleagues[17] and Mandelbaum and colleagues[15] observed an increase in peripheral vascular resistance with NP perfusion but neither Ritter[19] nor Paquet[18] could confirm this.

In earlier experiments we showed that the success of NP perfusion depended upon the perfusion pressure applied: 20 mm. Hg proved particularly favorable.[10] The flow rates achieved at this low pressure are surprisingly high and absolutely comparable to those obtained with P perfusion at higher mean pressures. The minimum flow rate with NP perfusion should be approximately 0.8 ml. per gram of kidney weight per minute, which is the value required by others for P perfusion,[4, 14, 22] and our results show that this rate can be achieved at 20 mm. Hg. This removes the main objection to NP perfusion.

Other objections to NP perfusion include elevated vascular resistance and edema formation of the kidney.[3] At the pressure we applied, however, the perfusion pressure did not increase during preservation and the kidney weight gain was unimportant. We believe that edema formation during preservation depends on the composition of the perfusion fluid: the osmolality should reach at least 330 mOsm. per kilogram and the sodium concentration should not exceed 140 to 145 mEq. per liter.[8] Furthermore, a high protein content (6 Gm. per 100 ml.) was used.

It is difficult to compare various preservation methods because the results are influenced by the composition of the perfusate, the pretreatment of the recipient, the reimplantation time, the cold and warm ischemia time of the organ, and other factors. This leads to contradictory statements of results. The experimental model we have developed allows a true comparison to be made between two methods and it can be used in other investigations as well. The perfusate was the same for both kidneys; the perfusion circuits consisted of the same materials, differing only in the pumps; the transplantation times were almost identical. Any technical errors that might creep in during the performance of the experiments (e.g., disease of donor or recipient animal, intraoperative circulation fluctuations, unduly long operation time, wrong composition of the perfusate, insufficient oxygenation of the perfusion medium) would affect both groups equally. The fact that the first transplanted kidney showed somewhat smaller clearances than the second did not influence the P vs. NP results.

CONCLUSIONS

1. Successful 48 hour canine kidney preservation is possible with the use of either pulsatile or nonpulsatile perfusion and there is sufficient immediate posttransplant function of the organ with either.
2. During perfusion there is no elevation in vascular resistance and only slight enzyme release and kidney weight gain.
3. The P- and NP-perfused kidneys do not differ in either perfusion behavior or organ function.
4. NP perfusion is technically simpler and less expensive than other comparable systems. Oxygenation of the perfusate by compressed air *only* is sufficient and it is not necessary to monitor the pH during perfusion.
5. When roller pumps are used the flow during perfusion can be easily evaluated because it corresponds linearly to the turns of the pump.

REFERENCES

1. Abouna, G. M., Lim, F., Cook, J. S., Grubb, W., Craig, S. S., Seibel, H. R., and Hume, D. M.: Three-day canine kidney preservation, SURGERY **71:** 436, 1972.
2. Belzer, F. O., Ashby, B. S., and Dunphy, J. E.: 24-hour and 72-hour preservation of canine kidneys, Lancet **2:** 536, 1967.
3. Belzer, F. O., Ashby, B. S., Huang, J. S., and Dunphy, J. E.: Etiology of rising perfusion pressure in isolated organ perfusion, Ann. Surg. **168:** 382, 1968.
4. Belzer, F. O., Reed, T. W., Pryor, J. P., Kountz, S. L., and Dunphy, J. E.: Cause of renal injury in kidneys obtained from cadaver donors, Surg. Gynecol. Obstet. **130:** 467, 1970.
5. Gesell, R. A.: On the relation of pulse pressure to renal secretion, Am. J. Physiol. **32:** 70, 1913.
6. Goodyer, A. V. N., and Glenn, W. W. L.: Relation of arterial pulse pressure to renal function, Am. J. Physiol. **167:** 689, 1951.
7. Grundmann, R., Landes, Th., and Pichlmaier, H.: 48-72 Stunden Konservierung von Hundenieren durch hypotherme, nicht-pul-

sierende Perfusion, Klin. Wochenschr. **50:** 1141, 1972.

8. Grundmann, R., Landes, Th., and Pichlmaier, H.: Hypothermic pulsatile perfusion of dog kidneys: factors limiting successful preservation time, Transplantation **14:** 742, 1972.
9. Grundmann, R., and Pichlmaier, H.: LDH-release in various experimental conditions as criterion for viability of the hypothermic perfused kidney, Res. Exp. Med. **159:** 298, 1973.
10. Grundmann, R., and Pichlmaier, H.: Preservation of canine kidneys wtih hypothermic nonpulsatile perfusion, Arch. Surg. **106:** 301, 1973.
11. Hooker, D. R.: A study of the isolated kidney—the influence of pulse pressure upon renal function, Am. J. Physiol. **27:** 24, 1910.
12. Johnson, R. W. G., Anderson, M., Flear, C. T. G., Murray, S. G. H., Taylor, R. M. R., and Swinney, J.: Evaluation of a new perfusion solution for kidney preservation, Transplantation **13:** 270, 1972.
13. Lokkegaard, H., Gyrd-Hansen, N., Iversen Hansen, R., Hasselager, E., Nerstrom, B., and Rasmussen, F.: Kidney preservation with pulsatile and non-pulsatile hypothermic serum perfusion, Acta Med. Scand. **188:** 245, 1970.
14. Lokkegaard, H., Gyrd-Hansen, N., Iversen Hansen, R., Hasselager, E., Nerstrom, B., and Rasmussen, F.: Further experience with kidney preservation for 24 hours using continuous hypothermic perfusion, Acta Med. Scand. **191:** 191, 1972.
15. Mandelbaum, I., Berry, J., Silbert, M., Burns, W. H., and Rothe, C.: Regional blood flow during pulsatile and nonpulsatile perfusion, Arch. Surg. **91:** 771, 1965.
16. Many, M., Soroff, H. S., Birtwell, W. C., Giron, F., Wise, H., and Deterling, R. A.: The physiologic role of pulsatile and nonpulsatile blood flow. II. Effects on renal function, Arch. Surg. **95:** 762, 1967.
17. Nakayama, K., Tamiya, T., Yamamoto, K., Izumi, T., Akimoto, S., Hashizume, S., Limori, T., Odaka, M., and Yazawa, C.: High-amplitude pulsatile pump in extracorporeal circulation with particular reference to hemodynamics, SURGERY **54:** 789, 1963.
18. Paquet, K. J.: Experimentelle Untersuchungen zur Funktion der isolierten Niere bei pulsatorischer und kontinuierlicher Perfusion, Bruns Beitr. Klin. Chir. **211:** 463, 1965.
19. Ritter, E. R.: Pressure flow relations in the kidney. Alleged effects of pulse pressure, Am. J. Physiol. **168:** 480, 1952.
20. Shephard, R. B., Simpson, D. C., and Sharp, J. F.: Energy equivalent pressure, Arch. Surg. **93:** 730, 1966.
21. Ssentjurin, B. S.: Über die Wirkung von Giften auf die Gefäße des isolierten Ohrs bei konstantem und pulsierendem Flüssigkeitsstrom, Pflügers Arch. Physiol. **215:** 683, 1927.
22. Sterling, W. A., Pierce, J. C., Lee, H. M., Hume, D. M., Hutcher, N. E., and Mendez-Picon, G.: Renal preservation by hypothermic storage plus pulsatile perfusion, Surg. Gynecol. Obstet. **135:** 589, 1972.
23. Woods, J. E.: Successful three- to seven-day preservation of canine kidneys. Immediate life-sustaining function, Arch. Surg. **102:** 614, 1971.

Microvascular anastomosis: A device for holding stay sutures and a new vascular clamp

R. D. Acland, F.R.C.S., *Bearsden, Glasgow, Scotland*

This paper describes an instrument for holding the stay sutures of a microvascular anastomosis. In this instrument, the position of the stay sutures in relation to the vessel is unalterable, so that unwanted movements are eliminated. A new microvascular clamp is also described.

From the Regional Plastic Surgery Centre, Canniesburn Hospital, Bearsden, Glasgow, Scotland

STAY SUTURES are a valuable aid in microvascular anastomosis. They stretch out the vessel edges, display the lumen, and enable the surgeon to judge exactly the position of all the remaining sutures. In spite of their value, stay sutures are a potent source of trouble throughout the procedure. They take up space where space is limited. Their tension must be precisely judged and constantly maintained. At any point, the slightest accidental tugging on a stay suture can tear it out and ruin the anastomosis. Whenever the vessel is turned over, the stay sutures must be turned over with it, one going above, and one beneath.

Previous workers have described varying ways of handling stay sutures. They can be handed to an assistant to hold.[2, 4] They can be attached to weights which are hung over the edge of the wound,[1] or they can be fastened to fixed points at the edge of the operative field. These methods all carry a grave danger of sudden unwanted movement. They are all cumbersome, especially when the vessel has to be turned over.

To overcome these problems, the author has developed a simple device for holding stay sutures; this device is incorporated as an integral part of his double anastomotic clamp (Fig. 1).* The stay sutures are held by two minute "cleats," made of fine wire. These work on the principle of the nautical cleat: the thread is wound round and becomes jammed fast in a narrow tapering gap. The cleats are on opposite sides of a square frame of steel wire, and the two clamps are fixed to this frame.

In use, the vessel ends are first brought together and held, one in each clamp. The first suture is put in and tied. One of its ends is left long and is wound round one of the cleats and gently pulled to fasten it. The second suture is put in one third of the circumference distant from the first, as described by Cobbett.[3] The long end of the second suture is fastened to the other cleat, under just enough tension to "spread" the anastomosis slightly (Fig. 2). The stay sutures are thus firmly fixed and can be moved only if they are deliberately unwound from their cleats. The position of the stay sutures in relation to the vessel is unalterable (Fig. 3). When the instrument moves, the stay sutures

Accepted for publication Sept. 7, 1973.

*This instrument is available from: Spingler-Tritt Chirurgische Nadeln, 7893 Jestetten/BRD, West Germany.

Fig. 1

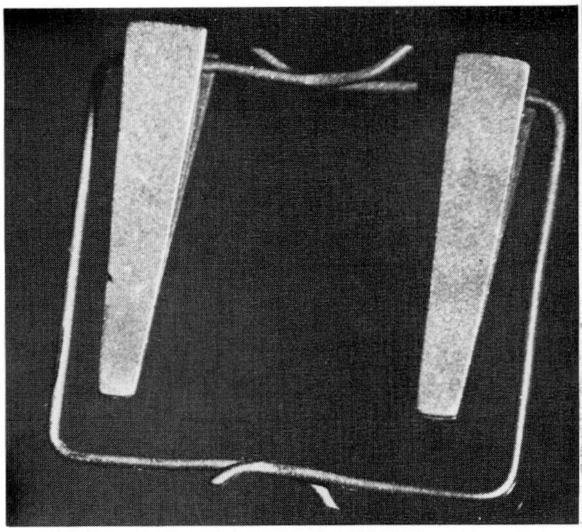

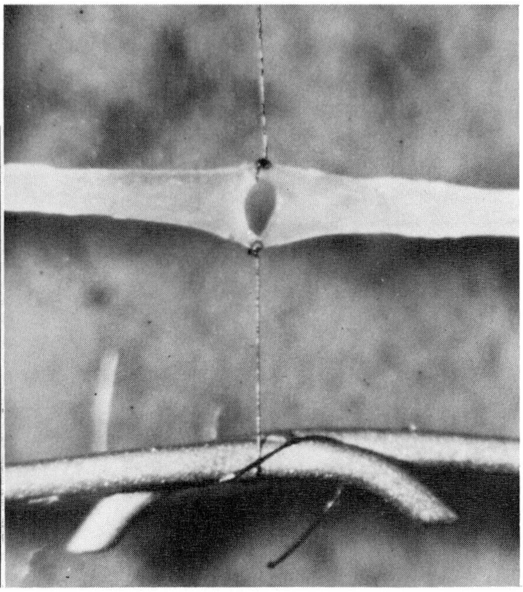

Fig. 2

Fig. 1. Double clamp, incorporating two crossed-wire "cleats" to hold stay sutures.

Fig. 2. Anastomosis of a 0.5 mm. artery in progress, showing one of the cleats and the way in which the stay sutures are held.

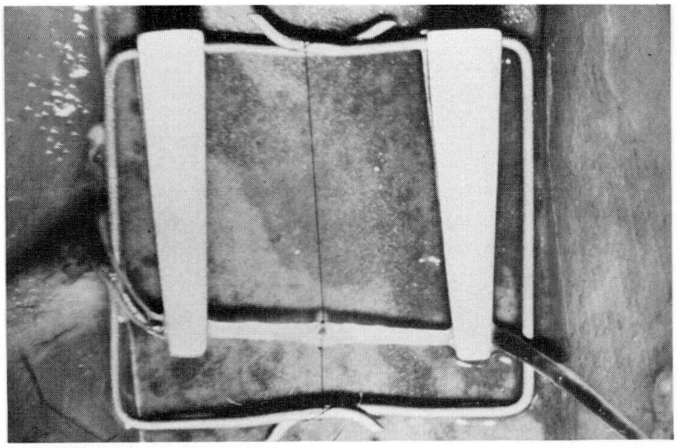

Fig. 3. The instrument lies free in the wound. It can be moved about and turned over, without any change in tension of the stay sutures.

move with it. The instrument is turned over in a single movement, and the stay sutures go over with it automatically, without a change in tension and without risk of accidental pulling.

The instrument is 1 by 1 cm. in over-all size and weighs 120 mg. A larger version is also made.

NEW MICROVASCULAR CLAMP

The clamps of this instrument are also made singly. They are of a new design. Most of the microvascular clamps available have been developed as permanently occluding clips for cerebral aneurysms. As temporary occluders of fine vessels, they have several faults. All exert an unnecessary amount of pressure. Most are bulky and heavy and tend to fall about in the wound. Many have pronounced teeth, which are likely to produce intimal shearing in fine vessels, with an increased risk of thrombus formation. Several types require an unwieldy applying instrument.

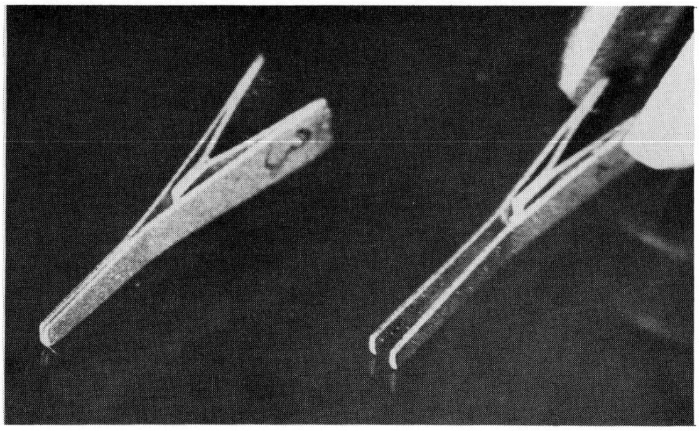

Fig. 4. Single vascular clamps, 8 mm. in over-all length.

The clamp devised by the author is light and compact (Fig. 4). The over-all length is 8 mm. It has a closing force which is the measured minimum needed to keep a vessel closed against an arterial pressure of 200 mm. Hg. The jaws of the clamp are treated by grit-blasting in order to produce a fine roughening. This gives enough grip to prevent displacement of the clamp. The outer faces are similarly treated to eliminate glare. The clamp is applied with a simple flat-jawed forceps. The hingeless welded spring design provides parallel opening of the jaws.

I am very much indebted to Mr. Ardelle Glaze of Fort Wayne Metals Research Products Corporation for his advice and to Messrs. Spingler and Tritt for their cooperation in developing these instruments.

REFERENCES

1. Buncke, H. J., and Schulz, W. P.: The suture repair of one millimetre vessels, *in* Donaghy, R. M. P., and Yasargil, M. G., editors: Microvascular surgery, The C. V. Mosby Company, St. Louis, Mo., 1967, pp. 24-35.
2. Chase, M. D., and Schwarz, S. I.: Suture anastomosis of small arteries, Surg. Gynecol. Obstet. **117:** 44, 1963.
3. Cobbett, J. R.: Small vessel anastomosis, Br. J. Plast. Surg. **20:** 16, 1967.
4. O'Brien, B. McC., Henderson, P. N., Bennett, R. C., and Crock, G. W.: Microvascular surgical technique, Med. J. Aust. **1:** 722, 1970.

Treatment and prevention of acute hepatic encephalopathy by intravenous levodopa

O. Abramsky, M.D., *and* **Z. Goldschmidt, M.D.,** *Jerusalem, Israel*

The results of the treatment and the possible prevention of acute hepatic encephalopathy by the intravenous administration of levodopa to cirrhotic patients with gastrointestinal bleeding are described. In all four patients there was a striking improvement of the comatose state together with a reversion to normal of the previously abnormal electroencephalogram within several hours. The improvement of hepatic coma by the administration of levodopa and other clinical and experimental evidence suggest that there may be a disturbed dopaminergic transmission in this condition.

From the Department of Neurology and Department of General Surgery A, Hadassah University Hospital and Hebrew University Hadassah Medical School, Jerusalem, Israel

THE PATHOGENESIS of the metabolic disorder responsible for the coma of acute hepatic failure remains obscure. Three clinical factors are involved in this condition: a portal systemic shunt, either surgical or spontaneous, hepatocellular failure, and increased nitrogen intake resulting from either increased dietary protein, ammonium salt, or gastrointestinal bleeding. As a result of the failure of the liver to detoxify nitrogenous substances of intestinal origin, blood ammonia levels are generally elevated and may be reflected in the state of cerebral function. This encephalopathy of liver failure may be related to disordered neurotransmission at the synapses in the brain as a result of changes in the production, accumulation, and balance of neurochemical transmitters. The arousal reaction in the electroencephalogram (EEG)[7, 17] and the improvement of hepatic coma with levodopa[9, 10, 14, 16] suggest that dopaminergic transmission is disturbed in this condition.

Accepted for publication Sept. 11, 1973.

The aim of this paper is to describe the results of the treatment and the possible prevention of acute hepatic encephalopathy by the intravenous administration of levodopa to patients with liver failure and gastrointestinal bleeding.

PATIENTS AND RESULTS

Case 1. Z. M., a 65-year-old woman, was admitted to the hospital with a seven-year history of liver cirrhosis. In the last two years, she had had six episodes of confusional states. On this occasion she was admitted because of severe upper gastrointestinal bleeding which began three days prior to admission. Examination revealed a thin, jaundiced, well-oriented female. Blood pressure was 95/70, and pulse rate was 120 beats per minute. A systolic blowing murmur, Grade 4/6, was heard at the base of the heart, the liver palpable 3 cm. and spleen 2 cm. Laboratory findings on admission: normal serum electrolytes and gases; blood pH, 7.37; hemoglobin, 8.3 Gm. percent; hematocrit, 25 percent; blood urea nitrogen (BUN), 48 mg. percent, bilirubin, 3.5 mg. percent, serum glutamic oxaloacetic transaminase (SGOT), 150 I.U.; serum albumin, 3.1 Gm. percent; globulin, 4.7 Gm. percent; prothrombin time, 50 percent; arterial blood ammonia, 60

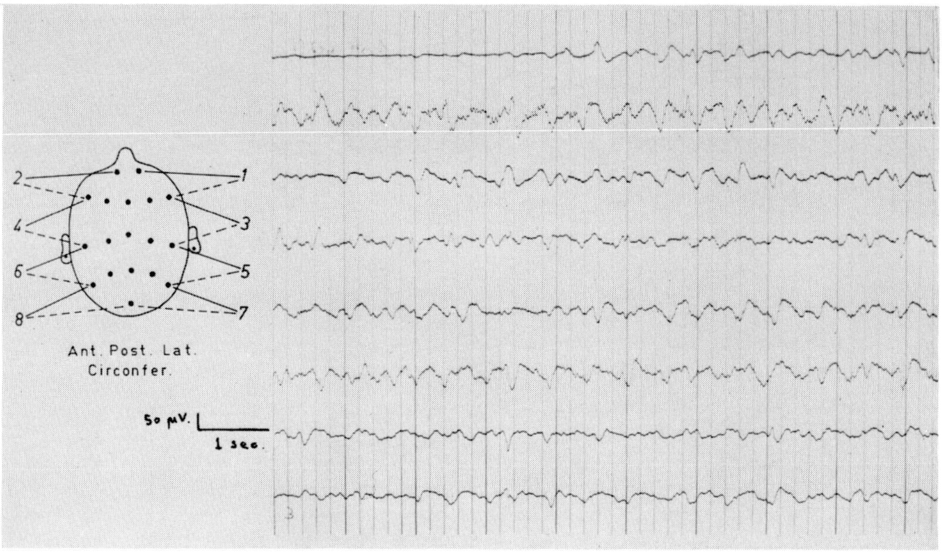

Fig. 1. Case 1. EEG of hepatic encephalopathy in the acute comatose state before levodopa treatment. There are diffused, poorly formed, synchronous and asynchronous low- to moderate-amplitude slow delta waves (2 to 3 cps). Some typical sharp ("triphasic") waves are presented in frontal and temporal areas.

mEq. per liter. X-ray study of the upper gastrointestinal tract revealed a duodenal ulcer without esophageal varices.

The patient was treated by blood transfusion, fluid infusion, and gastric drainage. After a few hours, the patient became stuporous with flapping tremor, fetor hepaticus, and urinary incontinence. The EEG recording showed a severe disturbance with a slow activity typical to the comatose state of acute hepatic encephalopathy (Fig. 1). Levodopa (0.1 in 0.9 percent saline solution) was administered intravenously in a dose of 600 mg. a day.* Thirty minutes after onset of therapy the EEG improved, and it became normal in one hour (Fig. 2). After two hours, the patient aroused from her stupor, was mildly confused for another four hours, and then returned to her previous normal mental state. Laboratory examinations during this period revealed raised levels of bilirubin and SGOT, 8.4 mg. percent and 250 I. U., respectively, without change of the electrolytes, blood gases, pH, and ammonia.

The levodopa infusion was continued for a period of five days, together with neomycin enemata. The patient remained in normal mental state and was discharged after ten days with recommendation for neomycin 4 Gm. taken orally, per day.

Case 2. M. H., a 52-year-old man, was admitted to the hospital because of severe fatigue, generalized wasting, and abdominal distention. Physical examination revealed a thin, conscious, plethoric man with mild jaundice, wasted musculature, ascites, hepatosplenomegaly, and distended veins of the anterior abdominal wall. The main laboratory findings were: hemoglobin, 21 Gm. percent; hematocrit, 60 percent, red blood cell (RBC) mass, 83 ml. per kilogram; total proteins, 6.2 Gm. percent; albumin, 2.1 Gm. percent; bilirubin, 4.0 mg. percent, vitamin B_{12}, 2,000 pg. per milliliter; SGOT, 250 I.U.; serum glutamic pyruvic transaminase (SGPT), 16 I.U. The clotting mechanism was normal. The levels of BUN, blood sugar, electrolytes, blood gases, and pH were normal. The ECG revealed a healed anterior wall infarct. The patient was diagnosed as having polycythemia vera causing hepatic vein thrombosis with a full-blown picture of Budd-Chiari syndrome. Liver biopsy showed centrolobular fibrosis compatible with hepatic vein thrombosis.

On the seventh day of hospitalization, the patient suddenly had a voluminous hematemesis followed by hypovolemic shock with a blood pressure of 70/40. A Blakemore tube was introduced and neomycin washings begun through the tube. After several hours the bleeding stopped, and hemodynamics stabilized. Laboratory examinations after blood replacement revealed: hemoglobin, 16.6 Gm. percent; hematocrit, 52 percent; normal clotting and bleeding times. Blood sugar, electrolytes,

*For intravenous use, levodopa was given 1 mg. per milliliter (0.1 percent) in 0.9 percent saline solution. The maximal concentration we obtained was 0.5 percent levodopa solution in 0.9 percent saline, but this solution was not adjusted to isotonicity (the maximal theoretical solubility of levodopa in water is 0.66 percent). We have not used the Ro 5-4759/B-4, ampules of 25 mg. levodopa (0.5 percent in 5 ml.).

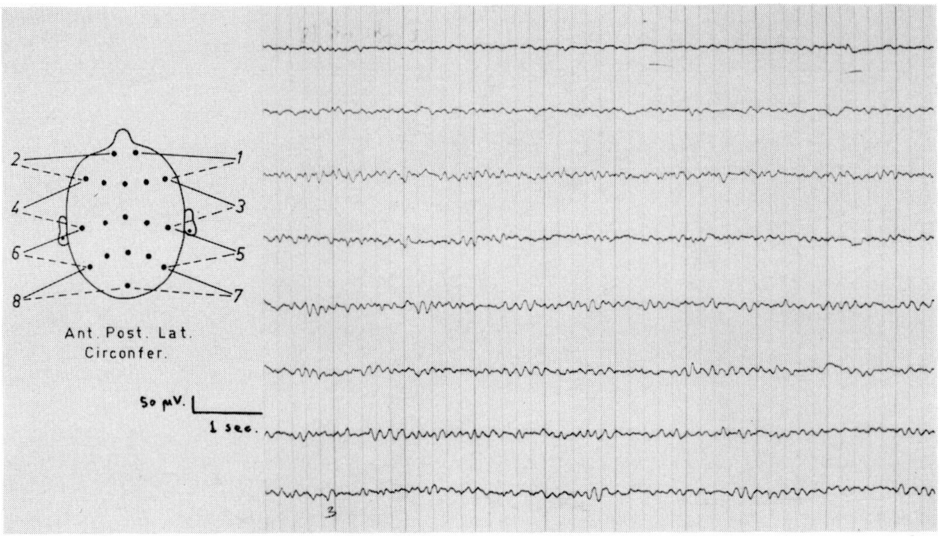

Fig. 2. Case 1. Normal EEG one hour after the beginning of levodopa treatment. There is a well-developed alpha rhythm (8 cps) posteriorly; alpha activity, mixed with minimal beta activity (more than 15 cps), is also presented anteriorly.

gases, and pH levels remained normal. Total bilirubin raised to 7.2 mg. percent; direct bilirubin was 1.8 mg. percent. The SGOT was 250 I.U., alkaline phosphatase was 240 U., calcium was 8.2 mg. percent, phosphorus was 3.0 mg. percent, magnesium was 2.0 mg. percent, uric acid was 6.4 mg. percent, and arterial ammonia was 80 mEq. per liter. On the following day, the patient became confused and rapidly sank into a profound coma. The EEG recording correlated with the comatose state and showed severe disturbances with a slow background activity. Levodopa (0.1 percent in 0.9 percent saline solution) was administered intravenously in dose of 600 Gm. a day.* Three hours after beginning this treatment the EEG reverted almost to normal and after five hours the patient aroused from coma. He was restless and remained confused for another 24 hours, but following this episode, he returned to his normal mental state. The values of main laboratory findings, including that of blood ammonia, were at this time without a significant change from those of the laboratory findings before and during the comatose state.

The levodopa infusion continued for three days, together with enemas of neomycin and intravenous infusions of arginine (25 Gm. a day), potassium, and albumin and lasix in order to alleviate the ascites. After another two weeks, the patient was discharged with recommendation for lasix and low-protein diet.

Case 3. E. A., a 55-year-old woman, was admitted to the hospital with a four-year history of progressive fatigue, weight loss, huge hepatosplenomegaly, ascites, and peripheral pitting edema. A diagnosis of liver cirrhosis with portal hypertension and esophageal varices had been established. One year previously she had had an episode of severe upper gastrointestinal tract bleeding, and after a period of preparation a side-to-side portacaval shunt was successfully performed. Two weeks after the operation, she developed behavioral disturbances which progressed toward severe confusion, disorientation, and finally coma. Laboratory findings then revealed: bilirubin, 7 mg. percent; total protein, 7.5 Gm. percent; albumin, 2.9 Gm. percent, normal SGOT, vitamin B_{12}, 1,100 pg. per milliliter; ammonia in arterial and venous blood, 75 and 55 mEq. per liter, respectively. She was treated with intravenous fluids and albumin, diuretic agents, and neomycin. Gradually over a period of seven days, she came out of her coma and slowly improved.

Two months later the patient was readmitted with signs of melena and acute hepatic encephalopathy with the same clinical picture of confusion progressing to coma. The laboratory findings were almost the same as in the previous episode, except for arterial and venous levels of ammonia which were 160 and 100 mEq. per liter, respectively. The EEG recording, showing high voltage paroxysmal slow activity with bilateral synchronous delta waves, was typical to hepatic coma. Levodopa (0.1 percent in 0.9 percent saline solution) was intravenously administered in a dose of 1,200 mg. per day.* One hour after the beginning of

*See explanatory footnote on p. 189.

*See explanatory footnote on p. 189.

treatment the EEG was normal, and after three hours, the patient emerged from her coma and became rapidly oriented to her surroundings. Blood ammonia remained on the same level.

Levodopa infusion was administered for another three days, together with neomycin, to be taken orally, aldactone, lasix, and a low-protein diet. The patient remained in normal mental state and was discharged from the hospital after ten days.

Case 4. T. S., a 30-year-old man, was diagnosed a year before the present admission as having liver cirrhosis and portal hypertension caused by a congenital persistent obstructive membrane of the inferior vena cava. After a trial to perform caval membranectomy failed, a shunt of the splenic vein to the right atrium was accomplished with the use of a free venous graft.[8] During the postoperative course following the first operation, the patient had two episodes of hepatic coma which followed massive hemorrhages from esophageal varices. These episodes of coma responded very slowly to treatment with neomycin, arginine, fluids, and diuretic agents.

Six months after operation, the patient had a repeat massive gastrointestinal tract hemorrhage. The bleeding was controlled by the introduction of a Blakemore tube. Five pints of blood and fluids were required to restore a stable hemodynamic state. Twenty-four hours later the patient gradually sank into coma. Laboratory findings showed: normal electrolytes and blood gases; normal calcium and phosphorus; pH, 7.42; total bilirubin, 19 mg. percent; direct bilirubin, 6.2 mg. percent; serum albumin, 2.3 Gm. percent; SGOT, above 2,500 I.U.; alkaline phosphatase, 150 U.; vitamin B_{12}, 3,000 pg. per milliliter; prothrombin time, 38 percent, BUN, 45 mg. percent, uric acid, 9.5 mg. percent, arterial blood ammonia, 120 mEq. per liter. The EEG recording showed slow activity correlated with the comatose state. Levodopa (0.1 percent in 0.9 percent saline solution) was administered intravenously in a dose of 1,000 mg. per day.* Two hours after the beginning of levodopa treatment, the EEG was almost normal. Four hours after the onset of treatment, the patient recovered from coma, became irritable, and after twelve hours was in his normal mental state, while all the laboratory findings, including ammonia, still remained severely disturbed.

After the patient became lucid he was treated with levodopa infusions and enemas of neomycin for five days. Blood ammonia and BUN levels gradually became normal, while bilirubin and SGOT levels remained abnormal (3.1 mg. percent and 150 I.U., respectively).

Half a year later, the patient was readmitted because of massive hematemesis with hemoglobin of 10 Gm. percent. Bleeding was controlled with a Blakemore tube. Since following each previous event of massive gastrointestinal bleeding, this patient had developed hepatic encephalopathy, he was given 1,000 mg. levodopa intravenously in addition to blood and fluids in order to stabilize his hemodynamic state. Although on this occasion nine pints of blood were required in order to maintain the hemodynamic state, he developed no confusional signs. Liver functions remained stable: bilirubin, 2.9 mg. percent; albumin, 2.5 mg. percent; SGOT, 165 I.U.; prothrombin time, 60 percent; arterial blood ammonia, 55 mEq. per liter. After stopping the intravenous treatment, we continued with the oral administration of levodopa (3 Gm. a day), and the patient was sent home with this treatment for another two weeks.

*See explanatory footnote on p. 189.

DISCUSSION

In 1963, Tsukiyama and associates[17] showed that dopa causes an arousal reaction in the EEG of patients with hepatic coma. Noting their observations, Parkes and coworkers[10] gave 5 Gm. of levodopa orally to five patients in stupor or coma caused by acute hepatic failure; in three patients the drug produced temporary improvement with striking improvement in the previously abnormal EEG. Fisher and James[2, 9] administered 3 Gm. of levodopa by way of a nasogastric tube to eight comatose patients with alcoholic cirrhosis; four patients awakened from coma within three to four hours. Sarrazin and colleagues[14] and Stefanini and associates[16] reported similar results. The levodopa administration in all these investigations was carried out orally and this represents a severe limitation in the therapy in patients after operation or with gastrointestinal bleeding.

Noting previous observations[4, 13] made in instances in which levodopa was given intravenously in Parkinsonism, its intravenous use was attempted in cirrhotic patients with stupor or coma resulting from gastrointestinal bleeding. Levodopa, 0.1% in 0.9% saline solution, was administered intravenously in four patients in doses of 600 to 1,200 mg. a day,* with striking and rapid improvement of the comatose state. Within two to five hours the patients had recovered their nor-

*See explanatory footnote on p. 189.

mal mental state. In one of these patients in the presence of a recurrent episode of massive gastrointestinal bleeding, the expected encephalopathy could be prevented by giving prophylactic intravenous levodopa. In all of these cases improvement was not temporary, where treatment was continued for three to five days. In all four patients, there was a striking improvement in the EEG 30 minutes after the onset of therapy, with a reversion to normal or almost normal in one to three hours (Figs. 1 and 2). Although the depth of coma and the EEG changes may indeed fluctuate in acute hepatic coma, it is most unlikely that the rapid clinical and EEG improvement described in these small series was spontaneous, particularly since neurological improvement occurred in the presence of a deteriorating general condition. There was no correlation between the improvement in the EEG and in the mental state and between the blood ammonia levels. Here, as shown by Silverman,[15] high blood ammonia levels were not inconsistent with a normal EEG.

The improvement of hepatic coma by the administration of levodopa, the precursor of both norepinephrine and dopamine, suggests that there may be a defect in cerebral neurochemical transmission in this condition. Some clinical and experimental evidences for this hypothesis have been noted by several investigators. The catecholamines (norepinephrine, and dopamine) play an important role in the regulation of normal synaptic transmission in the brain,[5] and disturbances in consciousness and brain functions may be a result of disturbances in these transmitters. Levodopa can produce an arousal reaction in the EEG of animals[7] and reduction in dopamine synthesis, induced in man by alpha-methyl-p-tyrosine, results in deep drowsiness.[6] Certain neurological manifestations occasionally seen in chronic hepatic encephalopathy (namely, akinesia, rigidity, and tremor) are also common to Parkinson's disease, in which dopamine depletion in the striatum and substantia nigra is proved.[1] The possibility of disturbed dopaminergic transmission in hepatic encephalopathy may be inferred from the fact that improvement of this condition is achieved only with levodopa and not with adrenaline, noradrenaline, 5-hydroxytryptophan, or drugs affecting cholinergic transmission.[10]

The encephalopathy as well as some of the cardiovascular and renal complications of hepatic insufficiency may be the results of disordered neurotransmission at synapses in the central and peripheral nervous system. They may be related to decreased production of normal neurochemical transmitters, such as epinephrine and dopamine, to the accumulation of false adrenergic neurochemical transmitters such as octapamine, and to altered ratio between normal and false transmitters. False transmitters are usually catabolized by the liver. But, when hepatic function is impaired and blood is shunted away from the liver, these amines accumulate and may replace normal endogenous transmitters by competition and result in a generalized derangement of cerebral function. Octapamine appears to increase in the brain as the severity of coma increases.[2, 3] The precursor of octapamine is tyramine which is produced by bacterial amino acid decarboxylase in the gut. Levels of ammonia, S-adenosylumethionine in the brain, and methionine in the blood may also be elevated during liver failure.[11]

Levodopa is the precursor of the normal transmitters norepinephrine and dopamine. According to Fischer and James,[2, 3, 9] when given in hepatic coma, levodopa is flooded into the system, shifting the equilibrium. The existing imbalance between normal and false transmitters is thus quickly reversed and the coma improves. Another possibility is that levodopa reduces the raised brain level of S-adenosylmethionine,[10] for it has been shown that levodopa can combine with S-adenosylmethionine in the brain and reduce its concentration.[18]

According to Read and associates,[12] if the serial EEG is showing progressive deterioration in a patient prone to develop hepatic encephalopathy (particularly after portacaval anastomosis), this should be an indication for treatment with neomycin and protein restriction. According to the recent investigations showing the value of levodopa in the treatment of acute hepatic encephalopathy, this drug should be administered early whenever coma or neuropsychiatric changes occur or are anticipated in the patients with liver disease.

The authors wish to thank Prof. N. J. Saltz, Head, Department of General Surgery A, and Prof. Z. Eyal from the Department of General Surgery A, for their help and advice.

REFERENCES

1. Engelman, K., Horwitz, D., Jéquier, E., and Sjoerdsma, A.: Biochemical and pharmacologic effects of alpha-methyl tyrosine in man, J. Clin. Invest. **47:** 577, 1968.
2. Fischer, J. E., and James, J. H.: Mechanism of action of L-dopa in hepatic coma, Surg. Forum **123:** 220, 1971.
3. Fischer, J. E., and James, J. H.: Treatment of hepatic coma and hepatorenal syndrome, Am. J. Surg. **123:** 222, 1972.
4. Gerstenbrand, F., Pateisky, K., and Prosenz, P.: Erfahrungen mit L-dopa in der therapie des Parkinsonismus, Psychiatr. Neurol. (Basel) **146:** 246, 1963.
5. Glowinski, J., and Baldessarini, R. J.: Metabolism of norepinephrine in the central nervous system, Pharmacol. Rev. **18:** 1201, 1966.
6. Heuser, G., Buchwald, N. A., and Wyers, E. J.: The "caudate-spindle." II. Facilitatory and inhibitory caudate-cortical pathways, Electroencephalogr. Clin. Neurophysiol. **13:** 519, 1961.
7. Kadzielawa, K., and Widy-Tyszkiewicz, E.: Electroencephalographic analysis of the central effect of dihydroxyphenylalanine, Electroencephalogr. Clin. Neurophysiol. **28:** 259, 1970.
8. Luttwak, E. M., Harousi, I., Licht, A., Fround, H., and Borman, J. B.: Emergency splenic vein–right atrium shunt for massive esophageal hemorrhage with cirrhosis of liver and inferior vena cava occlusion, Ann. Surg. **177:** 411, 1973.
9. Medical News.: Levodopa arouses patients from hepatic coma, J. A. M. A. **218:** 1127, 1971.
10. Parkes, J. D., Sharpstone, P., and Williams, R.: Levodopa in hepatic coma, Lancet **2:** 1341, 1970.
11. Phear, E. A., Rrebner, B., Sherlock, S., et al.: Methionine toxicity in liver disease and its prevention by chlortetracycline, J. Clin. Sci. **15:** 93, 1965.
12. Read, A. E., McCarthy, C. F., Ajdukiewicz, A. B., and Brown, G. J. A.: Encephalopathy after portacaval anastomosis, Lancet **2:** 999, 1968.
13. Roes, B. E., and Steg, G.: The effect of L-3,4-dihydroxyphenylalanine and dL-5-hydroxytryptophan on rigidity and tremor induced by reserpine and chlorpromazine, Life Sci. **3:** 351, 1964.
14. Sarrazin, A., Emerit, J., Oliver, L., Rebelo, F., and Bousquet, O.: Traitement du come hépatique par la L-dopa, Press Med. **79:** 2226, 1971.
15. Silverman, D.: Some observations on the EEG in hepatic coma, Electroencephalogr. Clin. Neurophysiol. **14:** 53, 1962.
16. Stefanini, M., and Hetherington, E. N.: Levodopa in hepatic failure, J. A. M. A. **220:** 1247, 1972.
17. Tsukiyama, K., Omura, I., Sekihara, T., et al.: Provocation of abnormal EEG by intravenous administration of ammonium chloride in patients with hepatic disease, Med. J. Osaka Univ. **14:** 151, 1963.
18. Wurtman, R. J., Rose, C. M., Mathysse, S., Stephenson, J., and Baldessarini, R.: L-dihydroxyphenylalanine: Effect on S-adenosylmethionine in brain, Science **169:** 395, 1970.

Intravenous infusion of hydrochloric acid for treatment of severe metabolic alkalosis

George M. Abouna, M.D., F.R.C.S.,* Philip R. Veazey, M.D., *and*
Daniel B. Terry, Jr., M.D., *Augusta, Ga.*

The acid-base balance of eight patients with severe metabolic alkalosis who failed to respond to treatment with potassium and sodium chloride infusion was successfully restored to normal by the intravenous infusion of hydrochloric acid. Prior to HCl administration, ammonium chloride, arginine hydrocholride, hemodialysis, and exchange blood transfusions were also given but had failed to correct the alkalosis. Each patient received from 150 to 1,200 mEq. of acid over a period of six hours to three days. Isotonic or hypertonic HCl solutions were given through a central venous catheter. No serious complications were encountered during this treatment. It is postulated that in cases of severe alkalosis particularly when associated with hypochloremia, direct infusion of hydrogen ion is desirable to neutralize the excess plasma bicarbonate, and sufficient chloride ion must be delivered in order to interrupt the vicious cycle of bicarbonate reabsorption and hydrogen ion secretion by the renal tubules. It is suggested that hydrochloric acid infusion is safe, and it should be administered to patients with hypochloremic alkalosis particularly after failure of conventional treatment.

From the Department of Surgery, Eugene Talmadge Memorial Hospital, and the Medical College of Georgia, Augusta, Ga.

WHILE METABOLIC acidosis has been recognized for many years as a dangerous acid-base complication, its treatment has become a standard and routine procedure which is often extremely effective. Alkalosis, on the other hand, has been recognized only very recently as a clinical problem and although it is less dangerous than acidosis, it has a more complicated etiology and it is much more difficult to treat.[19, 29] It has been recently recognized also that patients with gastric outlet obstruction and patients with cirrhosis and hepatorenal failure often develop severe metabolic and hypochloremic alkalosis which may become refractory to standard therapy.[8, 23, 26]

During the past four years, we have studied eight patients with a variety of complicated clinical problems in whom severe alkalosis persisted despite all conventional measures. These patients were successfully treated and acid-base balance was restored to normal by the intravenous infusion of hydrochloric acid. This paper is a report of our experience with this form of therapy.

PATIENTS AND METHODS

The eight patients studied were aged between 13 and 63 years. Two patients were in hepatic coma resulting from fulminant acute and subacute hepatitis. Two patients had severe hepatorenal failure caused by

Accepted for publication Sept. 14, 1973.

Reprint requests: Dr. George M. Abouna, Department of Surgery, University of Calgary Medical School, Foothills Hospital, Calgary, Alberta, Canada.

cirrhosis. One patient had received an orthotopic liver homograft for hepatorenal failure, and another patient developed sepsis and intestinal obstruction after bilateral pretransplant nephrectomy. The seventh patient developed peritonitis, gastric bleeding, and intestinal obstruction, while the eighth patient developed bowel fistula, ileus, and gastrointestinal hemorrhage following severe gunshot wounds of the abdomen (Table I).

When severe metabolic alkalosis developed treatment was first begun along conventional lines by infusion of sodium and potassium chloride solutions according to the estimated water and electrolyte deficit. In addition, intravenous arginine hydrochloride was given to two patients, ammonium chloride to two others, and exchange blood transfusion with heparinized fresh whole blood to three, and hemodialysis was the form of treatment for one patient. Intravenous hydrochloric acid was given only when all these measures had failed to correct the alkalosis. Blood gas analysis, pH, Po_2, Pco_2, plasma bicarbonate, and base excess were carried out at least once daily and at four-hour intervals during hydrochloric acid infusion. Plasma electrolytes, blood urea nitrogen, a full blood count, and in some cases urinary electrolytes were measured at these intervals with the use of standard laboratory techniques. Before hydrochloric acid treatment, the patients had blood pH of 7.58 to 7.71, plasma bicarbonate of 33 to 44 mEq. per liter and base excess of +8 to +18 mEq. per liter. Four patients had severe hypochloremia with plasma chloride concentration of 65 to 88 mEq. per liter.

The quantity and rate of hydrochloric acid administration was calculated from the estimated chloride and/or hydrogen ion deficit. The chloride deficit was calculated from the plasma chloride concentration and the chloride space (80 percent of the sodium space or 20 percent of body weight). The hydrogen ion deficit was calculated from the plasma base excess and the hydrogen ion space (total body water or 60 percent of body weight). An attempt was made to provide 100 percent replacement of the chloride deficit and 50 percent replacement of the hydrogen ion deficit during each 12 hour period of hydrochlric acid infusion. The rate of infusion was adjusted according to the patient's clinical status, usually over 12 to 24 hours. Hydrochloric acid was usually given as an isotonic solution containing 150 ml. of one normal HCl or 300 mEq. of H^+ and Cl^- in one liter of sterile water. In some cases hypertonic solution containing 200 ml. of normal HCl or 400 mEq. of H^+ and Cl^- per liter was used. Acid infusion was done through a central venous catheter. In addition to HCl infusion, daily requirements of fluid, sodium, and potassium were also given to each patient.

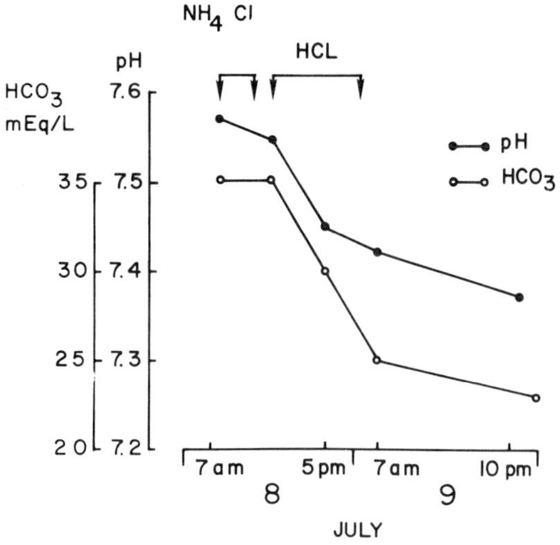

Fig. 1. Restoration of normal acid-base balance by hydrochloric acid infusion in Patient 6 (R. M.). Note that administration of ammonium chloride failed to correct the metabolic-hypochloremic alkalosis in this patient. Following infusion of 150 mEq. of intravenous hydrochloric acid, plasma bicarbonate and blood pH were returned to normal levels within 12 hours. Some overcorrection with drift of pH to 7.37 and base excess to −1.2 was noted a few hours later.

CASE REPORTS

Detailed case histories of four of these patients are given below.

Case 4. A 48-year-old Caucasian man was admitted to the Medical College of Virginia in October, 1970, with hepatic failure resulting from posthepatic cirrhosis and unsuspected hepatoma. He was evaluated and prepared for liver transplantation. After successful orthotopic liver

Table I. *Clinical and biochemncal data on the eight patients treated by intravenous HCl for severe*

Patient No.	Age (yr.)	Clinical state	Degree of alkalosis: pH	HCO₃	Base excess
1	(M. B.) 22	Hepatorenal failure; Ileus, nasogastric suction	(1) 7.62 (2) 7.71	42 44	+12 +16
2	(D. J.) 13	Fulminant hepatic coma; gastrointestinal bleeding; nasogastric suction	7.6	36	+ 8
3	(K. J.) 23	Chronic active hepatitis; coma, ileus, nasogastric suction	7.58	35	+ 9
4	(G. W.) 48	Orthotopic liver transplantation	7.63	40	+17
5	(L. G.) 32	Hepatorenal failure, terminal cirrhosis, pneumonia	7.62	33	+10
6	(R. M.) 15	Anephric intestinal obstruction; nasogastric suction	7.57	35	+11
7	(L. M.) 63	Biliary obstruction and cirrhosis choledochostomy; bleeding duodenal ulcer—pyloroplasty; intestinal obstruction; gastrojejunostomy; gastrostomy	(1) 7.63 (2) 7.62	44 36	+18 +13
8	(S. W.) 19	Multiple abdominal trauma; bowel fistula; bleeding stress ulcer; gastrostomy; nasogastric suction; tracheostomy; sepsis	(1) 7.58 (2) 7.62	40 36	+16 +13

*Note that these patients had failed to respond to treatment with NaCl, KCl, arginine, and ammonium chloride.

Table II. *Blood gas analysis and serum electrolyte in Patient 4 (G. W.) before and after treatment with hydrochloric acid**

	November 5	6	7
Blood gas analysis:			
pH	7.63	7.59	7.45
P_{CO_2}	39	50	36
HCO_3	40	38	27
Base excess	+17	+15	+1
Serum electrolytes:			
Cl	85	86	97
K	4.5	3.8	3.7
Na	143	140	134
BUN	32	31	34
Treatment:			
NaCl (mEq./day)	185	185	
KCl (mEq./day)	80	100	
Arginine (Gm.)	25	—	
HCl (mEq./day)	—	400	

*Note rapid correction of the alkalosis and the hypo- with intravenous infusion of 150 mEq. of acid.

transplantation on Nov. 5, 1970, he became very alkalotic with a pH of 7.63, a P_{CO_2} value of 39; a plasma bicarbonate value of 40; and a base excess of +17 mEq. per liter. In addition he developed postoperative ileus and was having moderately large volumes of nasogastric tube drainage. His serum electrolyte level showed moderate hypochloremia, but with normal potassium and sodium (Table II). Treatment was begun with infusion of sodium and potassium chloride to which arginine (25 mg., intravenous) was later added. However, there was very little response after 12 hours of this treatment, and the P_{CO_2} increased. Hypertonic hydrochloric acid (400 mEq. per liter) was infused slowly during the next 24 hours. During this treatment, the blood pH gradually returned to normal, base excess was reduced to +1, and the hypochloremia was corrected. He made satisfactory postoperative recovery and was discharged three months after transplantation with normal liver and renal function. Details of his clinical course are reported elsewhere.[12]

Case 6. A 15-year-old boy was admitted to the Medical College of Georgia, Augusta, in June, 1972, for pretransplant nephrectomy. Since the age of 3, he had had reflux pyelonephritis with renal failure caused by congenital urethral valves and bilateral nephrostomy tube drainage, which had been maintained for the previous 11 years. Following bilateral nephrectomy, he developed sepsis and intestinal obstruction. He was treated with chemotherapy, nasogastric suction, intravenous fluids and hemodialysis, but he developed severe hypochloremic alkalosis which could not be corrected by infusion of sodium chloride, potassium chloride, or dialysis. A slow intravenous infusion of 50 mEq. of ammonium chloride over a period of six hours caused drowsiness, tachycardia, and hypotension, and there was no improvement in alkalosis (Table III). Hydrochloric acid infusion was therefore started at a concentration of 300 mEq. per liter. He was given 500 ml. of this solution over a period of 12 hours. At the end of this time, the pH gradually fell to 7.37, the *metabolic alkalosis**

Serum electrolyte: Cl	K	Na	BUN	Previous treatment given
97	3.6	150	50	KCl, exchange transfusion
87	4.7	139	70	NaCl, KCl, arginine
88	3.8	145	10	NaCl, KCl, Exchange transfusion
90	4.0	150	19	NaCl, KCl, Exchange transfusion
85	4.5	143	32	NaCl, KCl, arginine
90	4.3	137	27	NaCl, KCl, dialysis
65	3.4	143	82	NaCl, KCl, NH_4Cl
75	4.7	150	72	NaCl, KCl, NH_4Cl
91	4.2	139	54	NaCl, KCl
91	4.4	143	45	NaCl, KCl
98	4.6	145	51	NaCl, KCl

plasma bicarbonate to 23, the base excess to –1.2, and serum chloride rose to 88 mEq. per liter (Fig. 1). During the next few days, the obstruction and sepsis gradually resolved, and he was eventually discharged. He has since received a successful renal allograft from his mother.

Case 7. A 63-year-old Caucasian man was admitted to the Medical College of Georgia in May, 1972, with a one-year history of obstructive jaundice and biliary cirrhosis. Percutaneous transhepatic cholangiogram demonstrated biliary calculi and common duct obstruction. After a preliminary choledochostomy, he underwent choledocholithotomy, cholecystectomy, and a feeding-gastrostomy. In the postoperative period, hepatorenal failure, ileus, and large gastric and biliary drainage developed and gave rise to severe hypochloremic metabolic alkalosis (Table IV). Treatment with 6 to 8 L. of sodium chloride and 140 to 230 mEq. of potassium per 24 hours, while maintaining normal serum potassium, failed to correct the hypochloremic metabolic alkalosis. Ammonium chloride infusion was then given but caused respiratory depression, hypoxia, and drowsiness.Intravenous hydrochloric acid infusion was thereforefore started at a rate of 300 mEq. per day for three days. Following this, the alkalosis and hypochloremia were gradually corrected (Fig. 2). He remained well for the next eight days, when sudden and severe hemorrhage insued from a large posterior duodenal ulcer. Emergency antrectomy, suture of the ulcer bed, ligation of the gastroduodenal artery and gastrojejunostomy were carried out. During this episode he received over 12 units of ACD (acid citrate dextrose)

Table III. *pH, blood gas analysis, and serum electrolyte in this child with renal failure (Patient 6)**

	July 8, 11 A.M.	July 8, 5 P.M.	July 9, 7 A.M.	July 9, 10 A.M.
Blood gas analysis:				
pH	7.57	7.55	7.45	7.37
P_{CO_2}	44	45	44	39
HCO_3	35	35	30	23
Base excess	+11	+10	+6	-1.2
Serum electrolytes:				
Cl	65	67	75	88
K	3.4	3.3	3.3	3.4
Na	143	144	138	136
BUN	82	83	91	99
Treatment:				
NaCl (mEq.)	50	77		
KCl (mEq.)	20	20		
NH_4Cl (mEq.)	50	—		
HCl (mEq.)	—	150		

*Note the rapid correction of the hypochloremic alkalosis with intravenous infusion of 150 mEq. of acid.

blood and once again he developed hepatorenal failure, ileus, and severe metabolic alkalosis. Treatment with intravenous infusion of hydrochloric acid was repeated and continued slowly over the

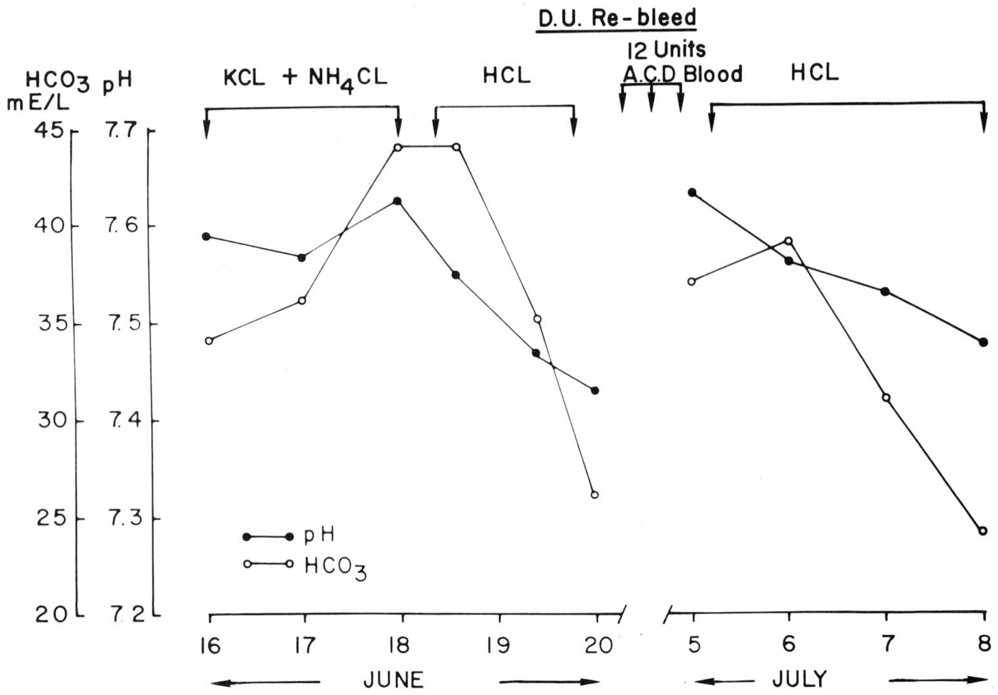

Fig. 2. Changes in blood pH and plasma bicarbonate during HCl infusion in Patient 7 (L. M.). Note how metabolic alkalosis continued despite administration of potassium and ammonium chloride for three days. Correction of acid-base balance was successfully achieved with intravenous HCl. Note also that when alkalosis followed administration of large quantities of ACD blood, this too, was reversed with HCl infusion.

Table IV. *Biochemical data on Patient 7 (L. M.) before and after two episodes of hydrochloric acid therapy**

	June						*July*			
				19						
	16	*17*	*18*	A.M.	P.M.	*20*	*5*	*6*	*7*	*8*
Blood gas analyses:										
pH	7.59	7.57	7.63	7.59	7.47	7.43	7.63	7.56	7.53	7.48
Pco_2	56	42	41	57	49	40	39	42	37	32
HCO_3	34	36	44	44	35	26	36	38	31	24
Base excess	+12	+13	+18	+17	+10	+2	+13	+13	+8	+2
Serum electrolytes:										
Na	144	148	150	147	147	147	139	141	142	135
K	4.4	4.4	4.7	5.3	5.5	6.0	4.2	4.7	5.3	4.0
Cl	88	78	75	80	101	102	91	90	101	96
BUN	72	77	77	80	82	83	54	51	37	30
Treatment:										
NaCl (mEq./day)	200	300	350	300	300	300	—	300	450	300
KCl (mEq./day)	140	230	200	120	100	100	110	260	180	340
NH_4Cl (mEq./day)	200	120	240	—	—	—				
HCl (mEq./day)	—	—	—	600	300	100	250	300	300	400

*Note that in the first episode, administration of large quantities of sodium, potassium, and ammonium chloride failed to correct existing hypochloremic metabolic alkalosis. This was completely corrected with 1,000 mEq. of HCl given for three days. In the second episode, severe metabolic alkalosis associated with large transfusion of citrated blood was again corrected with intravenous HCl.

next four days, during which time he received over 1,200 mEq. of acid. As a result, metabolic alkalosis was again corrected (Fig. 2). However, ten days later signs of duodenal stump leak were noted. This became profuse and he died from sepsis and pneumonitis two months after admission.

Case 8. A 19-year-old Caucasian man was referred to the Medical College of Georgia in July, 1972, from another hospital where he had received emergency splenectomy, left nephrectomy, transverse cholostomy, suture of gastric perforation, and tracheostomy for severe gunshot injury to the abdomen. This was complicated with sepsis and multiple abdominal abscesses. On admission to this hospital, emergency drainage of subphrenic and pelvic abscesses and repair of leaking gastrostomy suture line were carried out. On the third postoperative day, he developed ileus, pneumonitis, and severe metabolic alkalosis, and there were large quantities of gastrointestinal fluid drainage from bowel fistula (Table V). He was given 200 mEq. of hydrochloric acid over a period of 12 hours and his alkalosis was successfully controlled. Treatment was continued with chemotherapy, intravenous hyperalimentation, and positive pressure respiration. During the following two weeks, he appeared to be progressing satisfactorily when a sudden and severe hemorrhage developed from a duodenal stress ulcer. In view of the abdominal sepsis, it was elected to treat him with blood transfusion and intra-arterial infusion of vasopressin through an indwelling catheter in the celiac axis. After three days of this treatment and with 14 units of ACD blood all bleeding stopped. However severe metabolic alkalosis recurred (Table V). He was given 400 mEq. of intravenous hydrochloric acid over the next seven hours and the alkalosis was corrected. During the next six weeks, he remained in fluid, electrolyte, and acid-base balance; his clinical condition remarkably improved; his wounds and his fistulas healed; and he appeared to be making satisfactory recovery. Unfortunately, a sudden and catastrophic intratracheal hemorrhage developed as the result of erosion by the tracheotomy tube into the innominate artery. He died in a short time, six weeks after last receiving hydrochloric acid.

Table V. *pH, blood gas analysis and electrolyte in Patient 8 (S. W.)**

	July			
	25		*26*	
	6 A.M.	*3:50* P.M.	*2:30* A.M.	*9* P.M.
Blood gas analyses:				
pH	7.58	7.47	7.62	7.4
Pco_4	42	42	34.5	29
HCO_3	40	30	36	30
Base excess	+16	+5	+13	+4
Serum electrolytes:				
Cl	91	98	98	95
K	4.4	4.7	4.6	4.6
Na	143	142	145	141
BUN	45	42	51	57
Treatment:				
NaCl (mEq./day)	450		180	
K (mEq./day)	160		80	
HCl (mEq./day)	200		400	

*Severe metabolic alkalosis was corrected on two separate occassions with IV hydrochloric acid.

RESULTS

The results of hydrochloric acid infusion in the eight patients studied are shown in Table VI. It is seen that in all patients, acid infusion was effective in correcting the alkalosis and in restoring normal acid-base balance. In most cases, adequate correction was achieved within 24 hours except in Case 7 where treatment had to be continued for two to four days. In three patients, hydrochloric acid therapy had to be repeated for recurrent episodes of metabolic alkalosis.

No serious complications were encountered. There was one minor complication in Case 5; because of leakage around the intravenous catheter in the external jugular vein, a small and superficial area of skin necrosis occurred. This, however, healed spontaneously after discontinuation of hydrochloric acid therapy. In all patients, the hematocrit remained constant during and after treatment, and there was no evidence of hemolysis (Table VI). Examination of the urine which was carried out in some of these patients showed inconsistent results with paradoxical aciduria seen in some of the patients in whom there was a large chloride deficit.

DISCUSSION

There are only a few and scattered reports on the use of hydrochloric acid for the treatment of metabolic alkalosis in man.[3] The study reported in this paper demonstrates the effectiveness and the safety of hydrochloric acid administration as the spe-

Table VI. *Results of treatment of metabolic alkalosis with intravenous hydrochloric acid in eight patients**

Patient No.	pH		Total HCl (mEq.)	Duration of HCl therapy	Hematocrit		Complications
	Before treatment	After treatment			Before treatment	After treatment	
1	7.62	7.47	200	24 hr.	36	34	None
	7.71	7.45	250	20 hr.	41	39	None
2	7.6	7.41	150	12 hr.	38	39	None
3	7.58	7.44	200	16 hr.	41	40	None
4	7.63	7.45	350	36 hr.	42	41	None
5	7.62	7.46	400	24 hr.	33	32	Slight skin necrosis at site of catheter
6	7.55	7.37	150	12 hr.	30	28.5	None
7	7.63	7.43	1,000	2 days	49	46.5	None
	7.62	7.48	1,200	4 days	42	42.4	None
8	7.58	7.47	200	9 hr.	34	38	None
	7.62	7.42	400	16 hr.	33	32	None

*Note rapid restoration of acid-base balance in each case with 150 to 1,200 mEq. of HCl and no serious complications were seen in these patients. Note that there was no fall in the hematocrit after HCl therapy, indicating absence of hemolysis.

cific therapy for hypochloremic metabolic alkalosis. We believe that the rationale for the use of this form of therapy is based on sound biochemical and physiological mechanisms. Normally, the concentration of hydrogen ion in the extracellular fluids is maintained within relatively narrow limits by the chemical buffers of the blood, by the lungs, and by the kidneys, in that order. Although most metabolic processes generate excess hydrogen ion, the body is very efficiently geared for the active removal of hydrogen ion and for the retention of bicarbonate.[9, 22] Unfortunately, the mechanisms available for combating alkalosis are much less efficient than those available for combating acidosis and because of this, alkalosis is much more difficult to treat than acidosis.[19, 29]

Metabolic alkalosis is likely to occur under any condition causing excess hydrogen ion secretion or increased bicarbonate reabsorption. In clinical practice, this can occur in any of the following conditions: loss of upper gastrointestinal content; excessive alkali intake; administration of large quantities of citrated blood; hepatic cirrhosis and liver failure[23, 26]; excessive loss of potassium due to diarrhea, diuretic therapy, and ion exchange resins; primary hyperaldosteronisms and Cushing's disease; hypovolemic states, trauma and surgical stress[6, 19, 29]; hypercalcemic states, spontaneous or vitamin D induced[11, 13]; traumatic, hemorrhagic, and septic shock which often cause a mixed respiratory and metabolic alkalosis[19, 20, 29]; and following orthotopic liver transplantation.[1, 2] In the patients reported in this series, more than one of these conditions were present and despite diligent treatment by accepted and conventional methods including the administration of sodium and potassium chloride, alkalosis could not be corrected. One of the factors which makes treatment of metabolic alkalosis difficult is the fact that this form of alkalosis is rarely, if ever, completely compensated for by respiratory mechanisms.[10, 19] Respiratory compensation was almost completely absent in our patients.

The role of potassium deficiency in the genesis of metabolic alkalosis has given rise to much debate and confusion.[24, 28] It is now known[14-16] that while metabolic alkalosis is often accompanied by hypokalemia, potassium deficiency can exist in the presence of normal or even acid pH. Kassirer and coworkers[15] and Schwartz and colleagues[24] have shown that hypochloremic-hypokalemic alkalosis can be corrected by infusion of chloride alone but not by potassium alone, provided that the total body potassium deficit is less than 300 to 400 mEq.

Although alkalosis is less dangerous than

acidosis, severe hydrogen ion deficit with a pH greater than 7.55 has been shown to be harmful and even dangerous.[7, 18] In a recent study by Wilson and colleagues[29] involving 177 severely alkalotic surgical patients, a significant correlation was present between mortality and degree of alkalosis. Thus, with a pH of 7.54 to 7.56, there was a death rate of 40 percent while at pH 7.65 to 7.7 the mortality rate rose to 80 percent.[29]

The treatment of alkalosis depends, of course, on removing the cause. However, this is often difficult and treatment must begin by appropriate correction and replacement. When alkalosis is mild, correction can usually be achieved by infusion of sodium and potassium chloride within the limits of the patient's fluid intake and urinary output. However, in patients with uremia or hepatorenal failure, infusion of large volumes of sodium and potassium salts may be extremely dangerous. Also, when alkalosis is severe or when the chloride deficit is very marked, such as following large upper gastrointestinal fluid loss, correction with sodium and potassium chloride may prove very difficult. Arginine hydrochloride and ammonium chloride have been used by several investigators, but these may be dangerous in patients with hepatic or renal failure.

In conclusion, we believe that severe metabolic alkalosis which is refractory to conventional therapy should be treated by hydrochloric acid infusion until the acid-base balance is corrected. The infusion should be given over a period of 6 to 24 hours and during therapy, repeated measurements of pH, blood gas analysis, plasma electrolyte, and blood urea nitrogen should be carried out at four- to six-hour intervals. The acid should be preferably given in an isotonic solution which is prepared by adding 150 ml. of 1 normal HCl to one liter of sterile water. In most cases, alkalosis can be corrected after infusion of 1 to 2 L. of this solution over a period of 24 hours. If alkalosis recurs, there should be no hesitation in repeating the hydrochloric acid therapy until the underlying cause of alkalosis has been removed.

REFERENCES

1. Abouna, G. M., Aldrete, J. A., and Starzl, T. E.: Changes in serum potassium and blood pH during clinical and experimental orthotopic liver transplantation, SURGERY **69:** 419, 1971.
2. Aldrete, J. A., and Starzl, T. E.: Experience in hepatic transplantation, Philadelphia, 1969, W. B. Saunders Company, pp. 83-111.
3. Beach, F. X. M., and Jones, E. S.: Metabolic alkalosis treated with intravenous hydrochloric acid, Postgrad. Med. J. **47:** 516-520, July, 1971.
4. Bleich, H. L., Tannen, R. L., and Schwartz, W. B.: The induction of metabolic alkalosis by correction of potassium deficiency, J. Clin. Invest,. **45:** 573, 1966.
5. Bradham, G. B.: The intravenous use of hydrochloric acid in the treatment of severe alkalosis, Am. Surg. **34:** 551, 1968.
6. Cohen, J. J., and Ellis, J. H.: Correction of metabolic alkalosis by the kidney after isometric expansion of extracellular fluid, J. Clin. Invest. **46:** 1558, 1967.
7. Cook, W. A., Watts, R. W., and Metin, O. U.: Myocardial function capacity in response to compensated and uncompensated respiratory alkalosis, Surg. Forum **16:** 186, 1965.
8. Ghose, R. R.: The need for chloride replacement in the correction of metabolic alkalosis due to vomiting, Br. J. Clin. Pract. **21:** 570, 1967.
9. Giebisch, G.: Coupled ion and fluid transport in the kidney, N. Engl. J. Med. **287:** 913, 1972.
10. Goldring, R. M., Cannon, P. J., Heinemann, H. O., and Fishman, A. P.: Respiratory adjustments to chronic metabolic alkalosis in man, J. Clin. Invest. **47:** 188, 1968.
11. Heinemann, G. O.: Metabolic alkalosis in patients with hypercalcemia, Metabolism **14:** 1137, 1965.
12. Hume, D. M., Wolk, F., Lee, H. M., Abouna, G. M.: Liver transplantation in man, Transplant. Proc. **4:** 781, 1972.
13. Irvin, G. L., Gittes, R. F., and Gibbs, M. F.: Influence of acid-base disturbance on total plasma calcium and evidence for a homeostatic role of thyrocalcitonin, Ann. Surg. **164:** 1073, 1966.
14. Isaacs,M., and Vanamee, P.: The importance of the etiology of hypokalemic alkalosis in determining replacement therapy, Metabolism **14:** 1169, 1965.
15. Kassirer, J. P., and Schwartz, W. B.: Correction of metabolic alkalosis in man without repair of potassium deficiency, Am. J. Med. **40:** 19, 1966.
16. Kassirer, J. P., and Schwartz, W. B.: The re-

sponse of normal man to selective depletion of hydrochloric acid, Am. J. Med. **40:** 10, 1966.

17. Kassirer, J. P., Appleton, F. M., Chazan, J. A., and Schwartz, W. B.: Aldosterone in metabolic alkalosis, J. Clin. Invest. **46:** 1558, 1967.
18. Kilburn, K. H.: Shock, seizures and coma with alkalosis during mechanical ventilation, Ann. Intern. Med. **65:** 977, 1966.
19. Lyons, J. H., and Moore, F. D.: Post traumatic alkalosis incidence and pathophysiology of alkalosis in surgery, SURGERY **60:** 93, 1966.
20. MacLean, L. D., Mulligan, G. W., McLean, A. P. H., and Duff, J. H: Alkalosis in septic shock, SURGERY **62:** 655, 1967.
21. Mulhausen, R. O., and Blumentals, A. S.: Metabolic alkalosis, Arch. Intern. Med. **116:** 729, 1965.
22. Pitts, R. F.: Physiology of the kidney and body fluids, Chicago, 1972, Year Book Medical Publishers Inc., p. 179.
23. Riberon, E., Abtahi, H., Kukral, J. C., Zeineh, R. A., and Henegar, G. C.: Syndrome of metabolic alkalosis, hypokalemia, and hyperammonia in patients with cirrhosis, Surg. Forum **18:** 341, 1967.
24. Schwartz, W. B., de Strihou, C. V. Y., and Kassirer, J. P.: Role of anious in metabolic alkalosis and potassium deficiency, N. Engl. J. Med. **279:** 630, 1968.
25. Seldin, D. W., and Rector, F. C.: The generation and maintenance of metabolic alkalosis, Kidney International **1:** 306, 1972.
26. Sloop, R. D., and Orloff, M. J.: An important syndrome of metabolic alkalosis in patients with cirrhosis, bleeding varices, and portacaval shunt, Surg. Forum **17:** 37, 1966.
27. Tannen, R. L., Bleich, H. L., and Schwartz, W. B.: The renal response to acid loads in metabolic alkalosis; an assessment of the mechanisms regulating acid excretion, J. Clin. Invest. **45:** 562, 1963.
28. Walker, W. G., and Jost, L. J.: Relative roles of potassium and chloride in correction of hypokalemic, hypochloremic alkalosis, Johns Hopkins Med. J. **120:** 148, 1967.
29. Wilson, R. F., Gibson, D., Percinel, A. K., Ali, M. A., Baker, G., LeBlanc, L. P., and Lucas, C.: Severe alkalosis in critically ill surgical patients, Arch. Surg. **105:** 197, 1972.

Elevation in host splenic and in allograft parenchymal and capsular histidine decarboxylase activity and weights following renal allografting in rats

Thomas C. Moore, M.D., *Torrance, Calif.*, **Michael C. Sinclair, M.D.**, *and* **Carlos A. E. Lemmi, M.A.**, *Los Angeles, Calif.*

An elevation in host splenic and in allograft parenchymal and capsular histidine decarboxylose (HDC) activity and weights occurred following renal allografting in 54 rats in comparison with normal values and with those found after renal isografting. Splenic HDC elevation peaked at four days after allografting, whereas renal allograft parenchymal HDC activity did not become elevated significantly until the second five days after grafting and did not reach its maximum elevation until ten days after grafting. A steady increase in capsular weight occurred after grafting. Capsular elevation in HDC activity was biphasis with major elevations at 24 hours and ten days. The findings suggest a role of importance for HDC activity in both the afferent and efferent arcs of the immune response to organ allografting. The difference in renal allograft capsular and parenchymal HDC activity may reflect a difference in the response of non-sensitized animals to allografted tissue in contact with antigenically foreign tissue over a wide surface area for bulk in comparison with that exposed only to the antigenically foreign cellular elements of circulating blood.

From the Division of Pediatric Surgery and Renal Transplantation, UCLA–Harbor General Hospital, Torrance, Calif., and the Department of Surgery, University of California, Los Angeles, Los Angeles, Calif.

An increase in the urinary excretion of histamine has been observed following skin, heart, and kidney allografting in rats, dogs, and man.[4, 7, 8, 10] These elevated levels of urinary histamine excretion suggest an increase in histamine formation and release in association with sensitization to and rejection of organ allografts. They do not, however, provide evidence relative to the organs or tissues involved in the accelerated formation and/or release of histamine.

Histamine is formed intracellularly through the activity of the histidine decarboxylase (HDC) enzyme. A marked elevation in the activity of this enzyme has been found in allografted rat skin during rejection.[5] This elevation was as high as 33 times normal levels and reached its peak ten days following allografting. At this time, the levels of autografted skin were essentially those of normal skin. The sharp increase in histidine decarboxylase (HDC) activity of the allografted skin occurred five days after grafting with a peak elevation at ten days.

The reticuloendothelial system also has been found to be an area of accelerated histamine formation following antigenic challenge. An increase in splenic histidine

Supported by grants from The John A. Hartford Foundation, Inc., National Institutes of Health (AM-10373-01), and The Los Angeles County Heart Association.

Accepted for publication Oct. 10, 1973.

decarboxylase activity has been observed following skin allografting in rats.[6] The major increase took place in the initial five days after grafting. An increase in splenic histidine decarboxylase also has been found to occur following sheep red blood cell (SRBC) immunization of rats.[9] The peak elevation of enzyme activity in this system occurred four days after SRBC immunization. This was one day prior to the peak elevation in antibody-forming activity as determined by the Jerne blood agar plaque assay. An increase in lymph node HDC activity occurring after the administration of Freund's complete adjuvant has been reported by Schayer.[12]

The present report concerns alterations in splenic and in renal allograft parenchymal and capsular HDC activity which occur following renal allografting between inbred strains of rats. This model makes possible the acquisition of data concerning the effect of immediate revascularization on central reticuloendothelial (splenic) and allograft target organ HDC activity, a type of data not obtainable with skin allografting. It also provides a means of separating the reactions of the allograft capsule which is in immediate contact over wide area with "foreign" tissue from those of the allograft parenchyma which is exposed only to recipient blood.

MATERIAL AND METHODS

Male Brown-Norway (BN) inbred rats were used as kidney allograft donors and male Lewis rats were used as allograft and isograft recipients and as isograft donors. Male rats were selected for this study because of a difference in histamine metabolism between male and female rats and the comparatively large size of the male rats. Brown-Norway donor rats weighed approximately 280 grams, and the Lewis donor and recipient rats weighed approximately 360 grams.

Ether cone anesthesia was used. Renal transplantation was performed by the rat technique described by Lee.[2] The renal vein or a patch of inferior vena cava with renal vein was anastomosed end to side into the inferior vena cava of the recipient animal. A segment of donor aorta was anastomosed to recipient abdominal aorta for the transplant renal arterial perfusion and a small segment of donor urinary bladder with the donor kidney ureter was used for urinary tract reconstitution. At least one recipient kidney was left intact. The animals were fed a standard rat lab chow diet with water ad libitum postoperatively.

Fifty-four renal allografts and 29 renal isografts were performed. Eleven ungrafted BN kidneys and five ungrafted Lewis kidneys were used as normal control experiments. The majority of grafted animals were put to death during the initial ten days following operation. Five allografted animals were killed on each postoperative day from one through ten after the transplant procedure was performed. At death, the renal capsule of the transplanted kidney was separated from the kidney parenchyma. The allograft renal capsule and parenchyma and the spleen were weighed separately and were quick-frozen with dry ice and acetone or liquid nitrogen for storage at 87° C. in an ultra-deep freezer for later analysis.

HDC activity was determined by the method of Schayer.[11] This method involves the incubation of ^{14}C histidine and pyrodoxal-5-phosphate with a known weight of tissue for a three-hour period at 37° C. under nitrogen in a Dubnoff metabolic incubator. The ^{14}C histamine produced is converted to benzenesulfonyl histamine (BSH). The BSH is purified by repeated recrystalizations over a period of five days. The HDC activity, corrected for tissue blank, background activity, and recovery of BSH, is calculated and expressed as disintegrations per minute (dpm) per 100 mg. of BSH per gram of tissue.

RESULTS

Spleen. Spleens from 50 BN to Lewis renal allografted rats were used in this study. Five rats were killed on each of the first ten days following allografting. The HDC activity of five spleens from non-

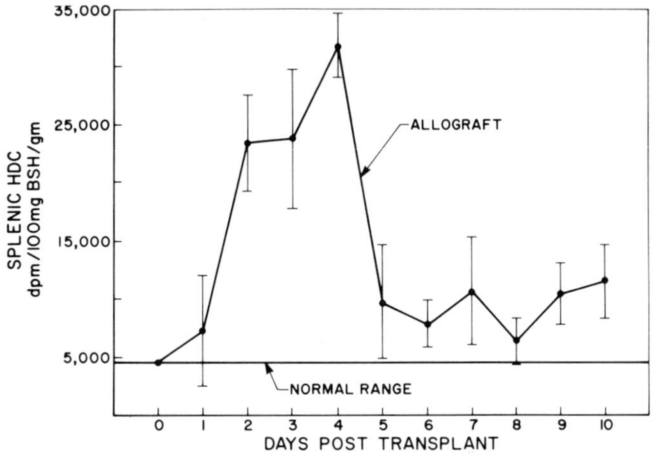

Fig. 1. Graph showing mean splenic histidine decarboxylase (HDC) activity expressed as dpm/100 mg. of BSH per gram of spleen from five rats killed on each of the first ten days following renal allografting (BN to Lewis) of 50 rats.

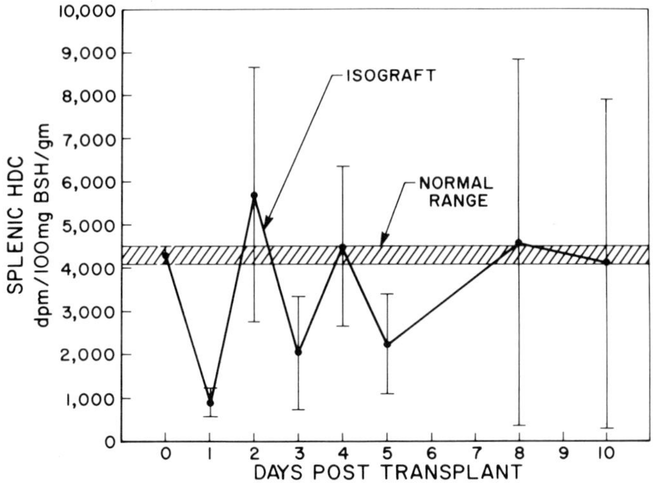

Fig. 2. Graph demonstrating mean HDC activity of recipient (Lewis) spleens per gram of spleen at death at intervals following isografting.

grafted animals was 4,223 ± 193 dpm per 100 mg. of BSH per gram of tissue. The major elevation of splenic HDC activity following allografting occurred in the initial five days following operation (Fig. 1). Although a mild elevation had occurred within 24 hours after operation, the most marked elevation per gram of splenic tissue took place in the two- to four-day period following grafting. The peak elevation of 31,603 ± 2,759 dpm per 100 mg. of BSH per gram of tissue was found four days after allografting. This peak elevation was significantly above the HDC activity of normal, ungrafted spleens ($P < 0.005$), an approximate eightfold elevation above normal levels. There was a rapid fall toward normal levels per gram of tissue in the second five days, which began at the fifth posttransplant day.

Splenic renal isografts (Lewis to Lewis) were performed in 29 rats. Varying numbers of rats were killed daily from one through five days after allografting and at eight and ten days after grafting. The concentration of determinations in the initial five days was because of the peak allografting elevation in splenic HDC activity during this period. At 24 hours after renal isograft-

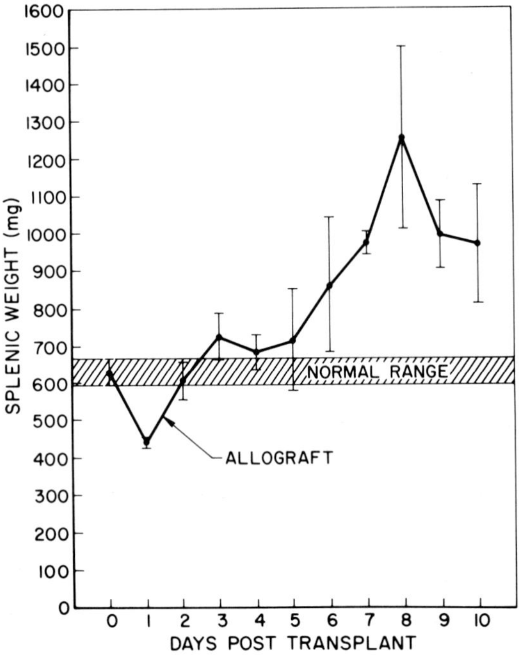

Fig. 3. Graph showing mean recipient splenic weights at death at intervals following allografting.

ing, recipient splenic HDC activity was depressed to 896 ± 323 dpm per 100 mg. of BSH per gram of tissue from the normal Lewis spleen level of 4,323 ± 193 (Fig. 2). This depression in activity contrasted with the mild elevation following allografting at 24 hours. There was no significant elevation of splenic HDC activity following isografting. At four days, when the peak elevation following allografting to 31,603 ± 2,759 occurred, the HDC activity of isografted Lewis spleens was 4,482 ± 1,843. The elevation of splenic HDC activity four days after allografting was significantly elevated above that of isografted spleens at four days ($p < 0.005$).

Mean splenic weight of allografted rats fell within 24 hours from a normal value of 630 ± 39 to 442 ± 16 mg. (Fig. 3). Thereafter, a steady rise in mean splenic weight occurred. A peak elevation to 1,255 ± 249 mg. was observed at eight days following allografting. This was significantly above normal mean splenic weights ($P < 0.01$). At this time, splenic weight had approximately doubled.

Twenty-four hours after isografting, mean

Table I. *Effect of allografting and isografting on rat renal capsular mean weights*

Posttransplant day	*Allografts: BN to Lewis (mg.)*	*Isografts: Lewis to Lewis (mg.)*
Normal	20	21
1	36	18
2	88	
3	86	
4	107	
5	108	20
6	143	
7	260	
8	534	13
9	710	
10	1,126	21

splenic weight was depressed even more than after allografting; it was depressed to 360 ± 120 mg. (Fig. 4). This was almost one-half the normal mean weight. Mean splenic weights remained depressed below normal levels in the initial ten days following renal isografting.

When total splenic HDC activity is considered (dpm per gram times splenic weight in grams), the major elevation following allografting still is found in the initial five days (Fig. 5). The peak elevation remains at four days. The differential between allografting and isografting is even greater when total splenic HDC activities are compared. At most intervals after grafting, the allografted rat spleen mean total HDC activity tended to be in the range of ten- to seventeenfold greater than that of the spleens of isografted animals.

Renal capsule. Renal capsular weights at day zero represent the normal mean weights of rat renal capsules from ungrafted animals. For allografts, the capsular weights are based on the mean weights of 11 BN rat renal capsules (donor rats in BN-to-Lewis allografting) and on the mean weights of Lewis rat renal capsules (donor rats in Lewis-to-Lewis isografting). The capsular weights of normal, ungrafted rats are quite similar (Table I). The 50 rat renal allografts were performed first to determine the daily alterations in capsular weight (based on five allograft recipient rats killed on each postgraft day

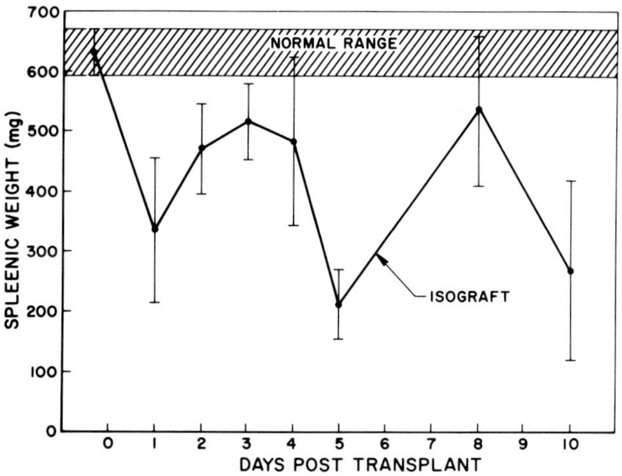

Fig. 4. Graph showing mean recipient splenic weights at death at intervals following isografting.

for the initial ten days). This data served as a comparison with the weight of normal, ungrafted BN rat capsular weights and as information for the timing of the subsequent sequence for the killing of isografted rats.

The immediately revascularized allografted kidney capsules which were exposed over a wide surface area for their weight and bulk to antigenically foreign living tissue showed a prompt increase in mean capsular weights thereafter. The weights of the capsules of allografted rats was increased more than fiftyfold above the mean weights of normal, ungrafted rat capsules and above the mean weights of isografted rat capsules. The major part of the increase in allografted capsular weight appeared to be due to the intense innflammatory reaction and the accumulation of immunoinflammatory interstitial edema fluid.

The mean HDC activity of normal, ungrafted capsules was quite low and comparable for BN and Lewis rat capsules. Within 24 hours (first day after grafting), the HDC activity of allografted capsule had increased almost one-hundred fold (Fig. 6). A marked increase also had occurred in isografted capsules. By weight of allografted capsule, the HDC activity decreased thereafter.

Since HDC activity is an intracellular enzymatic response and because of the major

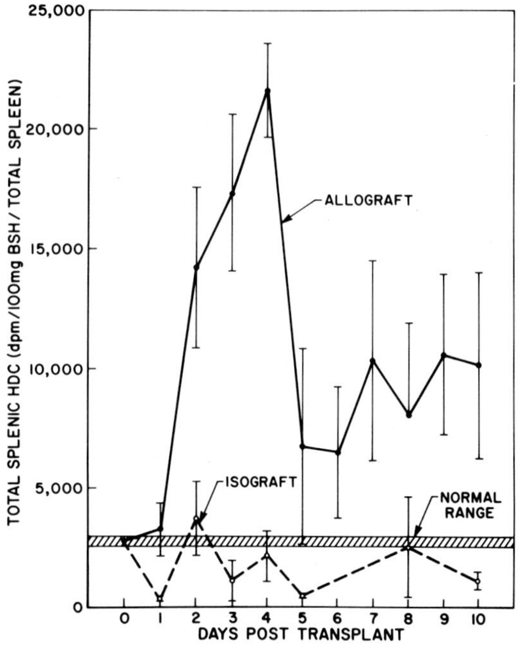

Fig. 5. Graph illustrating differences in a mean total splenic HDC activity of recipient spleens at intervals following allografting and isografting.

contribution of immunoinflammatory fluid accumulation to the increase in capsular weight, it seemed appropriate to consider the changes in HDC activity within the framework of total capsular HDC activity. Total HDC activity of allografted capsules was markedly increased within 24 hours and remained essentially at this level until the

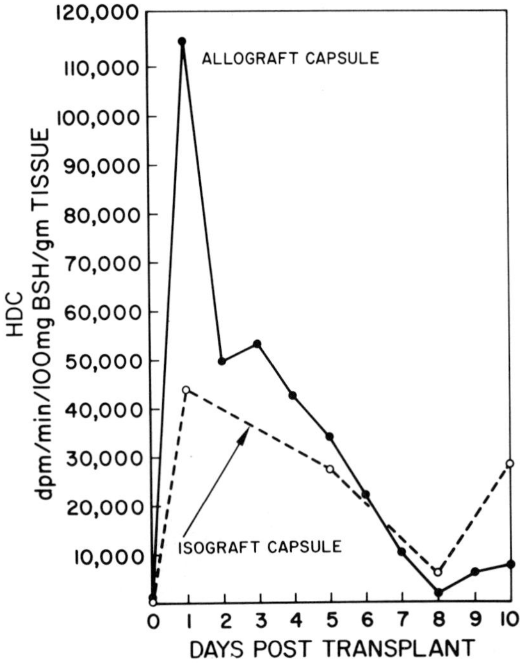

Fig. 6. Graph showing increase in rat renal capsular HDC activity per gram of grafted capsular tissue at intervals following renal allografting and isografting.

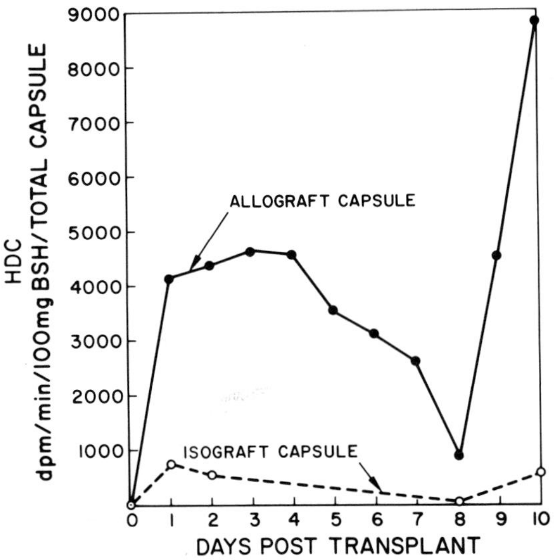

Fig. 7. Graph showing changes in rat renal capsular HDC activity per total grafted capsule at intervals following allografting and isografting. Total capsular HDC activity reflects both the level of HDC activity per gram of tissue and the alterations in capsular weight which occur. The secondary rise in allograft capsular HDC activity reflects the marked increase in capsular weight which occurred.

tenth day after grafting when a substantial increase occurred (Fig. 7). This mean HDC activity of isografted capsules, both per gram of tissue and per total capsule was greatest in the first 24 hours after grafting. At ten days after allografting, the increase in mean allografted capsule HDC activity was approximately fifteenfold greater than that of mean isografted capsule HDC activity.

Renal parenchyma. Renal parenchymal mean weights were essentially unchanged in the initial five days following allografting (Fig. 8). In the second five days, there was a progressive increase in mean parenchymal weight with the maximum increase in the eight- to ten-day period.

Renal parenchymal HDC activity in the normal, ungrafted kidney was quite low. Mean renal parenchymal HDC activity per gram of tissue remained comparatively low in the initial five days following allografting. Parenchymal allografted tissue was in contact only with the limited cellular elements of circulating blood. Renal parenchymal HDC activity became progressively elevated in the second five days following allografting (Fig. 9). The finding of peak elevation in parenchymal HDC activity at ten days after allografting in the initial 50 renal allografts led to an assessment of parenchymal HDC activity in the post–ten-day period in four additional allografts. By 12 to 14 days, it had fallen to the comparatively low mean level of 200 and 2,000. Renal isograft parenchymal activity remained comparatively unchanged with respect to the increase in allograft parenchymal activity in the second five days following grafting.

In view of the increasing mean parenchymal weights from immunoinflammatory edema fluid accumulation in the second five days following allografting, a more meaningful assessment of intracellular histamine formation from HDC activity may be obtained by considering the total parenchymal HDC activity in the second five days following allo-

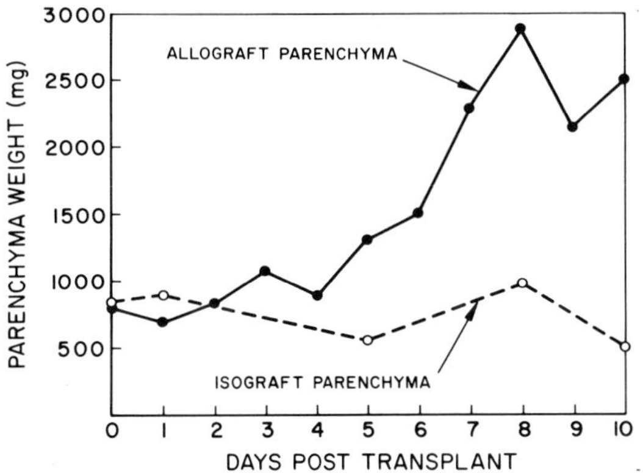

Fig. 8. Graph demonstrating increase in grafted rat renal parenchymal weights following renal allografting in comparison with renal isografting. Day 0 represents the mean weights of normal, ungrafted rat renal parenchyma for BN and Lewis rats.

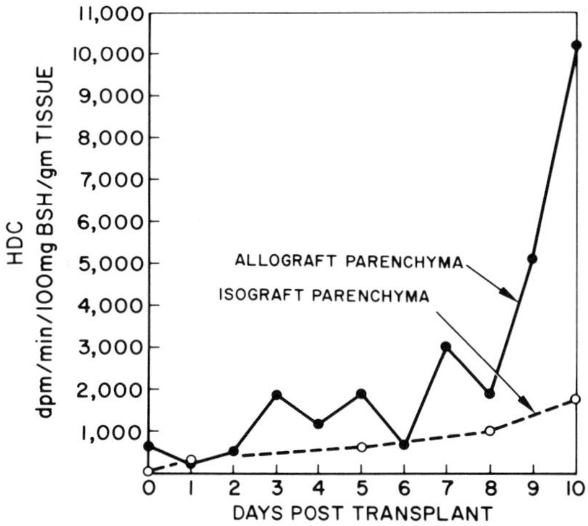

Fig. 9. Graph showing elevation in grafted rat renal allograft parenchymal HDC activity per gram of tissue in the second five-day posttransplant period in comparison with normal (day 0) and isograft levels.

grafting. Here a progressive increase in mean total parenchymal HDC activity occurred (Fig. 10). Mean parenchymal HDC activity following isografting remained comparatively low. At ten days following grafting, the HDC activity of total renal parenchyma following allografting was approximately twenty-seven fold greater than that found in the mean parenchymal activity following isografting.

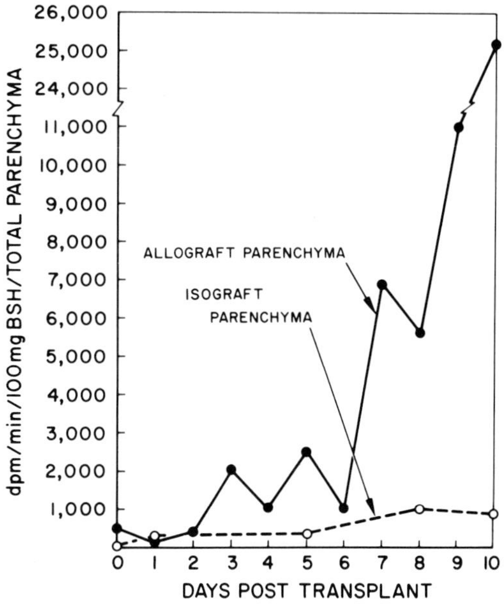

Fig. 10. Graph illustrating the marked elevation in grafted rat renal allograft parenchymal HDC activity per total kidney parenchyma in the second five-day posttransplant period in comparison with normal (day 0) and isograft levels.

DISCUSSION

This study presented a unique opportunity to dissect the immune response to allograft tissue as mirrored in tissue weights and HDC activity with respect to host spleen and to the immediately revascularized tissue components (renal capsule) exposed over an unusually wide area for mass and weight to antigenicly foreign tissue and the response of a much larger bulk of immediately revascularize tissue (renal parenchyma), exposed only to the limited number of cells in non-sensitized circulating blood.

HDC activity of the spleens of renal allografted rats was increased substantially in the initial five days following grafting. The major increase per gram of splenic weight was in the two- to four-day period after grafting with a peak eightfold increase at four days. The splenic HDC activity of kidney isografted animals did not increase after grafting.

Both isografted and allografted animal spleens lost weight 24 hours following operation. The magnitude of loss was greater for the isografted animal spleens. While the spleens of isografted animals remained at normal or subnormal weights, there was a progressive increase in the weights of the spleens of allografted animals. The peak elevation at eight days was to approximately double normal splenic weight.

The period of peak elevation in splenic HDC activity following renal allografting was similar to the finding of Moore and Schayer[5] following rat skin allografting. The peak was clearer cut, and the magnitude of increase above normal and above isograft-autograft levels was much greater following renal allografting. The immediate revascularization, with continuing maintenance of tissue metabolic competency at near normal levels, and the immediate exposure of the allograft to the elements of circulating blood, including immunocompetent cells and immunologically involved substances and enzymes, likely played an important role in the splenic HDC response to renal as compared with skin allografting.

It is of interest that splenic HDC activity peaked at day four whereas the weight increase did not peak until day eight. Increased HDC activity of the spleen may have played an important role in the recruitment of immunologically competent cells to the spleen and in a greater capability to respond immunologically. Histamine plays a role in promoting hyperemia and in increasing lymph flow. It also increases vascular permeability. Majno and associates[3] have shown the site of histamine action in producing increased vascular membrane permeability to be in the postcapillary venule area.

In the capsule and parenchyma part of this study, the larger bulk of renal allograft parenchymal tissue was protected from direct exposure to a large amount of antigenically foreign tissue by a "protective" capsule. The nature of these antigenic challenges was different from that presented by full-thickness skin allografting where a period of time was required for revascularization.

A prompt and steady increase in capsular weight occurred. An increase in parenchymal weight did not take place until the second five days following allografting. The capsular and parenchymal weights of isografted kidneys remained essentially unchanged in the ten days following grafting. The major part of the fiftyfold increase in mean allografted capsular weight appeared to be due to the progressive immunoinflammatory response with the accumulation of substantial amounts of interstitial edema fluid. Cellular invasion from circulating blood cells via the transplant renal artery and direct invasion by cells and blood vessels from the adjacent antigenically foreign living tissue also contributed to the marked increase in mean allograft capsular weight.

The comparatively stable capsular weight of isografted kidneys suggests a limited immunoinflammatory response. The increase in capsular HDC activity of isografted kidneys likely represents the normal HDC response found by Kahlson[1] to occur in fresh tissue wounds and in granulation tissue. Under these circumstances, Kahlson found peak elevations in wound and granulation in tissue HDC activity at one and five days following injury. Kahlson[1] also found elevated HDC activity in rapidly growing rat fetal and tumor tissue and regarded elevated HDC activity as a component of rapid tissue growth.

Allograft parenchymal weights remained essentially unchanged in the initial five days following grafting with a substantial increase in the second five-day period. The approximate threefold increase in rat renal allograft parenchymal weight was similar to the increase in allograft weight at ten days following renal allografting in dogs.

The major increase in parenchymal HDC activity also took place in the second five-day period following allografting. The later (12 to 14 days) reduction in parenchymal HDC activity probably was a result of tissue ischemia associated with a reduction in allograft blood flow secondary to an occlusive extravascular accumulation of edema fluid.

These findings of a peak increase in reticuloendothelial tissue (splenic) HDC activity in the initial five-day period following allografting suggest a period of delay for circulating blood elements to become sensitized and to produce the immunoinflammatory response to the delayed hypersensitivity type of rejection. These findings also suggest that the circulating cells initiating and mediating this response likely are of host origin.

The early response of allograft capsule with respect to weight gain and increase in HDC activity appear to be related to the extensive surface area exposure per mass of tissue to living, antigenicly foreign host tissue. Sensitized cellular element may play a role in later changes both by capsular perfusion from the transplant renal artery and by direct contact and vascular ingrowth from adjacent host tissue. The second rise in total allograft capsule HDC activity in the second five-day period after transplant with a ten-day posttransplant peak elevation was similar to posttransplant HDC activity response of allograft parenchyma during the second five-day period.

Appendical HDC activity of 50 of the renal allografted rats was assayed and did not change in the ten days after allografting. Thymus HDC activity also was assayed in 50 allografted rats and was significantly depressed from comparatively high normal levels of approximately 20,000 dpm per gram tissue to the 3,000 to 4,000 dpm per gram of tissue from the second posttransplant day throughout the initial ten posttransplant days involved in this study. Thymic HDC levels also were depressed postoperatively in isografted animals.

Knowledge of the role played by intracellular histamine formation and release in the afferent and efferent arcs of the immune response may be of considerable value in controlling and regulating the responses.

Furthermore, the importance of other vasoactive substances which release and are released by histamine should not be overlooked. These substances include serotonin, bradykinin, and prostaglandin E^1. They exert their vascular permeability effect on postcapillary venules, like histamine, and their action may be partially blocked by antihistamine therapy. In this regard, it may be of interest that we recently have observed a peak five-day postrenal allografting increase in rat plasma kallikrein activity,[10a] and with B. M. Jaffe,[4a] we have found a six-day postallografting peak increase in prostaglandin E^1 activity of coronary sinus blood of allografted rat hearts.

SUMMARY

Renal allografting and isografting were performed between and within inbred strains (BN and Lewis) in 83 rats. Host splenic and allograft capsule and parenchymal histidine decarboxylase (HDC) activity were assayed by a radioisotope method.

Splenic HDC activity of allografted rats increased sharply in the initial five days after allografting with a peak eightfold elevation at four days ($P < 0.005$). Splenic HDC activity of isografted rats was not altered significantly from normal levels.

Splenic weights increased following allografting with a peak twofold increase at eight days. Splenic weights following isografting remained in the normal or subnormal range.

A prompt and progressive increase in allograft capsular weight was observed and was associated with a marked early elevation in allograft capsular HDC activity. At ten days, mean total allograft capsular HDC activity was approximately 15 times greater than that of isografted capsules. Isograft capsular weights did not change.

Allograft parenchymal weights increased threefold in the second five-day period after grafting. An increase in allograft parenchyma HDC activity occurred in the second five days after grafting with a ten-day twenty-seven fold elevation above isograft parenchymal levels.

These findings may be contrasted with the failure of appendiceal HDC activity to change following renal allografting in rats and with the depression of rat thymic HDC activity following both renal allografting and isografting.

The results of this study suggest that increased intracellular histamine formation and release may be involved in an important way in both the afferent and efferent arcs of the immune response to organ allografting.

The earlier increase in weight and HDC activity of allograft capsular tissue as compared with allograft parenchymal tissue suggests a difference in the immunoinflammatory response over a wide surface area for bulk to antigenically foreign living tissue from the response to immediately revascularized allografted tissue exposed only to the cellular elements in circulating blood.

REFERENCES

1. Kahlson, G.: New approaches to the physiology of histamine, Perspect. Biol. Med. **5:** 179, 1962.
2. Lee, S.: An improved technique of renal allografting in the rat, SURGERY **61:** 771, 1967.
3. Majno, G., Palade, G. E., and Schoefl, G. I.: Studies on inflammation. II. The site of action of histamine and serotonin along the vascular tree: A topographical study, J. Biophys. Biochem. Cytol. **11:** 607, 1961.
4. Moore, T. C., and Chang, J.: Urinary histamine excretion in the rat following skin homografting and autografting, Ann. Surg. **167:** 232, 1968.

4a. Moore, T. C., and Jaffe, B. M.: Unpublished data.

5. Moore, T. C., and Schayer, R. W.: Histidine decarboxylase activity of autografted and allografted rat skin, Transplantation **7:** 99, 1969.
6. Moore, T. C., and Schayer, R. W.: Histidine decarboxylase activity of the rat spleen following skin allografting, Ann. Surg. **171:** 609, 1970.
7. Moore, T. C., Thompson, D. P., and Hayes, M.: Correlation of renal blood flow indices and histamine metabolism data after canine renal allografting, Arch. Surg. **101:** 45, 1970.
8. Moore, T. C., Cleveland, R. J., Thompson, D. P., and Nelson, R. J.: Vasoactive amine metabolism following canine and human heart transplantation, Ann. Surg. **174:** 51, 1971.
9. Moore, T. C., Lemmi, C. A. E., Orlando, J. C., and Pinkerton, W.: Correlation of splenic histidine decarboxylase activity and antibody formation following SRBC immunization, Transplantation **11:** 347, 1971.
10. Moore, T. C., Thompson, D. P., and Glassock, R. J.: Elevation in urinary and blood histamine following clinical renal transplantation, Ann. Surg. **173:** 381, 1971.

10a. Moore, T. C., Sinclair, M. C., and Lemmi, C. A. E.: Elevation of rat plasma kallikrein activity following renal allografting, Am. J. Surg. In press.

11. Schayer, R. W.: Formation and binding of histamine by rat tissues in vitro, Am. J. Physiol. **187:** 63, 1956.
12. Schayer, R. W.: Role of histamine in Freund's adjuvant action (abstract), Fed. Proc. **29:** 617, 1970.

Successful reversal of lethal carbon monoxide intoxication by total body asanguineous hypothermic perfusion

Juan C. Agostini, M.D., Ruben G. Ramirez, M.D., Solomon N. Albert, M.D., Leo R. Goldbaum, Ph.D., *and* **Karel B. Absolon, M.D., Ph.D.,** *Washington, D. C.*

Total body asanguineous hypothermic perfusion proved successful as a treatment of otherwise acute lethal carbon monoxide intoxication in dogs. The technique may prove the therapy of choice in human carbon monoxide poisoning. The rapidity with which carboxyhemoglobin can be removed and replaced with normal hemoglobin containing red blood cells and the technical safety of the procedure warrants its clinical exploration in suitable cases.

From the Departments of Surgery of the Washington Hospital Center, The George Washington University, and the George Hyman Research Foundation and the Department of Toxicology of the Armed Forces Institute of Pathology, Washington, D. C.

Rapid reversal of anoxia due to carbon monoxide toxicity should be the aim of therapy in carbon monoxide poisoning.[12] In the search for clinical applications of total body asanguineous hypothermic perfusion (TBHP), it was thought that severe systemic hypoxia resulting from carbon monoxide intoxication could be reversed by the rapid removal of the circulating carboxyhemoglobin. Replacement with normal blood should, in theory at least, restore normal oxygen transport. Furthermore, cooling of the subject would reduce the oxygen demands of body tissues, minimizing the anoxic damage caused by carbon monoxide.

At present, the commonly accepted method of treatment of carbon monoxide poisoning is hyperbaric oxygenation at a pressure of up to two atmospheres.[11] Even if the elaborate equipment is available, the procedure usually takes from one to six hours before the toxic concentration of carboxyhemoglobin is reduced to a level compatible with survival. Smith and Sharp's[10] report indicates that hyperbaric oxygenation often is unsuccessful. In two patients in their series, in spite of six and five hours of treatment with hyperbaric oxygen, autopsy showed typical cerebral ischemic lesions of the globus pallidus. Oxygen toxicity is another potential drawback of hyperbaric oxygen therapy in a critically ill patient.[9]

The present communication concerns observations on TBHP in normal dogs and dogs poisoned with carbon monoxide inhalation. Normothermic and hypothermic dogs given carbon monoxide and receiving the same treatment except for TBHP served as control subjects.

MATERIALS AND METHODS

Adult male, mongrel dogs, weighing 15 to 20 kilograms, were used and divided into four groups of five dogs each.

Group I. The animals in the first group were anesthetized with intravenous Sodium Nembutal, intubated endotracheally, and kept on positive pressure ventilation with

Accepted for publication Oct. 10, 1973.

Table I. *Average values of hemodynamic and biochemical indices*

*Indices**	*Prior to washout*		*During early washout*	
	Average	*Range*	*Average*	*Range*
Normal dogs + TBHP				
B/P	110/80	80/60–130/80	97/53	40/20–100/45
Temp. (° C.)	37	35–40	35	34–38
CVP (mm./H_2O)	7	1–15	12	5–22
Po_2 (mm./Hg)	269	91–550	525	450–750
Pco_2 (mm./Hg)	21.5	15.5–26	22.1	15–40
pH	7.37	7.32–7.41	7.32	7.2–7.4
Hct. (%)	35	28.4–47.1	17.5	10.5–19.6
Hbg. (Gm. %)	12	9.9–16.0	4.6	3.3–6.0
RCV (ml.)	551	282–770	—	—
PV (ml.)	1,203	832–1,719	—	—
TBV (ml.)	1,754	1,144–2,407	—	—
C. O. (L./min.)	2.5	2.2–2.6	—	—
CO intoxication + TBHP				
B/P	108/64	80/40–120/90	66/28	60/40–80/20
Temp. (° C.)	37.4	37–38	30.2	27–33
CVP (mm./H_2O)	7.2	4–10	16	10–20
% CO (%)	72.8	52–86	38	10–60
Po_2 (mm./Hg)	153	55–405	—	—
Pco_2 (mm./Hg)	36.25	22–57	—	—
pH	7.37	7.23–7.5	—	—
Hct. (%)	34.95	26.7–42.7	10.76	8.6–14.7
Hbg. (Gm. %)	12.14	8.8–14.6	3.76	3.1–5.1
RCV (ml.)	670	250–950	—	—
PV (ml.)	1,056	750–1,450	—	—
TBV (ml.)	1,726	1,000–2,180	—	—
ECF (ml.)	5,433	4,145–6,874	—	—
C. O. (L./min.)	2.4	2.1–2.6	—	—

*CVP, Central venous pressure; Hct., hematocrit; Hbg., hemoglobin; RCV, red cell volume; PV, plasma volume; TBV, total blood

30 percent oxygen. Catheters were inserted in the aorta and superior vena cava through femoral and neck vessels for direct monitoring of arterial and venous pressures. Electrodes attached to the extremities followed heart rate and rhythm. A rectal probe constantly monitored the core temperature.

Cannulation of the femoral vessels was performed with the use of a No. 18 Fr. venous cannula, 30 cm. in length, for drainage of blood, and a No. 12 Fr. arterial cannula was inserted in the artery for infusion. Blood samples were taken for complete blood counts and blood gases. Cardiac output measurements were obtained before and after total body perfusion with the use of the dye dilution technique. Blood volumes and extracellular fluid studies were obtained pre- and postoperatively by means of Cr^{51}-tagged red cells, I^{131} human serum albumin, and S^{35}. Cr^{51}-labeled red cells measures primarily the red cell compartment whereas radioactive iodinated serum albumin measures primarily the plasma volume compartment. Extracellular fluid was measured as a sulfate space with S^{35}, sodium sulfate. Radioanalysis for S^{35} was performed by liquid scintillation technique as described by Albert.[2] TBHP and replacement with donor blood was accomplished by the use of a heart-lung pump and three oxygenators for drainage and fluid or blood replacement, all of which were integrated by appropriate circuitry.

The circulatory exchange was initiated after injection of 2 mg. of heparin per kilogram of body weight. The animals were exanguinated into one reservoir, while simultaneous infusion of the asanguineous perfusate was started.

The perfusate was composed of a 1:1 dilution of Ringer's lactate and dextran 70 solutions, cooled to 27° C., and buffered to a pH of 8 with Tham (tromethamine). The input and the output of the system was

End of washout		*After washout*	
Average	*Range*	*Average*	*Range*
65/30	70/40–100/60	90/40	80/60–120/80
28	25–35	33	31–37
24	7–40	13	4–30
460	300–450	322	250–490
7.3	0–17	17.2	0–34
7.27	7.15–7.5	7.48	7.3–8.0
3.3	1.0–4.5	15.5	9.8–21.9
1.0	0–4	5.2	3.7–7.5
—	—	283	132–390
—	—	1,699	1,019–1,935
—	—	1,982	1,300–2,260
—	—	2.1	1.8–2.3
90/50	80/40–100/60	104/60	100/40–110/70
31.8	29–34	35.8	35–36
9.2	8–12	7.3	5–10
19.48	5–29	8.12	1–15
328.75	160–500	262.75	82–460
35	25–51	32.25	24–37
7.29	7.25–7.35	7.34	7.32–7.38
7.97	5.2–10.7	21.25	19.8–23.1
2.88	1.8–3.6	7.54	6.7–8.7
—	—	394	240–450
—	—	1,252	750–1,620
—	—	1,646	1,000–2,060
—	—	5,562	5,895–10,244
—	—	2.74	2.6–2.76

volume; ECF, extracellular fluid; C.O., cardiac output.

controlled so as to maintain close balance.

Samples for hemoglobin and hematocrit determinations were drawn periodically. The exanguination was continued until the venous return appeared diluted enough to ensure almost complete replacement of the dog's original circulating blood volume. Whole fresh, warm donor blood (acid citrate dextrose blood) was infused at this stage through the arterial line. Venous drainage was continued as long as the fresh blood reserve in the pump was considered safe to allow the maximum possible replacement of the perfusate with blood.

Uncross-matched blood was obtained for the final exchange from healthy mongrel dogs which had been lightly anesthetized with ketamine hydrochloride (5 mg. per kilogram). Five hundred milligrams of methylprednisolone was administered to obviate allergic reactions. At the end of the procedure, 5 mEq. per kilogram of sodium bicarbonate and 90 mg. of calcium gluceptate were added. The animals were kept on partial bypass until the core temperature reached normal values. At the completion of the procedure, the cannulas were removed and the wounds were closed. This first group of dogs served as operated control subjects and standardization of TBHP technique.

Group II. The second series of normothermic dogs were anesthetized with Sodium Nembutal, intubated with a cuffed endotracheal tube, and were left breathing spontaneously while monitored and sampled as the other experimental dogs.

A ten percent mixture of carbon monoxide and room air was delivered for three minutes through the endotracheal tube, connected to a closed-circuit five-liter balloon, after which room air was administered. Blood samples for carboxyhemoglobin levels were taken at regular intervals after poisoning until death. The percentage of carboxyhemoglobin was

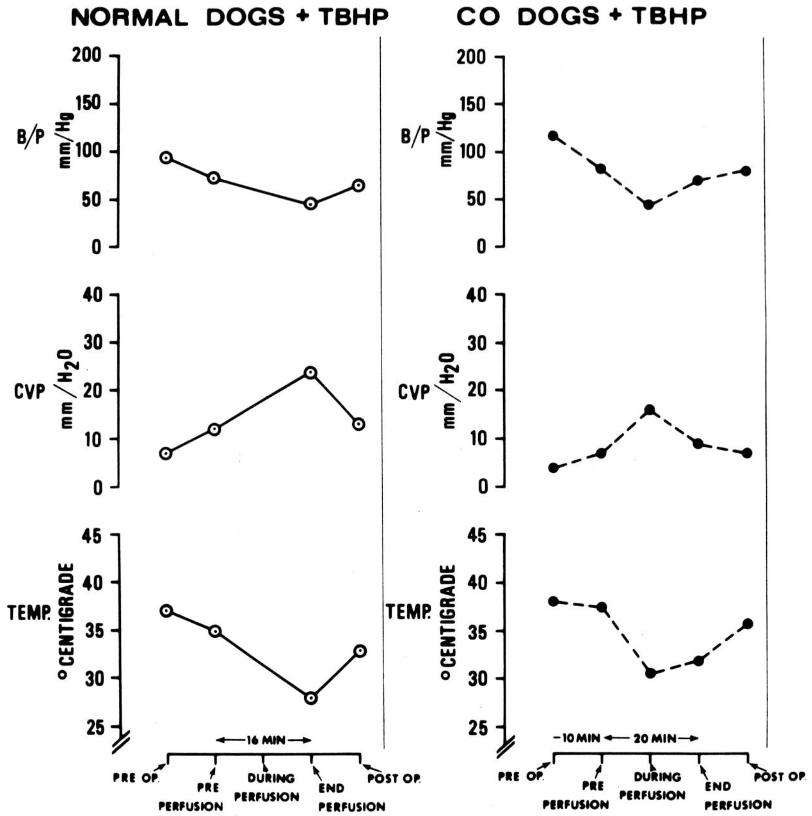

Fig. 1. Blood pressure, central venous pressure, and temperature traced for Group I (normal dogs plus TBHP) and Group III (carbon monoxide–intoxicated dogs plus TBHP).

determined by first analyzing the carbon monoxide content of the blood by a gas chromatographic procedure; then the total hemoglobin concentration of the sample was determined by the cyanmethemoglobin method.[13]

Group III. In the third group of hypothermic dogs with core temperature averaging 28.9° C. (range, 28–30° C.), carbon monoxide was administered in the same manner as the previous series. Subsequently, they were sampled periodically for COHb levels. They also received the same medication as Group I.

Group IV. In the fourth group, the same parameters as in the above series were studied. Carbon monoxide intoxication was accomplished as in the control series. These animals were treated with TBHP. The average time from intoxication to perfusion was 9.5 minutes (range, 4 to 15 minutes).

RESULTS

The five normal dogs in Group I subjected to TBHP and the five dogs intoxicated with carbon monoxide in Group II treated by TBHP survived. Gross and microscopic tissue examinations four weeks later showed no abnormalities.

Hemodynamic variations during TBHP for Groups I and III are summarized in Table I. Blood pressures tended to drop at the beginning of the procedure, reaching the lowest values at the peak of the hypothermic asanguineous stage, returning toward normal after replacement with whole blood and rewarming. The trend in blood pressure changes was the same in both series; however, the preperfusion mean pressures were much higher in Group III, suggesting a hypoxia-triggered hypertensive reaction. Central venous pressure was the adequate index of volume balance.

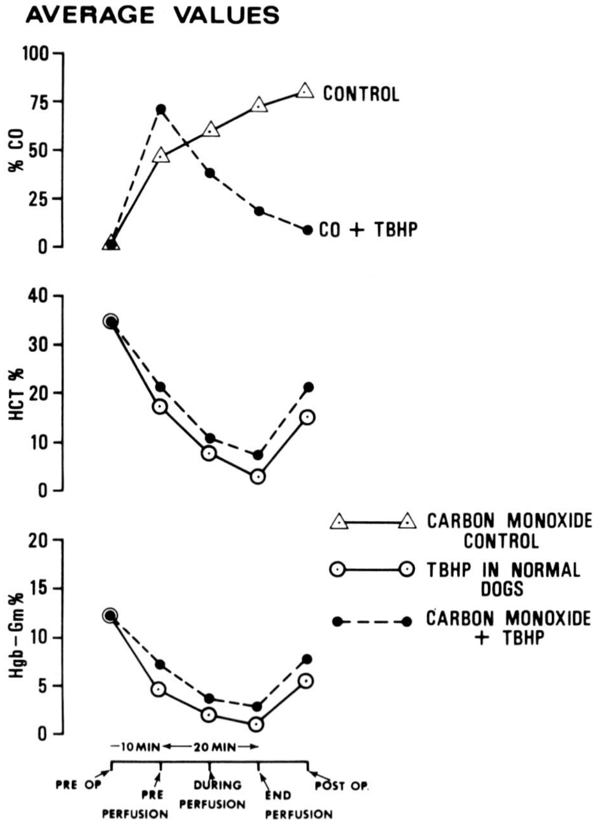

Fig. 2. Average values for carbon monoxide control dogs, TBHP in normal dogs, and carbon monoxide–intoxicated dogs plus TBHP.

In both Groups I and III, the drop in the blood pressure correlated with a rise in central venous pressure and a decrease in cardiac output after TBHP (Fig. 1). The hematocrit values decreased to an average low of 3.3 percent (range, 1.0 to 7.1 percent), returning to an average of 15.5 percent (range, 9.8 to 21.9 percent) in normal control subjects. In dogs intoxicated with carbon monoxide, the lowest average hematocrit was 7.97 percent (range, 5.2 to 10.7 percent) returning to an average of 21.5 percent (range, 19.8 to 23.1 percent) (Fig. 2). Cardiac outputs measured before the initiation of the exchange in normal animals and in the experimental series showed a slight decrease after TBHP in the normal animals from 2.35 to 2.00 L. per minute, in contrast to a slight increase (2.4 to 2.74 L. per minute) in carbon monoxide intoxicated dogs.

Blood volumes in Group I increased on the average 13 percent. Plasma volume was expanded to an average of 41 percent, while the red cell volume decreased 48 percent. In Group III, the average blood volume recorded a deficit after TBHP of 80 ml. (4.6 percent) from the preoperative value. The red cell mass was reduced to an average of 276 ml. (41 percent) from the preoperative value, and the plasma volume was expanded to an average of 204 ml. (16.4 percent). Extracellular fluid determinations showed a minimal expansion after TBHP from 5,433 to 5,562 ml. The total fluids exchanged in normal dogs was on the average 6,175 c.c. (range, 2,900 to 8,300 c.c.), consisting of an average of 17 percent blood (range, 13 to 20 percent) during the blood for fluid exchange. In dogs poisoned with carbon monoxide, the total washout averaged 4,940 c.c. (range, 4,500 to 5,300 c.c.); the blood exchange phase amounted to an average of 32 percent (range, 22 to 40 percent).

The most conspicuous electrocradiographic changes were S-T segment depression and T wave inversion observed in three dogs of Group I and all of the animals of Group III throughout the duration of the asanguineous state, which returned to normal within one hour after the completion of the exchange.

All of the animals of Group II subjected to carbon monoxide poisoning without resuscitative measures died within 65 minutes after exposure to the gas. The immediate responses to exposure to the gas consisted of a marked increase in the systolic and diastolic pressures accompanied by severe sinus bradycardia followed by sinus tachycardia, multiple extrasystoles, heart block, and finally cardiorespiratory arrest. The initial bradycardia usually changed to sinus tachycardia when the administration of the carbon monoxide was discontinued. Carbon monoxide blood levels in the control series average 80 percent (range, 70 to 100 percent).

All of the hypothermic animals of Group III subjected to carbon monoxide poisoning died in an average time of 132 minutes (range, 15 minutes to 10 hours). The average COHb concentration in this group was 64.6 percent (range, 54 to 73 percent).

In the five surviving dogs of Group IV, carbon monoxide concentrations of 72.8 percent (range, 52 to 86 percent) were reduced to an average of 8.12 percent (range, 1 to 15 percent) following TBHP. Average duration of the TBHP was 19.8 minutes (range, 14 to 30 minutes).

DISCUSSION

Total body asanguineous hypothermic perfusion provides a rapid method of removing various toxic substances from the circulation. This technique should prove especially useful for materials that cannot be dialized because of their low water solubility or a very strong chemical bond.

The method proved to be safe in normal dogs[1, 7] and patients suffering of liver failure.[4-6]

Carbon monoxide is a rather frequent cause of suicidal and accidental deaths.[8] The toxicity of carbon monoxide is due to its ability to block oxygen transport in the blood and tissues. Rapid distribution of carbon monoxide occurs in animals subjected to toxic concentrations of the gas toward binding sites other than hemoglobin, namely myoglobin and possibly the cytochrome system.[3, 8]

The carbon monoxide bound to the cellular metalloproteins theoretically should be displaced following the law of mass action, if a high concentration of oxyhemoglobin is readily available at the tissue level. This may be induced to some extent with hyperbarically administered oxygen but certainly is more effective through the agency of normal oxyhemoglobin.

In the present study, deeply comatose and hypoxic dogs with carbon monoxide levels well above a lethal dose could be resuscitated by TBHP and returned to a stable physiologic status in an average time of 19.8 minutes. The reduction in red cell mass observed in both normal and carbon monoxide–intoxicated dogs after TBHP was due to resulting hemodilution and did not affect the well-being of the animals. Interestingly a 50 percent carboxyhemoglobin-induced concentration had a detrimental effect, while a 50 percent reduction of the red cell mass was well tolerated. In normal dogs, hemodilution as part of the TBHP was spontaneously corrected in a 48 hour period.

Hypothermia plus steroids and heparinization proved to prolong survival time slightly; however as the only treatment, this combination was inefficacious in salvaging these animals.

In the present communication, carbon monoxide–intoxicated dogs were subjected to TBHP soon after exposure. Experiments to evaluate the usefulness of the method at different time intervals after carbon monoxide intoxication and its clinical applicability is under investigation.

The technical assistance of Mrs. Faye Totero, Mrs. Florence Dent, and Valerie Andrews is gratefully acknowledged.

REFERENCES

1. Agostini, J. C., Basu, A. P., Albert, S. N., and Absolon, K. B.: Total body asanguineous hypothermic perfusion and blood exchange in dogs, Ann. D. C. Med. Soc. **42:** 1, 1973.
2. Albert, S. N.: Blood volume and extracellular fluid, ed. 2, Springfield, Ill., 1971, Charles C Thomas, Publisher, pp. 224-227.
3. Coburn, R., Wallace, H., and Abboud, R.: Redistribution of body carbon monoxide after hemorrhage, Am. J. Physiol. **200:** 868, 1971.
4. Klebanoff, G., Hollander, D., Cosini, A., Standford, W., and Kennerer, W.: Asanguineous hypothermic total body perfusion in the treatment of Stage IV hepatic coma, J. Surg. Res. **12:** 7, 1972.
5. Klebanoff, G., Armstrong, R., Cline, R., Powell, J., and Bedingfield, J.: Resuscitation of a patient in Stage IV hepatic coma using total body washout, J. Surg. Res. **13:** 159, 1972.
6. Kokane, G., and Shuler, S.: Carbon monoxide poisoning, Arch. Surg. **96:** 211, 1968.
7. Neely, W. A., Turner, M. D., and Haihing, J. L.: Survival after asanguineous total body perfusion, SURGERY **54:** 244, 1963.
8. Omura, T., et al.: Function of cytochrome. P-450 of microsomes, Fed. Proc. **24:** 5, 1965.
9. Schilling, C. W., and Adams, B. H.: A study of the convulsive seizure caused by breathing oxygen at high pressures, U.S. Nav. Med. Bull. **33:** 327, 1935.
10. Smith, G., and Sharp, R.: Treatment of carbon monoxide poisoning with oxygen under pressure, Lancet **2:** 905, 1960.
11. Smith, G.: The treatment of carbon monoxide poisoning with oxygen at two atmospheres absolute, Ann. Occup. Hyg. **5:** 259, 1962.
12. Smith, G.: Carbon monoxide poisoning, Ann. N. Y. Acad. Sci. **117:** 684, 1965.
13. Tha, A., Schloegel, C. A., Domansk, E. L., and Goldbaum, L. R.: Gas chromatography procedure for the determination of carboxyhemoglobin in post mortem samples, J. Forensic Sci. **12:** 529, 1967.

Effect of adenosine triphosphate–magnesium chloride administration in shock

Irshad H. Chaudry, Ph.D., Mohammed M. Sayeed, Ph.D., *and*
Arthur E. Baue, M.D., *St. Louis, Mo.*

Hemorrhagic shock was produced in conscious rats by bleeding the animals to a mean arterial pressure of 40 mm. Hg which was maintained for 1 1/2 hours. The animals were then treated by various means. Intravenous infusion of ATP–$MgCl_2$ (adenosine triphosphate-magnesium chloride) before, during, or after a prolonged period of shock proved beneficial in the treatment of shock whereas ATP alone was beneficial only when given in early shock. Animals receiving ATP-$MgCl_2$ had an 83 percent survival rate, whereas those receiving ATP alone or ADP-(adenosine diphosphate–), AMP-(adenosine monophosphate-), or adenosine–$MgCl_2$ or Ringer's lactate had 100 percent mortality rate when treated after prolonged shock. The beneficial effect of high-energy phosphate compounds was specific to ATP–$MgCl_2$. The effect of ATP–$MgCl_2$ does not appear to be through vasodilatation alone since more potent vasodilating agents, such as ADP or AMP failed to produce any beneficial effect.

From the Division of Cell Physiology, Department of Surgery, Washington University School of Medicine and The Jewish Hospital of St. Louis, St. Louis, Mo.

PREVIOUS WORK from this laboratory[7] and by other investigators[19, 20, 23, 26] has shown depletion of liver and kidney ATP (adenosine triphosphate) during shock. Further evidence now indicates that this is a progressive change during shock with not only a decrease in ATP, but with dephosphorylation of ADP (adenosine diphosphate), AMP (adenosine monophosphate), and creatine phosphate, as well. We[8] have recently found that ATP-$MgCl_2$ (adenosine triphosphate–magnesium chloride) given intravenously to animals in shock rapidly restored the tissue ATP levels in the liver and kidney. This did not occur when blood alone, blood plus Ringer's lactate, ADP-$MgCl_2$, or AMP-$MgCl_2$ were given. Although the above-mentioned work suggests that ATP replenishment or priming the system could be helpful in the treatment of shock, such an approach has received little attention since the original work of Talaat, and associates[32] and of Sharma and Eiseman.[29]

The critical place of ATP in carbohydrate metabolism and tissue respiration,[21] as an energy supplier for various intracellular reactions and in muscle contraction[16, 18] is well recognized. In the work reported here, we have demonstrated that infusion of ATP-$MgCl_2$ before, during, or after a prolonged period of shock proved beneficial in the treatment of shock. This effect of ATP-$MgCl_2$ on survival was not shared by ADP-, AMP-, or adenosine-$MgCl_2$ or by ATP alone.

This investigation was supported by United States Army Contract No. DADA-17-69-9165 and United States Public Health Service Grant No. 5 RO 1 HL 12278-05.

Accepted for publication Oct. 10, 1973.

Reprint requests: Dr. Irshad H. Chaudry, Dept. of Biochemistry, Concordia University, 1455 de Maisonneuve, Montreal, Canada.

METHODS

ATP-$MgCl_2$ prior to hemorrhage. Albino Holtzman rats, weighing 250 to 280 grams were fasted for 16 hours prior to the experiment but were allowed water ad libitum. The animals were injected either intraperitoneally or intramuscularly with a mixture of ATP-$MgCl_2$ (0.25 ml., total; final concentration, 25 mM. each) and were placed back in the cage. In certain experiments, along with ATP-$MgCl_2$ phosphoenol pyruvate (20 mM.) and pyruvate kinase (4 U.) were also injected intramuscularly.

One hour after the intraperitoneal or intramuscular injection of ATP-$MgCl_2$ and other compounds as described above, the rats were lightly anesthetized with ether at room temperature and restrained in a supine position. Both femoral arteries were cannulated with polyethylene tubing (PE-50), and heparin (400 U.) was injected into each artery. One of the cannulas was connected to a 1.75 M. long PE-50 tubing, calibrated in millimeters of Hg, for monitoring arterial blood pressure. The above method of measuring blood pressure was compared to another method in which a Hewlett-Packard pressure transducer (Model No. 267BC) and a Sanborn 150 recorder were used, and blood pressure was found to be identical both under control conditions (i.e., prior to bleeding) as well as at various stages of shock. The other cannula was connected to a 10 ml. heparinized glass syringe which served as a blood reservoir. The animals were then allowed to awaken. The duration of anesthesia was about 45 minutes. Following this, they were bled rapidly within ten minutes to a mean arterial pressure of 40 mm Hg. Small amounts of blood were removed from time to time in order to maintain the blood pressure (B.P.) at 40 mm. Hg during the first 30 minutes. Maximal bleedout occurred in about 30 minutes following the onset of bleeding. Usually about 45 minutes from the onset of bleeding, the pressure began to fall below 40 mm. Hg and, approximately, 50 percent of the shed blood had to be returned slowly to maintain the B.P. at 40 mm. Hg for a total time of 1½ hours.

At the end of 1½ hours, the remaining blood in the reservoir was slowly returned (1 ml. in two to three minutes). The cannulas were removed, the vessels were ligated, the incisions were closed, and the rats were placed back in the cage. Food and water was then allowed ad libitum.

ATP-$MgCl_2$ intravenously at various stages of shock. In this set of experiments, the left femoral vein was also cannulated along with the femoral arteries. The protocol for bleeding was carried out as described above, except that ATP-$MgCl_2$ (0.25 ml., 0.1 ml. at two-minute intervals) was given intravenously either (1) following maximum bleedout, (2) thirty minutes following maximum bleedout, or (3) at the end of 1½ hours at 40 mm. Hg. Following the infusion at ATP-$MgCl_2$, the B.P. rapidly dropped from 40 mm. Hg to approximately 30 mm. Hg and then increased after approximately 30 seconds to above 40 mm. Hg; additional blood had to be removed to maintain the B.P. at 40 mm. Hg. At the end of 1½ hours, the remaining blood in the reservoir was slowly returned (1 ml. in two to three minutes). The cannulas were removed, the vessels were ligated, the incisions were closed, and the rats were placed back in the cage. Food and water was then allowed ad libitum.

ATP or $MgCl_2$ intravenously at various stages of shock. In these experiments, ATP or $MgCl_2$ (25 mM., 0.25 ml.) alone was given intravenously either 30 minutes following maximum bleedout or at the end of 1½ hours of shock.

ADP, AMP, or adenosine along with $MgCl_2$ after 1½ hours of shock. In this set of experiments, either ADP-$MgCl_2$ (0.25 ml., 25 mM. each), AMP-$MgCl_2$ (0.25 ml., 25 mM. each), or adenosine-$MgCl_2$ (0.25 ml., 10 mM. each) were given after 1½ hours of shock, followed by return of the remaining shed blood.

Blood plus Ringer's lactate after 1½ hours of shock. In this set of experiments, the animals received the remaining shed blood plus Ringer's lactate (equal to the maximum

Table I. *Effect of ATP administration**

Conditions†	*Mean body Weight (Gm.)*	*No. of survivors*	*No. of deaths*	*Survival rate (%)*
ATP-$MgCl_2$ I.M. or I. P. before shock	266	37	7	84.1
ATP-$MgCl_2$, PEP and PK I. M. before shock	272	10	2	83.3
ATP-$MgCl_2$ I. V. following MBO	261	28	6	82.4
ATP-$MgCl_2$ I. V. 30 min following MBO	260	10	2	83.3
ATP-$MgCl_2$ I. V. after 90 min	264	15	5	75
ATP alone I. V. 30 min following MBO	267	4	6	40
ATP or $MgCl_2$ alone I. V. after 90 min	274	0	20	0
Blood + Ringer's lactate	265	0	7	0
Controls (receiving saline)	262	0	23	0

*Control animals were run concurrently with the treatment groups on the same day. ATP-$MgCl_2$ was administered either I.P. or I.M. before hemorrhage. In another set of experiments, ATP-$MgCl_2$ was given I.V. following MBO, 30 minutes following MBO, or at the end of the experiments. In some experiments, ATP or $MgCl_2$ separately were given. Control animals received saline (0.25 ml.) and in the second set of control animals, the animals received blood + Ringer's lactate (approximately 8 ml.). For details, see "Methods" section.

†I.M., Intramuscularly; I.P., intraperitoneally; I.V., intravenously; MBO, maximum bleedout; PEP, phosphoenol pyruvate; PK, pyruvate kinase.

bleedout volume) at 1½ hours and were then treated as described above.

Control animals. Control animals were prepared and bled in the same way and received 0.25 ml. of saline before hemorrhage or at various stages of hemorrhagic shock as described above with the blood returned after 1½ hours.

Criteria for survival. An animal was considered to survive if he lived at least 24 hours following the termination of the experiment. Many animals were allowed to survive for longer periods of up to two months and showed no ill effects.

RESULTS

ATP-$MgCl_2$ before and during shock. As shown in Table I, administration of ATP-$MgCl_2$ intramuscularly or intraperitoneally before bleeding, following maximum bleedout (MBO) or 30 minutes after MBO proved beneficial for survival of the animals. The survival rate produced by such administration was 83 percent as compared to the 100 percent mortality rate in animals receiving saline, i.e., the control animals and animals receiving blood plus Ringer's lactate.

ATP-$MgCl_2$ at the end of shock period. The beneficial effect of ATP-$MgCl_2$ administration was apparent even when this complex was given at the end of the shock period, i.e., 1½ hours from the onset of bleeding. The percentage survival in these animals was 75 percent (Table I). The infusion of ATP by itself without $MgCl_2$ at 30 minutes following the onset of bleeding did have some beneficial effect; however, the animals failed to survive shock when ATP or $MgCl_2$ were given separately at the end of the 1½ hour shock period.

ADP-, AMP-, or adenosine-$MgCl_2$ infusion. Since ATP is degraded rapidly in the blood, and by tissues, it is possible that the beneficial effect of ATP seen above could have been due to one or all of the breakdown products of ATP rather than to ATP specifically. In order to test this, ADP, AMP, or adenosine along with $MgCl_2$ was infused at the end of the shock period. As shown in Table II, the mortality rate was 100 percent in animals receiving the breakdown products of ATP.

Groups of animals other than those receiving ATP-$MgCl_2$ died within one to three hours while the majority of those receiving ATP-$MgCl_2$ survived for two months at which time they were killed.

Effect of ATP-$MgCl_2$ treatment on bleedout volume. Table III shows that an average of 8.4 ml. of blood was removed from control rats in order to maintain them at 40 mm. Hg (maximum bleedout volume).

However, when ATP-$MgCl_2$ was given intramuscularly before bleeding, more blood had to be removed in order to maintain the animals at the above pressure. However, the situation was different when ATP-$MgCl_2$ was administered intraperitoneally. Intramuscular injection of ATP-$MgCl_2$ resulted in increased maximum bleedout whereas intraperitoneal injection resulted in a slightly decreased maximum bleedout.

The over-all effect of ATP-$MgCl_2$, when given intravenously, was to increase the maximum bleedout volume. Immediately after the infusion, there was a transient decrease in arterial pressure to about 30 mm. Hg. Within 30 seconds, the pressure increased above 40 mm. Hg, and further blood had to be removed to maintain this pressure. This occurred when ATP-$MgCl_2$ was given after maximum bleedout or 30 minutes after maximum bleedout (Table IV). When ATP was given alone without $MgCl_2$, the blood pressure decreased and stayed below 40 mm. Hg, and additional blood had to be returned in order to maintain this blood pressure.

DISCUSSION

It has been proposed by many investigators that depletion of tissue energy stores below a critical level is the primary mechanism for the ultimate collapse and death of animals in various forms of shock.[10, 20, 23] The difficulty is that no one knows what a critically low level of ATP or other nucleotides is. It has generally been thought that as long as any ADP or AMP remains, it can be phosphorylated back to ATP. Although we have demonstrated low levels of ATP, ADP, and AMP in shock,[7] we do not know if these are below some critical level. If the hypothesis is valid that critically low levels of energy are reached in severe shock, then if by some means the tissue ATP levels could be restored, the animal may survive shock.

There are many ways in which one may attempt to restore the levels of tissue high-energy phosphate compounds. The work of Triner and associates[33] showed that the

Table II. *Effect of ADP, AMP, and adenosine administration**

Conditions	*Mean body weight (Gm.)*	*No. of survivors*	*No. of deaths*	*Survival rate (%)*
ADP-$MgCl_2$	274	0	8	0
AMP-$MgCl_2$	268	0	6	0
Adenosine-$MgCl_2$	270	0	6	0

*Either ADP, AMP or adenosine along with $MgCl_2$ was given intravenously at the end of the shock period (1½ hours). For details, see "Methods" section.

Table III. *Maximum bleedout volume in various groups**

Conditions	*Maximum bleedout (ml.)*	*Blood remaining in syringe at 90 min.*
Control animals	8.4 (3.20 ml./100 Gm. body weight)	4.3
ATP-$MgCl_2$ I. M. 1 hr. before bleeding	10.6 (3.98 ml./100 Gm. body weight)	5.1
ATP-PEP-PK-$MgCl_2$ I. M. 1 hr. before bleeding	9.8 (3.60 ml./100 Gm. body weight)	5.4
ATP-$MgCl_2$ I. P. before bleeding	8.0 (3.00 ml./100 Gm. body weight)	4.6

*ATP–$MgCl_2$ (25 mM. each, 0.25 ml. volume) was given I.M., intramuscularly, I.P., intraperitoneally or I.V., intravenously as described above. Control animals received 0.25 ml. of saline.

administration of glucose prolonged immediate survival following hemorrhagic shock in rabbits. Subsequently, it was reported by Moffat and colleagues[24] that administration of hypertonic glucose during the stage of physiologic decompensation enhanced tolerance to hypovolemia in dogs. Similar results in humans have been reported by McNamara and co-workers.[22] The above investigators[22, 24, 33] proposed that exogenous glucose prolongs survival by providing energy substrate. This is in agreement with the hypothesis that increased ATP synthesis resulting from stimulation of glycolysis plays an important role in adaptation to acute hemorrhage. The proposal that exogenous glucose prolongs survival by providing

Table IV. *Blood volume in syringe before and after treatment*

Conditions	*Maximum bleedout (ml.)*	*Volume before treatment (ml.)*	*Volume after treatment (ml.)**	*Blood remaining in syringe at 90 minutes*
ATP-$MgCl_2$ I. V. after MBO	8.3 (3.18 ml./100 Gm. body weight)	8.3	9.0	7.0
ATP-$MgCl_2$ I. V. 30 minutes after MBO	8.3 (3.19 ml./100 Gm. body weight)	7.0	7.6	6.2
ATP alone I. V. 30 minutes after MBO	8.4 (3.14 ml./100 Gm. body weight)	7.1	3.9	2.3
ATP-$MgCl_2$ I. V. at 90 min	8.5 (3.21 ml./100 Gm body weight)	4.4		4.4

*Infusion of ATP–$MgCl_2$ following maximum bleedout or 30 minutes following maximum bleedout resulted in raising the B.P. above 40 mm. Hg, and additional blood had to be removed to maintain the B.P. at 40 mm. Hg. This is referred to as volume after treatment.

energy does not appear to be true in view of the studies of Stoner and colleagues.[31] These investigators showed that the oxidation of ^{14}C-glucose to $^{14}CO_2$ was decreased by 48 percent in the shocked rats as compared to the control animals. Decreased $^{14}CO_2$ production from ^{14}C-glucose in dogs subjected to hemorrhagic hypotension was also reported by Gump and co-workers.[17] The above studies[17, 31] suggest that the beneficial effect of glucose seen by other investigators[22, 24, 33] was not through provision of energy since oxidation of glucose to CO_2 is decreased during shock. It is much more likely that the beneficial effect of glucose could have been due to hemodynamic effects produced by hypertonic glucose. Subsequently, it was reported by Chick and co-workers[9] that administration of Krebs-cycle intermediates increased 24 hour survival in rabbits, and they postulated that increased survival was due to stimulation of ATP synthesis. These workers, however, did not measure the tissue ATP levels, and thus it is possible that administration of Krebs-cycle intermediates produces vasodilation[14] rather than increased ATP synthesis.

Perhaps the most direct approach for raising ATP levels of a tissue is to infuse ATP rather than administer agents which would stimulate ATP synthesis. This approach has been used by Talaat and associates[32] and Sharma and Eiseman[29] who showed that ATP was protective if given prior to bleeding but also that it was not protective if it was administered thereafter. The present studies extended the observations of the above workers[29, 32] and showed that administration of ATP-$MgCl_2$ before, during, or even after a period of severe shock, had a beneficial effect on the survival of rats. The essential difference between the present studies and those of others[29, 32] is that we gave $MgCl_2$ along with ATP rather than ATP alone. ATP is a biologically complexing agent[25,28] and, when given alone, may chelate divalent cations from the vascular system and produce a different hemodynamic effect. Such undesirable effects may be eliminated by giving equimolar amounts of $MgCl_2$ along with ATP. Moreover it has been shown that Mg in vitro and in vivo inhibits the deaminiation and dephosphorylation of ATP by tissue.[16] Thus, by giving ATP along with $MgCl_2$, higher concentration of ATP could be available to tissues as compared to when ATP is given alone. The experiments described in Table I indicate that ATP when given alone is protective if given during the early stages of shock but not if given thereafter. This is in agreement with the observations of Sharma and Eiseman.[29] However, the beneficial effect of ATP was seen even in a later stage of shock when ATP was given in combination with $MgCl_2$, i.e., ATP-$MgCl_2$ complex. Although the survival was measured over 24 hours, the majority of the rats receiving ATP-$MgCl_2$ survived for more than two months without any noticeable side effects.

Since ATP is susceptible to degradation by enzymes in the body, the possibility existed that the beneficial effect of ATP seen above was due to one or more than one of the breakdown products of ATP. In order to test this, ADP-, AMP-, and adenosine-$MgCl_2$ were infused; however, none of these had any beneficial effect. The beneficial effect of the nucleotide therefore resides in the terminal phosphate of ATP.

The administration of ATP to animals could produce vasodilatation[11] and other hemodynamic effects or provide ATP directly to tissues in which ATP levels were lowered or both. The possibility that ATP in the present experiments in combination with $MgCl_2$ produced beneficial effects through vasodilatation alone does not seem to hold true because of the fact that when (1) ATP-$MgCl_2$ was given, more blood was removed rather than given to maintain the same pressure (Table IV), and (2) agents such as ADP and AMP which are more potent vasodilators had no beneficial effect. However, when ATP was given alone, the blood pressure dropped and stayed low, and blood had to be returned to maintain the B.P. at 40 mm. Hg (Table IV). These findings strongly suggest that the action of ATP-$MgCl_2$ was not through vasodilatation but that ATP alone does act as a vasodilating agent, since its infusion without $MgCl_2$ resulted in spontaneous take-back of shed blood. Another possible explanation is that ATP-$MgCl_2$ has a beneficial effect on the circulation, on microcirculatory blood flow, or regional perfusion which was not provided by returning blood plus Ringer's lactate. These animals failed to survive shock when blood plus Ringer's lactate was given.

The possibility that the beneficial effect of ATP-$MgCl_2$ in the present experiments is through provision of energy is much more attractive but also very controversial. Although it is a popular belief that ATP does not cross the cell membrane,[3, 15] there are many experimental observations which contradict this concept. Buchthal and associates[4, 5] have shown that ATP added to the medium bathing isolated muscle fibers induced their contraction. Thus, however, could be a surface effect. More recently, Abood and colleagues,[1] Boyd and Forrester,[2] and Forrester[13] have provided evidence that ATP is released from active skeletal muscle and Chaudry and Gould[6] have shown that [^{14}C] ATP can enter skeletal muscle cells. The evidence presented by the above investigators[1, 2, 6, 13] strongly suggests that the release and uptake of ATP is a physiological process. In view of this information, it appears that the beneficial effect of ATP seen in the present experiments could be through a "priming effect" of this compound on the resynthesis of cellular ATP. It is recognized that the amount of ATP administered is small as compared to total ATP of the organism. The experiments of Ely[12] and Sharma and Eiseman[29] have shown that administered ATP is selectively taken up by liver, spleen, heart, and kidney. More recently, Ziegelhoffer and colleagues[34] have demonstrated that small amounts of exogenous ATP (1 mM.) but not ADP or IMP (inosine monophosphate) increased the ATP and total of adenine nucleotides of the myocardium of the hypoxic dog. We have previously shown severe depletion of liver and kidney ATP during shock.[7] It is possible, therefore, that administered ATP in our experiments raised the ATP levels of liver and kidney and was, therefore, protective to the shocked animals. Preliminary experiments have indicated that the infusion of ATP-$MgCl_2$, but not ADP- or AMP-$MgCl_2$ restored the nucleotide contents of liver and kidney.[8] It should be noted that the amount of ATP given to animals in the present experiments was approximately 6 mg. per 100 G. of body weight which is much less than the lethal dose described by Green and Stoner.[16]

Preliminary experiments from our laboratory have shown that ATP-$MgCl_2$ added to the whole blood in vitro did not cause platelet aggregation even after two hours.* However, it is well known that ADP causes the aggregation of platelets.[27, 30] The fact

*Chaudry, I. H., Sayeed, M. M., and Baue, A. E.: Unpublished observations.

that ADP and not ATP causes platelet aggregation may also explain why ATP and not ADP infusion was beneficial to animals in shock. This is on the assumption that platelet aggregation is harmful to the survival of animals. Moreover, it is also possible that ATP slowly breaking down in the bloodstream might have a different effect from that of exogenous ADP, AMP, or adenosine administered directly.

The idea that ATP may have some specific salutary effects on shock is controversial because: (1) ATP is thought to be rapidly broken down or degraded when given into the blood; (2) ATP has been thought not to be able to cross cell membranes; and (3) ATP has profound hemodynamic effects. The present study provides evidence that ATP does have a salutary effect. Potential explanations for this effect and speculation about its mode of action are presented. Future studies using labeled ATP may help to better define how it works and the fate of the ATP which was injected.

The authors wish to thank G. J. Planer, D. Buls, and L. Fishman for excellent technical assistance, and for their skill and assistance in typing of this manuscript, we wish to thank Ms. Gail Perry and Ms. Mary J. Hunt.

REFERENCES

1. Abood, L. G., Koketsu, K., and Miyamato, S.: Outflux of various phosphates during membrane depolarization of excitable tissues, Am. J. Physiol. **202:** 469, 1962.
2. Boyd, I. A., and Forrester, T.: The release of adenosine triphosphate from frog skeletal muscle *in vitro,* J. Physiol. **199:** 115, 1968.
3. Boyle, P. J., and Conway, E. J.: Potassium accumulation in muscle and associated changes, J. Physiol. **100:** 1, 1941.
4. Buchthal, F., Deutsch, A., and Knappies, G. G.: Release of contraction and changes in birefringence caused by adenosine triphosphate in isolated cross-striated muscle fibers, Acta Physiol. Scand. **8:** 271, 1944.
5. Buchthal, F., Deutsch, A. and Knappies, G. G.: Further investigation on the effect of adenosine triphosphate and related phosphorus compounds on isolated striated muscle fibers, Acta Physiol. Scand. **11:** 325, 1946.
6. Chaudry, I. H., and Gould, M. K.: Evidence for the uptake of ATP by rat soleus muscle *in vitro,* Biochim. Biophys. Acta **196:** 320, 1970.
7. Chaudry, I. H., Sayeed, M M., and Baue, A. E.: Alterations in adenosine nucleotides in hemorrhagic shock, Surg. Forum **23:** 1, 1972.
8. Chaudry, I. H., Planer, G. J., Sayeed, M. M., and Baue, A. E.: ATP depletion and replenishment in hemorrhagic shock, Surg. Forum **24:** 77, 1973.
9. Chick, W. L., Weiner, R., Cascarano, J., and Zweifach, B. W.: Influence of Krebs-cycle intermediates on survival in hemorrhagic shock, Am. J. Physiol. **215:** 1107, 1968.
10. Crowell, J. W., Jones, C. E., and Smith, E. E.: Effect of allopurinol on hemorrhagic shock, Am. J. Physiol. **216:** 744, 1969.
11. Drury, A. N., and Gyorgyi, S. A.: The physiological activity of adenine compounds with special reference to their action upon the mammalian heart, J. Physiol. **58:** 213, 1929.
12. Ely, J. O.: Distribution in the rat of injected radioactive "muscle shock factor" of Green, J. Franklin Inst. **238:** 378, 1944.
13. Forrester, T.: An estimate of adenosine triphosphate release into the venous effluent from exercising human forearm muscle, J. Physiol. **224:** 611, 1972.
14. Frohlich, E. D.: Vascular effects of the Krebs intermediate metabolites, Am. J. Physiol. **208:** 149, 1965.
15. Glynn, I. M.: Membrane adenosine triphosphatase and cation transport, Br. Med. Bull. **24:** 165, 1968.
16. Green, H. N., and Stoner, H. B.: Biological actions of the adenine nucleotides, London, 1950, H. K. Lewis & Co. Ltd.
17. Gump, F. E., Long, C. L., Wong, M., and Kinney, J. M.: Exogenous glucose as an energy substrate in experimental hemorrhagic shock, Surg. Gynecol. Obstet. **136:** 611, 1973.
18. Hajuda, S., and Gyorgyi, S. A.: Action of DOC and serum on the frog heart, Am. J. Physiol. **168:** 159, 1952.
19. LePage, G. A.: Biological energy transformations during shock as shown by tissue analyses, Am. J. Physiol. **146:** 267, 1946.
20. Loiselle, J. M., and Denstedt, O. F.: Biochemical changes during acute physiological failure in the rat. II. The behavior of adenine and pyridine nucleotides of the liver during shock, Can. J. Biochem. **42:** 21, 1964.
21. Long, C.: The *in vitro* oxidation of pyruvic and ketobutyric acids by ground preparations of pigeon brain: The effect of inorganic phosphate and adenine nucleotide, Biochem. J. **37:** 215, 1943.
22. McNamara, J. J., Molot, M. D., Dunn, R. A., and Stremple, J. F.: Effect of hypertonic glucose in hypovolemic shock in man, Ann. Surg. **176:** 247, 1972.

23. McShan, W. H., Potter, V. R., Goldman, A., Shipley, E. G., and Meyer, R. K.: Biological energy transformations during shock as shown by blood chemistry, Am. J. Physiol. **145:** 93, 1945.
24. Moffat, J. G., King, J. A. C., and Drucker, W. R.: Tolerance to prolonged hypovolemic shock: Effect of infusion of an energy substrate, Surg. Forum **19:** 5, 1968.
25. Ohnishi, T., and Ebashi, S.: Spectrophotometrical measurements of instantaneous calcium binding of the releasing factor of muscle. J. Biochem. (Tokyo) **54:** 506, 1963.
26. Rosenbaum, D. K., Frank, E. D., Ruttenberg, A. M., and Frank, H. A.: High energy phosphate content of liver tissue in experimental hemorrhagic shock, Am. J. Physiol. **188:** 86, 1957.
27. Salzman, E. W., Neri, L. L., Chambers, D. P., and Ashford, T. P.: Regulation of platelet volume, *in* Deutsch, E., Gerlach, E., and Moser, H., editors: Metabolism and membrane permeability of erythrocytes and thrombocytes, Stuttgardt, 1968, Georg Thieme Verlag, p. 274.
28. Sanui, H., and Pace, N.: Effect of ATP, EDTA, and EGTA on the simultaneous binding of Na, K, Mg and Ca by rat liver microsomes, J. Cell Physiol. **69:** 11, 1967.
29. Sharma, G. P., and Eiseman, B.: Protective effect of ATP in experimental hemorrhagic shock, SURGERY **59:** 66, 1966.
30. Spaet, T. H., and Zucker, M. B.: Mechanism of platelet plug formation and the role of adenosine, diphosphate, Am. J. Physiol. **206:** 1267, 1964.
31. Stoner, H. B., Heath, D. F., and Collins, O. M.: The metabolism of [^{14}C] glucose, [^{14}C] fructose and [2-^{14}C] pyruvate after limb ischemia in the rat, Biochem. J. **76:** 135, 1960.
32. Talaat, S. M., Massion, W. H., and Schilling, J. A.: Effects of adenosine triphosphate administration in irreversible hemorrhagic shock, SURGERY **55:** 813, 1964.
33. Triner, L., Mraz, M., and Chemelarova, M.: The favourable effect of glucose and glucose with insulin administered in dextran solution on the course of hemorrhagic shock in rabbits, Physiol. Bohemoslov. **13:** 87, 1964.
34. Ziegelhoffer, A., Fedelesova, M., and Kostolansky, S.: Specific ATP action on metabolism of isolated heart. Influence of pH, divalent cation concentration and stability of complexes, Acta Biol. Med. Germ. **28:** 893, 1972.

Experiences in the management of surgically correctable biliary atresia

Eitoku Arima, M.D., Eric W. Fonkalsrud, M.D., *and* **Robert C. Neerhout, M.D.,**
Los Angeles, Calif.

Ten patients with surgically correctable extrahepatic biliary atresia have undergone surgical biliary-enteric drainage at the UCLA Hospital during the past 16 years. During the same period, 39 additional patients underwent biopsy or other operative procedures for intrahepatic atresia. Three categories of "correctable" atresia are identified: Type A with a large cystic dilatation of the proximal duct; Type B with a moderately dilated proximal common duct measuring 4 to 12 mm. in diameter; and Type C with a blindly ending proximal duct less than 3 mm. in diameter. The prognosis for long-term survival with resolution of cirrhosis is good in patients with Types A and B atresia, provided biliary-enteric drainage is established before the age of four months. Five of the eight patients in the present study who underwent biliary-to-intestinal anastomosis before the age of four months are still alive and well. Choledochojejunostomy is less likely to be complicated by obstruction or cholangitis than is drainage to the duodenum. Patients with Type C atresia may occasionally benefit from jejunal anastomosis to the hepatoduodenal ligament if performed before the age of three months. A few patients may have a combination of intrahepatic and extrahepatic atresia.

From the Departments of Surgery and Pediatrics, UCLA School of Medicine, Los Angeles, Calif.

CONGENITAL biliary atresia, although uncommon, remains one of the most disappointing and controversial malformations of early infancy. The average survival time of infants with this condition is only 19 months unless some form of permanently effective drainage can be established surgically between the biliary ductal system and the gastrointestinal tract.[5] Since the report by Ladd[7] in 1935 of the first successful surgical correction in a patient with biliary atresia, methods to establish the diagnosis and to determine the optimal time for treatment of this malformation have been a source of extensive discussion between pediatricians and surgeons. Although Thaler and Gellis[12] expressed the opinion that a delay until four months of age should occur before an exploratory laparotomy is performed for obstructive jaundice, most surgeons disagree with this view, since cirrhosis may become irreversible by four to five months of age, even when adequate surgical drainage is established at that time.

The surgically correctable extrahepatic form of atresia has been reported to be present in 5 percent to 20 percent of patients with biliary atresia. In a survey of its mem-

Supported by the United States Public Health Service Grant No. HL 14333.

Presented at the Sixth Annual Meeting of the Pacific Association of Pediatric Surgeons, San Diego, Calif., April 18-20, 1973.

Accepted for publication Oct. 10, 1973.

Table I. *Summary of ten patients with correctable biliary atresia*

Patient No.	*Sex*	*Date of birth*	*Type of atresia*	*Age at operation*	*Type of operation*	*Complications*	*Present age*
1	F	8/31/56	B	6 wk.	Choledochoduodenostomy	Cholangitis, biliary obstruction	
				13 mo.	Choledochojejunostomy	Biliary obstruction	
				4½ yr.	Revision of choledochojejunostomy	Mild cirrhosis	17 yr., 1 mo.
2	F	4/24/58	C	6 mo.	Tube drainage of duct	Cholangitis, sepsis	Died at 1 yr., 8 mo.
3	F	3/27/59	B	6 wk.	Choledochoduodenostomy	Cholangitis	
				6 mo.	Revision of choledochoduodenostomy	Cholangitis	
				5 yr.	Splenectomy for hypersplenism	Hepatomegaly, varices	14 yr., 6 mo.
4	F	6/ 5/59	B	4 mo.	Choledochoduodenostomy	Cholangitis	
				6 mo.	Revision of choledochoduodenostomy	Intestinal obstruction	
				14 yr.	Mesocaval shunt for varices		14 yr., 3 mo.
5	F	6/10/60	C	8 wk.	Choledochoduodenostomy	Cholangitis	
				6 mo.	Hepaticoduodenostomy	Died postoperatively with hepatic failure and sepsis	Died at 6 mo.
6	M	5/ 6/62	C	2½ mo.	Longmire procedure	Biliary obstruction	
				6 mo.	Persistent jaundice		
				3 yr.	Revision of Longmire procedure	Enteric fistula	
				3⅓ yr.	Closure of enteric fistula	Sepsis, hepatic failure	Died at 3 yr., 5 mo.
7	F	8/31/69	B	6 wk.	Open-liver biopsy		
				7 mo.	Choledochojejunostomy	Ascites and sepsis	Died at 10 mo.
8	M	10/20/69	C	3 mo.	Hepaticojejunostomy	Persistent jaundice	
				3½ mo.	Catheter drainage of duct	Cholangitis and sepsis	Died at 11 mo.
9	F	7/19/72	A	4 mo.	Choledochojejunostomy	Mild ascites	1 yr., 3 mo.
10	M	8/ 3/72	C	2 mo.	Hepaticojejunostomy	Transient ascites	1 yr., 2 mo.

bers conducted by the Surgical Section of the American Academy of Pediatrics in 1966, only 102 of 843 collected cases of biliary atresia were considered to have been correctable (12 percent), and very alarming was the observation that only 53 of these patients were alive at the time of the survey.[9] Shiraki and associates[10] reported 62 cases of biliary atresia, with successful establishment of biliary drainage to the intestinal tract in only four of the 11 patients who were considered correctable. Long-term patient survival after operations for extrahepatic biliary atresia has been recorded infrequently in the literature.

The present study was undertaken to summarize the experience at the UCLA Hospital with ten patients who have undergone biliary-enteric anastomosis for extrahepatic biliary atresia during the past 16 years. This review is concerned with (1) the relationship of age at the time of surgical drainage to long-term survival and (2) the correlation between type of biliary-enteric anastomosis and incidence of postoperative morbidity.

CLINICAL MATERIAL

During the period from 1956 through 1972, 49 infants with biliary atresia under-

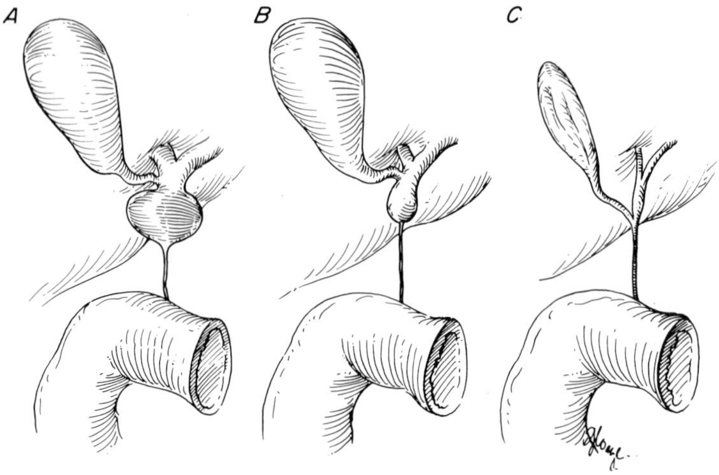

Fig. 1. Three types of correctable biliary atresia observed in the present study. *A,* Type A: marked dilatation of the common hepatic duct, almost cystic in appearance, with an atretic segment extending to the duodenum. *B,* Type B: moderate dilatation of the common hepatic duct. *C,* Type C: small common hepatic duct with atretic segment extending to the duodenum.

went a variety of operations at the UCLA Hospital, including liver biopsy, exploration of the hepatoduodenal ligament, biliary ductal or lymphatic drainage to the intestine, and liver allotransplantation. Ten of the 49 patients (20 percent) were considered to have a "surgically correctable" extrahepatic form of atresia with some bile-containing ductal structure present in the hepatoduodenal ligament. This report is concerned primarily with an analysis of the course of these ten patients, seven of whom were female (Table I).

Three types of proximal bile duct anatomy have been described in children with biliary atresia[9] and were recognized in these patients. A large cystic dilatation 2½ cm. in diameter at the confluence of the major hepatic ducts with an atretic fibrous strand extending to the duodenum (Type A) was identified in one patient (Patient 9); no intrahepatic ductal obstruction was observed on the liver biopsy (Fig. 1, *A*). A moderately dilated remnant of common bile duct, 4 to 12 mm. in diameter (Type B), was present in Patients 1, 3, 4, and 7 (Fig. 1, *B*). A small common hepatic duct less than 3 mm. in diameter (Type C) was present in Patients 2, 5, 6, 8, and 10 (Fig. 1, *C*). The gallbladders were atretic in all patients with Types B and C atresia. Four of the five patients with the Type C external atresia died within the first four years of life, and each was noted at autopsy to have severe biliary cirrhosis with a few distended intrahepatic ducts and spaces filled with bile sludge. The histologic appearance of the liver in each case suggested fewer intrahepatic ducts than are normally seen and some degree of intrahepatic atresia. One of the patients (Patient 10) is alive and free of jaundice ten months after a central hepaticojejunostomy.

Three of the four patients with Type B atresia are currently alive, and each is more than 14 years old. Each of these three patients underwent biliary-enteric anastomosis at four months of age or earlier. In contrast, the fourth patient with Type B atresia (Patient 7) underwent biliary drainage at age seven months and died three months later with severe cirrhosis and no drainage of bile from the duct. This patient had a dense plug of bile sludge in the gallbladder and the distended common bile duct. One of the three surviving patients (Patient 1) was available for recent evaluation; results of her liver function studies showed mild elevation of alkaline phosphatase but normal bilirubin, although the liver extends 3 cm. below the right costal margin. Patient 4 experienced repeated episodes of cholangitis with fever and jaundice and developed esophageal varices with repeated hemorrhage. A mesocaval shunt was performed at age 14 years, and choledochojejunostomy is planned because of repeated cholangitis. A liver biopsy at the time of operation showed moderate periportal fibrosis with chronic inflammation adjacent to the major bile ducts.

The patient with Type A ductal obstruction experienced gradual relief from her jaundice and transient ascites during the first six months after choledochojejunostomy. She has remained anicteric and has grown and developed above the seventy-fifth percentile.

Four patients underwent choledochoduodenostomy as the primary biliary drainage procedure; each has since required at least one revision of the anastomosis. One has undergone conversion to a choledochojejunostomy and is now 17 years of age (Patient 1). Another was converted to a hepaticoduodenostomy because of severe cholangitis and sepsis and died postoperatively (Patient 5). The two others (Patients 3 and 4) are still alive, but both have experienced repeated episodes of cholangitis and have developed cirrhosis with bleeding esophageal varices; each has required at least one operation for treatment of portal hypertension.

Although the experience with Roux-en-Y choledochojejeunostomy in patients with extrahepatic atresia in this series is limited (Patients 1, 7, 8, 9, and 10), the data suggest that anastomotic complications and cholangitis are less likely to occur with this procedure than when the biliary anastomosis is made to the duodenum. One of the patients who underwent choledochojejunostomy for Type B atresia (Patient 1) is alive, as are the one patient with Type A atresia (Patient 9) and one patient with Type C atresia (Patient 10). In Patient 8 with Type C atresia who had an initial Roux-en-Y jejunal segment placed over the hepatoduodenal ligament with insertion of a drainage tube into the tiny proximal bile duct, sepsis developed after a second operation to reinsert the drainage catheter; however, this does not necessarily reflect a complication of choledochojejunostomy since the patient had intrahepatic atresia of moderately severe degree. Tube drainage was eventually followed by death in Patient 2 who did not undergo an exploratory operation until six months of age, by which time severe cirrhosis was present.

DISCUSSION

Not until the recent report by Lou and associates,[8] which provided a 37-year follow-up study on the fourth patient with biliary atresia to be operated upon by Ladd, was a well-documented report available of a long-term surviving patient with biliary atresia. This case and that reported by Cameron and Bunton[1] indicated that when satisfactory biliary-enteric drainage is established before nine weeks of age, reversal of cirrhosis, liver regeneration, and production of normal bile are likely to occur within three years. Although late liver biopsies are not available for the three long-term surviving patients in the present study, a biopsy of Patient 1 taken at 4½ years of age showed minimal evidence of cirrhosis in contrast to the marked periportal scarring seen on the initial biopsy obtained at six weeks of age.

Further evidence is presented in this study to support the view that when drainage is established before the age of four months in a patient with a correctable form of biliary atresia, long-term survival is possible. Moderate-to-severe cirrhosis has been detected in infants with atresia as young as six weeks of age. One infant with atresia in our institution had moderate cirrhosis when a biopsy specimen was taken at the age of one week. Five of the eight patients who underwent biliary-to-intestinal drainage before the age of four months are still alive. On the other hand, when drainage is deferred an additional few months, as occurred in Patients 2 and 7, biliary cirrhosis becomes irreversible, minimal quantities of bile may be drained, and early death usually results. Previous studies have shown that when the common bile duct of the primate is completely occluded for more than two months before enteric drainage is established, cirrhosis may be fatal.[3] Five infants with neonatal hepatitis underwent liver biopsy under general anesthesia at the UCLA Hospital during the past 16 years; none experienced a progression of cirrhosis or died as a result of complications attributable to the operation or anesthetic.

Since adequate permanent biliary-enteric drainage has been so difficult to achieve in infants with extrahepatic atresia, it is our opinion that a Roux-en-Y choledochojejunostomy should be used as the initial drainage procedure. Catheter stents may be used to support the anastomosis and to maintain patency when feasible. Cholangitis and obstruction are more common after choledochoduodenostomy, as has been noted previously in our experience with patients who have undergone enteric drainage of choledochal cysts. These complications are not well tolerated in an infant with a cirrhotic liver.

Kasai and associates,[6] Suruga and colleagues,[11] and others have indicated that anastomosis of a Roux-en-Y jejunal segment to the hepatoduodenal ligament might provide sufficient biliary drainage in the majority of patients with intrahepatic as well as extrahepatic biliary atresia if performed when the infant is less than three months of age. These reports are encouraging and may have particular application to the patients with Type C atresia described in this report, all of whom had a combination of intrahepatic and extrahepatic atresia. One of the two patients who underwent this operative procedure (Patient 10) is alive ten months postoperatively and is free of jaundice. Thin watery bile-stained fluid usually drains from the hepatoduodenal ligament in infants with either intrahepatic or extrahepatic biliary atresia after surgical exploration. This has suggested that in certain instances the surgeon may not be able to differentiate easily between a dilated lymphatic channel and an atretic bile duct in the hepatoduodenal ligament. Previous experience in our hospital with five infants demonstrated that when a hepaticojejunal anastomosis is performed beyond the age of six months in patients with intrahepatic atresia, cirrhosis progresses rapidly, and the infants usually die under the age of two years.[4] It has been difficult to delineate clearly between intrahepatic and extrahepatic atresia, or combinations of both, in many infants; consequently, results of different types of operations have been difficult to evaluate. Some of these patients may represent a group of cases with potentially curable biliary atresia with both small intrahepatic and extrahepatic ducts (hypoplastic), similar to that described by Danks and asscociates.[2]

REFERENCES

1. Cameron, R., and Bunton, G. L.: Congenital biliary atresia, Br. Med. J. **2:** 1253, 1960.
2. Danks, D. M., Clarke, A. M., Jones, P. G., et al.: Extrahepatic biliary atresia: Further comments on potentially operable cases, J. Pediatr. Surg. **3:** 584, 1968.
3. Draz, S., Barajas, L., and Fonkalsrud, E. W.: Reversibility of biliary cirrhosis due to bile duct obstruction, J. Pediatr. Surg. **6:** 256, 1971.
4. Fonkalsrud, E. W., Kitagawa, S., and Longmire, W. P., Jr.: Hepatic lymphatic drainage to the jejunum for congenital biliary atresia, Am. J. Surg. **112:** 188, 1966.
5. Hays, D. M., and Snyder, W. H., Jr.: Lifespan in untreated biliary atresia, SURGERY **54:** 373, 1963.
6. Kasai, M., Kimura, S., Asakura, Y., et al.: Surgical treatment of biliary atresia, J. Pediatr. Surg. **3:** 665, 1968.
7. Ladd, W. E.: Congenital obstruction of the bile ducts, Ann. Surg. **102:** 742, 1935.
8. Lou, M. A., Schmutzer, K. J., and Regan, J. F.: Congenital extrahepatic biliary atresia, Arch. Surg. **105:** 771, 1972.
9. Pickett, L. K.: Liver and biliary tract, *in* Mustard, W. T., Ravitch, M. M., Snyder, W. H., Jr., et al., editors: Pediatric surgery, Chicago, Ill., 1969, Year Book Medical Publishers, p. 732.
10. Shiraki, K., Okamoto, Y., and Takatsu, T.: A follow-up study of prolonged obstructive jaundice in infancy, Pediatr. Univ. Tokyo **12:** 41, 1966.
11. Suruga, K., Nagashima, K., Kohno, S., et al.: A clinical and pathological study of congenital biliary atresia, J. Pediatr. Surg. **7:** 655, 1972.
12. Thaler, M. M., and Gellis, S. S.: Studies in neonatal hepatitis and biliary atresia. IV. Diagnosis, Am. J. Dis. Child. **116:** 280, 1968.

Identification of vagal structures at the esophageal hiatus

John E. Skandalakis, M.D., Ph.D., F.A.C.S., Joseph S. Rowe, Jr., M.D., Stephen W. Gray, Ph.D., *and* **John A. Androulakis, M.D.,** *Atlanta, Ga.*

The levels of the esophageal vagus plexus, the descending vagal trunks, the truncal divisions and their branches were examined in 100 adult cadavers. The number of vagal structures appearing at the hiatus is related to variations in the level of the lowest part of the esophageal plexus and the level at which the vagal trunks separate into the four divisions. In 88 percent of the cadavers, the plexus ended above the hiatus and the truncal divisions were formed below the hiatus. Two vagal trunks passed through the hiatus. In the remaining cases, plexus elements, divisions or branches of divisions were present at the hiatus, resulting in four or more vagal structures.

From the Departments of Surgery and Pathology, The Piedmont Hospital, and the Department of Anatomy, Emory Medical School, Atlanta, Ga.

To THE surgeon planning a vagotomy, truncal or complete, the pattern of the vagus nerves at the esophageal hiatus is important. The basic configuration and the variations of the vagus have been described by Dragstedt and colleagues[2] and others,[1, 4-6] but the thoracic pattern is not visible to the abdominal surgeon and he must proceed on the basis of the nerve structures that he can see emerging with the esophagus through the hiatus.

The variations of the vagus ("the wanderer") are such that no rules will fit every case that may be encountered, but we have attempted to provide a guide for the identification of vagal structures seen at the abdominal side of the esophageal hiatus. We have not concerned ourselves with variations of the branches of the vagal divisions within the abdomen.

Accepted for publication Oct. 10, 1973.

MATERIALS AND METHODS

The course of the vagus nerves and their branches within the thorax and through the esophageal hiatus of the diaphragm was studied in 100 adult cadavers of both sexes. Eighty-nine were cadavers in the dissecting room, and eleven were necropsy specimens.

FINDINGS

Two vagus nerves, left and right, descend parallel to the esophagus and form an esophageal vagal plexus between the level of the tracheal bifurcation and the level of the diaphragm. From this plexus two vagal trunks, anterior and posterior, are formed. Each trunk then divides to form two divisions.

From the anterior trunk the *hepatic* division passes to the right in the lesser omentum, branching before it enters the liver. One such branch turns downward to reach the pylorus and the first part of the

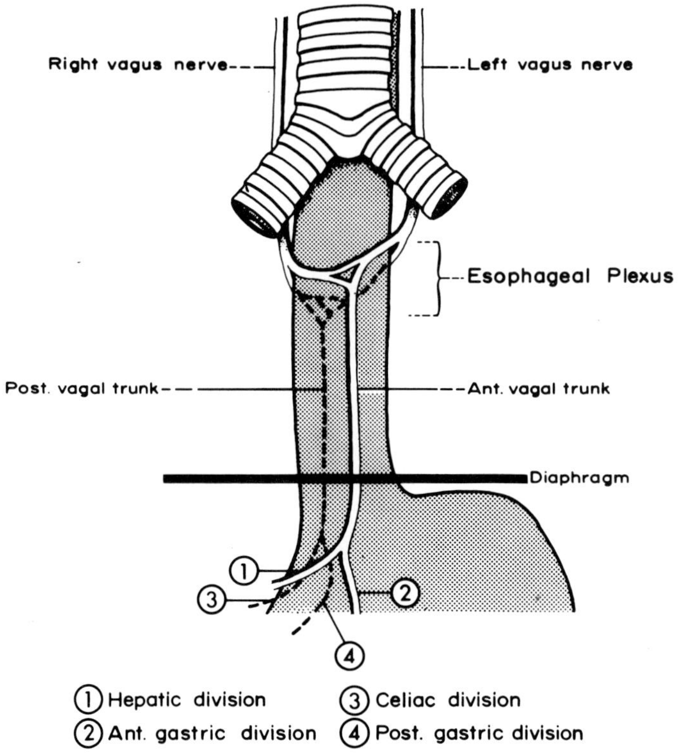

Fig. 1. Two vagal nerve structures (trunks) are present at the hiatus of the diaphragm. The esophageal plexus is "high" and the bifurcation of the trunks is below the diaphragm. This is the most common pattern.

duodenum. The second division, the *anterior gastric,* descends along the lesser curvature of the stomach, giving off branches to the anterior gastric wall.

The posterior trunk forms the *celiac* division passing to the celiac plexus, and the *posterior gastric* division which branches to supply the posterior gastric wall. Occasionally gastric branches arise serially so that a true gastric division never exists.[6]

NUMBER OF VAGAL STRUCTURES AT THE HIATUS

Table I shows the number of vagal structures emerging into the abdomen through the hiatus in our 100 specimens. We use the term "vagal structures" since they may be trunks, divisions, branches of divisions, or portions of the esophageal plexus.

Two structures (vagal trunks). This is the simplest and the most frequently encountered condition (Fig. 1). The esophageal plexus, from which the anterior and posterior trunks arise, lies well above the hiatus and the anterior and posterior trunks separate into divisions well below the hiatus.

Although the trunks are called anterior and posterior, they are not symmetrically placed with respect to the esophagus. Among 88 of our dissected specimens, 91 percent of anterior trunks and 86 percent of posterior trunks were to the right of the midline (Fig. 2). The remainder were to the left. This shift to the right was observed by Griffith.[4] He stated that the trunks always assume the right posterior and right anterior positions, but in our material a few trunks were found to the left of the midline of the esophagus.

After passing through the esophageal hiatus, the anterior vagal trunk lies closer to the esophagus than does the posterior trunk (Fig. 2). Griffith[4] found cases in which the posterior trunk was closer to the esophagus than to the aorta. In our material, it was always closer to the aorta.

Four structures (vagal divisions). If the

esophageal vagal plexus is high on the esophagus, the anterior and posterior vagal trunks may divide above the hiatus. In this case, four truncal divisions may emerge into the abdomen (Fig. 3, *A*).

More than four structures (branches of vagal divisions or the esophageal vagal plexus). In a small number of specimens more than four nerve structures emerge from the hiatus. Two distinct possibilities must be kept in mind: (1) The vagal trunks have formed divisions, one or more of which have already branched before entering the hiatus. Such branches will not reunite on the surface of the abdominal esophagus (Fig. 3, *B*).

(2) More than four nerve structures may also be found if the esophageal plexus itself extends below the hiatus; they may branch and anastomose. In such cases the anterior and posterior vagal trunks lie entirely within the abdomen (Fig. 3, *C*). If truncal vagotomy is to be performed, the surgeon must seek the truncal divisions and their branches well below the level of the hiatus.

DISCUSSION

The two factors that control the pattern of vagal sructures at the hiatus are (1) the level of the esophageal plexus and (2) the level of the separation of the vagal trunks into their divisions. The plexus may be "high," with all elements lying above the diaphragm or "low," extending through the hiatus on the abdominal esophagus. The truncal bifurcation may be "high," within the thorax or "low," within the abdomen. If the esophageal plexus is "low," the bifurcation must, of course, be "low." Both levels can vary considerably, but in the majority of individuals, the plexus is "high" (thoracic) and the truncal division is "low" (abdominal) (Fig. 1).

We cannot agree with Griffith's[4] view that it is the level of the diaphragm that varies with respect to the esophageal plexus. Such variations do of course occur in congenital short esophagus which is rare[3] and in hiatal hernia which may not be obvious at necropsy because the ascended stomach tends to return to the normal position after death. Both

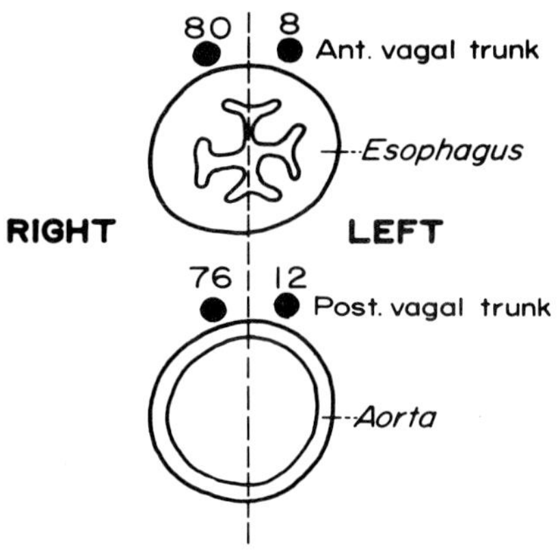

Fig. 2. Number of specimens with vagal trunks lying to the right or left of the midline. In most, but not all of the 88 specimens the trunks lay to the right. Note that the anterior trunk is closer to the esophagus than is the posterior trunk.

Table I. *Number of vagal structures passing through the esophageal hiatus*

No. of hiatal vagal structures	*No. of speci-mens*	*Terminology of hiatal vagal structures*
2	88	Vagal trunks
4	7	Divisions
> 4	2	Divisions and/or branches of divisions
> 4	3	Elements of the esophageal plexus
Total	100	

conditions could result in an apparent high plexus and high level of bifurcation. Aside from these variations the level of the diaphragm is relatively constant.

Nerve structures at the hiatus in addition to the usual two have sometimes been called "accessory." The validity of such a term is questionable. Accessory vagus structures (termed nerves) above the esophageal plexus have never been described. Any true accessory structures at the hiatus must originate from the plexus and descend parallel with the anterior and posterior vagal trunks, making no further communication with them. These would be "accessory vagal trunks." In our experience, all such parallel descending fibers rejoin the normal trunks proving them to be part of the esophageal plexus

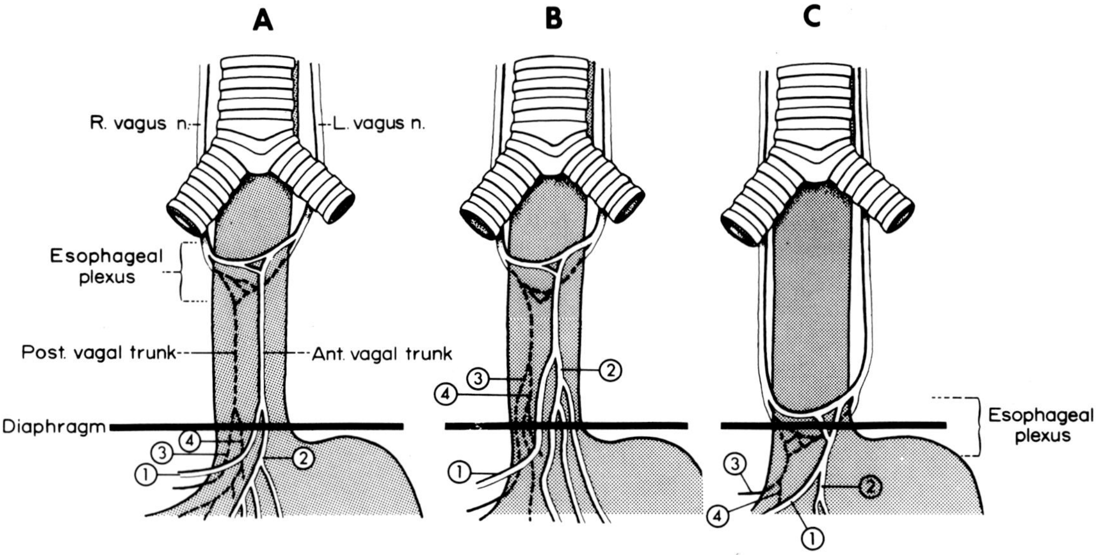

Fig. 3. *A,* Four vagal nerve structures (divisions) are present at the hiatus of the diaphragm. The bifurcation of the vagal trunks is above or at the diaphragm. *B,* More than four vagal nerve structures (divisions and/or their branches) are present at the hiatus of the diaphragm. The bifurcation of the vagal trunks is above the diaphragm. *C,* More than four vagal nerve structures (esophageal plexus) are present at the hiatus of the diaphragm. The esophageal plexus is "low" and extends below the diaphragm and the vagal trunks lie entirely in the abdomen. ①, Hepatic division; ②, anterior gastric division; ③, celiac division; ④, posterior gastric division.

rather than true accessory fibers. At least one drawing in the literature[6] shows a true accessory trunk. Weinberg and asssociates[6] qualify this in their text by stating "there may be small intercommunicating branches between the two." It is not clear whether he means that communicating fibers are sometimes present or that he did not verify their presence or absence in such cases. No accessory trunks appeared in our material.

The possibility of "accessory" divisions or "accessory" branches of divisions remains. In our diagrams, it appears that each vagal trunk divides neatly into two single and identifiable divisions which subsequently give off branches. Such is not the case. Jackson's diagrams[5] of the branches of the posterior trunk will illustrate the problem. Among his fifty cases, there were only two in which the posterior gastric division originated as a single trunk. In only 19 of the fifty cases was there a principal bundle of fibers that could be strictly called a posterior gastric division. As the gastric fibers are difficult to categorize into divisions and branches, there appears to be no point in calling some fibers "accessory divisions" or "accessory branches." We did not examine the distribution of branches of the divisions in our material.

SUMMARY

Vagal structures emerging from the esophageal hiatus of the diaphragm have been examined in 100 subjects. The structures may be identified by the number present at the hiatus.

Two vagal structures only. These are the *anterior* and *posterior vagal trunks* which have not yet formed the typical four divisions. Both are usually to the right of the midline of the esophagus. This is the most frequent pattern (88 percent).

Four vagal structures only. These are the four *divisions* of the vagal trunks. The trunks have divided above the diaphragm (seven percent).

More than four vagal structures. These may be: (1) divisions and/or *branches of* *divisions,* in which case the vagal trunks are entirely within the thorax. (Two percent); (2) elements of the esophageal *vagal plexus,* in which case the vagal trunks are entirely within the abdomen (three percent).

REFERENCES

1. Crow, R. W., Schulte, W. J., Ellison, E. H., and Winship, D. A.: Selective versus truncal vagotomy, Am. J. Surg. **121:** 684, 1971.
2. Dragstedt, L. R., Fournier, H. J., Woodward, E. R., Tover, E. B., and Harper, P. V., Jr.: Transabdominal gastric vagotomy: A study of the anatomy and surgery of the vagus nerves at the lower portion of the esophagus, Surg. Gynecol. Obstet. **85:** 461, 1947.
3. Gray, S. W., and Skandalakis, J. E.: Embryology for surgeons, Philadelphia, 1972, W. B. Saunders Company, p. 90.
4. Griffith, C. A.: A new anatomic approach to the problem of incomplete vagotomy, Surg. Clin. North Am. **44:** 1239, 1964.
5. Jackson, R. G.: Anatomic study of the vagus nerves, Arch. Surg. **57:** 333, 1948.
6. Weinberg, J. A., Campbell, G. W., and Voelker, R. B.: Vagus nerve section in the treatment of peptic ulcer, J. Thorac. Surg. **17:** 743, 1948.

"Smooth loop" arteriovenous fistulas for hemodialysis

Allastair M. Karmody, M.B., Ch.M., F.R.C.S. (Eng. and Edin.), *and*
Neil Lempert, M.D., F.A.C.S., *Albany, N. Y.*

A new type of arteriovenous fistula for chronic hemodialysis is described in this paper. This consists of the formation of a smooth arterial or venous loop runoff designed to ensure streamlined flow. Forty-six "smooth loop" fistulas have been created in 42 patients. There has been a primary failure rate of 4.3 percent and an over-all failure rate of 8.6 percent. These figures compare favorably with other reported series. All working fistulas have been used within one week of construction and the flow rates obtained have been uniformly high. The construction of the "smooth loop" fistula is simple and few local problems have been encountered.

From the Department of Surgery, Albany Medical College of Union University, Albany, N. Y.

THE AVAILABILITY of easily accessible arterial and venous channels has revolutionized the fate of countless individuals suffering from end-stage renal disease. The process began with the innovative external shunts pioneered by Quinton, Dillard, and Scribner[13] which subsequently underwent many modifications. Since 1966, the internal arteriovenous (A-V) fistula first described by Brescia and associates[1] has solved many of the problems of the external shunt, the majority of which were primarily related to the presence of an intravascular transcutaneous foreign body.[9] However, there is mounting evidence in the literature that there are some unsatisfactory features of the Brescia-Cimino (side-to-side) A-V fistula, and this is supported by a poor personal experience. In view of this, we have devised a method of fistula construction based on the principles of flow mechanics. This has proved to be simple while providing a high rate of blood flow and a low incidence of failure.

The project was supported by a grant from the James Hilton Manning and Emma Austin Manning Foundation.
Accepted for publication Oct. 10, 1973.

METHOD

The principle used in these fistulas consists of the construction of a smooth loop which gives a sreamlined runoff for the arterial inflow (Fig. 1). In patients with intact radial and ulnar arteries, the radial artery at the wrist was used to form the loop (Fig. 2, *A*). In cases where one wrist artery was not available because it had been used for a previous external shunt or a fistula which had failed, the vein was used to form the loop (Fig. 2, *B*) to ensure continuation of arterial flow into the hand (Fig. 3). In either event, the end of the vessel forming the loop was anastomosed to the side of that vessel which was left "in situ." In all radial artery fistulas, the cephalic vein was close enough to the artery to allow the use of a single longitudinal or transverse incision. In three of 11 ulnar artery fistulas, the position of the basilic vein necessitated the use of a second

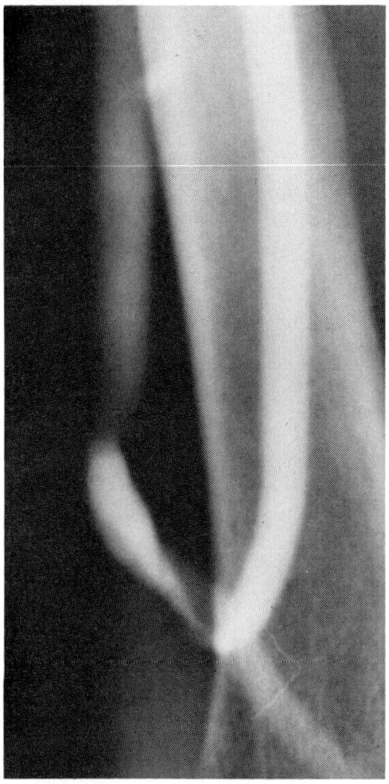

Fig. 1. Arteriogram of arteriovenous loop at the wrist. The radial artery forms the loop and is anastomosed to the cephalic vein.

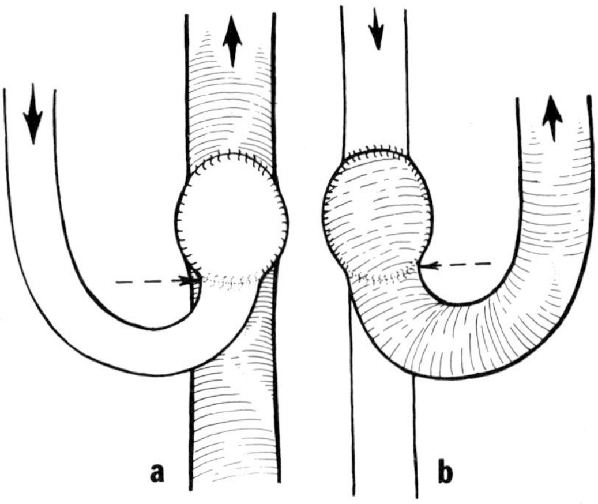

Fig. 2. Diagrams to illustrate the construction of "smooth loop" fistulas. *A,* The artery is looped and anastomosed to the "in situ" vein, e.g., radial artery to cephalic vein. *B,* The vein is looped and anastomosed to the "in situ" artery, e.g., basilic vein to ulnar artery. Symbols: →, Direction of flow; - - - →, area of technical difficulty.

longitudinal or a transverse incision to mobilize the vein adequately.

The greatest technical difficulty in these anastomoses was encountered at the inner aspect of the distal corner (Fig. 2). Accordingly, this area is sutured first when the vessels are easy to manipulate, relative to each other, in order to facilitate accurate suture placement.

In patients with small vessels, and particularly in children, the use of magnifying loupes and fine ophthalmic instruments was helpful. Two double-armed Dacron No. 6-0 sutures were initially used for the anastomoses but in the last 19 cases, the use of a special "high visibility" suture (Ethicon) was an important technical aid.[8]

RESULTS

The smooth loop fistula has been created 46 times in 42 patients (37 adults and five children). In 35 instances, the radial artery was anastomosed to the cephalic vein. In the remaining 11, the basilic vein was anastomosed to the ulnar artery because of previous use of the radial artery. In none of the patients with ulnar-basilic fistulas have ischemic symptoms of the hand appeared. This finding is in contrast to previous experience with external shunts in which interference with both wrist arteries has often resulted in digital ischemia. Primary operative failure occurred in two patients as a result of a poor choice of veins. One vein was sclerotic while the other was occluded proximal to the anastomosis. In a third patient, failure occurred three months after the original operation, because of involvement of the vein by disseminated lupus, the original cause of the patient's renal failure (Fig. 3). This patient also developed a small aneurysm in a forearm vein at a puncture site well removed from the arteriovenous anastomosis. In a fourth patient, primary arterial thrombosis occurred proximal to the anastomosis after one month (Fig. 4). This fistula was salvaged by open arterial thrombectomy and application of an onlay vein patch.

We have been able to use all patent fistulas within one week of their creation and the flow obtained has been uniformly high (220 to 400 ml. per minute). These fistulas have been in continuous use for periods ranging from 22 months to one month.

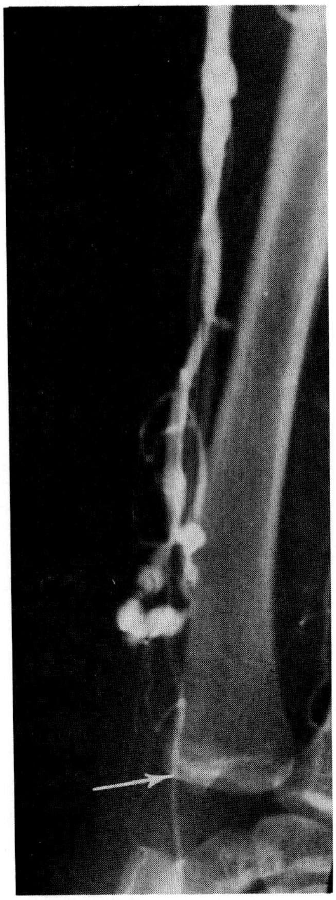

Fig. 3. Arteriogram of ulnar-basilic fistula in patient with disseminated lupus. The lupoid basilic vein is beaded and irregular. Spontaneous thrombosis later occurred. Arrow indicates patient distal ulnar artery.

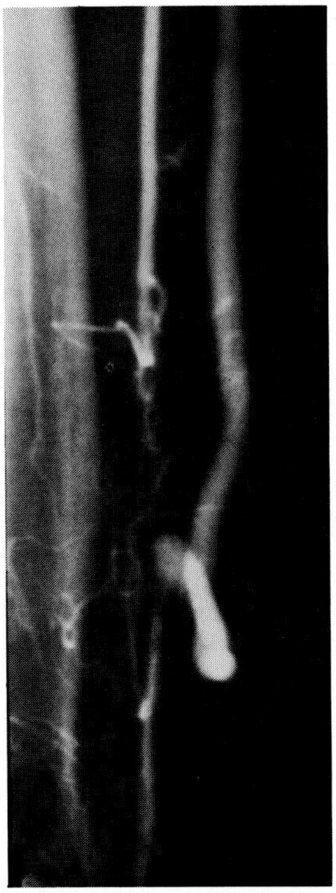

Fig. 4. Arterial thrombosis proximal to the A-V anastomosis. The limbs of the loop are superimposed. Fistula is salvaged by open arterial thrombectomy and onlay vein patch.

DISCUSSION

As a general principle of fluid mechanics, increasing the angle of flow causes correspondingly greater kinetic energy losses. Therefore, when flow is abruptly reversed, energy losses are maximal and at the point of transition, laminar flow is completely replaced by turbulence. These physical principles indicate the main hemodynamic problems with the side-to-side A-V fistulas as originally described.[1] In this system, blood flow has to negotiate a sharp, almost 360 degree turn at the upper angle of the fistula. The effect of this is the creation of very turbulent flow and eddy currents,[14] resulting in an increased tendency to intraoperative or early postoperative thrombosis. In addition, the smallest angle of flow and therefore the path of least resistance is toward the distal venous limb (Fig. 5, *A*). This may lead to significant diversion of arterial flow from the fistula into the veins of the hand[3, 4] and is responsible in part for the noticeably slow maturation of these fistulas.

A number of modifications of the side-to-side fistula have, therefore, been proposed. One consists of ligation of the distal venous limb of the fistula so that a "straight limb" end-to-side fistula results (Fig. 5, *B*). Another modification consists of the use of a split bifurcation "venous bell"[4] or "funnel"[7] (Fig. 5, *C*). The latter technique is certainly preferable but suffers from the disadvantages that it is not always possible to find a bifurcation precisely where required, flow is still angular and not fully streamlined, and the more open, lower angle may theoretically allow easier flow into the vein from the distal arterial limb. The smooth loop fistula is designed to overcome these objections. The principles of this vascular anastomosis are similar to those presently employed in the femoropopliteal venous bypass graft which is constructed to best ensure a streamlined flow-path (Fig. 5, *D*).

These features can also be obtained by the end-to-end anastomosis, provided that a smooth circuit is created.[10] However, leaving one vessel in situ allows the surgeon to concentrate on the prevention of torsion in only the second vessel. This is particularly important if the vein is to be detached to form the loop since it is prone to twisting. Experience has shown that anastomosis to a vessel which lies in its natural orientation is usually more satisfactory, and this is reflected in better long-term function.

The use of the smooth loop fistula has avoided or reduced many of the problems reported by other investigators. Thrombosis rates of 23 percent were reported by Tellis and associates[15] and 12 percent by Lytton and colleagues[11] within one week of side-to-side fistula construction. In the former series, there was a nearly 50 percent (11 of 24) primary failure rate in women. Goldberg and associates[7] have reported a 22 to 42 percent failure in their series of "funnel" fistulas. Our results are an immediate failure of 4.3 percent for the over-all series and 11 percent for females (one of nine). Aneurysm formation at the site of side-to-side anastomosis has been reported by Lytton and colleagues[11] and Tellis and co-workers[15] and has also been observed by us. The pathological basis for this complication has been demonstrated experimentally by Fallon and Stebhens.[5] A delay in dilatation of the forearm veins is a common experience with the side-to-side technique and was one of the reasons why Ehrenfeld and colleagues[4] preferred the immediate use of saphenous vein grafts for fistula construction. The satisfactory performance of the smooth loop fistulas has circumvented the much more extensive procedure involved in the transposition of autologous saphenous vein to the forearm.[6] We have used these vein grafts only for "problem" patients, e.g., women with obese arms

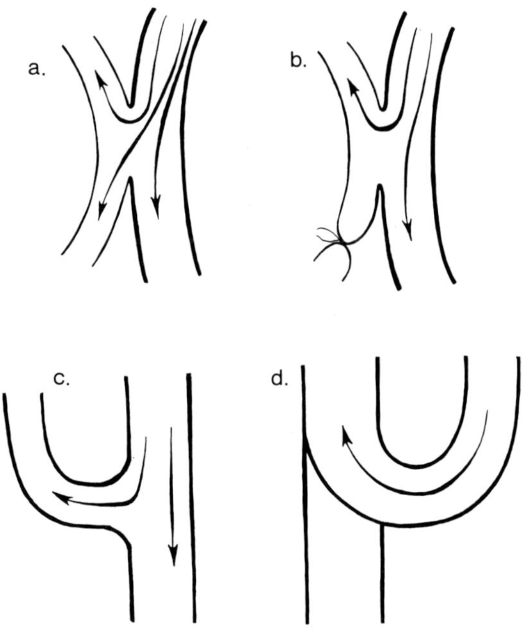

Fig. 5. Diagrams of fistulas in common use. *A,* Brescia-Cimino side-to-side A-V fistula showing directions of flow. *B,* Side-to-side fistula as in *(A)* with ligation of distal venous limb. In both *A* and *B,* the acute proximal angle of flow creates turbulence, thus predisposing to early and late failure. *C,* The "venous bell" anastomosis is a hemodynamic improvement, but flow is still subject to more turbulence than that in the "smooth loop" run-off, as illustrated in *(D)*.

or inadequate veins or those patients who have had several previous external shunts.

Bussell and associates[3] have described the radial steal syndrome in seven patients with side-to-side fistulas. Symptomatic ischemia of the hand was present in each case. Digital gangrene was reported in three similar patients by Buselmeier and colleagues.[2] There was agreement by both of these groups of authors that the mechanism of steal consisted of flow into the arterialized vein both from the proximal part of the artery and from the distal artery via the palmar arch. The flow characteristics of the smooth loop fistula effectively prevents steal phenomena. The most likely reason for this is that retrograde flow from the distal artery into the loop would have to negotiate a very acute angle in competition with an already well-established laminar flow pattern. Even the use of a

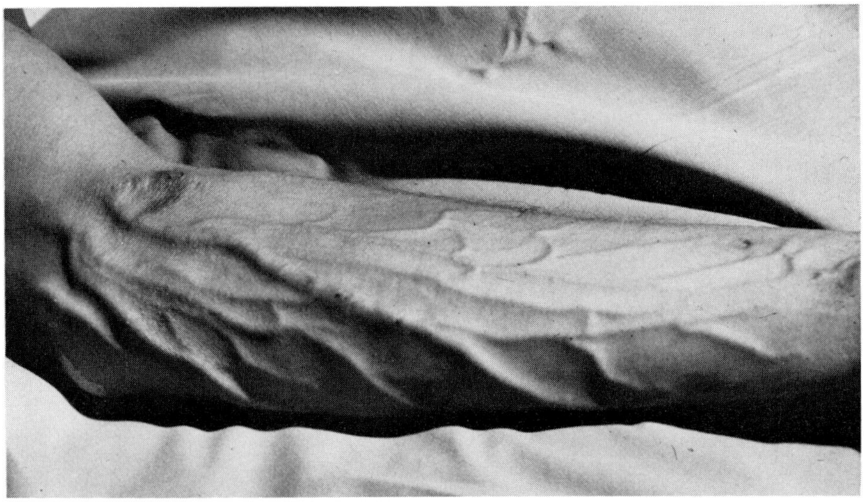

Fig. 6. Typical appearance of forearm with smooth loop fistula.

single remaining wrist artery has not caused symptoms of hand ischemia in any of the 11 patients so treated.

The soundness of the theoretical principles upon which the "smooth loop" fistula is based is confirmed by its low primary failure rate, rapidity of maturation, and high flow rate. Both radiocephalic and ulnar-basilic fistulas have been satisfactory in providing a sufficient number of veins of adequate caliber for repeated hemodialysis (Fig. 6). Complications of this procedure have been few with respect to technical failures and late local problems, e.g., thrombosis or aneurysm formation.

REFERENCES

1. Brescia, J. J., Cimino, J. E., Appel, K., and Hurwich, B. J.: Chronic hemodialysis using venipuncture and surgically created arteriovenous fistula, N. Engl. J. Med. **275:** 1089, 1966.
2. Buselmeier, T. J., Simmons, R. L., Rattazzi, L. C., et al.: A-V fistulas and the diabetic: Ischemia and gangrene may result in amputation, Trans. Am. Soc. Artif. Intern. Organs **19:** 49, 1973.
3. Bussell, J. A., Abbott, J. A., and Lim, R. C.: A radial steal syndrome with arteriovenous fistula for hemodialysis, Arch. Intern. Med. **75:** 387, 1971.
4. Ehrenfeld, W. K., Grauz, H., and Wylie, E. J.: Subcutaneous arteriovenous fistulas for hemodialysis, Am. J. Surg. **124:** 200, 1972.
5. Fallon, J., and Stebhens, W. E.: Venous endothelium in experimental arteriovenous fistulas in rabbits, Circ. Res. **31:** 546, 1972.
6. Giradet, R. E., Hackett, R. E., Goodwin, N. J., and Friedman, E. A.: Thirteen months' experience with the saphenous vein graft arteriovenous fistula for maintenance hemodialysis, Trans., Am. Soc. Artif. Intern. Organs **16:** 285, 1970.
7. Goldberg, E. M., Hill, W., Kanter, A., and Ooi, B. S.: A new vascular prosthesis for chronic hemodialysis, Trans. Am. Soc. Artif. Intern. Organs **18:** 441, 1972.
8. Karmody, A. M., and Lempert, N.: A new high visibility vascular suture. Submitted for publication.
9. Kurivila, K. C., and Beven, E. G.: Arteriovenous shunts and fistulas for hemodialysis, Surg. Clin. North Am. **51:** 1219, 1971.
10. Lawton, R. L., and Sharzer, L. S.: Vascular access for patients on maintenance dialysis, Surg. Gynecol. Obstet. **135:** 279, 1972.
11. Lytton, B., Goffinet, J. A., May, C. J., and Weiss, R. M.: Experience with arteriovenous fistula in chronic hemodialysis, J. Urol. **104:** 512, 1970.
12. May, J., Tiller, D., and Johnson, J.: Saphenous vein arteriovenous fistula in regular dialysis treatment, N. Engl. J. Med. **280:** 770, 1969.
13. Quinton, W. E., Dillard, D. H., and Scribner, B. H.: Circulation of blood vessels for prolonged dialysis, Trans. Am. Soc. Artif. Intern. Organs **6:** 104, 1960.
14. Stebhens, W. E.: Blood vessel changes in chronic experimental arteriovenous fistulas, Surg. Gynecol. Obstet. v. 127, p. 327, 1968.
15. Tellis, V. A., Veith, F. J., Soberman, R. J.: Internal arteriovenous fistula for hemodialysis, Surg. Gynecol. Obstet. **132:** 866, 1971.

Investigations of the enterobiliary metabolism of lecithin

Ronald K. Tompkins, M.D., *and* **William King, III, A.B.,*** *Los Angeles, Calif.*

Simultaneous sampling in pigs of thoracic duct lymph, portal and vena caval blood, and common duct bile after intestinal administration of ^{14}C-lecithin showed a rapid and progressive rise in the concentration of radioactivity in lipid fractions of the bile extracts. Analyses of the distribution of lipid radioactivity demonstrated triglycerides to be the major form of transport in lymph and blood, whereas 70 percent of the radioactivity in bile was in the lecithin (phosphatidyl-choline) fraction eight hours after isotope administration. The data demonstrate that dietary lecithin contributes to biliary lecithin secretion probably by way of its intestinal hydrolytic products. Animals with intact thoracic ducts showed the same cumulative rise in biliary lipid radioactivity as did those with thoracic duct fistulas, suggesting that the intestinal precursors of biliary lecithin synthesis may reach the liver by a route other than the thoracic duct.

From the Department of Surgery, Biliary Research Laboratory, UCLA School of Medicine, Los Angeles, Calif.

THE PRECIPITATING event in the formation of human cholesterol gallstones is a biochemical change that renders cholesterol insoluble in bile. Although the parameters of this change are not yet completely defined, several observations have been made. Two major classes of compounds, the bile acids and phospholipids (chiefly lecithin), are necessary for the maintenance of biliary cholesterol in solution. Previous studies have shown that the concentration of phospholipids in gallbladder bile is significantly less in humans with cholesterol gallstones than in those with normal biliary tracts.[2, 23] Although the bile salt pool has been calculated to be reduced in patients with cholesterol cholelithiasis,[28] the proportional amounts of bile acids of such patients have not been shown to differ significantly in individual bile samples from those of normal subjects.[1, 26]

Nutritional studies in humans have demonstrated that ingestion of lecithin in combination with a low-fat, low-cholesterol diet results in an increase in the hepatic bile phospholipid concentration[25] that is proportionately greater than that of the cholesterol concentration. The resultant elevation of the phospholipid: cholesterol (P/C) ratio is associated, in turn, with a proportionate rise in the cholesterol-holding capacity of the bile.[24] The mechanism by which dietary lecithin contributes to biliary lecithin concentrations has not been well defined.

Supported by grants from The John A. Hartford Foundation, Inc., New York, N. Y., and The U. S. Public Health Service (FR-05354).

Portions of this study were presented at the Annual Meeting of the American Gastroenterological Association, May, 1971,[8] Surgical Forum of American College of Surgeons, Oct., 1971,[26] and The Deuel Lipid Conference, March, 1972.[25]

Accepted for publication Oct. 10, 1973.

*Fellow in the Department of Pathology and Recipient of The American Gastroenterological Association Student Research Award, 1971.

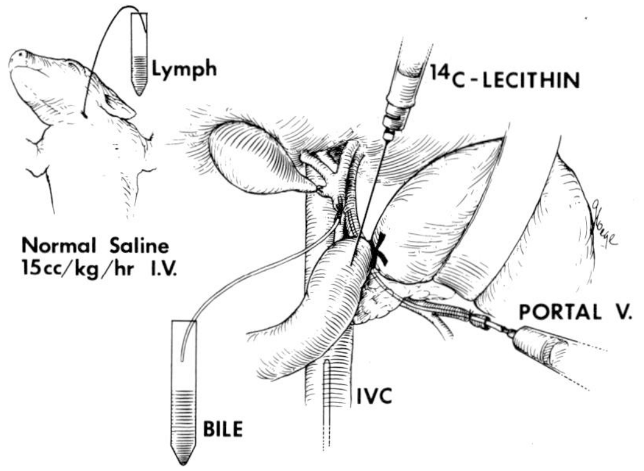

Fig. 1. Diagram of animal preparation. The ^{14}C-lecithin has been dissolved in fresh bile aspirated from the gallbladder of each pig.

The present study was undertaken to analyze simultaneously samples of blood, lymph, and bile obtained from pigs after intestinal administration of labeled lecithin in order to determine whether dietary lecithin contributes to biliary lecithin production and, if so, to what extent.

MATERIALS AND METHODS

A uniformly labeled lecithin [^{14}C-(U)-lecithin]* was chosen to trace possible breakdown products after intestinal administration of the isotope. The lecithin was prepared biosynthetically from *Chlorella pyrenidosa* grown in an atmosphere containing ^{14}C-carbon dioxide. Radiochemical purity of the compound was greater than 99 percent, and specific activity was 1.846 curies per millimole of phosphorus. Major fatty acids in lecithin obtained from another species of *Chlorella* (vulgaris) are linoleic (52 percent), oleic (16 percent), and palmitic (11 percent).[10]

Animal preparation. Four 2-month-old fasting pigs, weighing an average of 7.5 kilograms, were anesthetized with phenobarbital (150 mg. per kilogram of body weight), administered intravenously, and hydrated continuously during the study with normal saline (15 ml. per kilogram per hour) through a right external jugular vein cannula. To evaluate the effects of diversion of thoracic duct lymph, the thoracic duct was isolated in the left neck of two animals and cannulated with polyethylene tubing (inside diameter, 1.14 mm.). The thoracic duct was left intact in the other two animals. A midline abdominal incision was then made, the spleen was removed, and the splenic vein was cannulated with silicone rubber tubing (inside diameter, 2.0 mm.) until the proximal tip lay in the portal vein. The pylorus was occluded with umbilical tape, and the cystic duct was ligated with silk ligature. The common bile duct was cannulated with silicone rubber tubing (inside diameter, 2.0 mm.) just above the duodenum. Another silicone rubber catheter of the same size was passed into the infrahepatic vena cava via a cutdown in the right femoral vein. Both venous catheters were connected to three-way stopcocks, and dilute heparin saline was used to flush the tubing after sample collection.

At least 5 ml. of bile was aspirated from the gallbladder of each pig and used to dissolve 50 μCi of ^{14}C-(U)-lecithin (Fig. 1). After collection of base-line lymph, bile, and blood samples, the dissolved radioactive lecithin was introduced into the duodenal lumen. Samples of lymph, bile, and blood were collected at 5, 15, and 30 minutes and at 30 minute intervals thereafter for up to 8½ hours. Samples were collected in ice baths and centrifuged at 2,000 rpm for 20 minutes in an International centrifuge.* The supernatants were pipetted and frozen until extraction.

Chemical analyses. Two milliliters of supernatant from each sample were partitioned between chloroform and methanol-water by the method of Folch and associates.[5] An aliquot of the lower, lipid phase (chloroform) was evaporated to a residue (Fig. 2). Fifteen milliliters of 2:1 toluene: ethanol, containing 0.4 percent diphenyloxazole (PPO) and 0.01 percent para-bis-[2-(5-phenyl-oxazolyl)] benzene (POPOP), were added as the scintillation fluid and the

*New England Nuclear, Boston, Mass.

*Model No. HN-3, International Equipment Company, Needham Heights, Mass.

solutions were counted in a liquid scintillation spectrophotometer.* After initial counting, 10 μl of ^{14}C-toluene† were added to each vial as an internal standard, and the samples were recounted to calculate the amount of quenching. After correction for background, quenching, and dilution, the concentration of lipid radioactivity was expressed as counts per minute per milliliter of supernatant.

A second aliquot of the total lipid extract (lower phase) was evaporated under continuous gentle nitrogen flow in a 50° C. water bath, and the residue was dissolved in 0.1 ml. hexane for chromatographic analysis. Thin-layer plates (20 by 20 cm.) were spread with silica gel G‡ to a thickness of 250 μ and developed in a multi-solvent system after application of a streak of the sample at the origin. Thin-layer chromatographic standards used were cholesterol§; lysolecithin, sphingomyelin, lecithin, and phosphatidyl ethanolamine‖; mono-, di-, and tri-palmitate, triolein, oleic acid, and cholesterol oleate.¶

The plates were placed initially into chloroform:methanol:water (65:25:4 by volume) and developed to a height of 8 cm. to separate the phospholipid fractions. After being air dried for 60 seconds, they were placed into hexane:diethyl ether:acetic acid (70:20:4 by volume) and developed to a height of 12 cm. to separate mono- and diglyceride fractions. Again the plates were air-dried for 60 seconds and placed into a final tank containing hexane:diethyl ether: acetic acid (85:15:1 by volume) to aid in separating cholesterol esters and triglyceride fractions. Iodine vapor detected the lipid bands of the samples as well as the standards. Bands with Rf values greater than 0.5 (neutral lipids) were eluted with Folch reagent. Bands with Rf values below 0.5 (phospholipids) were eluted consecutively with the following four solvent systems of 5 ml. each: chloroform:methanol (2:1 by volume); chloroform:methanol (1:1 by volume); absolute methanol; and chloroform: methanol:acetic acid:water (25:15:1:4 by volume). Eluting solvents were then evaporated, and the residue of each band was suspended in scintillation fluid as above. Internal standards of ^{14}C-toluene were added after initial sample counting as before. After correction for background and quenching, lipid fraction radioactivity was expressed as corrected counts per minute. The percentage of the total lipid radioactivity contributed by each lipid fraction was calculated by dividing the counts of the individual bands by the total counts in all bands.

In one animal with a thoracic duct fistula, the pylorus and rectosigmoid junction were ligated at the completion of the study, and the entire intestine was removed. The luminal contents were removed by manual evacuation, and the lumen was rinsed twice with normal saline. The luminal contents were added to the saline rinses and then submitted to partitioning in Folch reagent. An aliquot of the lipid phase was evaporated and counted in a liquid scintillation counter as described above. A second aliquot of the lipid phase was submitted to thin-layer chromatography for separation of lipid fractions.

RESULTS

In all pigs, the bile became radioactive within the first 30 minutes, and radioactivity increased rapidly during the course of the experiment. Lymph radioactivity increased slowly over the first 90 minutes and then rose more rapidly during the last hours of the study. Portal and systemic venous radioactivity remained at lower levels throughout the study, with portal vein activity consistently higher than inferior vena caval activity.

Lipid extracts. In the two animals prepared with thoracic duct fistulas, the concentrations of radioactivity of the bile and lymph increased steadily after isotope ad-

*Packard Tricarb Model No. 4322, Packard Instrument Co., Inc., Downers Grove, Ill.

†New England Nuclear, Boston, Mass.; specific activity 4.26×10^5 dpm/ml.

‡Brinkman Instruments, Inc., Westbury, N. Y.

§Bureau of Standards, United States Department of Commerce, Washington, D. C.

‖Applied Science Laboratories, State College, Pa.

¶Generous gift of Dr. James Mead, Department of Biochemistry, University of California, Los Angeles.

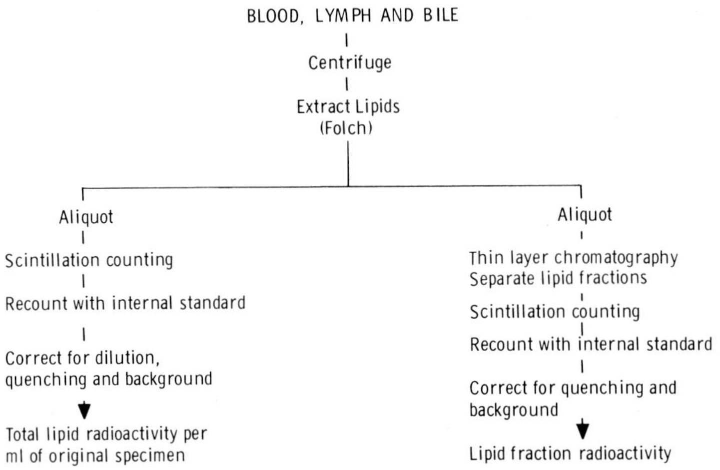

Fig. 2. Flow diagram of analyses of total lipid and lipid fraction radioactivity in blood, bile, and lymph.

Table I. *Mean lipid radioactivity in pigs with thoracic duct fistulas**

Time after administration of 50 μCi ^{14}C-lecithin (min.)	*Sample*			
	Thoracic duct lymph	*Common duct bile*	*Portal vein plasma*	*Inferior vena cava plasma*
5	0	—	9	0
15	0	4	38	4
30	11	42	37	6
60	37	135	58	19
90	72	248	76	30
120	124	326	80	44
150	150	443	121	65
180	241	539	168	67
210	512	920	184	68
240	—	1,168	171	76
270	—	1,003	—	166
300	—	1,335	271	100
330	870	1,430	260	91
360	1,015	1,628	220	105
390	—	1,465	250	98
420	3,411	—	229	139

*CPM/ml. of sample, corrected for background, dilution, and quenching.

ministration and continued to rise over the entire study period (Table I and Fig. 3). The concentration of radioactivity in portal and systemic venous blood increased only slightly over the study period, the portal blood always being higher in activity than the systemic circulation. In the animals without thoracic duct lymph fistulas, similar findings were obtained (Table II, Fig. 4). A consistent and rapid rise in bile radioactivity was noted throughout the course of the experiment with slight increases in radioactivity of the portal and systemic venous blood, the portal blood again being more active than systemic blood.

It was recognized that the content of radioactivity in the lymph and bile was in part dependent upon volume of flow; therefore, the volumes of each collection were measured and multiplied by the concentration of radioactivity in each specimen to obtain the total radioactivity per sample (Tables III and IV). The cumulative activity collected from bile and lymph at succeeding periods of time was calculated by summation of the total activity values. Evi-

Table II. *Mean lipid radioactivity in pigs without thoracic duct fistulas**

Time after administration of 50 μCi ¹⁴C-lecithin (min.)	Sample		
	Common duct bile	Portal vein plasma	Inferior vena cava plasma
5	0	8	4
15	0	10	0
30	119	17	12
60	105	30	15
90	258	43	17
120	544	53	30
150	576	61	38
180	722	87	50
210	843	94	61
240	857	182	90
300	834	188	130
360	971	363	224
390	1,318	359	291
435	1,435	439	296
480	1,713	528	399
525	1,843	430	380

*CPM/ml. of sample, corrected for background, dilution, and quenching.

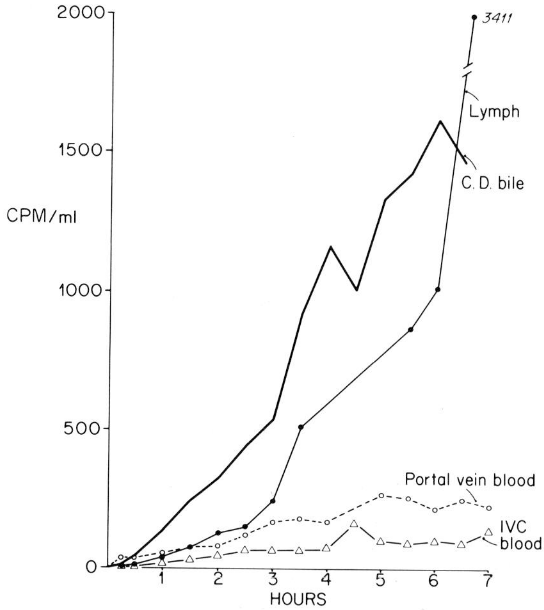

Fig. 3. Mean lipid radioactivity in blood lymph and bile and two animals with constant thoracic duct drainage.

dence for the reproducibility of the experimental preparation is found in the close agreement of the cumulative radioactivity curves for common duct bile in all four animals (Fig. 5). It was surprising that essentially no difference in cumulative bile activity was found between animals with lymph circulation intact and those with lymph diverted via thoracic duct fistulas.

Distribution of radioactivity among lipid fractions. Although radioactive phosphatidylcholine (lecithin) was found in the transport systems of lymph and portal and systemic blood, the activity of this lipid fraction tended to decrease with time and contributed one quarter or less of the total lipid radioactivity to any of these systems (Table V). The triglyceride fraction of lymph and portal and systemic blood contained the highest percentage of radioactivity, and the contribution of this fraction to total radioactivity increased with time.

In contrast, the phosphatidyl-choline (lecithin) fraction contributed the highest percentage of lipid radioactivity in common duct bile, an effect that increased steadily throughout the study.

Analysis of radioactivity in the intestinal contents at the termination of the experiment demonstrated that only 18 percent of the radioactivity administered remained in lipid soluble products. Free fatty acids accounted for 55 percent of this activity, lecithin for 23 percent, and lysolecithin for 22 percent.

DISCUSSION

The importance of lecithin for the solubilization of cholesterol in bile has been established by the studies of Isaksson[6] and further elucidated by the studies of Small,[16] Neiderhiser and associates,[9] and Swell and associates,[18] as well as those performed in this laboratory.[26] A marked decrease in lecithin concentration in gallbladder bile[23] and in biliary phospholipid excretion[19] have been observed in patients with cholesterol gallstones. The mechanism whereby bile becomes deficient in lecithin is not known; however, decreased lecithin in bile has been associated with a decreased bile salt pool in patients with cholelithiasis.[19] Other studies of Nilsson[11] and Balint and associates[3] have

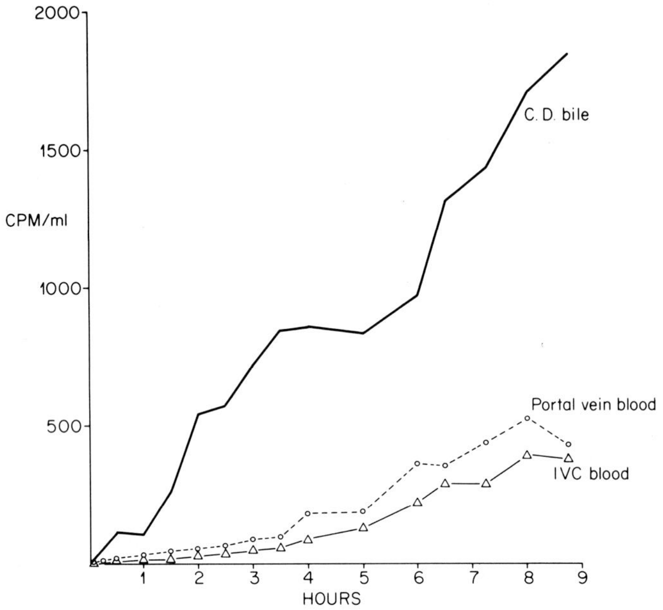

Fig. 4. Mean lipid radioactivity in blood and bile of two animals without interference with thoracic duct.

Table III. *Mean lymph and bile lipid radioactivity in pigs with thoracic duct fistulas*

	Lymph				*Bile*			
Time (min.)	*Volume (ml.)*	*Radioactivity concentration (CMP/ml.)*	*Radioactivity output (CPM)*	*Cumulative activity (CPM)*	*Volume (ml.)*	*Radioactivity concentration (CPM/ml.)*	*Radioactivity output (CPM)*	*Cumulative activity (CPM)*
15	7.0	0	0	0	2.2	4	9	9
30	7.5	11	83	83	2.6	42	109	118
60	8.5	37	315	398	2.4	135	324	442
90	7.5	72	540	938	3.0	248	744	1,186
120	8.3	124	1,029	1,967	3.2	326	1,043	2,229
150	5.7	150	855	2,822	2.8	443	1,240	3,469
180	7.3	241	1,759	4,581	2.7	539	1,455	4,924
210	8.5	512	4,352	8,933	2.9	920	2,668	7,592
240	9.3	—	—	—	2.9	1,168	3,387	10,979
270	6.8	—	—	—	2.5	1,003	2,508	13,487
300	12.0	—	—	—	1.5	1,335	2,003	15,490
330	13.0	870	11,310	—	1.0	1,430	1,430	16,920
360	15.0	1,015	15,225	—	1.5	1,628	2,442	19,362
390	14.5	—	—	—	0.7	1,465	1,026	20,388
420	17.5	3,411	59,693	—	1.3	—	—	—

shown that intestinal administration of bile salts is capable of increasing biliary phospholipid levels. Recent studies by Thistle and Schoenfield[20] indicate that oral chenodesoxycholic acid is the only bile acid capable of elevating significantly the lecithin:cholesterol ratio in human duodenal bile.

The relatively high incidence of patient intolerance to orally administered bile salts necessitates the investigation of other approaches to nonsurgical management of cholesterol cholelithiasis. Previous studies in humans fed low-fat (50 Gm. per day), low-cholesterol (400 mg. per day) diets supple-

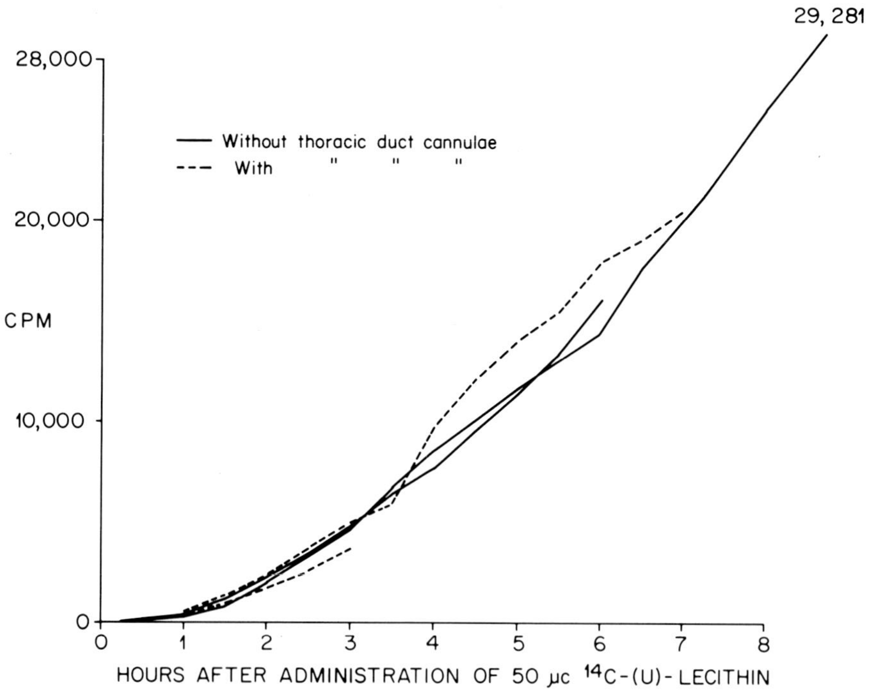

Fig. 5. Cumulative lipid radioactivity in common duct bile of each animal. Note that there is no difference between the animals with thoracic duct fistulas and those in which the thoracic duct circulation was intact.

mented with commercial soybean lecithin (10 Gm. per day) demonstrated that the phospholipid concentration and the phospholipid:cholesterol (P/C) ratio of hepatic bile were increased significantly over those values in a control group of patients given the same diet without lecithin.[25] The cholesterol-holding capacity of this phospholipid-enriched bile was thereby proportionately increased.[24] Studies by Scow and associates,[15] Saunders and associates,[14] and Nilsson and Borgstrom[12] have shown that intestinal lecithin is hydrolyzed to lysolecithin in the gut lumen, and a portion of this lysolecithin is absorbed and reacylated to lecithin in the intestinal mucosal cells and transported as lecithin in the thoracic duct lymph chylomicra. These data, obtained in rats with thoracic duct fistaulas, did not include simultaneous measurements of lymph, blood, and bile for more detailed analysis of the pathways of enterobiliary metabolism of lecithin. The present study was designed to clarify some of the mechanisms whereby intestinally administered lecithin might contribute to

Table IV. *Mean bile lipid radioactivity in pigs without thoracic duct fistulas*

Time (min.)	*Volume (ml.)*	*Radioactivity concentration (CPM/ml.)*	*Radioactivity output (CPM)*	*Cumulative activity (CPM)*
15	2.0	0	0	0
30	1.6	119	190	190
60	3.3	105	347	537
90	2.9	258	748	1,285
120	2.4	544	1,306	2,591
150	2.4	576	1,382	3,973
180	2.3	722	1,661	5,634
210	2.4	843	2,023	7,657
240	2.1	857	1,800	9,457
300	2.9	834	2,419	11,876
360	2.9	971	2,816	14,692
390	2.5	1,318	3,295	17,987
435	2.5	1,435	3,588	21,575
480	2.5	1,713	4,283	25,858
525	2.0	1,843	3,686	29,544

biliary lecithin production.[8, 22] The data demonstrate a rapid and progressive contribution to biliary lecithin synthesis from the intestinal lecithin molecule. The findings that the majority of lipid radioactivity in the transport systems (lymph and blood) is in

Table V. *Distribution of recovered lipid radioactivity among major lipid fractions*

Sample source	*Lipid fraction (percent of lipid radioactivity)* Phosphatidyl-choline	Lysophosphatidyl-choline	Phosphatidyl ethanolamine	Triglyc-erides	Free fatty acids	Other*
Four and one-half hours after isotope administration						
Vena cava (plasma)	13.5	0.9	0.0	42.7	8.4	34.5
Portal vein (plasma)	18.4	1.9	6.1	25.5	6.9	41.2
Thoracic duct (lymph)	25.2	0.4	0.1	36.9	5.3	32.1
Common duct (bile)	59.7	2.5	0.6	0.3	0.4	36.5
Eight hours after isotope administration						
Vena cava (plasma)	11.2	0.4	0.0	68.8	2.4	17.2
Portal vein (plasma)	15.1	2.1	0.0	42.3	16.7	23.8
Thoracic duct† (lymph)	11.7	0.6	2.7	72.8	0.0	12.2
Common duct (bile)	70.3	3.3	0.0	1.6	0.0	24.8

*Includes mono- and diglycerides, sterol esters, pigments (bile), and other phospholipids.

†Six-hour sample.

the triglyceride fraction and that approximately one half of the lipid radioactivity remaining in the gut lumen is in the form of free fatty acids support the observations by Saunders[13] that extensive intestinal hydrolysis of the lecithin molecule occurs in humans with biliary fistulas. Saunders concluded that there is no significant enterobiliary circulation of *intact* lecithin molecules, but he did not study the effect in these patients of ingestion of large amounts of lecithin upon biliary lecithin concentrations.

It is evident from the present study that intestinally administered lecithin does contribute to the biliary lecithin pool, probably through the agency of one or more of the hydrolytic products of intestinal lecithin which become precursors of biliary lecithin synthesis. The observation that cumulative lipid radioactivity in the bile is not diminished by diverting the thoracic duct lymph suggests that the responsible precursors reach the liver, and hence the bile, by a route other than thoracic duct lymph, possibly by lymphovenous shunts or, more likely, via the portal circulation. In this regard, it must be pointed out that the rapid circulation time in the portal system may result in the delivery of a large quantity of the radioactive portions of the intestinal lecithin molecule to the liver, despite the low concentration of radioactivity found in the portal vein at any one sampling period. Similarly, water-soluble portions of the lecithin molecule, such as choline and glyceryl phosphorylcholine, may also contribute considerably to biliary lecithin production, and these compounds would be expected to be transported mainly via portal circulation. Future studies will be directed toward determining the effects of administration of these various precursors upon biliary lecithin secretion.

The clinical importance of studies directed toward methods of increasing biliary phospholipid concentrations in patients with, or at high risk of developing, cholesterol cholelithiasis must be emphasized. Clinical experiments in which humans have ingested bile acids have met with some success, notably the disappearance of gallstones in one patient.[4] However, the reported side effects of abdominal cramping, diarrhea, and possible hepatotoxicity are difficult to reconcile to the patient with relatively asymptomatic gallstones who seeks a nonsurgical therapeutic modality. Others have raised more serious questions about the safety of prolonged use of bile acids and their effects on lipid metabolism and hepatic function.[7, 17]

In contrast, long-term ingestion of as much as 48 Gm. daily of a commercial soybean lecithin* has been well tolerated by patients and has not been associated with any abnormalities of thyroid, hepatic, or renal function as measured by serum chemistry tests. Phospholipid concentrations have been increased in the duodenal bile of these patients, and cholesterol crystals, present before lecithin was begun, have disappeared from the bile.[21] Of even greater interest is the finding that, in three patients (all male) with serum lipoprotein abnormalities (Type II and Type IV), the electrophoretic pattern has reverted to normal on this high phospholipid diet with the return to normal of the serum cholesterol and triglyceride levels.[27] Thus, a growing body of objective and subjective data supports the safety of long-term lecithin ingestion.

Continued studies of the enterobiliary metabolism of lecithin and the precursors of biliary lecithin synthesis may well disclose a more efficient and even better tolerated method of increasing biliary lecithin concentration. This type of change in human bile would increase the cholesterol-dissolving capacity of the bile and hasten the development of a medical treatment for cholesterol cholelithiasis.

*ALCOLEC, The American Lecithin Co., New York, N. Y.

REFERENCES

1. Admirand, W. H., and Small, D. M.: The physicochemical basis of cholesterol gallstone formation in man, J. Clin. Invest. **47:** 1043, 1968.
2. Anderson, F., and Bouchier, I. A. D.: Phospholipids in human lithogenic gallbladder bile, Nature **221:** 372, 1969.
3. Balint, J. A., Beeler, D. A., Kyriakides, E. C., and Treble, D. H.: The effect of bile salts upon lecithin synthesis, J. Lab. Clin. Med. **77:** 122, 1971.
4. Danzinger, R. G., Hofmann, A. F., Schoenfield, L. J., and Thistle, J. L.: Dissolution of cholesterol gallstones by chenodeoxycholic acid, N. Engl. J. Med. **268:** 1, 1972.
5. Folch, J., Lees, M., and Sloan-Stanley, G. H.: A simple method for the isolation and purification of total lipids from animal tissues, J. Biol. Chem. **226:** 497, 1957.
6. Isaksson, B.: On the lipid constituents of bile from human gallbladder containing cholesterol gallstones: A comparison with normal human bladder bile, Acta Soc. Med. Ups. **59:** 277, 1954.
7. Isselbacher, K. J.: A medical treatment for gallstones? (editorial), N. Engl. J. Med. **286:** 40, 1972.
8. King, W., III, and Tompkins, R. K.: Rapid biliary secretion of intestinal ^{14}C-lecithin, Gastroenterology **60:** 746, 1971.
9. Neiderhiser, D. H., Roth, H. P., and Webster, L. T.: Studies on the importance of lecithin for cholesterol solubilization in bile, J. Lab. Clin. Med. **68:** 90, 1966.
10. Nichols, B. W., James, A. T., and Breuer, J.: Interrelationships between fatty acid biosynthesis and acyl-lipid synthesis in Cholerella vulgaris, Biochem. J. **104:** 486, 1967.
11. Nilsson, S.: Synthesis and secretion of biliary phospholipids in man, Acta Chir. Scand. Suppl. **405:** 1, 1970.
12. Nilsson, A., and Borgstrom, B.: Absorption and metabolism of lecithin and lysolecithin by intestinal slices, Biochim. Biophys. Acta **137:** 240, 1967.
13. Saunders, D. R.: Insignificance of the enterobiliary circulation of lecithin in man, Gastroenterology **59:** 848, 1970.
14. Saunders, D. R., Parmentier, C. M., and Ways, P. O.: Metabolism of lysolecithin by rat small intestine, Gastroenterology **54:** 382, 1968.
15. Scow, R. O., Stein, Y., and Stein, O.: Incorporation of dietary lecithin and lysolecithin into lymph chylomicrons in the rat, J. Biol. Chem. **242:** 4919, 1967.
16. Small, D. M.: Physicochemical studies of cholesterol gallstone formation, Gastroenterology **52:** 607, 1967.
17. Small, D. M.: Prestone gallstone disease—Is therapy safe? (editorial), N. Engl. J. Med. **284:** 214, 1971.
18. Swell, L., Entenman, C., Leong, G. F., and Holloway, R. J.: Bile acids and lipid metabolism. IV. Influence of bile acids on biliary and liver organelle phospholipids and cholesterol, Am. J. Physiol. **215:** 1390, 1968.
19. Swell, L., Bell, C. C., Jr., and Vlahcevic, Z. R.: Relationship of bile acid pool size to biliary lipid excretion and the formation of of lithogenic bile in man, Gastroenterology **61:** 716, 1971.
20. Thistle, J. L., and Schoenfield, L. J.: Induced alterations in composition of bile of persons having cholelithiasis, Gastroenterology **61:** 488, 1971.

21. Tompkins, R. K.: Oral communication, Deuel Lipid Conference, Carmel, Calif., March 2, 1972.
22. Tompkins, R. K., and King, W., III: Contribution of intestinal lecithin to biliary lecithin excretion, Surg. Forum **22** 381, 1971.
23. Tompkins, R. K., Cornwell, D. G., Sprecher, H. W., and Zollinger, R. M.: Role of biliary phospholipids in the formation of human gallstones, Surg. Forum **18:** 411, 1967.
24. Tompkins, R. K., Burke, L. G., Cornwell, D. G., and Zollinger, R. M.: Enhancement of the cholesterol-holding capacity of human hepatic bile, Surg. Forum **19:** 344, 1968.
25. Tompkins, R. K., Burke, L. G., Zollinger, R. M., and Cornwell, D. G.: Elevation of phospholipid concentrations in human bile by feeding lecithin, Fed. Proc. **27:** 573, 1968.
26. Tompkins, R. K., Burke, L. G., Zollinger, R. M., and Cornwell, D. G.: The relationship of biliary phospholipid and cholesterol concentrations to the occurrence and dissolution of human gallstones, Ann. Surg. **172:** 936, 1970.
27. Tompkins, R. K., Corlin, R. F., Parkin, L. G., and King, W., III: Induced alterations in human serum lipids by prolonged phospholipid ingestion, Clin. Res. **21:** 276, 1973.
28. Vlahcevic, Z. R., Bell, C. C., Jr., Buhac, I., Farrar, J. T., and Swell, L.: Diminished bile acid pool size in patients with gallstones, Gastroenterology **59:** 165, 1970.

Factors affecting survival from acute subdural hematoma

T. Richards, M.D., *and* **J. Hoff, M.D.,*** *San Francisco, Calif.*

Of 100 patients who required operation for severe head injury with acute subdural hematoma, 25 survived. Fourteen survivors recovered completely. Seventy-five patients died. Few factors distinguished the postinjury course of those who lived from that of those who did not. Advanced age, preoperative shock, large bilateral subdural hematomas, gross disruption of brain, and inadequate removal of hematoma through burr holes were more often associated with death. An accurate forecast of outcome was not possible from the preoperative neurologic signs. Consequently, we favor early diagnostic studies including angiography when time permits, thorough removal of the hematoma usually by craniotomy, and vigorous postoperative management often including angiography and a second operation.

From the Departments of Surgery and Neurological Surgery, San Francisco General Hospital, University of California School of Medicine, San Francisco, Calif.

THE SURGICAL treatment of subdural hematoma began nearly fifty years ago.[16] Since that time, the disease has been classified as acute, subacute, and chronic according to the interval from injury to treatment,[4] and the surgical approach has included a spectrum from simple trephination[9, 16] on one end to radical calvariectomy on the other.[3, 10, 17] During that half-century, the surgical attack has evolved to simpler procedures for chronic hematomas[18] and more extensive operations for acute hematomas[6, 17] Thus burr holes for chronic subdural hematoma have become standard practice with an expected mortality rate of about 20 percent.[4, 18] On the other hand, morbidity and mortality rates from acute subdural hematoma remain high despite modern refinements in radiographic, surgical, and postoperative techniques.[2, 4, 5, 8, 9, 12, 14, 17, 19]

We reviewed the records of 100 patients with acute subdural hematoma treated at San Francisco General Hospital from 1963 to 1971. We sought to identify some of the factors that affect survival in these patients with acute hematomas and to reassess the effect of current therapy. This hospital, a primary care unit for patients who sustain severe injuries, is located within a low-income housing, industrial area of San Francisco, adjacent to two major highways.

CASE MATERIAL

Eighty-six patients were male; fourteen were female. The average age was 47 years (range two to 80 years). Twenty-nine percent of the injuries resulted from traffic accidents, 37 percent resulted from falls, 11 per-

This work was supported in part by Trauma Center Program Project Grant No. GM-18470 and NINDS Training Grant No. 5593.

Accepted for publication Oct. 10, 1973.

Reprint requests: Julian T. Hoff, M.D., Department of Neurological Surgery, University of California School of Medicine, San Fancisco, Calif. 94122.

*Dr. Hoff is recipient of Teacher-Investigator Award No. NS 11051 NSRB.

Table I. *Physical signs before operation in 100 patients*

Physical signs	*Percent*
Level of consciousness:	
Alert	0
Stupor	79
Coma	21
Decerebrate posturing	34
Abnormal respirations	24
Hemiplegia	26
Unilateral fixed pupil dilatation	57
Bilateral fixed pupil dilatation	13
External sign of head trauma	92
Other major injuries	13

cent were caused by assault, and 23 percent resulted from unknown causes. The time period between injury and operation averaged seven hours (range, one to 24 hours), during which a "lucid interval" was observed in 37 percent of the patients and seizures occurred in 17 percent.

Diagnosis. Physical signs prior to operation are listed in Table I. The most common sign leading to urgent evaluation was profound disturbance of consciousness that failed to improve promptly. Most were stuporous, i.e., unresponsive but arousable by vigorous and repeated stimuli. Some were comatose, or unresponsive and unarousable.[15] Among other signs, unilateral pupillary dilatation and decerebrate posturing were considered indications for either emergency angiography, operation, or both. Neurologic function deteriorated during the brief interval from admission to operation in 69 patients, while 31 patients failed to change during that time. Nine patients were in shock when first examined; three had sustained major abdominal or thoracic injuries; three had incurred extensive facial and scalp lacerations; two had obstructed airways; and one was hypotensive, presumably secondary to impairment of brain stem function. Breathing patterns were often impossible to assess accurately because assisted ventilation was frequently required immediately after admission.

In 88 patients, skull roentgenograms were obtained before operation, and 60 percent revealed a fracture. Plain skull films were normal in 20 cases, and a pineal shift was evident in seven. Cerebral angiography, performed in 31 patients, consistently demonstrated an extracerebral mass of varying size in the standard projections. Parenchymal contusions beneath the subdural hematoma were evident occasionally, particularly when in the frontal or parietal lobes, but more often they were not seen because of gross distortion from the overlying mass.

Treatment. Either assisted ventilation or general anesthesia was employed in all cases. Seventy-six patients underwent multiple burr holes as the initial procedure, and 24 had a unilateral craniotomy. Indications for craniotomy in preference to exploratory burr holes included inadequate hemostasis, insufficient removal of the hematoma through burr holes, an associated intracerebral hematoma, and the demonstration of an extracerebral mass by preoperative angiography. Unilateral subdural hematomas were present at operation in 70 patients, while the clot was bilateral in 30. The hematoma was either fresh clot admixed with liquid blood (73 percent) or tenacious and firm (27 percent). The hematomas removed varied in volume from 50 to 400 c.c. in the 85 patients in whom a volume estimate was made; 42 percent exceeded 100 c.c. and 20 percent exceeded 200 c.c. Hemorrhagic, swollen cortex was evident at operation in 57 percent of the patients, and temporal lobe contusion was sufficiently severe to require resection of pulped brain in 23 patients. In general, the craniotomy bone plate was replaced after removal of the hematoma (66 percent). In 50 of the 100 patients, the subdural space was drained for 24 hours after operation.

Postoperative treatment included supportive care, steroids for 71 percent, and hypothermia (33 to 35° C.) for 47 percent. All patients had either an endotracheal tube or tracheostomy until an adequate airway was self-maintained. Osmotic diuretic agents (mannitol, urea) were seldom used after operation, but 47 patients were so treated before or during the operative procedure.

Survival. Twenty-five patients (25 percent) survived. During the early recovery period, a second operation for recurrent subdural hematoma was necessary in seven survivors (28 percent). The diagnosis of recurrence was made either clinically on the basis of deterioration after a period of initial improvement, or angiographically when a patient's postoperative condition failed to improve. In each of the seven patients with recurrent hematomas, burr holes had been the initial operative procedure; in five the subdural space had been drained for 24 hours after operation. Other complications were infrequent among survivors. Fourteen patients had resumed their preinjury occupations at an average follow-up interval of 2.5 years (range, 0.5 to 7 years). The remaining eleven survivors required variable degrees of assistance in their daily lives. Four patients had recurrent seizures requiring anticonvulsant medication.

Seventy-five patients (75 percent) died. Fifty patients died within three days of operation. Two patients underwent a second operation for a recurrent hematoma, but both died subsequently. Only 16 percent of those who died showed transient clinical improvement after removal of the hematoma. Sepsis and pulmonary complications developed in the majority of patients dying after the third postoperative day.

Pathology. The extent of brain injury underlying the subdural hematoma in 74 patients who died is shown in Table II. The frequency of gross disruption of brain tissue—lacerations (61 percent), necrotic frontal and temporal lobes (49 percent)—is noteworthy. With two exceptions, parenchymal hematomas were contiguous with the subdural collection. The frequency of subdural hematomas present at autopsy is also of interest. The total of the 54 patients who had retained hematomas at death and the seven surviving patients requiring operation for a recurrent clot demonstrated that at least 61 percent of all patients treated surgically for acute subdural hematoma had postoperative retention or reaccumulation of significant hematomas (volume of 50+ c.c.).

Table II. *Autopsy findings in 74 patients*

Findings	*No.*	*Percent*
Cortical petechiae, perivascular hemorrhage	66	89
Leptomeningeal hemorrhage	53	72
Subdural hematoma (> 50 c.c.)	54	73
Cortical laceration	45	61
Hemorrhage and necrosis, frontal and temporal lobes	36	49
Ventricular hemorrhage	12	16
Primary parenchymal hematoma (temporal)	2	3

Table III. *Preoperative physical signs in survivors (25) and nonsurvivors (75) in the series of 100 patients*

Preoperative physical signs	*Survivors (25)*		*Nonsurvivors (75)*	
	No.	*Percent*	*No.*	*Percent*
Stupor	20	80	59	78
Coma	5	20	16	22
Decerebration	8	32	26	35
Abnormal respirations	5	20	19	25
Hemiplegia	8	32	18	24
Unilateral fixed pupil dilatation	15	60	42	56
Bilateral fixed pupil dilatation	3	12	10	13
External signs of head injury	24	96	68	90
Other major injuries	3	12	10	13
Shock	0		9	12

Comparison of survivors and nonsurvivors. Substantial differences between survivors and nonsurvivors were few. Surviving patients were only slightly younger (average age, 36 years) than nonsurvivors (average age, 51 years),[13] and a lucid interval, contrary to the experience of others,[4, 14] was more often associated with a fatal outcome (40 percent) than with recovery (28 percent). A comparison of physical signs present before operation in the two groups of patients is shown in Table III. The likelihood of death was greater in the presence of fixed pupillary dilatation,[5] and all patients in shock at initial examination died.[20]

Of more interest than the few differences was the striking similarity of other signs observed in both survivors and nonsurvivors. Preoperative seizures, the level of conscious-

Table IV. *Operative procedure and findings in the survivors and nonsurvivors*

		Survivors		Nonsurvivors	
	No.	No.	Percent	No.	Percent
Operative procedure					
Burr holes	76	16	21	60	79
Craniotomy	24	9	38	15	62
Operative findings					
Size of hematoma (operative estimate):					
Over 100 c.c.	35	7	20	28	80
Under 100 c.c.	50	18	36	32	64
Unilateral hematoma	70	23	33*	47	67
Bilateral hematoma	30	2	7*	28	93

*$\chi^2 = 28.7$, $p < 0.01$.

ness immediately prior to operation, decerebration, abnormal respirations, hemiplegia, unilateral or bilateral fixed pupillary dilatation, associated major injuries, and external signs of head injury were common to both groups of patients.

Findings at operation differed between the two groups (Table IV). While the average estimated size of hematoma removed per patient was nearly identical (126 c.c. average for survivors and 122 c.c. for nonsurvivors), the amount of clot removed did reflect a difference in survival rate.[1] When the hematoma was less than 100 c.c., 36 percent of the patients survived, but when the hematoma was more than 100 c.c., only 20 percent survived, suggesting that the size of the hematoma provided some index of prognosis. The presence of bilateral subdural hematomas exceeding 50 c.c. per side clearly indicated a poorer chance (7 percent) of survival than the presence of a unilateral hematoma (33 percent). Patients who underwent craniotomy as the initial procedure survived more often (38 percent) than those patients treated initially by burr holes (21 percent).[6, 11, 17]

Additional information emerged from analysis of the postoperative course. First, the mortality rate for the 71 patients treated during and after operation with steroids was 73 percent. The mortality rate for the entire group of 100 patients was 75 percent. Second, clinically evident recurrent hematomas were confined to patients in whom only burr holes had been performed initially. Third, drainage for 24 hours after operation failed to prevent reaccumulations in five of the seven patients who developed clinical recurrences. Finally, the mortality rate for patients treated without drainage (74 percent) was not significantly different from that for patients treated with drainage (76 percent).

DISCUSSION

This review of severe head injury during a recent eight-year period identified certain factors that influenced survival and some that did not. Advanced age, preoperative shock, large bilateral subdural hematomas, gross disruption of brain, and inadequate removal of clots through burr holes were frequently associated with fatal hematomas. Conversely, youth, minimal brain injury, a unilateral hematoma, and thorough removal of the clot by craniotomy favored survival. Some observations deviated from reported experience, e.g., a lucid interval after injury did not assure recovery, and some factors appeared to have little if any influence upon outcome, e.g. steroid therapy.

The primary brain injury in our patients was severe, indicated by the high incidence of cortical lacerations, necrosis, and parenchymal hemorrhage. The surprising frequency of recurrent or persistent subdural hematoma in both survivors and nonsurvivors probably reflects the widespread intracranial injury as well as the short-

Table V. *Comparison of mortality rates from acute subdural hematoma: 1938-1973*

Source	No. of patients	Time from injury to operation	Mortality rate
Kaplan[9] (1938)	100+	< 24 hr.	96
Laudig and associates[12] (1941)	24	< 24 hr.	83
Browder[2] (1943)	51	< 24 hr.	82
Echlin and associates[4] (1956)	93	< 7 days	72
McLaurin and Tutor[14] (1961)	90	< 24 hr.	73
Gurdjian and Thomas[5] (1966)	—	< 24 hr.	90
Ransohoff and associates[17] (1971)	40	< 48 hr.	85
	35	< 48 hr.	60
Talalla and Morin[19] (1971)	100	< 72 hr.	68
Jamieson and Yelland[8] (1972)	207	< 24 hr.	63
Richards and Hoff (1973)	100	< 24 hr.	75

comings of current surgical treatment, particularly of simple burr hole drainage.

The mortality of our patients was high despite the combined benefits of emergency diagnosis, prompt surgical treatment, and vigorous postoperative care in a neurosurgical unit. Similar results of therapy for this disease have been reported before (Table V).[2, 4, 5, 8, 9, 12, 14, 17, 19] It seems likely that current therapy, essentially unchanged from that of previous decades, will continue to yield similar results in the future. We believe the choice of craniotomy as the initial procedure for acute subdural hematoma may reduce our current high mortality rate.

This review attempted to identify those patients who were unlikely to survive their head injury. While some factors were often associated with death, an accurate forecast of outcome was not possible from the factors studied. Because of our inability to consistently predict outcome, particularly from physical signs present before operation, the current practice of emergency diagnosis and treatment will continue to be the standard approach for acute head injury with subdural hematoma regardless of the severity of presenting neurologic deficits. Our findings also argue for more frequent selection of craniotomy as the initial operation and a policy of angiographic investigation of patients whose unfavorable postoperative course may be attributable to a retained or recurrent hematoma.

REFERENCES

1. Aronson, S. M., and Okazaki, H.: A study of some factors modifying response of cerebral tissue to subdural hematoma, J. Neurosurg. **20:** 89, 1963.
2. Browder, J.: A resume of the principal diagnostic features of subdural hematoma, Bull. N. Y. Acad. Med. **19:** 168, 1943.
3. Clark, K., Nash, T. M., and Hutchinson, G. C.: The failure of circumferential craniotomy in acute traumatic cerebral swelling, J. Neurosurg. **29:** 367, 1968.
4. Echlin, F. A., Sordillo, S. V. R., and Garvey, T. Q.: Acute, subacute, and chronic subdural hematoma, J. A. M. A. **161:** 1345, 1956.
5. Gurdjian, E. S., and Thomas, L. M.: Chapter V: Surgical management of the patient with head injury, Clin. Neurosurg. **12:** 56, 1966.
6. Hoff, J. T., Grollmus, J., Barnes, B., and Margolis, T.: Clinical, angiographic, and cisternographic observations after removal of acute subdural hematoma, J. Neurosurg. In press.
7. Jamieson, K. G.: Extradural and subdural hematoma, J. Neurosurg. **33:** 632, 1970.
8. Jamieson, K. G., and Yelland, J. D. N.: Surgically treated traumatic subdural hematomas, J. Neurosurg. **37:** 137, 1972.
9. Kaplan, A.: Subdural hematoma, acute and chronic, with some remarks about treatment, SURGERY **4:** 211, 1938.
10. Kerr, F. W. L.: Radical decompression and dural grafting in severe cerebral edema, Proc. Mayo Clinic **43:** 852, 1968.
11. Kjellberg, R. N., and Prieto, A.: Bifrontal decompressive craniotomy for massive cerebral edema, J. Neurosurg. **34:** 488, 1971.
12. Laudig, G. H., Browder, E. J., and Watson, R. A.: Subdural hematoma, Ann. Surg. **113:** 170, 1941.

13. McKissock, W., Richardson, A., and Bloom, W. H.: Subdural hematoma, Lancet **1:** 1365, 1960.
14. McLaurin, R. L., and Tutor, F. T.: Acute subdural hematoma, J. Neurosurg. **18:** 61, 1961.
15. Plum, F., and Posner, J. (Eds.) Stupor and coma, Philadelphia, 1972, F. A. Davis, Company, p. 286.
16. Putnam, T. J., and Cushing, H.: Chronic subdural hematoma: Its pathology, its relation to pachymeningitis hemorrhagica and its surgical treatment, Arch. Surg. **11:** 329, 1925.
17. Ransohoff, J., Benjamin, M. V., Gage, E. L., Jr., and Epstein, F.: Hemicraniectomy in the management of acute subdural hematoma, J. Neurosurg. **34:** 70, 1971.
18. Rosenbluth, P. R., Arias, B., Quartetti, E. V., and Carney, A. L.: Current management of subdural hematoma, J. A. M. A. **179:** 759, 1962.
19. Talalla, A., and Morin, M. A.: Acute traumatic subdural hematoma: A review of one hundred consecutive cases, J. Trauma **11:** 771, 1971.
20. Wilson, C. B., Vidrine, A., and Rives, J. D.: Unrecognized abdominal trauma in patients with head injuries, Ann. Surg. **161:** 608, 1965.

The academic surgeon and the emergency department

Robert B. Rutherford, M.D., F.A.C.S., *Denver, Colo.*

More than materialistic incentives will be necessary to attract or retain qualified academic surgeons to serve as directors of the Emergency Departments of teaching hospitals in the future. The necessary ingredients appear to include a more effective functional separation of ambulatory and emergency health care problems within the institution if not the community, an opportunity for academically rewarding professional experiences, sufficient at least to balance the administrative and service obligations of the job, and the administrative and faculty support, and the authority, to get the job done. Time is of the essence, for the rate of turnover of surgeon-E.D. directors in teaching hospitals is already high and for many academic surgeons their hospital's E.D. has already become a matter of "flight or fight."

From the Department of Surgery, University of Colorado School of Medicine

The emergency facilities of hospitals throughout the United States and Canada are currently the scene of great change and unrest. Major quantitative and qualitative changes in the patient populations of these emergency "rooms" or departments have forced equally major adjustments to be made. Many if not most Emergency Department (E.D.) directors have become intimately involved with such matters as E.D. design, physician staffing plans, categorization, triage, screening or walk-in clinics, poison control, drug abuse, crisis intervention, emergency communication systems, heliport specifications, ambulance design, etc. It may be legitimately asked, what has all this to do with surgery and particularly academic surgery, since approximately three fourths of the E.D. directors in our teaching hospitals are still surgeons.

The surgeon's role as E.D. director is a legacy of the days when these facilities functioned almost exclusively for the care of the seriously ill or injured. But now the academic surgeon, originally drawn into the E.D. out of a natural interest in trauma and other surgical emergencies, often finds himself being drawn farther and farther afield from purely surgical interests, or indeed from any traditionally recognized academic pursuits. As the demands of the director's position grow with the size of the E.D., the surgeon may find that he can no longer do justice to both it and his other clinical and academic interests. Many academic surgeons still feel strongly that the E.D. should be surgical territory and that it takes the surgical approach to emergency problems to assure effective E.D. operations. Others, while resenting the intrusion of minor medical and other ambulatory care problems in the E.D., neverthe-

Presented in part as a Presidential Address at the Third Annual Meeting of the University Association for Emergency Medical Services, McMaster University, Hamilton, Ontario, Canada, May 25, 1973.

Accepted for publication Oct. 11, 1973.

Reprint requests: Dr. Robert B. Rutherford, Department of Surgery, University of Colorado Medical Center, 4200 E. Ninth Ave., Denver, Colo. 80220.

Table I. *Clinical interests of surgeon-E.D. directors*

	Listed (%)	Primary interest (%)	Relative rank*
Trauma	95	49	0.67
General surgery	74	26	0.48
Emergency medical services	60	13	0.34
Vascular surgery	31	8	0.17
Thoracic surgery	13	—	0.08
Transplantation	8	4	0.06
Pediatric surgery	5	—	0.05
Burns	5	—	0.05
Orthopedics	3	—	0.05

*Unity would be achieved if the same interest had been listed first by all respondees.

less feel that public pressures are irresistible and that E.D.'s will never be the same again, and are unwilling to fight to restore or retain the status quo. Many an academic surgeon will become involved in these issues, if he has not already. As departmental chairman, as chief of service of a teaching hospital, or as an E.D. director or future candidate for this position he should be—or become—vitally concerned with the function of today's E.D.

Recently, a survey was conducted among surgeons serving as directors of E.D.'s in teaching hospitals in order to better define the present and future role of academic surgeons in the E.D. A multiple-part questionnaire was sent to 68 E.D. directors who were listed as being surgeons by the University Association for Emergency Medical Services (EMS). Forty-six replies were received which were sufficiently complete for group analysis and they form the basis for this report.

FINDINGS

The "average" academic surgeon-E.D. director responding to the questionnaire was 42 years of age, nine years out of residency, and had held the position for almost four years. Nine percent held instructor's rank, 38 percent were assistant professors, 33 percent were associate professors, and 20 percent were full professors. A ranked list of their major professional interests is presented in Table I and reveals a wide range of clinical pursuits, led by trauma and general surgery. EMS ranked third, but more significantly was listed as the major professional interest by only 13 percent and was not listed at all by 40 percent.

The respondees spent an average of 14 hours a week physically present in the E.D. and an additional eight hours "outside" attending to E.D. matters. More than 75 percent were present in their E.D. less than 10 hours a week. The mean total effort represented approximately 30 percent of an average 70 hour week. Of the total time devoted to E.D. problems, an average of 50 percent was spent on administrative matters, 25 percent in teaching, 20 percent in patient care, and five percent in clinical research. Seventy-six percent indicated that they would not wish to continue as E.D. director if they were required to spend a minimum of 50 percent of their time in the E.D. Indeed, 58 percent stated that they would not continue if their degree of involvement in other surgical activities had to be significantly reduced in response to increasing demands from the E.D.

Eighteen percent of the respondees indicated that they received little or no professional satisfaction from their position as E.D. director and an additional 18 percent indicated a low level of satisfaction; 28 percent were moderately satisfied, and 36 percent were well satisfied. The source of professional satisfaction for the 64 percent who felt significantly rewarded for their activities as E.D. director are listed in Table II and the reasons for professional dissatisfaction listed by the other 36 percent are tabulated in Table III. Sixty percent of these surgeon-E.D. directors found the job frustrating and annoying much of the time, although only 12 percent admitted that they would quit if there were "a reasonable way out." Only 36 percent enjoyed the position enough that they had given no thought to quitting. Four percent had mixed feelings.

The main reasons listed for remaining on as E.D. director were: the enjoyment of running an active E.D. (58 percent), expectation of major future improvements (44 percent), a feeling of obligation to their departmental chairman (40 percent), and the lack of a qualified replacement (29 percent). Frequently multiple reasons were given. Seventy-three percent of the respondees indicated a willingness to continue on as director of the E.D. if it were given departmental status or its functional equivalent. Fifty-one percent indicated that they would be willing to step down if another qualified faculty member offered to take the job. Thirty-one percent indicated that they would not stay on as director if they became convinced that their E.D.'s situation was not going to improve significantly and 21 percent stated that they would not remain if they become convinced that major improvements in the total system of providing emergency medical services were not imminent.

Surprisingly, in view of the above findings, 64 percent of the respondees felt that a surgeon was still the most appropriate faculty physician to direct a university hospital E.D. Eighteen percent were in favor of "anyone interested and motivated," 12 percent recommended a full-time "emergency physician," and six percent favored an internist or family practitioner. Those favoring a surgeon as director picked as their major reasons that (1) "trauma and surgical emergencies were still the E.D.'s most important clinical problems" (55 percent) and (2) "the surgical personality is usually necessary to get the job done" (45 percent). Of the remaining 36 percent who felt that a surgeon was *not* the most appropriate E.D. director, opinions were fairly evenly divided between (1) "the job of E.D. director requires more time and effort than most academic surgeons can spare" (35 percent), (2) "today's E.D.'s have become ambulatory care facilities filled predominantly with general medical problems" (30 percent), and (3) "the complexities of today's E.D. require full-time 'emergency physicians' rather than someone from a traditional specialty which only partly covers the problems of emergency health care" (35 percent).

Table II. *Sources of professional satisfaction of surgeon-E.D. directors*

	Listed (%)	*Primary source (%)*	*Relative rank**
1. Service to patients and institution	97	39	0.76
2. Teaching experiences	95	28	0.76
3. Challenge of running an important clinical service	78	21	0.56
4. Personal clinical experiences	75	12	0.56
5. Clinical research opportunities	48	—	0.32
6. Increased financial rewards	40	—	0.19

*Unity would be achieved if the same source had been listed first by all respondees.

Table III. *Sources of professional dissatisfaction among surgeon-E.D. directors*

	Listed (%)	*Primary source (%)*	*Relative rank**
1. Lack of academic recognition for E.D. activities	69	37	0.59
2. Administrative impediments to running the E.D.	62	37	0.50
3. Lack of opportunity to do clinical research in E.D.	50	6.5	0.33
4. Impediments to developing good educational programs	41	6.5	0.30
5. Lack of personal clinic experience in E.D.	41	0	0.29
6. Lack of time to spend on E.D. problems	12	13	0.12

*Unity would be achieved if the same source had been listed first by all respondees.

The respondees listed and ranked the changes which would most significantly improve their situation as E.D. directors. The results are tabulated in Table IV. A more effective means of keeping nonemergency, general medical problems out of the E.D. received the highest ranking and several who did not list it acknowledged it as a very important objective, but one which

Table IV. *Changes which would most improve position of E.D. director*

	Listed	*Primary objective*	*Relative rank**
1. Effective means of keeping non-emergency, general medical problems out of the E.D.	68	20	0.73
2. Departmental status or its functional equivalent	75	20	0.66
3. Greater faculty support of E.D. policies and programs	82	13	0.62
4. An enlarged E.D. facility	70	5	0.56
5. Greater administrative support of E.D. policies and programs	68	5	0.50
6. A better coordinated regional EMS program	70	2	0.44
7. Facilities and funds for clinical research in E.D.	68	2	0.43
8. A separate trauma or acute surgical service under his direction	48	11	0.37
9. Increased salaries	50	—	0.29
10. More trauma and other surgical emergencies coming to the E.D.	41	2	0.29
11. A more cooperative, responsible house staff	41	2	0.28
12. A greater personal clinical experience in the E.D.	25	—	
13. Full time faculty coverage in the E.D. (write-in)	5	2	0.14 0.03

*Unity would be achieved if the same change had been listed by all respondees.

they had already achieved. In the same vein, 41 percent desired more trauma and other surgical emergencies coming to their E.D. and 54 percent felt that the educational value of their E.D. rotation was significantly diminished by the high percentage of uninstructive, minor medical problems which their house staff were required to see.

The desire for departmental status or its functional equivalent (i.e., representation on governing committees of the institution, budgetary control, hiring and firing privileges, etc.) ranked a close second. In answer to another set of questions, 93 percent felt that the E.D. director-should be represented on the governing body of the hospital medical staff or at least always be directly consulted on all matters affecting the E.D.; only 64 percent had this representation. Eighty-two percent felt that the director needed to play a major role in developing his E.D.'s budget; only 31 percent had this involvement. Sixty percent felt that the E.D. director should have "hiring and firing privileges" over the nurses, paramedical, and clerical personnel in the E.D.; only 20 percent held this authority.

Although ranked third, widespread institutional support of E.D. programs and policies was the most frequently listed change desired. In this regard, the respondees listed as most lacking in support of their E.D.: their dean (44 percent), the clinical faculty (42 percent), heads of other (nonsurgical) departments and services (36 percent), their hospital administrator (27 percent), and house staff (27 percent). Only 11 percent claimed lack of support from their own department head and only nine percent felt that their nursing service was not giving them adequate support.

Although over two thirds of the respondees desired an enlarged emergency facility and greater administrative support of their E.D. programs, only five percent listed either of these as their most desired improvement. A better coordinated regional EMS system and adequate facilities and funds for performing clinical research in the E.D. also ranked high (68 to 70 percent). Almost half listed a separate trauma or acute surgical service under their direction but this goal ranked fourth as a primary objective. Less than half of the respondees listed increased salaries, a greater trauma load, a more cooperative, responsible house staff, a greater personal clinical experience, and full-time staff physician coverage.

In answer to a question on financial incentive, 36 percent indicated they were receiving more income than they would have otherwise because of their position as E.D. director, but 60 percent of these felt that the amount received was not sufficient incentive. Of the majority who received no particular recompense for their efforts as E.D. director, 63 percent felt that this job justified some financial incentive.

In regard to faculty coverage and supervision, 67 percent had supervision from an on-call list of faculty who came to the E.D. only when called so that, for practical considerations, most of the supervision of the E.D. house staff was provided by other more senior house officers. Twenty-four percent had full-time, salaried, emergency physicians working alongside their house staff and nine percent had a panel of faculty on duty and physically present in the E.D., at least during the day and evening hours. The latter coverage was preferred by 44 percent of the respondees, coverage by full-time "emergency physicians" was the choice of 40 percent, and only 16 percent were satisfied with the most common type of coverage cited first above. Eighty-two percent felt that their house staff received less educational value from their E.D. rotation than they deserved because of lack of faculty involvement and supervision. Seventy-six percent felt that their house staff should have careful personal supervision by faculty and 64 percent felt that the house officers rotating through their E.D. should be more experienced than the usual level of first-year postgraduate training.

COMMENT

Admittedly, a certain degree of bias is automatically introduced into a survey such as this, just in the selection and wording of the questions. Nor is it easy to exclude bias from the interpretation of the answers to such a questionnaire. The author freely admits these biases. However, the responses to this questionnaire should speak for themselves and, in the final analysis, the reader must draw his own conclusions—particularly in regard to the importance of the underlying problems and their most appropriate solutions. Hopefully, few will dismiss the entire matter as simply a reflection of today's society where so many groups seem to be organizing for greater recognition, a sense of identity, more authority, greater self-determination, and better compensation. Even allowing for such motives, there appears to be sufficient cause for concern here and significant issues are involved that should not go unheeded. I will address my remaining comments to only a few of these.

First, there is undeniable evidence for widespread dissatisfaction among academic surgeons with the position of E.D. director. Most spend relatively little time in their E.D.'s and are unwilling to make a greater commitment of time and effort to the job of director unless it is made more attractive to them, administratively, clinically, and/or academically. Many are apparently staying on only because of the lack of a qualified replacement or out of a feeling of obligation to their department chairman. On the other hand, the majority apparently derive some measure of professional satisfaction from the job, feel that a surgeon is the most appropriate faculty member for this position, and would stay on under more desirable circumstances. For many of them, the main issue appears to be less one of whether surgeons should be directing the E.D.'s of teaching hospitals but how the position can be made more professionally satisfying and attractive to the academic surgeon. Based on this survey and personal experience, several recommendations appear worthy of consideration.

Of all the suggested changes designed to improve their lot as E.D. director, an effective means of diverting nonemergency traffic from the E.D. ranked highest. It is becoming difficult to defend the E.D. of a teaching hospital as "surgical territory" when neither surgical nor even emergency problems constitute a majority of those being treated there. In another survey of 50 university hospital E.D.'s, the author found that an average of only 29 percent of the presenting problems were classified as true emergencies and only 35 percent were surgical in nature. In spite of significant increases in trauma, it is the nonemergent, general medical problems which are overloading our E.D.'s. These facilities, originally designed, equipped, and staffed to care for the acutely ill and injured, now find themselves inundated with patients with relatively minor problems, who either have not established a functioning relationship with a physician practicing in the community, find it more convenient to use the E.D., were unable to reach their physician, were sent there by him, or simply find the E.D.'s always-open door to be their only reasonable point of access into today's health-care delivery system.

No one wishes to deny these particular patients appropriate medical care at reasonable cost and convenience, but the wisdom of allowing them to continue to clog up emergency care facilities, where they must suffer long treatment delays when forced to compete for medical attention with more urgent, higher priority problems, must be seriously challenged. The use of an E.D. for the management of nonurgent, general medical problems ends up being "episodic, ineffective, and expensive" medical care. But even if this trend can be reversed by a resurgence of general or family practice, the development of health maintenance organizations or other improvements in the "system," more adequate and accommodating ambulatory care facilities will be needed in many if not most of our hospitals.

An effective approach, in major population centers at least, would be the establishment of trauma and emergency care centers in selected *teaching* hospitals through a process of categorization of each hospital's capabilities followed by cooperative regional planning. This might even result in a shifting of nonemergency patients to hospitals which are not adequately equipped, staffed, or even motivated to manage the *seriously* ill or injured. Unfortunately, reactions to perceived threats to prestige or economy may seriously impede acceptance of this otherwise logical solution. The development of trauma and emergency care centers would not only improve emergency medical care but would also provide a sound basis for a major career interest and professional commitment to this field by an academic surgeon and stimulating educational experiences for surgical trainees and the other faculty who supervise them.

Failing the adoption of the above, the E.D. should at least be restored to its original function, reducing the number of nonemergency patients by providing alternative ambulatory care facilities elsewhere in the institution or community which stay open on evenings and weekends. If these ambulatory care facilities must share space with those devoted to emergency medical care, every effort should be made to have them functionally separate but adjacent, with a good triage or screening operation fronting the entire complex. In this manner, the administrative and noneducational service requirements of the E.D. could be reduced to a level which could be adequately managed on a part-time basis while allowing time for the academic surgeon to pursue other satisfying clinical and academic interests. This survey suggests that few surgeons with serious academic aspirations will be willing to continue on as director of an ever-expanding ambulatory care facility whose operation demands an inappropriately large expenditure of his time in proportion to the professional satisfaction and academic recognition he received in return for his efforts. Unless these objectives can be achieved, academic surgeons cannot be expected to provide the kind of motivated leadership a teaching hospital E.D. deserves.

Since lack of academic recognition for their E.D. activities was the greatest listed source of professional dissatisfaction in this survey, being acknowledged as a significant problem by 67 percent and as the primary source of dissatisfaction by 37 percent, it deserves additional comment. Certain questions naturally arise: What do we really mean by "academic recognition" and what sort of E.D. activities *will* provide a reasonable degree of academic recognition for the surgeon? "Academic recognition" means different things to different people. Some may measure it in terms of promotion, that is rank and tenure achieved in exchange for years of service. This survey indicates that the rate of academic promotion was not the reason for the expressed dissatisfaction with lack of academic recognition. To the contrary, because of the strong competition for qualified faculty to fill positions as E.D. directors in university hospitals, neither faculty rank nor salary should pose the problem they might have in the past when the job of E.D. director was considered just "another hat to wear," and a minor one at that.

To look further into the meaning of "academic recognition," we might do well to look at synonyms of the word "recognition." When we think of academic recognition, more emphasis needs to be placed on "commendation" and "appreciation" than simply on "identification" and "acknowledgement." Surgeons, rightly or wrongly, appear to recognize each other mainly for such things as technical skills, clinical judgment, operative innovations, and surgical research; while most surgeons will readily acknowledge the importance to their institutions of the services of a good E.D. director, most of his activities are not the sort that usually evoke respect and admiration among surgeons. Therefore the solution for the academic surgeon-E.D. director lies, not in trying to get his colleagues to appreciate him for his "nonsurgical activities" in the E.D. but in establishing a better base in the E.D. for his surgical activities. If, as recommended above, the E.D. can be made into a major referral center for trauma and other surgical emergencies, and therefore provide sufficient case material for personal clinical experiences, for a stimulating teaching program, and for clinical investigative studies, then it can provide an adequate basis for a major career commitment to the management of trauma and surgical emergencies, and if the academic surgeon can take advantage of these opportunities without becoming inundated with the administrative aspects of directing the E.D., academic recognition should take care of itself.

While the foregoing may be considered to be of essential importance to the academic surgeon, these changes alone may fail to produce a completely satisfying environment for the academic surgeon in the teaching hospital E.D. However, most of the other changes recommended by this survey would be considered desirable by any E.D. director, regardless of his professional background. This survey indicates that administrative impediments and the lack of widespread institutional support of E.D. programs and policies are other major sources of frustration and job dissatisfaction for the E.D. director. This is evident in the expressed desire for hospital departmental status or its functional equivalent, better coverage by supervisory faculty, more support from their dean and those clinical chiefs other than their own department head, and the opportunity to develop better educational programs for the house officers and medical students assigned to the E.D. It is equally clear that although an enlarged E.D. facility, a better coordinated regional EMS program, facilities and funds for clinical research in the E.D. and increased financial incentives are all listed as desirable improvements by the majority of these E.D. director, their individual lack does not constitute a major source of job dissatisfaction, since a combined total of less than 10 percent of the repondees listed any one of these as their primary objective.

Relative secretion of cholesterol-4-^{14}C in the bile and upper and lower small intestinal washings of the bile fistula rabbit

Henry Buchwald, M.D., Ph.D., Roger L. Gebhard, M.D., *and* **Richard L. Varco, M.D., Ph.D.,** *Minneapolis, Minn.*

The secretion of circulating labeled cholesterol by a total biliary fistula, by the isolated upper half of the small intestine, and by the isolated lower half of the small intestine was measured in 21 anesthetized rabbits over an average time of 13 hours. From the secreted radioactivity, ratios were calculated and the three key average radioactivity excretion ratios were: bile counts per minute (cpm)/combined total number of counts per minute (bile counts per minute + upper small intestinal counts per minute + lower small intestinal counts per minute), 0.5470; bile counts per minute/total number of small intestinal counts per minute, 1.4948; and jejunal-ileal counts per minute/distal ileal counts per minute, 1.6031. The measured average jejunal-ileal/distal ileal length ratio was 1.338. It is concluded that in the rabbit under the acute conditions of this experiment: (1) the cholesterol that is secreted in the bile is 1½ times the amount secreted by the small intestinal mucosa. (2) Small bowel mucosal cholesterol secretion, on the basis of comparison of the jejunal-ileal/distal ileal counts per minute and length ratios, does not appear to be localized to either the upper or the lower half of the small intestine. (3) Bowel mucosal cholesterol secretion is independent of the presence of bile salts in the intestinal lumen.

From the Department of Surgery, University of Minnesota Medical School, Minneapolis, Minn.

CHOLESTEROL absorption can occur in the entire small intestine but appears to be preferentially localized to the distal bowel by secondary factors, e.g., preparation time, bile salt absorption localization, and other factors.[4, 6, 8, 12] An attempt to study the corollary phase of the intestinal turnover cycle, namely, cholesterol secretion, is herein presented.

Cholesterol was found in gallstones as early as 1789,[10] and in 1824 Chevreul[9] established that cholesterol is secreted into the small intestine in the normal bile flow. In 1929, Burger and Oeter[7] and Beumer and Hepner[2] postulated that cholesterol is not only secreted in the bile but is secreted directly through the intestinal mucosa. These authors, however, considered the large intestine the intestinal site of cholesterol secretion. It was Sperry[17] and Schoenheimer and Sperry,[14] who presented definite experimental evidence for the intestinal secretion of cholesterol, when they showed that coprostanol was not only present in the intestines of animals subjected to total biliary diversion but, indeed, seemed to increase. When radioactive isotopes became available, Siperstein and Chaikoff[15] traced the C-4 ring carbon of the cholesterol molecule and found this atom to be eliminated from the rat almost

This work supported by a grant from the National Heart and Lung Institute HL11901-01, a grant from the Minnesota Heart Association, and a grant from the Graduate School of the University of Minnesota.

Accepted for publication Oct. 10, 1973.

Reprint requests: Dr. Henry Buchwald, Box 290, University of Minnesota Hospitals, Minneapolis, Minn. 55455.

entirely by way of the feces. On analyzing the fecal content for the C-4 label, they found 90 percent of the C-4 ring carbon in the saponifiable fraction and only ten percent in the non-saponifiable fraction, i.e., cholesterol, dihydrocholesterol, and coprostanol. Of this non-saponifiable fraction, half seemed to be secreted by the intestinal wall and half seemed to be secreted via the bile.

In 1953, Byers and associates[8] presented data on specific intestinal localization of cholesterol secretion. They showed that the total sterols secreted by colectomized rats were essentially equal to the amount excreted by intact control animals; however, the amount of free cholesterol contained in the excretum of the colectomized rats was 122 percent above that of the control animals, whereas the coprostanol fraction from the colectomized animals was less than 50 percent of the amount found in the control animals. These data indicated that the major site of cholesterol secretion is above the level of the large intestine and that the large intestine is primarily responsible, through the action of its bacterial flora, for the conversion of cholesterol to coprostanol. There are no published data giving evidence for or against a specific or predominant site for cholesterol secretion along the length of the small intestine.

The purpose of this experiment was to explore the capability of the isolated small intestine to secrete cholesterol, to determine the possible localization of cholesterol secretion to a segment of the small intestine, and to calculate the relative amounts of cholesterol secreted in the bile and in small intestinal washings. The experimental approach consisted of measuring the relative radioactivity of cholesterol-4-^{14}C in upper and lower small intestinal washings and in bile after the intravenous injection of 4 μCu of cholesterol-4-^{14}C in 21 rabbits with previously established total biliary fistulas.

MATERIALS AND METHODS

Animal surgery was performed under sodium 5-allyl-5(1-methlybutyl)-2-thiobarbiturate* anesthesia; two to three ml. of a 2.5 percent solution were injected via the ear vein. A total biliary fistula was established in each rabbit by ligation of the common bile duct with two ligatures of No. 4-0 silk just above its entry into the duodenum and placement of a No. 320 polyethylene cannula with a flanged tip into the dome of the gallbladder through a stab wound. The cannula was secured in place with a No. 5-0 silk purse-string suture reinforced by a No. 3-0 silk tie. The polyethylene tubing was led through the right upper quadrant and subcutaneously to the animal's back to prevent chewing of the tube. All animals received electrolyte and dextrose solutions by clysis until they resumed their oral intake. Animals were included in test groups only upon full and uncomplicated recovery from surgery and resumption of normal feeding patterns.

The biliary fistula rabbits, 10 to 14 days after operation, were injected via the ear vein with 4 μCu of cholesterol-4-^{14}C in 3.5 mg. carrier cholesterol suspended in 1 ml. of alcohol and 4 ml. of saline. Twenty-four hours after injection, the rabbit was anesthetized (drug and dosage as above) and the abdomen was opened. The small intestine was tied just distal to the first part of the duodenum, at the approximate middle of the small intestine and just above the ileocecal valve, so that the upper and lower small intestinal segments were separated from the rest of the bowel. At the entrance and at the exit of both isolated small intestinal segments, standard intravenous tubing was introduced through stab wounds in the wall of the intestine and held in place by No. 3-0 silk purse-string ties. An irrigating 0.9 percent saline solution (in some of the experimental runs, the saline contained 17 percent bile by volume) was dripped into each of the segments by the afferent cannula at a rate of 25 ml. per hour. The efferent cannulas were allowed to drain by gravity into test tubes alongside the operating table. Separate hourly collections were taken. The collections were continued until the animal

*Surital, Parke, Davis & Co., Detroit, Mich.

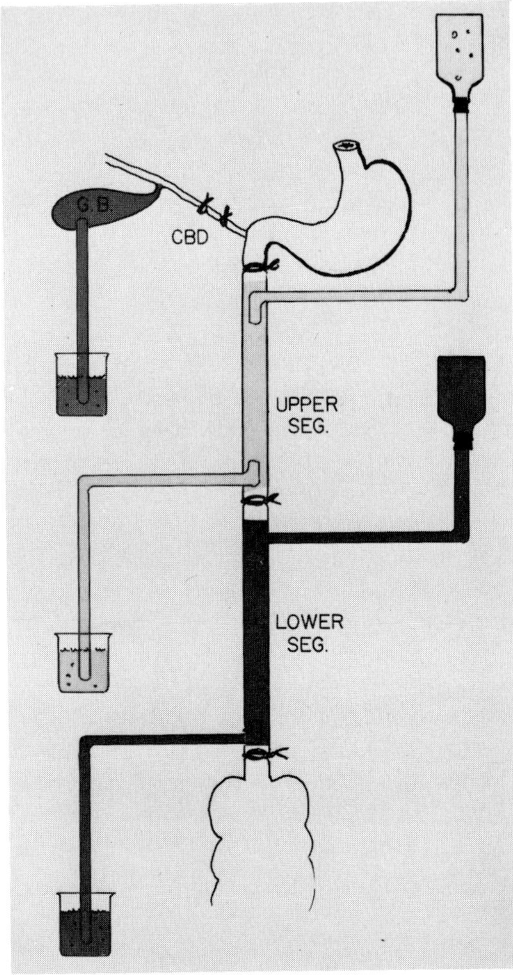

Fig. 1. Schematic representation of experimental design: ligature isolation of the upper and lower small intestinal segments; intestinal wash-through collections by timed gravity drip; gallbladder (G.B.) bile collections by gravity from previously constructed total biliary fistula (cholecystostomy) with ligation of the common bile duct (CBD).

died. The drip was then stopped and the fluid retained within each bowel segment was gently milked-down into the efferent cannula. The entire small intestine was subsequently removed and the precise lengths of the upper and lower segments were determined. Throughout the experimental run, bile was collected hourly into test tubes by gravity flow via the cholecystostomy cannula. Schematic representation of the test situation is given in Fig. 1.

The 21 rabbits employed in this experiment were divided into three groups.

Group 1. This group was composed of the eight rabbits in which the intestinal content radioactivity was analyzed by measuring the radioactivity in a 1 ml. aliquot of a homogenate of the fluid prepared in a Waring blender. Thus, when the counts per minute per milliliter (cpm/ml.) of the aliquot had been corrected for background, they were multiplied by the total number of milliliters for that hour of collection.

Group 2. This group consisted of eight rabbits in which intestinal content radioactivity analysis was carried out by extraction of a residue plug spun down in a centrifuge at 1,500 rpm. Utilization of this means of extraction provided far higher counts for an analyzed aliquot, since the radioactivity was concentrated in the insoluble residue. This gave greater counting accuracy in the spectrometer and eliminated the necessity of multiplication by the total number of milliliters in the hourly fluid sample.

Group 3. This group consisted of five rabbits in which the intestinal contents were analyzed by the homogenate method as above, but the 25 ml. per hour of irrigating fluid used to perfuse the isolated loops contained 17 percent rabbit bile by volume. The bile had been previously collected from the same animal before the injection of the tracer cholesterol. The bile was added in an attempt to elute the water-insoluble cholesterol which may not have been washed off the villi of the mucosa by the saline alone.

In all three groups, 1 ml. of the hourly bile samples collected from the cholecystostomy cannulas was extracted, with multiplication of the determined radioactivity by the total number of milliliters in the sample.

The bile and the intestinal washout extractions were carried out by a modification of the method of Abell and associates[1]; alcoholic potassium hydroxide saponification extraction of the non-saponifiable sterols into petroleum ether (b. p., 30 to 60° C.), and nitrogen stream evaporation of the ether. This method separates the sterols (for practical purposes, cholesterol only) in the bile extract from the bile salts. Radioactivity was determined in a Packard automatic tri-carb liquid-scintillation spectrometer with 0.3 percent 2,5-diphenyloxazole in 10 ml. of toluene as the fluor. Corrections were made for background and for machine variation (with use of a sealed cholesterol-4-^{14}C standard).

RESULTS

Experimental design permitted calculation of the relative secretion of labeled cholesterol from the circulating cholesterol pool in the bile, by the upper part of the small intestine and by the lower part of the small intestine. The only radioactivity from cholesterol-4-^{14}C present within the lumen of the small intestine had to originate within the mucosa of the small intestine, since the biliary fistulas had been constructed prior to the intravenous injection of radioactive cholesterol, thus permitting no flow of bile into the intestinal tract after the animal's cholesterol pool had been labeled.

Test analysis of excretion was carried out 24 hours after injection of the radioactive cholesterol, since this was the determined time of peak circulating radioactivity: In two animals, blood samples were taken immediately after injection of the radioactive test dose and hourly thereafter. After an initial blood radioactivity value between 500 and 800 cpm per milliliter, cholesterol-4-^{14}C was rapidly cleared from the blood (presumably by the liver), as evidenced by a drop of counts per minute per milliliter to about 200. Only ten hours after the giving of the test dose did the activity rise again (to 400 to 500 cpm per milliliter). Maximum values were achieved at approximately 24 hours, with counts as high as 6,300 cpm per milliliter. This was followed by a gradual exponential decline of blood radioactivity.

The bile flow varied from hour to hour and, since the amount of intestinal content also varied each hour with the final milked-down fluid often containing the maximum radioactivity, it was deemed impossible to construct any meaningful curve or steady state diagram of secretion for either the bile or the intestinal wall. Comparison evaluation was, therefore, carried out by calculation of the total radioactivity secreted for the entire duration of the life of the animal under the experimental conditions. Thus, for each animal the total number of counts per minute of bile cholesterol, the total number of counts per minute of cholesterol radioactivity in the upper small intestinal (jejunal-ileal segment) washings, and the total radioactivity of cholesterol-4-^{14}C in the lower small intestinal (distal ileal segment) washings were determined. From this, the total intestinal secreted cholesterol radioactivity was calculated. Several ratios of relativity were constructed from these data: (1) bile counts per minute/combined total number of counts per minute; (2) jejunal-ileal counts per minute/combined total number of counts per minute; (3) distal ileal counts per minute/combined total number of counts per minute; (4) bile counts per minute/total number of intestinal counts per minute; and (5) jejunal-ileal counts per minute/distal ileal counts per minute. In addition, from the measured postmortem lengths of small intestine, a jejunal-ileal/distal ileal length ratio was calculated for each animal.

The total secreted radioactivity and the comparison ratios for the eight rabbits in Group 1, in which the homogenate was used for analysis, are presented in Table I. The average ratio for bile counts per minute/combined total number of counts per minute was 0.5018, the average ratio for bile counts per minute/total number of intestinal counts per minute was 1.1428, and the jejunal-ileal counts per minute/distal ileal counts per minute ratio was 1.6428. The segmental length ratio of jejunal-ileal/distal ileal for this group was 1.494, and the average running time of the experiment for these rabbits was 15.25 hours. In a similar fashion, the values are represented for Group 2, the residue analysis group, in Table II; some of the sample material from two rabbits was partially lost and complete values for these animals could not be determined. Average ratios in this group were 0.6228 for bile counts per minute/combined total number

Table I. *Individual and average values for the counts per minute and the comparison ratios of*

Rabbit No.	Total counts per minute				
	Bile	Jejunal-ileal	Distal ileal	Total intestinal	Bile + intestinal total
143	15,180	10,890	3,617	14,507	29,687
153	5,451	3,441	1,785	5,226	10,677
202	16,980	3,384	2,633	6.017	22,997
208	9,188	4,235	4,776	9,011	18,199
226	11,613	9,614	3,218	12,832	24,445
242	12,459	9,983	11,870	21,853	34,312
257	17,076	4,863	10,517	15,380	32,456
261	6,668	6,768	3,888	10,656	17,324
Average	11,826	6,647	5,288	11,935	23,762

Table II. *Individual and average values for the counts per minute and the comparison ratios of*

Rabbit No.	Total counts per minute				
	Bile	Jejunal-ileal	Distal ileal	Total intestinal	Bile + intestinal total
272	7,536	2,032	1,682	3,714	11,250
271	4,894	1,681	2,284	3,965	8,859
866	14,152	6,791	2,142	8,933	23,085
875		1,050	645	1,695	
871		3,632	2,824	6,456	
877	5,396	1,959	1,359	3,318	8,714
885	29,289	3,665	1,301	4,966	34,255
895	329	187	254	441	770
Average	10,266	2,625	1.561	4,186	14,489

Table III. *Individual and average values for the counts per minute and the comparison ratios o*

Rabbit No.	Total counts per minute				
	Bile	Jejunal-ileal	Distal ileal	Total intestinal	Bile + intestinal total
287	42,014	7,298	10,879	18,177	60,191
288	5,854	8,742	2,872	11,614	17,468
868	30,725	7,880	6,698	14,578	45,303
876	11,911	20,759	9,209	29,968	41,878
878	37,415	10,356	10,190	20,546	57,961
Average	25,584	11,007	7,970	18,977	44,560

of counts per minute, 2.1862 for bile counts per minute/total number of intestinal counts per minute, and 1.5451 for jejunal-ileal counts per minute/distal ileal counts per minute. The jejunal-ileal/distal ileal length ratio was 1.176. The average experimental running time for this group was 11.81 hours. The data derived from the bile washout and homogenate analysis for the animals in Group 3 are presented in Table III. The average ratio for bile counts per minute/combined total number of counts per minute was 0.5282, the average ratio for bile counts per minute/total number of intestinal counts per minute was 1.2283, and the average ratio for jejunal-ileal counts per minute/distal ileal counts per minute was 1.6323. The average length jejunal-ileal/distal ileal ratio was 1.350, and the average survival time of the animals in this group was 11.50 hours. Combined average ratios for the entire 21 rabbits in the experiment are presented in Table IV, with the over-all values of 0.5470 for bile counts per minute/combined total number of counts per minute, 1.4948 for bile counts per minute/total number of intestinal *the eight rabbits in Group 1: Homogenate analysis*

Ratios					Length ratio: Jejunal-ileal/ distal ileal	Time (hr.)
Bile/total	Jejunal-ileal/total	Distal ileal/ total	Bile/intestinal	Jejunal-ileal/ distal ileal		
0.5113	0.3668	0.1218	1.0464	3.0107	2.696	8.00
0.5105	0.3223	0.1672	1.0431	1.9277	1.154	18.00
0.7384	0.1471	0.1445	2.8220	1.2852	1.333	23.00
0.5049	0.2327	0.2624	1.0196	0.8867	1.119	16.00
0.4751	0.3933	0.1316	0.9050	2.9876	1.237	12.00
0.3631	0.2909	0.3459	0.5701	0.8410	1.116	22.00
0.5261	0.1498	0.3240	1.1102	0.4624	1.115	9.00
0.3849	0.3907	0.2244	0.6258	1.7407	2.182	14.00
0.5018	0.2867	0.2152	1.1428	1.6428	1.494	15.25

the eight rabbits in Group 2: Residue analysis

Ratios					Length ratio: Jejunal-ileal/ distal ileal	Time (hr.)
Bile/total	Jejunal-ileal/ total	Distal ileal/ total	Bile/intestinal	Jejunal-ileal/ distal ileal		
0.6699	0.1806	0.1495	2.0290	1.2080	1.308	9.50
0.5524	0.1898	0.2578	1.2343	0.7360	1.325	15.50
0.6130	0.2942	0.0928	1.5842	3.1704	1.444	19.00
				1.6279	1.268	3.50
				1.2861	0.975	14.00
0.6192	0.2248	0.1560	1.6263	1.4415	1.355	15.00
0.8550	0.1070	0.0380	5.8979	2.8171	1.071	14.00
0.4272	0.2429	0.3299	0.7460	0.7360	0.661	4.00
0.6228	0.2066	0.1707	2.1862	1.5451	1.176	11.81

the five rabbits in Group 3: Homogenate analysis with bile washout

Ratios					Length ratio: Jejunal-ileal/ distal ileal	Time (hr.)
Bile/total	Jejunal-ileal/ total	Distal ileal/ total	Bile/intestinal	Jejunal-ileal/ distal ileal		
0.6980	0.1212	0.1807	2.3114	0.6708	0.816	13.00
0.3351	0.5005	0.1644	0.5040	3.0439	1.341	4.00
0.6782	0.1739	0.1478	2.1076	1.1765	1.283	11.00
0.2844	0.4957	0.2199	0.3974	2.2542	1.719	14.00
0.6455	0.1787	0.1758	1.8210	1.0163	1.590	15.50
0.5282	0.2940	0.1777	1.2283	1.6323	1.350	11.50

counts per minute, and 1.6031 for jejunal-ileal counts per minute/distal ileal counts per minute. The combined average length ratio was 1.338, and the average experimental running time was 13.00 hours.

The bile washout technique employed in the Group 3 rabbits did not increase the cholesterol radioactivity obtained from the intestinal segments. The differences between the counts-per-minute and length ratios for the jejunal-ileal to distal segments in the three test groups individually and combined are not significant. Thus, from the combined data it would seem (1) that the cholesterol secreted in the bile averages 1½ times the amount secreted by the small intestine and (2) that the small bowel mucosal secretion of cholesterol, on the basis of comparison of the jejunal-ileal/distal ileal counts per minute and length ratios, does not appear to be localized to either the upper or lower half of the small intestine. Furthermore, since in the experimental preparation bile is absent from the intestinal lumen, it follows that bowel cholesterol secretion is independent of luminal bile salts.

Table IV. *Average comparison ratios of the 21 rabbits in the combined test groups*

Counts per minute ratios					*Average length ratio: Jejunal distal ileal*	*Average time (hr.)*
Bile/total	*Jejunal-ileal/total*	*Distal ileal/total*	*Bile/intestinal*	*Jejunal-ileal/distal ileal*		
0.5470	0.2633	0.1913	1.4948	1.6031	1.338	13.00

DISCUSSION

We believe the work presented in this paper complements the findings of other authors[8, 14, 15, 17] in showing that cholesterol is secreted by the small intestine. The finding that cholesterol secretion in the small intestine is not localized to either the upper or lower half but appears to occur uniformly as a function of intestinal length is new. Our means of obtaining the secretion data is direct and not one of inference, namely, isolated small intestinal loop perfusion and recovery of circulating cholesterol radioactivity from intestinal segments previously deprived of bile contact. We have thus also shown that, even though intestinal luminal bile salts are essential for cholesterol absorption,[5, 16] cholesterol secretion by the small intestine is independent of the presence of luminal bile salts.

The ratio of bile to intestinal cholesterol secretion determined in this experiment may be dependent on the preparation—an animal with a total biliary fistula and isolated intestinal segments. We would, therefore, caution against the use of this ratio in calculating the relative cholesterol secretion in the intact rabbit. Furthermore, in the intact animal, some of the secreted cholesterol would be reabsorbed in the presence of intestinal bile salts and the contribution to cholesterol balance of the secretion mechanism, independently explored in this experiment, would undoubtedly be different.

Is the cholesterol secreted by the small intestine actually cholesterol extruded by the mucosal cell, or the product of apical cellular desquamation, or a combination of these processes? Because of the relatively short period of intestinal perfusion, the care taken to avoid intestinal wall damage, and the high radioactivity of the samples, we believe the main source of the secreted cholesterol is from cellular transport into the lumen of the bowel. In this experiment, this question has not been resolved, and we suggest that these data be regarded as indicative of total cholesterol secretion only.

Small intestinal mucosal cell cholesterol turnover is the product of several factors. We know that the intracellular mucosal cholesterol exists in a free state; however, the passage of cholesterol in and out of the cell involves esterification.[18] The esterification process from the intestinal lumen into the mucosal cell is mediated by the presence of bile salts within the intestinal lumen.[13] It has been demonstrated that transfer of cholesterol from within the mucosal cell into the intestinal lumen occurs and is independent of the presence of bile salts. The intracellular cholesterol can come from the circulating capillary bloodstream as the transfer of radioactivity in this study has shown. In addition, there is no reason to presume that the cellular-lymphatic transport of cholesterol is unidirectional; under the proper conditions, cholesterol should be able to enter the mucosal cell from the circulating lacteal lymph. Transport of cholesterol between the mucosal cell and the capillary bed is, on the other hand, probably unidirectional, because of the insolubility of cholesterol in the aqueous blood media with the cholesterol in the plasma existing in protein-bound complexes. Thus, cholesterol may enter the cell from the intestinal lumen, from the circulating lymph, from the circulating plasma, and it is, in addition, synthesized within the cell.[11, 19] Cholesterol is excreted from the cell to the lymph or, from the other side of the cell, into the intestinal lumen. Total mucosal cell turnover appears to be slow under ordinary conditions.[3]

From the data presented in this paper and in a previous publication,[4] we believe that the cholesterol absorption-secretion mechanism is not localized per se to any given segment of the small intestine, with the probability that the preferential localization of cholesterol absorption to the ileum is due to secondary factors. We would also like to suggest that the multi-directional flux of cholesterol in and out of the mucosal cell of the small intestine is regulated by a single cellular mechanism, sensitive to the relative cholesterol concentration within and on either side of the mucosal cell; the presence of bile salts in the intestinal lumen; and other, as yet unexplored, regulatory factors. Whether this mechanism is one of simple passive diffusion or one of active transport remains to be more definitively determined; however, the need for esterification for cholesterol transport in and out of the cell, the time lag within the cell, and the poor or non-absorption of structurally similar compounds all favor the presence of an active transport system.

REFERENCES

1. Abell, L. L., Levy, B. B., Brodie, B. B., and Kendall, F. E.: A simplified method for the estimation of total cholesterol in serum and demonstration of its specificity, J. Biol. Chem. **195:** 357, 1952.
2. Beumer, H., and Hepner, F.: Über die Ausscheidungswege des Cholesterins, mit freundlicher Unterstutzung der Notgemeinschaft, Z. Ges. Exp. Med. **64:** 787, 1929.
3. Borgstrom, B., Lindhe, B. A., and Wlodawer, P.: Absorption and distribution of cholesterol-4-C^{14} in the rat, Proc. Soc. Exp. Biol. Med. **99:** 365, 1958.
4. Buchwald, H., and Gebhard, R.: Effect of intestinal bypass on cholesterol absorption and blood levels in the rabbit, Am. J. Physiol. **207:** 567, 1964.
5. Buchwald, H., and Gebhard, R. L.: The essential role of bile in the intestinal absorption of cholesterol, Surgery **61:** 791, 1967.
6. Buchwald, H., and Gebhard, R. L.: Localization of bile salt absorption in-vivo in the rabbit, Ann. Surg. **167:** 191, 1968.
7. Burger, M., and Oeter, H. D.: Über den Cholesteringehalt der menschlichen Darmwand, Z. Physiol. Chem. **182:** 141, 1929.
8. Byers, S. O., Friedman, M., and Gunning, B.: Observations concerning the production and excretion of cholesterol in mammals. XI. The intestinal site of absorption and excretion of cholesterol, Am. J. Physiol. **175:** 375, 1953.
9. Chevreul, M. E.: Note sur la présence de la cholesterine dans la bile de l'homme, Mem. Museum Nat. Hist. Nat. Paris **11:** 239, 1824.
10. DeFourcroy: De la substance feuillettée et cristalline contenue dans les calculs biliaries, et de la nature des concretions cystiques cristalisées, Ann. Chim. **3:** 242, 1789.
11. Dietschy, J. M., and Siperstein, M. D.: Cholesterol synthesis by the gastrointestinal tract: Localization and mechanism of control, J. Clin. Invest. **44:** 1311, 1965.
12. Gebhard, R. L., and Buchwald, H.: Cholesterol absorption after reversal of the upper and lower halves of the small intestine, Surg. Forum **19:** 304, 1968.
13. Mueller, J. H.: The mechanism of cholesterol absorption, J. Biol. Chem. **27:** 463, 1916.
14. Schoenheimer, R., and Sperry, W. M.: Sterol secretion and coprosterol formation, J. Biol. Chem. **107:** 1, 1934.
15. Siperstein, M. D., and Chaikoff, I. L.: C^{14}-cholesterol III excretion of carbons 4 and 26 in feces, urine, and bile, J. Biol. Chem. **198:** 93, 1952.
16. Siperstein, M. D., Chaikoff, I. L., and Reinhardt, W. O.: C^{14}-cholesterol. V. Obligatory function of bile in intestinal absorption of cholesterol, J. Biol. Chem. **198:** 111, 1952.
17. Sperry, W. M.: A study of the relationship of the bile to the fecal lipids with special reference to certain problems of sterol metabolism, J. Biol. Chem. **71:** 351, 1926-1927.
18. Swell, L., Trout, E. C., Jr., Field, H., Jr., and Treadwell, C. R.: The role of lymph cholesterol in the regulation of endogenous cholesterol and cholesterol ester synthesis, J. Biol. Chem. **230:** 631, 1958.
19. Swell, L., Trout, E. C., Jr., Hopper, R., Field, H., Jr., and Treadwell, C. R.: The mechanism of cholesterol absorption, Ann. N. Y. Acad. Sci. **72:** 813, 1959.

Clinical review

Problems associated with the massive transfusion of stored blood

John A. Collins, M.D., *St. Louis, Mo.*

A new look at an old subject based on: (1) experience with massive transfusion in Vietnam, (2) the development of improved analytic techniques, and (3) awareness of major new problems related to massive transfusion.

From the Department of Surgery, Washington University School of Medicine, St. Louis, Mo.

THE PATIENT who requires massive transfusions of blood to sustain life represents the most severe challenge to blood banking as a science and an art. Any shortcomings in supply, distribution, storage, preservation, and administration will be greatly magnified. The results obtained with massively transfused patients can serve as guidelines to progress in blood banking. The problems associated with the massive transfusion of stored blood have been reviewed periodically through the years. Different periods tended to emphasize different areas, but even recent reviews have shown considerable disagreement as to what are the clinically important problems.[1-10] Unfortunately, detailed studies in patients undergoing massive transfusion have been rare, so that many of the potential problems have still not been adequately investigated. The clinical situation of massive transfusion is particularly ill suited to the requirements of careful documentation of events and the orderly, rational, and unobtrusive obtaining of necessary samples. The requirements for massive transfusion continue to grow, however, led by the worsening endemic of trauma in our society.

Three recent developments warrant this new look at an old subject. First was the war in Vietnam, where massive transfusion of blood reached an intensity of use never before approached. An abundance of clinical experience and a few careful studies in transfused patients were accumulated, and further clinical and experimental studies were stimulated. Second has been the development of improved analytic techniques which have made practical the more accurate study of some of these alleged problems: blood gas analysis, enzymatic methods for biochemical analysis on small samples, direct measurement of calcium ion activity, rapid analysis of oxyhemoglobin dissociation characteristics, more detailed and sophisticated analysis of the components of the clotting system, and others. Finally, major new problems related to massive transfusion have been proposed, problems hardly or not

Supported by Contract No. DADA 17-68-C-8006, United States Army Medical Research and Development Command, and by Contract No. NHL171-2106, National Institutes of Health.

The Twenty-sixth John G. Gibson, II, Lecture, presented at the College of Physicians and Surgeons, Columbia University, New York, N. Y., April 10, 1973. The Gibson Lecture is supported by a grant from Fenwal Laboratories, Morton Grove, Ill.

Accepted for publication Oct. 31, 1973.

Reprint requests: Dr. John A. Collins, Associate Professor of Surgery, Washington University School of Medicine, St. Louis, Mo. 63108.

at all considered as recently as five years ago, yet potentially overshadowing almost all the problems that haunted the consciousness of the blood bankers, clinicians, and investigators for the first 40 years of clinical blood banking.

PROBLEMS RELATED TO THE AMOUNT OF BLOOD TRANSFUSED

Some of the major problems that may be associated with massive transfusion are listed in Table I. Three of these are more closely related to the total volume of blood transfused than to the rate of transfusion and will not be our primary concerns today. Each of these is an important consideration, however. The transmission of disease is probably the major toxicity in stored bank blood today, and hepatitis is the single leading cause of death from transfusion. The incidence of hepatitis may be decreased by screening blood for hepatitis-associated antigen, by efforts to eliminate high-risk commercial donor pools, and by extensive washing of red cells, and the clinical severity of transfusion-induced hepatitis may be decreased by better characterization and use of immune globulin fractions, but none of these steps will eliminate the hepatitis problem.[11-14] Active immunization appears to offer the best chance for effective control. Other diseases transmitted by stored human blood continue to be identified. Cytomegalovirus and Ebstein-Barr virus may be transmitted relatively commonly, but the clinical significance in nonimmunosuppressed recipients is not clear.[15-17] Malaria and various respiratory viruses occur in stored blood on a seasonal and geopolitical basis. The list of transmitted diseases will vary and will certainly grow, and considerable uneasiness may occur as more tumor-related viruses are identified in human blood.

Although the chance of an immunologic mismatch must be considered proportional to the total amount of blood given, there is no doubt that under the stress of a massive transfusion situation errors in typing, crossmatching, identification, and administration are more likely to occur. The problem of interdonor incompatibility is, of course, accentuated during massive transfusion.[18] Similarly, immunization of the recipient is more likely to occur in massive transfusion because packed or washed cells are usually not used in an exsanguinating patient.

Table I. *Some potentially deleterious effects of the massive transfusion of stored blood*

Volume related:
Transmisison of disease
Immunologic mismatch
Immunization of recipient
Rate and volume related:
Altered hemoglobin affinity for oxygen
Coagulation abnormalities
Acid-base imbalance
Citrate toxicity
Hypothermia
Microembolization
Impaired red cell deformability
Infusion of plasticizers
Infusion of denatured proteins
Infusion of vasoactive substances
Elevated potassium, phosphate, ammonia levels
Hemolyzed blood products
Impaired antibacterial defenses
Graft-vs.-host reactions
Toxicity of new additives

PROBLEMS RELATED TO RATE AND VOLUME OF TRANSFUSION

Our main focus of interest will be on the problems that are related to a rapid and sustained rate of tranfusion. These problems largely reflect imperfections in methods of preserving and storing human blood for transfusion. Understanding the mathematics of exchange transfusion is essential for evaluating many of these potentially harmful effects insofar as they are related to the degree of replacement of cells or plasma with the stored product, so this will be considered first. Specific problems will then be considered individually, beginning with the most prominent.

Mathematics of exchange transfusion. The mathematics of exchange transfusion have been worked out in connection with the treatment of hemolytic disease of the newborn.[19, 20] The calculations can be kept fairly simple if a number of assumptions are

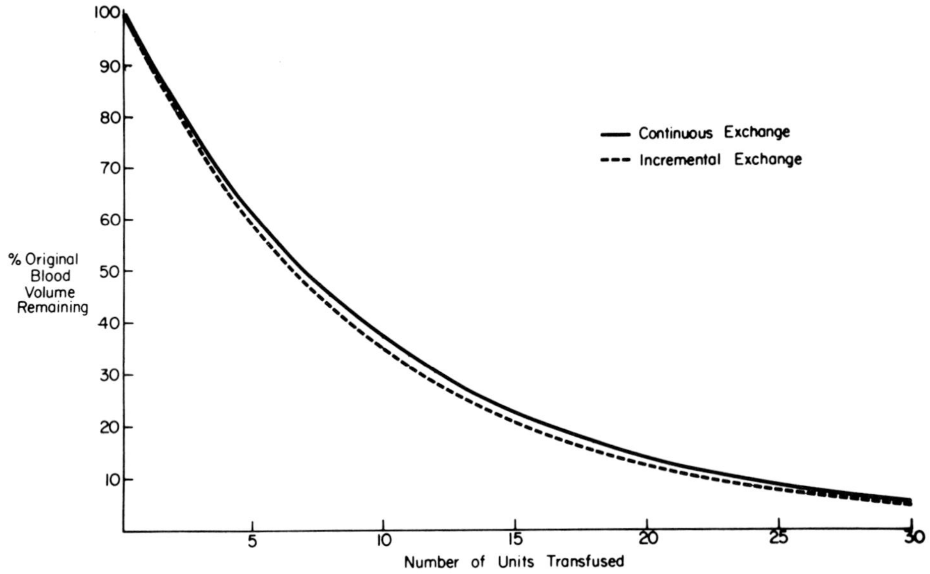

Fig. 1. Calculated original blood volume remaining after exchange transfusion of indicated number of units of blood in a patient wtih a 5 L. blood volume, assuming 500 ml. volume for each unit of blood. Solid line represents calculations for continuous exchange, broken line for incremental change according to formulas and assumptions described in the text. There is little difference in the results obtained by these two methods of calculation under clinically applicable circumstances.

made: mixing in the recipient is instantaneous and complete, the blood volume at completion equals the initial blood volume, the transfused blood is constant in composition, and the recipient is a closed system so that no substance in question is otherwise added or removed during the exchange and only the blood volume is involved in the exchange. When the exchange is performed in a stepwise or incremented manner, calculation is simplified to formula (1) if: the volume infused equals the volume withdrawn for each step, each step begins with withdrawal, infusion begins only after withdrawal is completed, and each step is equal in volume.

$$X_n = X_0 \left(1 - \frac{b}{v}\right)^n \qquad (1)$$

where X_n = the amount or concentration of the substance in question remaining in the recipient's blood after n units of blood; X_0 = the amount or concentration of the substance in question in the recipient's blood before transfusion; b = the volume of a unit of blood; v = the recipient's blood volume; n = the number of units of blood transfused.

For a situation of continuous exchange, if we assume that infusion and withdrawal occur simultaneously and at equal rates so that blood volume remains constant, then formula (2) applies:

$$X_t = X_0 e^{-\frac{b}{v}t} \qquad (2)$$

where X_t = the amount or concentration of the substance in question remaining in the recipient's blood after time t; t = the time (duration) of the transfusion; b = the blood volume infused in time t.

If time t is defined in terms of the time necessary to transfuse n units of blood, then (1) and (2) can be used in similar circumstances and (2) can be used even when the rate of transfusion varies, assuming that the rate of infusion always equals the simultaneous rate of withdrawal.

Under clinically applicable circumstances, there is little difference between the incremental and continuous exchange methods of calculation. The results that would ob-

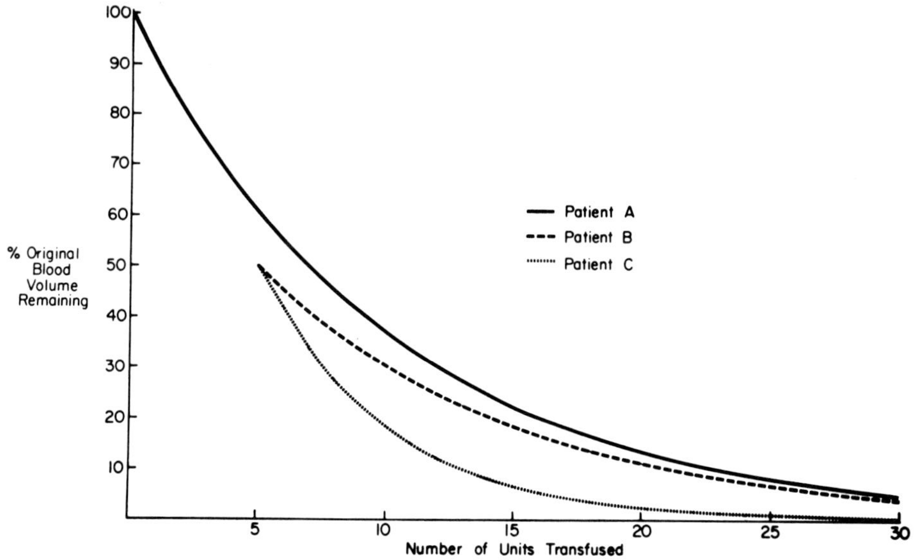

Fig. 2. Percent of original blood volume remaining in each of three hypothetical recipients, all beginning and ending with a blood volume of 5 L., assuming each unit of blood contains 500 ml., and using formulas and assumptions for continuous exchange as explained in text. Patient A remains normovolemic throughout. Patient B and C sustain a loss of half their normal blood volume before transfusion begins. In patient B this loss is replaced immediately and subsequent hemorrhage and transfusion occur with a normal blood volume. In patient C the initial loss is replaced only after hemorrhage has stopped.

Table II. *Percent of original blood volume remaining in the three hypothetical patients illustrated in Fig. 2 after hemorrhage and transfusion as indicated*

Patient	*Percent of original blood volume remaining**		
	1 blood volume (10 units)	*2 blood volumes (20 units)*	*3 blood volumes (30 units)*
A	36.8 (34.9)	13.5 (12.2)	5 (4.2)
B	30.4 (29.5)	11.2 (10.3)	4.1 (3.6)
C	18.4 (16.4)	2.5 (1.8)	0.4 (0.2)

*Computations based on continuous exchange formula; results with incremental exchange formula indicated in parentheses.

tain in an adult with a 5 L. blood volume exchanged either continuously or incrementally in 500 ml. steps, assuming a unit of blood contains 500 ml., are shown in Fig. 1. If we began with infusion before withdrawal, the line for incremental exchange would be an equal distance above the line for continuous exchange.

Far more significant is a variable that is very likely to occur clinically. In Fig. 2 are shown the theoretical results using the continuous exchange formula in three different hypothetical patients, each with the same blood volume (5 L.) and each transfused with the same amount of blood. In patient A, transfusion begins at a normal blood volume and keeps pace with hemorrhage throughout. In patient B, transfusion begins after an initial loss of half the blood volume, but this initial loss is rapidly replaced and further loss and transfusion occurs with the blood volume at 5 L. throughout. Patient C also sustained an initial loss of half the blood volume, but this is not replaced. Further hemorrhage and transfusion occur with a blood volume of 2.5 L. Blood volume is restored to normal only after the hemorrhage has stopped. These three patients, then, begin and end with the same blood volume and receive the same amount of stored blood, but with very different effects (Table II). Thus, one cannot precisely predict the

Table III. *P_{50} (mean values) as determined by correction of pH by standard correction factors (CF) vs. correction of pH by titration to 7.40 with 5 percent sodium bicarbonate or 1M Tris buffer, or by repeated washing with fresh heparinized plasma**

Day of storage	P_{50} of blood stored 3 to 4 weeks in ACD (N = 24)			
	CF	$NaHCO_3$	Tris	Plasma
In ACD (N = 24)				
21-28	14.3	17.3	17.4	17.0
In CPD (N = 5)				
0	24.8	25.1	25.2	
1	24.1	24.8	24.9	
2	25	25.1	25.6	
3	24.3	25.5	25.5	
7	22.4	23.1	23.5	
14	17.1	19.1	19.8	
21	15.9	18.3	18.3	
28	15.5	18.8	19.1	

*Based on unpublished data of Collins, J. A., and Kaplan, H. L.

amount of exchange or replacement, even knowing the recipients' starting and finishing blood volumes and the volume of blood administered. On computational terms only and completely ignoring physiologic considerations, *early complete replacement of blood volume in the massively bleeding patient lessens the impact of exchange transfusion with stored blood.*

Altered hemoglobin function. Undoubtedly the most interesting and exciting of the "new" considerations of the toxicity of massive transfusion involves the resulting alterations in oxygen delivery. The affinity of hemoglobin for oxygen increases markedly in blood stored in ACD,* and more slowly and not as extensively in blood stored in CPD.* These changes correlate with changes in 2,3-DPG (2,3-diphosphoglyceric acid) during storage.[21-24] The recipients of large amounts of stored blood exhibit a corresponding shift in oxyhemoglobin dissociation characteristics.[21, 25-31] It is apparent from these published studies and from our own data, however, that very large amounts of blood are necessary to drive the recipients' P_{50}† to 20 mm. Hg or below, and that shifts below 18 mm. Hg are almost never seen, despite truly massive amounts of transfused blood and extremely low 2,3-DPG levels. With total transfusions less than one or two blood volumes in 24 hours, the P_{50} usually remains well above 20 mm. Hg. This is to be expected from the demonstrable difficulty in totally exchanging the recipient's red cell mass with stored cells, and the rate with which 2,3-DPG is regenerated after transfusion.[31-33] In addition, a potential error arises from the application of standard correction factors for pH in measuring the P_{50} of stored blood. We have found that correction of pH with sodium bicarbonate, Tris (Tris [hydroxymethyl] aminomethane) buffer, or fresh heparinized plasma yields a P_{50} for stored ACD blood that is 3 mm. Hg higher than is obtained by using standard correction factors.[34] Massively transfused patients thus approach the true P_{50} of stored blood and P_{50} values below 18 mm. Hg should not be expected. We have investigated this phenomenon in prospective studies on blood stored in CPD and have found the same error (Table III). The magnitude of the error is related to the degree of depletion of 2,3-DPG in blood stored in either ACD[138] or CPD. We can thus predict that the P_{50} of the recipient after massive transfusion with blood stored in CPD should not go much below 20 mm. Hg despite the apparently lower P_{50} of the stored blood. Such data on patients heavily transfused with blood stored in CPD are not yet available.

*ACD, acid-citrate-dextrose anticoagulant for stored human blood (U.S.P. formula A). CPD, citrate-phosphate-dextrose anticoagulant for stored human blood (U.S.P.).

†P_{50}, oxygen tension in millimeters of mercury at which hemoglobin is half saturated with oxygen at 37° C. and pH 7.40.

Table IV. *Rats were exchange transfused 20 percent of estimated blood volume × 10 with rat blood stored in ACD 4 hours (fresh) or over 2 weeks (stored) in three hematocrit ranges obtained by adding citrated rat plasma, then hemorrhaged in a standardized manner, and treated with the same blood used for exchange (mean values)*

Blood	P_{50} (mm. Hg)	2,3-DPG (μM/Gm. Hgb)	Hematocrit	Deaths
Fresh	35	14.4	36	5/11
			31	4/11
			21	4/11
Stored	24	1.2	35	5/11
			30	7/11
			19.5	9/11

Even more pertinent is the question of the pathophysiologic effects of an acutely increased oxygen affinity for hemoglobin in critically ill patients. Despite the theoretical disadvantages,[139, 140] actual in vivo detrimental effects have been hard to document. The most supportive study so far has been that of Oski and associates,[35] in which patients with similar degrees of anemia but with dissociation curves shifted in opposite directions were studied under conditions of rest and exercise. The patient with the increased hemoglobin-oxygen affinity had a lower exercise tolerance, a higher cardiac output, and lower mixed venous Po_2 under similar conditions. Huggins and colleagues[36] reported an increased mortality rate in rats given stored human red cells depleted of 2,3-DPG compared to those given cells rich in 2,3-DPG when exchange-transfused to severe anemia with dextran. Several authors have shown a decrease in tissue or mixed venous Po_2 when animals were exchange-transfused with old stored blood.[37, 38] On the other hand, Woodson[39] found no difference in exercise tolerance in rats exchange-transfused with blood depleted of 2,3-DPG compared with those exchange-transfused with fresh blood. We are studying rats exchange-transfused to about 90 percent replacement with either fresh or stored blood (ACD), then challenged with a standard hemorrhagic shock model (Table IV). With hematocrits near normal, there was no difference in mortality rate in the groups treated with fresh vs. stored blood, despite achievement of a nearly 50 percent mortality rate. As hematocrit was lowered, however, the animals exchange-transfused with fresh blood clearly had better survival than those with stored blood. This is pertinent in view of the results reported above. Woodson found no effect of acutely shifting the oxyhemoglobin dissociation curve at normal hematocrits, while the studies of Oski and of Huggins showing the advantages of lower hemoglobin affinity for oxygen were performed at low hematocrits. It may be that in the resilient oxygen delivery system of healthy adults, a normal hematocrit level will protect against some of the impairment due to depletion of 2,3-DPG. Conversely, resuscitation methods involving hemodilution should be careful to preserve 2,3-DPG levels. With massive transfusion with blood stored in ACD, it is certainly easier to preserve hematocrit than to preserve 2,3-DPG levels.

The complexities of hemoglobin-oxygen affinity tend to be hidden by the use of P_{50} as the sole indicator.[40] This value eliminates pH and temperature as variables, thereby unduly emphasizing such factors as 2,3-DPG. We have studied the relative roles of 2,3-DPG and pH in influencing oxygen delivery in vivo in seriously ill patients with significant acid-base alterations[41] by measuring arterial–central venous oxygen saturation differences. Three values were used. The oxygen saturation differences were measured directly in the patient's blood samples ("actual"), and were derived using the measured oxygen tensions as an oxyhemoglobin dis-

Table V. *The relative effects of changes in pH and temperature vs. changes in 2,3-DPG on oxygen delivery in vivo were estimated as described in the text. Group A had A-V pH differences less than 0.4 pH units, Group B greater than 0.4 pH units (mean values)*

Patient group	No. of patients	Arterial pH	P_{50} (mm. Hg)	Change in O_2 delivery due to: pH and temp. (%)	Change in O_2 delivery due to: 2,3-DPG (%)
A	10	7.52	26.5	−22.8	−1
B	8	7.51	28.1	−9.2	+2.3
C	9	7.35	25.6	+36.3	−10

sociation curve constructed from the patient's blood with standard corrections for pH and temperature ("individual") and the universal human dissociation curve ("universal"), which presumably eliminates all variables.

$$\frac{\text{Actual-individual}}{\text{Universal}} \times 100 =$$

Percent change in O_2 delivery due to deviation of pH and temperature from normal;

$$\frac{\text{Individual-universal}}{\text{Universal}} \times 100 =$$

Percent change in O_2 delivery due to deviation of 2,3-DPG from normal concentrations.

When 2,3-DPG concentrations changed in the direction expected from changes in pH, thereby exerting an opposite effect on hemoglobin-oxygen affinity, the effect of pH usually predominated. Most alkalemic patients failed to raise 2,3-DPG levels and shift P_{50} to compensate for the Bohr effect. Such compensation has been demonstrated to be almost complete in normal adults[42] but was very incomplete or lacking in most of the sick patients we studied.

In acidemic patients, on the other hand, use of the P_{50} curve led to a gross underestimation of in vivo oxygen delivery. Several other factors were also important in determining oxygen delivery in vivo, but are not reflected in derived curves. Arteriovenous (A-V) pH differences were large enough in some patients to increase oxygen delivery. This effect was independent of the position of the curve. Hypoxemia, on the other hand, lessened the impact of a shifted curve on oxygen delivery by moving arterial values toward the steep portion of the curve. As a result, oxygen delivery in vivo was significantly different from that indicated by simple consideration of the P_{50} curve (Table V). In six of ten patients studied within 10 hours of extensive transfusion, the impairment in oxygen release caused by the alkalosis that is so commonly seen in these patients was quantitatively greater than that caused by the shift due to 2,3-DPG depletion. When studied at the time of maximum 2,3-DPG levels following transfusion, the relative effect of pH was of course even greater (Table VI). Obviously, considerations of oxygen delivery in vivo must include the relevant factors other than 2,3-DPG, especially pH, even in massively transfused patients. One immediate clinical corollary of these findings is that unnecessary alkalinization during massive transfusion should be avoided, as the effects of alkalosis and 2,3-DPG depletion are additive in impairing oxygen release by hemoglobin.

These considerations do not imply that 2,3-DPG is of no concern in the massively transfused patient. They are brought out rather to emphasize the complexities of oxygen delivery in vivo. Rather sweeping statements have been made about the lack of function of stored red cells, based on considerations of 2,3-DPG and P_{50} alone. Proposals for changes in clinical blood banking practices based on these assumptions could be disruptive and almost impossibly burdensome to most blood banks. It appears to us that not enough is known about the clinical importance of 2,3-DPG in massive transfusion to justify either the statements or the disruptions.

The situation may be more critical in children, especially in the newborn. Kevy and

Table VI. *The relative effects of changes in pH and temperature versus changes in 2,3-DPG on oxygen delivery were estimated after extensive transfusion. Values within 24 hours of transfusion (lowest 2,3-DPG levels) are contrasted with those following transfusion when 2,3-DPG reached the highest recorded levels*

Patient No.	Transfusion (units/hr. before study)	P_{50}	2,3-DPG (M:/Gm. Hgb)	Arterial pH	Change in O_2 delivery due to: pH and temp. (%)	Change in O_2 delivery due to: 2,3-DPG (%)
1	15/22	26	11	7.59	−22.4	−3.5
	(3 days later)	28.5	17.8	7.49	−6.7	+12.1
2	10/20	23.5	8.1	7.58	−18.3	−18.4
	(3 days later)	29	16	7.56	−21.6	+15.2
3	12/6	25	6.9	7.59	−23.7	−12.1
	(3 days later)	28	14.8	7.50	−8.8	+10.3
4	20/20	24	4.5	7.51	−23.8	−15.5
	(following day)	28	17.9	7.59	−19.6	+5.7
5	14/20	26	10.3	7.53	−28	−2.4
	(following day)	28	18.5	7.51	−11.2	+7
6	18/22	24	9.6	7.48	−8.1	−16
	(following day)	28	19.6	7.48	−5.2	+10.9
7	10/22	26	11.1	7.65	−21.5	−1.9
	(two days later)	28.5	20.4	7.48	−6.8	+8.7
8	22/35	23.5	7.2	7.54	−14.8	−16.5
	(three days later)	28	16.1	7.58	−24.2	+5.6
9	10/19	27.5	13	7.57	−42.3	+4.7
	(died)					
10	20/23	23	3.8	7.43	+1	−18.9
	(following day)	26	7.9	7.21	+48.7	−8.7
	(died)					

co-workers[43] reported a fall in muscle surface pH during massive transfusion that seemed greater in children given old blood. Exchange transfusion of piglets with fresh adult blood produced an increase in the mixed venous Po_2.[44] A prospective study of exchange transfusion with fresh adult blood in infants with respiratory distress syndrome is under way.[45]

Theoretically, the heart should be the organ most vulnerable to an acute increase in the affinity of hemoglobin for oxygen because its mixed venous Po_2 is already near the minimal functional level. If the ability of the coronary vessels to dilate is impaired, the affinity of hemoglobin for oxygen theoretically could become critical for survival. There have been no pertinent studies. Chance[46] found that constant perfusion of an isolated heart preparation with fresh vs. old blood made no difference in the redox state measured by surface fluorescence, but the oxygen loading pressure was so low (30 mm. Hg) that no difference in oxygen delivery could be expected even with markedly different affinities of hemoglobin for oxygen. In the clinical situation, patients with serious coronary disease usually do not survive the kind of blood loss that requires massive transfusion, so a certain element of preselection is operative. Nevertheless, there may well be a population with subclinical coronary disease in whom the affinity of hemoglobin for oxygen may become critically important at some point during resuscitation. Almost all experimental work and most clinical studies to date have dealt with a generally healthy young adult population.

Fortunately, 2,3-DPG levels are maintained near normal during the first week of storage in CPD, making preservation of 2,3-DPG levels in massively transfused patients more easily attainable with the impending change to CPD in the United States. Methods for generating high levels of 2,3-DPG in stored cells create the possibility of raising P_{50} above normal in transfused patients, if this is thought necessary.[47] One must not lose sight of the entire oxygen delivery system, however, as certain elements may vary in importance as other related elements are changed by treatment or disease.

Coagulation. Abnormal bleeding is one of the abnormalities traditionally attributed to massive transfusion. A major transfusion reaction can trigger an episode of intravascular coagulation and fibrinolysis. Stored blood itself is an imperfect clotting package, lacking platelets and ionized calcium, and with low levels of Factors V and VIII. Many of the bleeding problems after transfusion are often attributed to a dilutional effect.

It is assumed that cardiac standstill will occur before ionized calcium levels become low enough to interfere with clotting, but several examples have been reported of improvement in laboratory clotting tests coinciding with administration of ionized calcium.[48] We studied one such patient just prior to cardiac arrest during massive transfusion.[49] Even if true, this must be a very unusual situation.

Platelet levels fall significantly during transfusion, most likely because of a dilutional effect.[9, 49-55] In most reported series, platelet counts do not often fall below 50,000 per cubic millimeter even with transfusion of several blood volumes. Several groups, however, have concluded that dilutional thrombocytopenia or some impairment of platelet function is the cause of any observed bleeding tendencies,[50, 53-55] in spite of the fact that platelet counts at this level are ordinarily not associated with pathologic bleeding. The reported benefits of fresh blood remain essentially undocumented, and accounts of markedly increased platelet counts after transfusion of a few units of fresh blood are not compatible with the arithmetic involved. Studies on platelet function after massive transfusion have been very few. A wide variation in platelet agglutinability following trauma and extensive transfusion was reported recently.[55] Certain platelet breakdown products may inhibit platelet function (J. H. Joist, personal communication). If confirmed this bears obvious implications for massive transfusion practices. Depressed ionized calcium and alterations in pH and temperature also inhibit platelet function[56] and such abnormalities may occur transiently during transfusion. Plasticizers from the storage bag may also affect platelet function.[110] Studies of bleeding after massive transfusion will almost certainly focus on platelet function for the next few years at least.

Changes in intermediary clotting factors often reflect the dilutional effects of transfusion but may vary independently.[9, 49-55] Most studies have shown no easily identifiable pattern. We studied coagulation changes serially on a large number of combat casualties before, during, and after resuscitation.[49] The results were very varied and are not easily summarized. In general, the most seriously injured exhibited the most abnormal clotting patterns. Some casualties presented a typical picture of disseminated intravascular coagulation either before or during transfusion, with marked depletion of various clotting elements and the appearance of fibrin degradation products. In these patients, clotting studies were usually better during transfusion of stored blood but worsened when transfusion ceased. This finding is in contrast to the results reported by the Naval Surgical Research Team, which related abnormal findings solely to the volume of blood transfused.[53] Most patients in our series exhibited simple dilutional changes, approaching the values for stored blood during massive transfusion, then slowly improving after. These changes did not seem sufficient to cause major clinical bleeding problems. Once transfusion ended, a cyclical instability of various clotting tests became apparent in many of those with serious complications or persisting hypotension. Thus, these vigorous young adults tended to compensate very well for the clotting deficiencies of stored blood unless resuscitation was incomplete or complicated. Those with the most abnormal clotting studies usually showed evidence of desseminated intravas-

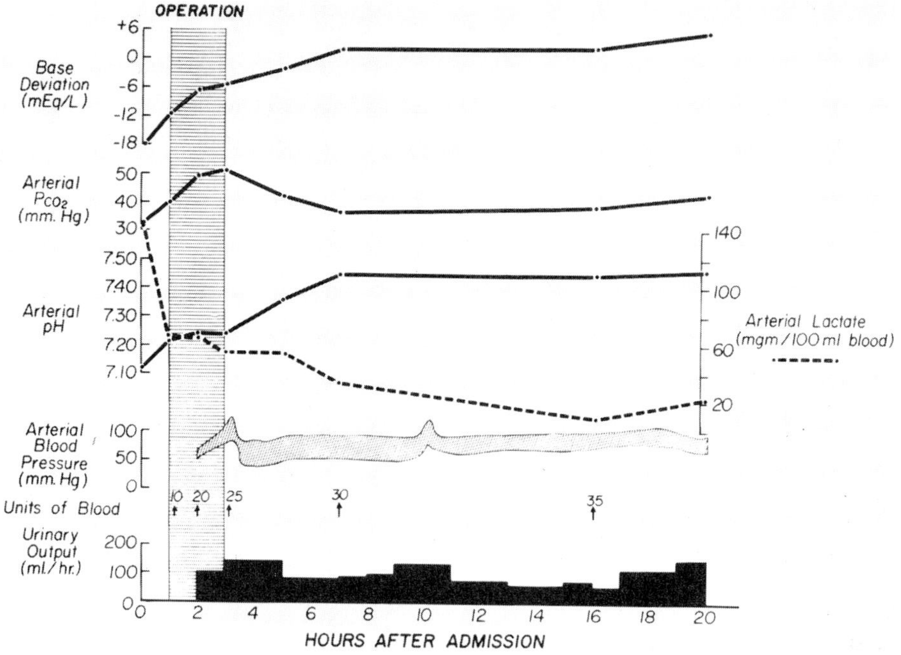

Fig. 3. Combat casualty with multiple blast amputations and penetrating wounds of all body cavities admitted with unobtainable blood pressure but with spontaneous respirations. Intra-abdominal hemorrhage required laparotomy before blood pressure was restored. Rapid transfusion of large amounts of stored blood combined with excellent transportation and management by multiple experienced teams in a hospital organized for this type of care led to an uncomplicated recovery. (Reprinted with permission from Collins, J. A., et al.: Ann. Surg. 173: 6, 1971.)

cular coagulation, often before much blood was given. In some, abnormal bleeding may have caused massive transfusion.

Once again, early and complete resuscitation probably prevented a complication usually attributed to massive transfusion, but more detailed studies of platelet function may indicate an induced defect and a need for replacement therapy with platelet packs above a certain level of transfusion. Patients with preexisting clotting defects, especially those with serious liver disease, may benefit from routine administration of fresh frozen plasma during transfusion. Routine use in otherwise intact patients should be done with awareness of the exchange mathematics involved: There should be little need during the first transfused blood volume. Emphasis, instead, should be placed on stopping the hemorrhage and restoring perfusion so as to prevent or terminate disseminated intravascular coagulation, which may be the greater culprit in many of the pathological bleeding states that arise during massive transfusion.

Acid-base imbalance.* Stored bank blood contains an appreciable acid load. Patients who require rapid and sustained transfusions are likely to have a pre-existing metabolic acidosis. Concern for the acid-base status of such recipients is reasonable, and several experiments indicate that the acid load of stored blood can be lethal to dogs. Many authors have, therefore, proposed the routine administration of alkalinizing solutions on an empiric basis in clinical situations of extensive transfusion, supporting this suggestion with uncontrolled clinical observations.

The excess acidity of stored blood is due mainly to the citric acid of the anticoagulant and the lactic acid generated during storage. Both of these organic acids are normal intermediary metabolites and are rapid-

*For a more detailed description and bibliography, cf. Collins et al.[57]

ly metabolized under normal conditions. The pre-existing metabolic acidosis of the recipient is also an organic acidosis which is rapidly reversed when blood volume is restored, an effect that is to be expected from the transfusion of stored blood. The impact of transfusion on the acid-base status of the recipient is, therefore, not a simple one of buffering and titration in a closed system, but rather a complex one involving rates of administration, rates of metabolic removal, and the changing circulatory efficiency of the recipient.

We studied in detail the acid-base changes in 36 heavily transfused casualties in Vietnam during and after transfusion (see Fig. 3).[57] They were divided into a group transfused rapidly (mean 15.4 units in 1.9 hours) and a group given a large volume of blood as a continuous transfusion (mean 28.7 units in 9.1 hours). The results were then studied according to lowest blood pressure observed, initial base deficit, or blood pressure at the end of transfusion. The last proved the most informative. Patients whose blood pressure was restored by transfusion and some of those who remained hypotensive easily handled the infused acid load of the transfusion and reversed pre-existing metabolic acidosis, when present. Those in whom hemorrhage was not controlled exhibited worsening acidemia that was probably due to shock as much as to transfusion. Administration of alkalinizing agents to this group was futile.

The routine administration of alkalinizing solutions during transfusion would have been unnecessary for most of these casualties. The failures of resuscitation were clinically evident. Failure was not due to the acid load of the stored blood but rather to uncontrolled hemorrhage. Unnecessary alkalinization in this group would have worsened the impairment of oxygen delivery induced by the stored red cells, would have resulted in a very large additional sodium load in patients prone to retain salt and water, and might have impaired the ability to mobilize ionized calcium during rapid transfusion. In the absence of need, the routine use of alkalinizing solution seems unwise. It must be acknowledged that these were healthy young adults, that resuscitation was well performed and monitored, and that the high ambient temperature prevented the development of hypothermia in the transfused patients. Nevertheless, it seemed to us that those who exhibited a worsening acidosis could be easily detected on clinical grounds, and that hypoperfusion rather than acidosis was their main problem. The Naval Research Team subsequently reported their studies in heavily transfused casualties, which were in agreement with ours.[58] We hope the practice of routine administration of alkalinizing solutions will be replaced by a more individualized and, whenever possible, objective approach based on blood gas analysis.

Citrate toxicity. One of the oldest and still most controversial aspects of massive transfusion revolves around the occurrence and importance of citrate toxicity. The commonly used anticoagulants for stored bank blood contain a planned excess of citrate to ensure complete anticoagulation. Recipients of blood in massive amounts over short periods of time can be expected to develop hypercitremia and hypocalcemia. This is easily produced in animals and studies on patients and volunteers indicate its occurrence clinically. The administration of calcium can itself be dangerous, however, and the documentation of hypocalcemia has been very difficult.

The older methods of estimating ionized calcium levels in blood may have been imprecise.[59, 60] The relationship between massive transfusion and ionized calcium changes in the recipient involves at least three variables: the rate of citrate administration in relation to its rate of metabolic removal, the rate at which calcium is mobilized from skeletal stores in response to needs, and the effect of simultaneous changes in blood pH on both calcium and citrate metabolism. In considering the biologic effect of hypocalcemia on the patient, it may be necessary to also consider elevations in plasma potassium, which may be additive,[61] and the less marked but real calcium-binding effects of lactate and phosphate. Potassium, lactate, and phosphate are all elevated in stored blood.

Citrate has long been known to be rapidly metabolized and to become toxic only at high rates of administration.[62] A number of clinical studies have documented elevated citrate levels in patients rapidly transfused or being infused with citrate solutions.[62-65] More than moderate elevations were usually found only at transfusion equivalents greater than one unit every five minutes for a 70 kilogram recipient. Howland and associates[64] reported a patient infused for 20 minutes at the citrate equivalent of 25 units of blood per hour for a 70 kilogram recipient. The arterial citrate level dropped from 80 to 15 mg. percent during the 20 minutes after cessation of the infusion. Drucker and associates[66] found no impairment of citrate metabolism during or after elective operations under general anesthesia without significant blood loss. Bunker and associates[63] detected impaired citrate metabolism in only one of six severely hypotensive patients, but always detected severe impairment when hypotension was combined with diffuse liver disease or hypothermia. Howland and coworkers[64] seemed to find more evidence of impairment in severe shock. This critical point has been minimally documented and clearly needs more extensive study in clinical situations.

We accumulated indirect evidence on the rate of citrate metabolism in our studies of acid-base changes in combat casualties during massive transfusion.[57] The relationship between the blood level of lactate and the blood base deficit changed constantly during rapid transfusion, with the base deficit becoming progressively smaller in relation to the lactate level. Since these casualties were not given exogenous alkali, this presumably represented the continuous metabolism of citrate-yielding alkali from the 15 mEq. of sodium citrate per unit of blood. In addition, the consistency with which acid-base balance was maintained in these patients during rapid transfusion and the rapidity with which they metabolized lactate implied a rapid metabolism of citrate.

Although citrate is the main cause of hypocalcemia during transfusion, the relationship between citrate levels and ionized calcium levels is probably not simple because of the rapidity with which calcium can be mobilized from skeletal stores.[67] Studies on calcium mobilization during severe hypotension are lacking, however. Blood flow to bone is sharply reduced in hemorrhagic hypotension[68, 69]; this must result in impaired mobilization of calcium. Saffran and Denstedt[70] demonstrated that high blood citrate levels can be accompanied by normal ionized calcium levels. It is conceivable that the rate of increase of the blood citrate level is more important than the absolute blood level itself.

Blood pH is another variable in the citrate–ionized calcium relationship. Alkalosis increases the binding of ionized calcium by plasma proteins. Studies with pure albumin in solution indicate that this substance alone does not nearly account for the changes observed in whole blood in vivo.[59, 60] Perhaps even more important, alkalosis produces a decrease in total calcium in the blood of intact animals.[71-73] Acidosis has the opposite effects. The often-quoted clinical experiments of Bunker, in which he related clinical signs and symptoms of hypocalcemia to absolute blood levels of citrate, included estimations of ionized calcium that were made without regard to pH changes.[63, 74] Sodium citrate was the anticoagulant solution and produced a marked alkalemia in the recipients. Many of the patients exhibited a decline in serum total calcium despite the citrate infusion. Other investigators have observed much less change in human volunteers at similar rates of anticoagulant infusion, using standard anticoagulant infusions instead of sodium citrate.[64, 75]

Acid-base balance may also influence citrate metabolism. Renal excretion of citrate is increased in alkalosis.[76-78] Renal excretion is a rather minor pathway for removal of citrate in man, however, even though most urinary citrate comes from plasma citrate.[79] Alkalosis decreased citrate oxidation by renal cortex in rats, and the renal metabolism of citrate is a major site of metabolic removal, but this impairment did not occur elsewhere in the body.[77] The overall effect of acid-base alterations on the rate of removal of infused citrate in man is not known. Modest alkalosis in rats appeared not to influence the rate of production and removal of citrate.[79]

Interest in citrate toxicity has been reawakened by the development of the calcium ion–sensitive electrode, which permits practical and accurate measurement of ionized calcium levels in blood.[59] Based on the use of this instrument, a few clinical studies have been reported. Perkins and colleagues[80] have studied four patients undergoing cardiopulmonary bypass with citrated blood. All patients exhibited moderate hypocalcemia. Pittinger and associates[81] reported three rapidly transfused patients, with spectacular hypocalcemia in one (0.2 mM. per liter) and modest depression of ionized calcium in the other two. Interestingly, the patient with severe hypocalcemia received no supplemental calcium yet did not exhibit tetany, emphasizing the incompleteness of our knowledge concerning the proper management of calcium changes during extensive transfusion. Hinkle and Cooperman[82] found acute decreases of about 23 percent in the ionized calcium levels in six patients during moderate transfusions. Recovery was very rapid after transfusion ceased. Gershanik and associates[141] studied ten term infants during exchange transfusion with ACD blood and concluded that supplemental calcium was not necessary. Many reviews of massive transfusion in clinical practice indicate that supplemental calcium is often not given routinely, without apparent detriment.[9, 57, 83] Objections to the routine use of calcium have been raised on the basis of indirect evidence and sporadic case reports of apparent iatrogenic hypercalcemia,[84] but the problem is still handled in an empiric manner because of lack of data.

Despite the impending change to CPD as the most commonly used anticoagulant for blood banking in the United States, we could find no studies on its effects on ionized calcium levels during infusion. We are contrasting ACD with CPD in rapid, sustained infusions in rabbits. At comparable rates of infusion, ACD produced a greater metabolic acidosis, lower ionized calcium levels, and a lower percentage of total calcium in the ionized form. Despite extremely low ionized calcium levels, death or tetany was rare in these unanesthetized animals. Animals given sodium bicarbonate in doses according to published suggestions for massive transfusion exhibited slower recovery of ionized calcium levels compared to controls given sodium chloride, indicating that such iatrogenic alkalosis may indeed interfere with the body's defense of plasma ionized calcium levels.

The development of the calcium ion–sensitive electrode hopefully will allow us to finally answer the old questions about citrate toxicity. The complexities of the clinical transfusion situation are so great that it seems self-evident that conclusions relating to patient care can be drawn only on the basis of clinical investigations.

Hypothermia. The specific heat of blood is about 0.9.[85] Thus, warming 10 L. of blood from 4° to 37° C. would require nearly 300 Kcal. While this number is not very large in itself, if the blood were given over a two-hour period this would represent an added caloric requirement of 150 Kcal. per hour, which is double the normal resting caloric expenditure. Looked at another way, 300 Kcal. represents an hour of moderately heavy muscular work. 300 Kcal., if supplied by the oxidation of glucose with complete conversion to heat, would require 54.6 L. of oxygen (STP). With the usual postabsorptive respiratory quotient, 62 L. of oxygen would be required.[86] This added requirement comes precisely at the worst time, when oxygen supply and energy consumption are being severely stressed.

Many studies have established the propensity of the heavily transfused patient to become hypothermic if the blood is not warmed, especially if transfusion occurs in the operating room.[87, 88] Apart from significantly increasing oxygen and energy requirements, hypothermia interacts with many of the other alterations induced by massive transfusion in a detrimental way. Thus, hypothermia impairs the metabolism of citrate and of lactate, increasing the chances of developing hypocalcemia and metabolic acidosis. Cold promotes the release of potassium from the intracellular space, which would also be increased by the acidosis resulting from the impaired metabolism of organic acids. Cold increases the affinity of hemoglobin for oxygen, an effect already produced by the storage of red cells in ACD. Cold seems to impair clotting, but the mechanisms are not known. This would presumably be additive to the various clotting factor depletions already discussed. Cold may further impair red cell deformability, but it is not clear how much temperature change is required to produce a significant effect. The metabolism of anesthetic agents or of administered narcotics is impaired by cold, as is the ability to detect a major transfusion reaction during operation. The danger of arrhythmias at levels below 30° C. is well known. It is conceivable that rapid transfusion through central venous catheters could differentially cool certain areas of the heart and worsen this problem. Looking at the problem of massive transfusion as a whole, hypothermia is uniquely active in worsening many of the other problems that might otherwise be adequately handled by the body. There are technical problems in warming blood safely because the margin between normal body temperature and hemolysis by heat is small,[89] but the disadvantages of hypothermia are so great as to require a satisfactory solution to this relatively minor technical problem.

Microembolization. Stored blood contains a considerable amount of clot and debris which easily pass the filters in common use. One of the research teams in Vietnam measured up to 4 Gm. wet weight of particles per unit of stored blood which could be removed by a 170 micron filter.[90] Considerably more can be removed by using finer filters, which are now available commercially. The technical problem is one of maintaining acceptably rapid flow through such relatively efficient filters, but the newer designs look promising.

Seriously injured and transfused patients exhibit an increase in resistance of the flow of their blood through a relatively coarse screen (screen filtration pressure).[91] This phenomenon was studied by several of the research teams in Vietnam.[92, 93] Interpretation and physiologic significance are uncertain, but mixture of the recipient's blood with stored blood caused "microaggregation" of the recipient's blood.[94] Use of an efficient filter lowered the screen filtration pressure of stored blood.[95]

Hypoxemia after resuscitation has been related to the amount of blood transfused and by implication to embolization from transfusion.[93] The problem with such studies is that the most seriously injured patients receive the most blood. We grouped casualties by types of injury and examined the relation between transfusion and hypoxemia within similarly injured groups. There was no correlation. Hypoxemia was much more closely related to the type of injury.[96,97] These were vigorously healthy young adults, however, who could probably tolerate a significant load of infused debris without developing hypoxemia. Particulate debris can be found in the pulmonary capillaries after extensive transfusion in man and animals.[98, 99] If flow can be maintained at the necessary levels, the use of more effective filters during extensive transfusion certainly appears to be desirable.

Red cell deformability. Because the human red cell is significantly larger than the lumen of the average capillary, the ability of individual red cells to deform during passage through capillaries is one of the single most important elements determining the resistance of blood to flow in vivo.[100] Stored red cells change toward a spherical shape and become much more rigid as cellular levels of ATP (adenosine triphosphate) decline.[101-103] The loss of deformability is very marked. As ATP is regenerated these changes reverse. The regeneration of ATP occurs fairly rapidly after transfusion,[32] but studies on red cell deformability after transfusion have not yet been done. Decreased red cell ATP levels in severe hypophosphatemia have been associated with increased rigidity, spherocytic morphology, and decreased red cell survival.[104] Red cell deformability can now be quantitated by a variety of widely different methods,[100, 105] and the elements of membrane vs. internal viscosity changes can be studied by viscosimetry at different hematocrits.[106] With the evident importance of red cell deformability and the marked changes that occur during storage, studies on massively transfused patients are clearly needed.

Plasticizers. Plasticizers diffuse from the plastic bag into stored blood.[107, 108] The amount of plasticizer that accumulates in blood stored in plastic bags is surprisingly large—0.25 mg. per 100 ml. per day. Toxicity has been reported in various studies in tissue culture with much smaller amounts,[109] but the toxicity to adult animals is not clear. Plasticizers may strongly influence the agglutinability of platelets in vitro[110]; in vivo effects are unknown.

Phthalate esters have been found in appreciable quantities in the blood and tissues of heavily transfused patients.[111] There were some inconsistencies in this report, and the controls seemed inadequate. A better designed study now in progress indicates that these ubiquitous plasticizers can also be found in non-transfused controls.[142] Nevertheless, these are clearly disturbing findings and further investigation is urgently needed.

Denaturation of proteins. Denaturation of plasma proteins during storage has received less attention than it deserves. The exposure of blood to foreign surfaces and to gas before infusion has a marked effect on the mortality rate of hemorrhaged animals.[112, 113] There are a number of reports in which the reinfusion of shed blood is more deadly than no treatment at all or use of simple salt solutions[114, 115]; these are characterized by harsh handling of the blood. Toxic effects of protein denaturation have long been postulated for bubble oxygenators,[116, 117] and this is one of the main incentives to develop newer surfaces to separate blood from gas during oxygenation for cardiopulmonary bypass. Unfortunately, protein denaturation is difficult to control and to measure with quantitative accuracy. The pathophysiologic effects have not been extensively studied. Some protein fractions may be much more harmful than others.

Vasoactive substances. Serotonin levels increase in plasma during storage of whole blood.[118] It is likely that histamine is released also. I am not aware of any measurements of the kinin systems during storage, but it would not be surprising if some conversion of kininogens to kinins occurred as a result of activation of Factor XII by foreign surface contact. Prostaglandin levels have not been measured during storage. The addition of PGE_1 facilitates the harvesting of platelets,[119] so at least some types of blood for clinical use may soon contain iatrogenically elevated prostaglandin levels. In relatively small amounts, this does not seem to have any marked physiologic effects.[120] Other as yet unidentified vasoactive substances may also accumulate during storage.[121]

Potassium, ammonia, phosphate. These substances become elevated in the plasma of stored blood[122] and deleterious effects have been postulated, especially in certain high-risk patients. Potassium has received the most attention because of its potential for cardiovascular toxicity and because of the impressively high concentrations in stored blood. Even at a level of 25 mEq. per liter, however, a liter of stored blood contains only 15 mEq. of plasma potassium, and of this only 12.3 mEq. is in excess of normal plasma levels. Moreover, most of this excess potassium has leaked from viable red cells, which gradually take back potassium after infusion into the recipient.[32] Studies on potassium levels during and after massive transfusion have revealed hypokalemia to be more common than hyperkalemia, probably because of the metabolic and respiratory alkalosis that these patients manifest.[9, 63, 123] Most of the hyperkalemic patients have been incompletely resuscitated, with persistent hypotension and acidosis. A major concern with elevated potassium levels in stored blood is the additive effect that would occur between transient hyperkalemia and hypercitremia. This has been discussed previously.

Ammonia levels can become very high during storage. Again, however, this is a high level in a small volume relative to the volume of total body water. Furthermore, this represents accumulation during storage and not impaired ability of the recipient to metabolize ammonia. Fresh blood is often recommended for use in patients with serious liver disease, but with little documentation of beneficial effects on the blood ammonia levels of recipients.

Phosphate levels become elevated during storage but not markedly so. Use of CPD as an anticoagulant increases these levels somewhat, but very little data are available on the changes in plasma phosphate levels during massive transfusion with blood preserved in CPD or even in ACD. The main toxicity is expected to be binding of calcium ion. Experimental comparisons with ACD already referred to have been reassuring. As with potassium, phosphate is largely an intracellular ion so that these infused quantities represent a relatively small addition to the total body store.

Miscellaneous. Hemolysis during storage can cause serious problems during transfusion. These problems were probably erroneously attributed to hemoglobin, which in pure form appears to be well tolerated.[124] Red cell stromal lipids, however, can produce intravascular coagulation and marked circulatory and renal impairment. Hemolysis during storage does not appear to be a major problem with modern blood banking methods.

There may be significant changes in antibacterial defenses caused by transfusion. Homologous blood appears to impair the antibacterial defenses of heavily transfused dogs.[125] Washed red cells produced little change in reticuloendothelial function in dogs, but transfusion with whole blood, either autologous or homologous, impaired clearance of aggregated albumin.[126] An impairment of antibacterial defenses in massively injured patients seems very apparent clinically. It is not clear if transfusion contributes to this.

A graft-vs.-host reaction has been proposed to explain some of the pulmonary problems encountered following cardiopulmonary bypass.[127] It appears that the lymphocytes in stored blood remain viable for several weeks.[128, 129] Fresh blood can certainly cause serious graft-vs.-host reactions in immunosuppressed recipients,[130] but there has been essentially no direct evidence to support such an event in immunologically intact recipients.

Hypoglycemia has been reported after exchange transfusion in newborn infants and has been correlated with a persistence of high insulin levels triggered by the elevated glucose concentrations of the stored blood.[137] This must be very unusual in heavily transfused adults, but illustrates the principle that infants are less able to compensate for many of the metabolic challenges inherent in massive transfusion and that many such problems remain undiscovered.

TOXICITY OF NEW ADDITIVES

In the search for better methods of storing red cells, a number of additives have been found that offer clear advantages over the present rather simple anticoagulant system based on citrate and glucose. Adenine clearly improves ATP levels in stored human red cells and produces a commensurate increase in storage time with acceptable viability.[131] A metabolic product, 2,8-dioxyadenine, has been found precipitated in the renal tubules of animals given large amounts of adenine, however.[132] Considerable clinical experience with the use of stored blood containing adenine has been gained in Europe, but the number of carefully studied massively transfused patients has been low. Rapid infusion of large amounts of anticoagulant containing adenine was well tolerated by normal volunteers, but urinary function tests were minimal.[75] Studies in primates have been rather reassuring.[133, 134] Adenine causes a decrease in 2,3-DPG levels but this can be offset by adding inosine.[135] A combination of inosine, pyruvate, and phosphate can restore 2,3-DPG in stored, depleted cells, and even raise levels to well above normal.[47, 136] Infusion of inosine, however, causes elevated blood uric acid levels. Some form of washing the red cells avoids the potential toxicities of these additives, but this becomes operationally difficult because of short survival after washing. Extensive reliance on "universal donor" blood for emergencies could reduce this problem considerably, but it is not clear if the over-all benefits outweigh the added risks and expenses.

Other substances appear less likely to enter into widespread use as additives. Guanosine offers little advantage over inosine or adenine. Dihydroxyacetone and ascorbic acid[144] provide energy substrates and preserve 2,3-DPG levels, but no better or even less well than other additives. Considerations of toxicity, however, may increase their usefulness as additives.

CONCLUSION

This has been an impressive list of potential hazards to the recipient due to imperfections in the process of storing human blood for use when needed. Apparent contradictions abound: on a computational basis, the more blood that is used early, the less the over-all impact on the massively bleeding patient because exchange then occurs wtih a full blood volume. Giving acidic blood to an acidotic patient more often than not results in alkalosis, because the acids are organic and are rapidly burned up when perfusion is restored. Hyperkalemic blood often produces a mild hypokalemia in the recipient because of the alkalosis that commonly results. The most striking apparent contradiction of all, however, is clinically the most important: many of the serious toxicities attributed to the massive transfusion of stored blood are often due to giving too little blood or giving it too late. Acidosis, hypercitremia, hyperkalemia, disseminated intravascular coagulation, and the degree of replacement with stored blood are all worsened by allowing the recipient to remain hypovolemic during hemorrhage and transfusion. *An intact circulation is a very good defense against the metabolic problems of massive transfusion.*

Significant improvements are in sight for storing blood and for transfusing large amounts rapidly. CPD is clearly a more physiologic anticoagulant than ACD, and produces less disturbance in oxygen-hemoglobin affinity, acid-base balance, and calcium metabolism. Better filters and warmers are becoming available. Real control of hepatitis is hopefully imminent, and will represent the greatest single advance in blood banking since Landsteiner and Lewisohn. Blood components and even the red cells themselves can now be harvested and functionally altered for special purposes. Frozen blood is free of many of the disadvantages of conventionally stored blood for massive transfusion but is not now available rapidly enough. There are still many potential problems requiring better definition, such as the status of platelet function after massive transfusion, the importance of transmitted diseases other than hepatitis, the toxicity of plasticizers, the whole array of biologic effects that can result from alteration of proteins during storage, and there is still an urgent need for better documentation in patients of some of the classical and newly defined metabolic disadvantages of massive transfusion. A host of others are undoubtedly still unsuspected.

A more ideal pattern of massive transfusion would involve use of red cells with normal or high 2,3-DPG levels and good post-transfusion survival, extensively washed to remove many of the potentially hazardous substances present in stored plasma. Albumin and salt water can be used as volume replacement. When one to two blood volumes are exceeded, fresh frozen plasma and platelet concentrates can be added to provide clotting elements. All this is currently possible, but highly impractical. It is certain that liquid stored whole blood will continue to be relied upon for the foreseeable future in situations of exsanguinating hemorrhage.

In spite of all the problems with liquid stored whole blood, we have a product that usually works well. Historically, as new problems associated with massive transfusion have been defined, they have almost always been grossly overstated. One need only consider extraordinary experiences with massive transfusion such as occurred in Vietnam to gain a sense of proportion. The Military Blood Program Agency is now carefully collating and checking the records of blood utilization in American military hospitals in Vietnam. I hope these figures will be published soon because they are very impressive for a number of reasons. A spot check of 1,776 transfused combat casualties by Gen. R. M. Hardaway revealed that 16 per cent received more than one blood volume in transfusion, 5 per cent more than 2.5 blood volumes, and 2 per cent more than five blood volumes, most of this during the period of resuscitation. When one considers the great numbers of transfused casualties, the low mortality rate, and the fact that most such deaths were due to uncontrolled bleeding from combat injuries, the value of even our presently imperfect product in saving lives from massive hemorrhage becomes evident. The casualty whose resuscitation is shown schematically in Fig. 3 is a dramatic but not unusual example of the efficacy of massive transfusion with stored blood when the basic principles of resuscitation from trauma were observed by well-trained and experienced teams under enviable conditions of organization, transportation, and supply, even though in the middle of a jungle. Stored blood is useful and effective, even when it must be given rapidly in large amounts. There is considerable room for improvement and a number of promising recent developments, but change must occur in terms of proved, not assumed progress.

REFERENCES

1. Ballinger, W. F., and Cohn, H. E.: The preservation of whole blood, Surg. Gynecol. Obstet. **112:** 411, 1961.
2. Baue, A. E., Hermann, G., and Shaw, R. S.: A study of bank blood toxicity, Surg. Gynecol. Obstet. **113:** 40, 1961.
3. Boyan, C. P., and Howland, W. S.: Problems related to massive blood replacement, Anesth. Analy. **41:** 497, 1962.
4. Howland, W. S., and Schweizer, O.: Physiologic compensation for storage lesion of bank blood, Anesth. Analg. **44:** 8, 1965.
5. Bunker, J. P.: Metabolic effects of blood transfusion, Anesthesiology **27:** 446, 1966.
6. Vogel, A. P., Frederickson, E. L., and Holder, T. M.: Massive blood replacement, Arch. Surg. **95:** 38, 1967.
7. Gruber, U. F.: Blood replacement, Berlin, 1969, Springer-Verlag.
8. Rudowski, W. J.: Complications associated with blood transfusion, Progr. Surg. **9:** 78, 1971.
9. Wilson, R. F., Mammen, E., and Walt, A. J.: Eight years of experience with massive blood transfusions, J. Trauma **11:** 275, 1971.
10. Mollison, P. L.: Blood transfusion in clinical medicine, ed. 5, London, 1972, Blackwell Scientific Publications.
11. Grady, G. F., and Bennett, A. J. E.: Risk of post-transfusion hepatitis in the United States, J. A. M. A. **220:** 692, 1972.
12. Vyas, G. N., Perkins, H. A., and Schmid, R.: Hepatitis and blood transfusion, New York, 1972, Grune & Stratton, Inc.
13. Prince, A. M., Szmuness, W., Woods, K. R., and Grady, G. F.: Antibody against serum hepatitis: Prevalence and potential use as immune serum globulin in prevention of serum-hepatitis infections, N. Engl. J. Med. **285:** 933, 1971.
14. Conrad, M. E.: Prevention of HAA-positive hepatitis with serum gamma globulin, N. Engl. J. Med. **285:** 1486, 1971.
15. Kaariainen, L., Klemola, E., and Palohuimo, J.: Rise of cytomegalovirus antibodies in an infectious-mononucleosis-like syndrome after transfusion, Br. Med. J. **1:** 1270, 1966.
16. Henle, W. H., Henle, G., Scriba, M., et al.: Antibody responses to the Ebstein-Barr virus and cytomegaloviruses after open-heart and other surgery, N. Engl. J. Med. **282:** 1068, 1970.
17. Prince, A. M., Szmuness, W., Millian, S. J., et al.: A serologic study of cytomegalovirus infections associated with blood transfusions, N. Engl. J. Med. **284:** 1125, 1971.
18. Franciosi, R., Awer, E., and Santana, M.: Interdonor incompatibility resulting in anuria, Transfusion **7:** 297, 1967.
19. Wiener, A. S., and Wexler, I. B.: The use of heparin when performing exchange blood transfusions in newborn infants, J. Lab. Clin. Med. **31:** 1016, 1946.
20. Marsaglia, G., and Thomas, E. D.: Mathematical consideration of cross circulation and exchange transfusion, Transfusion **11:** 216, 1971.
21. Valtis, D. J., and Kennedy, A. C.: Defective gas transport function of stored red blood cells, Lancet **1:** 119, 1954.
22. Akerblom, O., de Verdier, C. H., Garby, L., et al.: Restoration of defective oxygen transport function of stored red blood cells by

addition of inosine, Scand. J. Clin. Lab. Invest. **21:** 245, 1968.
23. Bunn, H. F., May, M. H., Kocholaty, W. F., et al.: Hemoglobin function of stored blood, J. Clin. Invest. **48:** 311, 1969.
24. Dawson, R. B.: The hemoglobin function of blood stored at 4° C. in ACD and CPD, Clin. Res. **17:** 323, 1969.
25. Gullbring, B., and Strom, G.: Changes in oxygen-carrying function of human hemoglobin in cold acid-citrate-dextrose solution, Acta Med. Scand. **155:** 413, 1956.
26. O'Brien, T. G., and Watkins, E.: Gas-exchange dynamics of glycerolized frozen blood, J. Thorac. Cardiovasc. Surg. **40:** 611, 1960.
27. Sugerman, J. H., Davidson, D. T., Vibul, S., et al.: The basis of defective oxygen delivery from stored blood, Surg. Gynecol. Obstet. **131:** 733, 1970.
28. Broennle, A. M., Tung, C. K., Buchman, B., et al.: Oxyhemoglobin dissociation following massive transfusion in man, Fed. Proc. **29:** 329, 1970.
29. Valeri, C. R., and Collins, F. B.: Physiologic effects of 2,3-DPG-depleted red cells with high affinity for oxygen, J. Appl. Physiol. **31:** 823, 1971.
30. McConn, R., and Derrick, J. B.: The respiratory function of blood: Transfusion and blood storage, Anesthesiology **36:** 119, 1972.
31. Kopriva, C. J., Ratliff, J. L., Fletcher, J. R., et al.: Biochemical and hematological changes associated with massive transfusion of ACD-stored blood in severely injured combat casualties, Ann. Surg. **176:** 585, 1972.
32. Valeri, C. R., and Hirsch, N. M.: Restoration in vivo of erythrocyte adenosine triphosphate, 2,3-diphosphoglycerate, potassium ion, and sodium ion concentrations following the transfusion of acid-citrate-dextrose-stored human red blood cells, J. Lab. Clin. Med. **73:** 722, 1969.
33. Beutler, E., and Wood, L.: The in vivo regeneration of red cell 2,3-diphosphoglyceric acid (DPG) after transfusion of stored blood, J. Lab. Clin. Med. **74:** 300, 1969.
34. Severinghaus, J. W.: Oxyhemoglobin dissociation curve correction for temperature and pH in human blood, J. Appl. Physiol. **12:** 485, 1958.
35. Oski, F. A., Marshall, B. E., Cohen, P. J., et al.: Exercise with anemia: The role of the left-shifted or right-shifted oxygen-hemoglobin equilibrium curve, Ann. Intern. Med. **74:** 44, 1971.
36. Huggins, C. E., Suzuki, H., and Grove-Rasmussen, M.: Life support by liquid and frozen blood, Presented at 24th Ann. Meeting, Am. Assoc. of Blood Banks, Chicago, Sept. 12-16, 1971.
37. Riggs, T. E., Shafer, A. W., and Guenter, C. A.: Clinical significance of acute change in the oxyhemoglobin dissociation curve, J. Lab. Clin. Med. **78:** 1011, 1971.
38. Balcerzak, S., Buy, J., Metz, E., et al.: Studies on the ability of stored blood to transport oxygen in vivo, Adv. Exp. Med. Biol. **28:** 433, 1972.
39. Woodson, R. D., Wranne, B., and Detter, J. C.: Oxygen delivery to exercising muscle: Effect of increased blood oxygen affinity, *in* Preservation of red blood cells, Washington, D. C., 1973, National Academy of Science, p. 97.
40. Laver, M. B.: A fable of our time: Oxygen transport, or does the Emperor have new clothes? Anesthesiology **36:** 105, 1972.
41. Collins, J. A., and Kaplan, H. J.: Relative importance of pH and 2,3-DPG in determining oxygen delivery in seriously ill patients, Presented at 127th Meeting, Society of Clinical Surgery, St. Louis, Nov. 7-9, 1972.
42. Bellingham, A. J., Detter, J. C., and Lenfant, C.: Regulatory mechanisms of hemoglobin oxygen affinity in acidosis and alkalosis, J. Clin. Invest. **50:** 700, 1971.
43. Kevy, S. V., Button, L. N., and Filler, R. M.: The effect of massive transfusion of stored blood on oxygen transport—A preliminary report, Adv. Exp. Med. Biol. **28:** 511, 1972.
44. Delivoria-Papadopoulos, M., Morrow, G., and Oski, F. A.: Exchange transfusion in the newborn infant with fresh and "old" blood: The role of storage on 2,3-diphosphoglycerate, hemoglobin-oxygen affinity, and oxygen release, J. Pediatr. **79:** 898, 1971.
45. Delivoria-Papadopoulos, M., Oski, F. A., Miller, L. D., and Forster, R. E.: The pathophysiology of exchange transfusion of the newborn with regard to O_2 transport, *in* Preservation of red blood cells, Washington, D. C., 1973, National Academy of Science, p. 137.
46. Chance, B., and Salkovitz, I. A.: Intracellular oxygen requirements, *in* Preservation of red blood cells, Washington, D. C., 1973, National Academy of Science, p. 73.
47. Duhm, J., Deuticke, B., and Gerlach, E.: Complete restoration of oxygen transport function and 2,3-diphosphoglycerate concentration in stored blood, Transfusion **11:** 147, 1971.
48. Aggeler, P. M., Perkins, H. A., and Watkins, H. B.: Hypocalcemia and defective hemostasis after massive blood transfusion. Report of a case, Transfusion **7:** 35, 1967.
49. Simmons, R. L., Collins, J. A., Heisterkamp, C. A., et tal.: Coagulation disorders in combat casualties, Ann. Surg. **169:** 455, 1969.
50. Krevans, J. R., and Jackson, D. P.: Hemor-

rhagic disorders following whole blood transfusions, J. A. M. A. **159:** 171, 1955.
51. Scott, R., and Crosby, W. H.: Changes in the coagulation mechanism following wounding and resuscitation with stored blood, blood **9:** 609, 1954.
52. Gollub, S., Ulin, A. W., Winchell, H. S., et al.: Hemorrhagic diathesis associated with massive transfusion, SURGERY **45:** 204, 1959.
53. Miller, R. D., Robbins, T. O., Tong, M. J., et al.: Coagulation defects associated with massive blood transfusions, Ann. Surg. **174:** 794, 1971.
54. McNamara, J. J., Burran, E. L., Stremple, J. F., et al.: Coagulopathy after major combat injury: Occurrence, management, and pathophysiology, Ann. Surg. **176:** 243, 1972.
55. Lim, R. C., Olcott, C., Robinson, A., and Blaisdell, F. W.: Platelet response and coagulation changes following massive blood replacement, J. Trauma **13:** 577, 1973.
56. Rogers, A. B.: The effect of pH on human platelet aggregation induced by epinephrine and ADP, Proc. Soc. Exp. Biol. Med. **139:** 1100, 1972.
57. Collins, J. A., Simmons, R. L., James, P. M., et al.: Acid-base status of seriously wounded combat casualties. II. Resuscitation with stored blood, Ann. Surg. **173:** 6, 1971.
58. Miller, R. D., Tong, M. J., and Robbins, T. O.: Effects of massive transfusion of blood on acid-base balance, J. A. M. A. **216:** 1762, 1971.
59. Moore, E. W.: Ionized calcium in normal serum, ultrafiltrates and whole blood determined by ion-exchange electrode, J. Clin. Invest. **49:** 318, 1970.
60. Jacobs, N. S., Hattner, R. S., and Bernstein, D. S.: Physico-chemical study of calcium-albumin aggregation employing a calcium specific electrode, Clin. Chim. Acta **31:** 467, 1971.
61. Smith, N. T., and Corbascio, A. N.: The interaction of potassium and calcium on the isolated guinea pig atrium, Fed. Proc. **23:** 326, 1964.
62. Salant, W., and Wise, L. E.: The action of sodium citrate and its decomposition in the body, J. Biol. Chem. **28:** 27, 1916.
63. Bunker, J. P., Stetson, J. B., Coe, R. C., et al.: Citric acid intoxication, J. A. M. A. **157:** 1361, 1955.
64. Howland, W. S., Bellville, J. W., Zucker, M. B., et al.: Massive blood replacement. V. Failure to observe citrate intoxication, Surg. Gynecol. Obstet. **105:** 529, 1957.
65. Ludbrook, J., and Wynn, V.: Citrate intoxication: A clinical and experimental study, Br. Med. J. **2:** 523, 1958.
66. Drucker, W. R., Craig, J., Kingsbury, B., et al.: Citrate metabolism during surgery, Arch. Surg. **85:** 557, 1962.
67. Nakasone, N., Watkins, E., Jr., Janeway, C. A., et al.: Experimental studies of circulatory derangement following the massive transfusion of citrated blood, J. Lab. Clin. Med. **43:** 184, 1954.
68. Kita, R., Witoszka, M. M., Hopkins, R. W., et al.: Bone marrow pressure and blood flow and resistance in experimental hemorrhagic shock, Am. J. Surg. **123:** 380, 1972.
69. Yu, W., Shim, S., and Hawk, H. E.: Bone circulation in hemorrhagic shock, J. Bone Joint Surg. **54A:** 1157, 1972.
70. Saffran, M., and Denstedt, O. F.: Effect of intravenously injected citrate on the serum ionized calcium in the rabbit, Can. J. Med. Sci. **29:** 245, 1951.
71. Irvin, G. L., Gittes, R. F., and Gibbs, M. F.: Influence of acid-base disturbances on total plasma calcium and evidence for a hemeostatic role of thyrocalcitonin, Ann. Surg. **164:** 1073, 1966.
72. Kaplan, E. L., Hill, B. J., Locke, S., et al.: Acid-base balance and parathyroid function: Metabolic alkalosis and hyperparathyroidism, SURGERY **70:** 198, 1971.
73. Hoffken, B., Parkinson, D. K., Storms, P., et al.: Effects of alterations of blood pH on calcium ion activity in rat plasma, Clin. Orthop. **78:** 30, 1971.
74. Bunker, J. P., Bendixen, H. H., and Murphy, A. J.: Hemodynamic effects of intravenously administered sodium citrate, N. Engl. J. Med. **266:** 372, 1962.
75. Shields, C. E., Dennis, L. H., Eichelberger, J. W., et al.: Rapid infusion of large quantities of ACD adenine solution into humans, Transfusion **7:** 133, 1967.
76. Gamble, W., Orten, J. M., and Smith, A. H.: Citric acid cycle in certain alterations of acid-base balance in human subjects, J. Appl. Physiol. **16:** 593, 1961.
77. Simpson, D. P.: Regulation of renal citrate metabolism by bicarbonate ion and pH observations in tissue slices and mitochondria, J. Clin. Invest. **46:** 225, 1967.
78. Szilagyi, G.: Effect of acidification and alkalinisation on calcium and citrate metabolism in normal and parathyroidectomized dogs, Acta Physiol. Acad. Sci. Hung. **38:** 281, 1970.
79. Gordon, E. E.: Effect of acute metabolic acidosis and alkalosis on acetate and citrate metabolism in the rat, J. Clin. Invest. **42:** 137, 1963.
80. Perkins, H. A., Snyder, M., Thacher, C., and Rolfs, M. R.: Calcium ion activity during rapid exchange transfusion with citrated blood, Transfusion **11:** 204, 1971.
81. Pittinger, C., Chang, P. M., and Faulkner, W.: Serum ionized calcium: Some factors

influencing its level, South. Med. J. **64:** 1211, 1971.
82. Hinkle, J. E., and Cooperman, L. H.: Serum ionized calcium changes following citrated blood transfusion in anaesthetized man, Br. J. Anaesth. **43:** 1108, 1971.
83. Howland, W. S., Schweizer, O., and Boyan, C. P.: Massive blood replacement without calcium administration. Surg. Gynecol. Obstet. **118:** 814, 1964.
84. Wolf, P. L., McCarthy, L. J., and Hafleigh, B.: Extreme hypercalcemia following blood transfusions combined with intravenous calcium, Vox Sang. **19:** 544, 1970.
85. Mendlowitz, M.: The specific heat of human blood, Science **107:** 97, 1948.
86. White, A., Handler, P., Smith, E. L., et al.: Principles of biochemistry, ed. 2, New York, 1959, McGraw-Hill Book Company, Inc.
87. Boyan, C. P.: Cold or warmed blood for massive transfusions, Ann. Surg. **160:** 282, 1964.
88. Dybkjaer, E., and Elkjaer, P.: The use of heated blood in massive blood replacement, Acta Anaesth. Scand. **8:** 271, 1964.
89. Arens, J. F., and Leonard, G. L.: Danger of overwarming blood by microwave, J. A. M. A. **218:** 1045, 1971.
90. Moseley, R. V., and Doty, D. B.: Changes in the filtration characteristics of stored blood, Ann. Surg. **171:** 329, 1970.
91. Swank, R. L., Seaman, G. V., Hissen, W., et al.: Physicochemical changes in blood induced by trauma, Surg. Gynecol. Obstet. **123:** 251, 1966.
92. Berman, I. R., Gutienez, V. S., Burran, E. L., et al.: Intravascular microaggregation in young men with combat injuries, Surg. Forum **20:** 14, 1969.
93. McNamara, J. J., Molot, M. D., and Stremple, J. F.: Screen filtration pressure in combat casualties, Ann. Surg. **172:** 334-341, 1970.
94. Ashmore, P. G., Swank, R. L., Gallery, R., et al.: Effect of Dacron wool filtration on the microembolic phenomenon in extracorporeal circulation, J. Thorac. Cardiovasc. Surg. **63:** 240, 1972.
95. McNamara, J. J., Burran, E. L., and Suehiro, G.: Effective filtration of banked blood, Surgery **71:** 594, 1972.
96. Collins, J. A., Gordon, W. C., Hudson, T. L., et al.: Inapparent hypoxemia in casualties with wounded limbs: Pulmonary fat embolism? Ann. Surg. **167:** 511, 1968.
97. Collins, J. A.: The causes of progressive pulmonary insufficiency in surgical patients, J. Surg. Res. **12:** 685, 1969.
98. Moseley, R. V., and Doty, D. B.: Death associated with multiple pulmonary emboli soon after battle injury, Ann. Surg. **171:** 336, 1970.
99. Connell, R. S., and Swank, R. L.: Pulmonary microembolism after blood transfusions: An election microscopic study, Ann. Surg. **177:** 40, 1973.
100. Braasch, D.: Red cell deformability and capillary blood flow, Physiol. Rev. **51:** 679, 1971.
101. Haradin, A. R., Weed, R. I., and Reed, C. F.: Changes in physical properties of stored erythrocytes: relationship to survival in vivo, Transfusion **9:** 229, 1969.
102. LaCelle, P. L.: Alteration of deformability of the erythrocyte membrane in stored blood, Transfusion **9:** 238, 1969.
103. Longster, G. H., Buckley, T., Sikorski, J., et al.: Scanning electron microscope studies of red cell morphology: Changes occurring in red cell shape during storage and post transfusion, Vox Sang. **22:** 161, 1972.
104. Jacob, H. S., and Amsden, T.: Acute hemolytic anemia with rigid red cells in hypophosphatemia, New Engl. J. Med. **285:** 1446, 1971.
105. Hochmuth, R. M., and Hohandas, N.: Uniaxial loading of the red-cell membrane, J. Biochem. **5:** 501, 1972.
106. Chien, S., Usami, S., and Bertles, J. F.: Abnormal rheology of oxygenated blood in sickle cell anemia, J. Clin. Invest. **49:** 623, 1970.
107. Guess, W. L., Jacob, J., and Autian, J.: Blood bag assemblies. I. Alteration or contamination of ACD solutions, Drug Intell. **1:** 120, 1967.
108. Marcel, Y. L., and Noel, S. P.: Contamination of blood stored in plastic packs, Lancet **1:** 35, 1970.
109. Jaeger, R. J., and Rubin, R. J.: Plasticizers from plastic devices: Extraction, metabolism, and accumulation by biological systems, Science **170:** 460, 1970.
110. Bowie, E. J., and Owen, C. A.: Some factors influencing platelet retention in glass bead columns including the influence of plastics, Am. J. Clin. Pathol. **56:** 479, 1971.
111. Jaeger, R. J., and Rubin, R. J.: Migration of a phthalate ester plasticizer from polyvinyl chloride blood bags into stored human blood and its localization in human tissues, N. Engl. J. Med. **287:** 1114, 1972.
112. Rush, B. F., and Wilder, R. J.: Mortality and renal tubular necrosis in hemorrhagic shock in dogs: The effect of blood handling, Surg. Forum **14:** 1, 1963.
113. Hardaway, R. M., Johnson, D. G., Houchin, D. N., et al.: The influence of extracorporeal handling of blood on hemorrhagic shock in dogs, Exp. Med. Surg. **23:** 28, 1965.
114. Drucker, W. R., Holden, W. D., Kingsbury, B., et al.: Metabolic aspects of hemorrhagic shock. II. Metabolic studies on the need for erythrocytes in the treatment of hypovolemia

due to hemorrhage, J. Trauma 2: 567, 1962.
115. Brand, E. D., Suh, T. K., and Avery, M. D.: Reversal of postoligemic shock in the cat by hypervenobaric massive fluid therapy, Am. J. Physiol. **211**: 1232, 1966.
116. Lee, W. H., Krumhaar, D., Fonkalsrud, E. W., et al.: Denaturation of plasma proteins as a cause of morbidity and death after intracardiac operations, SURGERY **50**: 29, 1961.
117. Dobell, A. R., Mitri, M., Galva, R., et al.: Biologic evaluation of blood after prolonged recirculation through film and membrane oxygenators, Ann. Surg. **161**: 617, 1965.
118. Strauss, H. W., Smith, R. B., Polimeni, P., et al.: Plasma serotonin levels in stored human blood, Angiology **18**: 535, 1967.
119. Shio, H., and Ramwell, P. W.: Prostaglandin E_1 in platelet harvesting: An in vitro study, Science **175**: 536, 1972.
120. Valeri, C. R., Zaroulis, C. G., Rogers, J. C., et al.: Prostaglandins in the preparation of blood components, Science **175**: 539, 1972.
121. Bohr, D. F., and Johansson, B.: Contraction of vascular smooth muscle in response to plasma: Comparison with response to known vasoactive agents, Circ. Res. **19**: 593, 1966.
122. Schechter, D. C., and Swan, H.: Biochemical alterations of preserved blood, Arch. Surg. **84**: 269, 1962.
123. Schweizer, O., and Howland, W. S.: Potassium levels, acid-base balance and massive blood replacement, Anesthesiology **23**: 735, 1962.
124. Rabiner, S. F., Hlebert, J. R., Lopas, H., et al.: Evaluation of a stroma-free hemoglobin solution for use as a plasma expander, J. Exp. Med. **126**: 1127, 1967.
125. Ollodart, R., and Mansburger, A. R.: The effect of hypovolemic shock on bacterial defense, Am. J. Surg. **110**: 302, 1965.
126. Wilson, J. D., Taswell, H. F., and Didisheim, P.: Effects of washed-cell and whole-blood transfusion on reticuloendothelial function in dogs, Transfusion **9**: 289, 1969.
127. Melrose, D. G., Nahas, R., Alvarey, D., et al.: Postoperative hypoxia after extracorporeal circulation: A possible graft against host reaction, Experientia **21**: 47, 1965.
128. Petrakis, N. L., and Politis, G.: Prolonged survival of viable, mitotically competent mononuclear leukocytes in stored whole blood, N. Engl. J. Med. **267**: 286, 1962.
129. McCullough, J., Benson, S. J., Yunis, E. J., et al.: Effect of blood-bank storage on leucocyte function, Lancet **2**: 1333, 1969.
130. Collins, J. A., Hechtman, H. B., Theobald, T. J., et al.: Treatment by transfusion of severe general radiation injury in dogs, Transfusion **6**: 134, 1966.
131. Simon, E. R.: Adenine and purine nucleosides in human red cell preservation: A review, Transfusion **7**: 395, 1967.
132. Philips, F. S., Thiersch, J. B., and Bendich, A.: Adenine intoxication in relation to *in vivo* formation and deposition of 2,3-dioxyadenine in renal tubules, J. Pharmacol. Exp. Ther. **104**: 20, 1952.
133. Siegel, D. C., Reed, P. C., Fresquez, V., et al.: Renal effects of massive infusions of adenine during resuscitation from hemorrhagic shock in the baboon, Ann. Surg. **174**: 932, 1971.
134. Shields, C. E., Lopas, H., and Beindorf, N. I.: Investigation of nephrotoxic effects of adenine and its metabolic product, 2,8-dioxyadenine, on primates (Macaca irus), J. Clin. Pharmacol. **10**: 316, 1970.
135. Dawson, R. B., and Ellis, T. J.: Hemoglobin function of blood stored at 4° C. in ACD and CPD with adenine and inosine, Transfusion **10**: 113, 1970.
136. Valeri, C. R., and Zaroulis, C. G.: Rejuvenation and freezing of outdated human red cells, Adv. Exp. Med. Biol. **28**: 457, 1972.
137. Schiff, D., Aranda, J. V., Colle, E., et al.: Metabolic effects of exchange transfusion. II. Delayed hypoglycemia following transfusion with citrated blood, J. Pediatr. **79**: 589, 1971.
138. Wranne, B., Woodson, R. D., and Dotter, J. C.: Bohr effect:interaction between H^+, CO_2, and 2,3-DPG in fresh and stored blood, J. Appl. Physiol. **32**: 749, 1972.
139. Finch, C. A., and Lenfant, C.: Oxygen transport in man, New Engl. J. Med. **286**: 407, 1972.
140. Brewer, G. J., and Eaton, J. W.: Erythrocyte metabolism: Interaction with oxygen transport, Science **171**: 1205, 1971.
141. Gershanik, J. J., Levkoff, A. H., and Duncan, R.: Serum ionized calcium values in relation to exchange transfusion, J. Pediatr. **82**: 847, 1973.
142. Rubin, R. J., and Nair, P. P.: Plasticizers in human tissues, New Engl. J. Med. **288**: 915, 1973.
143. Brake, J. M., and Deindoerfer, F. H.: Preservation of red blood cell: 2,3-diphosphoglycerate in stored blood containing dihydrooxyocetone, Transfusion **13**: 84, 1973.
144. Wood, L., and Beutle, E.: The effect of ascorbic acid on the 2,3-diphosphoglycerate (2,3-DPG) level in stored blood, Clin. Res. **20**: 186, 1972.

Starch pleuritis: A postthoracotomy syndrome possibly caused by surgical glove powder

Andrew L. Warshaw, M.D., *and* **Lawrence J. Mills, M.D.,** *Boston, Mass.*

This report describes a patient who developed transient pleuritic chest pain, fever, wound induration, and a sterile pleural effusion eight days after thoracotomy. Thoracentesis yielded sterile fluid which contained many mononuclear leukocytes and many starch granules. Control pleural fluid from asymptomatic postthoracotomy patients did not contain starch. These circumstances are precisely analogous to those in starch peritonitis. We suggest that this patient's symptoms were due to starch pleuritis.

From the General Surgical Services, Massachusetts General Hospital, and the Department of Surgery, Harvard Medical School, Boston, Mass.

SURGICAL GLOVE powder can produce a granulomatous peritonitis manifested by fever and abdominal pain one to four weeks after laparotomy.[1] The diagnosis may be facilitated by aspiration of characteristic ascitic fluid, which is sterile and contains many mononuclear leukocytes and starch granules.[4, 5] An analogous syndrome may occur after thoracotomy.

CASE REPORT

A 44-year-old man had a right lower lobectomy for carcinoma. Anterior and posterior drainage tubes were removed one and three days later. A chest roentgenogram on the fourth postoperative day showed pleural thickening (Fig. 1). On the eighth day he complained of pleuritic pain and increased discomfort in the wound. His temperature rose from normal to 102.4° F. The wound was swollen and indurated. The peripheral leukocyte count was 12,000 per cubic millimeter. Roentgen examination of the chest showed a large pleural effusion (Fig. 2). Thoracentesis was performed by the use of a disposable plastic syringe and a sheathed plastic cannula inserted through a needle (Intracath). No gloves were worn during the procedure. The pleural fluid was serosanguinous and contained 10,000 leukocytes per cubic millimeter, 70 percent of which were mononuclear. Abundant granules with Maltese-cross birefringence, characteristic of starch, were present upon microscopical examination under polarized light (Fig. 3). Bacterial cultures were sterile. A posterior chest tube was inserted, resulting in drainage of 300 ml. of fluid, and it was removed the following day. Three days later, the fever was gone, the wound was normal in appearance, and a chest roentgenogram showed residual pleural thickening, but no effusion. He remained well thereafter.

Pleural fluid obtained from two patients with congestive heart failure and six patients one to seven days after uncomplicated thoracotomy did not contain starch granules.

Accepted for publication Nov. 16, 1973.

Reprint requests: Dr. A. L. Warshaw, Massachusetts General Hospital, Boston, Mass.

DISCUSSION

Although the presence of starch granules in the pleural effusion of this patient does not prove their etiologic importance, the clinical symptoms, including pain, fever, wound induration,[3] and a sterile effusion arising after a latent period of well-being, are strikingly

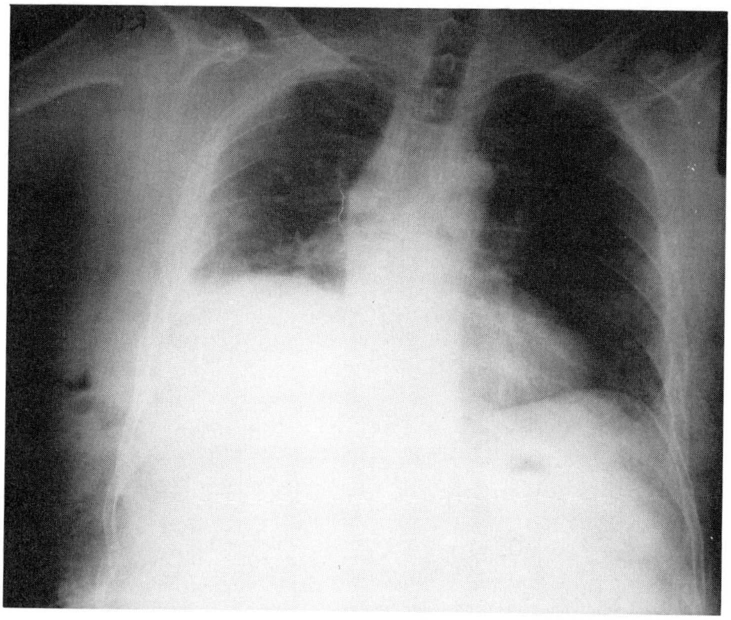

Fig. 1. Upright roentgenogram of the chest on the fourth postoperative day. There is minimal pleural thickening and appropriate elevation of the right hemi-diaphragm.

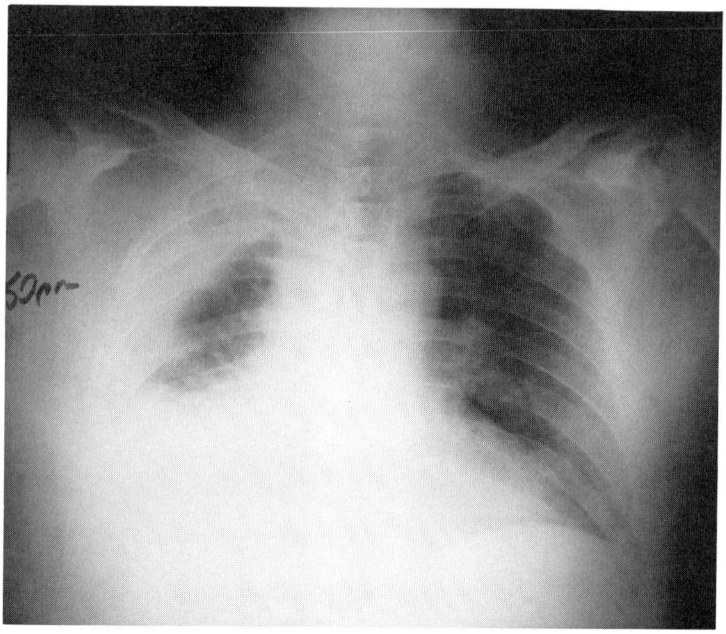

Fig. 2. Upright roentgenogram of the chest on the eighth postoperative day. There has been a marked increase in the amount of pleural fluid and of pleural thickening since the previous study.

similar to the features of the starch peritonitis syndrome.[1, 5] No alternative explanation is apparent. Starch granules have been previously reported in a postthoracotomy pleural effusion,[2] but accompanying clinical features were not given.

We propose that postthoracotomy starch pleuritis exists as a recognizable syndrome,

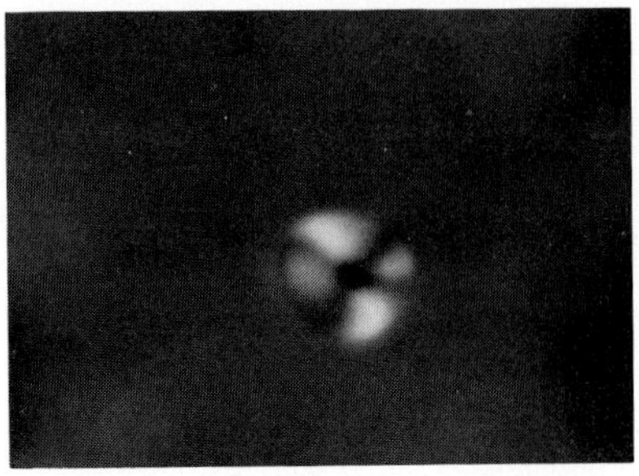

Fig. 3. Polarized-light photomicrograph of a starch granule, showing the Maltese-cross pattern of birefringence. Starch granules range in size from 10 to 20 μ.

the diagnosis of which may be substantiated by thoracentesis performed carefully to avoid artifactual introduction of starch from gloves or instruments. If the analogy to starch peritonitis is valid, the reaction should subside spontaneously, but evacuation of the effusion may hasten the process. The usefulness of anti-inflammatory drugs such as corticosteroids[1] or indomethacin[5] is unknown.

REFERENCES

1. Ignatius, J. A., and Hartmann, W. H.: The glove starch peritonitis syndrome, Ann. Surg. **175:** 388, 1972.
2. Sobel, H. J., Schiffman, R. J., Schwarz, R., et al.: Granulomas and peritonitis due to glove starch powder, Arch. Pathol. **91:** 559, 1971.
3. Soderberg, C. H., Jr., Lou, T. Y., and Randall, H. T.: Glove starch granulomatous peritonitis, Am. J. Surg. **125:** 455, 1973.
4. Warshaw, A. L.: Diagnosis of starch peritonitis by paracentesis, Lancet **2:** 1054, 1972.
5. Warshaw, A. L.: Management of starch peritonitis without the unnecessary second operation, SURGERY **73:** 681, 1973.

A simplified correction of subclavian steal syndrome

Harry H. LeVeen, M.D., Vincent A. Piccone, Jr., M.D., Carlos Diaz, M.D., George Christoudias, M.D., Walter Slade, M.D., *and* **Iris Norstrand, M.D.,** *Brooklyn, N. Y.*

A simple cross-axillary artery bypass is being proposed as therapy for the subclavian steal syndrome. In subclavian artery occlusion, blood flows retrogradely through the vertebral artery to supply blood to the arm, thus stealing blood from the head and causing brain ischemia. The problem is to supply blood to the arm and subclavian artery with sufficient pressure to profuse the arm and, in addition, provide prograde flow in the vertebral artery. A vein graft or prosthesis is attached to the good axillary artery and brought across the chest to the contralateral side. The second and third parts of the axillary artery are exposed at the shoulder. The bypass is anastomosed to the third part of the axillary artery on each side. The graft is pulled through a split in the pectoralis major muscle and through a subcutaneous tunnel created on the chest wall to the opposite side. Operations performed in the neck and behind the clavicle utilize the good ipsolateral carotid artery as the source of blood for revascularization of vertebral or subclavian artery. Intrathoracic operations may be of more serious consequence than the disease. Even the clavicle-splitting operations are of appreciable magnitude and produce prolonged disability. Utilization of the good carotid artery imposes the added risk of serious brain ischemia during surgery and postoperatively. The simplicity of the procedure and the excellent long-term clinical result obtained with axillary-to-axillary artery bypass makes it the procedure of choice.

From the Departments of Surgery and Neurology, Veterans Administration Hospital and State University of New York, Downstate Medical Center, Brooklyn, N. Y.

SURGICAL RELIEF of the subclavian steal syndrome generally is achieved by transthoracic endarterectomy, bypass, or graft interposition.[3, 8, 12] These procedures have an excellent record in re-establishing prograde flow in the vertebral artery with a low mortality rate[8, 12] and of providing dramatic relief of ischemic cerebral symptoms.[8, 12] However, with the exception of reversed vertebral flow from proximal subclavian trauma[15, 16] or palliation of a tetralogy,[5] the subclavian steal syndrome usually occurs in older patients in whom the risk of thoracotomy is increased. The danger of major surgery has been diminished by the transcervical approach to subclavian endarterectomy,[17] again with good results. The lack of enthusiasm for Wheeler's[17] technique stems from poor proximal control close to the aorta and the poor exposure of the subclavian artery compared with that offered by thoracotomy. Introduction of a carotid-subclavian bypass by North and associates,[10] subclavian artery transposition by Parrott,[11] and vertebral artery transposition by Clark and Perry[1] retained the basic appeal of the nonthoracic approach and overcame the danger of endarterectomy of the proximal subclavian artery from a

Accepted for publication Nov. 20, 1973.

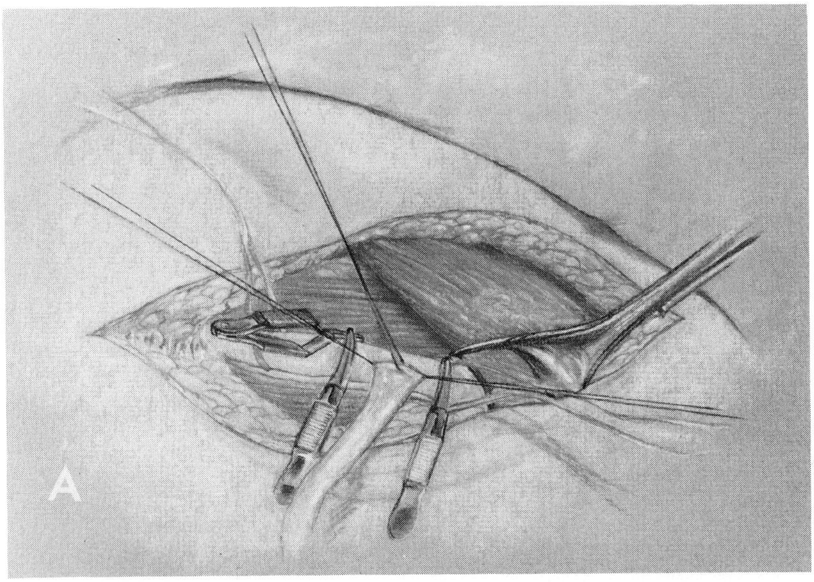

Fig. 1*A*. Demonstration of the exposure of the axillary artery (by retracting pectoralis major) and the anastomosis of vein graft.

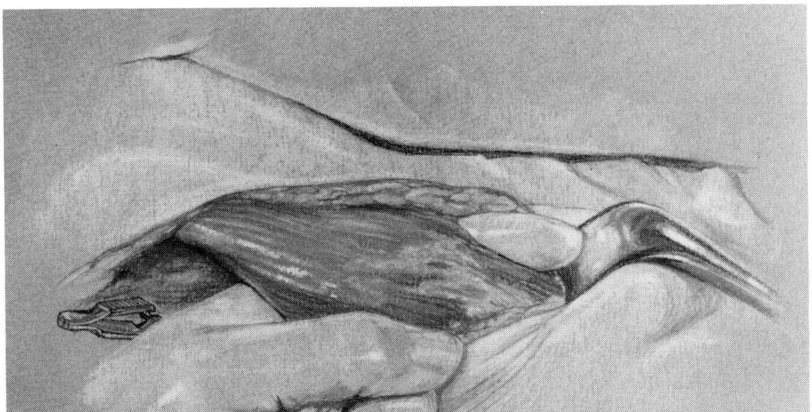

Fig. 1*B*. Demonstration of tunnel for vein graft to pass through pectoral muscle.

cervical incision. However, Dumanian and associates[4] and others[6] experimentally demonstrated decreased flow to the left common carotid artery distal to the anastomosis of the bypass graft. While clinical results of carotid-subclavian bypass and transposition operations do not appear to bear out the experimental objections,[1, 7, 10, 11] an alternate possibility which does not present these disadvantages has become evident.

A bypass graft from one axillary artery to the other corrects the pathophysiology of the subclavian steal syndrome without thoracotomy, without any occlusion of a major extra-

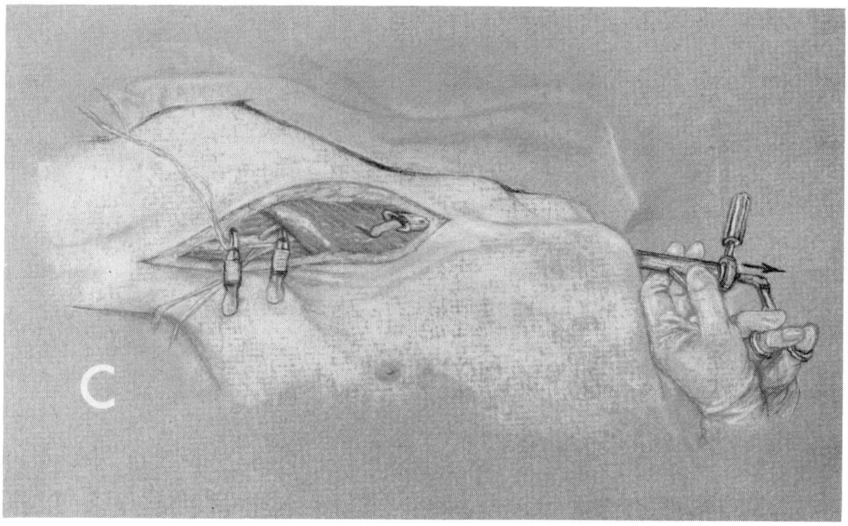

Fig. 1*C*. Demonstration of vein graft brought through bronchoscope to avoid kinking or twisting of the graft in the tunnel.

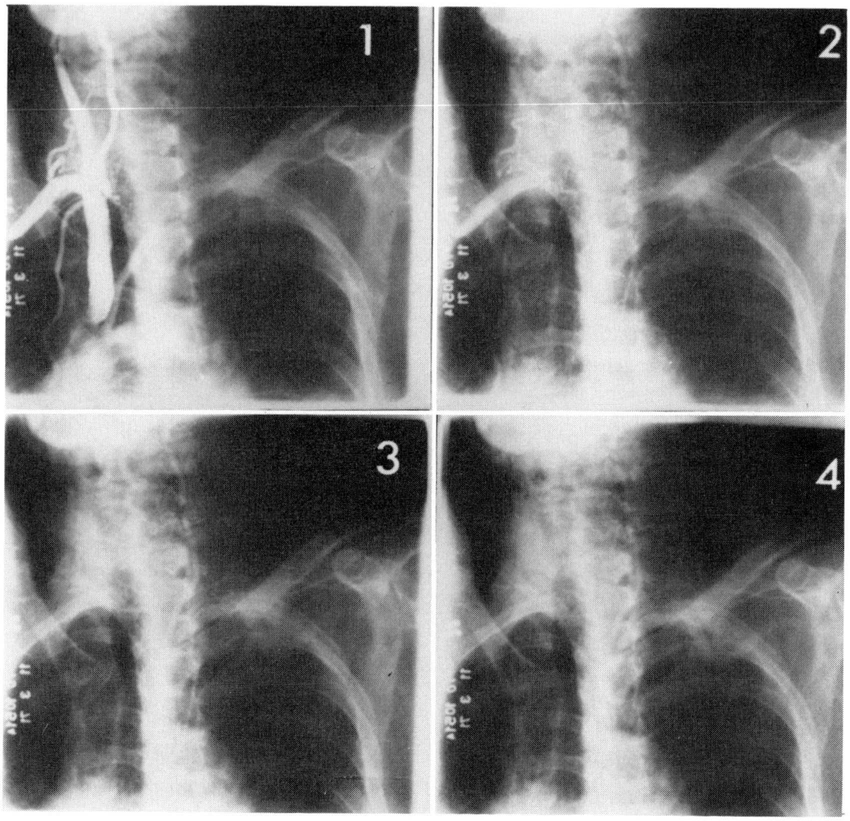

Fig. 2. Total occlusion of the left subclavian had been demonstrated on arch aortography. The above films resulted when the right brachial artery was injected with contrast medium. The contrast medium traversed up the right carotid and vertebral arteries and then passed down the left vertebral artery and filled the left subclavian artery.

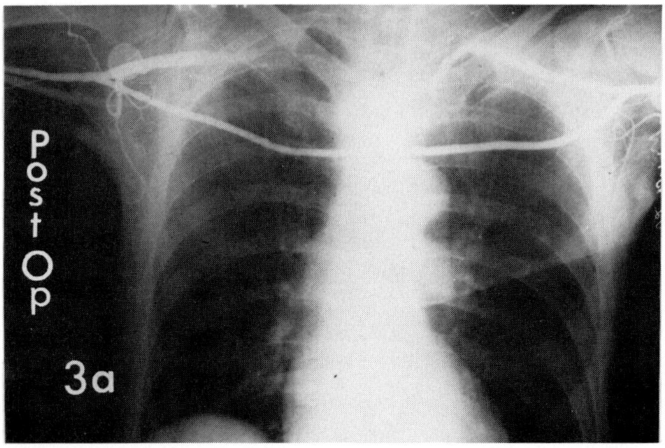

Fig. 3*A*. This illustration shows the excellent flow of contrast medium from the right subclavian artery to the left subclavian artery via the bypass graft.

cranial cerebral vessel, with simple exposure and minimal trauma. It is ideally suited for the elderly patient.

Experience with a single patient in September, 1971, proved so much simpler than our experience with the intrathoracic procedures,[13] that the authors were prompted to describe the technique as a feasible alternative to the more standard procedures.

TECHNIQUE

A linear incision is made over the base of the arm just under the edge of the biceps and continued over the axillary fold produced by the pectoralis major. The incision is deepened to expose the axillary artery surrounded by nerve bundles. The distal portion of the axillary artery is isolated with tapes. The saphenous vein is removed and heparin is administered. The graft is sutured in place in an end-to-side fashion with four traction sutures to give the arteriotomy a diamond configuration (Fig. 1*A*). Continuous sutures are used but the vessel edges are maintained under constant traction to prevent the purse-string effect with tightening of the suture line. The course of the bypass is simulated with the index finger, and the pectoralis major muscle is pierced at a place which will allow the graft to lie in direct line across the chest (Fig. 1*B*). A tunnel is created in the subcutaneous tissue to the contralateral axilla with the use of an "olive on a stick" instrument. Some difficulty may be encountered at the midline where the skin is adherent to the sternum. The vein graft is drawn over to the contralateral axilla through a bronchoscope (Fig. 1*C*). An end-to-side anastomosis of vein to axillary artery identical to that on the other side is repeated.

CASE REPORT

A 63-year-old white male was admitted on Sept. 22, 1971, complaining of recurrent headaches and dizziness of seven months' duration. These had increased in severity two weeks prior to admission. Physical examination showed weak radial pulse on the left and a significantly lower blood pressure in the left arm. Neurological examination was essentially negative. The clinical impression of a subclavian steal syndrome was corroborated by an arch aortogram and brachial arteriogram (Fig. 2). On Nov. 8, 1971, an axilloaxillary bypass was performed with the use of the saphenous vein. The postoperative period was uneventful and prograde flow was restored in left vertebral artery (Figs. 3*A* and 3*B*). All symptoms disappeared, the blood pressure became equal in both arms, and a normal left radial pulse was restored. On discharge on Dec. 3, 1971, he was completely asymptomatic. He has been followed periodically at the clinic for the past two years and has remained in good health. The neurological complaints have not recurred. The pulsating subcutaneous bypass is easily palpated and demonstrates long-term patency of the vein graft.

DISCUSSION

Past opinion has been divided as to the surgical management of the subclavian steal

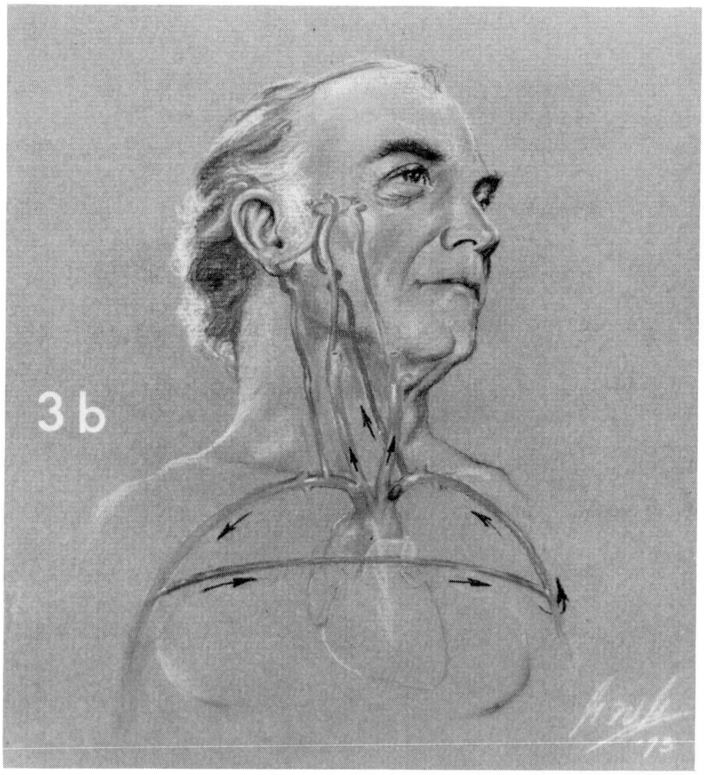

Fig. 3*B*. Diagrammatic presentation of the operative correction of the steal.

syndrome, especially in poor-risk patients. Simple ligation of the vertebral artery[14] will prevent the reversal of flow and relieve ischemia, but it also may cause (1) cerebellar infarction caused by thrombosis[9] and (2) ischemic damage to the ipsilateral upper extremity.[16] Surgery required to restore prograde flow has been of greater magnitude. The posterolateral thoracotomy has been used with occlusions of the left subclavian artery while sternal splitting incisions have been used for the innominate artery and right subclavian artery. Even more minimal operations such as removing a section of the clavicle for the subclavian approach can produce disabling symptoms. Operations performed on the neck and behind the clavicle with the use of a bypass from the ipsilateral carotid artery impose the added risk of serious brain ischemia with postoperative neurological deficits. Transthoracic endarterectomy of the subclavian artery, besides posing a major challenge for the patient, may occasionally be complicated by an intimal flap closing the vertebral ostium and thereby achieving no more than vertebral artery ligation.[13]

The axilloaxillary bypass approximates the length of the long femoropopliteal bypass, is on the anterior chest wall where it is exposed to trauma, and passes across bone. However, a collective review[12] reveals the intrathoracic approach to the arteries carries a 3.4 percent failure rate and a 3.4 percent mortality rate for endarterectomy and about three percent mortality rate for bypass grafts. In the case reported, an excellent clinical result was obtained with very minimal surgery. The simplicity of the axilloaxillary approach warrants further use, especially in very poor-risk patients.

REFERENCES

1. Clark, K., and Perry, M. D.: Carotid vertebral anastomosis: An alternate technique for repair of the subclavian steal syndrome, Ann. Surg. **163:** 414, 1966.
2. Craddock, D. R., and Logan, A.: The sub-

clavian steal and its surgical management, Br. J. Surg. **53:** 926, 1966.
3. Daicoff, G. R., Lancaster, J. R., Ranniger, K., and Moulder, P. V.: Rationale for aorto-subclavian artery bypass, J. Thorac. Cardiovasc. Surg. **49:** 945, 1965.
4. Dumanian, A. V., Frahm, C. J., Pascale, L. R., Teplinsky, L. L., and Santschi, D R.: The surgical treatment of the subclavian steal syndrome, J. Thorac. Cardiovasc. Surg. **50:** 22, 1965.
5. Folger, G. U., and Shah, K. D.: Subclavian steal in patients with Blalock-Taussig anastomosis, Circulation **31:** 241, 1965.
6. Harper, J. A., Golding, A. L., Mazzei, E. A., and Cannon, J. A.: An experimental hemodynamic study of the subclavian steal syndrome, Surg. Gynecol. Obstet. **124:** 1212, 1967.
7. Javid, H., Julian, O. C., Dye, W. S., and Hunter, J. A.: Management of cerebral arterial insufficiency caused by reversal of flow, Arch. Surg. **90:** 634, 1965.
8. Killen, D. A., Foster, J. H., Gobbel, W. G., Jr., Stevenson, S. E., Collins, H. A., Billings, F. T., and Scott, H. W., Jr.: The subclavian steal syndrome, J. Thorac. Cardiovasc. Surg. **51:** 539, 1966.
9. Murray, D. S.: Post-traumatic thrombosis of the internal carotid and vertebral arteries after non-penetrating injuries of the neck, Br. J. Surg. **44:** 556, 1957.
10. North, R. R., Fields, W. S., De Bakey, M. E., and Crawford, E. S.: Brachial-basilar insufficiency syndrome, Neurology **12:** 810, 1962.
11. Parrott, J. C.: The subclavian steal syndrome, Arch. Surg. **88:** 661, 1964.
12. Piccone, V. A., Jr., and LeVeen, H. H.: Collective review. The subclavian steal syndrome, Ann. Thorac. Surg. **9:** 1, 1970.
13. Piccone, V. A., Karvounis, P., and LeVeen, H. H.: The subclavian steal syndrome, Angiology. In press.
14. Rob, C.: Incipient strokes: Technique of surgical therapy, *in* Millikan, C. H., Siekert, R. G., and Whisnant, J. P., editors: Cerebral vascular diseases, New York, 1961, Grune & Stratton, Inc., p. 112.
15. Rojas, R. H., Levitsky, S., and Stansel, H. C.: Acute traumatic subclavian steal syndrome, J. Thorac. Cardiovasc. Surg. **51:** 113, 1966.
16. Webb, W. R., and Burford, T. H.: Gangrene of arm following use of subclavian artery in a pulmonosystemic anastomosis, J. Thorac. Surg. **23:** 199, 1952.
17. Wheeler, H. B.: Surgical treatment of subclavian artery occlusions, N. Engl. J. Med. **276:** 711, 1967.

A simple and inexpensive tunneler for use in peripheral vascular surgery

Robert M. Blumenberg, M.D., *and* **Michael L. Gelfand, M.D.,** *Schenectady, N. Y.*

A simple and inexpensive tunneler has been employed in arterial grafting encompassing femoropopliteal, aortofemoral, and axillofemoral bypass procedures. This is fashioned from the polyethylene containers used to store Argyll chest and sump drainage tubes. This technique is recommended because of its simplicity, ready availability, lack of expense, and relative safety.

From the Departments of Surgery, Ellis Hospital, Schenectady, N. Y., and the Albany Medical College, Albany, N. Y.

PERIPHERAL arterial bypass procedures performed with the use of synthetic prostheses or reversed autogenous veins are common modalities of arterial reconstruction. Indications range from disabling claudication to limb salvage. A point of technique, obvious to the success of these procedures, is the prevention of twisting or kinking of the graft as it is brought through the various tunnels between the proximal and distal anastomoses. For instance, the route preferred by most peripheral vascular surgeons in performing a femoropopliteal bypass operation is the subsartorial tunnel. An unavoidable "blind area" along the midportion of such a tunnel has engendered a variety of elaborate and relatively expensive devices designed for the purpose of creating the tunnel and preventing twisting of the graft.[1, 2] We routinely employ a simple and inexpensive technique using materials which are readily available and often discarded in most operating rooms. The instrument utilized is actually a container, used to store a variety of Argyll* catheters such as chest drainage and sump tubes.

Accepted for publication Dec. 10, 1973.

*Sherwood Medical Industries, 1831 Olive St., St. Louis, Mo. 63103.

MATERIALS AND METHOD

The outer polyethylene casings, which contain the Argyll tubes, are saved after their contents have been used. The tubes are soaked clean of their labels and stored in the operating room vascular cart until they are needed for the bypass procedure. At the time of surgery, the tube and cap are autoclaved along with the surgical tray. The bullet-shaped cap is placed on the tube at the operating table and held in place by two through-and-through sutures of No. 2-0 silk passed through the plastic by a relatively heavy needle (Fig. 1). The tube is trimmed to a length slightly shorter than the graft by cutting off the blunt closed end with a heavy scissors after tube placement. After the tunnel has been started by finger dissection, the "tunneler" can be passed either proximally or distally. The rounded cap of the tube easily opens up the tunnel with a minimum of tissue trauma. Mild pliability of polyethylene is superior to more rigid materials in avoiding serious damage to surrounding vital structures which might be

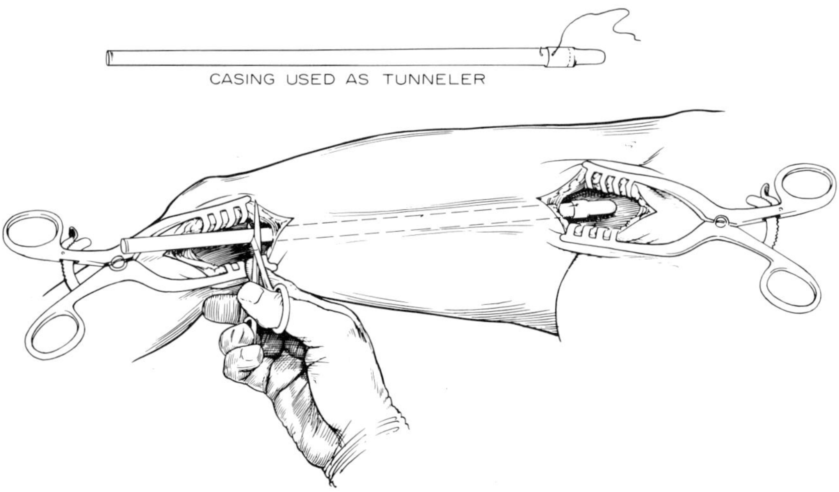

Fig. 1. Cap is sutured to casing with No. 2-0 silk. Tunneler placed in subsartorial canal with emergence at popliteal level. Excess trimmed with heavy scissors.

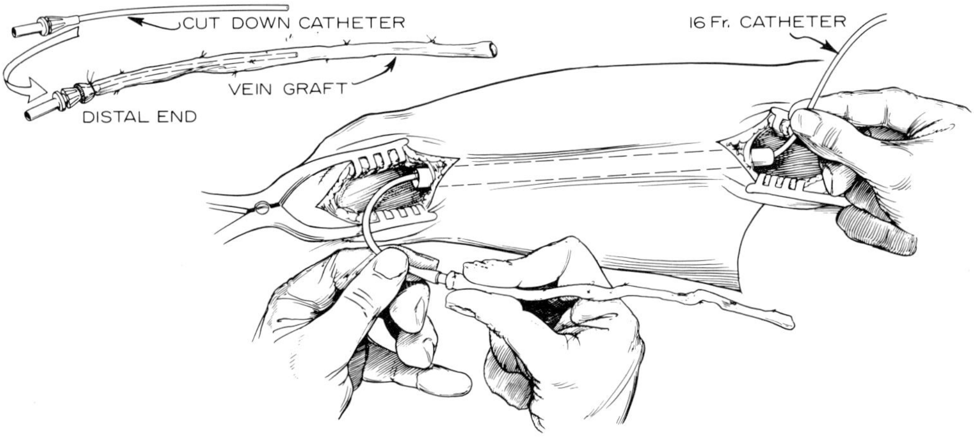

Fig. 2. A polyethylene cutdown catheter, temporarily fixed within the lumen of the reversed saphenous vein, is closed with its "plugged tip," and a No. 16 Fr. catheter is attached to this tip.

incurred by injudicious "forcing" of the tunneler. When the tube has come to lie in the position, the silk sutures are cut, the cap removed, and the closed end of the tube transected at the desired length (Fig. 1). A No. 16 Fr. red rubber catheter is attached to the end of a cutdown catheter previously placed within the vein or Dacron graft, and it is passed into the plastic tunneler (Fig. 2). This allows for direct observation of the graft as it disappears into the tunnel. Additionally, the lettering on the rubber catheter can be observed as it emerges from the tunneler to ensure that the catheter itself has not rotated. When the graft has been drawn through the tunneling device, it is then dilated with heparinized solution and properly positioned for the performance of both anastomoses (Fig. 3). The tunneler is then gently withdrawn. The caliber of the tunneler significantly exceeds the graft diameter so that it can readily be withdrawn without fear of damage to the graft as it comes to lie independent of the tunnel. The tunneler is then discarded, and the procedure continues in standard fashion.

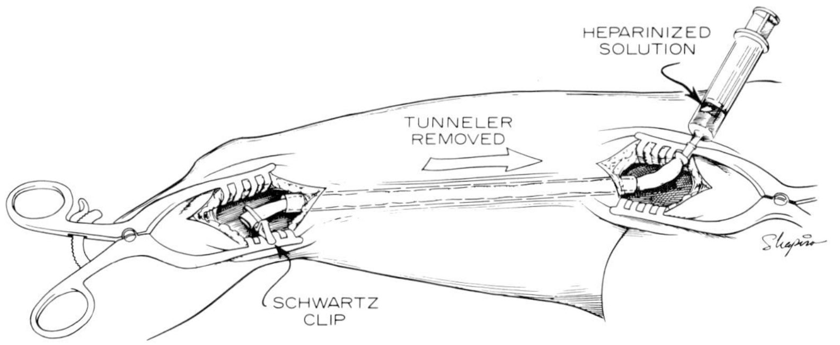

Fig. 3. The rubber catheter and attached reversed vein graft are gently pulled through the tunneler without twisting. Following rubber catheter detachment, heparinized solution is used to distend the graft. Following gentle removal of the tunneler, the anastomoses are performed in routine fashion.

COMMENT

The authors have utilized the above technique in well over 100 bypass procedures. In our hands, it is routinely used to develop the subsartorial tunnel in the performance of femoropopliteal and femorotibial bypass operations. Moreover, it has greatly simplified aortofemoral grafting via the retroperitoneal space, as well as axillofemoral shunting. The relative safety, simplicity, ready availability, and lack of expense recommends this technique for common usage in peripheral vascular reconstructive procedures.

REFERENCES

1. Parsonnet, V., and Driller, J.: A tunneler for bypass vascular surgery, Arch. Surg. **106:** 236, 1973.
2. Rob, C. G., and DeWeese, J. A.: Tunneler for arterial bypass grafts, SURGERY **62:** 393, 1967.

Editorials

How to be an adequate vagotomist

John Alexander-Williams, *Birmingham, England*

From The United Birmingham Hospitals

MANY TRAINEE surgeons are being taught vagotomy and many surgeons who once used partial gastrectomy have learned to perform vagotomy with pyloroplasty or antrectomy as the standard operation for duodenal ulcer disease. The technique is neither self-evident nor simple and there is no obvious anatomic end-point that tells the surgeon when he has achieved an adequate vagotomy.

After a partial gastrectomy more than half the patient's stomach is sent to the pathologist, and the surgeon can be confident that there is a more than 95 percent chance of his having cured the ulcer, but the surgeon may send three or more portions of vagus nerve tissue to the pathologist and still have left intact sufficient vagal nerve fibers to permit an early recurrence. What is an adequate vagotomy is difficult to determine and no final answer to the question has yet been given, although the subject has recently been reviewed in detail.[1] It is certain that we should abandon the old all-or-none concept of a positive or negative insulin test indicating a complete or incomplete vagotomy. Some vagotomy operations are more "complete" than others and some are certainly *inadequate* as means of preventing recurrent ulcer. Today we no longer assume that a surgeon cuts either all or none of the vagal fibers to the stomach. No secretory value can be defined as the dividing line between complete and incomplete vagotomy but it is probable that the higher the rise in acid secretion after insulin the more vagal fibers remain intact. The advantage of Hollander's[2] criteria is that they are the most widely investigated and understood but we should remember that "Hollander negative" does not mean that every vagal fiber to the stomach is divided nor does "Hollander positive" necessarily mean that the vagotomy is inadequate to cure the ulcer.

Johnston and Goligher[3] surveyed the vagotomy achievements of a number of their colleagues and their own department in Leeds and found that some surgeons were consistently better than others at achieving an adequate vagotomy as judged by the early postoperative insulin test. The success rate was not necessarily related to experience or seniority.

How do most surgeons discover whether or not they are a "good vagotomist"? I suspect that most do so by performing a large number of vagotomies and then waiting to see whether many of their patients complain of recurrent symptoms. This approach is unlikely to give a true impression since the dissatisfied patients of the most consistent incomplete vagotomist may seek a second opinion about their recurrent symptoms while the first surgeon blithely continues to practice his faulty technique in the belief that all his patients "seem to do well."

Accepted for publication May 1, 1973.

Reprint requests: Mr. John Alexander-Williams, The United Birmingham Hospitals, Steelhouse Lane, Birmingham B4, 6NH, England.

It is one thing to pay lip service to the need to ensure that our vagotomy technique is adequate but another to take effective steps toward this goal. We can test for the adequacy of vagotomy *during* operation by one of a number of techniques or we may test *after* operation by the insulin test or by calculating the decrease in the stimulated peak acid output. It is clearly preferable to test during operation so that any inadequacies can at once be remedied.

To achieve universal acceptance, intraoperative tests for adequacy of vagotomy should be simple, speedy, safe, inexpensive, reliably reproducible, and, above all, effective. With so many different criteria to fulfill it is not surprising that none is as yet universally used. The intraoperative tests so far devised rely on one of three principles: (1) specific staining of nerve fibers, (2) demonstration that the efferent motor nerves in the vagus have been divided, or (3) the confirmation that the efferent secretory fibers have been divided.

In the search for a vital stain for nerve fibers, Lee[4] claimed success using leuko-methylene blue. Methylene blue is colorless in a solution of ascorbic acid but turns blue in the presence of oxygen. It is claimed that nerve fibers have more available oxygen than muscle or connective tissue and that this makes leuko-methylene blue change color and stain nerve tissue blue. In theory, if the dye is applied to the surface of the esophagus and then rapidly washed off with saline, the nerve fibers remain bluer than the surrounding tissue, thus aiding their identification. In practice the method certainly results in many fine blue strands of tissue being stained. Unfortunately it is unreliable in that major nerve trunks are not always stained (not necessarily a serious defect) and that if all the blue fibers identified are submitted to histologic examination only about half of them prove to be nerve fibers.[5-7] Grassi and Orecchia, in this issue of SURGERY, indicate that, out of 30 patients considered to have a "complete" vagotomy after the leuko-methylene blue test, nine (23 percent) were shown to be "incomplete" by other intraoperative and postoperative tests. A similar failure rate was found on postoperative insulin testing by Frimer and associates.[6] While the leuko-methylene blue test may be of value in reminding surgeons of the need to be meticulous in looking for very fine nerve fibers in or around the lower esophagus it does not ensure an adequate vagotomy.

The electrical stimulation test designed by Burge and Vane[8] relies on detection of muscular contraction of the stomach when the vagus is stimulated electrically. When the stimulating electrode is placed round the lower esophagus, including the vagus nerves, the current produces a muscular contraction in the air-filled stomach that can be measured manometrically. An absence of contraction is thought to indicate that the vagotomy is "complete."

The test is based on sound principles, if we accept that secretory nerve fibers are also motor nerves. Furthermore, there is no doubt that the originator and main protagonist of the test achieves a high rate of adequate vagotomy and a low rate of recurrent ulcer that are the envy of most vagotomists.[9] It is by no means certain, however, that this success is due entirely to the use of the electrical stimulation test nor that if all surgeons used the test they would achieve results as good as those of Burge. On the contrary, there is evidence that their results would be no better even if the test were used.[10, 11] Furthermore, the test is inconvenient and time consuming and requires the unswerving cooperation of the anesthetist (and indeed also the patient) in avoiding any anticholinergic medication before and during the operation. Although Hollanders[12] has reported results that show that the test is effective in Burge's hands the difficulties just mentioned obviously influence many surgeons, as a survey of the vagotomy practice of 132 surgeons in the United Kingdom and the United States showed that only four used the electrical stimulation test and even then they used it only occasionally.[13]

The intraoperative test described by Grassi[14] is based on the assumption that the secretory response of the parietal cells to a circulating stimulant (pentagastrin or histamine) is dependent, at least in part, on the "cholinergic tone" resulting from an intact vagal nerve supply. When the vagal nerve supply is interrupted there is an immediate rise in the threshold of excitability of the parietal cells so that a stimulus that hitherto would have evoked secretion no longer has this effect. The test involves mapping out the area of acid-secreting cells in the stomach by an electrode or pH-sensitive dye such as Congo red. It is claimed that when the vagal nerve supply is divided the acid secretion is so reduced that the pH does not fall below 3.5. If any area retains its vagal innervation as the result of an undivided fiber continued acid secretion will be detected by a fall in the intragastric pH to below 3.5.

A variation of this principle is proposed by Cole,[15] who has evolved a test used so far only in experimental animals. He employs 2-desoxy-D-glucose as a vagal stimulant and parenteral neutral red as a pH-sensitive dye that is secreted by the parietal cells. In the presence of vagal innervation of the parietal cell area both drugs administered intravenously cause the outpouring of a purple secretion from the gastric glands of the body of the stomach. When all the vagal fibers are divided no colored secretion occurs.

The results reported by Grassi and Orecchia using the pH mapping technique are certainly impressive and seem to be better than those, in their hands, with either the leukomethylene blue or electrical stimulation tests. It must be emphasized, however, that this comparison is not strictly valid because the intraoperative pH test was the latest test applied by a team that has an extensive vagotomy experience. Their results would anyway be expected to improve with experience.

In patients with a "negative" response to the insulin test after operation the peak acid output in response to histamine or pentagastrin, although it is reduced compared with before operation, is certainly not abolished. In view of this finding the apparent success of the test is, in the authors' own words, perplexing. They postulate that after denervation there is an immediate loss of response that later recovers. Nevertheless the concept and apparent success of the test opens a new chapter in the search for a reliable intraoperative test for an adequate vagotomy. It has further merit in that, unlike the electrical stimulation test, it is applicable to the new types of vagotomy that denervate only the acid-secreting part of the stomach. It has the serious disadvantage that it involves opening the stomach, so destroying the benefit inherent in avoiding any opening of the gut in proximal gastric vagotomy with preservation of antral innervation. It remains to be seen whether the intraoperative pH test will significantly alter the vagotomy achievements of other surgeons and if so whether it fulfills sufficient of the criteria described earlier for it to gain widespread adoption.

Meanwhile, until intraoperative tests are proved to be simple, safe, and reliable, what should the aspiring vagotomist do? I suggest that he should not wait five or ten years to see how many recurrent ulcers develop in his patients; he should employ as meticulous a search for vagal fibers as he is able and use a postoperative acid-secretion test with pentagastrin or histalog and insulin as a stimulant and he should keep a record of his results.[16] If he cannot regularly ensure an adequate reduction in gastric acid secretion by vagotomy he should either adopt one or other of the intraoperative tests until he can do so or he should abandon vagotomy.

REFERENCES

1. Baron, J. H., and Alexander-Williams, J.: Gastric secretion tests, *in* Taylor, S., editor: Recent advances in surgery, London, 1973, Churchill-Livingstone, pp. 166-198.
2. Hollander, F.: The insulin test for the presence of intact nerve fibers after vagal operations for peptic ulcer, Gastroenterology **1:** 607, 1946.
3. Johnston, D., and Goligher, J. C.: The influence of the individual surgeon and of the type of vagotomy upon the insulin test after vagotomy, Gut **12:** 963, 1971.
4. Lee, M.: A selective strain to detect the vagus

nerve in the operation of vagotomy, Br. J. Surg. **56:** 10, 1969.
5. Cooke, W. M., Talbot, I. C., Welbourn, R. B., and Cox, A. G.: Leucomethylene-blue as an aid to vagotomy, Lancet **1:** 864, 1970.
6. Frimer, M. C., Cohen, M. M., Harrison, R. C., and Holubitsky, I. B.: The selective nerve strain leucomethylene blue as an intraoperative aid to achieving complete vagotomy, Gut **11:** 881, 1970.
7. Jensen, H. E., Kragelund, E., and Amdrup, E: Intraoperative studies of the stomach, Chir. Gastroenterol. **5:** 303, 1971.
8. Burge, H. W., and Vane, J. R.: Method of testing for complete nerve section during vagotomy, Br. Med. J. **1:** 615, 1958.
9. Burge, H., Maclean, C., Stedeford, R., Pinn, G., and Hollanders, D.: Selective vagotomy without drainage; an interim report, Br. Med. J. **3:** 690, 1969.
10. Lythgoe, J. P.: Comparison of the insulin and electrical stimulation tests for completeness of vagotomy, Br. Med. J. **1:** 1196, 1961.
11. Clarke, C. G., and Murray, J. C.: The Burge test for complete vagotomy, J. R. Coll. Surg. **8:** 212, 1963.
12. Hollanders, D.: Electrical stimulation and insulin tests used with bilateral selective vagotomy, Gut **12:** 629, 1971.
13. Williams, J. A.: *In* Williams, J. A., and Cox, A. G., editors: Current practice in after vagotomy, London, 1969, Butterworth & Co., Ltd., pp. 399-413.
14. Grassi, G.: A new test for complete nerve section during vagotomy, Br. J. Surg. **58:** 187, 1971.
15. Cole, R. E.: An operative test for the completeness of vagotomy, Am. J. Surg. **123:** 543, 1972.
16. Kay, A. W.: *In* Williams, J. A., and Cox, A. G., editors: After vagotomy, London, 1969, Butterworth & Co., Ltd., pp. 1-11.

Diminished surgical infection by systemic antibiotic administration in potentially contaminated operations

Hiram C. Polk, Jr., M.D., *Louisville, Ky.*

From the Department of Surgery and the Price Institute of Surgical Research, University of Louisville School of Medicine, Health Sciences Center, Louisville, Ky.

THE CAUSE and therefore the prevention of surgical infection, specifically that involving the surgical incision and the cavity subjected to operation, are largely dependent upon the nature of the operation. For example, it has been verified by Hart and Wright and their associates that reduction of air-borne bacteria by ultraviolet light reduces the frequency of infection occurring in refined clean operations, such as elective craniotomy. This reflects the extreme cleanliness of the organ operated upon and the ability to deal effectively with skin contaminants, thus leaving air-borne bacteria as the most likely pathogens. The converse is true in a colon resection, where the most likely source of bacteria leading to infection is from within the colon itself, microbes spilled at the time of operation. Indeed, elimination of all air-borne bacteria in this setting contributes little to the control of sepsis, no doubt due to the grossly disproportionate numbers of bacteria in the colon compared to those in the operating theater air. Control of infection by the use of intraluminal (oral) antimicrobial agents has not been demonstrated regularly, probably because of the relatively slight effect of such agents upon fecal microbial concentrations.

Accepted for publication Aug. 16, 1973.

Reprint requests: Dr. Hiram C. Polk, Jr., Department of Surgery, University of Louisville School of Medicine, Health Sciences Center, Louisville, Ky. 40201.

Precisely these circumstances led us to consider the role of systemic administration of an antimicrobial agent for the control of infection associated with elective operations upon the stomach, the small bowel, and the colon.

The experiments of Miles, Miles, and Burke indicated that the maximum influence of an agent upon a local bacterial infection is exerted before bacterial challenge, concomitant with challenge, or immediately thereafter. Prior clinical and laboratory studies of the prevention of wound infection by systemic antimicrobial therapy were peculiarly irreconcilable. Laboratory studies showed almost perfect protection by those antibiotics for bacteria sensitive to the agent. Clinical studies, largely retrospective in nature, failed to confirm such protection and occasionally showed such "prophylactic" antibiotic usage to be associated with increased rates of infection. Accordingly, a regimen was devised for the administration of an antibiotic to a patient just before an elective operation in which contamination and therefore infection were reasonably likely and for a short postoperative period to test prospectively in the clinic the conclusions of a multitude of animal experiments.

Subsequently, in a double-blind, controlled experiment, this regimen reduced a wound infection rate, which had been stable at more than 20 percent, despite a variety of other maneuvers, to six percent. This communication describes our experience in more than 600 additional patients (not in a double-blind experiment) with this particular regimen for the control of infection following operations in which the stomach, small bowel, and/or colon were opened.

Shortly after the completion of the double-blind portion of the study previously reported in this JOURNAL, the regular conduct of operations upon the stomach and small and large bowel on a surgical service at the principal teaching hospital of the University of Miami School of Medicine (Jackson Memorial Hospital) implemented the use of cephaloridine regularly. All patients were suitably prepared with diet and mechanical cleansing related to their anticipated operations. No antimicrobial agents were used in any form other than those described in the original protocol; specifically, no antibiotic bowel preparation was employed. On call to the operating room, 1 Gm. of cephaloridine was administered intramuscularly concomitant with the usual preanesthetic medication. Five hours after this injection an additional gram of cephaloridine was administered intramuscularly and seven hours later a final 1 Gm. dose was given. Intestinal operations were performed with standard open anastomoses of two layers, generally employing an inner layer of catgut and an outer layer of silk. No *special* precautions were taken to control wound contamination during these procedures. A wound protector which proves particularly satisfactory for isolation of skin and subcutaneous fat from the operative field is, however, now often utilized as described by Cole and Bernard.

A total of 630 consecutive operations were studied and clinically significant bacteriologic data recorded. The blood and wound antibiotic levels described in the original reports were not determined on the subsequent patients. The presence or absence of wound infection was established according to those criteria described in the National Research Council ultraviolet light study.

The wound infection rate in the patient population has remained at 7 percent. There was no significant variation from year to year on the service through July, 1971, at which time the study was discontinued. Of all infected wounds, 84 percent were cultured.

During this 3½ year period, with the use of a single antibiotic primarily on a single surgical ward, no change occurred in the evolution of surgical pathogens, except the occasional appearance of *Serratia marcescens* later in the study. The author feels that this is an artifact, reflecting the recognition of nonpigmented Serratia, which in the earlier years of the study were often called Enterobacter. During this period, isolates from this particular surgical service did not change with respect to their sensitivity to the antibiotic agent in question from that which existed on the ward before introduction of the cephaloridine.

One may take this as an extraordinary testimony of the efficacy of the drug. The author believes the extremely short course of antimicrobial therapy is more likely responsible than any specific characteristic of the drug in question. The brief administration of the drug is not only within safety limits described for cephaloridine *per se* but also allows a minimum opportunity for the selection of bacterial forms resistant to the antimicrobial agent.

One particular aspect of the original study needs further explanation. The bacteria identified as causing wound infection in both the placebo and treated group failed to include any organisms recognized as anaerobes. A specific inquiry was made to the laboratory personnel involved, following the appearance of numerous reports of anaerobic organisms as surgical pathogens. Although anaerobic cultures were undertaken on all of the patients in the double-blind segment of the study, we learned later that the personnel involved were not regularly capable of recognizing anaerobic organisms.

Indeed, the great preponderance of prospective studies of the influence of systemic antibiotics upon surgical infection now show a significant reduction of infection, provided that the antimicrobial agent is first administered prior to the time of operation. Whether the concept will be useful in operations in which contamination is of lesser magnitude remains to be demonstrated. It is now clearly the method most likely to control incisional and peritoneal sepsis for elective operations upon the stomach, small bowel, and colon.

The role of paramedical personnel in organ procurement

Folkert O. Belzer, M.D., *San Francisco, Calif.*

From the Department of Surgery, University of California Medical School, San Francisco, Calif.

A MAJOR problem in renal transplantation is the lack of sufficient cadaver organs to treat all patients with end-stage renal disease. Fortunately, because of the emphasis upon educating physicians and the public about the value of cadaver organ transplants, the number of cadaver donors is steadily increasing, and we must devise better methods for organ harvesting. Two approaches have been used. The first method is to have the members of the transplant team perform the donor nephrectomy. The team travels to the hospital of the donor, or the donor is transferred to the transplant center for nephrectomy.

In our transplant center, most of the nephrectomies have been performed by one of the senior members of the transplant team, and under these conditions, technical errors are greatly reduced. A team of technicians always travels with the surgeon to the donor hospital and preservation of the kidneys after nephrectomy is performed by these paramedical personnel.

In other medical centers, surgeons not associated with the transplant team perform the donor nephrectomy. These surgeons have often been given special training in donor nephrectomy by a transplant center.

Both of these methods have disadvantages. Although the first method undoubtedly produces kidneys of the highest quality,[1] the time invested by the transplant surgeons is often excessive. The second method has the disadvantage that few surgeons are willing to perform cadaver donor nephrectomies on a routine basis. Because of the inherent problems in both of these methods, we have been using a third approach for the last year which may prove to be the method of choice if the number of donor organs continues to increase.

Our technicians, Mr. Robert Hoffman and Mr. Kenneth Steiper, have been involved in organ procurement and preservation for the past five years, and one of them always acts as first assistant to the transplant surgeon during donor nephrectomy. Their training and technical ability in this difficult surgical procedure have been of much help to us. These technicians are also trained in the techniques of organ preservation, and all kidneys receive the uniform and optimum treatment necessary for function after transplantation.

Surgeons who have performed cadaver donor nephrectomy know that it can be a difficult procedure because it must be done quickly, and if anatomical variations are not recognized, kidneys may be removed which are unsuitable for transplantation. Even a well-qualified surgeon often finds that his first donor nephrectomy, when performed by himself alone, has disappointing results, but when he is assisted by a person skilled in this procedure, excellent kidneys will be obtained. We now send our team of technicians to outlying hospitals to act as first

Accepted for publication Nov. 20, 1973.

Reprint requests: Folkert O. Belzer, M.D., Department of Surgery, University of California Medical Center, San Francisco, Calif. 94143.

assistants to local surgeons during donor nephrectomy and the kidneys have usually been of excellent quality.

This method has several advantages. Donor nephrectomies performed by many different surgeons will still be performed with standard techniques. No one surgeon will be burdened by a heavy load of donor nephrectomies since many surgeons in one area can now perform this procedure, even without previous experience.

With adequate financial remuneration, it should be possible to find a surgeon in every community who is willing to perform the donor nephrectomy if a kidney becomes available. Many small hospitals receive only one or two potential donors a year. While it is important to obtain these kidneys, it would be a waste of time to train a surgeon in this procedure since the opportunity to perform it would arise only rarely.

If paramedical personnel are to become an integral part of a successful organ procurement team, their selection and training will be of the utmost importance. The technicians must be highly motivated, either by past experience in related medical fields or because of previous participation in research. The importance of their role in providing health care for transplant recipients must be recognized and they must be paid adequately. In addition to their base salary, additional incentive pay should be given for each kidney that is procured and transplanted. The salaries of the technicians are paid from the hospital charges made to the transplant recipients. The technicians must have specialized surgical skills as well as a thorough knowledge of anatomy. These skills can be obtained in the experimental surgical laboratory and the autopsy room and also by assisting surgeons skilled in the technique of donor nephrectomy. The technicians must be trained in the methods of preservation and if perfusion equipment is used, they must be familiar with the mechanical aspects of their equipment. Even though this will probably bring down upon me the wrath of Women's Lib, technicians probably should be males since perfusion equipment is heavy and difficult to move. It might be difficult for a private surgeon to accept the advice of a paramedical person on surgical techniques, and this problem would be amplified if the technician were female. However, we have found that surgeons in this community are usually willing to take advice from our technicians because they quickly recognize and appreciate their special training and skills. The quality and function of kidneys obtained in this manner have been usually as good as those obtained by the transplant surgeon working with the technicians.

In the future, nephrectomy may be done entirely by paramedical personnel, but at the present a physician must be involved in the actual organ procurement. The method outlined above has logistical and financial advantages and should allow us to obtain large numbers of organs of the high quality necessary for good results after transplantation.

REFERENCE

1. Belzer, F. O., and Kountz, S. L.: Experience with locally obtained kidneys, Transplant. Proc. **4:** 603, 1972.

Letters to the editors

Pulse-contour vs. dye-dilution methods

To the Editors:

The exhaustive and important study of Jurado, Matucha, and Osborn (Cardiac output estimation by pulse-contour methods: Validity of their use for monitoring the critically ill patient, SURGERY 74: 358, 1973) is impressive in its scope, but perhaps questionable in its conclusions. Since a dye-dilution technique was "used as the standard" against which cardiac output determinations by pulse contour were measured and compared, the assumption of accuracy by the "standard" is clear. Failure to find significant correlation between determinations by pulse-contour and dye-dilution methods except with the use of an error factor, called a "proportionality constant K" (which required "recalibration" with time and was therefore not a constant), raises a serious question: In which technique was the greater error, indicator dilution or pulse contour?

Dr. Jurado and his associates straightforwardly enumerate the theoretic and demonstrated difficulties inherent in cadiac output determinations based upon the "windkessel" assumption. However, similar treatment was not extended to their "standard," dye dilution. Although sophisticated hardware for indicator-dilution techniques is widely available, the number appearing on the digital face bears no necessary relationship to volume of blood flow except that correlation warranted by the validity of the assumptions underlying the basic method.

If we can eliminate all errors of technique, then several assumptions must be faced: (1) complete and uniform mixing occurs, (2) marker concentration is a linear function of solvent volume, (3) marker does not leave the vascular system nor combine with tissue, (4) optical density is a linear function of marker concentration and passes through the zero point, (5) no recirculation exists during the primary curve, (6) recirculation time permits meaningful logarithmic extrapolation, (7) "trapping" of the marker does not occur in low flow states, and (8) steady-state conditions prevail.

This last assumption is perhaps the most damaging. If blood flow is not *constant* (not steady state), but rather is pulsatile or periodic, samples from such systems are *time*-average samples, not volume-average samples. Visscher and Johnson,[1] in their elegant analysis, have shown that integration of time-average samples is mathematically improper unless either the flows or the marker concentrations are equal on both sides of the heart at *each* instant of time. Such conditions seem unlikely under the unpublished General Principle of Biologic Inconstancy.* Since marker concentration is integrated over time in the present method of calculation, the greater the deviation from constancy for flow and concentration at each instant, the greater the magnitude of error.

Some authors have attempted to justify indicator-dilution results by claiming close correlation with values obtained by the Fick principle.[2] However, these theoretic objections apply in sense to the Fick principle as well, and objectivity has not been furthered.

Marked discrepancies between actual flows and those obtained by dye-dilution techniques in carefully controlled pulsatile model systems have been reported.[3, 4] Poor correlation between results from electromagnetic flowmetry and dye dilution have been observed.[5] Whether these theoretic considerations are satisfactory explanations for the apparent discrepancy is unknown, as many of these objections remain untested.

One cannot help admiring the industry

*Corollary to Moriarity's Field Law: "If it can go wrong, it will."

of the authors but, on the basis of these thoughts, I remain uncertain as to the validity of their conclusions.

E. L. Bradley, III, M.D.
Department of Surgery
Emory University School of Medicine
69 Butler St., S.E.
Atlanta, Ga. 30303

REFERENCES

1. Visscher, M. B., and Johnson, J. A.: The Fick principle; analysis of potential errors and its conventional applications, J. Appl. Physiol. **5:** 635, 1953.
2. Grenvik, A.: Errors of the dye dilution method compared to the direct Fick method in determination of cardiac output in man, Scand. J. Clin. Lab. Invest. **18:** 486, 1968.
3. Jacobs, R. R., Schmitz, A., Heyden, W. C., et al.: A comparison of the accuracies in the electro-magnetic flow meter in the cardiogreen dilution blood flow measurement techniques in a model, Surg. Forum **19:** 113, 1968.
4. Carey, J. S., Williamson, H., and Scott, C. R.: Accuracy of cardiac output computers, Ann. Surg. **174:** 762, 1971.
5. Jacobs, R. R., Heyden, W. C., Williams, B. T., et al.: Cardiac output in the exercising dog: An evaluation of the dye dilution method using the electro-magnetic flow meter as the standard, J. Surg. Res. **10:** 25, 1970.

Length of residency

To the Editors:

That the discussion of proposed changes in a recent editorial[1] "has revealed considerable uncertainty about the wisdom of a four-year training program in Surgery" must be an understatement of the consensus feeling of surgical teachers. Interns, first-year bona fide general surgical residents, and "resiterns" of the modern first- or second-year echelon here at the Valley Medical Center of Fresno, are all graduates of the United States or Canadian class A medical schools, and some are A.O.A. members. They all recognize that five years after medical school is not too long. They also recognize that no bona fide first-year resident in Surgery is going to step aside and permit a "resitern" to "play through." Institutions providing graded, increasing clinical responsibility coupled with the sufficient case-load will always be able to attract candidates who will benefit from the long-range plan of the standard four-year residency.

My personal feeling is that General Surgery training could be much better if five full post-intern years were required. Living-wage stipends for residents are now the rule so that the economic hardship of the trainee is no longer a factor. Therefore, NO considerations other than the educational, judgment-ripening, and technical elegance parameters deserve a place in determination of the optimum duration of training.

Paul A. Carlson, M.D.
Chief of Surgery
Valley Medical Center
445 S. Cedar
Fresno, Calif. 93702

REFERENCE

1. Spencer, F. C., Reemtsma, K., and Ebert, P. A.: The surgical residency: Length and quality, SURGERY **74:** 791, 1973.

Volume 75 Number 3

SURGERY

MARCH, 1974

Original communications

Surgical preparation, perfusion techniques, and cryoprotectants used in successful freezing of the kidney

A. Eira Rebelo, M.D., Edmund F. Graham, Ph.D., Bo G. Crabo, D.V.M., Ph.D., Richard C. Lillehei, M.D., Ph.D., *and* **Ronald H. Dietzman, M.D., Ph.D.,*** *Minneapolis, Minn.*

Canine kidneys have been successfully frozen solid to −22° C. and have, after thawing, been capable of sustaining the dog's life following contralateral nephrectomy. This successful cryopreservation of the kidney depends upon four factors: (1) surgical preparation, (2) perfusion techniques, (3) cryoprotectants, and (4) freeze-thaw techniques. This paper focuses attention upon the first three factors. A nontraumatized, defatted kidney, capable of producing urine volumes greater than 2 ml. per minute prior to excision, is mandatory. A nonpulsatile perfusion system employing physiologic arterial and venous pressure has proved to be a satisfactory technique to deliver the perfusate. This study shows that hemoglobin-free, cryoprecipitated plasma was superior to Ringer's lactate or cryoprecipitated plasma containing hemoglobin. The latter two perfusates resulted in renal edema, reflected in the post-freeze renal weight gain. This edema results in vascular obstruction and nonuniform cryoprotectant distribution. The cryoprotectants were subdivided into two groups: general, consisting of two subgroups—penetrating and nonpenetrating—and specific, consisting of two subgroups—membrane-stabilizing and enzyme-modifying agents. The nonpenetrating cryoprotectants produced microcirculatory obstruction and were found unsuitable for protecting whole organs. The penetrating cryoprotectant, DMSO 12.5 per cent, offered the greatest protection when combined with the specific cryoprotectants, namely, the membrane-stabilizing drugs, methylprednisolone and isoproterenol, and the enzyme modifier, flurophenylalanine. With this combination the least freeze-thaw damage resulted and, in this group, kidneys were successfully preserved which were capable of sustaining the life of the dog.

From the University of Minnesota Health Sciences Center and Department of Animal Science, Minneapolis, Minn.

Accepted for publication Oct. 10, 1973.

Supported by: United States Public Health Service Grant No. PH 43-68-99, Freezing and Thawing Whole Organs, and the Commonwealth Electric Fund.

*Established Investigator, American Heart Association.

Reprint requests: Dr. Ronald H. Dietzman, Department of Surgery, University of Minnesota, Mayo Memorial Building, Box 148, Minneapolis, Minn. 55455.

As the initial phase in achieving cryopreservation of organs at liquid nitrogen temperatures for a prolonged period of time, we have investigated the problem of freezing and thawing the canine kidney. We have now established a protocol with which we can freeze the canine kidney to −22° C., and this kidney, upon thawing and reimplantation, will function sufficiently to sustain the dog's life following contralateral nephrectomy. It is the purpose of this paper to present in detail the experimental evidence in the areas of surgical preparation, perfusion techniques, and cryoprotectants that have led to the establishment of this successful freeze-thaw protocol.

METHODS

1. Surgical preparation.

Pre-excision. A total of 154 adult mongrel dogs (average weight, 18.1 kilograms) were used. All dogs were premedicated with morphine sulfate (1 mg. per kilogram), anesthetized with sodium thiamylal until depression of the corneal reflex, and intubated. An intravenous infusion of lactated Ringer's (1 L.) with mannitol (1 Gm.), furosemide (5 mg. per kilogram), and sodium bicarbonate (10 mEq.) was given at a rate of 40 drops per minute prior to renal excision and 85 drops per minute following transplantation. Methylprednisolone (30 mg. per kilogram) was given intravenously following induction. The right kidney was isolated through a right flank incision and the ureter transected in its distal one third. After the vessels were dissected free and following removal of all perinephric fat, we waited until the kidney was firm and the urine output exceeded 2 ml. per minute before it was excised.

Coarse vs. gentle manipulation. Renal cell damage due to routine handling of the kidney during excision, i.e., coarse handling, was compared to a technique of gentle manipulation—that is, extreme care was taken so that no visible vasospasm or change in renal parenchymal tone occurred. Unnecessary handling of the kidney and perivascular tissue dissection thus were minimal.

Post-thawing. All kidneys were reimplanted into a pocket created in the right neck with an end-to-end carotid–renal artery and external jugular–renal vein anastomosis and then a dependent cutaneous ureterostomy was created. In this location particular attention must be given to the venous anastomosis to prevent angulation and obstruction at the entrance of the jugular vein into the thorax.

Postoperative. The ureterostomy was cleansed twice daily with pHisoHex for five days until urine volume increased and urine protein decreased. On the first postoperative day the dogs were given 500 ml. of 5 percent dextrose in water with 20 mg. of furosemide. On the second, fourth, and sixth postoperative days they were given 20 mg. of furosemide intramuscularly. After the first day all dogs were fed meat and milk. Bicillin, 200,000 U., was given intramuscularly on the day of operation and every fifth day thereafter. A contralateral nephrectomy through a left flank incision was performed after two weeks, renal function of all surviving dogs was studied, and the dogs were put to death at the end of the third week for histologic examination of the previously frozen kidney.

2. Perfusion.

Perfusion technique. Following excision of the kidney, polyethylene cannulas were inserted into the renal artery and vein. The arterial cannula was flushed with 100 ml. of the defined perfusate (10° C.) at a gravity perfusion pressure of 80 mm. Hg. Following the flush, the kidney was weighed and the perfusion was continued by means of a non-pulsatile gravity system with a total of 800 ml. of perfusate. The perfusion time averaged 30 minutes. The perfusion pressure was maintained at 80 mm. Hg in the artery and at 8 mm. Hg in the vein. The venous pressure was controlled by the catheter diameter (the same diameter as the arterial catheter) and by elevation of the catheter tip. The venous effluent was collected in 20 ml. aliquots which were analyzed for LDH (lactic acid dehydrogenase) and GOT (glutamic oxalacetic transaminase). The kidney was weighed, frozen, and then thawed. Following thaw, the kidneys were perfused with one of the defined perfusates (10° C.), with the use of the pressure and analysis parameters described, and then weighed prior to implantation.

Perfusates. The perfusion solutions studied were: lactated Ringer's (Hartmann's solution) and cryoprecipitated plasma.[3, 4] The cryoprecipitated plasma was of two types; one contained more than 0.15 mg. per 100 ml. of hemoglobin (Hgb.) and the second contained no hemoglobin. These three perfusates were chosen after extensive study following a pilot project in which we demonstrated failures with other trial perfusates including egg yolk (five dogs) and boiled plasma (three dogs). Heparin (500 U.) and cryoprotectants were then added to these perfusates. Prior to freezing, the cryoprotectants used in the Ringer's vs. hemoglobin-containing cryoprecipitated plasma study were the general cryoprotectant, glycerol (7.5 percent), and the specific cryoprotectants, methylprednisolone (125 mg.) and procaine (50 mg.). In the hemoglobin-containing vs. hemoglobin-free cryoprecipitated plasma study, the general cryoprotectant added was dimethylsulfoxide (DMSO 12.5 percent) and the specific cryoprotectants were methylprednisolone (125 mg.), flurophenylalanine (2 mg.), and isoproterenol (1 mg.). Following thawing, in all groups, heparin (500 U.), methylprednisolone (40 mg.), and KCl (8 mEq.) were added to the perfusate (400 ml.). The pH was adjusted to 7.40 in each perfusate, just prior to use, with either $NaHCO_3$ or KH_2PO_4.

3. Cryoprotectants.

General cryoprotectants.[11, 12, 19]

PENETRATING (COLLIGATIVE) AGENTS. From a previous study in our laboratory of 88 potential penetrating agents tested with the use of single-cell suspensions, two were selected for study in the canine kidney—glycerol and DMSO.[15]

NONPENETRATING (POLYMERIC) AGENTS. Similarly, we previously have studied 78 potential nonpenetrating agents in single-cell suspensions (unpublished data). From this group, low molecular weight dextran (LMWD) and ascorbic acid were studied in the kidney.

Specific cryoprotectants.

MEMBRANE-STABILIZING AGENTS. From our previous studies in shock, we recognized the need for cellular protection during hypoxia and stress. These studies suggested that this protection could be afforded with high doses of the corticosteroid, methylprednisolone or dexamethasone.[8] At the dosages defined in our shock preparation, methylprednisolone (30 mg. per kilogram) or dexamethasone (6 mg. per kilogram) was given as a single intravenous bolus over a period of five minutes following anesthetic induction. To evaluate the effects of corticosteroids in the perfusate, dogs were studied in which no methylprednisolone was added to the perfusate, and in which methylprednisolone was added in dosage greater than 6 mg. per gram of kidney weight. Additionally, dexamethasone was evaluated in equivalent intravenous and perfusate dosages. Isoproterenol was added for its vasodilating, enzyme-modifying, and membrane electrical potential–stabilizing effects.[9, 17, 28]

ENZYME MODIFIERS. In addition to isoproterenol, flurophenylalanine was added for its inhibitory effect on the synthesis of the lysosomal hydrolase enzymes.[6]

4. Freeze-thaw process. The experimental work for the freeze-thaw parameters was described previously.[10, 24] Freezing was accomplished via conduction in a specially designed unit. The kidney was immersed in a fluorocarbon bath which was then cooled by liquid nitrogen vapor flowing through coils. The freezing rate was controlled by a specially designed valve system. The renal core temperature was monitored by a copper-constantan thermocouple connected to a recorder. The freezing rate was 1 to 2° C. per minute. We have shown previously that freezing rates of less than 1° C. per minute are not successful.[24] Thawing was accomplished in a modified microwave unit with the kidney positioned in the wave guide, the kidney being rotated slowly during the microwave radiation period in order to avoid the

Table I. *Comparative renal cell damage due to surgical manipulation*

Urine	Gentle manipulation, 6 dogs (2-6 ml./min.)			Coarse manipulation, 3 dogs (< 2 ml./min.)		
	Before	*After*	*p value*	*Before*	*After*	*p value*
LDH (U./ml.)	0.8	1.3	0.22	0.9	30.3	0.03
GOT (U./ml.)	1.6	1.4	0.38	0.9	17.6	0.005

Table II. *Perfusate: Comparative effects of cryoprecipitated plasma with or without free hemoglobin on renal viability*

	Plasma with hemoglobin	*Plasma without hemoglobin*	*p value*
Prefreeze:*			
No. of dogs	14	8	
LDH (U./ml./Gm.)	0.11	0.14	0.45
GOT (U./ml./Gm.)	0.03	0.03	0.50
Post-thaw:*			
No. of dogs	5	8	
LDH (U./ml./Gm.)	12.7	6.4	< 0.001
GOT (U./ml./Gm.)	4.3	1.7	< 0.001
ATN	Nonfunction	Function	

*Freeze rate, 1 to 2° C. per minute; depth, −22° C.; thaw rate, 70° C. per minute.

thermal runaway problem. The power of the unit was 500 watts at 2,400 MHz with a pulsatile power output control. We have previously shown that thawing rates of less than 70° C. per minute are not successful.[24]

5. Renal viability studies. Prereimplantation renal viability was assessed with the use of venous effluent LDH and GOT levels determined by an AutoAnalyzer.[1, 2, 18] Renal edema was evaluated by differential weight gain. Renal vascular changes were reflected in perfusion flow rates. In that arterial inflow and venous outflow pressures were held constant, perfusion time reflects change in the resistance to flow. The contralateral nephrectomy was performed two weeks following heterotopic reimplantation of the cryopreserved kidney. Renal damage was evaluated by means of standard light and electron microscopy techniques three weeks following reimplantation. Renal function was assessed by serum creatinine (milligrams per 100 ml.) and blood urea nitrogen (BUN) (milligrams per 100 ml.) levels. Preliminary results of these renal function studies have been summarized.[10]

RESULTS

1. Surgical preparation. With designed coarse manipulation, i.e., routine surgical excision of the kidney (three dogs) and its vessels, the kidneys became engorged and tense, and urine output did not exceed 2 ml. per minute for at least five minutes following completion of dissection. Coarse manipulation resulted in renal cell damage evidenced by a significant increase in urinary LDH ($p = 0.03$) and GOT ($p = 0.005$) levels. In contrast, with designed gentle manipulation, the kidneys (six dogs) did not become engorged and urine outputs, 2 to 6 ml. per minute, occurred in less than three minutes. Concurrently, less renal cell damage occurred, as evidenced by the insignificant increase in urine LDH ($p = 0.38$) and GOT ($p = 0.22$) levels (Table I). Urine flow began approximately ten minutes after reimplantation. The initial urine was usually pink in color and contained 2+ glucose and 4+ protein. Because of this protein, obstruction of the ureterostomy can occur; to avoid it, the ureterostomy must be cleansed daily with pHisoHex.

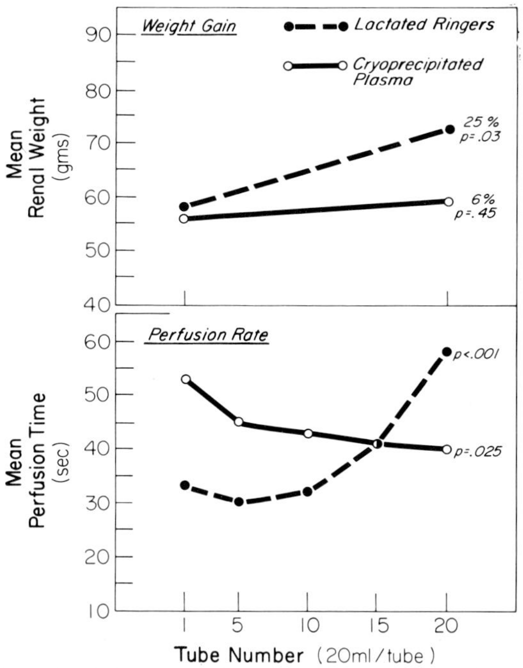

Fig. 1. Effect of perfusates on renal edema. Lactated Ringer's vs. cryoprecipitated plasma (cryoprotectants: glycerol 7.5%, methylprednisolone, and procaine). Alterations in renal weight gain, pre- and postperfusion rate. Note that as renal weight increases perfusion time increases concurrently.

2. Perfusion. Perfusion pressure was maintained in all kidneys at 80 mm. Hg. Hand flushing results in an inconsistent perfusion pressure and unnecessary and excessive renal edema and weight gain.

Three factors were important in predicting renal viability following perfusion before freezing: (1) renal weight gain, (2) perfusion rate, and (3) venous effluent GOT levels. Renal weight gain was greatest with lactated Ringer's solution. During perfusion with lactated Ringer's solution, mean renal weight (12 dogs) increased 25 percent ($p = 0.03$). When cryoprecipitated plasma was used, mean renal weight (13 dogs) increased only 6 percent ($p = 0.45$). During perfusion with the crystalloid, Ringer's, perfusion time increased significantly following the first 200 ml. ($p < 0.001$). In contrast, with the colloid, cryoprecipitated plasma, perfusion time decreased significantly ($p = 0.025$) (Fig. 1).

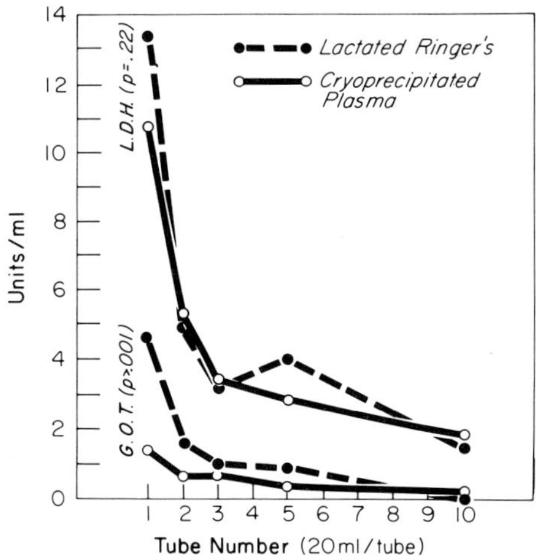

Fig. 2. Prefreezing renal venous effluent enzymes. Lactated Ringer's vs. cryoprecipitated plasma (cryoprotectants: glycerol 7.5%, methylprednisolone, and procaine). Note significantly greater renal cell damage evidenced by GOT elevation with lactated Ringer's perfusate.

The venous effluent GOT levels in the first sample following perfusion with the crystalloid were significantly greater than when using the colloid ($p > 0.001$) (Fig. 2). No significant difference was noted at this time in LDH levels ($p = 0.22$). Within one week of reimplantation all kidneys perfused with lactated Ringer's solution were either absorbed or markedly infected. Kidneys perfused with hemoglobin-free cryoprecipitated plasma did not resorb or become infected until the second week following reimplantation. Indeed, most kidneys simply demonstrated contraction due to fibrosis. We have subsequently demonstrated, using hemoglobin-free cryoprecipitated plasma and improved cryoprotection and freeze-thaw techniques, that these kidneys are capable of sustaining the dog's life following contralateral nephrectomy.[10] In contrast, if the cryoprecipitated plasma contained free hemoglobin obtained from hemolyzed blood, renal cell damage was demonstrated. This damage was not demonstrated prior to freezing but was clearly evident following thawing. The postthaw venous effluent LDH and GOT levels were significantly greater if the cryoprecipitated plasma contained free hemoglobin

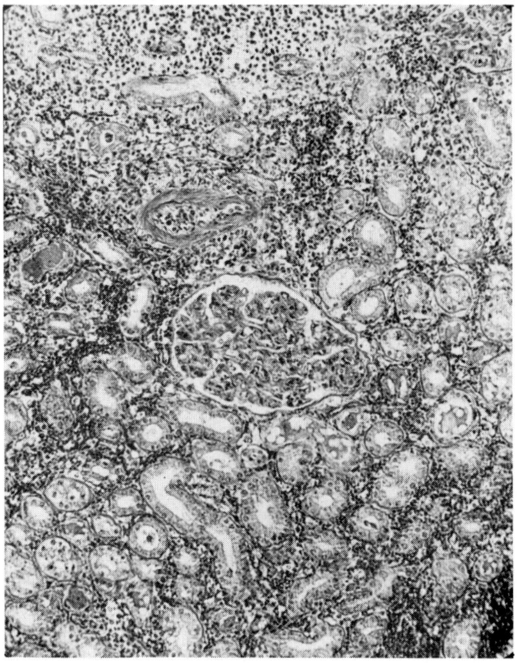

Fig. 3. Light microscopic hemotoxylin-eosin stain of dog kidney resected three days following reimplantation. This kidney was perfused with cryoprecipitated plasma obtained from hemolyzed blood. Note hemoglobin in lumen of tubules and cell damage.

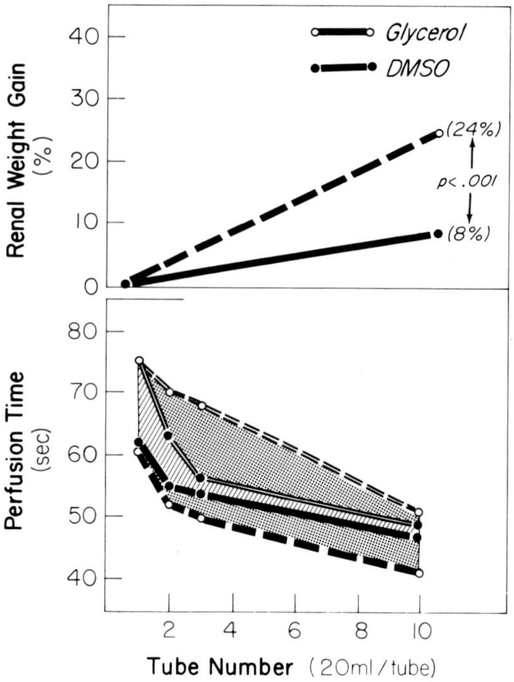

Fig. 4. Renal edema following cryopreservation (−22° C.). Comparative effects of glycerol and DMSO (12.5 percent). Note significant renal weight gain following freeze-thaw with glycerol. Additionally, note marked increase in perfusion time prefreeze (lower curves) to post-thaw (upper curves) comparing glycerol (heavy stippled area) to DMSO (light stippled area).

($p < 0.001$) (Table II). Hemoglobin was noted in the tubules of kidneys perfused with plasma containing free hemoglobin as shown in Fig. 3. In this study, the general cryoprotectant was DMSO 12.5 percent and the specific cryoprotectants were methylprednisolone, isoproterenol, and flurophenylalanine. All kidneys perfused with cryoprecipitated plasma containing hemoglobin developed acute tubular necrosis (ATN), failed to function, and, if left in situ, underwent autodigestion beginning on the fifth day after transplantation.

3. Cryoprotectants.

General cryoprotectants: Penetrating agents. We began our studies using glycerol (5 percent) in cryoprecipitated plasma to evaluate the amount of renal damage. When only this general penetrating cryoprotectant was used, there was marked renal damage. Following perfusion, prior to freezing, in kidneys from four dogs, the LDH was 0.5 and the GOT was 0.1 U. per milliliter per gram of renal weight in the initial 20 ml. of venous effluent. In contrast, following thawing, LDH rose to 243 and GOT rose to 99 U. per milliliter per gram of renal weight. All kidneys failed to function, became necrotic, and began autodigestion within two to three days.

In recognition of the need for additional cryoprotection, the membrane-stabilizing agents, methylprednisolone and isoproterenol, and the lysosomal enzyme synthesis inhibitor, fluorophenylalanine, were added. Concurrently, higher concentrations of glycerol were investigated and compared to equivalent concentrations of DMSO (Table III). From these results, we noted that at a concentration of 7.5 percent there was no difference between glycerol (10 dogs) and DMSO (five dogs) except for a significantly lower initial 20 ml. post-thaw venous effluent LDH ($p = 0.03$). In contrast, when the

Table III. *Renal viability following cryopreservation (–22° C.)*

	7.5 Percent			12.5 Percent		
	Glycerol (10 dogs)	DMSO (5 dogs)	p value	Glycerol (5 dogs)	DMSO (9 dogs)	p value
Prefreeze:						
LDH (U./ml./Gm.)	0.10	0.12	> 0.05	0.15	0.12	> 0.05
GOT (U./ml./Gm.)	0.04	0.04	> 0.05	0.04	0.03	> 0.05
Weight gain (%)	14	18	> 0.05	22	20	> 0.05
Post-thaw:						
LDH (U./ml./Gm.)	19.1	10.6	0.03	17.0	8.0	0.001
GOT (U./ml./Gm.)	4.9	3.4	> 0.05	4.8	2.1	0.006
Weight gain (%)	19	21	> 0.05	24	8	< 0.001

cryoprotectant concentrations were increased to 12.5 percent, there was a significantly lower venous effluent amount of LDH ($p = 0.001$) and GOT ($p = 0.006$) with DMSO (nine dogs) than with glycerol (five dogs). Additionally, renal vascular resistance was less, perfusion times improved, and renal weight gain was significantly less with DMSO (Fig. 4).

With the use of either glycerol or DMSO at a concentration of 7.5 percent with methylprednisolone, less than 6 mg. per gram of kidney weight (mean, 3.4), and isoproterenol (1.0 mg. per 800 ml. of perfusate), 50 percent of the kidneys became necrotic and autodigested within four to five days. The remaining 50 percent produced gradually decreasing amounts of urine for five days and then developed fibrosis over a period of 19 to 20 days. Of interest was the loss of medullary substance in association with hemorrhage in the glycerol group. The cortex was fibrotic in both groups.

When the concentration of glycerol and DMSO was increased to 12.5 percent, methylprednisolone to more than 6 mg. per gram of kidney weight (mean, 10.5), and flurophenylalanine (0.4 mg. per gram of kidney weight) were added in addition to the isoproterenol (1.0 mg. per 800 ml. of perfusate), urine output improved only in the group with DMSO. In the group with glycerol (12.5 percent) three out of five kidneys became necrotic within one week and, in the remaining two kidneys, renal cortical fibrosis was comparable to that observed at 7.5 percent; however, the loss of medullary substance and severity of hemorrhage was greater by the third week. Urine output in this group was not improved over that at 7.5 percent concentration. Five out of nine dogs with DMSO (12.5 percent) survived a minimum of 19 days. Of these, two were put to death on day 21 for study purposes (the other three died on day 19). In the two dogs that were killed the cryopreserved kidney was able to maintain BUN (17 and 21 mg. per 100 ml.) and creatinine (1.7 and 7.0 mg. per 100 ml.) and to produce adequate amounts of urine (50 to 100 ml. per hour with a volume challenge) to sustain the dogs' life. Light and electron microscopic photographs from one of these dogs are shown in Figs. 5 and 6. Of the remaining four dogs, surviving less than 19 days, one died of pneumonia, one of arteriovenous thrombosis, and two of ATN (acute tubular necrosis).

General cryoprotectants: Nonpenetrating agents. In recognition of the fact that additional cryoprotection was indicated, the nonpenetrating cryoprotectants, LMWD (900 m.w.) and ascorbic acid, were studied in six dogs. To 800 ml. of heparinized cryoprecipitated plasma with DMSO (12.5 percent), methylprednisolone (> 6 mg. per gram of kidney weight), isoproterenol (1.0 mg. per 800 ml. of perfusate), and flurophenylalanine (0.4 mg. per gram of kidney weight), we added LMWD (10 percent) and ascorbic acid (2.5 Gm.). Following freeze-thaw and reimplantation, all kidneys became congested and cyanotic immediately. The vein was transected. Venous flow was less than 5 ml. per minute, indicating significant intrarenal vascular obstruction.

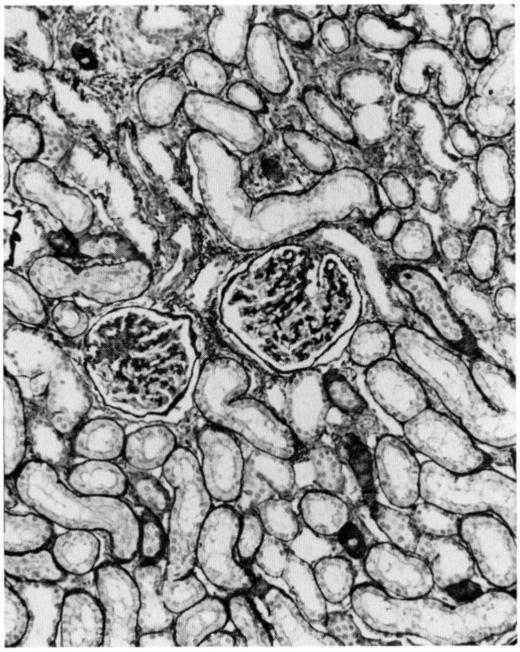

Fig. 5. Light microscopic (Hansen stains) photomicrograph demonstrating normal glomeruli and tubules three weeks following freeze-thaw and reimplantation and one week following contralateral nephrectomy.

Table IV. *Specific cryoprotectants (corticosteroids): Comparative effects of perfusate with or without methylprednisolone on renal viability*

	Without steroids	*With steroids (< 6 mg./Gm.)*	*p value*
No. of dogs	7	20	
LDH (U./ml./Gm.)	0.35	0.18	< 0.001
GOT (U./ml./Gm.)	0.06	0.03	< 0.001

Table V. *Specific cryoprotectants (corticosteroids): Comparative effects, small vs. large dosages methylprednisolone in perfusate on renal viability*

	<6 mg./Gm. (3.4)	*>6 mg./Gm. (10.5)*	*p value*
No. of dogs	10	10	
LDH (U./ml./Gm.)	0.17	0.07	0.002
GOT (U./ml./Gm.)	0.04	0.01	0.004

Specific cryoprotectants. To evaluate the effects of corticosteroids in the perfusate, seven dogs without steroids in the perfusate were compared with 20 dogs with less than 6 mg. per gram of methylprednisolone in the perfusate (Table IV). In this study, the perfusate was either cryoprecipitated plasma or lactated Ringer's solution to which were added glycerol (7.5 percent), isoproterenol (1.0 Gm. per 800 ml. of perfusate), and flurophenylalanine (0.4 mg. per gram of kidney weight). The renal venous effluent prefreeze contained significantly ($p < 0.001$) less LDH and GOT in the group with corticosteroids in the perfusate, indicating less renal cell damage. To study the effect of corticosteroid dosage on renal cell protection, methylprednisolone was added to the perfusate in dosages less than 6 mg. per gram (mean, 3.4) of kidney weight (10 dogs) and greater than 6 mg. per gram (mean, 10.5) of kidney weight (10 dogs) (Table V). In this study the perfusate was cryoprecipitated plasma to which was added DMSO (12.5 percent), isoproterenol (1.0 mg. per 800 ml. of solution), and flurophenylalanine (0.4 mg. per gram). Significantly less renal cell damage occurred in the group treated with more than 6 mg. per gram of methylprednisolone, indicated by the lower venous effluent LDH ($p = 0.002$) and GOT ($p = 0.004$) levels. Because of the differences in protection afforded by various corticosteroids in shock and the presence of fluoride in the steroid, dexamethasone in dosages equivalent to that of methylprednisolone was studied. Dexamethasone (6 mg. per kilogram intravenously and 2 mg. per gram of kidney weight in the perfusate) was used in three dogs. Significantly greater cellular protection was achieved using methylprednisolone ($p < 0.001$) (Table VI). The reason for this difference is not completely understood at present.

In an additional six dogs with DMSO (12.5 percent), methylprednisolone (< 6 mg. per gram), and flurophenylalanine (0.4 mg. per gram of kidney weight), isoproterenol was increased to 2.0 mg. per 800 ml. of

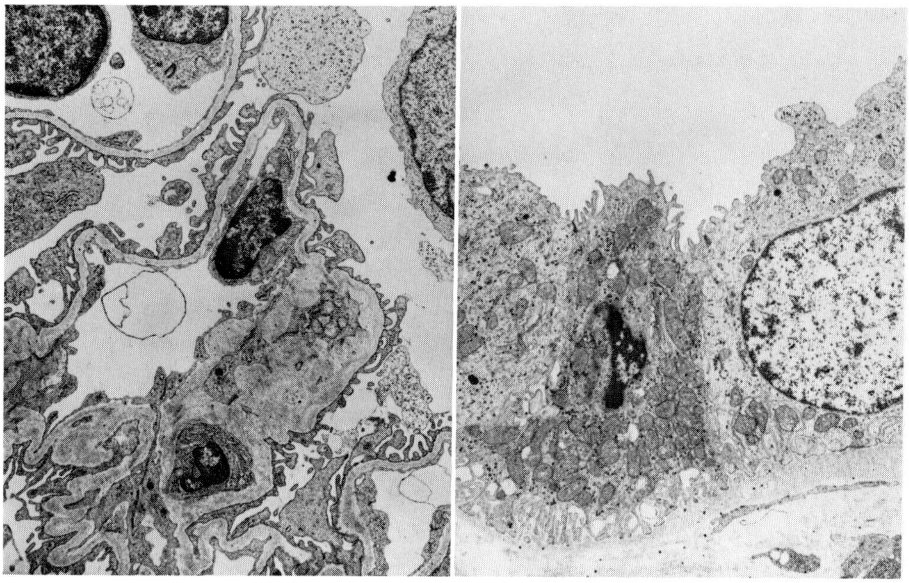

Fig. 6. Electron microscopic photomicrograph of kidney shown in Fig. 5 demonstrating *(left)* glomeruli and *(right)* distal tubule.

perfusate in an effort to further improve protection. In four of these dogs, arterial and venous thrombosis occurred within the kidney vessels distal to and unrelated to the anastomotic site. The ureters in all four were dark and avascular by the fourth to fifth day.

DISCUSSION

The critical parameters of surgical preparation, perfusion techniques, and cryoprotectants were studied to establish a protocol of freezing and thawing the canine kidney at –22° C.

1. Surgical preparation. Our results emphasize three major points: (1) It is important to excise a nontraumatized kidney with all perinephric fat removed, especially about the renal pelvis; (2) gentle manipulation of the renal artery and vein must be accomplished to avoid vasospasm; and (3) it is necessary to maintain a urine output of 2 to 6 ml. per minute prior to excision.

Perinephric fat. All perinephric fat must be excised prior to the freeze-thaw procedure. Fat becomes edematous during perfusion and fat also has a dielectric constant different from the renal parenchymal cells and ureter; consequently, thermal runaway occurs in fat-containing areas during thawing.[16] This is particularly important in the renal pelvis.

Table VI. *Specific cryoprotectants (corticosteroids): Comparative effects of dexamethasone and methylprednisolone in equivalent intravenous and perfusate dosages on renal viability*

	Dexamethasone	*Methylprednisolone*	*p value*
No. of dogs	3	10	
LDH (U./ml./Gm.)	0.29	0.07	< 0.001
GOT (U./ml./Gm.)	0.05	0.01	< 0.001

Manipulation. Traumatic manipulation of the kidney and its vessels results in vasospasm and hypoxia. Following restoration of blood flow, prior to excision, renal congestion occurs and accentuates the hypoxic cellular damage reflected, as shown above, by increased urinary LDH and GOT levels.

Urine output. Experimental transplantation studies have shown decreased ATN and better renal functional results when the pre-excision urine output exceeds 2 ml. per minute. This volume can be achieved by the gentle manipulation of the kidney combined

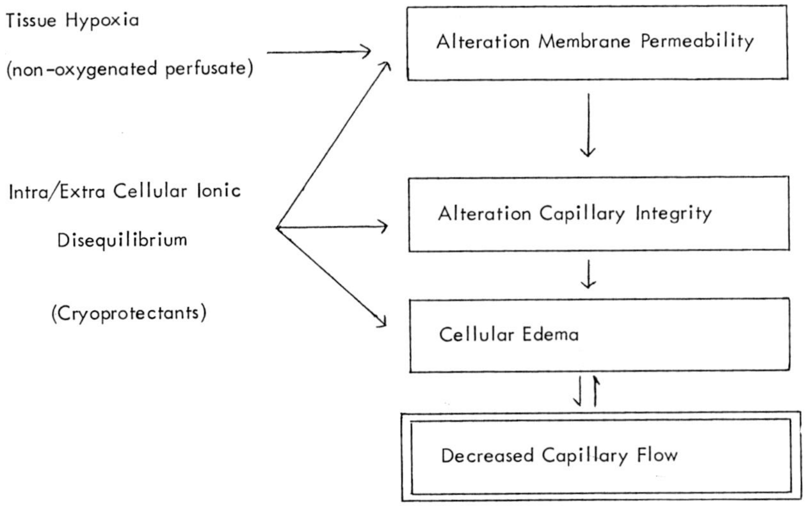

Fig. 7. Flow sheet.

with maintenance of an adequate systemic intravascular volume coupled with diuretic stimulation by mannitol and furosemide.[25] In general, principles followed in clinical renal transplantation must be faithfully applied to the preparation of the kidney.[20] If these principles are not applied to the cryopreserved kidney, the result is uniform failure.

2. Perfusion.

Perfusion technique. Three factors are of importance in renal cryopreservation: (1) perfusion pressure, (2) nonpulsatile flow, and (3) perfusate temperature.

PERFUSION PRESSURE. Arterial perfusion pressure, equivalent to 80 mm. Hg, has been used because it falls within the physiologic range for an excised kidney prior to transplantation.[7] For the same reason, venous pressure was maintained at 8 mm. Hg. Thus the cryoprotectants are delivered to the cells under nearly physiologic conditions.

NONPULSATILE FLOW. Nonpulsatile flow is easier to accomplish than pulsatile flow. Nonpulsatile flow is adequate for perfusion times of less than three hours.[26] Perfusion times for cryopreservation rarely exceed 30 minutes.

PERFUSATE TEMPERATURE. The kidney is perfused under ischemic conditions. To reduce organ temperature and cellular metabolism, the perfusate is cooled to 10° C. Following reimplantation, Van der Werf[27] has shown no adverse effects following perfusion at this temperature.

Perfusate. Two factors are of importance concerning perfusates: (1) the ideal perfusate would consist of a balanced salt solution with an appropriate oncotic pressure capable of delivering the cryoprotectants to all cells without producing damage, and (2) all organs, to be cryopreserved, must achieve this protection through the vascular system via perfusion.

1. We chose a crystalloid (lactated Ringer's solution) as a perfusate because we desire a slower and lower increase in nonpulsatile perfusion pressure during our short perfusion time. The viscosity of plasma increases with a reduction in temperature below 10° C.[5] With crystalloids, unfortunately, renal weight increased significantly and concomitantly perfusion time increased. Renal weight gain and significant prolongation of perfusion time were not observed with cryoprecipitated plasma.[3, 4] The reason for this edema with the perfusate/cryoprotectant is not completely understood, but appears to be as shown in Fig. 7. The purpose of cryoprecipitation is the removal of lipids and lipoproteins which, if not removed, aggregate and become embolic, thereby reducing capillary flow.[5] This lipid fraction is removed by means of a triple Millipore filter system and

the cryoprecipitated plasma is then used immediately before additional precipitation occurs.

2. In contrast to single-cell suspensions and thin tissue slices in which the structures to be frozen are bathed in the cryoprotectant media and diffusion and active transport alone permit the cryoprotectant to penetrate the cell, the whole organ depends upon its vasculature for cryoprotectant distribution. For this reason, any decrease in capillary flow due to edematous luminal narrowing or obstruction results in nonuniform cryoprotectant distribution; therefore, the perfusate of choice must produce the least amount of renal damage. Hemoglobin-free cryoprecipitated plasma appears at this time to be the perfusate of choice. As shown, cryoprecipitated plasma obtained from hemolyzed blood results in significant and fatal renal cell damage. We chose to study cryoprecipitated plasma containing hemoglobin because, unfortunately, this is the usual condition of plasma obtained from dogs bled into a glass reservoir under a vacuum. To obtain plasma-free hemoglobin, we had to use plastic bags containing heparin or acid-citrate-dextrose (ACD) and separate the plasma from the red cell mass immediately following removal of the blood from the dog.

3. Cryoprotectants. One of our initial problems in studying renal cryopreservation was the choice of appropriate cryoprotectants. From our previous studies with single-cell suspensions, 163 potential general cryophylactic agents were evaluated. Of these, 85 were considered penetrating and 78 nonpenetrating.[15]

Penetrating or colligative cryoprotectants bind water, thereby controlling the size and rate of ice crystal formation.[23] Following our initial investigation, these penetrating agents were subdivided into four groups: (1) chemical materials tested for cryoprotective activity but reacted by precipitation of protein; (2) chemical materials tested for cryoprotection, sustaining cell life, but showing low cryoprotective properties on freezing; (3) chemical materials tested for protection, not severely precipitating protein, but toxic to the cell; and (4) cryoprotective agents showing protection to the cell during freezing. In this latter group, 21 agents demonstrated one of two unique features; namely, the presence of at least two hydroxyl groups or one double-bonded oxygen. Of these 21 agents, two afforded the greatest protection to sperm cells —glycerol and DMSO; therefore, these two were selected for initial study in the kidney. From our previous studies using glycerol with sperm cells and our review of the literature, the cryoprotecting range appeared to lie between 5 and 20 percent. Our initial investigation of glycerol (5 percent) resulted in failure. Increasing the concentration of glycerol and comparing it to a like concentration of DMSO, we found no significant benefit at a concentration of 7.5 percent except for an apparent reduction in cell damage reflected by LDH. Increasing the concentration to 12.5 percent resulted in improved cryoprotection with both glycerol and DMSO, but the only significant improvement was with DMSO. We recognize that some of the DMSO is bound to the plasma proteins and that the total amount in the perfusate is not available to the cell.[13] We also recognize the fact that DMSO is better than glycerol in transforming the salt solution into a glasslike substance as temperature decreases, thus preventing the formation of eutectic concentration of salts.[14] Empirically, however, we noted that the 12.5 percent concentration level affords protection. This protection is dependent, in part, upon the cellular exposure time to the cryoprotectant. We found that a perfusate volume of 450 ml. was insufficient to afford protection and consequently we increased the volume to 800 ml. and thus the exposure time.

Concurrent to our recognition of the need to increase the concentration of the general cryoprotectant, we began our studies using the specific cryoprotectants. From our previous studies in shock, we were impressed that cellular protection could be gained by the use of membrane-stabilizing agents such as corticosteroids and beta-adrenergic–stimulating drugs. By adding these membrane-stabilizing agents, we were able to reduce renal autodigestion by 50 percent. Clearly, further protection was necessary to control autodigestion. One means of control, suggested by Persidsky,[22] was the modification of the lysosomal hydrolase enzymes. Based upon this concept and impressed by Cohn's[6] description of the ability of flurophenylalanine to reduce acid phosphatase synthesis of phagocytes, we chose to add this compound to our perfusate. The concept of specific cryoprotectants appears to be more important in organs rich in lysosomes in contrast to single-cell or thin tissue cryopreservation. This difference also may be attributed, in part, to the dependence upon the vasculature as a means of delivery of the cryoprotectant to the cell. Simply increasing the concentration of the general cryoprotectant in the perfusate may result in vascular endothelial cell damage with resultant alteration of its selective membrane permeability.

Nonpenetrating or polymeric cryoprotectants act by coating cell surfaces.[21] These agents have been useful in protecting single cells or thin tissue slices during freeze-thaw. However, because of their large molecular weight, they may never leave the vascular lumen. If this is the case, their role in cryopreservation of organs may be limited—limited to their protective effect upon vascular endothelial cells. This endothelial cell coating may significantly reduce lumen size at the capillary level. This resultant obstruction can explain our observation of the development of a congested, cyanotic kidney with a reduced venous flow using these nonpenetrating cryoprotectants, LMWD and ascorbic acid.

Other factors are important in considering cryoprotectants. Although we have been successful in freezing canine kidneys to –22° C., we have not yet solved the problem at lower temperatures. Recently, however, we have applied the same protocol used in our present study to the study of freezing two canine kidneys to –75° C. with freezing rates of 2° C. per minute from 0 to –22° C. and 2 to 4° C. per minute from –22 to –75° C. Although these kidneys did not function long enough to be able to sustain the dog's life following contralateral nephrectomy, we have been very encouraged to find that they did produce urine (10 ml. per hour) for 48 hours upon reimplantation.[10]

REFERENCES

1. Babson, A. L., Shapiro, P. O., Williams, P. A. R., and Phillips, G. E.: Clin. Chim. Acta **7:** 199, 1962.
2. Beisang, A. A., Graham, E. F., Lillehei, R. C., Dietzman, R. H., and Carter, J. R.: Transplant. Proc. **1:** 862, 1969.
3. Belzer, F. O., Ashby, B. S., and Dunphy, Y. E.: Lancet **2:** 536, 1967.
4. Belzer, F. O., Ashby, B. S., Huang, J. S., and Dunphy, J. E.: Ann. Surg. **168:** 382, 1968.
5. Belzer, F. O., Ashby, B. S., May, R. E., and Dunphy, Y. E.: *In* Norman, J. C., editor: Organ perfusion and preservation, New York, 1968, Appleton-Century-Crofts, p. 113.
6. Cohn, Z. A., and Benson, B.: Exp. Med. **121:** 279, 1965.
7. Collins, G. M., Bravo-Shugarman, M., and Terasaki, P. I.: Transplant. Proc. **8:** 821, 1969.
8. Dietzman, R. H., Castaneda, A. R., Lillehei, C. W., Ersek, R. A., Motsay, G. J., and Lillehei, R. C.: Chest **57:** 440, 1970.
9. Dietzman, R. H., and Lillehei, R. C.: *In* Schwartz, S. I., editor: Principles of Surgery, New York, 1969, McGraw-Hill Book Company, Inc., pp. 119-135.
10. Dietzman, R. H., Rebelo, A. E., Graham, E. F., Crabo, B. G., and Lillehei, R. C.: Surgery **74:** 181, 1973.
11. Doebbler, G. F.: Cryobiology **3:** 2, 1966.
12. Farrant, J., Walter, C. A., and Armstrong, J. A.: R. Soc. London Proc. **168:** 293, 1967.
13. Filo, R., Bell, T., Pessotti, R., Gartner, S., and Sen, K.: Proc. 9th Ann. Meet. Soc. Cryobiology, Washington, D. C., Abst. 48, 1972.
14. Greaves, R. I. N., and Davies, J. D.: Ann. N. Y. Acad. Sci. **125:** 548, 1965.
15. Graham, E. F., and Crabo, B. G.: 11th Int. Cong. Anim. Reprod. and A. I., Munich, 1972.
16. Karow, A. M., Jr., and Webb, W. R.: Surg. Gynecol. Obstet. **119:** 609, 1965.
17. Lambotte, L., Otto, J. B., and Kestens, P. J.: Europ. Soc. Exp. Surg., 7th Cong. Amsterdam, The Netherlands, p. 52, 1972.
18. Levy, A. L., Dalmasso, C., and Daly, J.: Automat. Anal. Chem. Technician Symp. 1965.
19. Meryman, H. T.: Cryobiology **8:** 173, 1971.
20. Najarian, J. S., Gulyassy, P. P., Duffy, G.,

Stoney, R. J., and Braunstein, P.: Ann. Surg. **164:** 398, 1966.
21. Nash, T.: *In* Meryman, H. T., editor: Cryobiology, New York, 1966, Academic Press, Inc., p. 179.
22. Persidsky, M. D.: Cryobiology **8:** 482, 1971.
23. Rapatz, G. T., and Luyet, B. J.: Cryobiology **5:** 18, 1968.
24. Rebelo, A. E., Graham, E. F., Crabo, B. G., Lillehei, R. C., and Dietzman, R. H.: J. Surg. Res. 1974.
25. Rikukawa, Y., and Lindsey, E. S.: *In* Norman, J. S., editor: Organ perfusion and preservation, New York, 1968, Appleton-Century-Crofts, p. 131.
26. Romolo, Y. L., Aryan, S., and Halasz, N. A.: Cryobiology **8:** 407, 1971.
27. Van der Werf, B. A. M.: Arch. Chir. Neerl. **23:** 1, 1971.
28. Webb, W. R., Wax, S. D., Jones, F. X., Kamiyama, T., Sugg, W. L., and Echer, R. R.: *In* Norman, J. C., editor: Organ perfusion and preservation, New York, 1968, Appleton-Century-Crofts, p. 121.

Surgery in the twenty-first century

J. Englebert Dunphy, M.D., F.A.C.S., *San Francisco, Calif.*

In exploring the future of surgery in the twenty-first century, the author sees the forthcoming developments in orthopedic surgery and neurosurgery, the possibility of pharmacological and physiological advances eliminating much of endocrine surgery, and the great changes awaiting vascular and cardiac surgery. He discusses the future elimination of congenital defects, the future developments possible for the cure of cancer, and the likelihood of little progress in the area of surgical infection. Advances in the control of hemorrhage and pain in operations and the care of the critically ill and critically injured patient are discussed as well as the changes in the physical structure of the hospital and the functions, qualifications, and composition of its medical and surgical personnel.

From the Department of Surgery, University of California, San Francisco, Calif.

BEFORE presenting revelations from my crystal ball, I must express my very deep appreciation to this great University for the honor and privilege of participating in this Symposium. My gratitude is exceeded only by my humility over the haziness of my predictions. In addition to my own reflections, I have sought the views of a number of my distinguished American colleagues. What I shall present, therefore, is a synthesis of my own vision and that of Professors Walter Ballinger, James Maloney, Francis Moore, Jonathon Rhoads, David Sabiston, and Robert Zollinger.

Since history repeats itself, a look at the past may enable us to see the future. The surgical arena has been repeatedly changed by advances in medicine. Tuberculosis and syphilis were leading chapters in surgical texts when I was in medical school. Orthopedic surgery found one of its major accomplishments in the wake of poliomyelitis. Sympathectomy for hypertension, total thyroidectomy for angina pectoris, tonsillectomy for tonsils, and hysterectomy for almost anything have all come and gone. What similar changes can we foresee in the twenty-first century?

Considering each of the surgical specialties, I would suggest that urological surgery will no longer be concerned with renal calculi. Prostatic surgery for benign hypertrophy also should no longer be required—sooner, rather than later, I hope. Indeed, if prostatism is not readily controlled by medical measures, we will face some interesting logistical problems in the twenty-first century. With a steadily aging population, thousands of old men reluctant to undergo surgery will be queued up for miles at football games and other sporting events. If medicine does not solve this one, it will become a challenging problem in crowding and pollution for the engineers.

Address presented at an International Symposium, "Medicine in the Twenty-first Century," Medical School Centenary, University of Manchester, England, September, 1973.

Accepted for publication Dec. 17, 1973.

Orthopedic surgery which has lost corrective operations for the ravages of poliomyelitis, is now on the verge of one of its finest eras. John Charnley of this University has opened the way to joint replacement which is becoming one of the great triumphs of surgery. It will remain a greatly needed operation in the latter part of this century and probably well into the next. On the other hand, with our increasing knowledge of immunologic mechanisms and the behavior of collagen and scar tissue, it is quite possible that rheumatoid arthritis at least will be controlled. Joint replacement, however, should continue to be required for an aging population with degenerative joint changes, and of course there will always be the problems of crippling injuries. For one entering the surgical arena, I would regard this as one if its most exciting and rewarding fields.

Neurosurgery also faces some exciting new frontiers. Revascularization of the brain by microsurgical techniques is almost certain to become practical and beneficial. Nerve grafting, nerve regeneration, and, quite likely, cord regeneration will be possible. Except for revascularization procedures, however, I predict that the brain will remain an untouchable area. The fantasy of brain transplants will be as impossible in the twenty-first century as it is ridiculous to consider in this century.

Endocrine surgery will be subject to major eliminations: Thyroidectomy for hyperthyroidism is an uncommon operation today. It probably will not be necessary at all in the twenty-first century, and pharmacological and physiological advances will lead to the control of hyperadrenalism, hyperinsulinism, and hyperparathyroidism. Surgery, however, will not lose everything in this field because deficiency states, including diabetes, will be effectively treated by tissue and organ transplantation, of which I shall have more to say later.

In my own field of general surgery, I am not so sanguine about major changes. Biliary surgery undoubtedly will be limited to cancer, tumors, and rare infections. Gallstones will either be prevented by appropriate diet or effectively dissolved, almost certainly without surgical intervention. One might hope for a major advance in the non-surgical management of duodenal and gastric ulcer, but I predict that despite antacids, anti-gastrins, and new pharmacological agents for control of vagal impulses, ulceration of the upper gastrointestinal tract will plague man in the twenty-first century. Hemorrhage, perforation, and obstruction will still occupy the attention of surgeons and there will be continuing debate as to which method of treatment is the most efficacious. Similarly, I do not seen any evidence that appendicitis, diverticulitis, and colitis in its various forms, will be treated any differently in the twenty-first century than today.

On the other hand, vascular and cardiac surgery almost certainly face great changes. By the twenty-first century, we should have learned enough about atherosclerosis either to control it or to treat it effectively. Cardiac surgery for coronary artery disease will reach its peak in the latter half of this century and then be replaced almost entirely by non-surgical methods. Similarly, with peripheral vascular disease, surgical procedures will rarely be required. Arteriosclerotic plaques will be detected early and treated either by medication, diet, or the infusion of solutions directly into the involved vessels. The surgeon may well be involved in some of these procedures but more likely it will be the radiologist who, with his ingenious catheters, will simply wash out the obstructed vessel. Cardiac surgery for arteriosclerotic heart disease will also be rarely required.

Congenital defects which now require intensive treatment by nearly all surgical disciplines may be preventable. The possibility of genetic engineering eliminating the defect is one consideration. An even more exciting vista is the concept of fetal surgery in which the defect is detected early and then corrected in utero, so that the child is born normal. As the geneticists point out, of course, such procedures will correct the defect but not the gene and the incidence of congenital problems would very likely increase. A more realistic and practical approach might be the detection of defects within the early weeks of pregnancy thus providing rational grounds for abortion, eliminating both the defect and the genes. I doubt that man will be any more rational in the twenty-first century than he is today. For example, a creature from another planet would find it hard to understand why at one end of my own campus perfectly healthy fetuses are destroyed every day while premature babies with the most incredible congenital anomalies are kept alive and their defects repaired with extraordinary ingenuity and skill and at fantastic expense. I suspect that this concern for the individual and lack of concern for the race will continue in the twenty-first century.

Thus far, I have said nothing about cancer, and truly I do not know what to say. This was the principal area in which my panel of advisors disagreed. About half were optimistic that chemotherapy and immunology would bring about an early and significant advance in the treatment of cancer. The others felt that, despite significant progress in what might be called local successes, the great biological variations of cancer would make it impossible to eliminate. In any given situation, as one cancer was controlled by some type of therapy, immunological or chemotherapeutic, another cancer would be released, much as we see in our attempts to control infection at the cellular level.

My own view is that we will inch forward as in the past. Bit by bit, one cancer or another will be effectively treated. We now have methotrexate for choriocarcinoma, an invariably fatal disease now curable in a very high percentage of cases. Rhabdomyosarcoma, another invariably fatal tumor, is now very successfully managed by a combination of surgery, chemotherapy, and irradiation. I suspect that malignant melanoma and a variety of other sarcomas will be similarly controlled.

One must surely hope that cancer of the lung, breast, and colon can be either prevented or treated more effectively than at present. Part of the difficulty is that man does not want to give up anything unless he is certain that he himself will benefit, as evidenced by the indifference of the public to the hazards of smoking tobacco. I suspect that if we could find evidence that roast beef properly cooked and served with roast potatoes and Yorkshire pudding was a principal factor in the growth of cancer of the colon, the dietary habits in the United States and Great Britain would change very little. On the other hand, if we were able by immunological or other testing to identify specifically potential victims of particular cancers, the response would be better. I am confident that the total outlook for the patient with cancer in the twenty-first century will be far better than today. Survival rates will be greatly increased and many cancers will be totally curable, but I believe that the problem of cancer, like the problem of aging, will still remain with us.

The other area where I think progress will be disappointing is surgical infection. Sepsis has been with us since before Pasteur and Lister. Each generation has had its hopes raised that man will at last conquer the microbe, but each generation finds the microbe still present, still elusive, and still deadly. Anti-sepsis, asepsis, antibiotic drugs, and theatre design still have not prevented or eliminated infection from our hospitals. Indeed, today we find our hospitals the very center of sepsis, and hospital-acquired infections present the same problem, only in a new form, as first recognized by Semmelweiss and Holmes. The use and overuse of antibiotic agents, although life-saving in selected cases, have in the long run contributed to rather than solved the problems of infection.

To be sure, much progress has been made in the prevention of infection in clean, elective surgical operations. Although we are on solid ground here, if one reviews the surgical literature, infection rates in clean operations still vary less than one percent to as high as ten percent, and the disability and mortality rates occasioned by infection in clean surgical wounds are still enormous. In the critically ill or critically injured patient, we find sepsis as the final common denominator in every fatal course. The greatest threat comes from the gram-negative organisms which predominate in our hospitals today. I see little hope of resolving the matter and will have more to say on this point with respect to hospital design and construction in the twenty-first century.

The practice of surgery has been founded on the control of sepsis, hemorrhage, and pain. Sepsis will remain a continuing, though changing, problem; but there will be incredible advances in the control of pain. Beyond acupuncture, the pain of surgical operations will be simply eliminated by taking a pill. This pharmacologic agent will produce total blockage of somatic nerve impulses without affecting the sympathetic nervous system and with no metabolic, respiratory, or circulatory effects. George Crile's dream of anoci-association will be realized. Progress in anesthesiology will eliminate the anesthesiologist. His principal role will be in the application of life support systems, computer monitoring, and the minute-to-minute care of the very critically ill. Of course, this will not eliminate the need for someone to talk to the patient. Anesthetists in the future, therefore, will carry on light or serious conversation with the patient rather than with each other or their residents. Indeed, since the conversational requirements of patients will vary, anesthesiologists will become the most cultured of physicians—experts on literature, art, economics, politics, history, and so on. They will be assigned to cases on the basis of their educational backgrounds. "What would you like to talk about during your operation, Mr. Jones? Sanskrit. Ah, well —that will be Dr. Smith." If the patient says that he wants to talk about nothing, one of the hospital barbers will be pressed into service!

Blood loss during operations will become a thing of the past, although hemorrhage may be massive because of the magnitude of certain operations and injuries. In the twenty-first century, the scalpel will have become obsolete and some type of cutting and coagulating current which divides tissue with a minimum of trauma and, at the same time, seals small vessels, will become available. The smallest amount of blood loss will be collected by a special sucking apparatus which will automatically and atraumatically pass blood through filters which will remove all debris, bacteria, damaged cells, and lipids. The blood will immediately be returned to the patient's circulation. This will constitute ideal replacement as the blood is lost. Those religious sects that have always opposed blood transfusions will at last have been vindicated, and all of the complications of transfusion, hepatitis, sensitization, and mismatching will be reduced to a minimum. Blood transfusions will only be required in the initial treatment of massive loss of blood from injuries or for blood diseases.

A major advance will be made in the case of the critically ill or injured patient. Trauma will undoubtedly be a surgical specialty and recovery from the most lethal injuries, including head injuries, will ensue. Respiratory and circulatory support systems will become very effective, miniaturized, and well tolerated. I doubt, however, that long-term cardiac or respiratory support will be provided by implantable systems. It will be possible to revive and to sustain patients in severe cardiac or respiratory failure by extracorporeal machines which will function satisfactorily for periods of weeks, so as to permit either the natural recovery of the heart or lung or allow for organ transplantation. It is in this area that computers will find their greatest use in surgery. Monitoring of every parameter of the critically ill patient with immediate feedback controls will be available. Fluid replacement, drug therapy, blood transfusion, nutritional needs, platelet transfusion, all will be monitored on a minute-to-minute basis. Anticoagulation with heparin, which at present is carried out in the crudest manner, will be monitored minute by minute with computerized feedback control. Perhaps heparin will no longer be used and a better anticoagulant will be available. New drugs sometimes lead to new diseases, some of which require surgical operation; the bleeding intestinal ulceration produced by certain potassium preparations or the postoperative adhesions caused by new kinds of powder for surgical gloves are two instances. The twenty-first century will undoubtedly provide us with new iatrogenic disorders, some of which may require surgical treatment. New diseases may arise or be recognized. Regional ileocolitis, the Zollinger-Ellison syndrome, and hyperaldosteronism were unrecognized in the early years of this century. Undoubtedly new diseases requiring surgery will appear in the twenty-first century.

Surgical care will also be enhanced by our ability to accelerate or decelerate the rate of wound healing. Indeed, it is likely that some substance can be infiltrated into the site of an operation to start the healing process a week or two before the incision is made. On the day after an operation, the wound would already be one or two weeks old. This will eliminate wound disruption and add one more helpful factor in the eternal struggle with infection.

The final frontier will be tissue and organ transplantation. Cardiac and renal transplants will become established and easily performed operations. I am less optimistic about hepatic transplants, only because organ preservation will become an essential part of organ transplantation. It seems quite likely that cardiac and renal preservation, for significant periods of time, will be possible. The complex function of the liver, however, makes it doubtful that it can ever be preserved for long periods. I have already mentioned that endocrine transplantation will become an accepted surgical procedure. Endocrine cells will be grown in tissue cultures, the antigenic properties removed, and huge clones will be transplanted and vascularized. Addison's disease, diabetes, hypothyroidism, hypoparathyroidism, and hypopituitarism will become disorders of the past. Retransplantation of limbs will be more successful because nerve regeneration will have been made effective and rapid, even over long segments as in the leg.

However, despite the spectacular advances of organ transplantation, the need will be less because of a general slowing down of the aging process and the elimination of vascular, cardiac, and metabolic disorders.

Hospital design will become greatly simplified. No longer will huge mausoleums of granite, brick, steel, or cement be built. Hospitals will be at the periphery of cities, not in the center. They will be close to major arteries of transport and all will be equipped with helicopter landing fields. There will be a return to the cottage type of hospital, largely because of the progressively increasing difficulties with sepsis and because the cottage-type ward will permit easy replacement or enlargement. Current emphasis on individual private rooms will be found impractical and undesirable. A single room is desirable only for the few who want to be alone and can afford and demand individual attention. Most people like to be with others, certainly during convalescence. In the twenty-first century, the behavioral scientists will have told us that the large, pleasant, well-lighted and companionable open 30 bed ward of the 1930's is what most people prefer. Being sick then becomes an interesting social experience. These practical cheerful facilities should be preserved in new hospitals even today and certainly will be demanded by the public in the twenty-first century. Thus, hospital construction in the twenty-first century will be very comparable to that of the emergency hospitals built in Great Britain in World War II or the Army hospitals so popular with both British and American armies in World Wars I and II. Solar energy will be used for heating at minimal expense.

Both the quality and the availability of surgical care will be vastly improved. In many countries there is still a substantial difference today between what might be called the very best and the very worst of surgical care. The National Health System in Great Britain has done a great deal to narrow this difference, but much remains to be done in the United States. Surgical care will be delivered exclusively by specialists and at varying levels of primary to tertiary care. Specialization will be even greater than at present so that the old-fashioned general surgeon of the past will disappear. Very difficult or complicated operations within the established specialties will be performed by super specialists in joint replacement, organ transplantation, and so forth. There is no doubt that the quality of technical surgery will be vastly improved. Maintaining the spiritual and humanitarian side of surgical practice in the twenty-first century will be as essential as ever. There is a hopeful trend. Women are entering the surgical field in increasing numbers and doing very well. Despite the efforts of Women's Lib to make females males, I predict that the lady surgeon of the future will be just as good a surgeon—but also a much nicer person—than her male colleague. It is my good fortune to have two superb young women among my residents. I can hardly wait for them to begin to write papers with me so I can take them to important surgical congresses as my scientific companions!

In closing, a word about education and research. Surgical research will continue much as today, mostly applied. The study of new drugs, new agents, new devices, new procedures, and new techniques for the advancement of surgical care will continue. Cancer, sepsis, and the metabolic problems of age will occupy the attention of surgical investigators. Shock, wound healing, and gastrointestinal, respiratory, and cardiac physiology will still be the subjects of study. The questions will be the same; but then the answers will be better.

Education will continue to be broad at its base but highly specialized at the senior levels. There will be a general recognition throughout the world of what is required for the proper education of the surgeon, and it will be comparatively easy to equate surgical education in one country with that in another. This development will take place first among the English-speaking colleges and will be accomplished long before the twenty-first century begins. In brief, a young man having his education in Edinburgh and fulfilling the qualifications for admission to the Edinburgh College would be immediately accepted for membership in the American College of Surgeons were he to move to the United States. The same recognition will exist among all English-speaking colleges, and by the twenty-first century this will be world-wide. I firmly believe that it will be necessary to make the spiritual and humanitarian aspects of surgery an integral part of surgical education. This must be done by the surgeon himself not by a psychiatrist or behavioral scientist. A tradition of humanitarian care can only be instilled by the teacher and leader in his own field. It cannot be delegated to anyone.

The ability of the surgeon to prolong life and indeed restore life will be so great that he must recognize that duty requires him only to alleviate suffering and maintain a happy and useful life. Euthanasia will not be required, but the withdrawal of support systems and cessation of ill-advised treatment must become natural and normal decisions. Lear's plea not to be stretched out longer on the rack of this world must be honored. As I have said elsewhere, "death far from being a tragedy for the individual, may be easeful and merciful. Living without life is more to be feared than death. It can be hell. Death is normal. It may be just, it can often be easeful and merciful, it should always be dignified. It might even be heaven."

In summary then, in the twenty-first century the world will be older and, hopefully, wiser. The surgical arena will have undergone dramatic changes, but surgery and the surgeon will still be on the scene. Let us trust that then as today his surgical science and skill will be matched by his responsibility to, and love for, his patient.

Transcholecystic extraction of residual calculi in common bile duct

Rodolfo M. Mazzariello, M.D., *Buenos Aires, Argentina*

The transcholecystic technique was used in 13 extractions of residual biliary stones; results were satisfactory in nine. Forceps, catheters, and sounds were used in the intubation and dilatation procedures followed by extraction of the stones. The number of sessions necessary ranged from three to 22; duration of treatment ranged from seven days to two months.

From the Surgical Department, Rivadavia Hospital

THE INSTRUMENTAL extraction of residual biliary calculi through drainage tube fistulas has proved a valuable complement to biliary surgery.

This technique was first introduced by Argentine surgeons.[1, 2, 11] My personal experience with it dates from 1964. Since then, adoption of more sophisticated instruments and the ever-increasing number of extractions have resulted in a rising percentage of successful results.[3-10]

Some patients with residual common bile duct stones have drainage tubes of varying diameters leading directly from the operative stump of the cystic duct; in others the drainage has been left with the object of carrying out postoperative studies. Most of these problems was satisfactorily solved by removing the stones through the cystic stump, even when this had to be accomplished by way of very fine drainage tubes.

This maneuver led me to consider the possibility of using the cholecystostomy opening for the removal of residual stones in the common bile duct; my first extraction of this type was in 1970. Since then, out of my total series of 348 cases of instrumental extraction of residual biliary stones without reoperation, 13 were done with the use of the transcholecystic technique and these are reported in this article.

Cholecystostomy is an emergency measure used in severely ill patients in whom a complete biliary exploration is impossible. Residual calculi in the common bile duct are not an unusual finding in postoperative cholangiography of these patients (Fig. 1). Not all of these patients are in a condition to undergo reoperation; most of them are elderly and have cardiovascular disorders, serious bronchopulmonary disease, diabetes, etc.

The first case which induced me to perform a transcholecystostomy extraction was that of a patient who had been under intensive care in another hospital for respiratory diseases caused by serious respiratory insufficiency. While he was in the hospital an episode of biliary obstruction had given rise to a severe septic condition. An emergency cholecystostomy was performed under local anesthesia and any additional operation involving the main biliary ducts would obviously have been dangerous. After several

Accepted for publication Sept. 11, 1973.

Reprint requests: R. M. Mazzariello, M.D., Republiquetas 6320, Buenos Aires, Argentina.

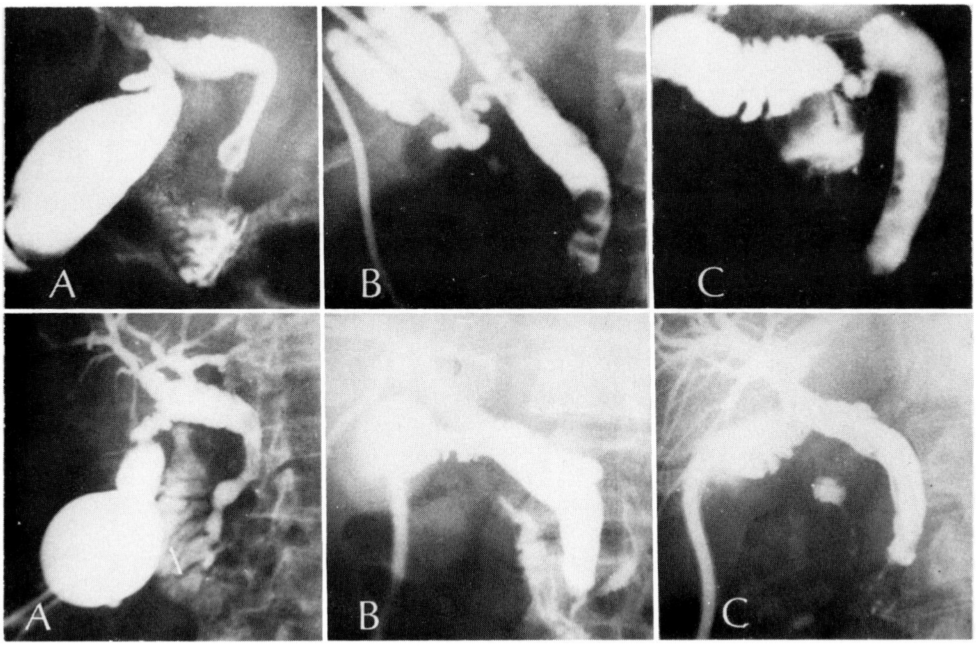

Fig. 1. Cholangiographies taken before and after treatment of cases 6 *(A)*, 7 *(B)*, and 9 *(C)* in which stone extraction proved arduous and time consuming due to long and winding cystic ducts and insufficient dilatation. In one of the patients the duct flowed into the internal border of the common bile duct *(B)*.

attempts the stones were extracted through the cholecystostomy opening.

METHOD

The general indications for instrumental extraction are basically identical to those for postcholedochotomy procedures. It is advisable to wait at least one month after the operation. There is no need to hospitalize the patient unless there has been a general deterioration in his condition. Usually no sedatives or analgesics are required.

The instruments used include forceps, basket-tipped catheters, ureteral catheters, and sounds of varying diameters and tips (perforated, conical and olivary, angulated, etc.).

Intubation and dilatation of the cystic duct. A prior cholangiographic study is necessary to determine the condition of the biliary ducts. The patient must be in the correct oblique position: in the anteroposterior projection the common bile duct usually looks short and thick but, when the patient is slowly rotated, the duct can be seen in all its extension, which facilitates the correct manipulation of the instruments.

The biliary duct should be filled with a concentrated contrast medium (aqueous solution of iodine in 40 to 50 percent concentration). Should reflux of the opaque solution occur upon withdrawal of the sound used for the injection, the lost amount must be replenished. The tract left by the sound is of varying length, depending upon the distance of the cholecystostomy opening from the skin surface. From this the width of the drainage tract and the work involved in the extraction maneuvers may be determined.

The first sounds are introduced up to the gallbladder in order to determine the degree of freedom of action possible. Should there be an impediment, this first tract is dilated, either immediately or by the daily introduction of sounds of progressively greater diameter.

After easy access to the gallbladder has been obtained, the cystic duct is dilated. This does not present any difficulty when the gallbladder outlet tapers smoothly into the cystic

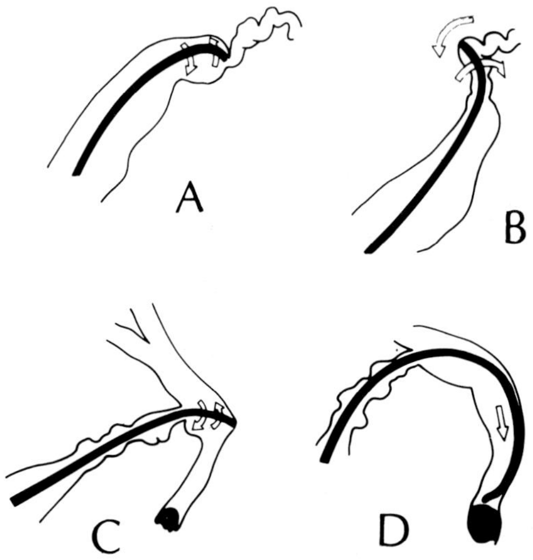

Fig. 2. Schematic representation of rotary maneuvers to reach the common bile duct through the gallbladder and the cystic duct.

duct but this outlet may be eccentrically located, it may be unusually small, or it may be valve shaped. A redundant Hartmann's pouch may hide the point of entry into the cystic duct or prevent its intubation owing to the sounds impinging against the wall before actually entering the duct. This may prove to be the crucial point of the procedure. From here on the extraction maneuvers need not encounter any other serious impediment. As a matter of fact, in the four cases which were failures, the failure was the result of inability to assure a satisfactory passage between the gallbladder and the cystic duct.

With the foregoing in mind, specific maneuvers to facilitate intubation of the duct will be considered. Outward traction at the level of the skin orifice may improve the layout of the involved area and its visualization can be facilitated by rotating either the patient or the fluoroscopic apparatus. It is most important to employ adequate sounds of progressively increasing diameter and different tips. Sometimes it is possible to introduce them without a stylet. The most useful sounds are those with a curved tip since they facilitate "hooking" the duct aided by a rotary movement (Fig. 2).

After entrance to the cystic duct has been achieved, no difficulty is experienced in threading through it—if it is free from pronounced valves or exaggerated curves. Such impediments may be overcome by rotating the sound while it is being pushed toward the common bile duct (Figs. 2 and 3). Very fine and soft catheters are required at times so that they may adapt themselves to the spiral-like course of the duct without becoming rolled up in the gallbladder. If such inconvenience does occur, it may be overcome by introducing the sound, held rigid by a stylet inside it but leaving the tip free and flexible. Another solution involves the introduction of the catheter into a semirigid sound reaching up to the entrance to the cystic duct. Also it is at times useful to grasp the catheter with a forceps at the level of the neck of the gallbladder and rotate it while achieving its gradual introduction (Fig. 6).

Once the sound has reached the common bile duct, it is indispensable to begin dilating its lumen, since it is most unlikely that its natural caliber will enable the eventual passage of the stones to be extracted (Fig. 3).

The great elasticity of the duct may enable it to return to its normal diameter while retaining its valves—a fact which should be kept in mind when undertaking the dilatation. In this connection it should be mentioned that sounds left *in situ* have been known to slip back into the gallbladder between sessions, causing retraction of the duct diameter. This renders indispensable reinitiation of the dilatation maneuvers with very fine sounds.

Dilatations should be initiated slowly and progressively after passing the first sound into the common bile duct (Figs. 6 and 7). It is advisable to leave this first sound as a guide, and to slip another sound with an open end over it. A stylet or catheter is inserted to increase the reach of the sound serving as a guide to allow the subsequent one to be slipped in without difficulty.

Every two or three days a larger sound is inserted until the required dilatation is obtained. Whenever a sound is replaced by a thicker one, as mentioned above, it is neces-

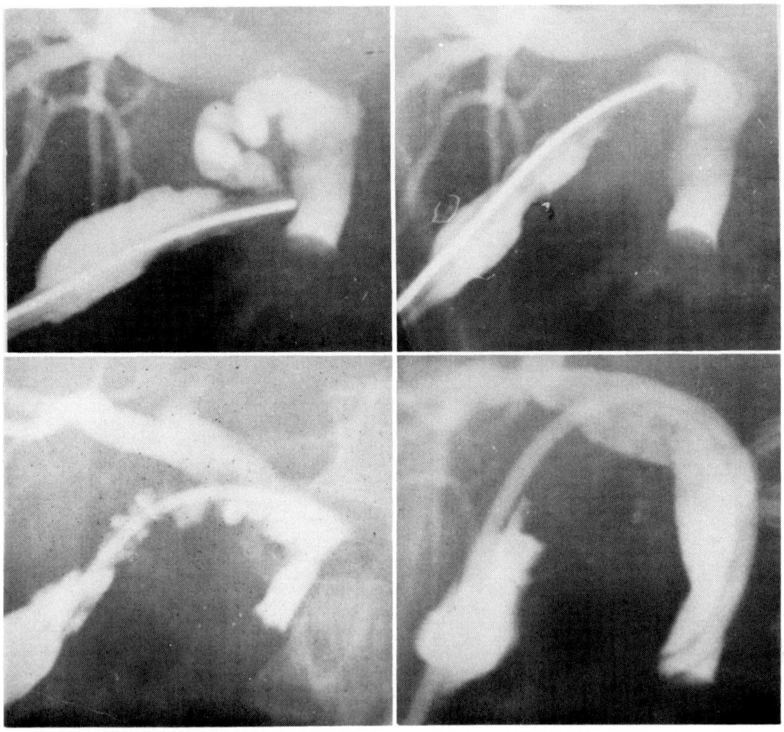

Fig. 3. Case 5. Radiographic sequence of transcholecystic extraction of a large residual calculus in the common bile duct. Intubation of cystic duct with stylet-guided sounds of fine diameter and progressive dilatation of the cystic duct with plastic sounds slipped over catheters to guide them.

sary to introduce the catheter serving as a guide to avoid the creation of a false passage.

Occasionally a partial introduction into the cystic duct is obtained and further progress is impossible despite the above-mentioned maneuvers. This may be attributed to the possible existence of a spiral-like obstruction or acutely bent passage. Under such circumstances it is advisable to leave the sound *in situ* until the next session. In order to avoid its slipping back, a Foley catheter can be introduced into the gallbladder and inflated to compress the sound or catheter to a degree sufficient to hold it firmly. This prevents stricture of the fistulous tract of the cholecystostomy as well. This maneuver in two of my patients enabled the sound to surmount the obstacle spontaneously (Fig. 7).

Gradually, the dilating sounds simplify the course of the cystic duct which, upon distension, becomes shorter while its valvular prominences turn smoother, thus facilitating the entrance to the common bile duct.

The degree of dilatation which can be obtained is surprisingly large, as evidenced by case 5, where the large size of the residual stone made it necessary to attain a diameter of over 15 mm. (Figs. 3 to 5). This dilatation having been reached, the elastic retraction is definitely overcome as shown by intravenous cholangiography after extraction of the stone (Fig. 5). A Foley catheter can be introduced into the cystic duct, facilitating dilatation by means of successive inflations of its balloon along its course.

It is most important that each of the sounds remain *in situ* for two or three days, taped to the skin. They should be examined daily because bile extravasation or gallbladder secretions may dampen the dressing and allow slipping of the sounds.

When the dilating sound reaches a diameter of 4 to 5 mm. this indicates that the

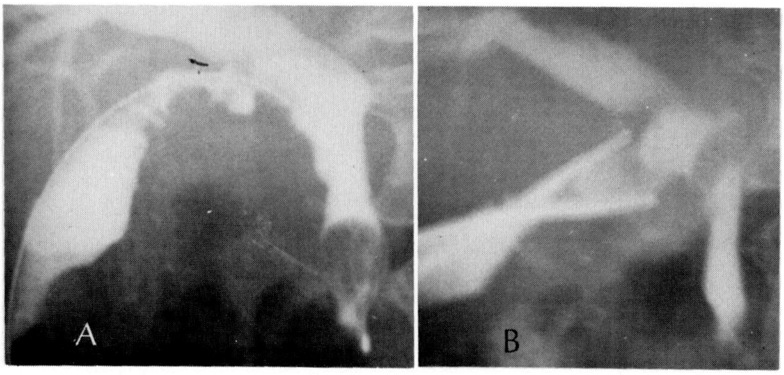

Fig. 4. Case 5. *A,* Basket-tipped catheter used in the stone extraction; *B,* forceps used in the extraction of large fragments of stones trapped in the cystic duct.

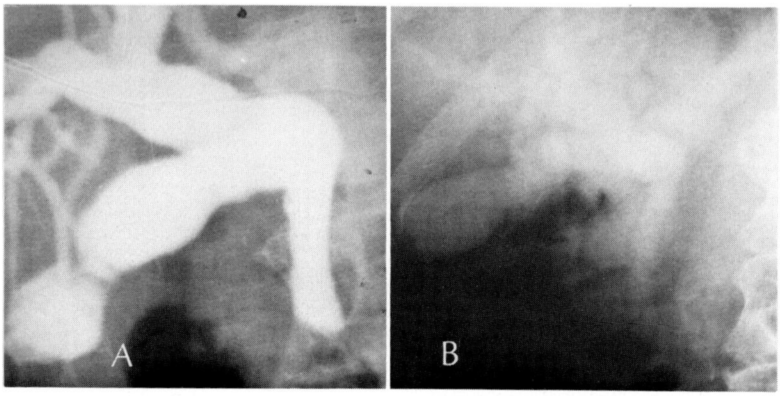

Fig. 5. Case 5. *A,* The stone extraction having been completed there remains an enormously dilated cystic duct; *B,* 10 months postoperatively, control cholangiography revealed no stones. The dilatation is still evident.

passage has been established for the introduction of larger sounds without further need of stylet guiding. Usually the diameter of the sounds can be increased at the rate of 1 mm. per session until the size of the stone to be extracted has been exceeded.

Permanent patency of the sounds is necessary to prevent such consequences of biliary hypertension as colics, septic conditions, or sound expulsion, as a result of calculous obstruction.

Stone extraction. Depending upon the anatomical structure of the confluence between the cystic and the common bile ducts, the instruments are likely to follow a course toward the lower area of the biliary ducts. Usually the choledochocystic angulation renders access to the upper biliary ducts from the gallbladder difficult unless there is unusual dilatation and shortening of the cystic duct.

My series of 13 patients submitted to the transcholecystostomy procedure presented lithiasis of the terminal portion of the common bile duct. When instrumental manipulation resulted in displacement of a stone to a position above the cystic opening, I either waited for its spontaneous descent or provoked it by aspiration lavage, the extraction maneuver being continued when the stone was in the terminal portion of the duct.

The actual extraction is made with forceps having three different types of curves or a basket-tipped catheter (Figs. 4 and 8). The former can be passed through a dilated cystic duct in order to grasp the stone, if it is not very far removed, and the curves of the duct are not very pronounced or wind-

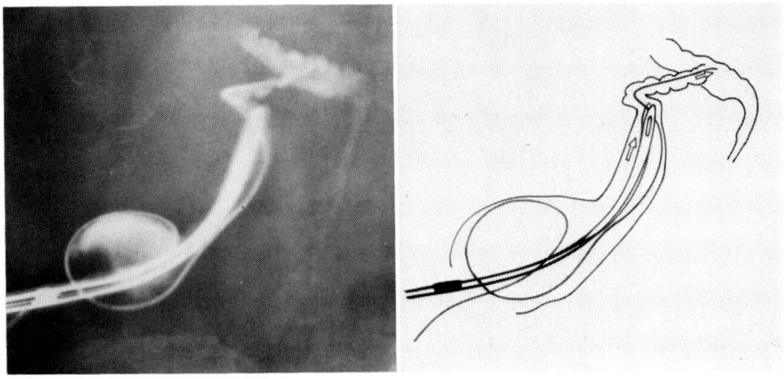

Fig. 6. Case 13. Guiding catheter directed by forceps introduced through the gallbladder.

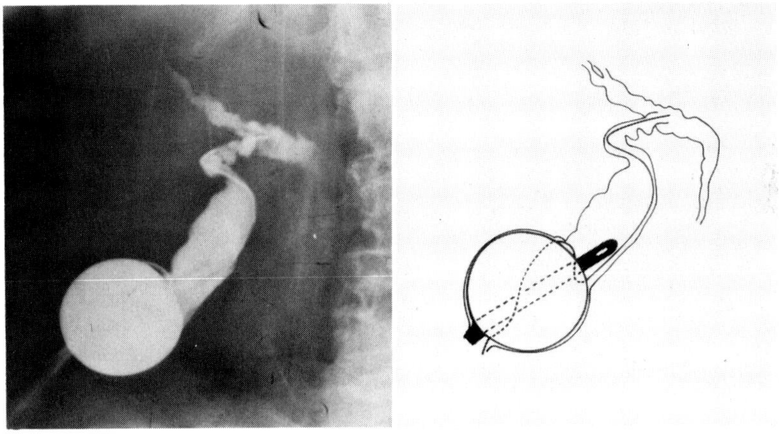

Fig. 7. Case 13. Dilating sound is retained in situ by the inflated balloon of a Foley catheter.

ing (Fig. 4). The advantage of using a forceps is that it enables fragmentation of the stone, thus facilitating its passage outward. The disadvantage is represented by the long —and at times complex—passage implicated by the transcholecystostomy extraction.

When confronted with such a situation it is advisable to employ the basket-tipped catheter, which must be used through open-end sounds to direct it. The technique has been fully described in a previous paper.[10]

Should a stone escape during the course of extraction there is no option but to repeat the maneuver. However, when the stone becomes detached within the gallbladder a forceps proves superior for the extraction because of the high mobility of the stone in that area and the short and direct access thereto.

On one occasion an abnormally large stone remained lodged in the terminal portion of the common bile duct. Upon reaching the opening of the cystic duct it became trapped within it, notwithstanding its prior dilatation. Firm traction on the already grasped stone resulted in its being sectioned by the basket wires of the catheter and no further difficulty then ensued in the extraction of the individual fragments (Fig. 4).

Of the nine successful extractions via the cholecystostomy opening, five were done with basket-tipped catheter, one with forceps, and three required the use of both types of instruments (see Figs. 6 to 8).

The transcholecystostomy approach also enabled dilatation of the sphincter of Oddi in order to eliminate residual fragments which had been carried down to the duo-

Table I. *List of patients submitted to transcholecystic extraction of residual calculi*

Case No.	*Sex, age*	*Operative diagnosis*	*Period after operation (days)*	*Type of cystic duct*
1	M, 58	Biliary lithiasis; serious bilioseptic condition	32	Long, winding
2	M, 65	Acute cholecystitis; pericholecystitis; lithiasis	40	Long, winding
3	F, 59	Acute cholecystitis; pericholecystitis; lithiasis	36	Fine, long, winding
4	M, 66	Cholelithiasis	31	Long, with folds
5	M, 79	Cholecystic empyema; lithiasis	65	Long, tortuous
6	F, 42	Empyema; pericholecystic induration; lithiasis	33	Fine, long, tortuous
7	M, 76	Bile peritonitis; ruptured gallbladder	45	Long, winding flexuous, anomalous opening
8	M, 43	Pericholecystitis; lithiasis; induration	34	Fine, tortuous; anomalous opening
9	M, 76	Empyema; lithiasis; pericholecystitis; pancreatitis	42	Long, tortuous
10	F, 84	Cholelithiasis, hepatomegaly	40	Fine, long, tortuous
11	M, 35	Cholecystic empyema; induration; lithiasis	20	Long, winding
12	F, 72	Bile peritonitis; lithiasis; pancreatitis	37	Short, thick
13	F, 71	Bile peritonitis; cholelithiasis	34	Fine, long, winding

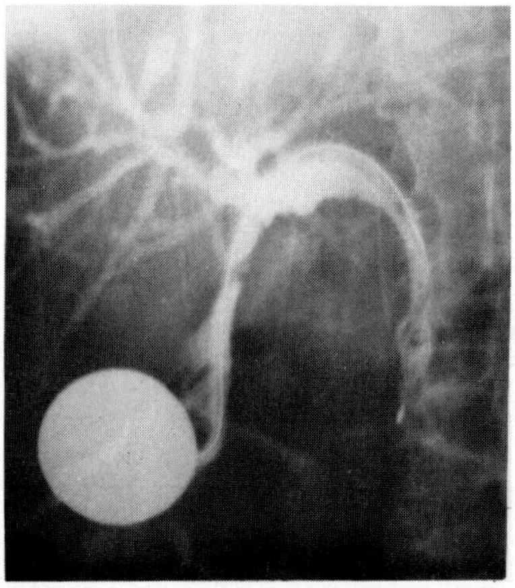

Fig. 8. Case 13. Extraction with the basket-tipped catheter after dilatation. Control filling through Foley catheter.

denum either through use of the catheter or of lavage.

RESULTS

The extraction of residual biliary stones proved successful in nine (69 percent) of 13 patients (Table I), as compared with an almost total absence of failure experienced at present with the extractions carried out through common bile duct drainage tubes (Table II).

The minimum number of sessions for the extractions amounted to three and the maximum to 22. The duration of the treatments ranged from seven days to two months, depending upon the anatomical structure, the diameter of the cystic duct, and the size of the stones.

The ages of the patients ranged from 35 to 84 years; most were elderly. Emergency operations were the rule, with severe biliary or biliary-pancreatic manifestations.

Chronic conditions, postoperative complications, dehiscences, wound infections, etc., were also often seen in these patients. Therefore, the fact that in 69 percent of the cases a satisfactory solution was obtained without morbidity or death attributable to the procedure speaks highly of its value in the extraction of residual biliary stones without reoperation.

It must be admitted, however, that some of the maneuvers proved both difficult and laborious and great care and patience were required to prevent injury to the ducts.

No. of sessions	*No. and size of stones (mm.)*			*Instruments used*	*Accidents and complications*	*Result*
6	4	6-8		Forceps	—	Success
12	4	5-10		Basket-tipped catheter; forceps	—	Success
2	1	8	(?)	—	—	Failure
1	1	10	(?)	—	—	Failure
22	1	20		Basket-tipped catheter	Transitory cholangitis	Success
4	1	6		Basket-tipped catheter	—	Success
21	5	8-12		Basket-tipped catheter	Basket tip became detached	Success
2	1	10	(?)	—	—	Failure
11	5	5-8		Basket-tipped catheter; impelling sounds	—	Success
2	1	10	(?)	—	—	Failure
6	1	5		Basket-tipped catheter	Transitory cholangitis	Success
3	1	12		Basket-tipped catheter	—	Success
11	1	8		Basket-tipped catheter	Damaged common bile duct	Success

There were practically no complications with the exception of two cases of slight transitory cholangitis.

On one occasion the basket tip of the catheter, with a stone inside, became detached inside the cystic duct. However, it was retrieved by means of a hooked wire protected by a rubber sound.

In another patient the use of a very fine plastic urinary catheter provoked a perforation of the common bile duct. A temporary drainage with a fine sound was established and no complications ensued.

The first patient with successful stone extractions died a few weeks later as a result of aggravation of his cardiorespiratory condition. The remaining eight patients continue to be free from biliary symptomatology, and cholangiographic control in three of them has confirmed the absence of disease notwithstanding the time elapsed (one to two years) since nonoperative treatment of their residual lithiasis.

Of the four failures, one (case 10) was submitted to reoperation and died nine days later of cardiovascular complications. During the operative procedure no lesion was found attributable to the unsuccessful extraction maneuvers. Two of the other failures were also reoperated upon without consequences. No follow-up data are available regarding the fourth patient.

Table II. *Nonoperative extraction of residual biliary stones: Analysis of results obtained with different accesses (1964-1973)*

Access	*No. of patients*	*Success*		*Failure*	
		No.	*%*	*No.*	*%*
Transcholedochal	330	316	95.8	14	4.2
Transcholecystic (choledochal stones)	13	9	69.0	4	31.0
Transcholecystic (gallbladder stones)	5	3	60.0	2	40.0
Totals	348	328	94.3	20	5.7

It is very likely that has all these cases successfully treated been submitted to reoperation the mortality rate would have been unduly high.

DISCUSSION

An analysis of these cases opens a new horizon to the method of instrumental extraction of residual biliary stones. Although the indications are not those in which we can practically foretell a successful result, the favorable experience gathered so far induces us to persevere under special circumstances which we dared not tackle before.

The possibility of extracting stones from the common bile duct via a cholecystostomy opening surprised me, especially since it was necessary to overcome ducts of a practically normal diameter with an intact valvular system.

When the spontaneous passage of stones from the gallbladder to the biliary ducts brings about a considerable dilatation and shortening of the cystic duct, this situation goes a long way toward facilitating the instrumental extraction of residual stones, as happened in case 12.

On other occasions, and notwithstanding the passage of stones, the duct proves long, winding, or tortuous, thus making the extractions more difficult. Occasionally it is even impossible to intubate the duct.

Although my transcholecystostomy stone extractions proved practically 70 percent successful, I would not recommend this approach unless the surgeon is thoroughly familiar with easy extractions via choledochotomy drainage; I would advise the new technique with favorable vesicocystic ducts, with regard to diameter and length, and provided the stones are not unduly large.

A diseased gallbladder could be the start of new infectious processes or calculi. It should be borne in mind that there are patients who obtain a definite cure after having undergone cholecystostomy. On the other hand, very elderly patients may die before further vesicular disease sets in.

Although the time elapsed since my patients were submitted to transcholecystostomy extractions is not too long, it should be noted that there has not been a repetition of their biliary disorder.

Intravenous cholangiography has revealed that enlargement of the cystic duct persisted for a long time in those cases in which considerable prior dilatation had been necessary. This means that once the parietal elasticity has been overcome the duct retains an appreciable diameter and that an ample and direct communication exists with the gallbladder, thus doing away with one of the causes of infection, stasis, and biliary precipitation. It is therefore logical to assume that good future prospects can be expected for these patients upon elimination of the main cause likely to bring about a repetition of their gallbladder disorder.

SUMMARY

The method of instrumental extraction of residual biliary stones can be used in special situations in which it was not originally indicated. Such is the extraction of stones in the common bile duct through a cholecystostomy opening or what may be denominated transcholecystic extraction.

As a rule, the technique is more laborious and demands more care and time than that carried out through choledochotomy openings. However, it enables the satisfactory solution of cases of residual common bile duct lithiasis in which an additional operation would have jeopardized the patient's life.

Thirteen patients were treated according to the transcholecystostomy technique with satisfactory results in nine.

Practically no morbidity and no deaths accompanied this procedure, and periodical examinations from 7 to 34 months have later revealed a perfect evolution.

REFERENCES

1. Del Valle, D., Moudet, A., and Figueroa, M. A.: Extracción incruenta en la litiasis residual del colédoco, Bol. Soc. Arg. Cir. **16:** 502, 1955.
2. Goñi Moreno, I.: Tratamiento de la litiasis residual de las vías biliares con la extracción instrumental; Bol. Soc. Cir. Bs. Aires **51:** 525, 1967.
3. Mazzariello, R.: La extracción instrumental de cálculos biliares residuales, Bol. Soc. Arg. Cir. **27:** 640, 1966; **27:** 709, 1966.
4. Mazzariello, R.: Tratamiento de la litiasis residual de las vías biliares en la extracción instrumental, Bol. Soc. Cir. Bs. Aires **51:** 516, 1967.
5. Mazzariello, R.: La extracción incruenta de

cálculos biliares residuales, Editor Martínez de Murguía, Buenos Aires, 1968.
6. Mazzariello, R.: Nuevos aportes a la extracción instrumental de cálculos biliares residuales, Bol. Soc. Arg. Cir. **29:** 404, 1968.
7. Mazzariello, R.: La extracción instrumental de cálculos biliares residuales, Prensa Med. Arg. **57:** 1855, 1970.
8. Mazzariello, R.: Removal of residual biliary tract calculi without reoperation, SURGERY **67:** 566, 1970.
9. Mazzariello, R.: Application of the Dormia catheter to the extraction of residual biliary tract calculi, Acta Gastroenterol. Lat. Am. **3:** 79, 1971.
10. Mazzariello, R.: Review of 220 cases of residual biliary tract calculi treated without reoperation. An eight-year study, SURGERY **73:** 229, 1973.
11. Mondet, A.: Técnica de la extracción incruenta de los cálculos en la litiasis residual del colédoco, Bol. Soc. Cir. Bs. Aires **46:** 278, 1962.

Experimental lobar pneumonia in canine lung grafts

Peter Schick, M.D., John R. Benfield, M.D., Bernard Gondos, M.D., Betty Hayakawa, M.A., Edwin Shors, B.S., Koichiro Shimada, M.D., *and* **Michael Peter, M.D.,** *Torrance and Los Angeles, Calif.*

Diplococcus pneumoniae type III was used to induce pneumonitis in the left lower lobes of unoperated dogs and in dogs with either autografted or allografted left lungs. Transbronchoscopic inoculation with an empirically derived dosage of inoculum was reliably successful in producing lobar pneumonitis amenable to penicillin therapy in six unoperated normals and immunosuppressed dogs. The same technique was generally lethal to lung graft recipients that were unable to confine the infection. Inocula delivered into peripheral segmental bronchi of lung grafts through bronchotomies at the time of lung grafting produced penicillin-curable localized experimental lobar pneumonias in nine autografts and allografts. For diagnosis, cultures from endobronchial specimens were less precise than cultures of tissue. The response to penicillin was eradication of D. pneumoniae from most specimens within four days after initiation of therapy. However, lung biopsy cultures at this time and for at least nine days thereafter, continued to grow other organisms which were predominantly gram-negative despite "clinical" and histologic evidence of resolution of the pneumonitis. It was concluded that experimental lobar pneumonitis can be induced transbronchoscopically in normal dogs. In lung graft recipients, the ability to confine the pneumonitis appears to be impaired. Diagnosis by lung biopsy is more precise than by bronchial brush cultures. The therapeutic response to a specific antibiotic is prompt eradication of sensitive organisms with prolonged lingering of other bacteria. The applicability of these data to the management of human lung transplant recipients has been discussed.

From the Departments of Surgery and Pathology, Harbor General Hospital, Torrance, and UCLA School of Medicine, Los Angeles, California.

THE POOR RESULTS from clinical lung transplants are in part the consequence of incomplete understanding of the manifestations of graft rejection in an organ which is particularly vulnerable to infection.[7] From our laboratory studies it has become apparent that the differentiation of the structural changes of rejection from nonspecific signs of pulmonary injury and from certain features of end-stage pneumonia may be difficult.[3] Our recent reports, therefore, have focused upon the immunologic, structural, and physiologic alterations of rejection,[1, 4] and the need for prospective laboratory studies of coexisting pneumonia and rejection was recognized. This report describes experimentally produced, successfully treated, bacterial pneumonia in transplanted dog lungs.

Supported by United States Public Health Service Research Grant No. HE-13077 from the Department of Health, Education and Welfare, National Institutes of Health, Heart and Lung Institute.

Accepted for publication Aug. 3, 1973.

Reprint requests: Dr. Benfield, Harbor General Hospital, 1000 W. Carson St., Torrance, Calif. 90509.

METHODS

Left lower lobe pneumonia was induced with penicillin-sensitive *Diplococcus pneumoniae* type III in mongrel dogs weighing

15 to 25 kilograms, with and without lung grafts.

Group I, consisting of dogs without grafts, was divided into equal subgroups. Group Ia was immunosuppressed with 0.5 mg. per kilogram of prednisolone and 2.0 mg. per kilogram of azathioprine commencing three days before inoculation and continued throughout the experiment. Group Ib received no immunosuppression.

Group II, consisting of dogs with left lung grafts, was divided into equal subgroups. Group IIa received left lung autografts and no immunosuppressives. Group IIb received randomly chosen allografts with immunosuppression on the same dosage schedule as that in the Group Ia controls.

Antibiotics were used only according to protocol.

Organisms and inocula. *Diplococcus pneumoniae* type III, sensitive to penicillin, was grown on sheep blood agar plates. After 22 to 24 hours of growth the organisms were washed off the plates and the resulting cell suspension was adjusted with sterile saline to approximate the turbidity of a fully grown broth culture. This suspension was added to brain-heart infusion broth (Difco Laboratories, Inc., Detroit, Mich.) which had been preheated in order to drive off dissolved oxygen in the proportion of 0.2 ml. of inoculum per 10 ml. of medium. The broth culture was incubated at 37° C. and it was harvested by centrifugation 22 to 24 hours later. The cells were washed once with saline and suspended in a volume of saline equal to $\frac{1}{40}$ of the volume of the growth medium. Then 5 ml. of this solution (approximately 2.9×10^9 cells by plate counts) were used to inoculate each dog in Group I. For the dogs in Group II the inocula were 1 ml. containing from 2.7×10^6 to 4.5×10^7 viable bacteria.

Inoculation and study procedures. Base-line studies included bronchoscopy with a flexible 5 mm. fiberscope (Machida Endoscope Co. Ltd., Tokyo, Japan). Left lower lobe washings were obtained for cultures. Left thoracotomies were performed and left lower lobe biopsies were taken for bacteriologic and pathologic examination.

Lung grafts were made with the use of the atrial cuff technique with 5-0 polyester suture for the atrium and bronchus and 6-0 suture for the pulmonary artery. All suture lines were by continuous technique interrupted at two points of the circumference.

In Group I, two days after the thoracotomies for base-line studies, percutaneous left lower lobe biopsies were taken via pneumatic power drill. Bronchoscopies were performed, left lower lobe cultures were taken, and left lower lobe pneumonias were induced by transbronchoscopic injection of the inocula via 36 inch 18 gauge polyethylene catheters into the left lower lobe bronchi.

The same inoculation method used for Group I was initially attempted but, for reasons described under "Results," the following method for inoculation evolved for graft recipients. The lung grafts were made immediately after base-line studies under the same anesthetic. Just before completion of the bronchial anastomoses, a 12 inch 18 gauge polyethylene catheter was introduced through the almost-completed suture line and passed into the medial segments of the left lower lobe of the grafted lung. The pneumococcal suspension was introduced. The pleural surface overlying the areas of inoculation, as identified by observing transient distension during injection of inocula, was tagged with felt mesh. The purpose of the marker was to identify the inoculated areas for future reference. The catheters were withdrawn and the bronchial anastomoses were completed.

Two days after induction of pneumonia all dogs had bronchoscopies in order to obtain brushings for culture from the left lower lobes. Immediately thereafter open left lower lobe biopsies were taken for cultures and pathologic examination. The graft recipients (Group II) had upper lobe biopsies in addition to the studies of lower lobe specimens.

Antibiotic therapy was withheld until after the biopsies were taken two days following induction of pneumonia. Then one million units of procaine penicillin were administered intramuscularly and continued twice daily for a period of seven days.

Table I. *Protocol schedule for experimental lobar pneumonia*

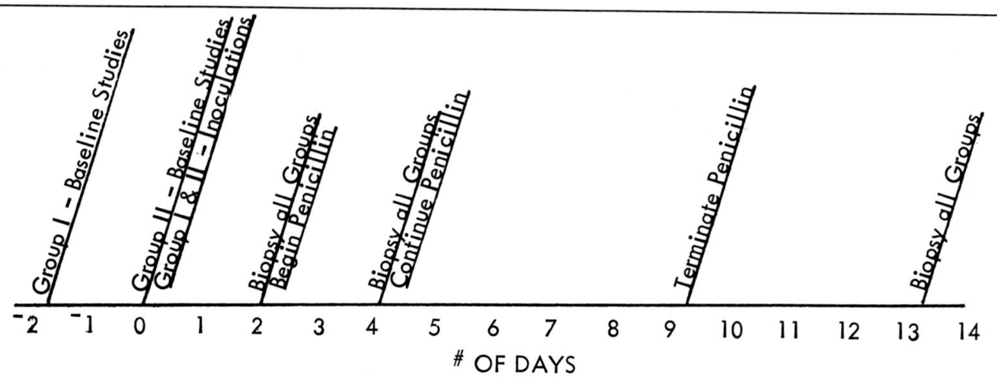

Group I = Without grafts: Ia = immunosuppressed; Ib = not immunosuppressed

Group II = With grafts: IIa = autografts; IIb = allografts

Four days after initiation of penicillin treatment all dogs had bronchoscopies and thoracotomies. Left upper and lower lobe biopsies were histologically examined and the lower lobe specimens were homogenated and cultured. Four days following cessation of penicillin therapy these procedures were repeated.

The protocol concerning the timing of biopsies, inoculation, and treatment of pneumonias is summarized in Table I.

Processing of bronchial brushings and tissue biopsies. The bronchial brushings were applied directly to five percent sheep blood agar plates and to a Levine Eosin Methylene Blue (EMB) plate. They were also used to inoculate thioglycollate medium. One blood agar plate was placed in an anaerobic jar and all media were incubated at 37° C. The plates were examined at 24 and 48 hours. Predominating organisms were picked for further study and identification.

Tissue biopsies were divided into two parts. One part was stained with hematoxylin and eosin and prepared for examination by light microscopy and the second part was manually ground in a mortar to which sterile glass beads had been added to aid in the homogenization of the tissue. Samples from the homogenates were then handled precisely like the brushing specimens.

Identification of D. pneumoniae. The type III organism used in this study characteristically produces very large, mucoid colonies on sheep blood agar, especially when incubated anaerobically with CO_2. These large alpha-lytic colonies were unlike any other type experienced in this study. Gram stains of the organisms revealed short chains of gram-positive cocci that were often paired in the chains. Within 24 hours they were often turning gram-negative. Optochin sensitivity and bile solubility were used definitely to identify these organisms as pneumococci. In some instances specific serologic typing was used to confirm the identification as *D. pneumoniae* type III.

RESULTS

Attempts at producing pneumonia were made in 47 dogs. Data from the 15 dogs in which lobar pneumonia was successfully produced and treated are summarized in Table II.

There were eight unoperated normals,

Table II. *Diplococcal left lower lobe pneumonia in canine lung grafts**

		Before inoculation		*2 Days after inoculation*			*During penicillin treatment*		*4 Days after penicillin stopped*	
Group	*Dog No.*	*LLL B*	*LUL T*	*LUL T*	*LLL B*	*LLL T*	*LLL B*	*LLL T*	*LLL B*	*LLL T*
Ia. Controls	677	0	GN rods		GN rods, +	+	GN rods		S	GN rods
	602	GN rods	GN rods		GN rods, +	+	0	GN rods, S	GN rods, S	0
	745	S	GN rods		GN rods, +, S	+	0	S	GN rods	GN rods
Ib. Controls with immunosuppression	688	GN rods, S	0		GN rods, +, S	GN rods, +, S	X	X	X	X
	765	0	0		+	+	GN rods	GN rods	GN rods	GN rods
	760	GN rods, S, Str	GN rods		GN rods, +	+	0	GN rods	GN rods	GN rods, S
IIa. Autografts	325	0	0	+	GN rods, +	+	GN rods, Str	0		GN rods, Str
	322	0	0	+, S	+, S	+	0	GN rods, S	GN rods, +, S	+, S
IIb. Allografts	200	0	0	+, S	+, S, GN rods	+, S	S, GN rods	+, GN rods		S, GN rods
	272	GN rods	GN rods	0	+, S, GN rods	+	S	S, GN rods		S, GN rods
	289	0	0	+	+, GN rods	+	GN rods	S, GN rods		S, GN rods
	239	GN rods	0	+	+, GN rods	+	GN rods	+, S, GN rods	+, S, GN rods	S
	247	0	0	+, Cl	+, GN rods	+, Cl	S, GN rods	GN rods	GN rods	S, GN rods
	221	GN rods	GN rods	+, GN rods	+, GN rods	+, GN rods	GN rods	GN rods	X	X
	218	GN rods	0	+, S	+, GN rods	+	GN rods	GN rods	X	X

*Abbreviations: LUL, left upper lobe; LLL, left lower lobe; B, bronchial brushing culture; T, culture of tissue; 0, no growth; +, *D. pneumoniae* cultured; Cl, clostridium; GN, gram-negative rods; S, staphylococcus; Str, streptococcus; X, dog died.

two of which did not develop pneumonia after inocula of 5.8×10^6 cells. Inocula of about 2.9×10^9 cells were finally found effective for Group I. One immunosuppressed normal (Dog No. 688) died of overwhelming pneumonia two days after inoculation. After exclusion of the dogs which did not develop pneumonia, the six dogs listed in Group I remained.

There were 39 graft recipients inoculated. The first 16 recipients, inoculated like the controls, died of overwhelming and widespread pneumonia shortly after lung grafting. The next six dogs, subjected to base-line thoracotomies and thereafter infected by bronchoscopy, received less potent (about 3×10^7 cells) doses. These dogs died of widespread pneumonia shortly after transplantation. The remaining nine dogs comprised Group II, in which there was experimentally induced pneumonia suitable for study in grafted lungs. Two of the allografts (Nos. 218 and 221) died before the end of the protocol but they are nevertheless included in the data summarized in Table II because they survived a sufficient portion of the protocol to provide meaningful data.

Henceforth, the isolation of *D. pneumoniae* type III shall be referred to as a *positive culture* and failure to isolate this organism shall be described as a *negative culture*. None of the bronchial brushings and lung biopsies obtained for base-line cultures from dogs which were later successfully inoculated was positive. All lungs appeared grossly normal at the time of first biopsies. All cultures of tissues were negative for the test organism, although six of them contained other orga-

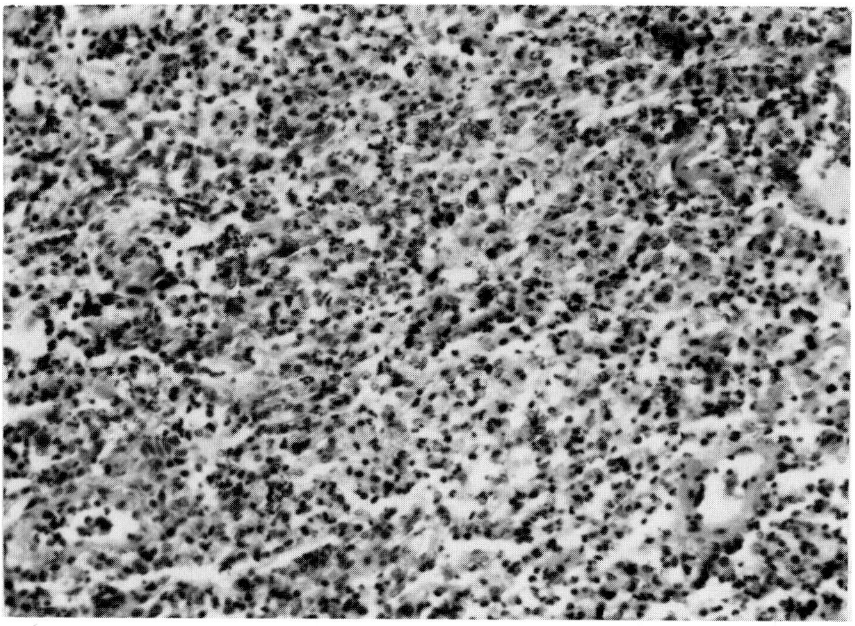

Fig. 1A. Acute pneumonia in control group with characteristic heavy polymorphonuclear infiltration two days after inoculation with *D. pneumoniae.* (Hematoxylin and eosin; ×150.)

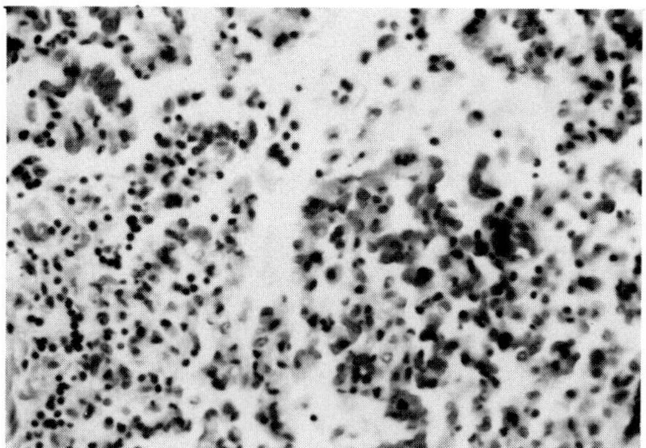

Fig. 1B. Intraalveolar accumulation of lymphocytes and macrophages four days following the beginning of penicillin treatment. Dog No. 602. (Hematoxylin and eosin; ×150.)

nisms which were gram-negative rods.

Considering the period after successful inoculation and prior to penicillin therapy, there were 30 left lower lobe cultures; 15 were cultures of tissue and the remainder were cultures from brushings. The histologic findings in the 15 tissue biopsies were consistently compatible with bacterial pneumonia. Endobronchial pus was uniformly seen on bronchoscopy.[4] All cultures taken from lower lobe biopsies were positive. Parallel bronchial brush cultures were also positive. However, while 11 of 15 cultures of tissue contained only *D. pneumoniae,* only one of 15 bronchial cultures was a pure positive ($p < 0.005$). The variety of bronchial brushing organisms included potential pathogens such as staphylococcus and gram-negative rods. These incidental organisms found within the bronchi could have been mistakenly considered responsible for the pneumonia were it not for the tissue biopsy cultures. Therefore, the biopsies of tissue were more precise than the brush biopsies in identifying the causative organism for the pneumonia.

Cultures taken from the left upper lobe biopsies in Group II were positive in eight of nine specimens. However, microscopic sections from all of these samples failed to to show evidence of pneumonia. Thus, by histologic and gross criteria, pneumonitis was reliably limited to the left lower lobes.

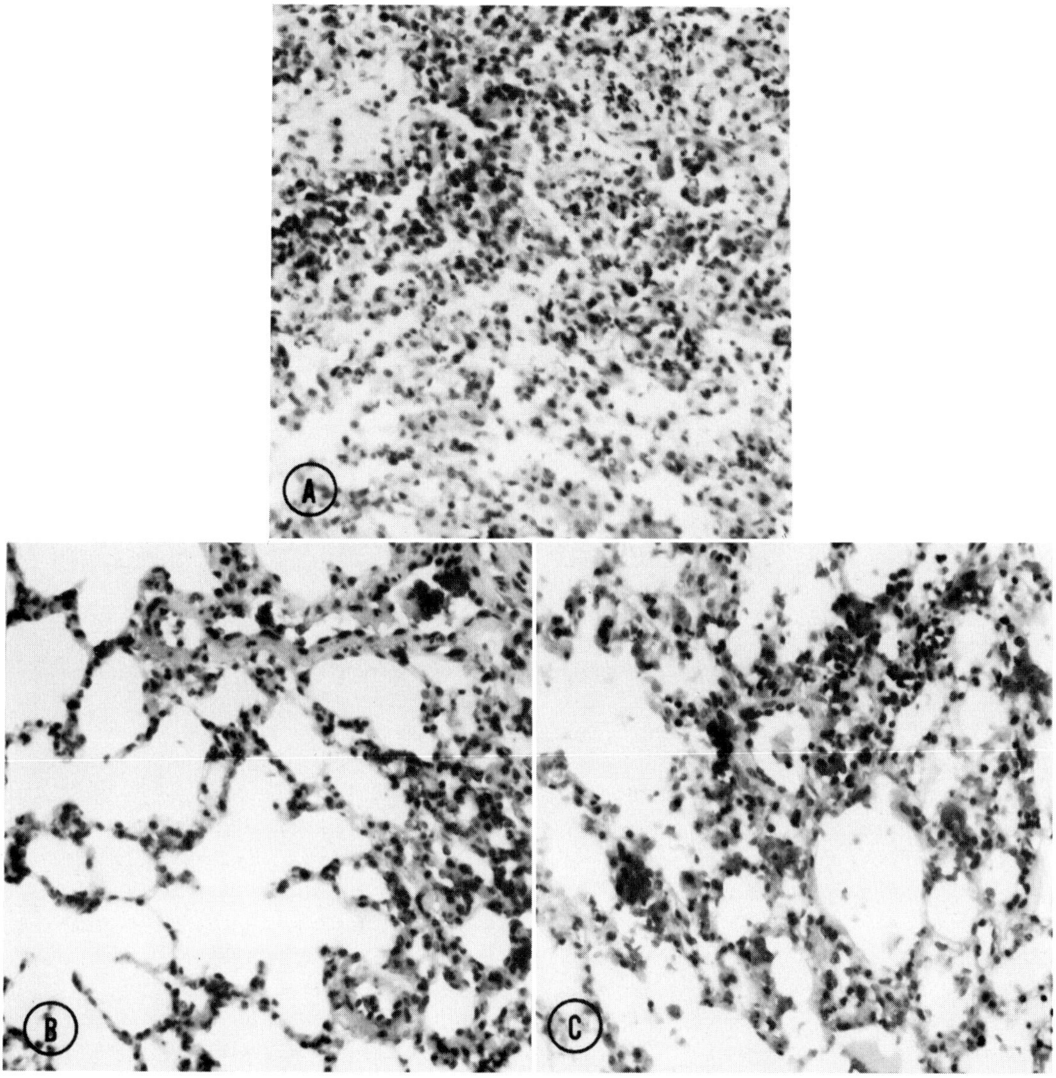

Fig. 2. *A,* Acute pneumonia in lower lobe of allograft two days after inoculation of lower lobe. *B,* Normal-appearing area in left upper lobe, biopsy taken from graft at same time as left lower lobe biopsy. *C,* Minimal perivascular infiltration, in different area from same upper lobe biopsy. Dog No. 218. (Hematoxylin and eosin; ×150.)

During penicillin therapy (four days after inoculation, two days after antibiotic was begun) all cultures from bronchial brushings were free of *D. pneumoniae* but two of the cultures from lung tissue remained positive. None of the positives was pure in that all of them grew out other organisms as well. The predominating other organisms were gram-negative rods.

After penicillin had been stopped there was pathologic evidence of resolving pneumonia. Cultures at this time were negative for *D. pneumoniae* except for the biopsy and bronchial brushing from Dog No. 322 and the brushing from Dog No. 239. Other organisms, still primarily gram-negative rods, remained in all but one of the tissue biopsies from the lower lobes of the 12 dogs which survived to the end of the protocol. The incidence of these other organisms after completion of the protocol was significanttly different as compared to base-line studies ($p < 0.01$).

Microscopic examination. Microscopic ex-

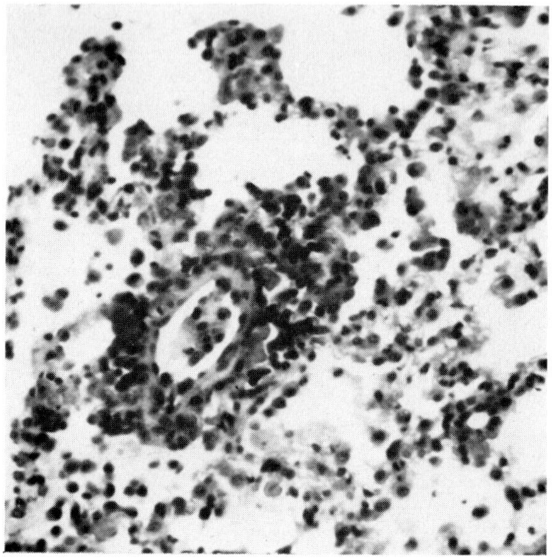

Fig. 3. Perivascular cuffing by mononuclear cells, following successful antibiotic therapy, left lower lobe. Dog No. 247. (Hematoxylin and eosin; ×150.)

amination of biopsies from Group I dogs revealed the following: Two days after inoculation all biopsies showed heavy polymorphonuclear infiltration. After four days of penicillin therapy, both immunosuppressed and nonimmunosuppressed dogs showed many macrophages and chronic inflammatory cells in alveolar spaces (Fig. 1). Two days later there was alveolar clearing, with only small infiltrates remaining. After one week there was complete resolution, with no difference between immunosuppressed dogs.

Microscopic examination of biopsies from Group IIa (autografts) showed normal findings before induction of pneumonia. Two days after inoculation all biopsies showed acute pneumonia, with a heavy polymorphonuclear infiltration. Following treatment and resolution findings were essentially the same as in Group I.

Biopsies from Group IIb (allografts) revealed the following: All lower lobe biopsies showed acute pneumonia following inoculation (Fig. 2, *A*). Upper lobe biopsies at this time either were normal (Fig. 2, *B*) or had minimal perivascular infiltration (Fig. 2, *C*). After four days of penicillin pneumonia had begun to clear in all but one of the dogs. In other animals there were patchy, perivascular infiltrates suggestive either of resolution of pneumonia or of early rejection (Fig. 3). Subsequent biopsies continued to show evidence of a chronic inflammatory process, localized particularly around blood vessels (Fig. 4) even long after the acute process of pneumonia had cleared. Thus, changes consistent with chronic inflammation or with early rejection persisted during the entire period of observation and well beyond the duration of such changes in any of the other experimental groups. Criteria definitively to differentiate rejection from chronic infection could not be developed.

DISCUSSION

Our technique to induce pneumonia is a modification of that used by Terrell, Robertson, and Coggeshall.[5] We found that 5.8×10^6 cells, as they suggested, did not suffice to produce pneumonia reliably in normal dogs. Instead we needed inocula of 2 to 3×10^9 cells to give reproducible pneumonia which was nevertheless generally amenable to therapy without overwhelming sepsis.

It is noteworthy that the technique for inducing pneumonia which was well tolerated and readily controlled by treatment in unoperated lungs was overwhelming to grafted lungs. The graft recipients inoculated like controls almost always died of pneumonia before the protocol could be completed. Even when the potency of the inocula was decreased, this was not tolerated. To overcome this we elected to proceed with grafting at the first operation in Group II after obtaining base-line specimens. We devised the technique to inoculate into a peripheral segment at operation in preference to the transbronchoscopic inoculation method used for the controls because the bronchoscopic method after grafting generally caused widespread pneumonias. Segmental inoculation at operation usually caused confined lower lobar pneumonias, as judged grossly and histologically. However, cultures from upper lobe biopsies often also contained *D. pneumoniae*. Unfortunately, comparable upper lobe cultures from controls are not available. Based primarily upon the fact that graft recipients suffered overwhelming widespread pneumonias more easily than controls,

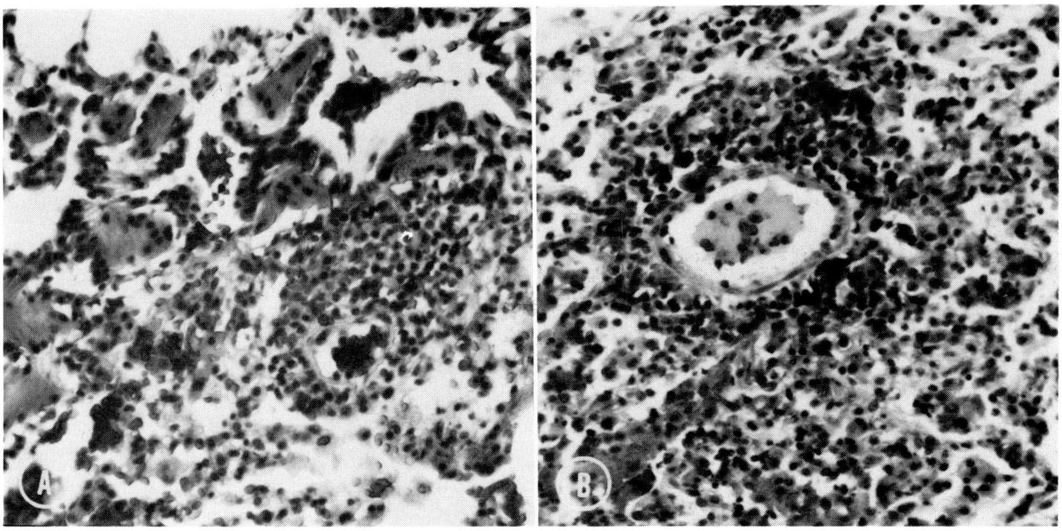

Fig. 4. *A,* Biopsy from left lower lobe of allograft showing chronic inflammation and scarring four days after completion of penicillin. *B,* Perivascular and intraalveolar chronic inflammatory cells. Dog No. 239. (Hematoxylin and eosin; ×150.)

we believe it likely that lung grafting interferes significantly with the ability to confine and resist infection.

The bronchial brushing cultures as compared to the cultures of tissue gave parallel results, in that both methods indicated the presence of *D. pneumoniae.* However, biopsies of tissue often yielded pure cultures of the test organisms while the brushing cultures almost always were mixtures of the Diplococci and other bacteria. Since it is clear that *D. pneumoniae* were the infectious organisms in these experiments, one can infer that cultures from tissue biopsies are more precise than endobronchial cultures with regard to identifying the causative organism for pneumonia.

Bronchoscopy can be useful for the diagnosis of pneumonia in ways other than cultures. It may reveal an endobronchial purulent exudate which is characteristic of pneumonia but absent in pure lung allograft rejection.[4] Thus bronchoscopy may help to differentiate rejection from infection after lung transplantation.

The replacement of *D. pneumoniae* with other organisms, predominantly gram negative, following penicillin therapy has important implications regarding the controversy which surrounds the use of prophylactic antibiotics after thoracic surgery. We cannot resolve that controversy with this study but the techniques we have presented may be useful toward that end in the future. We also cannot comment upon exactly how long after apparent "clinical cure" parenchymal bacteria persisted. Unfortunately, we neither continue to obtain serial lung biopsies until they became sterile nor were biopsy specimens always sterile at the time of base-line studies. However, we can say that penicillin therapy of induced *D. pneumoniae* pneumonitis promptly eradicated the inoculated organism from lung tissue while other bacteria persisted and flourished during apparent recovery.

With exception of the decreased resistance to dissemination found after inoculation in grafted lungs as compared to unoperated lungs, the bacteriologic pictures and susceptibilities to therapy were essentially the same in both groups of dogs once tolerable pneumonias were established. From the viewpoint of achieving clinical therapeutic success with lung transplantation, the decreased resistance to disseminated infection which appears to be a consequence of lung grafting is an important observation which stresses the importance of optimum antibiotic management.

We recognize that the organism selected

for this preparation is not a likely clinical problem, and the pneumonia model used in these experiments makes no pretense at precisely mimicking the clinical situation in lung transplant recipients who develop infections "spontaneously." Rather, we have used this preparation as a tool with which to study coexisting lung allograft rejection and pneumonia which is readily amenable to antibiotic cure in the laboratory. To our knowledge this is the first effort in this direction. Despite the limitations of the method to which we have just alluded, and the fact that we have not yet been able to develop microscopic criteria to differentiate rejection from chronic infection, we believe that our data have provided valuable information which may be applicable to clinical management of human recipients by inference.

What are the inferences one can make from this study in dogs regarding coexisting pneumonia and rejection in human lung transplants? First, because autografted infected lungs responded to antibiotic treatment like the controls, we inferred that denervation alone is not a serious deterrent to successful therapy of pneumonia. This inference must, however, be tempered with the realization that our experience also showed that grafted lungs are easier to infect with lesser inocula than unoperated lungs. We therefore believe that pneumonia will continue to be a significant but surmountable risk of lung transplant recipients.

The second major inference we can make from our data is that pneumonia coexisting with rejection can be successfully treated and identified. Certainly the experience of Derom[2] and Veith[6] and their co-workers support this contention. Our data add the knowledge that endobronchial specimens for culture are not as accurate in identifying the causative organisms as are biopsies of the graft parenchyma, and we have demonstrated that resolving pneumonia in lung allografts goes through the same stages as in lungs that have not been operated upon.

Our third inference is that we must still recognize that the stages of organization and resolution in allografted lungs present a special problem. As we and others have pointed out previously, perivascular mononuclear cell infiltration is also a feature of resolving pneumonia.[3] Extensive edema, hemorrhage, and necrosis may occur in terminal stages of rejection as well as in terminal pneumonia. The present study re-emphasizes the difficulty in distinguishing between resolving pneumonia and changes associated with pulmonary rejection. However, it also strongly suggests that occasionally lung biopsies in human lung transplant recipients may be the only way definitively to identify the causative organisms for pneumonia where there is coexisting rejection. Therefore, we believe that lung biopsies in the postoperative management of human transplant recipients will be indicated, but only relatively infrequently and primarily for the purpose of obtaining material for reliable cultures.

REFERENCES

1. Benfield, J. R., Beall, G. N., Gondos, B., Peter, M. E., Shimada, K., and Schick, P.: Serial observations on immunologically matched lung allografts, J. Thorac. Cardiovasc. Surg. **64:** 907, 1972.
2. Derom, F., Barbier, F., Ringoir, S., Versteck, J., Rolly, G., Berzseny, G., Vermeire, P., and Urints, L.: Ten-month survival after lung homotransplantation in man, J. Thorac. Cardiovasc. Surg. **61:** 835, 1971.
3. Gondos, B., White, P., and Benfield, J. R.: Histologic changes associated with rejection of canine lung transplants, J. Thorac. Cardiovasc. Surg. **62:** 183, 1971.
4. Shimada, K., Gondos, B., and Benfield, J. R.: Photofiberoptic bronchoscopic observations during lung transplant rejection, Arch. Surg. **106:** 774, 1973.
5. Terrell, E. E., Robertson, O. H., and Coggeshall, L. T.: Experimental pneumococcus lobar pneumonia in the dog, J. Clin. Invest. **12:** 393, 1933.
6. Veith, F. J., Koerner, S. K., Siegelman, S. S., Kawakami, M., Kaufman, S., Attai, L. A., Hagstrom, J. W. C., and Giedman, M. L.: Diagnosis and reversal of rejection in experimental and clinical lung allografts, Ann. Thorac. Surg. **16:** 172, 1973.
7. Wildevuur, C. H., and Benfield, J. R.: A review of 23 human lung transplantations by 20 surgeons, Ann. Thorac. Surg. **9:** 489, 1970.

Accelerated rejection of 36 immediate posttransplant functioning machine-preserved human cadaveric kidneys

Thomas C. Moore, M.D., Thomas V. Berne, M.D., *and* **Thomas S. English,** *Los Angeles, Calif.*

Accelerated rejection of 36 immediate posttransplant functioning machine-preserved human cadaveric kidneys of good quality from perfusion data was encountered in a group of 246 first and second transplants (15 percent). Accelerated rejection was more frequent in first transplants (16 percent) than in second transplants (seven percent). It occurred more frequently in adult than in pediatric age recipients (16 percent as opposed to three percent) and was encountered more frequently at transplant centers with lower incidences of recipient presensitization as judged by other early transplant function data. It was associated with prolonged hemodialysis prior to transplantation within intermediate length ranges and with intermediate incidences of recipient presensitization as determined by pretransplant antibody against the panel cytotoxicity assays. Accelerated rejection occurred between two and eight days after transplantation. Longer periods of pretransplant hemodialysis were associated with the earlier onset of accelerated rejection. It is suggested that an early transplant function (ETF) index may provide a useful clinical yardstick for the evaluation of the effectiveness and sensitivity of in vitro methods for the detection of recipient presensitization and that prolonged pretransplant hemodialysis may be a major factor in recipient presensitization. From the findings of this study, it is suggested that accelerated rejection of machine-preserved cadaveric human kidneys of good quality may be due to recipient presensitization with intermediate harmful titers of anti-transplant antibody.

From the Greater Los Angeles Mobile Preservation Unit, UCLA–Harbor General Hospital, and the Departments of Surgery, University of California, Los Angeles, and the University of Southern California.

In 1970, Lucas and associates[2] reported the association of early posttransplant failure and subliminal sensitization of human renal transplant recipients. They employed a sensitive radioimmunoassay for anti-HLA antibody and observed that low levels of antibody, not detectable to cytotoxicity assays, were rapidly destructive to human renal allografts. They found that the titer of antibody correlated with the severity of early renal transplant failure. High titers of antibody were associated with a hyperacute rejection type of immediate anuria. Intermediate titers were associated with immediate diuresis and with graft failure within 24 to 96 hours (accelerated rejection) and low titers were associated with mild impairment of transplant function suggestive of ischemic damage. Microscopy study by them of accelerated rejection kidneys revealed polymorphonuclear cell infiltration, interstitial hemorrhage, hemorrhagic necrosis, and extensive necrotizing vasculitis with thrombosis. They concluded that a substantial number of early posttransplant failures previously attributed

Supported by grants from California Regional Medical Programs and the California Transplant Foundation.

Accepted for publication Oct. 10, 1973.

Table I. *Perfusion-preservation and recipient data for accelerated rejection first transplant kidney*

Machine kidney No.	Duration dialysis (mo.)	Recipient sex	Recipient age (yr.)	Highest antibody before (%)	Highest antibody after (%)	No. of HL-A antigens mismatched (D → R)
125	0	F	11	8		2
43	1	F	34	0		3
3	2	F	45	0	0	3
239	2	M	17	3		1
246	2	F	43	0		2
228	4	M	27	1	1	4
243	5	F	52	0		4
4	6	M	44	1	5	2
241	6	M	33	0		3

*F (immediate and continued good function in initial 10 to 14 days); F^{AR} (immediate good function with accelerated rejection, AR initial 14 days); NF (essential non-function in initial 10 to 14 days); NF^{HA} signifies NF with hyperacute rejection (HA) observe

by others to obscure causes may have been due to harmful titers of antibodies not detected by routine cytotoxicity tests used for direct cross-matching and other studies.

In a recent review of a 24 month experience with machine preservation of 302 human cadaveric kidneys for transplantation, the authors[3] found a marked difference in the quality of early posttransplant function at the various transplant centers served by the preservation unit. The observed differences in function appeared to be related most clearly to the duration of hemodialysis prior to transplantation and to the level of presensitization as determined by the highest pretransplant recipient level of cytotoxic antibodies against a panel of cell donors.[4]

Of the 302 perfused kidneys, 254 (84 percent) were transplanted. Of this number, 246 were transplanted in the Greater Los Angeles metropolitan area of 10.2 million population. Thirty-six of the locally transplanted kidneys which functioned immediately after transplantation were observed to be affected by an accelerated rejection type of malfunction in the two- to eight-day posttransplant period (15 percent). The purpose of this report is to review the various factors associated with this early posttransplant accelerated rejection type of malfunction.

NATURE OF STUDY

The Greater Los Angeles Mobile Kidney Preservation Unit is based in the research laboratory of the senior author at the Harbor General Hospital campus of the UCLA School of Medicine. It serves ten transplant centers affiliated with four medical schools (UCLA, USC, UC Irvine, and Loma Linda). The Unit consists of two Belzer perfusion-preservation machines, a preservation machine transport truck, perfusate preparation, and monitoring equipment; it is staffed by five full- and part-time perfusion-preservation technicians and a full-time secretary for data accumulation and storage.

Regional harvesting responsibilities and organ distribution to transplant centers are based on guidelines established by the Organ Harvesting and Distribution Committee of the Los Angeles Transplant Society, a group of transplant-interested physicians, surgeons, and basic scientists founded in 1967 by P. I. Terasaki and R. J. Glassock. Communications and tissue typing are based in the laboratory of P. I. Terasaki on the Westwood campus of the UCLA School of Medicine. Antibody against the panel (AbAP) tests reported in this study were performed in Dr. Terasaki's laboratory by the standard two-stage cytotoxicity assay with 1½ hours of incubation.

Early function of machine-preserved kidneys, based on daily urine output and blood urea nitrogen and serum creatinine levels, was classified as F (immediate function and continuing good function in the initial ten to 14 day posttransplant period), F^{AR} (immediate function with accelerated rejection mal-

ransplanted into patients on hemodialysis 0 to 6 months

Day of accelerated rejection	Early function, other kidney*	Machine perfusion data			Ischemia time	
		Time (hr.)	Flow (ml./min.)	Pressure (mm. Hg)	Warm (min.)	Cold (hr.)
4	F	30	110	58/18	30	¼
6	F	19	200	80/18	0	½
6	NF^{HA}	21	100	60/20	0	⅙
6	F	14	130	58/18	15	½
5	NF	17	195	60/20	10	1
3	Not used	21	140	58/12	15	1
7	Not used	29	180	60/18	15	½
6	F	13	150	60/16	5	¾
6	F^{AR}	23	225	58/16	0	1¼

n two- to eight-day posttransplant period); SF (slow initial function with diuresis by 7 to 9 days with improving function thereafter in
t operation.

function in the two- to eight-day posttransplant period), SF (slow initial function with diuresis by the seventh posttransplant day and continuing improvement in function in the initial 10 to 14 day posttransplant period), and NF (essential non-function of the transplant in the initial 14 days following transplantation).

RESULTS

Because of the apparent role of length of hemodialysis prior to transplantation on the suitability of early posttransplant function, the presumed association of increasing levels of recipient presensitization with prolonged hemodialysis and the observations of Lucas and associates relative to the role of presensitization in accelerated rejection of human renal transplants, this experience with early posttransplant accelerated rejection (F^{AR}) of machine-preserved kidneys will be considered with respect to lengths of time of dialysis. First and second transplants will be considered separately. Period of dialysis groups have been selected as 0 to 6 months, 7 to 12 months, and over 12 months in this study.

First-transplant recipients on hemodialysis 0 to 6 months. Nine of the F^{AR} class early function first-transplant kidneys were transplanted into recipients who had been on hemodialysis in the 0 to 6 month period (Table I). This comparatively small number is of interest since nearly one half of the F class early function kidneys had been transplanted into this group (Table II). Two of

Table II. *Relationship between duration of hemodialysis and early posttransplant function of the F and F^{AR} classes*

Duration of dialysis (mo.)	Early posttransplant function class			
	F		F^{AR}	
	No.	Percent	No.	Percent
0– 6	42/88	48	9/33	27
7–12	29/88	33	12/33	36
Over 12	17/88	19	12/33	36

these F^{AR} class recipients in the 0 to 6 months dialysis group were women who had had pregnancy difficulties of a possible immunological nature. One had developed malignant hypertension in the later part of her pregnancy with rapid renal failure which required the initiation of hemodialysis. She was transplanted approximately one month after this episode. The other patient had had eight pregnancies, all of which had ended with miscarriages. A second transplant was placed in this recipient five months after the accelerated rejection of the first transplant. Mismatched HL-A antigens of both the first transplant and of her husband were avoided in the second transplant. This second transplant functioned immediately and has continued to function well for 2½ years. None of these 0 to 6 month dialysis recipients were observed to have cytotoxic antibodies against ten or more percent of the panel before or after transplantation. There were no unusual findings in the perfusion or ischemia times data. All of these kidneys had perfused well

Table III. *Perfusion-preservation and recipient data for accelerated rejection first transplant kidneys*

Machine kidney No.	*Duration dialysis (mo.)*	*Recipient sex*	*Recipient age (yr.)*	*Highest antibody before (%)*	*Highest antibody after (%)*	*No. of HL-A antigens mismatched (D → R)*
198	7	M	59	1		3
203	7	F	50	12		1
109	8	M	30	1	1	4
218	8	F	48	1	99	4
193	8	F	41	0	100	4
199	10	F	22	1		3
71	10	F	42	3		2
208	11	M	30		35	4
131	12	F	51	1		1
136	12	F	43	36	1	1
92	12	M	23	0	1	2
221	12	M	41	3		1

Table IV. *Perfusion-preservation and recipient data for accelerated rejection first transplant kidneys*

Machine kidney No.	*Duration dialysis (mo.)*	*Recipient sex*	*Recipient age (yr.)*	*Highest antibody before (%)*	*Highest antibody after (%)*	*No. of HL-A antigens mismatched (D → R)*
94	13	F	30	0		3
119	15	M	31	0	0	0
248	15	M	40	51		4
202	15	F	42	1	0	1
226	15	M	39	1	47	4
249	16	M	32	3		4
42	18	F	41	83	70	2
184	19	F	30	83	0	3
139	24	F	38			2
5	24	M	31	22		2
242	24	M	35	0		2
176	30	F	47	1		3

with good flows and low resistance as mirrored in systolic and diastolic pressures.

First-transplant recipients on hemodialysis 7 to 12 months. A larger number of F^{AR} class early function first-transplant kidneys were found in the 7 to 12 month dialysis group (Table III). Two of the 11 recipients in this group studied prior to transplantation were found to have antibodies against ten or more percent of the panel. In one, the determination was obtained nine months prior to transplantation. A second determination on this recipient four months prior to transplantation had revealed antibodies against zero percent of the panel. In the other, the determination (12 percent) was obtained on the day of transplantation. Antibodies against the panel were found in half of the six recipients studied in this group after transplantation. The two very high percents were obtained 11 and 25 days after transplantation. The 35 percent was found 61 days after transplant. Machine perfusion and ischemic times data were within customary limits.

First-transplant recipients on hemodialysis over 12 months. In the over 12 month dialysis group of first-transplant kidneys with F^{AR} early function, four of 11 studied before transplantation had elevated AbAP percents before transplantation (Table IV). In one of the two highest, the elevation was encountered on the day of transplantation. In the other, it was elevated to 83 percent 49 days before transplantation and was one percent 12 days before transplantation. The recipient with antibodies against 51 percent of the panel was studied nine months prior to transplanta-

transplanted into patients on hemodialysis 7 to 12 months

Day of accelerated rejection	Early function, other kidney	Machine perfusion data			Ischemia time	
		Time (hr.)	Flow (ml./min.)	Pressure (mm. Hg)	Warm (min.)	Cold (hr.)
6	NF	18	130	60/16	15	3
7	F	39	180	60/12	0	½
6	Only K perfused	16	200	60/34	15	¼
5	NF	18	90	60/12	1	2
5	F	18	215	56/14	0	2
6	Only K used	16	160	60/10	5	½
3	Only K used	13	150	72/28	60	½
7	F	28	210	60/16	15	½
7	F	38	85	62/26	30	⅙
3	F	18	165	60/10	15	2
2	NF	17	100	56/12	20	½
7	F	25	120	60/18	5	1¼

transplanted into patients on hemodialysis over 12 months

Day of accelerated rejection	Early function, other kidney	Machine perfusion data			Ischemia time	
		Time (hr.)	Flow (ml./min.)	Pressure (mm. Hg)	Warm (min.)	Cold (hr.)
5	F	33	150	60/20	45	1
6	NF	29	170	60/14	15	1
7	F^{AR}	18	120	58/12	5	¼
5	F	17	220	60/12	0	¾
4	F^{AR}	23	140	60/24	5	2
6	F^{AR}	45	115	60/10	5	½
2	F	22	180	78/20	20	½
3	NF	23	225	56/14	29	
2	NF^{HA}	45	110	62/16		
2	F	14	150	60/16	5	1
3	F^{AR}	26	225	60/16	0	1¼
4	NF	16	200	60/16	10	1

tion. Four subsequent studies, including the day of transplantation, were zero at two percent. In another recipient, antibodies against 22 percent of the panel were found nine months before transplantation and against zero percent 15 days before transplantation. AbAP percents after transplantation were increased in two of five studied. These studies were obtained ten and 22 days after transplantation. Machine perfusion and ischemic times data were considered to be within normal limits.

Second-transplant recipients. Three second-transplant kidneys experienced F^{AR} type early posttransplant function (Table V). It is of interest that all of these kidneys were transplanted at USC–County, the transplant center with the apparent lowest incidence of recipient presensitization as determined by other data from the general review of this total perfusion-preservation experience. None of these recipients had elevated AbAP percents before or after transplantation. Perfusion preservation and ischemic times were within normal limits.

The donor of one kidney with F^{AR} function was six years old. All other donors of kidneys in this F^{AR} class early function were 13 years of age or older. Recipient age was of particular interest. All but one of the recipients of F^{AR} kidneys were 22 years of age or older.

Increasing periods on hemodialysis prior to transplantation were associated with an increasing number of recipients with elevated AbAP percents (Table VI). AbAP studies were obtained prior to transplantation in 34 of the 36 recipients of F^{AR} early class function kidneys. Five recipients had one deter-

Table V. *Perfusion-preservation and recipient data for accelerated rejection second transplant kidneys*

Machine kidney No.	Duration dialysis (mo.)	Recipient sex	Recipient age (yr.)	Highest antibody before (%)	Highest antibody after (%)	No. of HL-A antigens mismatched (D → R)
188	15	M	29	0	0	3
225	19	M	31	1	1	4
129	26	F	29	3		4

Table VI. *Influence of duration of hemodialysis in first-transplant F^{AR} recipients on cytotoxic antibodies against panel of cell donors*

Duration of dialysis (mo.)	No. with antibodies against 10 or more percent of panel	Percent with antibodies against 12 or more percent of panel
0– 6	0/9	0
7–12	2/11	18
Over 12	4/11	36

Table VII. *Mean day of onset of accelerated rejection in first-transplant recipients of F^{AR} kidneys with respect to pretransplant interval of hemodialysis*

Duration of hemodialysis (mo.)	No. of F^{AR} kidneys	Mean day of onset of accelerated rejection
1– 6	8	5.6
7–12	12	5.3
13–18	6	5.5
18–30	6	2.7

mination prior to transplantation and 12 had two. Three determinations were obtained in six, four were obtained in two, five were obtained in three, and six had six or more.

AbAP determinations were obtained after first transplantation in 13 recipients of F^{AR} kidneys. In the one- to six-month dialysis group, AbAP percents were 1 and 0 at 12 and 13 days after transplant and five at 26 days. In the over six-month dialysis group, levels were 0 and one at two days and four months. They were 70, 100, 0, and 0 at 10, 11, 12 and 13 days, respectively, after transplant. Both determinations in the 20 to 30 day posttransplant period were elevated to 47 and 99 percent at 22 and 25 days. At 54 and 60 days, the levels were 1 and 35 percent.

Lucas and associates[2] found that recipients with accelerated rejection to renal transplants had radioisotope-binding antibody levels which fell markedly within hours to two days after transplant. The rate of disappearance of antibody correlated well with the rapidity of onset of oliguria. They found that the previous high levels of antibody had returned within 48 hours after removal of the graft. It is possible that in situ destruction of the graft by the accelerated rejection response might produce an effect similar to that achieved by operative removal of the graft.

It is possible, as suggested by Lucas and associates, that the rapidity of onset of the acceleration rejection may be influenced by the titer of antibody. The day of onset of accelerated rejection in our study appeared to be earlier in those recipients who had been on hemodialysis for extended periods of time and who may have been sensitized with higher antibody titers (Table VII).

There appeared to be no correlation with the number of donor HL-A antigens mismatched with the recipient. Six of the recipients had only one antigen mismatched, and one was a full-house zero antigen mismatch. The full-house zero mismatch recipient had been on hemodialysis for 15 months. He had been receiving 1 Gm. per day of methyl prednisolone in addition to azathioprine when his accelerated rejection started on the sixth posttransplant day. The rejection was severe and was reversed slowly only by seven days of heparin therapy. One year after this accelerated rejection episode,

Day of accelerated rejection	Early function, other kidney	Machine perfusion data			Ischemia time	
		Time (hr.)	Flow (ml./min.)	Pressure (mm. Hg)	Warm (min.)	Cold (hr.)
8	F	40	80	60/28	20	1½
6	F^{AR}	19	140	60/24	5	1½
3	F	24	100	60/24	5	2

Table VIII. *Comparison of F, F^{AR}, and NF class early function recipients with respect to percent with cytotoxic antibodies against ten or more percent of a panel of cell donors prior to transplantation in first transplants*

Early function class	No. with detected cytotoxic antibody	Percent with detected cytotoxic antibody
F	4/88	5
F^{AR}	6/31	19
NF	14/62	23

Table IX. *Comparison of F, F^{AR}, and NF class early function recipients with respect to percent with cytotoxic antibodies against ten or more percent of a panel of cell donors prior to transplantation in second transplants*

Early function class	No. with detected cytotoxic antibody	Percent with detected cytotoxic antibody
F	1/12	8
F^{AR}	0/3	0
NF	16/21	76

his transplant is functioning well with a blood urea nitrogen level of 22 mg. percent and a serum creatinine of 1.3 mg. percent.

There was a wide distribution in the donor to recipient mismatch histocompatability antigens. The most frequently mismatched HL-A antigens were 27 (ten times), 12 (eight times), nine (seven times), and two (seven times). None of the other mismatched donor antigens were encountered more than six times.

When AbAP data was used for comparison between the various types of early function, an influence of recipient presensitization in less than F early function was suggested. This influence was observed in both first-transplant recipients (Table VIII) and in second- and third-transplant recipients (Table IX). When AbAP percents were elevated above ten in second- and third-transplant recipients, the type of early transplant malfunction tended to be largely of the NF type.

F^{AR} early transplant function was encountered more frequently at transplant centers (USC and UCLA–Harbor) where the level of recipient presensitization appeared to be lower than at other centers from the relative incidence of F and NF types of early transplant function. Forty-eight percent of the 246 locally transplanted kidneys (117) were transplanted at the USC–County and UCLA–Harbor transplant centers. These two centers accounted for 64 percent of the F^{AR} transplants. The relation of F^{AR} early transplant function to duration of hemodialysis prior to transplantation and AbAP levels in comparison to F, SF, and NF classes of early transplant function for both first and second transplants at USC–County and UCLA–Harbor is presented in Tables X and XI. F^{AR} transplants were encountered largely (21 of 23, 91 percent) in the 4 to 26 month hemodialysis range. The only two transplants not falling into this dialysis duration range involved recipients cited earlier in which there was strong suggestive evidence of pregnancy-involved presensitization. A progressive deterioration in the level of early transplant function as indicated by early function of other than the F class was encountered with increasing long pretransplant periods of hemodialysis for both first and second transplants. Recipients on hemodialysis for more than 26 months tended to have NF or F function. Of 13 first- and second-transplant recipients in this group eight had

Table X. *Relation of F^{AR} early transplant function to duration of hemodialysis and AbAP levels in*

Duration of hemodialysis (mo.)	No. of transplants	Early						
		F				F^{AR}		
		No.	Percent	No.* AbAP↑	Percent AbAP↑	No.	Percent	No. AbAP↑
First transplant								
1– 3	11	11	100	1	9	0	0	
4– 6	10	8	80	0	0	2	20	0
7–12	27	17	63	1	6	6	22	2
13–26	18	6	33	1	17	4	22	2
Over 26	4	3	75	0	0	0	0	
Second transplant								
1– 3	0							
4– 6	1	1	100	0	0	0	0	
7–12	2	0	0			0	0	
13–26	4	0	0			3	75	0
Over 26	1	0	0			0	0	
Total	78	46	59	3	7	15	19	4

*Antibody against panel (AbAP) assay elevated to ten or more percent.

Table XI. *Relation of F^{AR} early transplant function to duration of hemodialysis and AbAP levels in*

Duration of hemodialysis (mo.)	Number of transplants	F				F^{AR}		
		No.	Percent	No.* AbAP↑	Percent AbAP↑*	No.	Percent	No. AbAP↑
First transpant								
1– 3	5	2	40	0	0	2†	40	0
4– 6	7	4	57	0	0	1	14	0
7–12	9	7	78	1	14	0	0	
13–26	6	0	0			5	83	1
Over 26	5	1	20	0	0	0	0	
Second transplant								
1– 6	0							
7–12	3	2	67	0	0	0	0	
13–26	1	0	0			0	0	
Over 26	3	0	0			0	0	
Total	39	16	41	1	6	8	21	1

*Antibody against panel (AbAp) assay elevated to ten or more percent.
†These two recipients were women with histories of pregnancy associated difficulties of possible immunological significance.

NF early transplant function, four had F function, and one had SF function. None of the four F transplants had elevated AbAP percents. This contrasted sharply with the seven of eight NF transplants (88 percent) with elevated AbAP percents. Six of the 13 recipients in the over 26 month hemodialysis group did not have elevated AbAP percents, and four of them (67 percent) achieved F class early transplant function. These findings suggest an intermediate level of recipient presensitization for F^{AR} recipients as judged by pretransplant durations of hemodialysis and AbAP levels.

DISCUSSION

Our experience with machine preservation of human cadaveric kidneys for transplantation has provided evidence that suggests that the early function of machine-preserved kidneys of good quality from perfusion data (flows and pressures) is adversely affected by prolonged periods of recipient hemodialysis prior to transplantation. It is likely that this is due to presensitization of the recipients to donor kidney histocompatability antigens. From the findings of our review of early function of 246 locally (Greater Los Angeles) transplanted machine-preserved kid-

comparison with F, SF, and NF function at USC–County Transplant Center

transplant function								
	SF				*NF*			
Percent AbAP↑	*No.*	*Percent*	*No. AbAP↑*	*Percent AbAP↑*	*No.*	*Percent*	*No. AbAP↑*	*Percent AbAP↑*
	0	0			0	0		
0	0	0			0	0		
3	2	7	0	0	2	7	0	0
50	2	11	0	0	6	33	3	50
	0	0			1	25	1	100
	0	0			0	0		
	1	50	1	100	1	50	0	0
0	1	25	1	100	0	0		
	0	0			1	100	1	100
27	6	8	2	33	11	14	5	45

comparison with F, SF, and NF function at UCLA–Harbor Transplant Center

	Early transplant function							
	SF				*NF*			
Percent AbAP↑	*No.*	*Percent*	*No. AbAP↑*	*Percent AbAP↑*	*No.*	*Percent*	*No. AbAP↑*	*Percent AbAP↑*
0	0	0			1	20	1	100
0	2	29	0	0	0	0		
	2		1	50	0	0		
20	0	0			1	17	1	100
	1	20	0	0	3	60	2	67
	1	33	0	0	0	0		
	0	0			1	100	0	0
	0	0			3	100	3	100
13	6	15	1	17	9	23	7	78

neys, it has been estimated that machine-preserved kidneys of good quality should, when transplanted into totally non-sensitized recipients, achieve F class early fnuction in approximately 95 percent of recipients, perhaps in more.

In support of this assumption, it was observed that 100 percent of 11 kidneys preserved by this Unit and transplanted into recipients on hemodialysis for one to three months at USC–County transplant center achieved F class early function. Progressive deteriorization in early function as represented by attainment of other than F class function at this center was found with increasingly long periods of hemodialysis. This was true for both first and second transplants.

It also appeared that accelerated rejection of transplants with immediate good function (F^{AR} class function) occurred more frequently at transplant centers with lower incidences of recipient presensitization as judged by the relative frequencies of F and NF types of function. At these centers, F^{AR} early function transplants were encountered almost exclusively in the 4 to 26 month hemodialysis group. The only exceptions were two women with histories of pregnancy-associated difficulties of possible immunological nature. This clustering of F^{AR} kidneys in this intermediate length hemodialysis range suggests a possible intermediate level of antibody recipient presensitization in this type of early posttransplant rejection response. Longer periods of pretransplant hemodialysis were associated with earlier posttransplant onset of accelerated rejection. This suggests a higher titer of presensitization in these recipients. Lucas and associates[2] found earlier onset of accelerated rejection in recipients with higher titer humoral antibody levels by their radioimmunoassay.

It was of interest that F^{AR} early function was found almost exclusively in adult recipients. Accelerated rejection involved only three percent of pediatric age recipient transplants in comparison to 16 percent for adult recipient transplants. Pediatric age recipients appeared to have lower levels of presensitization judged from early transplant function. This likely was related to shorter periods of pretransplant hemodialysis prior to transplantation and the transplantation of anatomically and functionally larger adult donor kidneys into approximately one half of the 33 pediatric age recipients (16 years of age and younger). These larger than needed adult kidneys presumably could absorb greater relative immunologic damage from these smaller recipients before showing early posttransplant malfunction of the accelerated rejection type.

A higher incidence of elevated antibody against the panel (AbAP) assays was encountered before transplantation in the recipients of F^{AR} kidney than was found in F transplant recipients. The incidence, however, was lower than that found in the recipients of NF kidneys.

Accelerated rejection occurred more frequently in first transplants (16 percent) than in second transplants (seven percent). It did not occur in third transplants. It also is of interest that all of the second transplant F^{AR} kidneys were transplanted at the center (USC–County) with the apparent lowest incidence of recipient presensitization. This was the only transplant center which made extensive use of the Kiil dialysis system for pretransplant hemodialysis. It was also the center which employed pretransplant splenectomy most frequently.

Although presensitization may come from a number of sources, the most frequently involved one appears to be prolonged hemodialysis. Terasaki's[4] group has shown increased sensitization with cytotoxic antibodies to histocompatability antigens with prolonged hemodialysis. Blood transfusions may play a role in this process. Hammond and associates[1] in a study of non-uremic patients given blood at weekly intervals, found antibodies by agglutinin and cytotoxicity assays for four to six months in almost every patient. The immunosuppressive effect of the uremic state appears to have diminished this response in hemodialysis patients with respect to the high titers required for cytotoxicity. Nonetheless, it is clear from clinical experiences such as this and others and from the studies of Lucas and associates[2] that significant presensitization also may occur in uremic patients, although detected less frequently and effectively by routinely employed cytotoxicity assays of the various types employed, including panel studies.

The intravenous administration of the bacterial and other antigens during hemodialysis also may play a role in presensitization. Some of these antigens may lead to the production of cross-reacting antibodies which react with transplant cellular antigens. Pregnancy is another recognized source of presensitization. Multiparous women provided much of the anti–HL-A antibodies used in the early stages of tissue typing.

Improvement methods for the detection of harmful levels of anti-transplant antibody in proposed recipients of human renal transplants are needed. Cytotoxicity assays in their various forms appear to be too insensitive for complete assurance of recipient non-presensitization. The standard two-stage cytotoxicity AbAP assay with 1½ hours of incubation used during the period of this study is less sensitive than some of the more recently employed modifications of the cytotoxicity assay (longer incubation and the use of trypsin, ficin, or antiglobulin reagents).

Early transplant function of machine-preserved cadaveric human kidneys of good quality from perfusion data (flows and pressures) may provide a useful index of the presence and level of recipient presensitization. This early transplant function (ETF) index may prove to be useful as a clinical yardstick for the evaluation of the effectiveness of in vitro assays of recipient humoral and cellular presensitization to random and specific donor transplant antigens.

The findings of this study of F^{AR} transplants suggest that accelerated rejection is probably due to recipient presensitization and that this presensitization is probably at intermediate levels of harmful anti-transplant activity.

Every effort should be made to avoid transplanting good kidneys into sensitized recipients. A major part of this effort should be to eliminate or, at least, to shorten markedly the period of hemodialysis in end-stage renal failure prior to renal transplantation.

REFERENCES

1. Hammond, D., Mattiuz, P. L., and Curtoni, E. S.: *In* Curtoni, E. S., et al. editors: Histocompatability testing 1967, Baltimore, 1967, The Williams & Wilkins Company, p. 325.
2. Lucas, Z. J., Coplon, N., Kempson, R., and Cohn, R.: Early renal transplant failure associated with subliminal sensitization, Transplantation **10:** 522, 1970.
3. Moore, T. C., Berne, T. V., and English, T.: Machine preservation of 302 human cadaveric kidneys for transplantation, Surg. Gynecol. Obstet. In press.
4. Terasaki, P. I.: Personal communication.

Prolonged survival of canine orthotopic small intestinal allografts preserved for 24 hours by hypothermic bloodless perfusion

Luis H. Toledo-Pereyra, M.D., Richard L. Simmons, M.D.,* *and* **John S. Najarian, M.D.,** *Minneapolis, Minn.*

Whole orthotopic small intestinal transplants were carried out into moderately immunosuppressed dogs. Survival time was compared between the dogs with fresh grafts and those with grafts preserved by hypothermic bloodless pulsatile perfusion for 24 hours. Two perfusates were used during preservation; (1) cryoprecipitated pooled dog plasma or (2) human plasmanate. Survival was significantly better in the dogs which received the preserved grafts. The best survival time was achieved in intestinal allografts perfused with human plasmanate (mean survival, 45 days, the longest being 67 days). These results suggest that significant prolongation of allograft survival in moderately immunosuppressed animals might be achieved by modification of the immunogenicity of grafts either by preservation or by binding with non-specific xenogeneic antibodies in a perfusate solution.

From the Department of Surgery, University of Minnesota, Minneapolis, Minn.

We have previously observed that the orthotopic small intestinal allotransplants preserved for 24 hours by hypothermic bloodless perfusion can maintain life for more than four weeks after transplantation.[45] Some transplants did not manifest the classical signs of rejection even after prolonged residence in immunologically normal hosts. It was important to compare the survival of preserved and fresh allotransplants to determine if perfusion can alter immunogenicity of the small bowel allograft.

MATERIALS AND METHODS

Adult mongrel dogs weighing between 15 and 24 kilograms were used as organ donors and recipients. All dogs were anesthetized with sodium methohexital for induction and with halothane for maintenance. Through a midline incision, the entire small bowel from the third portion of the duodenum to the ileocecal valve was resected. A short, wide, rubber tube was inserted into each end of the bowel to drain the intraluminal contents. The mesenteric vessels were skeletonized, ligated, and divided. The superior mesenteric artery was cannulated, and the small intestine was flushed with a cold (4° C.) Ringer's lactate solution containing heparin (10,000 U. per liter) and procaine (1 Gm. per liter) until the venous effluent was clear. The unrelated recipient dogs in Group I received fresh orthotopic small bowel transplants. The recipient dogs in Groups II and III received orthotopic transplants which had been perfused for 24 hours in a modified Mox-100 Minnesota preservation apparatus (Fig.1).[25] In Group II, the perfusate used was pooled cryoprecipitated canine plasma.[4] In Group

Supported by Grant No. 5-PO2-AM 13083-04 from the National Institutes of Health.

Accepted for publication Oct. 31, 1973.

Reprint requests: Dr. L. H. Toledo-Pereyra, Box 223, University of Minnesota Hospitals, Minneapolis, Minn. 55455.

*John and Mary Markle Scholar in Academic Medicine.

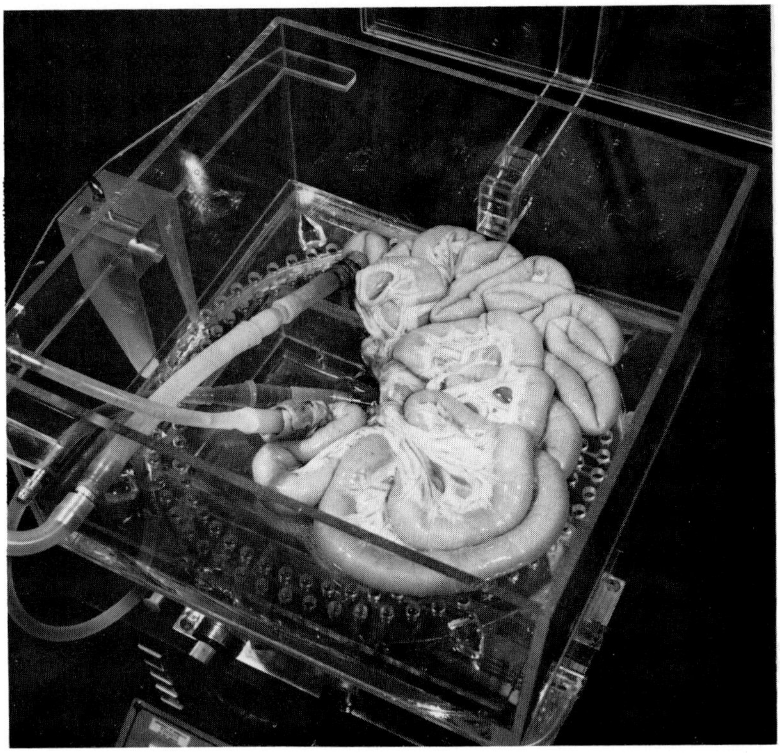

Fig. 1. Preservation technique for whole intestinal transplant. The entire small bowel from the third portion of the duodenum to the ileocecal valve rests in a special cassette. A tube is inserted into each end of the bowel to drain the intralumenal contents. The mesenteric artery is cannulated and perfused.

III, commercial human plasmanate (obtained from Cutter Laboratories, Inc., Berkeley, Calif.) was used without cryoprecipitation. Ampicillin (1 Gm. per liter), kanamycin (500 mg. per liter), methylprednisolone (500 mg. per liter), $MgSO_4$ (1 Gm. per liter), regular insulin (80 U. per liter), and phenosulfonphthalein (12 mg. per liter) were added to all the perfusates.

The perfusion system was primed with 750 ml. of perfusate. The temperature was set at 7° C., and gas mixtures were adjusted to pH of 7.4 and Po_2 of 200 mm. Hg. After the small bowel was placed in the circuit, the pulse rate was fixed at 60 beats per minute and the systolic mesenteric arterial pressure at 60 mm. Hg. The small bowel output through the distal ileum was monitored and if the perfusate decreased to critical levels, fresh perfusate was added to maintain sufficient circulating volume. The hemodynamic characteristics during perfusion and chemical composition of the perfusate[2, 9, 18, 30] were noted initially at 2, 6, 12, 18, and 24 hours. The absorptive capacity of the small bowel during perfusion was measured by administering 10 Gm. of D-xylose dissolved in 100 ml. of water into the cannulated proximal portion of the duodenum immediately after the start of perfusion and then at 12 and 24 hours. Samples for the D-xylose test were taken at 15, 30, 45, 60, 120, 180, 240, and 300 minutes following administration and determined according to standard techniques.[29] Intraluminal samples for total proteins, globulin, and electrolytes were determined every six hours.

Following preservation in Groups II and III or immediately after flushing in Group I, the small intestine was transplanted orthotopically into an unrelated dog according to standard techniques.[31] Eight inches were resected, however, from both proximal and distal ends of the small bowel before the

Table I. *Technical failures observed during preservation and following small bowel allotransplantation*

Causes	*No. of technical failures**		
	Group I	*Group II*	*Group III*
Surgical			
Hemorrhage	2 (15, 24)	1 (18)	1 (14)
Early vascular thrombosis	1 (23)	1 (28)	1 (19)
Anesthesia	1 (3)	0	1 (6)
Sepsis (generalized)	1 (15)	1 (22)	0
Dehydration	0	1 (29)	1 (40)
Total	5	4	4
Preservation			
Air emboli	0	0	1 (4)
Gram-negative contamination	0	1 (12)	1 (6)
Kinked loops	0	1 (9)	0
Total	0	2	2

*Number in parenthesis indicates time of death in hour post transplantation.

Table II. *Physical changes of small bowels perfused for 24 hours with either cryoprecipitated dog plasma or human plasmanate (mean values ± S.E.)*

Parameters	*Group II: Cryoprecipitated plasma*		*Group III: Human plasmanate*	
	Initial	*Final*	*Initial*	*Final*
Flow rate (ml./min./Gm.)	0.45 ± 0.08	0.40 ± 0.05	0.42 ± 0.09	0.40 ± 0.07
Perfusion pressure (mm. Hg)	55 ± 8.5	65 ± 4.5	55 ± 6.5	60 ± 5.4
Vascular resistance (dyne/sec./cm.$^{-5}$ × 10^3)	55.7 ± 10.6	62.8 ± 11.2	54.8 ± 10.8	64.7 ± 13.2
Fluid loss (L./24 hr.)	None	1.8 ± 0.8	None	1.0 ± 0.3
Weight gain (% from control)	None	10 ± 3.5	None	9.5 ± 3.0

intestinal anastomosis was performed. Immediately after the mesenteric anastomosis was completed and the clamps were released, methylprednisolone (1.0 Gm.) was given intravenously. Biopsy specimens were taken immediately after revascularization. Before the abdominal wall was closed, one Penrose drain was left in each side of the abdominal cavity. The drain was removed three days later. Kanamycin abdominal irrigations with 250 mg. were given every 12 hours until the drains were removed.

Neither the donor nor the recipient dogs were allowed to have solid food for five days prior to transplantation, and only fluids were supplied. Kanamycin (500 mg.) and neomycin (1 Gm.) three times a day were administered orally for four days prior to surgery. Following transplantation, azathioprine (2.5 mg. per kilogram per day) was given intravenously to recipient dogs until death. Parental hyperalimentation with glucose 10 percent (I L.), albumin 25 percent (50 ml.), and vitamin B complex (1 ml.) were given intravenously daily for one week according to the clinical state of hydration. Methylprednisolone (250 mg. every eight hours) was given intravenously for two days. Chloramphenicol (500 mg., intravenously, every eight hours) and kanamycin (500 mg., intramuscularly, every 12 hours) were given for three days, and then the dosage was decreased to once a day for one week. Oral feeding was begun by the seventh postoperative day. On several occasions, however, when the animal did not tolerate oral intake, intravenous feedings were maintained until better clinical state was attained.

All animals were examined daily until death. Values for hemoglobin, hematocrit, leukocyte count, serum electrolytes, total proteins, albumin, and globulins were determined every other day for the first week and once a week thereafter. The D-xylose absorption tests were performed at weekly in-

Table III. *Chemical and metabolic changes of small bowel perfusate during 24 hours perfusion with either cryoprecipitated dog plasma or human plasmanate (mean values ± S.E.)*

Determinations	Group II: Cryoprecipitated plasma		Group III: Human plasmanate	
	Initial	Final	Initial	Final
LDH (40-80 U./100 ml.)	39.5 ± 6.5	75.5 ± 15.5	49.7 ± 13.8	80 ± 10.2
SGOT (0-40 U./100 ml.)*	27.5 ± 12.7	35.8 ± 6.5	31.2 ± 6.7	40.5 ± 5.2
β-glucuronidase (80-120 U./100 ml.)*	93.7 ± 11.2	125 ± 15.2	100.3 ± 18.2	115 ± 10.5
Potassium (3.5-5.5 mEq./L.)*	3.9 ± 0.7	5.8 ± 1.5	4.1 ± 0.4	5.9 ± 0.9
Sodium (138-142 mEq./L.)*	139 ± 3.2	138 ± 6.5	138 ± 2.7	140 ± 4.5
Osmolarity (270-300 mOsm./L.)*	285 ± 12.5	295 ± 5.5	287 ± 13.2	282 ± 10.2
Oxygen consumption (ml./min./100 Gm.)	1.5 ± 0.09	1.3 ± 0.07	1.6 ± 0.08	1.4 ± 0.05
Lactic acid (10-20 mg./100 ml.)*	11.5 ± 6.2	18 ± 5.2	13.2 ± 7.1	20.6 ± 4.5
D-xylose (120 min.) (4-8 mg. %)*	5.6 ± 1.1	6.5 ± 2.1	5.9 ± 1.4	7.3 ± 1.9

*Normal values.

Table IV. *Proteins and electrolytes excreted from the small bowel lumen during perfusion (mean values ± S.E.)*

	Group II: Cryoprecipitated plasma		Group III: Human plasmanate	
	12 hr.	24 hr.	12 hr.	24 hr.
Total proteins (Gm. %)	3.6 ± 1.0	5.4 ± 1.5	4.2 ± 0.9	6.2 ± 2.3
Albumin (Gm. %)	2.0 ± 0.7	2.5 ± 1.3	1.7 ± 1.2	2.4 ± 1.7
Globulin (Gm. %)	1.6 ± 1.2	2.7 ± 1.1	2.5 ± 0.7	3.8 ± 1.4
Sodium (mEq./L.)	155.3 ± 17.5	162.5 ± 20.7	151.4 ± 23.7	171.6 ± 36.5
Potassium (mEq./L.)	7.5 ± 2.3	8.7 ± 2.8	8.2 ± 1.8	9.1 ± 2.3

tervals in all dogs in accordance with standard techniques.[29, 31] Vitamin A absorption tests were performed by giving 100,000 U. (62 mg.) of vitamin A orally and sampling venous blood at 0, 40, 80, 120, and 240 minutes. Vitamin A content of serum was determined by the technique of Sobel and Snow.[35] This test was performed weekly at the same time as the D-xylose absorption tests. Postmortem examinations were performed in all dogs.

All the animals with gross technical failures are listed in Table I. These dogs were eliminated from the final group for analysis. There were ten dogs in each group the deaths of which were not clearly related to technical failure, and these dogs are used for all subsequent data compilations.

RESULTS

Perfusion and preservation characteristics. The small bowels perfused with either cryoprecipitated plasma or plasmanate did not show significant changes during 24 hours preservation. The flow rate, perfusion pressure, and vascular resistance were very similar to each other during the entire perfusion (Table II). The fluid loss reached 2.6 L. in 24 hours in Group II and 1.3 L. in Group III. The weight gain after 24 hours was slightly increased in both groups. The perfusate concentrations of lactic dehydrogenase (LDH), serum glutamic oxaloacetic transaminase (SGOT), and β-glucuronidase were near the upper limits of normal. Similar results were observed for osmolarity, sodium, potassium, and lactic acid (Table III). The oxygen consumption and the D-xylose absorption were also not modified by 24 hours of bowel perfusion. In addition, a similar protein and electrolyte excretion pattern was observed at 12 and 24 hours after perfusion (Table IV).

The bowel from all groups immediately after grafting had active tone with some indirect signs of motility and minimal gross

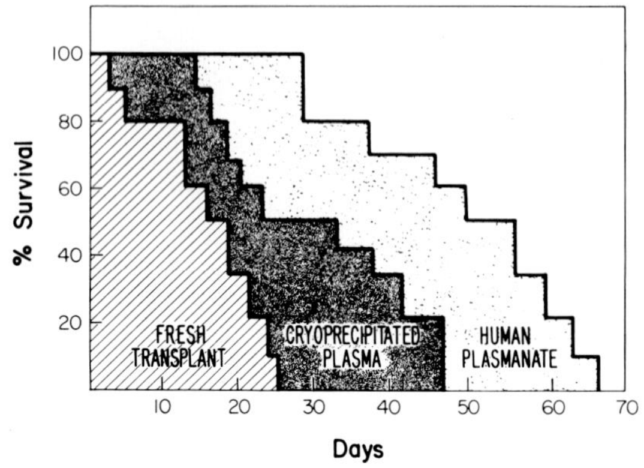

Fig. 2. Survival of the dogs allotransplanted with nonperfused small bowel and organs perfused with canine cryoprecipitated plasma and human plasmanate.

damage to the serosa, mucosa, or mesentery. There were no hemorrhagic areas. The appearance of the tissues on histologic examination was practically normal, and there was no evidence of villi necrosis or signs of hemorrhage. There was, however, minimal interstitial inflammation.

Survival. The survival of dogs receiving technically satisfactory graft is summarized in Fig. 2. The dogs with small bowel allotransplanted immediately after flushing, without perfusion, generally survived more than two weeks. The main causes of death were intestinal obstruction, cachexia, and vascular thrombosis. Classical microscopic signs of rejection were not observed except in one case. The dogs receiving small intestinal allotransplants after 24 hours of perfusion in Group II (cryoprecipitated plasma) and Group III (human plasmanate) survived for much longer periods of time than did fresh transplants (Fig. 2). The longest survival was observed in the dogs transplanted with small bowels perfused with human plasmanate (Group III). The cause of death among dogs of Group II and III were rejection (45 percent), cachexia (15 percent), late vascular thrombosis (10 percent), and obstruction (10 percent). Four dogs (20 percent) died of other causes such as: small bowel perforation (two), local peritonitis with abscess (one), and severe liver disease (one).

Except for the differences in survival, there were practically no clinical differences among the three groups of dogs (Fig. 3). All dogs lost weight at almost the same rate, and weight loss reached 30 percent in dogs which survived more than six weeks after grafting. Anemia and hypoproteinemia with hypoalbuminemia were constant features in all animals and preoperative values were not attained by any of the dogs, although slight improvement in serum protein and albumin levels were seen five weeks after transplantation in Group III. The best results of D-xylose absorption were observed five weeks after transplantation in dogs of Group III. It was evident, however, that longer periods of survival did not correct the weight gain, the anemia, or the hypoproteinemia. Furthermore, the improvements in D-xylose absorption at five weeks after grafting disappeared by six weeks after transplantation.

DISCUSSION

Most of the physiologic and morphologic observations on intestinal allografts have been performed on short heterotopic segments[3, 7, 13, 16, 26, 27, 43, 46] and thus cannot answer the question whether animals will survive for any period of time when the intestinal allograft is the sole source of absorption. Short heterotopic segments appear to undergo classic rejection in hosts which receive no immunosuppression.[7, 26] With the use of immunosuppression, such short heterotopic segments survived for prolonged periods.[13, 16, 22, 26, 43] In contrast, animals which receive total or near total orthotopic small intestinal transplants do not seem to undergo the classic changes of rejection.[31] Ruiz and associates[31] have suggested that the massive lymphatic transplant produces a graft-versus-host reaction in the recipient which complicates the clinical and pathological picture. In any case, recipients of total small bowel intestinal allografts rarely survive more than three weeks.[31] Only Ruiz and associates[31] have observed a mean survival in immunosuppressed dogs of two weeks with the longest single survivor living 42 days. The studies here present dogs

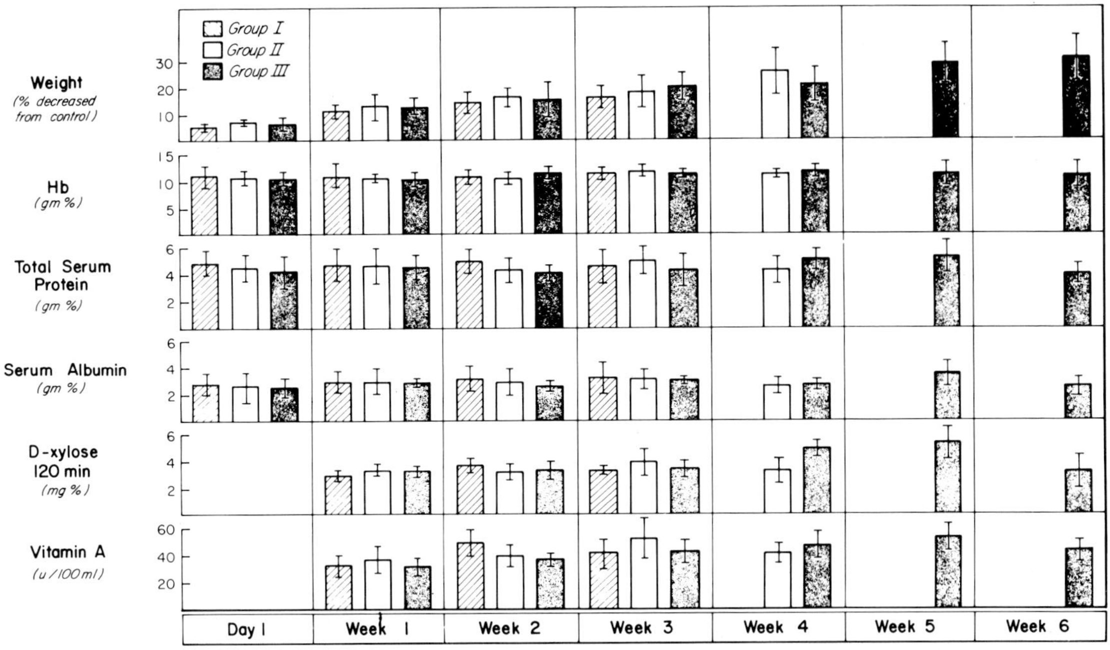

Fig. 3. Weight pattern, hematology, serum chemistries, and absorption values of all dogs following small bowel allotransplantation (mean values ± S.E.).

which survive longer than any other in the literature with a mean survival of 45 days and the longest animal living 67 days. The amount of azathioprine used in these animals is not generally sufficient to allow renal allograft survival between unrelated randomly chosen dogs more than ten to 12 days.[6]

To achieve such prolonged survival, certain modifications of the standard orthotopic allotransplantation technique were devised. Both donor and recipient intestinal tracts were treated vigorously with antibiotic agents for five days. Postoperative antibiotic agents both intraperitoneally and systemically were utilized, and small segments of bowel were removed from each end prior to anastomosis in order to alleviate mechanical problems involved in the anastomosis. With the use of these procedures plus the use of azathioprine, even fresh allotransplants show prolonged survival (mean, 14.5 days, the longest time being 25 days) when compared with our previous experience with intestinal allografts.[44]

Two groups of animals achieved even longer survival times. Both groups received grafts preserved for 24 hours by hypothermic bloodless perfusion with the use of two different perfusate solutions. Both perfusate solutions contained the same additives which include methylprednisolone which is known in some circumstances to reduce the immunogenicity of some allografts.[20, 21] In other respects, the perfusates were different. Pooled cryoprecipitated dog plasma (Group II) was utilized for one perfusate, and this prolonged the survival of intestinal allografts; the second perfusate (Group III) was human plasmanate which led to the greatest prolongation of allograft in dog survival.

Prolongation of allograft survival has been achieved in the past mainly by suppression of the recipients immune response. Fewer studies have been concerned with prolonging graft survival by inducing modification of the antigenicity or immunogenicity of allografts. Treatment of allografts *in vitro* with corticoids,[20, 21] thalidomide,[15] urethane,[5] radiation,[38] or electrophoresis,[10, 21] have prolonged the survival of some allografts to a greater degree than systemic administration of these same agents. In vitro treatment of grafts with streptokinase-streptodornase,[8] ribonucleic acid,[23] or with purified recipient transplantation antigens[14] results in lesser degrees of prolongation than results obtained from pharmacologic manipulations. Minimal or no immune reaction has been observed toward allografts treated *in vitro* with formalin,[36] cyanide,[11] or by freeze-drying.[1] Schechter[33] reports that mouse skin allografts treated in vitro with gluteraldehyde prolong their survival from 12.4 to 39.2 days has recently been shown to be due to death of the skin allograft in our laboratories.[17, 32] Ray and Simmons[28] have recently shown that it is possible to mask histocompatibility antigens on suspended lymphoid cells with substances which bind to those lymphocytes such as plant lectins. Lippman[24] has also shown that various glycoproteins such as condroitin sulphate and heparin will reduce the immunogenicity of grafts.

One of the most promising methods of reducing the immunogenicity of grafts have been the use of Fab fragments of antibodies directed against the histocompatibility antigens themselves.[39, 42, 47] These antibody fragments which lack the Fc (complement binding) portion of the antibody molecule might be expected to mask histocompatibility antigens on the grafts. A similar, but apparently non-specific effect has been found by Callender and associates[6] in our laboratories utilizing heterologous antilymphoblast globulin which apparently binds to kidney grafts, thereby reducing their immunogenicity. Most strikingly, Summerlin and colleagues[40, 41] have found that skin grafts in organ culture will loose their allograft immunogenicity permanently after transplantation, allowing permanent survival in unimmunosuppressed host.

The results presented here that whole organ intestinal allografts transplanted orthotopically to moderately immunosuppressed animals survive for longer periods of time than do fresh allografts support the idea that preservation of organs might result in lessened graft immunogenicity, with preservation of graft function. The prolongation might be attributable to (1) phenomena such as that described by Summerlin and colleagues[40, 41] by which preservation itself alters the immunogenicity of a graft, (2) the presence in the perfusate of different agents (i.e. heparin,[24] hydrocortisone,[21] methylprednisolone,[20] ampicillin, kanamycin, magnesium sulphate, insulin, or phenophthalein) which chemically alters the immunogens, (3) the perfusion itself may wash out passenger leukocytes[37] which are thought to provide a major immunogenic stimulus in any graft,[12, 37] (4) cryoprecipitated plasma may contain substances which bind non-specifically to graft surfaces, thereby reducing their immunogenicity.

The further prolongation of graft survival when human plasmanate was utilized is even more impressive. There is considerable evidence that animals and humans possess antibodies against the tissue antigens of xenogenic species.[34] It may be that human plasmanate contains such antibodies which bind at hypothermic temperatures, thereby interfering with the perception of allogenic antigens on the graft by unrelated dogs.

Since the process by which huge allografts of lymphoid containing organs such as intestines is not clear and since such interaction may include a degree of graft-versus-host reaction, it is possible that the interactions between perfusate and graft interfere with the graft-versus-host reaction rather than mask the tissue antigens. Whatever the case, these hypotheses are suitable for subsequent experimental verification or contradiction, but the results strongly suggest there is room for graft modification in the prolongation of whole organ grafts.

REFERENCES

1. Abbott, W. M., and Pappas, A. M.: Comparative studies on fresh and preserved skin: Fundamental biological differences in behavior as grafts, Ann. Surg. **172:** 781, 1970.
2. Amador, L. E., Dorfman, L. E., and Wacker, W. E. C.: Serum lactic dehydrogenase activity: An analytical assessment of current assays, Clin. Chem. **9:** 391, 1963.
3. Barnett, W. O., Truett, G., and Stone, J.: Experimental small bowel homografts, Am. J. Dig. Dis. **7:** 833, 1962.
4. Belzer, F. O., and Kountz, S. D.: Preservation

and transplantation of human cadaver kidneys: A two-year experience, Ann. Surg. **172:** 394, 1970.

5. Bonmassar, E., Francescori, G., Mansoni, S. C., and Prelli-Ercolini, M.: Chemical detection of histocompatibility antigens–Homograft survival of rat skin treated with "Urethan" *in vitro,* Nature **209:** 1141, 1966.
6. Callender, C. O., Santiago, E. A., Santiago, E. A., Sutherland, D. E., Howard, R. J., Toledo-Pereyra, L. H., Olson, L., Condie, R., Simmons, R. L., and Najarian, J. S.: Renal allograft prolongation after graft perfusion with heterologous ALG, Surg. Forum **24:** 306, 1973.
7. Cohen, W. B., Hardy, M. A., Quint, J., and State, D.: Absorptive function in canine jejunal autografts and allografts, SURGERY **65:** 440, 1969.
8. Dukes, C. D., and Blocker, T. G.: Studies on the survival of skin homografts. I. Prolongation of life of full-thickness grafts by the action of streptokinase-streptodornase, Ann. Surg. **136:** 999, 1962.
9. Fishman, W. H., and Bernfeld, P.: Colowick, S. P., and Kaplan, N. O., editors: Glucuronidases in methods in enzymology, New York, 1955, Academic Press, vol. I, pp. 262-269.
10. Gemahlich, M.: Ein neues Prinzip zur Verlangerung der Uberlebensdauer von Hauthomiotransplantaten, Bruns. Beitr. Klin. Chir. **210:** 245, 1965.
11. Grillo, H. C., and McKhann, C. F.: The acceptance and evolution of dermal homografts freed of viable cells, Transplantation **2:** 48, 1964.
12. Guttmann, R. D., and Lindquist, R. R.: Renal transplantation in the inbred rat. XI. Reduction of allograft immunogenicity by cytotoxic drug pretreatment of donors, Transplantation **8:** 490, 1969.
13. Hardy, M. A., Quint, J., and State, D.: Effect of antilymphocyte serum and other immunosuppressive agents on canine jejunal allografts, Ann. Surg. **171:** 51, 1970.
14. Hellmann, K., and Duke, D. I.: *In vitro* alteration of skin graft antigenicity, Transplantation **5:** 184, 1967.
15. Hellman, K., Duke, D. I., and Tucker, D. T.: Prolongation of skin homograft survival by thalidomide, Br. Med. J. **2:** 687, 1965.
16. Holmes, J. T., Yek, S. D. J., Winawer, S. J., Kawano, N., and Fortner, J. G.: Absorption studies in canine jejunal allografts, Ann. Surg. **174:** 101, 1971.
17. Im, H. M., and Simmons, R. L.: Mechanism for the prolonged survival of glutaraldehyde-treated skin allografts, Transplantation **14:** 527, 1972.
18. Karmen, A. J.: A note on the spectrophotometric assay of glutamic-oxalacetic transaminase in human blood serum, J. Clin. Invest. **34:** 131, 1955.
19. Klaue, P., and Jolley, W. B.: The comparative effectiveness of corticosteroids applied topically as pretreatment of rabbit skin allografts, SURGERY **70:** 718, 1971.
20. Klaue, P., and Jolley, W. B.: Prolongation of rabbit skin allograft survival following treatment of the skin with electrophoresis prior to transplantation, Transplantation **11:** 30, 1971.
21. Klaue, P., and Jolley, W. B.: Prolonged survival of rabbit skin allograft after treatment with locally applied triamcinolone acetonide in combination with small doses of systemic immunosuppressives, Transplantation **13:** 53, 1972.
22. Kunklin, A., Gaston, J. P., Shiu, M. H., Winawer, S. J., and Fortner, J. G.: The isolated allograft pouch: A useful method for monitoring small bowel allografts, Surg. Forum **23:** 237, 1972.
23. Lemperle, G.: Prolonged survival of skin allografts after incubation with recipient DNA or RNA, J. Surg. Res. **8:** 511, 1968.
24. Lippman, M.: Transplantation and cytotoxicity changes induced by acid mucopolysaccharides, Nature **219:** 33, 1968.
25. Moberg, A. W., Mozes, M. F., Santiago, E. A., Campos, R., Mason, R., and Najarian, J. S.: A new transplantable organ perfusion system: Experimental and clinical experience. Lancet **2:** 1403, 1971.
26. Preston, F. W., Macalalad, F., Wachouski, T. J., Randolph, D. A., and Apostol, J. V.: Survival of homografts of the intestine with and without immunosuppression, SURGERY **60:** 1203, 1966.
27. Quint, J., Hardy, M. A., and State, D.: Effects of antilymphocyte serum on absorptive function and survival of dog intestinal allografts. Surg. Forum **19:** 184, 1968.
28. Ray, P. K., and Simmons, R. L.: Masking of cellular histocompatibility antigens with phytomitogens, J. Immunol. **110:** 1693, 1973.
29. Roe, J. H., and Rice, E. W.: Photometric method for determination of free pentoses in animal tissue, J. Biol. Chem. **173:** 307, 1948.
30. Rosenberg, J. C., and Rush, B. F.: Enzymatic spectrophotometric determination of pyruvic and lactic acid in blood, Clin. Chem. **12:** 299, 1966.
31. Ruiz, J. O., Uchida, H., Schultz, L. S., and Lillehei, R. C.: Problems in absorption and immunosuppression after entire small bowel allotransplantation, Am. J. Surg. **123:** 297, 1972.
32. Santiago-Delpin, E. A., Yunis, E. J., Callender, C. O., and Najarian, J. S.: Effect of

glutaraldehyde on skin grafts, Proc. Soc. Exp. Biol. Med. **141:** 996, 1972.

33. Schechter, I.: Prolonged survival of glutaraldehyde-treated skin homografts, Proc. Natl. Acad. Sci. **68:** 1590, 1971.
34. Shons, A. R., Moberg, A. W., and Najarian, J. S.: Xenotransplantation, *in* Najarian, J. S. and Simmons, R. L., editors: Transplantation, Philadelphia, 1972, Lea & Febiger.
35. Sobel, A. E., and Snow, S. D.: The estimation of serum vitamin A with activated glycerol dichlorhydrin, J. Biol. Chem. **171:** 617, 1947.
36. Silverstein, P., Raulston, G. L., Walker, H., Foley, F. D., and Pruitt, B. A.: Evaluation of formalin-fixed skin as a temporary dressing for granulating wounds, Surg. Forum **22:** 60, 1971.
37. Steinmuller, D.: Allograft immunity produced with skin isografts from immunologically tolerant mice, Transplant. Proc. **1:** 593, 1969.
38. Steinmuller, D., Warden, G., Coleman, M., Lofgreen, J., and Reentsma, K.: Prolonged survival of rat heart and kidney allografts irradiated *in vitro,* Transplantation **12:** 155, 1971.
39. Stuart, F. P., Saitoh, T., Fitxh, F. W., and Spargo, B. H.: Immunologic enhancement of renal allografts in the rat, SURGERY **64:** 17, 1968.
40. Summerlin, W. T., Broutbar, C., Foanes, R. B., Payne, R., Stutman, O., Hayflich, L., and Good, R. A.: Acceptance of phenotypically differing cultured skin in man and mice, Transplant. Proc. **5:** 707, 1973.
41. Summerlin, W. T., Charlton, E., and Kanasek, M. J.: Transplantation of organ cultures of adult human skin, J. Invest. Dermatol. **55:** 310, 1970.
42. Sutherland, D. E. R., Howard, R. J., and Najarian, J. S.: Immunological enhancement of renal allografts in an outbred animal susceptible to hyperacute rejection, Fed. Proc. **32:** 971, 1973.
43. Taylor, R. M. R., Watson, J. W., Walker, F. C., and Watson, A. J.: Prolongation of survival of jejunal homografts in dogs treated with azathioprine (Imuran), Br. J. Surg. **153:** 134, 1969.
44. Toledo-Pereyra, L. H., and Najarian, J. S.: Small bowel preservation for allotransplantation, Surg. Gynecol. Obstet. **137:** 445, 1973.
45. Toledo-Pereyra, L. H., and Najarian, J. S.: Small bowel preservation: Comparison of perfusion and nonperfusion systems, Arch. Surg. **107:** 875, 1973.
46. Westbrook, D. L., Rothengatter, C., Vriesendorp, H. M., and van Rood, J. J.: Histocompatibility and heterotopic segmental small bowel allograft survival in dogs, Eur. Surg. Res. **2:** 401, 1970.
47. Wilson, R. E., Pippin, A., Dagher, R. K., Kinneart, P., and Bush, G. J.: Prolonged canine renal allograft survival after pretreatment with solubilized antigen, Transplantation **7:** 360, 1969.

Exposure of the tibial-peroneal arteries by a single lateral approach

Herbert Dardik, M.D., Irving Dardik, M.D., *and* **Frank J. Veith, M.D.,** *Bronx, N. Y.*

A lateral approach with fibular resection provides excellent exposure of the tibial and peroneal arteries of the upper leg. Bypass grafting to either of these vessels is feasible and suggested when preoperative angiograms show severe diffuse stenosis or occlusion of the popliteal artery or when intraoperative angiography or surgical exploration discloses unsuspected major occlusive disease of the distal popliteal artery. Delayed films will often show reconstitution of one or more of the leg vessels amenable to revascularization by the lateral approach.

From the Department of Surgery, Montefiore Hospital and Medical Center and the Albert Einstein College of Medicine, Bronx, N. Y.

THE MOUNTING evidence for the success of bypass grafting to the tibial and peroneal arteries in the lower extremity[4, 5, 9, 11, 12, 14] has focused on the need for improved exposure of these arteries. The standard medial approach as employed by Imperato and associates[7] provides ready access to the distal popliteal artery and only the upper portions of the tibial arteries. Tyson and Reichle[13, 15] also approach the posterior tibial and peroneal arteries by a medial incision placed just posterior to the tibia. These arteries can be easily dissected in the fascial plane deep to the soleus and flexor hallicus longus muscles, respectively. The peroneal artery lies lateral by this approach. A separate anterior incision is required for the anterior tibial artery. Minken and May[10] also described a medial approach to the posterior tibial and peroneal arteries. Evans and Bernhard and associates[1, 4] employ separate incisions for each of the leg arteries, vertical anterolateral for the anterior tibial, medial for the posterior tibial, and lateral for the peroneal. Rongeuring off the posterior half of the fibula is additionally recommended for exposure of the peroneal artery.

Accepted for publication Nov. 26, 1973.

Reprint requests: Dr. H. Dardik, 1555 Center Ave., Fort Lee, N. J. 07024.

Our interest in a single approach to all the vessels of the upper leg was stimulated by experience with a patient who sustained fractures of the proximal left tibia and fibula in an auto accident. Soon after initial evaluation, the left foot became severely ischemic with loss of pedal pulsations and marked swelling of the entire leg. Operation was performed by the lateral approach with resection of the fibula from the neck distally to the lower third. Copious hematoma was released and bleeding from distal sites appeared as the tense, swollen musculature was decompressed. The distal popliteal artery and its bifurcation into anterior tibial and tibioperoneal trunks were readily identified. The division of the latter could also be easily traced. We have since confirmed

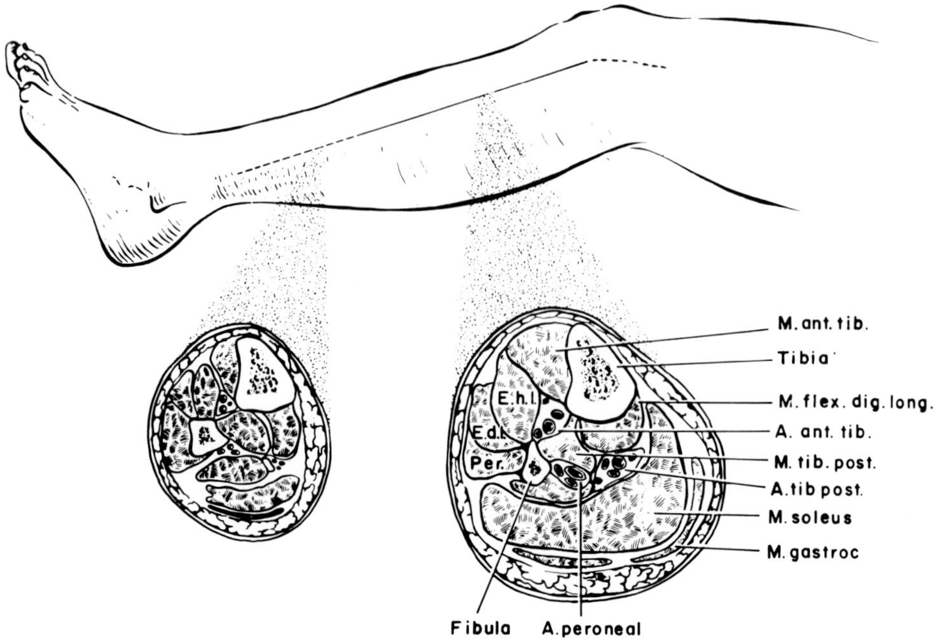

Fig. 1. Location of skin incision for lateral exposure of small vessels of leg. Cephalad extension enables resection of fibular head. Normal anatomic relationships at upper and lower third levels of leg are depicted in cross-section.

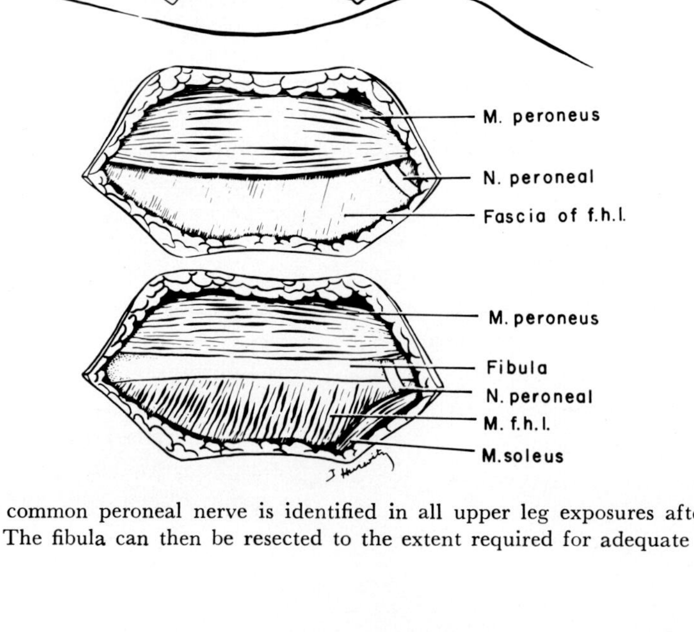

Fig. 2. The common peroneal nerve is identified in all upper leg exposures after incising the deep fascia. The fibula can then be resected to the extent required for adequate exposure.

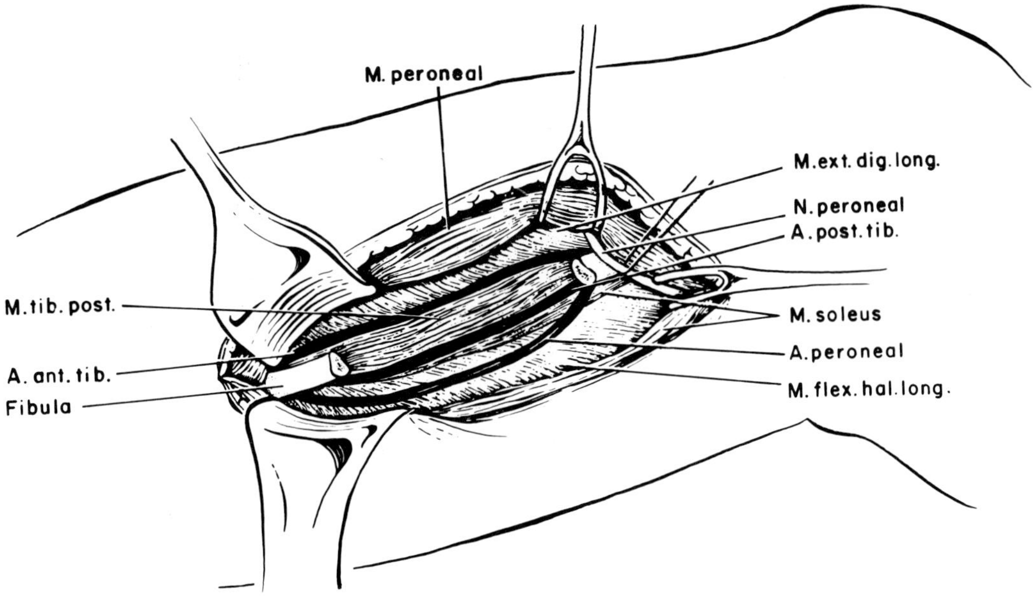

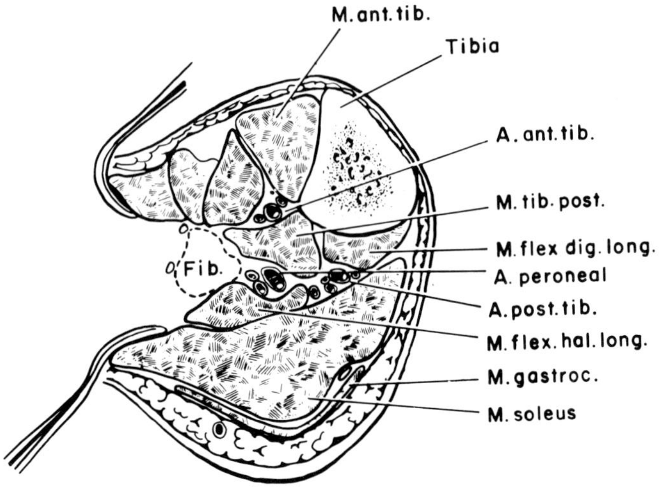

Fig. 3. Anatomic relationships of the three leg arteries to adjacent muscles in the upper leg. The opened cross-section depicts the mode of this approach.

the simplicity and adequacy of this approach by dissection of four amputated limbs.

TECHNIQUE

The patient is positioned with the involved extremity rotated medially and flexed approximately 60 degrees at the knee. The skin incision is placed over the fibula beginning at the head and carried distally 15 cm. or further if necessary (Fig. 1). If the head of the fibula must be resected to improve exposure of the distal popliteal artery, the incision is extended cephalad along the inferior margin of the biceps tendon. For implantation into the middle or lower one-third leg levels, the incision is centered directly over that segment of the fibula. After incising the skin, subcutaneous layer and deep fascia, the common peroneal nerve is identified and dissected in the upper angle of the operative field as it courses about the neck of the fibula (Fig. 2). The fascia between the peroneus longus and

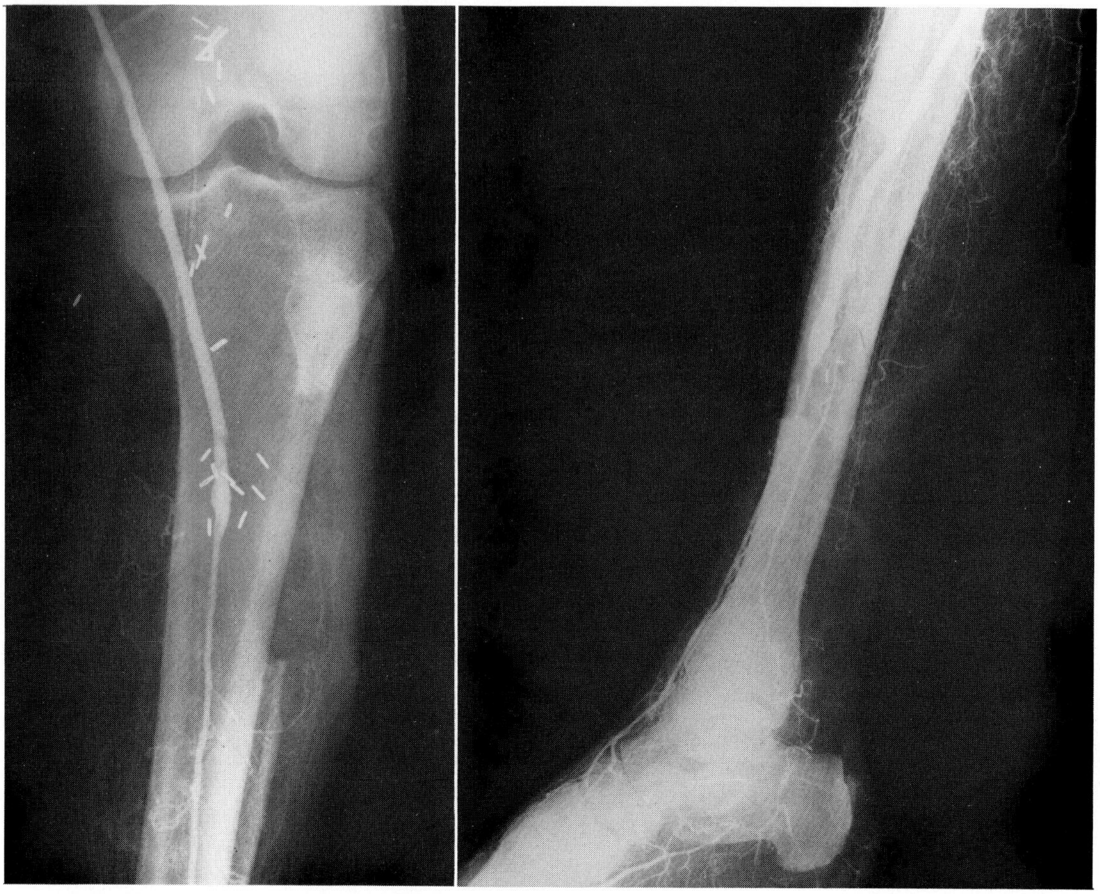

Fig. 4*A*. Intraoperative arteriogram of a femoroperoneal bypass graft. Note resected fibula segment.

Fig. 4*B*. Popliteal-anterior tibial bypass to lower leg level by lateral approach.

soleus muscles is divided along the length of the incision. As this intermuscular plane is developed, the lateral margin of the fibula is exposed by retracting the peroneus longus anteriorly and the soleus posteriorly. Subperiosteal resection of the fibula brings the tibialis posterior muscle into direct view in the center of the operative field. The anterior tibial artery is identified anterior to the tibialis posterior muscle and just behind the extensor digitorum longus. The peroneal artery is easily dissected on the surface of the flexor hallicus longus as the latter is retracted posteriorly (Fig. 3). The posterior tibial artery lies deep in the operative field but can be mobilized into it by separating the tibialis posterior and flexor hallicus longus muscles. The dissection is comparable at all levels of the leg except for the obvious care needed in dissecting the peroneal nerve at the upper level of the leg.

Each of the vessels can be prepared to accept a bypass graft by meticulous dissection of investing tissue. Often division of numerous venous channels that course with the artery is required. Hemoclips facilitate this phase of the operation. Elastic vessel loops are employed for both retraction and control of bleeding. Intraoperative angiograms are performed routinely (Figs. 4*A* and 4*B*). Wound closure consists simply of approximating deep fascia, subcutaneous tissue, and skin in separate layers. Suction catheter drainage is advocated for 24 to 48 hours, being cautious to place the catheter away from vascular structures. Postoperative angiography may be required to demonstrate graft patency and evolution of defects in the graft or runoff that may be amenable to operative correction (Fig. 5).

DISCUSSION

Exposure of the tibial and peroneal vessels by the lateral approach with fibular resection has been described by Elkin and Kelley[3] and by Henry.[6] Danese and Singer[2] called attention to its use for exposing the popliteal trifurcation and its application in three instances of bypass grafting to the anterior tibial artery. Jackson[8] also employed the lateral approach for bypass grafting to the anterior tibial artery in eight cases.

We have employed the lateral approach with fibular resection for vascular reconstruction in seventeen cases. This is in addition to its use for compartmental decompression of the leg and exploration of the distal popliteal artery in cases of trauma. Femoroposterior tibial bypasses were performed in two cases. Femoral or popliteal peroneal bypasses were performed in fourteen cases with one case of a popliteal anterior tibial bypass. Autogenous saphenous vein was used in all but one instance where a bovine heterograft was employed. For another one of the femoroperoneal bypasses, a composite was constructed of proximal bovine heterograft and distal autogenous saphenous vein. The dissection of the arteries proved simple and the exposure more than adequate. Intraoperative angiography can be performed prior to reconstruction to assess runoff and optimal site of the distal anastomosis. Repeat studies after all anastomoses are completed are important in order to demonstrate and correct potential technical problems.

Early patency (less than six months) was achieved in twelve of the seventeen cases (71 percent). All five failures occurred within the first week following surgery. Of six cases followed beyond six months and for as long as 1½ years, one femoral peroneal bypass failed at seven months. All six failures underwent successful below-knee amputations but hospitalization and rehabilitation were prolonged in three because of wound problems. Thus, failure of vascular reconstruction by this approach does not necessarily convert the potential below-knee amputation to an above-knee level.

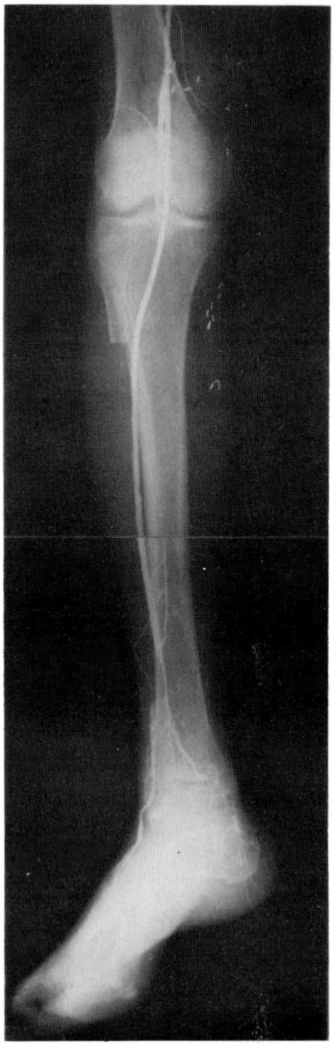

Fig. 5. Postoperative angiogram of a popliteal-peroneal bypass extending to lower leg level by lateral approach.

Patients selected for this approach should have demonstrated severe occlusive disease of the distal popliteal artery either preoperatively or during surgery. Often delayed films will show reconstitution of a tibial or peroneal artery that can serve for a distal vascular anastomosis by the lateral approach.

REFERENCES

1. Bernhard, V. M., Ashmore, C. S., Evans, W. E., and Rodgers, R. E.: Bypass grafting to distal arteries for limb salvage, Surg. Gynecol. Obstet. **135:** 219, 1972.
2. Danese, C. A., and Singer, A.: Lateral approach to the popliteal artery trifurcation, SURGERY **63:** 588, 1968.
3. Elkin, D. C., and Kelley, R. P.: Arteriovenous aneurysm: Exposure of the tibial and peroneal vessels by resection of the fibula, Ann. Surg. **122:** 529, 1945.
4. Evans, W. E., and Bernhard, V. M.: Tibial artery bypass for limb salvage, Arch. Surg. **100:** 477, 1970.
5. Garrett, H. E., Kotch, P. I., Green, M. T., et al.: Distal tibial artery bypass with autogenous vein grafts: An analysis of 56 cases, SURGERY **63:** 90, 1968.
6. Henry, A. K.: Extensile exposure, ed. 2, Baltimore, 1957, Williams and Wilkins Co.
7. Imperato, A. M., Kim, G. E., and Chu, D. S.: Surgical exposure for reconstruction of the proximal part of the tibial artery, Surg. Gynecol. Obstet. **136:** 453, 1973.
8. Jackson, B. B.: Anterior tibial artery in revascularization of the leg and foot, Am. J. Surg. **107:** 907, 1964.
9. Kaminski, D. L., Barner, H. B., Dorighi, J. A., et al.: Femoral-tibial bypass grafting, Arch. Surg. **104:** 527, 1972.
10. Minken, S. L., and May, A. G.: Use of peroneal artery for revascularization of the lower extremity, Arch. Surg. **99:** 594, 1969.
11. Noon, G. P., Diethrich, E. B., Richardson, W. P., and De Bakey, M. E.: Distal tibial arterial bypass: Analysis of 91 cases, Arch. Surg. **99:** 770, 1969.
12. Reichle, F. A., and Tyson, R. R.: Bypasses to tibial or popliteal arteries in severely ischemic lower extremities: Comparison of long-term results in 233 patients, Ann. Surg. **176:** 315, 1972.
13. Tyson, R. R., and Reichle, F. A.: Femorotibial bypass, Ann. Surg. **170:** 429, 1969.
14. Tyson, R. R., and Reichle, F. A.: Femorotibial bypass for salvage of the ischemic lower extremity, Surg. Gynecol. Obstet. **134:** 771, 1972.
15. Tyson, R. R., and Reichle, F. A.: Technique of femorotibial bypass, SURGERY **68:** 730, 1970.

Nonoperative closure of atrial septal defects

Terry D. King, M.D., *and* **Noel L. Mills, M.D.,** *New Orleans, La.*

Atrial septal defects (ASD) were created in 13 adult dogs. An experimental technique and apparatus have been developed for transvenous closure of the defects. The procedure employs a pair of interlocking umbrella-like components made of stainless steel and Dacron. The umbrellas are introduced and locked across the ASD's through an outer catheter introduced through the femoral vein. The defects can be closed within 30 minutes using this procedure. Physiologic closure was documented by repeat cardiac catheterization in the five animals in which the procedure was completed. Autopsy of these experimental animals proved complete anatomical closure of the ASD.

From the Departments of Pediatrics, Section on Pediatric Cardiology, and the Department of Surgery, Ochsner Clinic and Ochsner Foundation Hospital, New Orleans, La.

VARIOUS noninvasive techniques have been used for the diagnosis and treatment of congenital heart disease.[1, 4] Certain specific congenital heart lesions lend themselves especially to nonsurgical techniques for treatment due to current technologic advances and miniaturization. Herein is described our technique for closure of atrial septal defects (ASD's) during cardiac catheterization.

TECHNIQUE AND INSTRUMENTATION

The procedure is performed on dogs which are lightly anesthetized and breathing spontaneously. ASD's (1 to 2 cm. in diameter) are created 10 to 21 days earlier in the animals by means of a punch biopsy technique.[2] Systemic heparinization follows routine catheterization which confirms the presence and size of the ASD's.

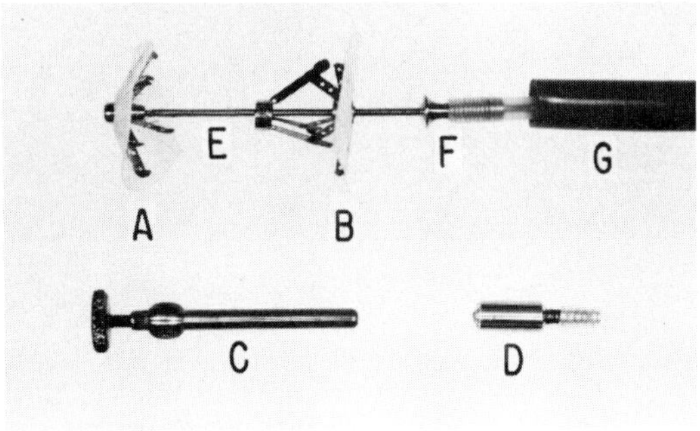

Fig. 1. Photograph of the catheter closure system showing: *(A)* left atrial umbrella, *(B)* right atrial umbrella, *(C)* T-piece, *(D)* opening cone and catheter, *(E)* threaded obturator guide wire, *(F)* locking catheter and cone, and *(G)* an outer catheter.

The device used to close the defects (Fig. 1) consists of a left atrial umbrella device, a right atrial umbrella device, a T-piece, opening cone and catheter, a threaded obturator guide wire, a locking catheter and cone, and an outer catheter.

This investigation was supported by the Alton Ochsner Medical Foundation and the Mrs. W. C. Feazel Research Award of the Louisiana Heart Association.

Accepted for publication Dec. 10, 1973.

Reprint requests: Terry D. King, M.D., Chairman, Department of Pediatrics, Ochsner Clinic, 1514 Jefferson Highway, New Orleans, La. 70121.

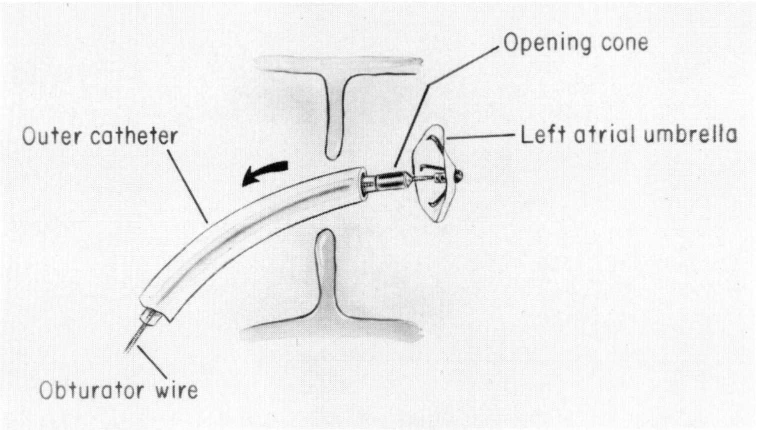

Fig. 2. The left atrial umbrella has been introduced into the left atrium and is only partially open. The opening cone and catheter will complete the opening to place the struts at right angles. The outer catheter and the obturator wire are withdrawn as the arrow indicates so as to approximate the left atrial umbrella against the left side of the interatrial septum.

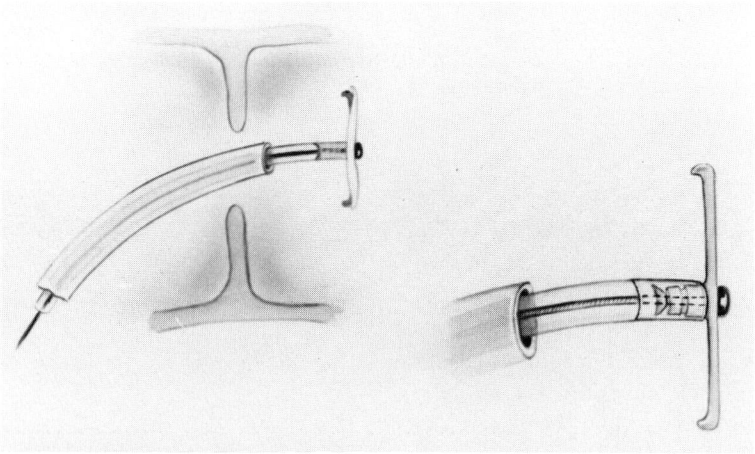

Fig. 3. The mechanism of action of the opening cone is shown. The enlarged version of the left atrial umbrella shows that the left atrial hub is actually allowed to slip inside the opening cone by means of an internal spring mechanism, thus elevating the struts to right angles.

The umbrellas are produced in sizes ranging from 1 to 3.5 cm. in diameter. A 2.0 cm. diameter locked umbrella device weighs 380 mg. The obturator wire is 1.1 mm. in diameter and 250 cm. in length.

The outer catheter is introduced via the femoral vein into the right atrium and subsequently across the ASD. The position is confirmed by oxygen data and selective cineangiocardiogram. The left atrial umbrella is advanced through the outer catheter across the ASD into the body of the left atrium and opened (Figs. 2 and 3). The outer catheter is withdrawn into the right atrium and the left atrial umbrella is fixed against the left side of the interatrial septum. The right atrial umbrella is advanced into the right atrium and opened (Fig. 4). With the locking catheter it is mated to the left atrial umbrella by a special internal locking device (Fig. 5). The T-piece is applied to the obturator wire, and with 5½ counterclockwise turns, the obturator wire is unscrewed from the locked umbrella

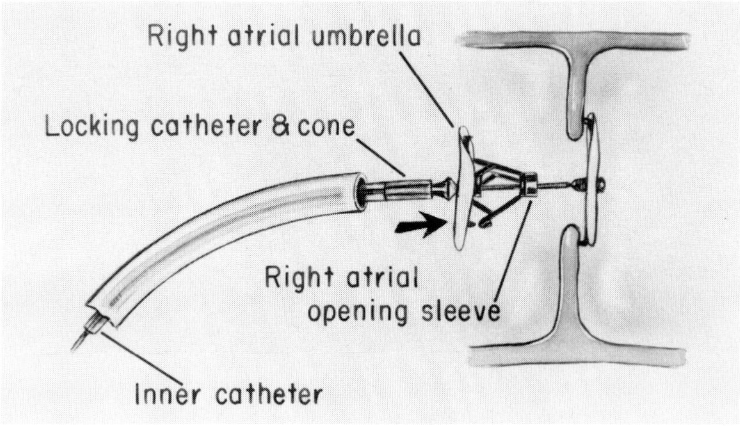

Fig. 4. The mechanism of action of the right atrial umbrella is shown. The left atrial umbrella is in place on the left side of the atrial septal defect. The right atrial umbrella and opening sleeve are being advanced toward the left atrial umbrella by the locking catheter as the arrow indicates. As the opening sleeve is advanced, the right atrial struts are elevated to a 90 degree angle.

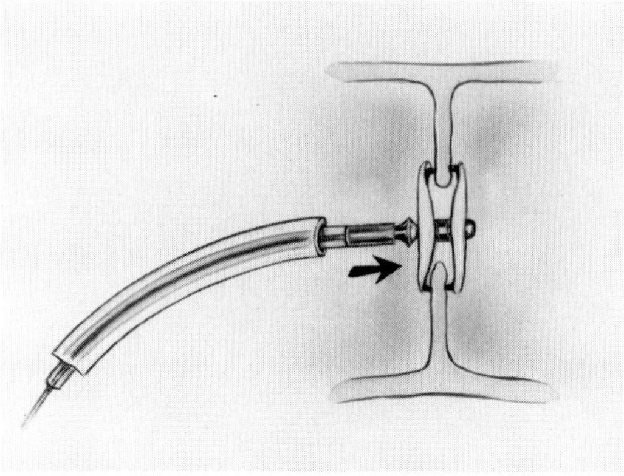

Fig. 5. The right and left umbrellas are approximated across the interatrial septal defect. With advancement of the locking catheter and with traction on the obturator wire, the locking device is engaged and the umbrellas permanently locked.

(Fig. 6). The catheters and obturator wire are withdrawn, leaving the locked umbrella device across the closed ASD (Fig. 7). The femoral vein and leg incision are closed routinely after neutralization of the heparin with protamine.

Electrocardiograms (ECG), chest x-rays, CBC's, and serum hemoglobin determinations are performed before creation of the ASD and at two-month intervals following atrial septal closure.

Table I. *Successful nonoperative closure of ASD's in five dogs*

Dog No.	*Results*
6	Killed 2 wk. after closure
12	Killed 10 mo. after closure
10	Alive and well 6 mo.
11	Alive and well 3 mo.
13	Alive and well 1 mo.

Table II. *Unsuccessful nonoperative closure of ASD's in eight dogs*

Dog No.	*Results*
1	Spontaneous closure of ASD
3	Spontaneous closure of ASD
9	Spontaneous closure of ASD
2	Failure of locking device
7	Failure of locking device
8	Failure to lock secondary to bolus of heartworms
4	Inappropriate umbrella size
5	Inappropriate umbrella size

RESULTS

The procedure has been performed on 13 adult dogs. There were five successful closures (Table I) and eight failures (Table II). Of the animals that had unsuccessful closure, three had spontaneous closure of

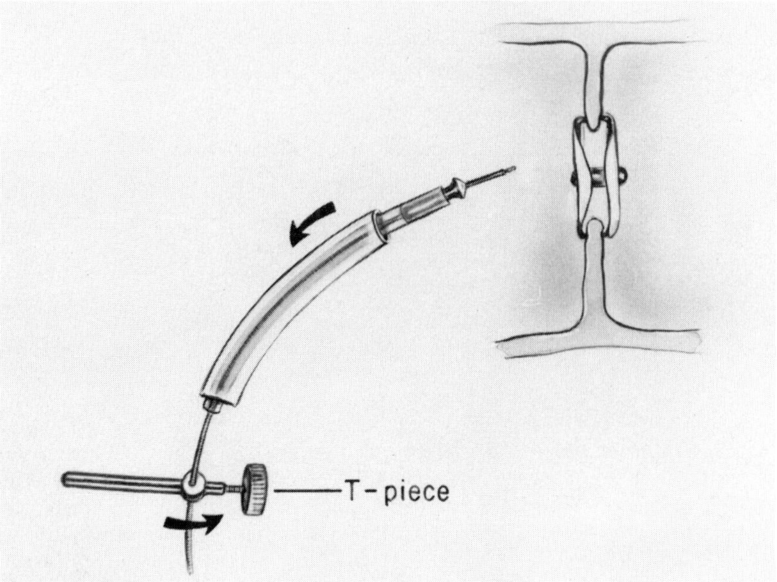

Fig. 6. With the use of the T-piece the obturator wire is unscrewed from the left atrial hub by 5½ counterclockwise turns. Once disengaged, the obturator wire and all catheters are withdrawn from the body.

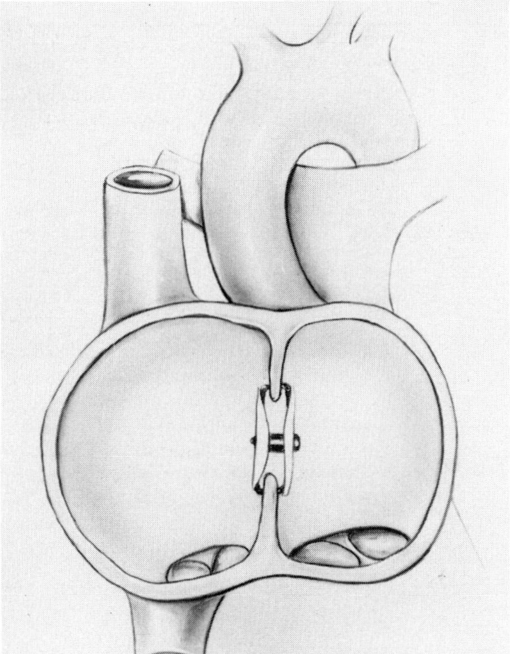

Fig. 7. An enlarged version of the right and left atria is shown with locked umbrellas in place. The total weight of a locked pair of umbrellas, 20 mm. in diameter, is approximately 380 mg.

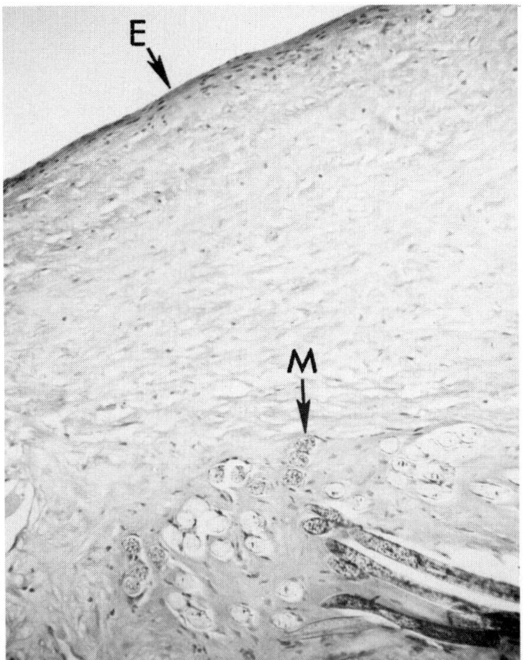

Fig. 8. Photomicrograph showing endothelialization *(E)* of the Dacron material *(M)* obtained at necropsy study of dog No. 12. (Hematoxylin and eosin; ×100.)

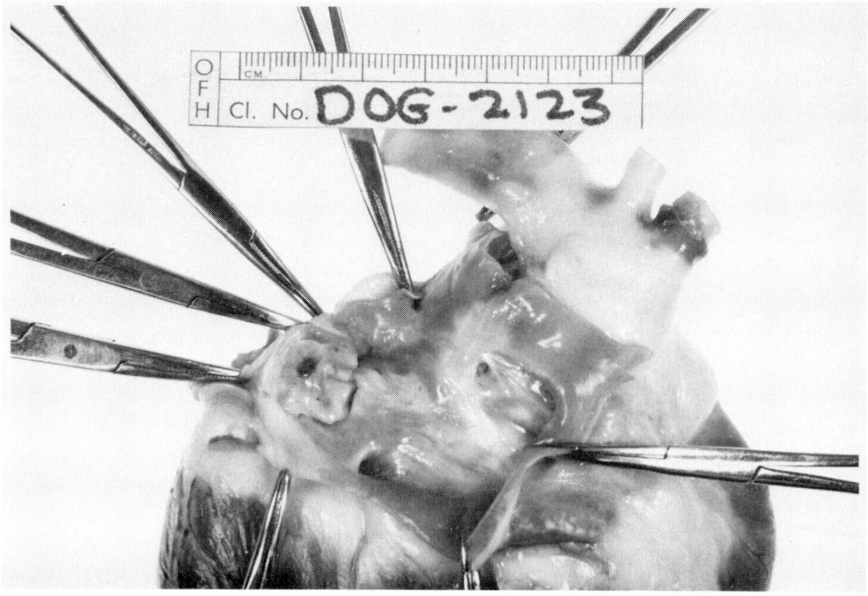

Fig. 9. Right atrial view of the successful closure of the atrial septal defect of dog No. 12 which was killed at 10 months following normal cardiac catheterization. The Dacron material is visible through the endothelial covering. The right atrial struts are also seen.

the ASD found at catheterization and proved at autopsy. We were not able to lock the umbrella device in dog No. 8 because a large bolus of heart worms *(Dirofilaria immitis)* prevented apposition of the umbrella components. In dogs Nos. 4 and 5 the left atrial umbrella diameters were of inappropriate size to be retained on the left atrial side of the defect. In dogs Nos. 2 and 7 the earlier prototype locking device failed to maintain apposition of the right and left atrial umbrellas. Systemic embolization to the aorta resulted in dog No. 7.

Five animals had complete closure of their ASD from the femoral vein. ECG's chest x-rays, serum hemoglobin determinations, and CBC's were taken at two-month intervals and revealed no significant change from control values. Dog No. 6 was put to death at two weeks and early endothelialization of the Dacron umbrellas was found. Dog No. 12 was killed at 10 months following a normal cardiac catheterization and at necropsy an intact atrial septum was found with endothelialization of the umbrellas (Figs. 8 and 9). Dogs Nos. 10, 11, and 13 are alive and well. Recatheterization, which included hydrogen electrode studies, revealed no shunt at the atrial level. All animals have gained weight and show no ill effects from closure of their ASD's with this device.

DISCUSSION

This investigation is part of an ongoing study of noninvasive closure of ASD's as well as other intercardiac shunts, such as ventricular septal defects[3] and patent ductus arteriosus. The technique is simple and reproducible. It has evolved from numerous trials with various prototype devices. The device uses only standard materials such as Dacron and stainless steel (300 series). These materials are routinely left within the heart in procedures for closure of defects and valve replacement.

We have tested the design, feasibility, and mechanism of this device in human patients during open-heart operations for routine closure of ASD's. Although we have not left these devices in place, it has been clearly demonstrated that they would be effective in closing the defects. More experimental data are necessary before application of this technique in patients in the cardiac catheterization laboratory. The initial prototype devices were less refined than the current models and clearly less reliable (Table II). Secure, reliable locking is insured with the present model and is readily appreciated at the time of mating of the umbrella components.

We are cognizant of the wide spectrum of size and configuration of ASD's encountered clinically. Certain defects, especially those associated with other anomalies, would not lend themselves to this procedure and technique. It is imperative that the size and location of the ASD be precisely determined before this type of device is used clinically. Experimentally, the ASD's can be sized by several techniques to avoid the problems encountered in dogs Nos. 4 and 5.

Experience as to the hematologic data, tissue incorporation, longevity, and arrhythmias has been extremely favorable and long-term results will be reported in the future. Further miniaturization will allow the installation of such a catheter closure system through smaller catheters and in smaller experimental animals. Our data demonstrate that transvenous closure of secundum ASD's can readily be performed as there were only four failures referable to the closure technique. With increased experience the ease and safety of this procedure has improved significantly, eliminating the early problems of sizing the defects and locking of the umbrellas.

REFERENCES

1. Forssmann, W.: Die Sonderrung des rechten Herrizens, Klin. Wochenschr. **8:** 2085, 1929.
2. May, A. G.: Technic for production of experimental ventricular septal defect, Am. J. Surg. **112:** 462, 1966.
3. Mills, N. L., Vargish, T., Kleinman, L. H., Bloomfield, D. A., and Reed, G. E.: Balloon closure of ventricular septal defect, Circulation **43** (Suppl. 1): 111, 1971.
4. Rashkind, W. J., and Miller, W. W.: Creation of an atrial septal defect without thoracotomy: A palliative approach to complete transposition of the great vessels, J. A. M. A. **196:** 991, 1966.

Transplantation and reimplantation in the arts

Bianca Tosatti, Ph.D. (**Literature**), *Genoa, Italy*

The artist draws inspiration for his work from the beautiful and the ugly, the cruel and the gentle, the unreal and the impossible. Medical miracles, falling in this category, have provided, during the centuries, inspiration for several masterpieces. This paper reviews some of the most impressive artistic creations dealing with the miraculous restoration of severed parts of the body. Since reimplantations, as the result of the progress of medical science, are today a practical reality, probably the subject has lost forever its appeal for the artist.

From the Facolta di Lettere, Genoa University, Genoa, Italy

Recently there has been a great deal of discussion in the medical literature and even more in the lay press of the extreme difficulty of performing organ grafts and of the unsolved problems for their success. By now, even the non-medical public has heard about the efforts to transplant organs such as the heart, kidney, lungs and liver, and also of the still bewildering success obtained in the reimplantation of severed limbs. Thanks to the recent advances of vascular surgery, arms, legs, and even fingers have been successfully reimplanted; successful reimplantation of a severed ear or nose has not been accomplished yet, probably because of the smallness of its arteries and veins.

One of the most dramatic reimplantations is the one recently described by Balas: A young Greek female arrived at the Hospital of Athens minus her right arm which was delivered wrapped in newspaper. This is a spectacular success; others have achieved equally good results and often in equally dramatic circumstances.

These cases have been fully reported in the medical literature and do not constitute the purpose of this presentation. What I would like to bring to your attention are the equally extraordinary operations never published in journals, medical or otherwise, but which have enjoyed masterful documentation by the hands of known and unknown masters of the arts. Unfortunately, for twentieth-century surgeons hoping to learn from their amazing abilities, the paintings and sculptures illustrating them concentrate mainly on the results, not on how the saints achieved them. However, I thought it interesting to show how the hard-won success of modern surgery had been anticipated hundreds of years ago, as the miracles of the past are becoming the scientific realities of today.

Scanty material exists in the pre-Christian era. Probably the most dramatic operation was the creation of woman. It was more than a transplant and really cannot be

Accepted for publication Sept. 7, 1973.

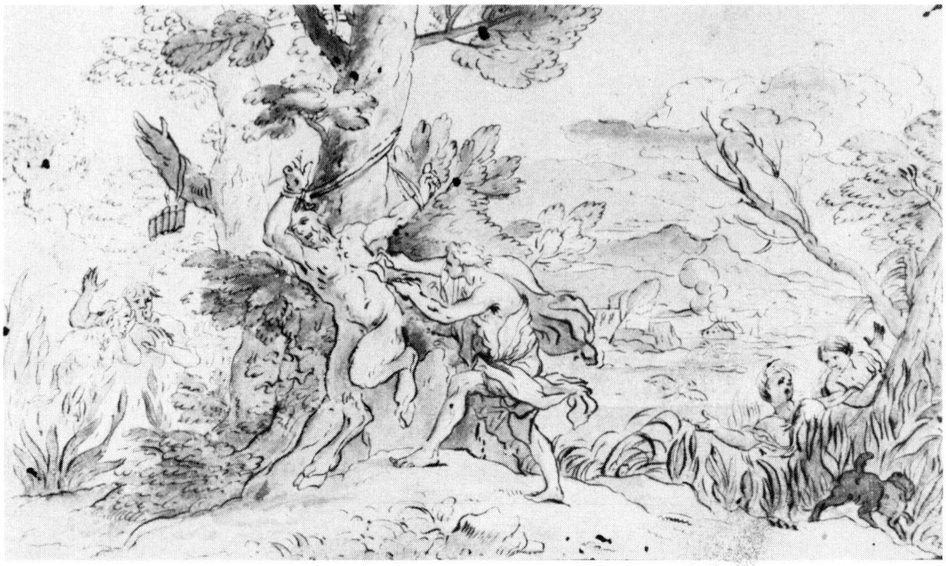

Fig. 1. *Mercury Removes a Piece of Skin from Marsyas,* Luca Giordano. Private collection, Genoa.

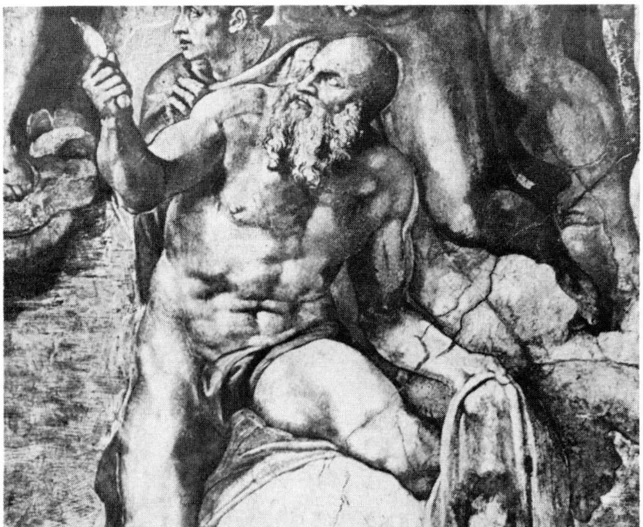

Fig. 2. Saint Bartholomew holding his own flayed skin, detail from the *Last Judgement* by Michelangelo, sixteenth century Italian painter. Sistine Chapel, Rome.

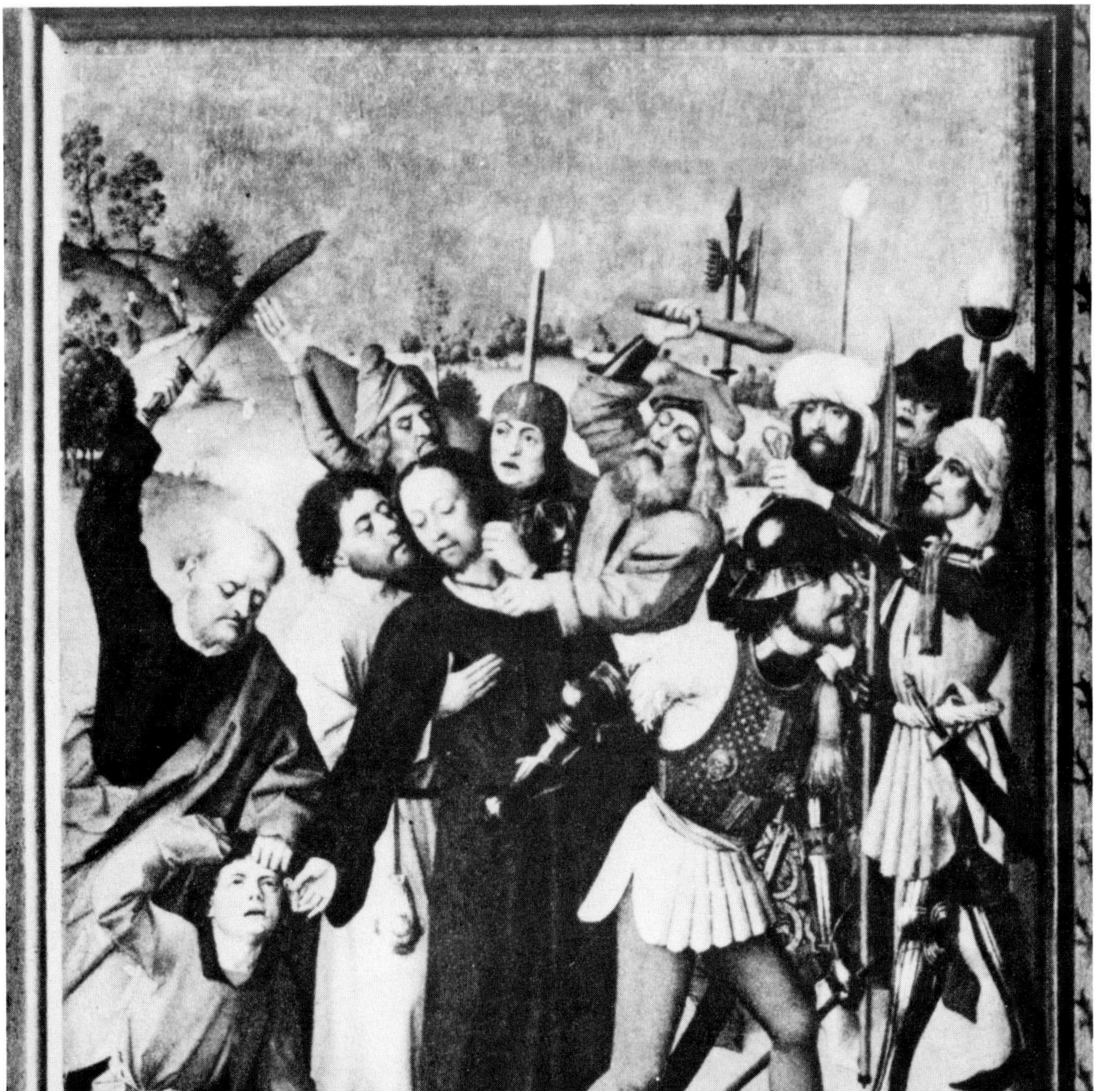

Fig. 3. *Arrest of Christ,* School of Dirc Bouts, fifteenth century Netherlandish painter. Museum: Wallraf-Richartz, Cologne.

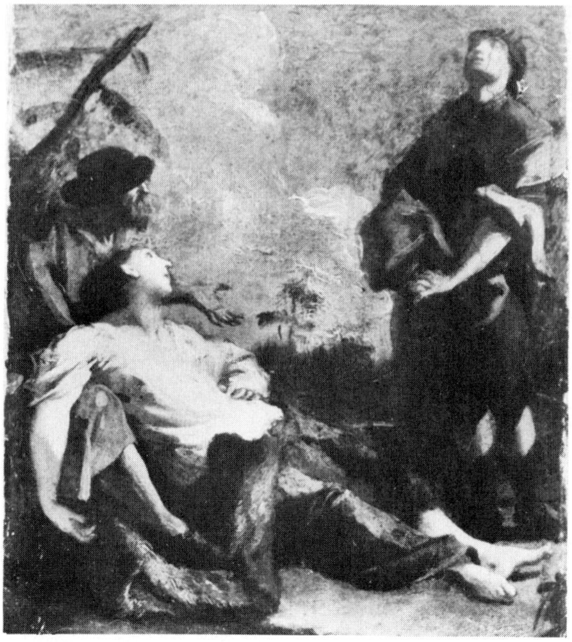

Fig. 4. *Saint Mark Reimplanting an Arm of a Soldier,* by G. B. Tiepolo, seventeenth century Italian painter. Genoese private collection.

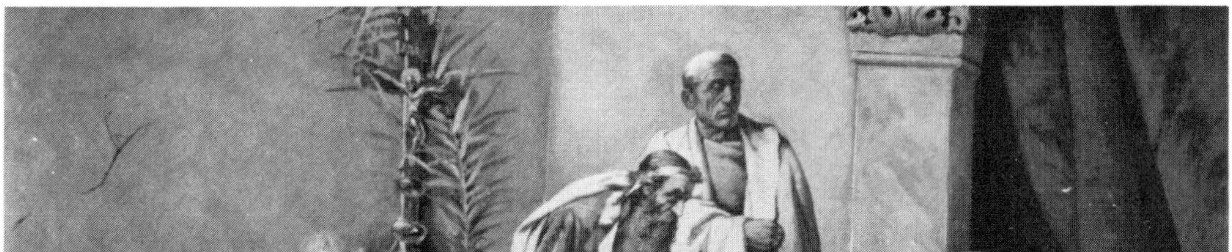

Fig. 5. *Saint Anthony of Padua Reimplanting the Boy's Leg,* by P. de Servi, nineteenth century Italian painter. Church of Lavagna, Genoa.

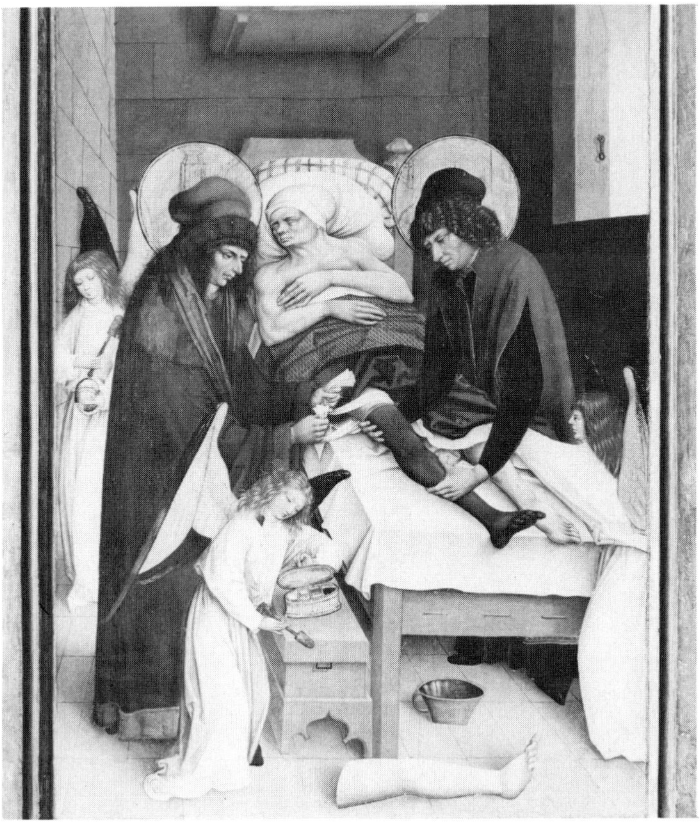

Fig. 6. *Saints Cosmas and Damian Transplanting a Leg,* by an unknown Netherlandish painter of the fifteenth century. Wurttembergisches Landesmuseum, Stuttgart.

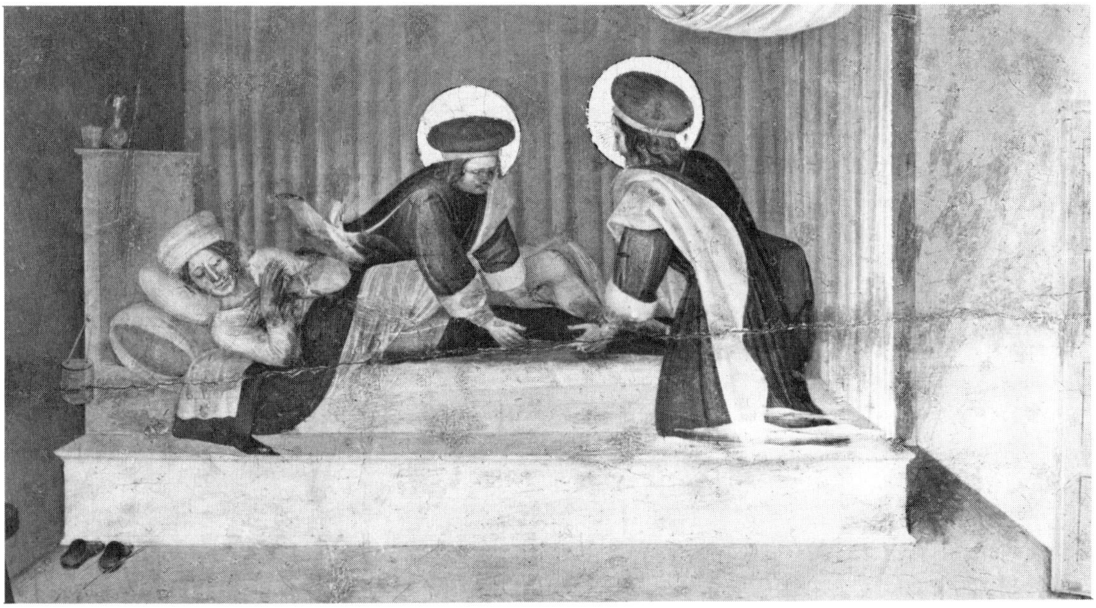

Fig. 7. *Saints Cosmas and Damian Transplanting a Leg,* by Fra Angelico, fifteenth century painter. Museum of the Church of San Marco, Florence.

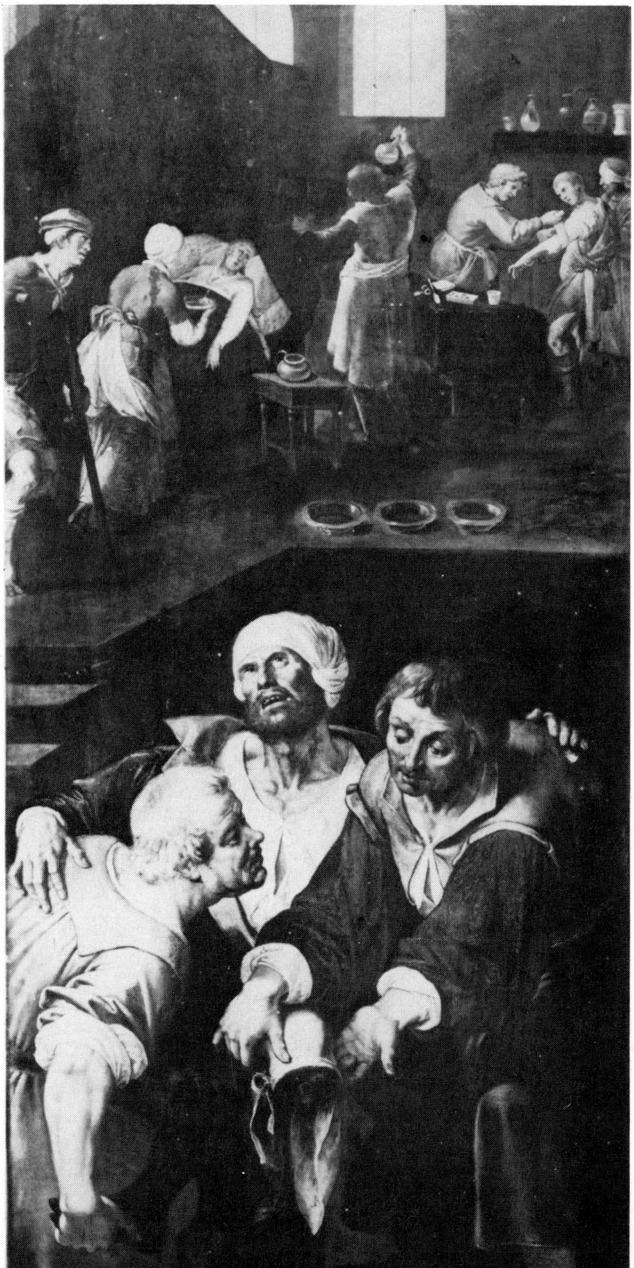

Fig. 8. *Saints Cosmas and Damian Transplanting a Leg,* by Ambrosius Francken the Older, seventeenth century Flemish painter. Koninklijk Museum voor Schoone Junsten, Antwerp.

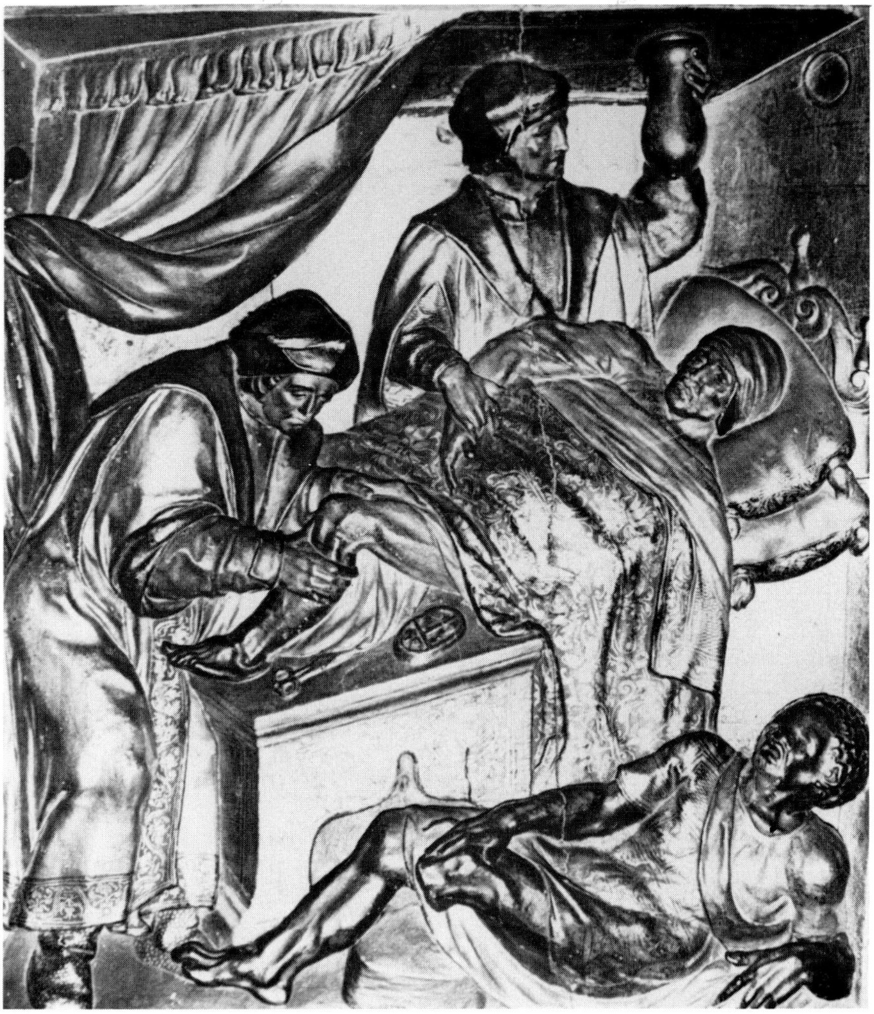

Fig. 9. *Saints Cosmas and Damian Transplanting a Leg,* by a sixteenth century Spanish sculpturer. Museo Nacional de Escultura Valladolid.

classified in modern surgical terminology; but from the account in the second book of Genesis, it appears that it was an operation carried out with all the rules, at least as far as the anesthesia and the handling of the wound is concerned: "And the Lord God caused a deep sleep to fall upon Adam and he slept. He took one of his ribs and he closed up the flesh instead thereof." There is no mention of whether an informed consent had been obtained and this is a flaw.

In Pagan times there were very few possible examples. Mercury removed a sheet of skin from Marsyas (Fig. 1), but it is unlikely that this was done for transplantation purposes. As a matter of fact, Pagans and Infidels, in general, although they acquired considerable skill in removing skin, never really used the removed part for medical purposes, and so St. Bartholomew, as Michelangelo saw it, on the Day of Judgement will be able to reclaim his skin which the Indians had masterfully flayed from his body (Fig. 2).

Not surprisingly, it was Christ who performed the first reimplantation. While Christ was being arrested by the Roman soldiers, Peter attacked a Jew who accompanied them and cut off his ear. Christ simply reached out and re-attached it (Fig. 3),

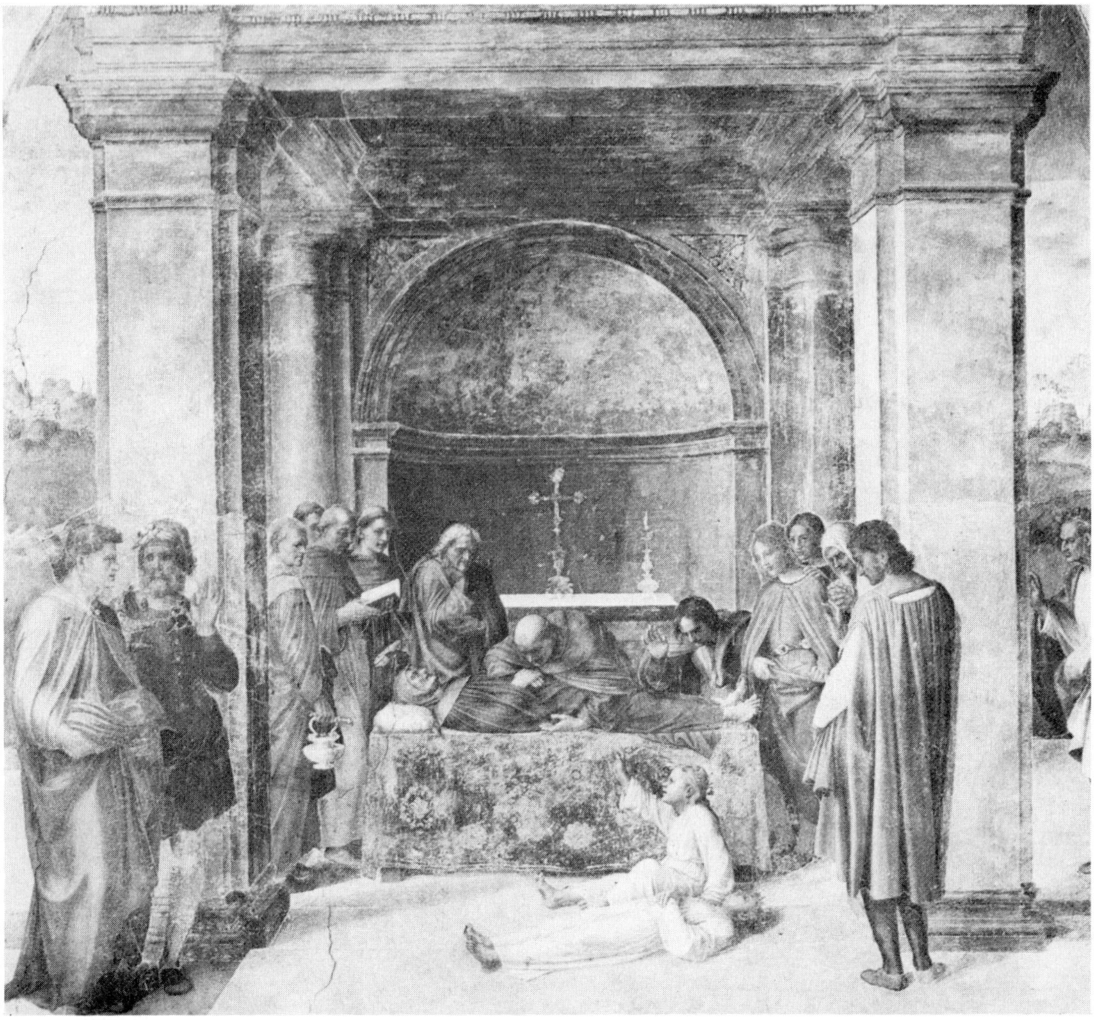

Fig. 10. *Resurrection of a Child,* by Philip Andrea del Sarto, sixteenth century Italian painter. Church of Santissima Annunziata, Florence.

bypassing any need for assistants, anesthesia, sterile conditions, etc. Having witnessed the miracle, St. Peter was able, later, to accomplish an even more dramatic one: When St. Agatha was cruelly tortured and her breasts were pulled off with pliers, St. Peter, pitying her and admiring her courage, reimplanted them.

St. Mark, who lived in the first century A.D., was referred a case of a soldier whose hand had been almost totally cut off in a battle. All the other doctors had advised amputation; St. Mark reimplanted it without ado (Fig. 4). One fifth-century saint, Pope Leo, cut off his own hand because a woman kissed it and aroused his ardor. Mary, the mother of Christ, appeared to him and reimplanted it as Pope Leo had, after all, resisted the temptation!

Inferior limbs also were reimplanted and transplanted as well. St. Anthony of Padua (1195-1231 A.D.) obtained a remarkable success in very demanding circumstances. Once when a young boy told him in confession that he had kicked his mother so hard that she had fallen over, the saint reproved him by saying that anyone who did that should have his leg cut off. The impressionable boy was so remorseful he did just that. It was only through the Saint's surgical skills that he regained his leg (Fig. 5). Saints Cosmas and Damian, themselves doctors and later honored as the patron saints of physicians, did one leg transplant which probably has been the best-documented instance of all. They replaced the cancerous leg of a faithful tower bell custodian with the sound leg of an Ethiopian. Most of the accounts of this transplant claim that the donor was already dead (Figs. 6, 7, and 8). However, at least one Spanish sculpture seems to suggest that the Ethiopian was not only still alive, but awake as well and probably, judging from his expression, somewhat confused about the happenings (Fig. 9).

From the various paintings and sculptures illustrated here, we can gain some idea of the saints' *modus operandi.* In some cases, the saints physically do the surgery (Figs. 3, 5, and 8); probably because Cosmas and Damian were doctors, surgical instruments and equipment including an angelic scrub nurse are present (Figs. 6, 7, and 8). However, in other operations, the saint is not at work but only gazing heavenward without touching the patient (Fig. 4). This attitude would be frowned upon by any surgical board or college, but probably in the life of any surgeon there will be a time when he would like to be able to call on that kind of back-up aid!

Then too, the saints had a last resort that today's doctors may envy. No matter how badly the operation went, they could always raise their patient from the dead (Fig. 10).

Thus, in some ways, today's surgical advances were surpassed long ago in the artists' conception of the power of the thaumaturgists. The twentieth-century physician cannot learn much from their methodology nor can they follow them all the way. However, it is inspiring to recognize the continuity of intent and to realize that many complex life-saving processes, once possible only through miracles, are now often within the reach of man.

The author is grateful to her father, Professor E. Tosatti, Chairman of the Department of Surgery, Medical School of Genoa University, for his encouragement in this project. She expresses thanks also to Sarah Wilk, Instructor in History of Art, at the City University of New York, and to Dr. C. A. Danese, Associate Professor of Surgery, the Mount Sinai School of Medicine, New York, for their help in translating and editing the manuscript.

Xenon-133 radiospirometry in electrophrenic respiration: Diaphragm pacing

Glenn S. Forbes, M.D., W. W. L. Glenn, M.D., *and* **R. C. Lange, Ph.D.,** *New Haven, Conn.*

The use of radioactive xenon scanning techniques for assessing ventilation and perfusion characteristics in patients using electrophrenic respiration (EPR) is described. Over 50 xenon dynamic studies including inhalation and intravenous techniques have been performed on 10 patients with radiofrequency phrenic nerve pacer units for central hypoventilation. Ventilation and perfusion fractions, washout times, and V/Q values have been calculated in individual lungs and regional lung fields for each of these patients with a unilaterally electrically stimulated diaphragm. The role of xenon radiospirometry in supplementing other conventional tests to study pulmonary function in these patients is discussed.

From the Department of Surgery, Section of Nuclear Medicine, Yale University School of Medicine, New Haven, Conn.

ALVEOLAR hypoventilation resulting from an abnormality in the central nervous system mechanism of respiratory control has become a well-recognized syndrome.[5, 9, 14-16, 19-21] The electrical stimulation of a phrenic nerve by means of transmission of radiofrequency (RF) impulses has been intensively investigated in patients with central hypoventilation.[6, 7, 11, 18, 22] Pulmonary function during electrophrenic respiration (EPR), or diaphragm pacing, has previously been evaluated with blood gases, conventional bronchospirometry, and instantaneous flow-volume curves. However, these are general tests which deal with the respiratory system as a whole unit. In patients having unilaterally stimulated phrenic nerves these methods have not separated the paced diaphragm from the unpaced diaphragm for a comparison of efficiency. Differential bronchospirometry would reveal differences in air distribution, and indeed did so in our first patient.[11] However, this is a difficult technique which has been superseded by radioisotope scanning techniques.

Supported by the National Institutes of Health, Education and Welfare, HL 04651.

Accepted for publication Oct. 10, 1973.

Reprint requests: Glenn S. Forbes, M.D., Department of Radiology, Mayo Clinic, Rochester, Minn. 55901.

Xenon-133 dynamic isotope scanning has recently been widely applied to the study of regional pulmonary ventilation and blood flow distribution under a variety of circumstances.[1, 2, 4, 8, 10, 12, 13] The usefulness of these scans for providing physiologic information and their specificity for regional lung function have made them a major tool in evaluating many cardiopulmonary situations.

METHODS AND MATERIALS

Radioactive xenon may be administered both as a solution injected intravenously and as a gas through a closed spirometer. When Xe-133 dissolved in saline is injected intravenously, over 95 percent of the isotope passes from the pulmonary capillary bed into the alveolar air spaces and is subsequently cleared by ventilation. The initial count rates over

Table I

Patient	Age (yr.)	Sex	Primary diagnosis	Implantation		Xenon study
				Date	Side	
A. A.	33	M	CVA; central respiratory depression	10/30/69	Left	2½ yr.
R. S.	52	M	Primary hypoventilation	5/25/73	Left	1 mo.
S. F.	47	M	Primary hypoventilation—Pickwickian	9/22/71	Left	1; 1½ yr.
E. D.	51	F	Primary hypoventilation	7/28/70	Left	2 yr.
E. K.	54	M	Central respiratory depression—post-encephalitis	3/11/69	Left	2; 1½; 3½; 4 yr.
M. M. (infant)	2	F	Primary hypoventilation—Leigh's disease	10/20/72	Left	1 mo.
A. D.	53	M	Primary hypoventilation	4/22/71	Left	1½ yr.
L. T.	38	M	Primary hypoventilation	1/16/73	Left	1 mo.
M. S.	47	F	Primary hypoventilation	6/31/72	Left	9 mo.
M. M. (adult)	39	F	Hypoventilation—surgical cordotomy; osteogenic sarcoma	4/17/72	Right	1 mo.

the chest picked up by a scintillation camera represent the regional perfusion in the pulmonary system with the maximum peak quantitating the distribution of pulmonary blood flow. The rate of disappearance of the radioactive xenon then measures the rate of regional air exchange of the perfused lung tissue. When the isotope is administered as a gas through a closed air-O_2 system, the relative distribution of ventilation is determined by similar monitoring of count rates over the chest. Disappearance rates during subsequent air breathing with the system open to exhaust then give the rate of air exchange in all ventilated areas. When concurrent intravenous studies and inhalation studies are performed together in a patient, ventilation-perfusion relationships can be determined over any selected region of the lung field.

The xenon dynamic scanning techniques were used to evaluate pulmonary function in 10 patients who were being treated by diaphragm pacing for central hypoventilation syndromes resulting from a number of different causes (Table I). The methods of phrenic nerve electrode implantation and diaphragm pacing have been reported previously.[3, 6, 17, 22] Patients are examined in the supine position using the posteroanterior view; the supine position is used because this is the position in which diaphragm pacing is customarily used and is most effective.

The isotope studies were done with a Pho-Gamma III Scintillation camera in conjunction with computer data retrieval equipment. Data were recorded on magnetic tape at two- and five-second intervals throughout the studies. The computer tabulates count rates and constructs decay curves for each lung region selected for the study. Maximum count rates after intravenous injection of xenon-saline represent the distribution of pulmonary blood flow. Inspirational peak counts were used for ventilation distribution and equilibrium counts after rebreathing for comparison of aerated lung volumes. Half-life times of the washout curves represented times needed to clear 50 percent of the isotope by ventilation ($T_{½}$). In these studies the computer tabulates counts within six designated regions representing right lung, left lung, RU, RL, LU, and LL lung fields. These data are reported on computer print-out cards and simple mathematical comparisons are made to quantitate the perfusion and ventilation ratios of each designated lung region. The values for each study are listed in Table II. These methods of computerized quantitation of regional lung perfusion and ventilation have been described previously.[8, 10, 12]

RESULTS

Over 50 xenon dynamic studies have been performed at various time intervals on 10 patients who were on diaphragm pacing implants. Typical radioactivity curves derived

Table II. *Results of studies in ten patients*

Patient	*Ventilation ratio*		*Perfusion ratio*		*50 percent washout time (sec.)*		*Ventilation/perfusion (V/Q)*	
	Right	*Left*	*Right*	*Left*	*Right*	*Left*	*Right*	*Left*
A. A.:								
Base	70	30	54	46	28	40	1.3	0.65
EPR	53	47	52	48	28	14	1.0	1.0
R. S.:								
Base	39	61	48	52	42	37	0.8	1.1
EPR	35*	65	47	53	42	30	0.7	1.2
(3/73) Base	43	57	44	56	120	90	1.0	1.0
(3/73) EPR	35†	65	44	56	50	30	0.8	1.1
S. F.:								
Base	55	45	53	47	15	23	1.0	0.96
EPR	48	52	52	48	28	25	0.9	1.1
EPR	46	54	48	52	33	25	0.9	1.0
(3/73) Base	55	45	59	41	18	18	0.9	1.1
(3/73) EPR	43	57	50	50	18	8	0.85	1.1
E. D.:								
Base	59	41			10	18		
EPR	49	51			25	12		
E. K.:								
Base	55	45	48	52	35	35		
EPR	35	65			35	18		
Base‡	52	48			35	35		
Base§	54	46			35	35		
M. M. (infant):								
Base	77	23			(T¼) 8	6		
					16	14		
EPR	51	49			(T½) 6	4		
					16	8		
A. D.:								
Base	57	43	49	51	40	52	1.1	0.85
EPR	51	49	53	47	30	30	0.9	1.0
L. T.:								
Base	58	42	53	47	30	30	1.1	0.9
EPR	45	55	51	49	40	40	0.9	1.1
M. S.:								
Base	54	46	51	49	75	75	1.0	0.9
EPR	45	55	50	50	80	60	0.9	1.1
(2/73) Base	54	46	55	45	75	80	1.0	1.0
(2/73) EPR	42	58	58	42	70	45	0.7	1.3
M. M. (adult):								
Base			46	54	42	35		
EPR			50	50	37	35		
Fatigue EPR			48	52	40	38		
(2/73) EPR	63	37						

*Upper lobe to lower lobe ratio = 3.

†Upper lobe to lower lobe ratio = 10.

‡Base (no pacing) study immediately after 10 hours simulation period (fatigue study).

§Base (no pacing) study after six hours of rest following above study.

from perfusion and inhalation studies are depicted in Figs. 1*A* and 1*B*. A comparison of the ventilatory clearance rates of each lung during normal breathing and during diaphragm pacing is illustrated in Fig. 2. Fig. 3 shows the scintiphotos of a patient during diaphragm pacing which correlate with the washout scans. In these pictures

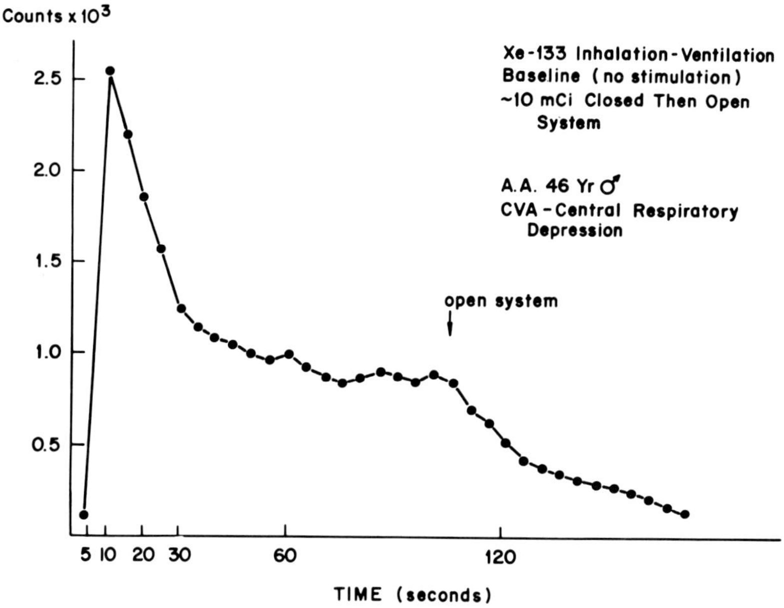

Fig. 1A. Lung activity of inhalation-ventilation study. Injection of 10 mCi. of Xe-133 gas into closed breathing system with subsequent breathing in system open to air and exhaust. Each point represents integration of all counts recorded over individual lung during five-second period.

the lung on the side stimulated during pacing quickly clears the isotope from the alveolar air space. The retention of tracer gas on the contralateral side is manifested by a prolonged ventilation clearance time. Such perfusion, ventilation, and isotope clearance curves may be constructed for each individual patient from the xenon studies. Ventilation ratios, perfusion ratios, ventilation clearance times, and V/Q were determined for individual lungs and regional lung fields.

Ventilation. The inhalation studies in ten patients revealed that, compared to during normal resting breathing (base study), during EPR (diaphragm pacing) a greater proportion of the total inspired air was exchanged by the lungs on the implant side than by the lungs on the contralateral side: $\overline{(V_i/V_n)}_{epr} = 1.22 \pm 0.03$ and $\overline{(V_i/V_n)}_b = 0.80 \pm 0.03$. In all cases there was a decrease of U/L ventilation ratio on the side of the implant during diaphragm pacing, indicating an increase of aeration of the base of the lung. In two patients decreased ventilation in the contralateral (nonstimulated) lungs' base during pacing was demonstrated (noted as decreased RL ventilatory flow and increased RU/RL ratio during pacing). In both patients the left diaphragm was stimulated. This has been attributed to paradoxical diaphragmatic motion which has been observed in these patients on fluoroscopy.

Eight of nine patients had an increased rate of isotope clearance (decreased half-life washout time) in the stimulated lung during diaphragm pacing (average change, 16.5 seconds). In one patient the rate remained the same within the limits of measurement of the scans. In all patients studied, the side of the implant had a higher rate of ventilatory clearance than the nonstimulated side during diaphragm pacing.

Perfusion. The distribution of pulmonary blood flow to each lung was within accepted normal limits during resting respiration, with perfusion ratios ranging from 46 to 54 per cent in each lung. The distribution remained unchanged in all patients during diaphragm pacing. The mean ratio during the base study, $\overline{(Q_i/Q_n)}_b$, was 0.97 ± 0.03 and during EPR, $\overline{(Q_i/Q_n)}_{epr}$, was 0.98 ± 0.03. Since all

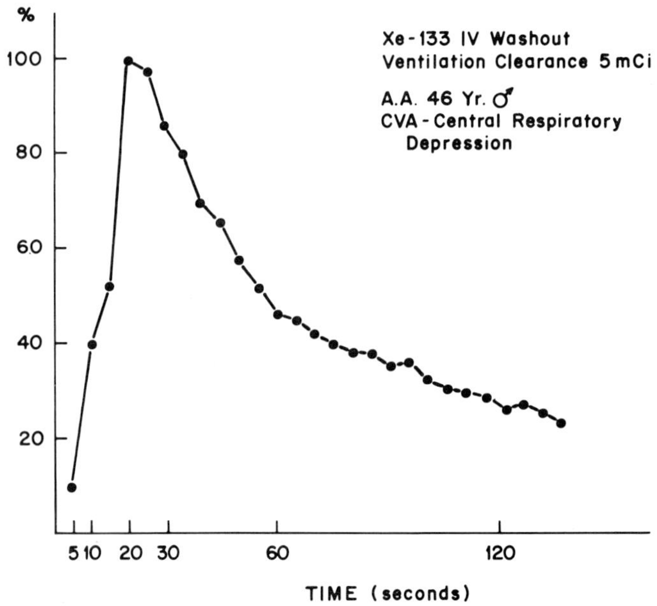

Fig. 1B. Lung activity of perfusion-ventilation study. Injection of 5 mCi. of Xe-133–saline solution intravenously with patient breathing in system open to air and exhaust. Peak of graph represents perfusion of individual lung with subsequent exponential decay curve representing washout of perfused areas (ventilatory clearance rate).

parameters were evaluated in the supine position, the perfusion gradient one might expect to see in the upright patient was not manifest in these studies. During diaphragm pacing the V/Q on the stimulated side increased in all patients. The V/Q of the contralateral lung dropped slightly, although it remained in the range of 0.90 to 1.05, except in one patient who had accessory muscle wasting due to hemiplegia on that side.

Fatigue studies. Several patients have been restudied at various time intervals after their implantations and initial radioisotope evaluations. In patients studied before and after a ten-hour period of continuous pacing, there was no evidence of significant diaphragm fatigue according to the ventilatory and perfusion indices after the pacing period (Table II, patients E. K. and M. M.). Patient E. K. demonstrated no significant changes in ventilation or perfusion two years after his initial xenon tests and about four years after implantation (see case report No. 1); patient M. S. showed no change in ventilation clearance rates or V/Q values over a nine-month period between implantation and restudy.

Clinical correlation. Four patients with obstructive lung disease had slightly decreased ventilation clearance rates during resting respiration compared to the other patients (average, 10.5 seconds). Nevertheless, the ventilatory clearance rate increased during pacing (average change, 13.5 seconds). Thus mild to moderate degrees of obstructive lung disease do not negate the benefits of increased ventilation with diaphragm pacing.

In all cases increased ventilation clearance rates were associated with lower arterial P_{CO_2} levels and higher O_2 levels during diaphragm pacing (Table II). No significant differences in perfusion ratios, V/Q, or clearance rates were noted in patients with elevated pulmonary arterial pressures on right heart catheterization; these patients could not be differentiated from other patients with the xenon scanning techniques.

CASE REPORTS

Case 1. E. K., a 54-year-old white man, was afflicted with encephalitis in 1958 and developed a hypoventilation syndrome with somnolence and

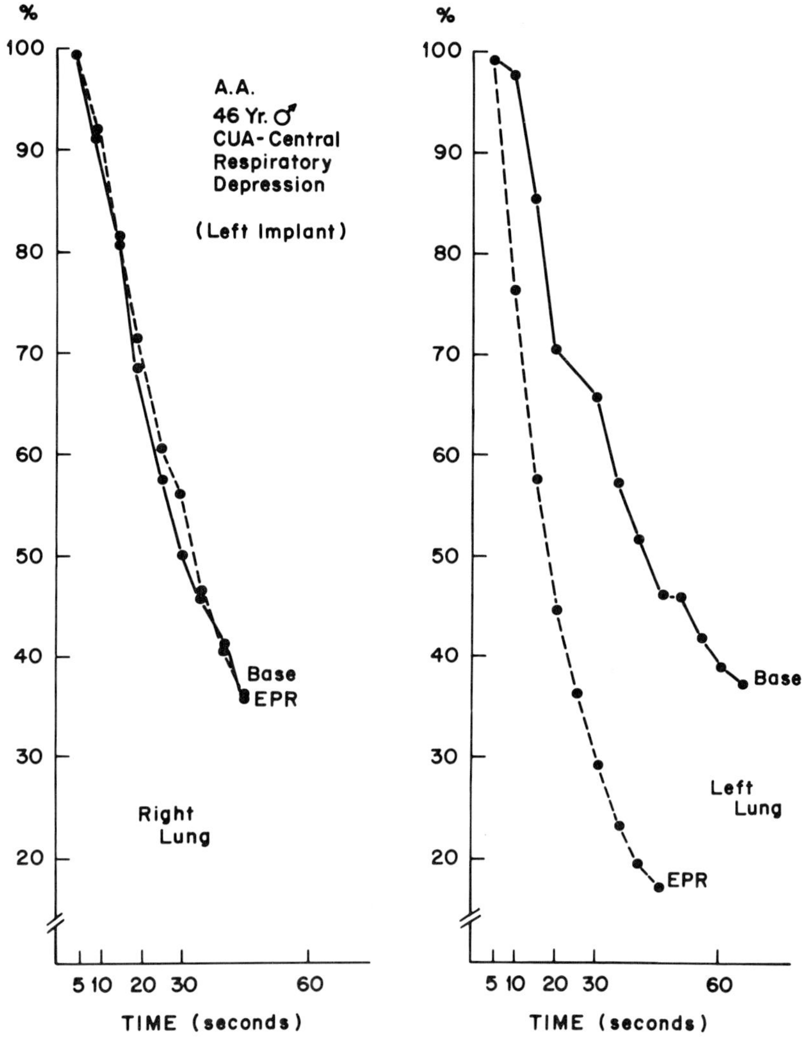

Fig. 2. Ventilatory clearance washout curves: normal respiration and EPR. During stimulation there is increased rate of ventilatory clearance on the left side but no change on the right side.

periods of apnea and cyanosis during sleep. After ten years' use of a rocking bed for sleep he received an RF-EPR pacing unit and has been paced satisfactorily now for about four years.

Isotope washout times indicated greater ventilation on the stimulated side during the first xenon studies 1½ years after implantation. Four years after implantation this patient was found to have had little change in ventilation clearance of either lung over the last two years of pacing (Fig. 4).

This patient was also studied immediately before and after a 10 hour period of pacing. Immediately after the 12 hour period, the ventilation ratio returned to the prestimulated values (52 percent R, 48 per cent L) and clearance rates returned to the base-line value (35 seconds). Studies repeated six hours after the pacing period again revealed no change (Fig. 4). There was no fatigue effect demonstrable in this patient with the xenon studies.

Case 2. S. F., a 47-year-old obese man, developed alveolar hypoventilation of unknown etiology complicated by excessive respiratory effort due to his weight problem. He received an RF-EPR pacing unit in September, 1971, and was discharged with marked improvement of his respiratory status with the aid of diaphragm pacing.

Xenon studies at 1 and 1½ years after implantation revealed improved pulmonary function with pacing. The ventilation distribution, isotope clearance, perfusion ratio, and V/Q values during stimulation remained unchanged after nine months of daily pacing (Table II). This patient manifested decreased isotope clearance, decreased

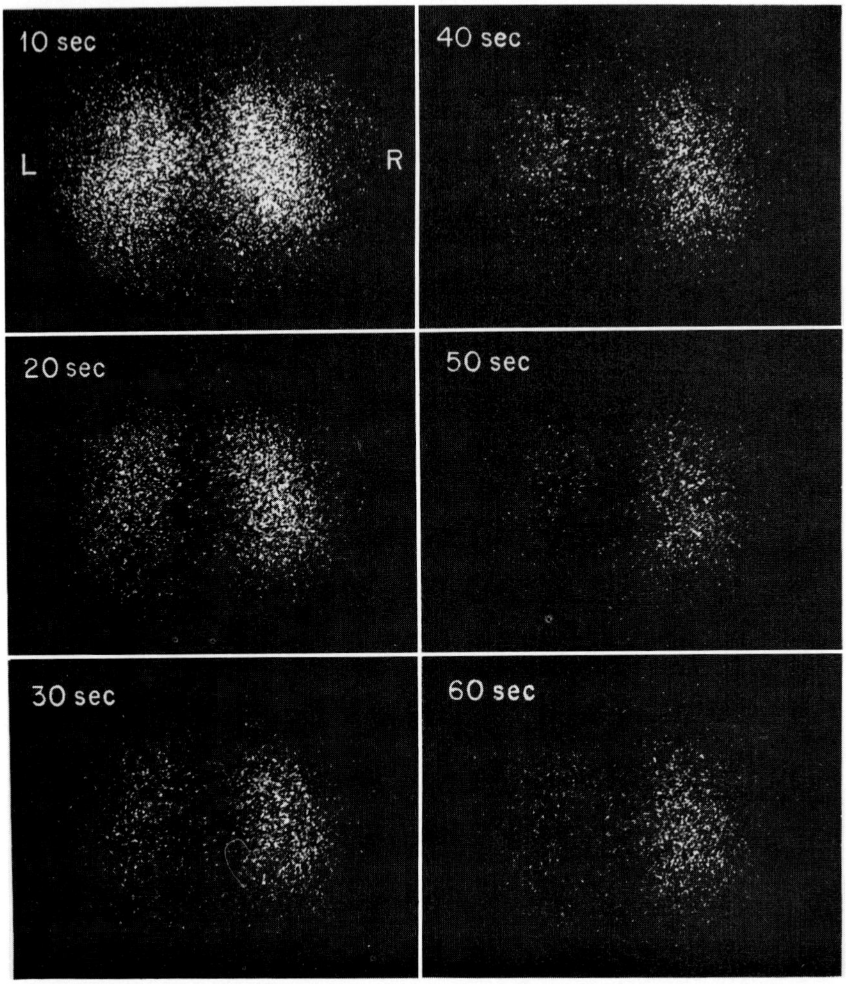

Fig. 3. Scintiphotos of xenon washout during electrophrenic respiration. Left diaphragm is being paced. Note rapid clearance of tracer gas from left lung compared to right. Washout is nearly complete within one minute in the left lung while a significant amount of isotope remains in the right lung.

ventilation, and poor basal ventilation in the contralateral lung during pacing. These changes correlated with paradoxical right diaphragmatic movement on fluoroscopy and are probably related to relatively high intra-abdominal pressure on the diaphragm in the supine position.

DISCUSSION

The chief benefit of xenon pulmonary studies in the management of patients with diaphragm pacemakers is the clinical information from the ventilation and perfusion data that cannot be obtained by other methods. The xenon studies add a new perspective to the evaluation of the pulmonary physiology and can be used to supplement the bronchospirometry data to assess pulmonary function. The following assessment of diaphragm pacing can be made from this investigation with xenon scanning:

1. There is an easily demonstrable increase in ventilation on the side of implantation during diaphragm pacing in all patients.

2. V/Q values are improved on the stimulated side during diaphragm pacing. Normal regional ventilation-perfusion ratios are usually maintained on the contralateral side on and off pacing.

3. There is no evidence of significant dia-

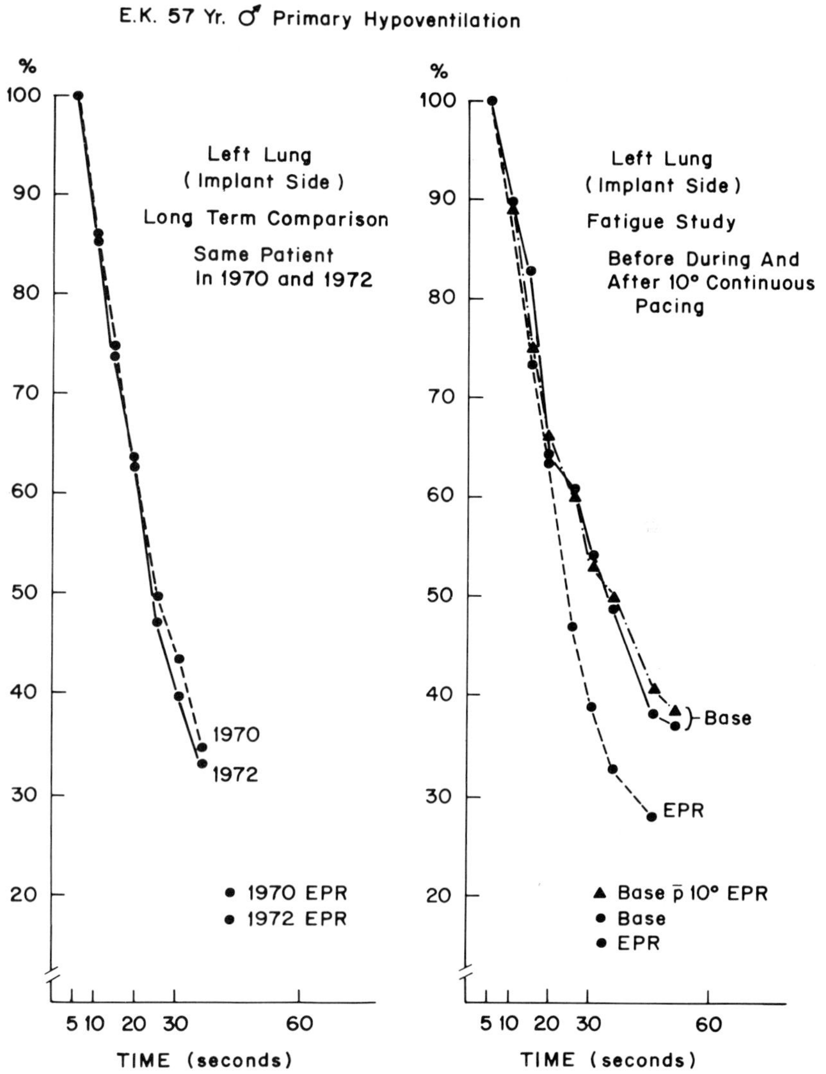

Fig. 4. Long-term and fatigue study. Left: Relative ventilatory clearance washout curves are shown in 1970 and 1972. Note little difference in rate of ventilation clearance in the two-year period. Right: The first curve represents study immediately before stimulation test period. Patient was then studied during ten-hour stimulation period with noticeable increase in ventilatory washout. Patient was then restudied (no stimulation) immediately after the ten-hour EPR period. There was no demonstrable change in ventilatory clearance before and after the stimulation period. (Note: The data in this illustration were presented in a different form before the American Association of Thoracic Surgery in April of 1973 and are published in the *Journal of Thoracic and Cardiovascular Surgery* 66: 505, 1973.)

phragm fatigue—as determined in several patients who were available for restudy. In the patient with the longest pacing in the series, the xenon scans have shown no change in ventilation or clearance rates over a two-year period of continuous pacing. This patient had been using a diaphragm pacer for about four years at the time of the latest xenon study.

4. There is no significant change in perfusion ratios or distribution in either lung during normal respiration or during electrophrenic respiration.

5. Xenon scanning was found to be a be-

nign and straightforward procedure; radiation from brief exposure to 5 and 10 mCi. dosages was negligible.

SUMMARY

Over 50 radioactive dynamic scans using xenon-133 gas and solution in conjunction with a scintillation camera and computer data retrieval equipment were employed to evaluate pulmonary function in ten patients who had diaphragm pacing for central hypoventilation syndrome from a number of causes. Measurements were made of various physiologic parameters in each lung, and in selected lung fields: ventilation and perfusion, V/Q, and ventilation clearance.

Increases in ventilation fractions, ventilation clearance rates, and improved V/Q ratios were readily demonstrated on the side of implantation during diaphragm pacing. No significant changes in perfusion ratio or distribution were found in either lung during pacing. Pulmonary changes correlated well with other clinical parameters in demonstrating improved respiration with pacing. The xenon data were found to be helpful in following the pulmonary function of several patients available for restudy. No significant ventilatory changes due to long-term pacing were demonstrated in the several patients evaluated for fatigue phenomena.

The xenon-133 studies were found to be benign and practical procedures which are well tolerated by the patients and have little or no side effects or risks. The parameters of selective lung ventilation and perfusion cannot be measured by other conventional methods. These isotope studies can be used along with the other tests of respiratory physiology to add a new perspective in evaluating pulmonary function in diaphragm pacing.

REFERENCES

1. Ball, W. C., Jr., Stewart, P. B., Newsham, L. G. S., and Bates, D. V.: Regional pulmonary function studies with Xe-133, J. Clin. Invest. **41:** 519, 1962.
2. DeNardo, G. L., Goodwin, D. A., Ravasini, R., and Dietrich, P. A.: The ventilatory lung scan in the diagnosis of pulmonary embolism, N. Engl. J. Med. **282:** 1334, 1970.
3. deVilliers, R., Nosé, Y., Meier, W., and Kantrowitz, A.: Long-term, continuous electrostimulation of peripheral nerve, Trans. Am. Soc. Artif. Intern. Organs **X:** 357, 1964.
4. Dittrich, F. A., and Goodwin, D. A.: Early recognition of chronic airway disease by the Xe-133 lung scan, J. A. M. A. **220:** 1120, 1972.
5. Fishman, L. S., Samson, J. H., and Sperling, D. R.: Primary alveolar hypoventilation syndrome (Ondine's curse), Am. J. Dis. Child. **110:** 155, 1965.
6. Glenn, W. W. L., Holcomb, W. G., Gee, B. L. J., and Rath, R.: Central hypoventilation; Long-term ventilatory assistance by radiofrequency electrophrenic respiration, Ann. Surg. **172:** 755, 1970.
7. Glenn, W. W. L., Holcomb, W. G., McLaughlin, A. J., O'Hare, J. M., Hogan, J. F., and Yasuda, R.: Total ventilatory support in a quadriplegic patient with radiofrequency electrophrenic respiration, N. Engl. J. Med. **286:** 513, 1972.
8. Goodrich, J. K., Jones, R. H., Coulam, C. M., and Sabiston, D. C., Jr.: Xe-133 measurement of regional ventilation, Radiology **103:** 611, 1972.
9. Grant, J. L., and Arnold, W., Jr.: Idiopathic hypoventilation, J. A. M. A. **194:** 119, 1965.
10. Jones, R. H., Coulam, C. M., Goodrich, J. K., and Sabiston, D. C., Jr.: Radionuclide quantitation of lung function in patients with pulmonary disorders, SURGERY **70:** 891, 1971.
11. Judson, J. P., and Glenn, W. W. L.: Radiofrequency electrophrenic respiration, J. A. M. A. **203:** 1033, 1968.
12. Mishkin, F. S., Brashear, R. E., and Reese, I. C.: Evaluation of regional perfusion and ventilation using Xe-133 and the scintillation camera, Am. J. Roentgenol. **108:** 60, 1970.
13. Murray, J. F., Davidson, F. F., and Glazier, J. B.: Modified technique for measuring pulmonary shunts using xenon-133 and indocyanine green, J. Appl. Physiol. **32:** 695, 1972.
14. Naeye, R. L.: Alveolar hypoventilation and cor pulmonale secondary to damage to the respiratory center, Am. J. Cardiol. **8:** 416, 1961.
15. Plum, F., and Brown, H. W.: The effect on respiration of central nervous system disease, Ann. N. Y. Acad. Sci. **109:** 915, 1963.
16. Rodman, T., Resnick, M. E., Berkowitz, R. D., Fennelly, J. F., and Olivia, J.: Alveolar hypoventilation due to involvement of the respiratory center by obscure disease of the central nervous system, Am. J. Med. **32:** 208, 1962.
17. Sarnoff, S. J., Hardenbergh, E., and Whitten-

berger, J. L.: Electrophrenic respiration, Am. J. Physiol. **155:** 1, 1948.

18. Sato, G., Glenn, W. W. L., Holcomb, W. G., and Wuench, D.: Further experience with electrical stimulation of the phrenic nerve: electrically induced fatigue, SURGERY **68:** 817, 1970.
19. Seriff, N. S.: Central alveolar hypoventilation syndrome, Trans. Am. Neurol. Assoc. **89:** 252, 1964.
20. Severinghaus, J. W., and Mitchell, R. A.: Ondine's curse. Failure of respiratory center automaticity while awake, Clin. Res. **10:** 122, 1962.
21. Tsitouris, G., and Fertakis, A.: Alveolar hypoventilation due to respiratory center dysfunction of unknown cause, Am. J. Med. **39:** 173, 1965.
22. van Heeckeren, D. W., and Glenn, W. W. L.: Electrophrenic respiration by radiofrequency induction, J. Thorac. Cardiovasc. Surg. **52:** 655, 1966.

Hemodynamics of the terminal vascular bed in canine hemorrhagic shock

Arnost Fronek, M.D., Ph.D., *and* **Thomas Witzel, M.Sc.,** *La Jolla, Calif.*

Reversible and irreversible hemorrhagic shock experiments ("single withdrawal") were performed in which the moment of retransfusion of shed blood was varied in 24 dogs: retransfusion in the "reversible" group was initiated after the arterial blood pressure dropped 20 percent from the peak compensated pressure while retransfusion over a 40 percent pressure drop resulted in an "irreversible" shock. Several hemodynamic functions were monitored, including the effective capillary pressure in the intact hindlimb. Pre- and postcapillary resistance and their ratio were calculated. Hematocrit and plasma protein determinations indicate massive fluid loss during the irreversible phase. However, no significant difference in pre- and postcapillary resistance ratios could be detected between the reversible and irreversible groups. The effective capillary pressure continuously declined in the irreversible group and returned close to control values in the reversible group. It is concluded that in this "single withdrawal" hemorrhagic shock model no intra- to extravascular fluid flux could be observed in the hind limb, while at the same time massive fluid losses occurred in the over-all circulatory system. Different probable sites of transcapillary fluid losses have to be therefore assumed.

From Ames-Bioengineering, University of California–San Diego, School of Medicine, La Jolla, Calif.

THE EXACT pathogenesis underlying the irreversible phase of the hemorrhagic shock is still obscure. Several possibilities are to be considered: myocardial depression, decreased vascular reactivity, and transcapillary fluid loss. The significance of the first possibility, which assumes a continuously declining cardiac performance, has not yet been clearly established. Evidence can be found in the literature supporting[2-4, 12, 13, 15, 17, 21, 23] and denying a significant participation of the cardiogenic factor in the irreversible phase of hemorrhagic shock.[1, 9, 10, 14, 16, 17, 20] The possibility of decreased vascular reactivity has been raised repeatedly, however, with contradictory conclusions.[1, 8, 25, 30] Most investigators agree that there is no significant decrease in peripheral resistance, at least in the initial period of the "irreversible" phase.[8] On the other hand, some vascular regions exhibit "trapping" of blood, demonstrated mainly in tissues amenable to microvascular studies.[29, 30] So far, there seem to be no reliable data regarding significant changes in permeability during the "irreversible" phase of shock.[18] We think, however, that fluid loss plays an important role under these circumstances.[9, 10, 14, 15, 24] It is generally assumed that transcapillary fluid shifts do occur during the irreversible phase in a number of vascular beds, and it is presumed that a significant role in this process is performed

Supported by National Heart and Lung Institute Grant No. 2 RO1 HL 12690-04.

Accepted for publication Oct. 19, 1973.

Reprint requests: Dr. A. Fronek, Ames-Bioengineering, Room 5028, Basic Science Building, University of California–San Diego, P.O. Box 109, La Jolla, Calif. 92037.

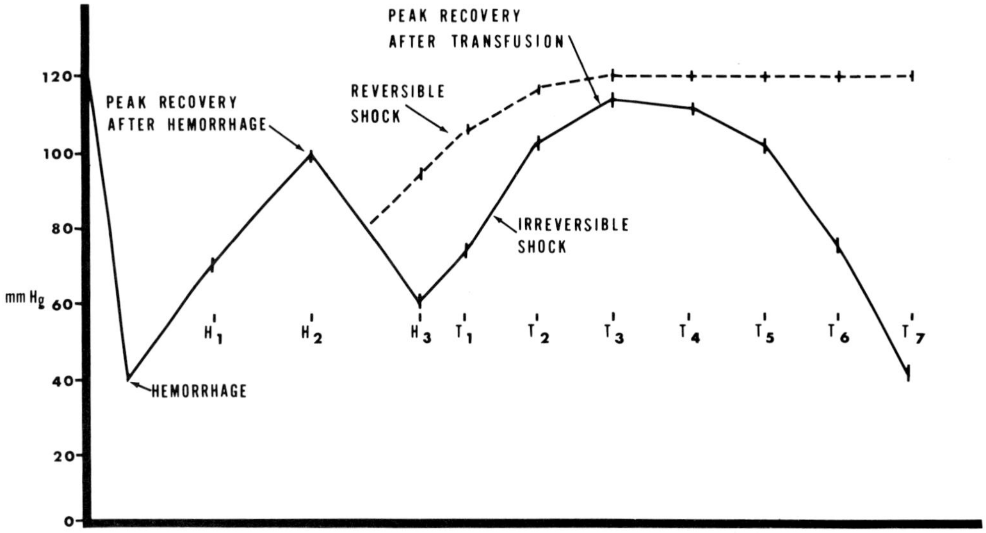

Fig. 1. Schematic time course of the "reversible" and "irreversible" shock experiments (broken line, "reversible"; unbroken line, "irreversible").

by the skeletal muscle system, mainly because of its large over-all volume. Mellander and Lewis,[16] Hollenberg and Nickerson,[9] and Hollenberg and associates[10] concluded from their experiments that most probably a decrease in pre- and postcapillary resistance ratio in the skeletal muscle circulation is responsible for the transcapillary fluid loss.

Since in their experiments the pre- and postcapillary resistance ratio (R_{pr}/R_{ps}) was estimated indirectly and capillary pressure (P_c) was not determined at all, we decided to study the dynamics of P_c, R_{pr}, and R_{ps} under hemorrhagic shock conditions. Capillary pressure determination requires either direct microscopic observation,[27, 31] which limits considerably the area of application or utilizes the "isogravimetric" procedure described by Pappenheimer and Soto-Rivera.[19] This technique requires, however, complete isolation of the observed vascular system; the investigated organ has to be completely isolated to obtain a continuous weight recording (in the case of the hindlimb, it must be amputated), and thus, it is also deprived of its nervous supply. The "isovolumetric" technique described recently[6] obviates these difficulties and was therefore applied in this investigation.

Wiggers' hemorrhagic shock model,[11, 26, 29] although highly reproducible and widely used, has the disadvantage of artificially maintaining a predetermined low level of arterial blood pressure. Spontaneous compensatory mechanisms cannot, therefore, properly develop and are continuously interfered with by the movement of blood into and out of the reservoir during the hypotensive period. In addition, the constant pressure model is far from a clinical reality. We developed, therefore, a "single withdrawal" hemorrhagic shock model which is fairly reproducible and, at the same time, provides an opportunity for the study of the spontaneous dynamics of the homeostatic mechanisms.

METHODS

Hemorrhagic shock model. The optimal conditions for a reproducible single withdrawal shock model were examined in a series of experiments on 17 dogs of either sex; they were anesthetized with Nembutal (30 mg. per kilogram of body weight). The procedure, partially utilizing the results reported by Ehrlich and associates[5] and Schmidt and Schmier,[22] is as follows: After an initial steady-state control period (C), blood is withdrawn at a rate of 30 ml. per minute, up to about 20 percent of the

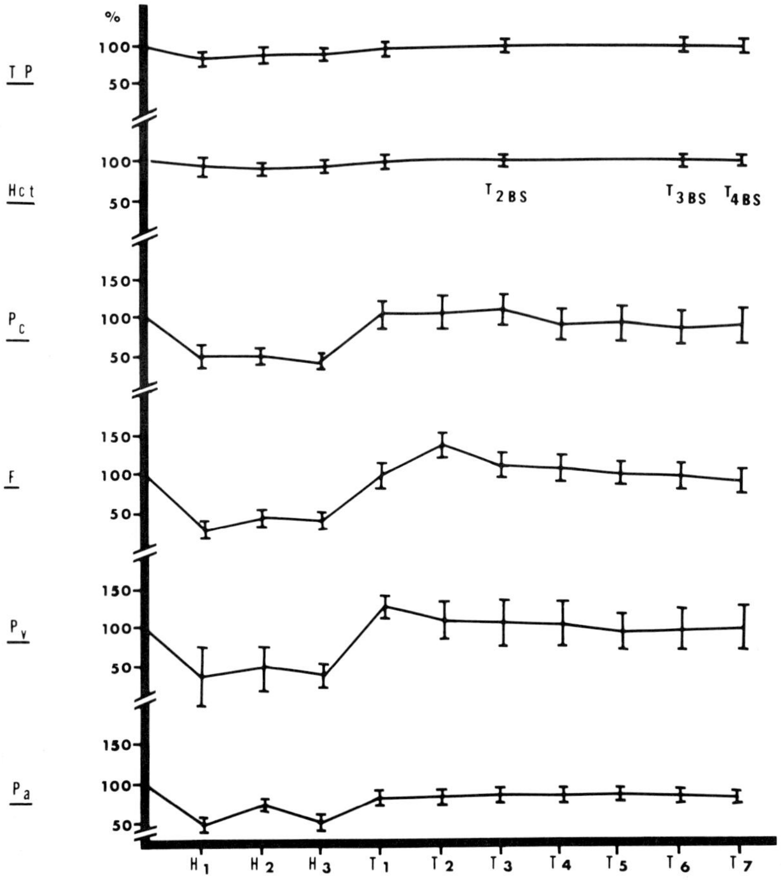

Fig. 2. "Reversible" shock, measured values (percent changes). *TP,* total proteins; *Hct,* hematocrit; P_c, effective capillary pressure; *F,* femoral artery flow; P_v, femoral vein pressure; P_a, arterial blood pressure. Absolute values (control) in Table I.

Table I. *Values for two shock groups*

	"Reversible"		*"Irreversible"*	
	Control	*S.E.*	*Control*	*S.E.*
P_a*	135.3	9.01	125.9	4.14
P_v	7.5	1.00	4.0	0.83
F	50.3	7.74	52.5	6.08
P_c	21.7	0.77	20.8	1.16
Hct.	39.0	2.22	41.1	1.28
T. P.	7.1	0.60	7.2	0.35
R. R.	2.6	0.71	2.4	0.84
R_{pr}	3.3	0.64	2.1	0.77
R_{ps}	0.57	0.07	0.49	0.13
R_{pr}/R_{ps}	4.7	0.55	4.3	0.64

*P_a = fem. art. blood pressure (mm. Hg); P_v = fem. venous pressure (mm. Hg); F = fem. art. blood flow (ml./min.); P_c = effective capillary pressure (mm. Hg); Hct = hematocrit (vol. %); T.P. = total plasma proteins (GM. %); RR = regional resistance $\left(\frac{\text{mm. Hg}}{\text{ml./min.}}\right)$; R_{pr} = precapillary resistance $\left(\frac{\text{mm. Hg}}{\text{ml./min.}}\right)$; R_{ps} = postcapillary resistance $\left(\frac{\text{mm. Hg}}{\text{ml./min.}}\right)$.

calculated blood volume (8.5 percent of body weight[5]). At this phase, the withdrawal rate is either increased or decreased as dictated by the arterial blood pressure. The ultimate goal is to reach an arterial blood pressure (P_a) of 40 mm. Hg and a total removal of 37.5 percent of the calculated blood volume. Usually this was achieved, but if one of the two criteria (40 mm. Hg or 37.5 percent of the calculated blood volume) was reached before satisfying the second criterion, the bleeding is discontinued and the spontaneous compensatory mechanisms could be observed. P_a usually rises and later starts to decline after having reached a transient peak P_a max. From this moment, two alternatives are available: to retransfuse the total amount of shed blood at 80 per-

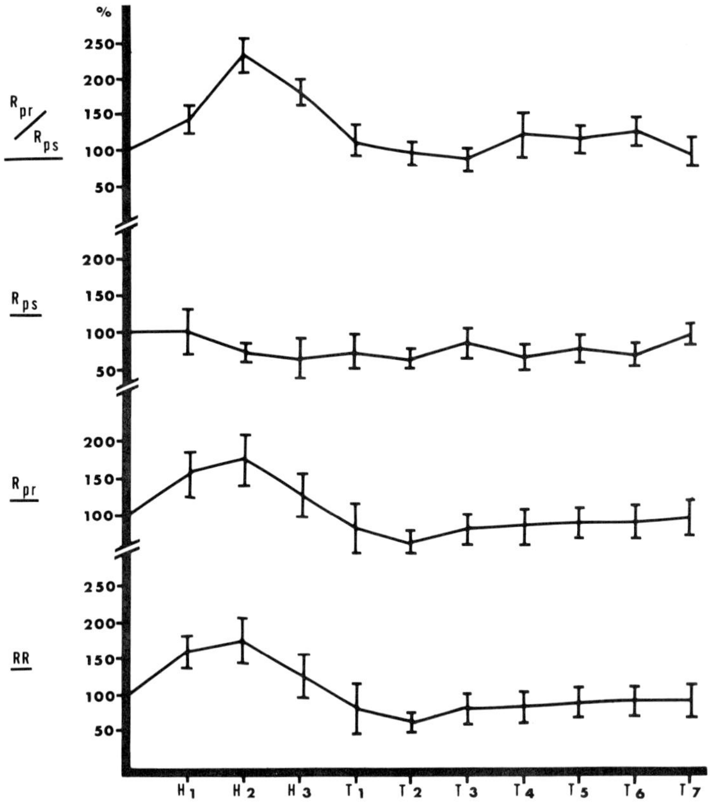

Fig. 3. "Reversible" shock, calculated values (percent changes). R_{pr}/R_{ps}, precapillary/postcapillary resistance ratio; R_{ps}, postcapillary resistance; R_{pr}, precapillary resistance; *RR*, regional resistance $= (P_a\text{-}P_v)/F$. Absolute values (control) in Table I.

cent of P_a max ("reversible group") or at 60 percent of P_a max ("irreversible group"). The animals are then observed over a period of six hours or until the death of the animal. The shed blood was heparinized (10 mg. of heparin per 100 ml. of blood) and stored in a glass beaker immersed in a constant temperature water bath. Blood was retransfused at a rate of 30 ml. per minute.

Effective capillary pressure determination.[6] The circumference of the intact hindlimb was continuously recorded by a mercury-in-rubber gauge,*[28] and the inflow and outflow pressures, together with the blood flow† were continuously recorded. In this modification, as in the original Pappenheimer and Soto-Rivera's[19] technique, the "isovolumetric" venous pressures are plotted against the respective flow values, and the extrapolation to zero flow yields the effective capillary pressure P_c. A rubber tourniquet, threaded under the femoral artery, vein, and nerve, is used to occlude the collateral circulation while the limb circulation is not affected. The first P_c determination after retransfusion was performed 20 minutes later. The subsequent determinations of hemodynamic functions were performed in 30 minute intervals and the last measurement was taken when P_a dropped to 40 percent of P_a max. Since the duration of the posttransfusion period was not uniform, all monitored and calculated values were graphed and the interpolated values, spaced at six equal periods (in addition to T_1), were used for statistical evaluation. The common evaluation periods are therefore as follows (Fig. 1): C, control period; H_1, 20 minutes after termination of blood withdrawal; H_2, the arterial blood

*Parks Electronics, Beaverton, Ore.

†Model No. M4001 electromagnetic flowmeter, Statham, Oxnard, Calif.

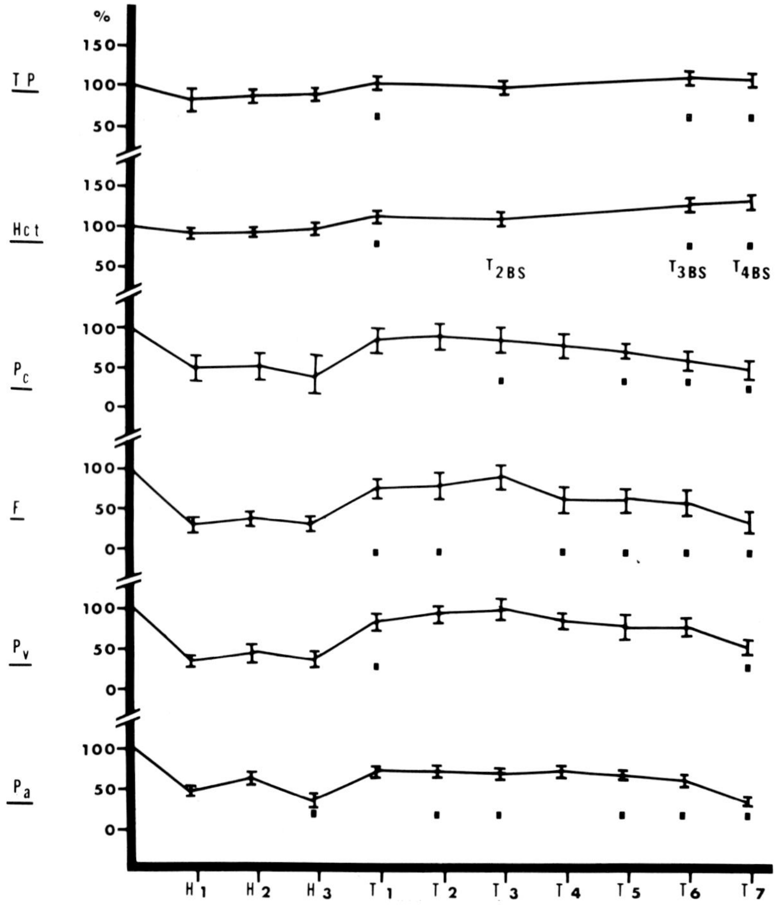

Fig. 4. "Irreversible" shock, measured values (percent change). Legend the same as for Fig. 2. The square (■) indicates satistically significant difference ($p < 0.05$ or better) as compared to corresponding values in Fig. 2.

pressure reaches the compensatory maximum (P_a max), H_3, prior to retransfusion; T_1, 20 minutes after completed retransfusion; T_2 to T_7, equally spaced periods, with T_7 representing the last experimental period (in the reversible series six hours after hemorrhage, in the irreversible series as described above). In addition, hematocrit and protein determinations were performed with the use of the microhematocrit and spectrophotometric (280 nm. absorption) techniques, respectively. Blood samples for these tests were taken at periods C, H_1, H_2, H_3, and T_1. In the reversible group, the next sample was taken about one hour after retransfusion (T_{2BS}); T_{3BS} was taken three hours after retransfusion. T_{4BS} was taken prior to the termination of the observation period. In the "irreversible" shock group, the T_{2BS} sample was taken at the peak of the P_a response, the T_{3BS} at 80 percent level, and T_{4BS} at 60 percent level. The amount of blood withdrawn for samples (2 ml. each) was immediately replaced by dextran (Rheomacrodex).

RESULTS

The initial (control) values for both groups are given in Table I and the following results during the experiments are expressed in percentage of the initial values.

Reversible hemorrhagic shock. Experiments were performed on seven dogs (12 to 20 kilograms) in which the shed blood was retransfused after the arterial blood pressure (P_a) dropped 20 percent from its P_a max.

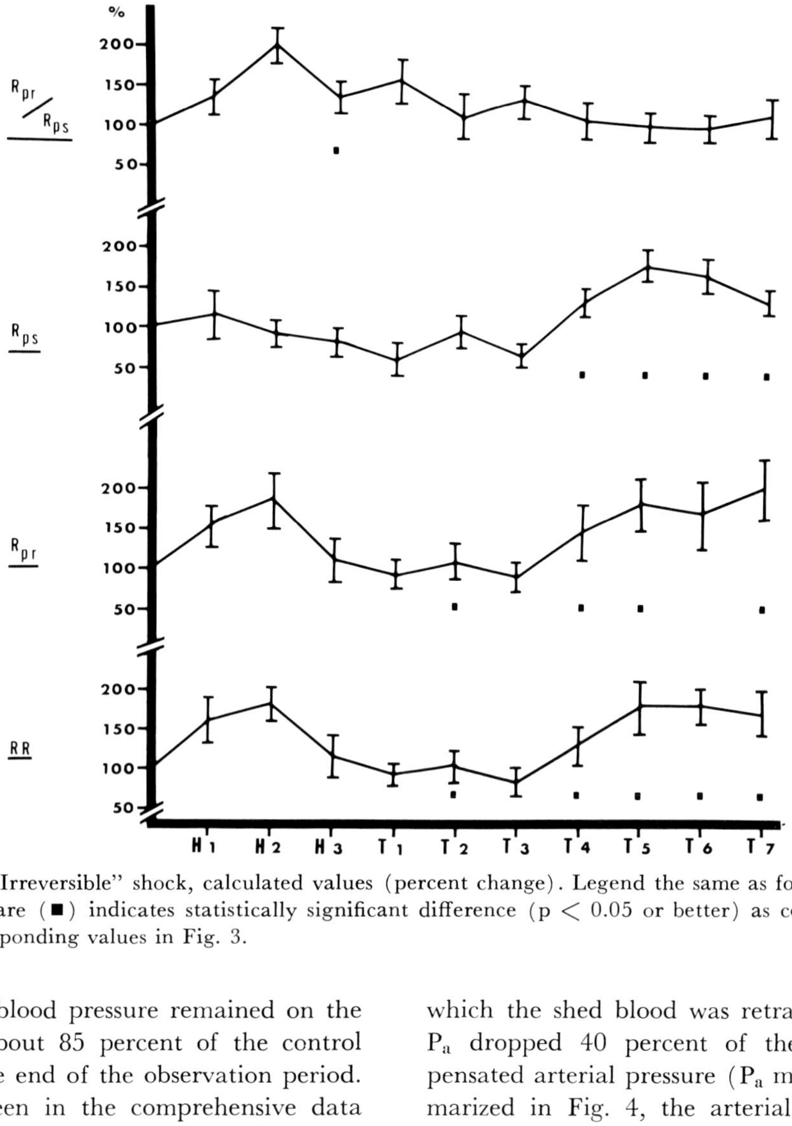

Fig. 5. "Irreversible" shock, calculated values (percent change). Legend the same as for Fig. 3. The square (■) indicates statistically significant difference ($p < 0.05$ or better) as compared to corresponding values in Fig. 3.

The arterial blood pressure remained on the average at about 85 percent of the control level until the end of the observation period. As can be seen in the comprehensive data graph (Fig. 2), the effective capillary pressure (P_c) in the posttransfusion period reached 100 percent of the control value and with minor oscillations remained relatively stable until the end of the observation period. Fig. 3 summarizes the dynamics of the calculated functions. It can be pointed out that the pre- and postcapillary resistance ratio did not change significantly throughout the posttransfusion period. Hematocrit values reached the control value after a transient drop and steady state could be observed until the end of the observation period.

Irreversible shock. Experiments were performed on 17 dogs (13 to 18 kilograms) in which the shed blood was retransfused after P_a dropped 40 percent of the peak compensated arterial pressure (P_a max). As summarized in Fig. 4, the arterial pressure increased transiently after retransfusion and started to decline after about 40 minutes. The average survival time from the moment of retransfusion was 163.3 (±95.0 S.D.) minutes.

Several functions behaved differently in this group as compared to the "reversible" shock group. Hematocrit increased continuously until the end of the experiment, while P_c after a transient peak (close to 90 percent of the control value) started to decline, and this trend continued toward the end of the experiment. As depicted in Fig. 5 the pre- and postcapillary resistance ratio did oscillate throughout the experiment but did not drop below the initial control value in the posttransfusion period in spite of the declining P_c and increasing hematocrit.

DISCUSSION

The shock model. It seems that the described "single withdrawal" shock model is closer to clinical reality than the generally used Lamm-Wiggers model.[11, 29] The essential difference represents the opportunity to study the inherent homeostatic mechanisms of the animal without influencing them by the siphoning effect of the reservoir. The 20 and 40 percent drop of P_a after P_a max seems to represent a reliable criterion which determines whether the experiment will end as a reversible or irreversible shock respectively (as defined in the methodical part).

The dynamics of the terminal vascular bed. In contrast to several previous reports in which the changes of the pre- and postcapillary resistance ratio in the hindlimb have been estimated indirectly,[10, 16] no significant changes could be detected in the posttransfusion period in spite of the fact that P_c continuously declined. A significant loss in transcapillary fluid in the observed hindlimb, as postulated previously,[10, 16] would require a decrease in pre- and postcapillary resistance ratio, especially in view of a declining P_c. In addition, the conditions favorable to filtration are not improved by an increase in colloid osmotic pressure of plasma which can be indirectly assumed in view of the increasing hematocrit and plasma protein concentration.

On the other hand, our results confirm that one of the most striking features of the irreversible hemorrhagic shock phase in this canine hemorrhagic shock model is a massive loss of fluids. We may, therefore, conclude that under our experimental conditions there is a significant loss of transcapillary fluid during the irreversible phase which, however, does not occur in the hindlimb, but most probably takes place in one or several other vascular regions, e.g., the intestinal or hepatic. Specifically designed experiments are planned to investigate these assumptions.

There are several possibilities to account for the differences between previous reports and our results. Species differences cannot be discarded when comparing Mellander and Lewis'[16] results since their experiments were performed in cats. Besides that, these authors did not determine pre- and postcapillary resistance directly but only the sensitivity of the terminal vascular bed was tested throughout hemorrhage and during the short retransfusion period so that actually no irreversible phase was observed.

Similarly, the experimental conditions described in the reports by Hollenberg and coworkers[9, 10] were also different. In this case the classical Wiggers technique was used, which may explain the delayed upswing of plasma protein concentration. This basic difference in the shock model may also explain the continuously increasing postcapillary pressure the authors observed in their experiments.

REFERENCES

1. Bond, R. F., Manley, E. S., and Green, H. D.: Cutaneous and skeletal muscle vascular responses to hemorrhage and irreversible shock, Am. J. Physiol. **212:** 488, 1967.
2. Crowell, J. W.: Cardiac deterioration as the cause of irreversibility in shock, *in:* Shock and hypotension, New York, 1965, Grune & Stratton, Inc., pp. 605-608.
3. Crowell, J. W., and Guyton, A. C.: Further evidence favoring a cardiac mechanism in irreversible hemorrhagic shock, Am. J. Physiol. **203:** 248, 1962.
4. Crowell, J. W., and Guyton, A. C.: Cardiac deterioration in shock, *in:* Hershey, S. G., editor: Shock, Boston, 1964, Little, Brown and Co.
5. Ehrlich, F. E., Kramer, S. G., and Watkins, E.: An experimental shock model simulating clinical hemorrhagic shock, Surg. Gynecol. Obstet. **129:** 1173, 1969.
6. Fronek, A., and Witzel, F.: Circumference measurement as a criterion for capillary pressure determination, Microvasc. Res. **6:** 1, 1973.
7. Gomez, O. A., and Hamilton, W. F.: Functional cardiac deterioration during developments of hemorrhagic circulatory deficiency, Circ. Res. **14:** 327, 1964.
8. Green, H. D.: Physiology of peripheral circulation in shock, Fed. Proc. **20:** 61, 1961.

9. Hollenberg, N. K., and Nickerson, M.: Changes in pre- and post-capillary resistance in pathogenesis of hemorrhagic shock, Am. J. Physiol. **219:** 1483, 1970.
10. Hollenberg, N. K., Waters, J. R., Toews, R. R., Davies, R. O., and Nickerson, M.: Nature of cardiovascular decompensation during hemorrhagic hypotension, Am. J. Physiol. **219:** 1476, 1970.
11. Lamson, P. D., and De Turk, W. E.: Studies on shock induced by hemorrhage. XI. A method for the accurate control of blood pressure, J. Pharmacol. Exp. Ther. **83:** 250, 1945.
12. Lefer, A. M.: Role of a myocardial depressant factor in the pathogenesis of circulatory shock, Fed. Proc. **29:** 1836, 1970.
13. Lefer, A. M., Craddock, G. B., Cowgill, R., and Brand, E. D.: Performance of papillary muscles isolated from cats in postoligemic shock, Am. J. Physiol. **211:** 687, 1966.
14. Lundgren, O., Lundwall, J., and Mellander, S.: Range of sympathetic discharge and reflex vascular adjustments in skeletal muscle during hemorrhagic hypotension, Acta Physiol. Scand. **62:** 380, 1969.
15. Martin, A. M., and Hackel, D. B.: Myocardium of the dog in hemorrhagic shock, J. Lab. Clin. Invest. **21:** 77, 1963.
16. Mellander, S., and Lewis, D. H.: Effect of hemorrhagic shock on the reactivity of resistance and capacitance vessels and on capillary filtration transfer in cat skeletal muscle, Circ. Res. **23:** 105, 1963.
17. Nickerson, M.: Vascular adjustments during the development of shock, Can. Med. Assoc. J. **17:** 853, 1970.
18. Nicoll, P., and Frayser, R.: Physiological considerations of the microcirculation as related to shock, Progr. Cardiovasc. Dis. **9:** 558, 1967.
19. Pappenheimer, J. R., and Soto-Rivera, A.: Effective osmotic pressure of the plasma proteins and other quantities associated with the capillary circulation in the hindlimbs of cats and dogs, Am. J. Physiol. **152:** 471, 1948.
20. Rothe, C. F.: Heart failure and fluid loss in hemorrhagic shock, Fed. Proc. **29:** 1854, 1970.
21. Rothe, C. F., and Selkurt, E. E.: Cardiac and peripheral failure in hemorrhagic shock in the dog, Am. J. Physiol. **207:** 203, 1964.
22. Schmidt, H. D., and Schmier, J.: Normotoner hemorrhagischer Schock, Pfluegers Arch. **298:** 336, 1968.
23. Schmier, J.: Das Herz im Shock, Langenbecks, Arch. Klin. Chirurgie **319:** 992, 1967.
24. Schwinghamer, J. R., Grega, G. J., and Haddy, F. J.: Skin and muscle circulatory responses during prolonged hypovolemia, Am. J. Physiol. **219:** 318, 1970.
25. Selkurt, E. E.: Status of investigative aspects of hemorrhagic shock, Fed. Proc. **29:** 1832, 1970.
26. Werle, J. M., Cosby, R. S., and Wiggers, C. J.: Observations on hemorrhagic shock, Am. J. Physiol. **136:** 401, 1942.
27. Wiederhielm, C. A., Woodbury, J. W., Kirk, S., and Rushmer, R. F.: Pulsatile pressure in the microcirculation of the frog's mesentery, Am. J. Physiol. **207:** 173, 1964.
28. Whitney, R. J.: The measurement of volume changes in human limbs, J. Physiol. **121:** 1, 1953.
29. Wiggers, C. J.: Physiology of shock, New York, 1950, Commonwealth Fund.
30. Zweifach, B. W.: Microcirculatory derangements as a basis for the lethal manifestations of experimental shock, Br. J. Anaesth. **30:** 466, 1958.
31. Zweifach, B. W., and Intaglietta, M.: Mechanics of fluid movement across single capillaries in the rabbit, Microvasc. Res. **1:** 83, 1968.

Method for maintaining the neonate's intraoperative core temperature

Walton K. T. Shim, M.D., F.A.C.S., F.A.A.P., *and* **Peter Halford, M.D.,** *Honolulu, Hawaii*

The sequelae of metabolic acidosis and respiratory depression following decreases of core temperature in the newborn period have been well documented. Although many methods of maintaining the intraoperative temperature have been suggested, none is entirely successful. Some of these have included the use of circulating warm water mattresses, wrapping the infant's extremities in insulating material and/or aluminum foil, packing the child in warm water–filled gloves, and transmission of radiant heat through a fiberoptic system in the operative field. This communication describes the adaptation of a commercially available IMI infant warmer for use in the operating room. It is suspended from an extruded aluminum light track and remains out of the congested surgical field. It has been effective in raising the core temperature even while the viscera are exposed to a high degree of evaporative heat loss and it has had great acceptance with the nursing and anesthesiology members of the team.

From the Department of Surgery, Kauikeolani Children's Hospital and the University of Hawaii School of Medicine, Honolulu, Hawaii.

THE BAD effects of allowing a newborn infant's temperature to fall have received much attention and are well documented,[1-4] but the problem of maintaining a newborn infant's intraoperative temperature has long plagued pediatric surgeons. Many techniques have been suggested, including wrapping the infant's extremities with aluminum foil to decrease radiant loss, surrounding the child in warm water–filled gloves,[5] and conveying radiant heat through a fiberoptic system.[6] Unfortunately, none of these methods is entirely satisfactory. It is the purpose of this communication to describe a mechanical adaptation of the radiant heat infant warmer which can be used in the operating room for maintaining the infant's core temperature.

Presented at the Pacific Association of Pediatric Surgeons meeting in San Diego, Calif., April 20, 1973.

Accepted for publication Oct. 31, 1973.

MATERIALS AND METHODS

A commercially available IMI infra-red heating unit is suspended from a standard surgical light track. The details for connecting the hood to the track are given in Fig. 1. The heating hood can be adjusted to the height of the operating table and can be retracted along the course of the track to the edge of the room out of the congested area. Double light tracks parallel the heater on both sides and the two operating lights are positioned on both sides of the heater. Figs. 2 and 3 demonstrate the unit in use.

RESULTS

The heater's effectiveness is demonstrated in Figs. 4 and 5. The infants had their intestines exposed, and without covering the gut or in any other way changing the surgical procedure the infant warmer was turned on. Immediate warming trends can be

Vol. 75, No. 3, pp. 416-420

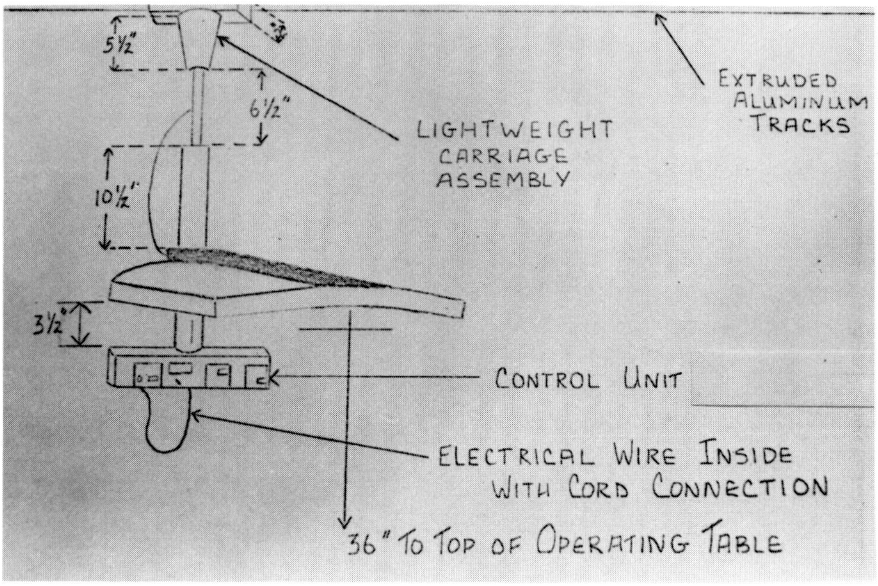

Fig. 1. Diagram showing details of mechanical suspension and electrical connection of the overhead infant warmer.

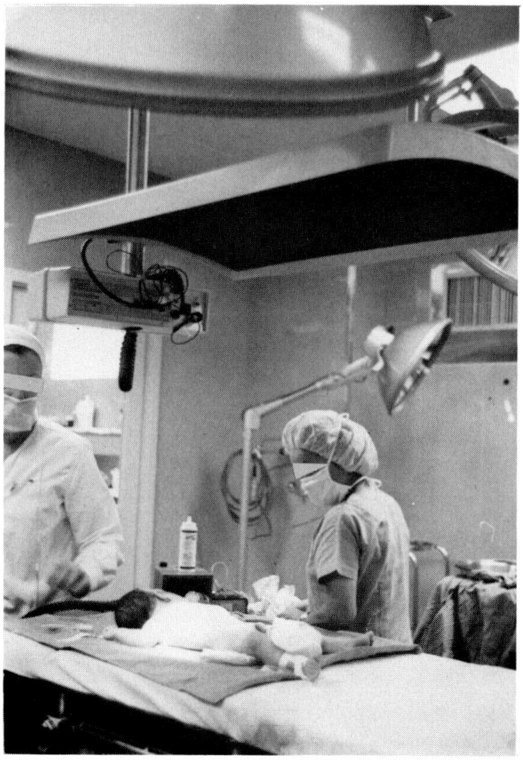

Fig. 2. The infant warmer suspended over the operating table. It is not obstructive to the surgical team or the light source.

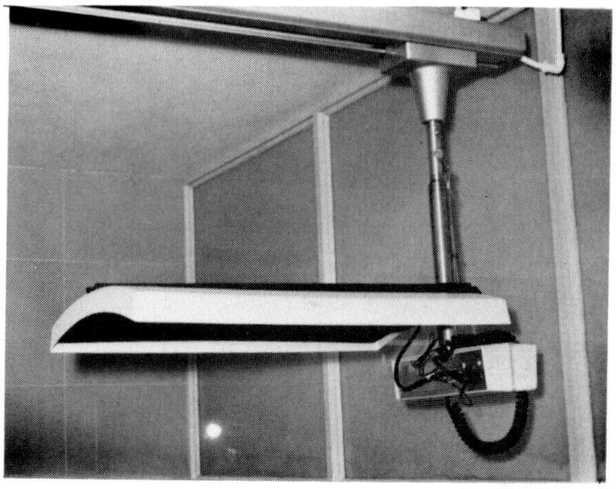

Fig. 3. The unit can be pushed to the edge of the operating room when not in use.

seen by the temperature curves, and normothermia is achieved within several minutes. Average room temperature is 23° C. and temperature under the heating unit is 34° C.

DISCUSSION

The two pathways for heat loss most likely to cause cooling in the cooled and dehumidified operating room are radiant loss

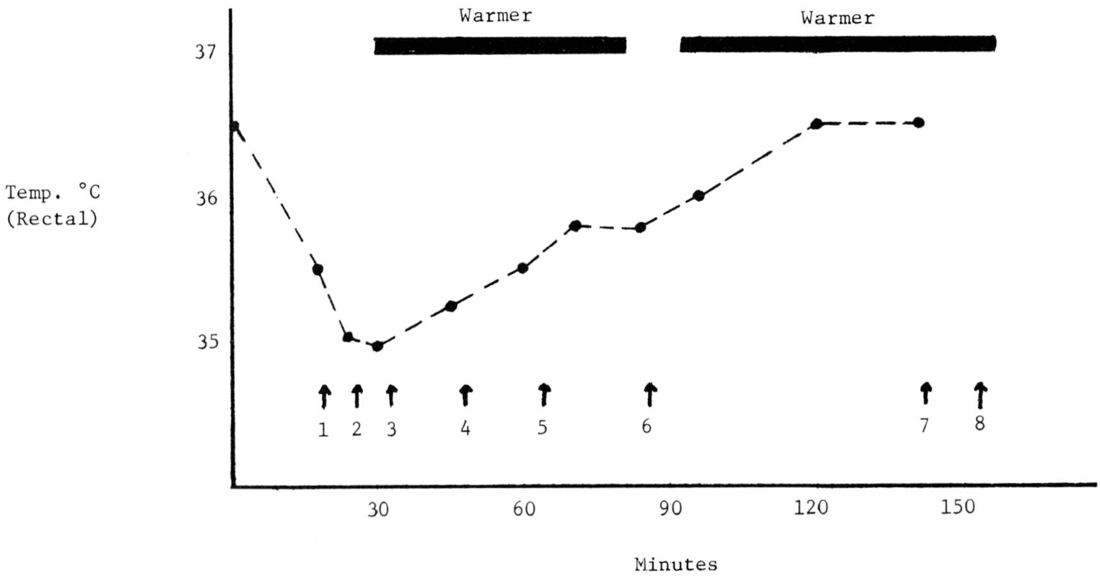

Fig. 4. Temperature curve of a neonate during exposure of his intestines for repair of duodenal atresia. Note the reversal of his temperature decrease by the use of the infra-red heat. Ambient room temperature was 23° C.; Temperature under heating unit was 34° C. Arrows: *1,* Cut-down; *2,* surgical preparation; *3,* draped; *4,* abdomen open; *5,* gastrostomy; *6,* duodenoduodenostomy; *7,* extubation; *8,* to ICU.

and evaporative loss. Radiant heat loss cannot be altered, but with the use of the infra-red heater, radiant heat gain will reverse the temperature drift. Evaporative heat loss is most likely to occur during the preoperative scrub when the skin is wet and also when the viscera are exposed to the drying effect of the ambient air. Once cooling has occurred the neonate's heat generating capacity is frequently inadequate to raise his core temperature without the addition of external heat. We have found that especially during the preoperative preparation and when the intestines are exposed, the radiant heater is an indispensable adjunct for maintaining the child's temperature. Since it is suspended above the surgeon's head, it is not in the way of the surgical procedure and does not provide great discomfort for those above whose heads it is positioned. Once the patient's temperature has been brought to a normal level, it can be turned off or moved out of the center

We have found that the circulating warm water mattress is insufficient to maintain the neonate's temperature during the preoperative preparation and when the serosal surfaces are exposed. Consequently, prior to our use of the suspended radiant heater, warm water–filled gloves were also packed around the infant. However, these usually cooled within a short time. Wrapping the infant's extremities with aluminum foil is likewise insufficient to maintain core temperature, and combining all three of these maneuvers is cumbersome and still not totally effective.

The greatest advance in the area of intraoperative heat control is the use of infra-red or radiant heat. Shaw's[6] use of his "hot pipe" system, for delivery is ingenious. Although we have not used this system, it seems that the mechanics of radiant energy delivery by "hot pipe" conductors within the sterile field would be cumbersome. However, using the same principle of infra-red heat application, we adopted the commercially available infant warmer to the operating room and have used it for about two years and in more than 100 operations. It has had great acceptance with the nursing team and anesthesiologists and is simple to use. No sterile

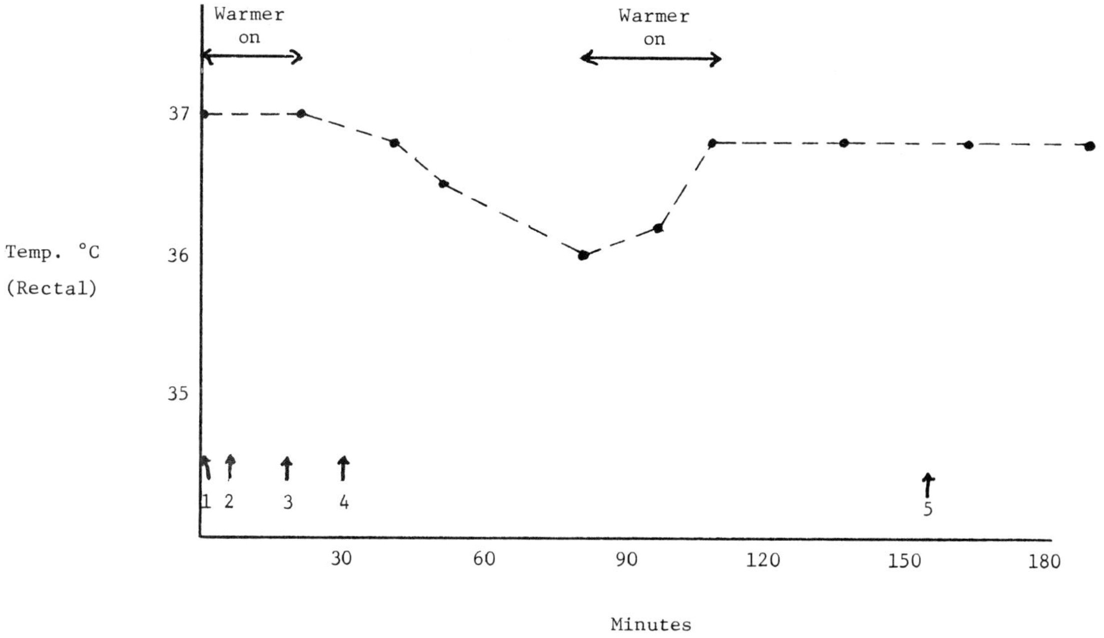

Fig. 5. Hirschsprung's disease with agangionosis to the jejunum. Procedure consisted of multiple biopsies with frozen section and the creation of a jejunostomy. Ambient room temperature was 23° C.; Temperature under heating unit was 34° C. Arrows: *1,* Induction; *2,* surgical preparation; *3,* incision; *4,* peritoneum open; *5,* abdomen closed.

equipment is necessary. The unit is always used in conjunction with a circulating warm water mattress.

No unusual increase in drying of the serosa was noticed, but this aspect was not precisely studied. As with operating in any dehumidified room, serosal drying had to be counteracted by wetting the bowel. Whether or not radiant energy causes injury to the bowel has not been determined, and its effect in the genesis of fibrous adhesions has not been studied.

The heating head is supplied with a thermistor which may or may not be used intra-operatively. We have not used this servo mechanism but have preferred to observe the child's core temperature and to switch the heating element on or off manually. We use a thermistor inserted into the rectum or esophagus attached to a telethermometer.

Since the use of the infra-red infant warmer intra-operatively, post-operative respiratory problems and acidosis have been less frequent and less severe. When combined with good anesthetic management, our infants awake and cry vigorously before leaving the operating room.

CONCLUSION

A detailed method for suspending a commercially available IMI infra-red infant warmer from a standard electrical track is presented. The warmer can be elevated and pushed out of the way when not in use. It is easily positioned by the circulating nurse and has been very effective in maintaining the intra-operative core temperature of surgical neonates when combined with a circulating warm water mattress.

Grateful acknowledgement is made to Mr. Isamu Takahashi, who designed the electrical and mechanical connections for the warmer and supplied the drawings for this communication.

REFERENCES

1. Du, Joseph N. H., and Oliver, T. K., Jr.: The baby in the delivery room: A suitable microenvironment, J. A. M. A. **207:** 1502, 1969.
2. Gandy, G. M., Adamsons, K., Jr., Cunningham, N., Silverman, W. A., and James, L. S.: Thermal environment and acid-base homeostasis in human infants during the first few hours of life, J. Clin. Invest. **43:** 751, 1964.

3. Miller, D. L., and Oliver, T. K., Jr.: Body temperature in the immediate neonatal period: The effect of reducing thermal losses, Am. J. Obstet. Gynecol. **94:** 964, 1966.
4. Oliver, T. K., Jr., Adams, F. H., Adamsons, K., Jr., Day, R. L., James, L. S., and Silverman, W. A.: Thermoregulation of the newly born; Supplement No. 2, Reports of Ross Conferences of Pediatric Research, 1964.
5. Shim, W. K. T.: Lateral plication of synthetic sac for large gastroschisis and omphalocele defects, J. Pediatr. Surg. **6:** 143, 1971.
6. Shaw, A., Franzel. I., and Bordiuck, J.: Prevention of neonatal hypothermia by a fiberoptic "hot pipe" system: A new concept, J. Pediatr. Surg. **6:** 354, 1971.
7. Silverman, W. A., and Sinclair, J. C.: Temperature regulation in the newborn infant, N. Engl. J. Med. **274:** 92, 1966.

Estimation of functional reserve of normal and regenerating dog livers

Layton F. Rikkers, M.D., *and* **Frank G. Moody, M.D.,** *Salt Lake City, Utah*

Maximal capacity for uptake of indocyanine green (ICG) by dog livers before and at intervals after 70 percent resection was compared to mass in an attempt to quantitate hepatic functional reserve. Removal rates of graded, submaximal ICG doses were compatible with Michaelis-Menten kinetics in approximately 80 percent of preoperative determinations, allowing calculation of maximal rate of uptake (R_{max}) and the Michaelis constant (K_m). R_{max} was reproducible preoperatively in 10 of 13 dogs. Since each value for R_{max} was derived from multiple individual studies done on separate days, this parameter could not be reliably measured during regeneration when hepatic mass was increasing. Only 32 percent of calculations obeyed Michaelis-Menten kinetics during the first six weeks after hepatectomy; however, removal rate of a single, near-maximal ICG dose (10 mg. per kilogram) paralleled restoration of liver mass during this early interval. R_{max} could be determined in 55 percent of cases in the last postoperative period (after six weeks) but revealed contrasting trends in the six dogs studied. In conclusion, R_{max} for ICG could be successfully measured in dogs in the stable state. During periods of rapid change, hepatic reserve could be estimated by removal rate of a single large ICG dose.

From the Department of Surgery, University of Utah School of Medicine, Salt Lake City, Utah

DIAGNOSIS and treatment of liver disease is compromised by lack of a technique which accurately assesses functional hepatic reserve. Although impaired uptake of organic anions such as sulfobromopthalein (BSP), rose bengal, and indocyanine green (ICG) has been one of the more sensitive indicators of liver disease, their removal rate in the usual doses employed has not been a quantitative measure of the degree of hepatic dysfunction. Soon after its introduction Hunton, Bollman, and Hoffman[4] showed that the uptake of ICG by normal dog liver approached a maximal rate limit when large doses were utilized. Paumgartner and coworkers[8] postulated that such a plateau in removal rate represented saturation of receptor sites for this dye and, therefore, might be a measure of hepatic reserve. These investigators successfully applied classical enzyme kinetic analysis to the estimation of the maximal rate of ICG uptake by both normal and abnormal rat and human livers from the removal rates of individual submaximal doses. In the present investigation this concept has been adopted for the evaluation of canine hepatic reserve in the stable state and during regeneration following partial hepatectomy.

Research supported by federal funds from Public Health Service Grant No. 7 R01 AM 16233-01.

Accepted for publication Oct. 31, 1973.

Reprint requests: Frank G. Moody, M.D., Department of Surgery, University of Utah College of Medicine, Salt Lake City, Utah 84112.

MATERIALS AND METHODS

Seventeen healthy adult mongrel dogs of either sex, 20 to 30 kilograms, were maintained on ad lib water and standard kennel rations and housed in individual runs throughout the study. During analysis with ICG* each dog was placed in a Pavlov frame and 19 gauge butterfly needles were inserted into the veins of both forelegs. From each, 5 ml. of blood to serve as a blank sample were withdrawn into a heparin-lined syringe. ICG in varying doses was then injected into one foreleg, while sequential samples were obtained from the opposite leg at 5, 10, and 15 minutes. ICG concentrations of the plasma fraction of these samples were determined spectrophotometrically† at a wavelength of 800 μ, after appropriate dilution with normal saline. Plasma disappearance rate (PDR), the percent of ICG plasma concentration removed by the liver per minute, was calculated as the slope of natural logarithm of plasma concentration versus time. PDR in doses of 0.5, 1.0, and 5.0 mg. of ICG per kilogram of body weight was measured in all dogs. Determinations were performed on separate days with a 24 to 48 hour interval between studies to allow for complete hepatic excretion. PDR of a 10 mg. per kilogram dose was calculated in 13 dogs. A 15 mg. per kilogram dose was administered to one dog (Control 1) in an attempt at approaching saturation of the ICG removal mechanism. All doses were prepared from 2 mg. per ml. ICG solutions, which were stabilized with 5 ml. of dog plasma and used on the same day. Individual solutions were compared for uniformity by measuring optical density (OD) of standard dilutions. The slope of OD vs. ICG concentration was 1.269 ± 0.004 mg. per 100 ml. per OD for the 29 solutions tested.

Partial hepatectomy and regeneration. With the use of the operative technique described by Sigel,[13] 70 percent hepatectomies were performed on 14 previously studied dogs. Following intravenous pentobarbital (20 to 30 mg. per kilogram) anesthesia, a generous midline abdominal incision was made. After dissection of the porta hepatis, hepatic ligaments, and hepatic veins, left and central division lobes as well as the papillary process of the caudate lobe were resected. To remove contained blood, excised lobes were perfused through the portal vein with normal saline. Segments were weighed following desiccation in a drying oven for seven days at 200° F. Dry weight of the liver prior to hepatectomy was calculated, assuming the resected specimen to represent 70 percent of hepatic mass (cf. Sigel,[13] p. 791[3]). The remaining three dogs were subjected to sham operation, during which all the above dissections were performed. Postoperatively all animals were maintained on water for the first 24 hours. They resumed preoperative diet thereafter as tolerated. Serum albumin, total bilirubin, alkaline phosphatase, and glutaminoxaloacetic transaminase (SGOT) were measured preoperatively and frequently after hepatectomy in five dogs. These determinations were performed with an SMA 1200 serum analyzer.* PDR in doses of 0.5, 1.0, 5.0, and 10 mg. per kilogram was measured at varying intervals, again allowing at least 24 hours between studies. The residual liver segment (consisting of right lateral and caudate lobes) was removed at autopsy and weighed following saline perfusion and dessication.

Kinetic analysis of ICG removal. The following equation[8] can be used to depict the interaction between ICG and a theoretical hepatic receptor which is responsible for extraction from sinusoidal blood:

$$(\text{ICG}) + (\text{H}) \underset{k_2}{\overset{k_1}{\rightleftharpoons}} (\text{ICG} - \text{H}) \xrightarrow{k_3} (\text{ICG})' + (\text{H})$$

where,

(ICG) = ICG dose,
(H) = hepatic receptor,
(ICG − H) = ICG − receptor complex,
(ICG′) = ICG released from the receptor for further processing by the cell,
k_1, k_2, and k_3 = association and dissociation constants of the complex.

If the assumption is made that the rate of ICG removal by the liver is proportional

*Indocyanine green (Hynson, Westcott & Dunning, Baltimore, Md.).

†Spectronic 70 (Bausch and Lomb, Rochester, N. Y.).

*Technicon Co., Tarrytown, N. Y.

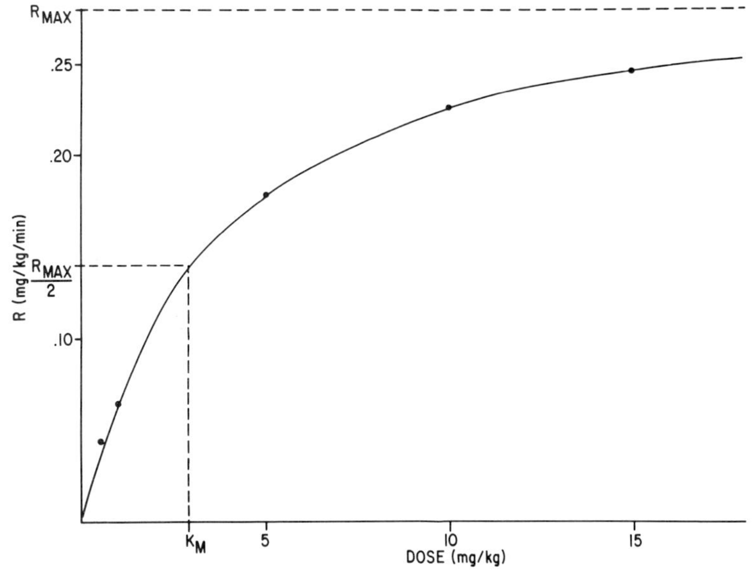

Fig. 1. Relationship between hepatic ICG removal rate (R) and dose administered in control dog 1. At high doses R approaches R_{max} (calculated by Scatchard analysis). The point on the X-axis at which $R = R_{max}/2$ is equal to the dissociation constant, K.

to concentration of its complex with hepatic receptors, the following derivation, which is the Michaelis-Menten equation,[7] applies:

$$R = \frac{R_{max}\ (ICG)}{K_m + (ICG)}$$

where,

R = PDR × dose = initial removal rate of an individual ICG dose,

R_{max} = initial maximal removal rate in milligrams per kilogram per minute or the removal rate when all receptors are complexed with ICG,

$K_m = (k_2 + k_3)\ k_1$ = Michaelis-Menten constant.

Representation of the above equation as a graph (Fig. 1) of dose vs. R inscribes a rectangular hyperbola with R asymptotically approaching R_{max} at high doses, and K_m representing the affinity of hepatic receptors for ICG, equalling the dose at which $R = R_{max}/2$. Since R_{max} and K_m are imprecisely estimated by such a curve, Scatchard[12] analysis, which is a linear transformation of the Michaelis-Menten equation, was utilized to determine these parameters. The conformity of each set of data to such a linear plot validates the application of these principles to those data. In the present study when an R_{max} determination resulted in a correlation coefficient (r) greater than 0.95 on Scatchard transformation, it was accepted as obeying Michaelis-Menten kinetics.

Preoperatively R_{max} and K_m were estimated from three-dose (submaximal doses of 0.5, 1.0, and 5.0 mg. of ICG per kilogram) and four-dose (addition of 10 mg. per kilogram dose) studies. Postoperatively hepatic reserve was measured in two ways: (1) determination of R_{max} by three-dose studies at varying intervals; and, (2) calculation of the removal rate of a single, near-maximal dose (10 mg. per kilogram) at 3, 6, 10, 14, and 42 days following partial hepatectomy. All computations were performed with a Monroe 1266 data processor. All means are presented ± their standard error. Student's t test was utilized to determine significant differences between groups of data. Paired data (e.g., three-dose and four-dose R_{max} and K_m calculations in the same dog) were analyzed with the paired test.

RESULTS

Preoperative. Hepatic removal of ICG was exponential at all doses with near perfect linearity of the PDR plot in 91 percent of individual dose studies. PDR decreased as

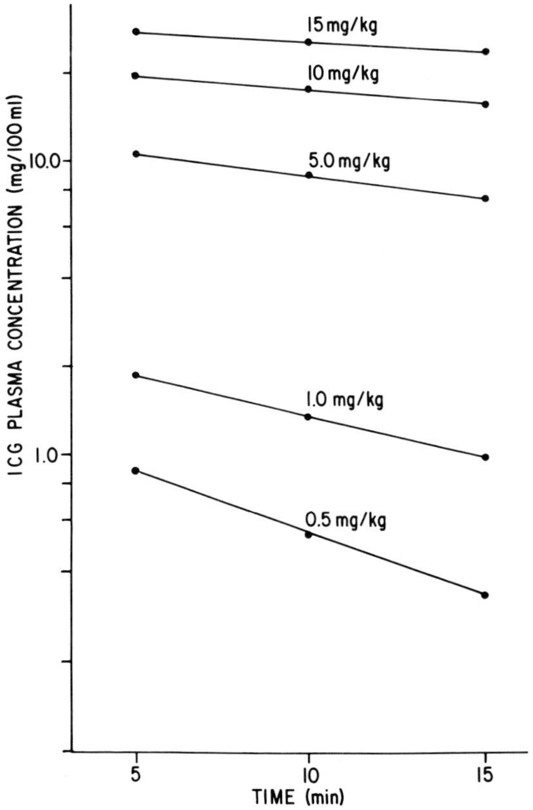

Fig. 2. The slope of ICG plasma concentration on a logarithmic scale vs. time after injection on a linear scale is equal to PDR. These sequential studies in control dog 1 indicate that, as dose of ICG is increased, PDR decreases. This results in a nonlinear increase in R (PDR × dose) which is graphically presented in Fig. 1.

dose of ICG increased (Fig. 2) resulting in a nonlinear increase in removal rate (R) with an approach to maximal removal rate (R_{max}) at high doses (Fig. 1). Thirty-four of the 45 three-dose (76 percent), 11 of 13 four-dose (85 percent), and the single five-dose (including 10 and 15 mg. per kilogram doses) studies obeyed Michaelis-Menten kinetics. These results are presented in Table I. All studies in which R_{max} could not be estimated with reasonable accuracy are excluded from further consideration. When three- and four-dose determinations done in the same dog are compared, the four-dose studies appeared to result in higher values for both R_{max} and K_m (0.236 ± 0.005 mg. per kilogram per minute and 2.599 ± 0.092 mg. per kilogram compared to 0.213 ± 0.007 mg. per kilogram per minute and 2.292 ± 0.137 mg. per kilogram), but differences were not significant ($p > 0.1$). In the single five-dose study R_{max} (0.281 mg. per kilogram per minute) was identical to the value obtained with four doses in that dog (control 1). Reproducibility of R_{max} was shown by sequential three-dose studies in 10 of 13 dogs with a mean difference between determinations of 11.3 ± 0.9 percent. One dog (control 1) studied five times over a six-month interval prior to operation was found to have a gradually increasing R_{max} from an initial value of 0.137 to 0.227 mg. per kilogram per minute just prior to sham operation.

Postoperative. Partial hepatectomy in 14 dogs resulted in an immediate mortality rate of 14 percent and an over-all mortality rate of 50 percent (Table II). The two intraoperative deaths were secondary to accidental ligation of the main portal vein and hepatic venous air embolism, respectively. All three of the sham-operated animals survived. Estimated preoperative dry liver weight in all dogs undergoing resection was 5.06 ± 0.5 Gm. per kilogram of body weight.

Most animals were awake and eating within 48 hours after operation. A mild weight loss, which was regained within two weeks, occurred in five of the seven long-term survivors. Two dogs had a marked reduction in weight of 6 and 9 Kg., respectively. The etiology of weight loss in one dog (No. 4) was never determined; the other dog (No. 2) had extrahepatic biliary obstruction as evidenced by markedly elevated serum total bilirubin (9.1 mg. per 100 ml.) and alkaline phophatase (4,020 I.U.) on the sixth postoperative day. While total bilirubin had returned to normal by four weeks, alkaline phosphatase was still elevated (300 I.U.) just before the animal was killed at 11 weeks after hepatectomy.

PDR of ICG was exponential in 87 percent of individual studies. However, R_{max} could not be reliably measured during the first six weeks of regeneration, with only seven of 22 studies (32 percent) being com-

Table I. *Preoperative R_{max} determinations*

Dog No.	Determination 1: PDR (% min.) of dose (mg./Kg.) 0.5	1.0	5.0	Determination 1: 3 dose R_{max} (mg./Kg./min.)	Determination 2: PDR (% min.) of dose (mg./Kg.) 0.5	1.0	5.0	10	Determination 2: 3 dose R_{max} (mg./Kg./min.)	4 dose R_{max} (mg./Kg./min.)
1	0.061	0.052	0.019	0.122	0.074	0.063	0.019		0.112	
2	0.124	0.109	0.036	0.229						
3	0.059	0.058	0.024	0.169	0.054	0.046	0.025		0.209	
4	0.097	0.070	0.026	0.154	0.087	0.077	0.030	0.025	0.206	0.257
5	0.078	0.057	0.024	0.153	0.073	0.060	0.024		0.164	
6	0.073	0.067	0.026	0.176	0.093	0.087	0.032	0.023	0.217	0.256
7	0.071	0.056	0.027	0.195	0.057	0.051	0.023	0.017	0.170	0.179
8	0.118	0.082	0.023	0.126						
9	0.123	0.078	0.024	0.130	0.122	0.088	0.034		0.207	
10	0.121	0.097	0.038	0.249	0.111	0.088	0.038	0.025	0.259	0.284
11	0.089	0.066	0.029	0.188	0.054	0.049	0.022	0.020	0.165	0.234
12	0.073	0.068	0.034	0.280	0.064	0.064	0.030	0.023	0.242	0.297
13*	0.089	0.066	0.034	0.242	0.062	0.051	0.035	0.016	0.349	0.241
14	0.064	0.057	0.025	0.179	0.056	0.054	0.024		0.176	
Control 1†	0.082	0.068	0.031	0.227	0.088	0.082	0.033	0.021	0.227	0.246
Control 2					0.099	0.069	0.027	0.017	0.165	0.183
Control 3					0.075	0.064	0.020	0.019	0.125	0.186

*A 3 dose R_{max} value not included in table was 0,201 mg./Kg./min.

†Three-dose (0.137, 0.176, and 0.177 mg./Kg./min.) and 4 dose (0.281 mg./Kg./min.) R_{max} values not included in table.

Table II. *Comparison of estimated preoperative and residual dry liver weights*

Time of death postop.	Dog No.	Cause of death	Est. preop. dry liver wt. (Gm./Kg.)	Residual dry liver wt. (Gm./Kg.)	Percent of preop. wt.
Day 1	6	Aspiration	5.52	1.95	35.36
Day 1	13	Gastric perforation	5.48	1.18	21.56
Day 2	7	Biliary obstruction	5.61	2.35	41.93
Day 3	8	?	4.83	3.04	62.89
Day 5	10	Gastric perforation	5.69	4.71	82.82
Day 6	A	Killed	5.58	3.25	70.57
Week 2	B	Killed	5.50	4.91	89.40
Week 6	11	Killed	4.62	5.80	125.63
Week 10	12	Killed	5.15	5.72	110.99
Week 11	2	Killed	—	7.44	—
Week 14	9	Killed	5.38	5.33	99.12
Week 16	4	Killed	3.98	5.31	133.41
Week 20	3	Killed	3.95	5.90	149.63
Week 21	1	Killed	4.56	7.75	169.93
Week 3	Control 2	Killed	—	4.85	100.00
Week 3	Control 3	Killed	—	6.59	100.00

patible with Michaelis-Menten kinetics. In contrast, the removal rate of a 10 mg. per kilogram ICG dose could be accurately determined and revealed a sharp initial reduction followed by a rapid increase in the first two weeks and more gradual return to preoperative values by the sixth week after hepatectomy (Fig. 3). The 10 mg. per kilogram R was also reduced at three days in the control animals but returned to preoperative levels by six days. The decrease in R at six days in the hepatectomized animals was significant at the 5 percent level when compared to operative controls. Beyond six weeks, hepatic uptake of ICG more closely obeyed Michaelis-Menten kinetics (12 of 22 determinations—55 percent) but revealed contrasting trends in the six dogs studied.

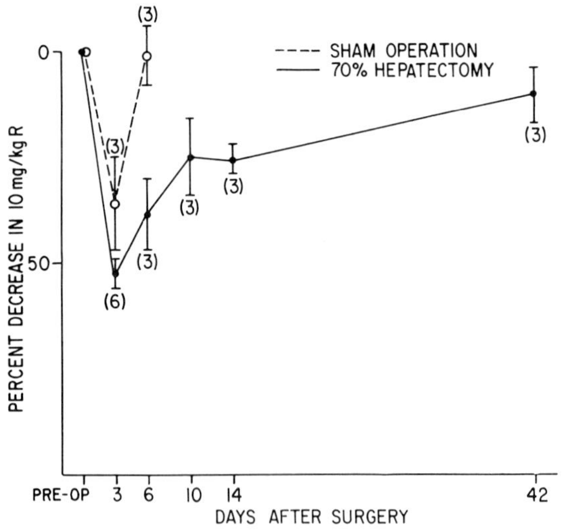

Fig. 3. Relationship between hepatic removal rate (R) of a 10 mg. per kilogram ICG dose and time after 70 percent hepatectomy or sham operation. Vertical bars represent standard error of the mean. Numbers in parentheses indicate the number of dogs analyzed at each interval.

Dogs 1 and 4 exceeded preoperative levels for R_{max} at eight and six weeks, respectively. At sacrifice, elevations of 40 and 41 percent in R_{max} were accompanied by an increase in dry weight of residual liver over estimated preoperative liver weights of 70 and 33 percent, respectively. Dog 2, despite the presence of biliary obstruction earlier in its course, exceeded its preoperative R_{max} by 15 percent at seven weeks. While residual hepatic mass appeared to have returned to normal, this could not be quantitated since preoperative liver weight had not been obtained. In contrast, dogs 3 and 12, after regaining preoperative R_{max} values, progressively deteriorated with respect to this parameter despite return to normal of standard liver function tests and apparent clinical well-being. Sacrifice at 20 and 10 weeks, respectively, revealed that residual dry liver weight was elevated by 50 percent in dog 3 and 11 percent in dog 12. Dog 9 took an intermediate course with an elevated R_{max} at seven and nine weeks followed by a decrease of 32 percent in this parameter at sacrifice, when residual liver weight had returned to the estimated preoperative level.

R_{max}, measured during the second week after sham operation, was similar to preoperative values in the three control animals. Liver weights from dogs sacrificed or dying from complications within the first two postoperative weeks revealed a rapid, though variable, restoration of hepatic mass during this early interval (Table II). Satisfactory liver weights were obtained in 12 of 14 hepatectomized dogs, two of three control dogs, and two additional dogs (A and B) which had not been studied with ICG.

Standard liver function test determinations which were performed in five dogs (Fig. 4) revealed an early brief increase in bilirubin and SGOT following hepatectomy. Serum albumin was decreased postoperatively with return to normal by six weeks. Levels of alkaline phosphatase remained significantly ($p < 0.05$) elevated even at ten weeks, with the highest values occurring during the first two weeks.

DISCUSSION

One major restriction to effective management of liver disease relates to an inability to accurately assess hepatic functional reserve. In the present study mass law was applied to the interaction between ICG and its hepatic uptake mechanism (receptor) in the normal and regenerating dog liver to estimate the maximal removal rate (R_{max}) for this dye. Since R_{max} respresents the rate of ICG extraction when all receptors are occupied, its determination has definite advantages over the disappearance rate of individual submaximal doses. First, since the value obtained for R_{max} depends on the total amount of receptors present, this parameter should be a good indicator of hepatic reserve at least as it relates to organic anion removal. If receptor mass is proportional to total liver mass, then R_{max} should parallel changes in liver weight such as occur following partial hepatectomy and during regeneration. Second, since saturation can potentially be attained despite decreased liver blood flow or the presence of competitors for removal such as bilirubin and other organic anions, R_{max} should be independent of these factors.[8]

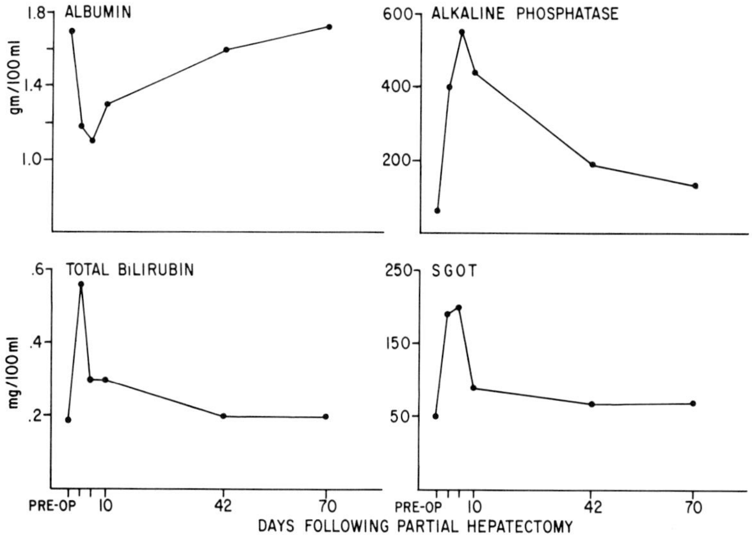

Fig. 4. Serum albumin, alkaline phosphatase, total bilirubin, and SGOT at various intervals following 70 percent partial hepatectomy in five dogs (Nos. 3, 4, 9, 11, and 12).

However, these variables do influence hepatic uptake of individual ICG doses and must remain constant throughout the multiple-dose studies for an R_{max} determination to be accurate. R_{max} could be reliably and reproducibly estimated in the preoperative period presumably because of a relatively steady state in these factors as well as in the hepatic mechanisms responsible for ICG removal. The mean value for four-dose studies (0.236 ± 0.005 mg. per kilogram per minute) was somewhat lower than the R_{max}'s determined from the data of Hunton and colleagues[4] for their two dogs (0.327 and 0.397 mg. per kilogram per minute). The reason for this discrepancy is not clear. Significantly higher values for R_{max} have been established in normal rat[8, 11] and man[8] (3 to 4 mg. per kilogram per minute), suggesting species differences with respect to this parameter.

In a previous study by us[11] R_{max} was successfully measured in rats during regeneration and was found to closely correlate with anatomic liver mass. Each rat was analyzed with a single ICG dose and several animals, all studied at the same interval after hepatectomy, contributed to an individual R_{max} determination. In the present experiment, which is analogous to the clinical situation, it was necessary to separate dose studies by 24 hours to allow for hepatic excretion. Thus, in all cases R_{max} was determined over a significant time interval and could have been subject to fluctuations in those physiologic factors which affect hepatic ICG extraction. In addition, following 70 percent hepatectomy, liver mass and presumably the quantity of ICG receptors were increasing, especially during the initial six weeks. This resulted in only 32 and 52 percent of determinations obeying Michaelis-Menten kinetics in the early and late postoperative periods, respectively.

In order to circumvent these problems, we utilized a single near-maximal dose for measurement of hepatic reserve during regeneration. Initial removal rate (R) of a 10 mg. per kilogram ICG dose did provide a good quantitative estimate of liver function during the first two weeks following resection, with return to near control at six weeks. Hepatic mass was restored at a similar pace, as judged by the few animals sacrificed during this period. Depression of the 10 mg. per kilogram R immediately following sham operation probably was secondary to anesthesia or operative trauma. The prompt return to preoperative levels by six days, however, suggested that these effects were transient and not related to changes in hepatic mass, although liver weights were not obtained at these intervals. The advantage of the single-dose test, especially in its clinical application, is its ability to approximate hepatic reserve during periods of rapid change. Disadvantages include cost and possible toxicity. The only untoward effect observed in our dogs was emesis, occurring 10 to 15 minutes after injection of a dose of 10 mg. per kilogram. In addition, previous studies have revealed cholestasis in experimental animals following the administration of ICG both as a constant infusion and in single large doses.[5]

The progressive increase observed in residual dry liver weight in five long-term dogs might be related to induction of ICG of various intracellular processes responsible for its uptake. Previous studies have shown the stimulating effect of phenobarbital and other drugs on the cytoplasmic "Y" proteins,[10] the in vitro metabolism of BSP,[6] and the canalicular transport processes,[6] respectively, with subsequent increased metabolism and excretion of various organic anions and other compounds. That an organic anionic dye, which is not metabolized such as ICG, can itself act as an inducing agent has not previously been described, to our knowledge. Induction, however, may account for both the overshoot in R_{max} and liver weight that occurred in several long-term dogs. The same phenomenon would explain the continually increasing preoperative R_{max} observed in one dog analyzed over a six-month period. Why some animals deteriorated in the late postoperative period with respect to R_{max} despite regaining or exceeding preoperative liver weight is not known.

The metabolic parameters evaluated postoperatively generally followed patterns similar to those previously reported for regenerating dog liver. However, the persistent elevation in serum alkaline phosphatase observed in our dogs through the tenth postoperative week is at variance with an earlier study in[2] which short-term increases in this enzyme after hepatectomy were thought to be secondary to anesthesia and operative trauma. Other investigators[9] have noted a large rise in activity of alkaline phosphatase in the plasma membranes of regenerating liver cells. They postulate that this enzyme facilitates transport of certain substances into the cell. Another recent report[3] indicates that alkaline phosphatase may be necessary for phosphorylation of certain histones prior to cellular division and, thus, might play a regulatory role in replication of regenerating hepatocytes.

The authors gratefully acknowledge the technical assistance of E. Jane Pipes and Stephen G. DeWitt.

REFERENCES

1. Aronsen, K. F., and Ericsson, B.: Metabolic changes following partial hepatectomy in dogs, Acta Chir. Scand. **134:** 282, 1968.
2. Aronsen, K. F., Hägerstrand, I., Nordén, J. G., and Pihl, B.: Enzyme histochemical studies of the liver remnant following partial hepatectomy in dogs, Acta Chir. Scand. **136:** 521, 1970.
3. Balhorn, R., Chalkley, R., and Granner, D.: Lysine-rich histone phosphorylation. A positive correlation with cell replication, Biochemistry **11:** 1094, 1972.
4. Hunton, D. B., Bollman, J. L., and Hoffman, H. N.: The plasma removal of indocyanine green and sulfobromophthalein: Effect of dosage and blocking agents, J. Clin. Invest. **40:** 1648, 1961.
5. Klaasen, C. D., and Plaa, G. L.: Plasma disappearance and biliary excretion of indocyanine green in rats, rabbits, and dogs, Toxicol. Appl. Pharmacol. **15:** 374, 1969.
6. Klaasen, C. D., and Plaa, G. L.: Studies on the mechanism of phenobarbital-enhanced sulfobromophthalein disappearance. J. Pharmacol. Exp. Ther. **161:** 361, 1968.
7. Michaelis, L., and Menten, M. L.: Die Kinetik der Invertinwirkung, Biochem. Z. **49:** 33, 1913.
8. Paumgartner, G., Probst, P., Kraines, R., and Leevy, C. M.: Kinetics of indocyanine green removal from the blood, Ann. N. Y. Acad. Sci. **170:** 134, 1970.
9. Pekarthy, J. M., Short, J., Lansing, A. I., and Lieberman, I.: Function and control of liver alkaline phosphatase, J. Biol. Chem. **247:** 1767, 1972.
10. Reyes, H., Levi, A. J., Gatmaitan, Z., and Arias, I. M.: Studies of Y and Z, two hepatic cytoplasmic organic anion-binding proteins:

Effect of drugs, chemicals, hormones, and cholestasis, J. Clin. Invest. **50:** 2242, 1971.
11. Rikkers, L. F., Brown, A. C., and Moody, F. G.: Kinetics of indocyanine green removal during hepatic regeneration (abst.), Gastroenterology **64:** 789, 1973.
12. Scatchard, G.: The attractions of proteins for small molecules and ions, Ann. N. Y. Acad. Sci. **51:** 660, 1949.
13. Sigel, B.: Partial hepatectomy in the dog, Arch. Surg. **87:** 788, 1963.

Parabiotic inhibition of murine sarcoma growth

Robert P. Feraci, M.D., *and* **Lionel Schour, M.D., F.A.C.S.,** *Bethesda, Md.*

Inbred mice bearing a methylcholanthrene-induced sarcoma were placed in parabiosis with normal mice or with mice previously immunized against the same tumor. After 15 days in parabiosis, tumor volumes in each group were less than half that observed in the control (single tumor-bearing) animals. Placement of animals in pseudoparabiosis, permitting duplication of physical restraint created by parabiosis without the development of cross-circulation, failed to affect tumor growth. Thus, the mechanism of parabiotic tumor growth inhibition is not related to physical restraint or non-specific factors accompanying the parabiotic state. Sarcoma challenge of previously normal mice, following separation from their tumor-bearing partners, revealed development of tumor immunity in a number of animals. Results of lymphocyte-mediated cytotoxicity studies paralleled the in vivo tumor challenge data. An immunological mechanism is postulated for the parabiotic inhibition of tumor growth.

From the Surgery Branch, National Cancer Institute, National Institutes of Health, Bethesda, Md.

PARABIOSIS, the union of two living animals with subsequent development of a common circulation, was utilized as early as 1908[9] for immunologic investigations. In 1909, Rous[7] was unable to demonstrate transfer of tumor immunity by parabiotic union of normal rats with tumor-resistant rats, and thus from his experiments, he concluded that circulating antibodies to cancer were not present. Although the results of early experiments were complicated by the use of non-syngeneic animals, recent investigators have utilized parabiosis in syngeneic tumor-host systems in order to study tumor immunity.

In 1968, Fisher and Hammond[4] demonstrated parabiotic protection against tumor challenge by passive transfer of tumor immunity from immune to normal mice. They also suggested that parabiosis had an inhibitory effect on the growth rate of a murine adenocarcinoma. The purpose of the present study was to determine the effect of parabiosis on the growth rate of a methylcholanthrene-induced sarcoma in C_{57} mice and to correlate this with in vitro lymphocyte-mediated cytotoxicity determinations.

Accepted for publication Nov. 8, 1973.

METHODS

An inbred strain of C_{57}Bl/6J female mice, obtained from the Laboratory Aids Branch, National Institutes of Health, was utilized in all experiments. The tumor employed was a sarcoma (MCA-10) induced by an injection of methylcholanthrene in a female C_{57}Bl/6N mouse and maintained by serial trocar transplantation.

Tumor cell suspensions were prepared by mincing tumor in 0.25 percent trypsin and agitating for 20 minutes. This was repeated twice, and the supernatant from the second trypsinization was centrifuged at 1,500 rpm at 4° C. for ten minutes. The cells were resuspended and counted in a hemocytometer. Viability was tested by ability to exclude 0.05 trypan blue, and cell suspensions of 80 to 90 percent viability were obtained.

Mice were immunized by subcutaneous injection of 1×10^6 tumor cells in the leg, followed by amputation of the tumor 14 days later. Ten days following amputation, mice were challenged by intramuscular injection of 1×10^3 tumor cells into the remaining hind limb. Using this technique, 100 percent incidence of immunity to tumor growth was achieved.

Parabiotic union was established with the use of the technique of Sauerbruch and Heyde[8] as modified by Bunster and Meyer.[2] Skin incisions were made from the base of the tail to the ear in each of two animals anesthetized with intraperitoneal pentobarbital. The peritoneum of each animal was incised from the iliac crest to the costal margin and all edges of peritoneum were sutured together to ensure firm union but prevent development of a common peritoneal cavity. The scapulas of the animals were sutured together and the skin edges were approximated with skin clips.

Pseudoparabiosis was achieved by placing heavy sutures through intact skin and scapulas of each animal and tying these over bolsters of polyethylene tubing. Sham-operated single animals underwent incision of skin from the base of the tail to the ear and the peritoneum from the iliac crest to the costal margin. The peritoneum was then resutured and the skin closed with clips.

Lymphocyte-mediated cytotoxicity studies were accomplished by routine methods.[6, 10] MCA-10 sarcoma cells were plated out in No. 3034 Microtest tissue culture plates* (approximately 100 cells per well) and 24 hours later, splenic lymphocytes were added at a ratio of 100:1 to target cells. The plates were incubated at 37° C. for 48 hours in a 5 percent CO_2, atmosphere, following which

*Falcon Plastics, Oxnard, Calif.

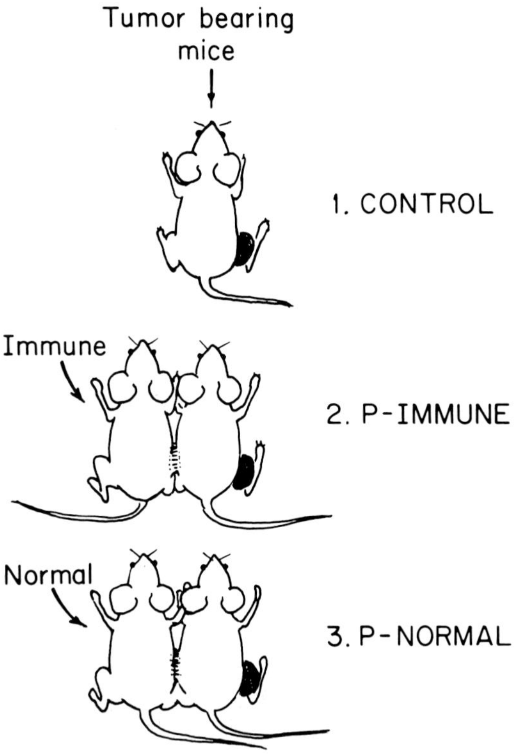

Fig. 1. Experiment 1. Designation of groups.

lymphocytes were removed, the plates were stained, and the remaining target cells were counted. Forty-two replicate wells were included for each test group. Cytotoxic indices were calculated for each replicate well by the following method.

$$CI = \frac{\text{No. of viable control cells} - \text{No. of viable test cells}}{\text{No. of viable control cells}}$$

A cytotoxic index of greater than 0.20 was significant ($p < 0.05$).

Experiment 1. Mice harboring tumors induced by intramuscular injection of 1×10^4 tumor cells into the right hind limb 14 days earlier were utilized. Tumors were measured in three dimensions with a vernier caliper, and volumes were calculated according to the method of Attia.[1] Animals were then divided into the following groups (Fig. 1).

Group 1. Parabiotic normal (P-Nrl): Tumor-bearing animals joined in paraboisis with normal mice (nine pairs).

Group 2. Control (Cont.); Tumor-bear-

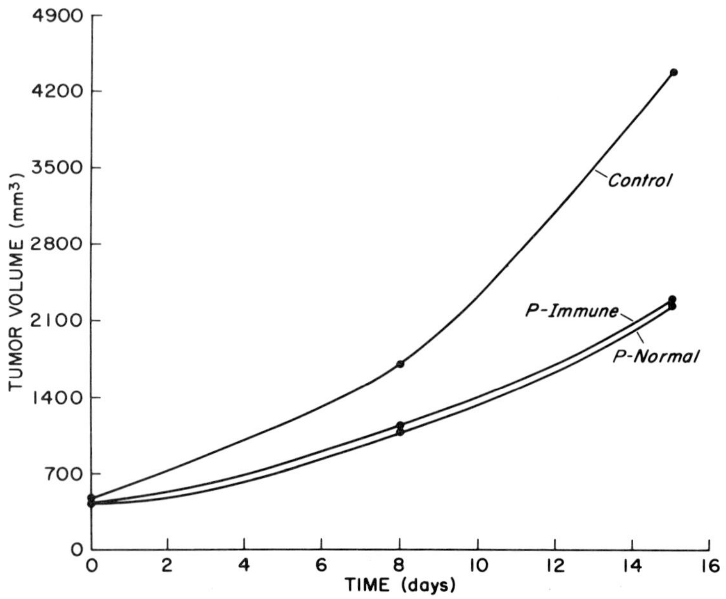

Fig. 2. Experiment 1. Average tumor volumes for each of the groups.

ing animals not undergoing parabiosis (13 animals).

Group 3. Parabiotic-immune (P-Imm): Tumor-bearing animals joined in parabiosis with immune mice (11 pairs).

Tumor volumes were measured on the day each animal was placed in parabiosis and again on days 7 and 15. Average daily growth rate was calculated by dividing tumor volume by the number of days in parabiosis. On day 15, surgical separation of the parabiotic pairs was carried out. At this point, 15 non-tumor-bearing animals separated from the P-Nrl group, 12 non-tumor-bearing animals separated from the P-Imm group, 14 normal $C_{57}Bl/6N$ mice, and 20 mice immune to the MCA-10 sarcoma were challenged with 1×10^4 tumor cells injected intramuscularly into the hind limb. Prior to tumor challenge, lymphocytes from representative animals from all of these groups were harvested by the ficoll-hypaque method[11] for use in the cytotoxicity assay.

Experiment 2. Animals bearing tumors which developed 14 days after intramuscular injection of 1×10^4 tumor cells were divided into three groups.

Group 1. Pseudoparabiosis: Tumor-bearing animals placed in pseudoparabiosis with normal mice (seven pairs).

Group 2. Sham operated: Tumor-bearing mice subjected to sham operation (ten mice).

Group 3. Control: Tumor-bearing mice not subjected to any surgical procedure (eight mice).

Tumor volumes were measured as in Experiment 1.

RESULTS

Fig. 2 shows the average tumor volumes recorded for each of the groups in Experiment 1. On day 15, the average tumor volume in control animals (4,400 $mm.^2$) was more than twice that of the P-Imm group (2,303 $mm.^2$) and the P-Nrl group (2,270 $mm.^2$). Average daily tumor growth rates of the P-Imm group (124 $mm.^2$ per day) and the P-Nrl group (122 $mm.^2$ per day) were similar, and both were significantly different ($p < 0.001$) from the control group (262 $mm.^2$ per day).

Non-tumor-bearing mice from the P-Nrl group (NTB-P-NRL), separated from their partners after 15 days in parabiosis and then challenged with tumor, showed a decreased tumor incidence (65 percent) compared with the control animals (93 percent).

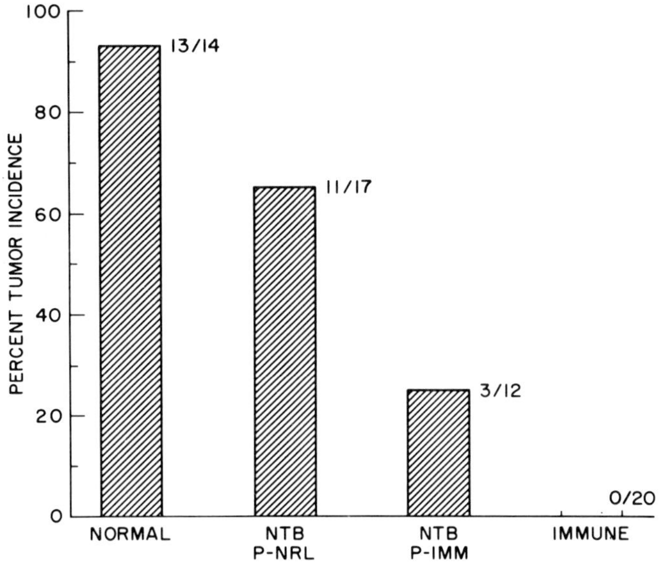

Fig. 3. Experiment 1. Sarcoma incidence in non-tumor-bearing animals following separation from parabiosis and intramuscular challenge with MCA-10 sarcoma. Control normal and immune animals are also included.

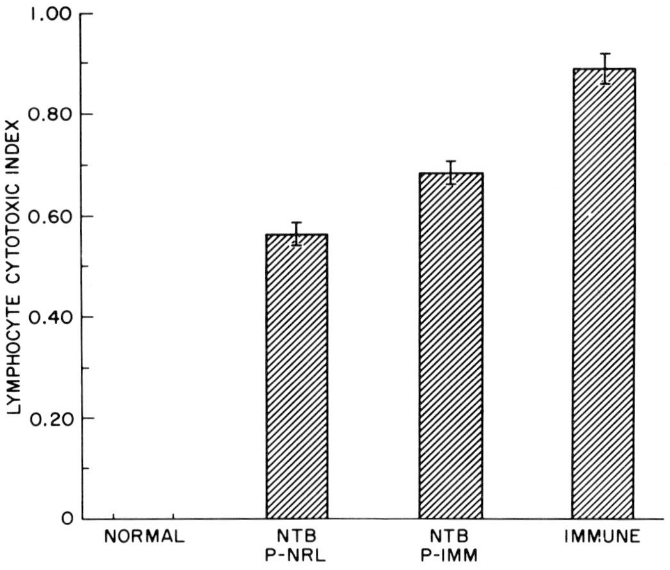

Fig. 4. Experiment 1. Results of lymphocyte-mediated cytotoxicity against MCA-10 sarcoma following separation from parabiosis for the groups included in Fig. 3.

Non-tumor-bearing mice from the P-Imm group (NTB-P-IMM) showed even lower tumor incidence (25 percent) following challenge, and mice immune to the MCA-10 sarcoma were completely resistant to tumor challenge (Fig. 3). Lymphocyte cytotoxicity studies revealed results paralleling those seen with the in vivo tumor challenge. Significant cytotoxicity ($p < 0.001$) was seen in all experimental groups and was greatest in the immune animals, followed by NTB-P-IMM animals and NTB-P-NRL animals, respectively (Fig. 4).

The results of Experiment 2 reveal no sig-

Table I. *Experiment 2. Average daily tumor (MCA-10 sarcoma) growth rates for each of the groups*

Experiment 2 groups	*Growth* (*mm.^{3}/day*)
Control	74
Pseudoparabiosis	66
Sham operated	76

nificant difference in average daily tumor growth rate among the pseudoparabiotic, sham-operated, and control groups (Table I).

DISCUSSION

The results demonstrate parabiotic inhibition of growth of a murine sarcoma and provide information about the mechanism of this inhibition. Parabiosis is a highly artificial and stressful state. Therefore, the hypothesis might be advanced that mechanical and physical factors (such as restraint, confinement, and interference with feeding) associated with parabiosis produce a decrease in tumor growth rate and volume as part of a generalized non-specific wasting of the experimental animals. Pseudoparabiosis permitted duplication of the physical restraint created by true parabiosis without the development of cross-circulation. The data in Experiment 2 demonstrates that pseudoparabiosis had no effect on the tumor growth rate compared with the control animals. Furthermore, it demonstrates that the surgical procedure, per se, had no effect on tumor growth rate since the findings in sham-operated and control groups were the same.

Passive transfer of immunity from the immune animal in the P-Imm group is probably responsible for the decreased growth-rate in the tumor-bearing partner. In support of this concept, previous work has shown that immunity can be transferred across the parabiotic barrier. Zaiman and associates[12] have demonstrated passive transfer of immunity to *Trichinella spiralis* across the parabiotic barrier as early as five days after injection of one of the partners. Falls and Kirschenbaum[3] have shown passive transfer of tumor immunity from immune to normal animals via parabiosis. In addition, passive transfer of tolerance to skin homografts in mice has been demonstrated using parabiosis.[5]

The striking finding in the present experiment is that this same phenomenon may be occurring in the P-Nrl group as well as in the P-Imm group. The data in Fig. 3 suggests that during the period of parabiotic union, the previously normal mice developed immunity to the MCA-10 sarcoma. This immunity could then act to inhibit sarcoma growth in the tumor-bearing parabiotic partner. Although the degree of immunity which the previously normal mice developed was not sufficient to result in 100 percent prevention of tumor growth when the mice were challenged following separation from parabiosis, it apparently was sufficient to cause the retardation of sarcoma growth noted in their tumor-bearing partners during the period of parabiotic union.

The in vitro lymphocyte-mediated cytotoxicity results parallel those of the in vivo tumor challenge data, and further support the concept of the development of immunity in the previously normal animals in the P-Nrl group. Fig. 4 shows that the cytotoxic index in the NTB-P-NRL animals (CI = 0.56) is highly significant ($p < 0.001$), although it is less than that of NTB-P-IMM animals (CI = 0.68) and immune animals (CI = 0.89).

The demonstration of resistance to tumor challenge and significant lymphocyte-mediated cytotoxicity in both the NTB-P-IMM and NTB-P-NRL animals suggests an immune mechanism by which tumor growth was retarded during the period of parabiosis. Clearly, the NTB-P-NRL animals developed immunity during parabiosis as evidenced by their ability to achieve 35 percent tumor rejection following challenge and their demonstration of significant lymphocyte-mediated cytotoxicity to MCA-10 target cells.

Although the in vivo immunity and in vitro cytotoxicity in the NTB-P-IMM animals was not as great as that seen in the

NTB-P-IMM animals and the single immune animals (Figs. 3 and 4), nevertheless, established sarcomas in the P-Nrl *group* demonstrated inhibition of tumor growth rate equal to that seen in the P-Imm *group*. These findings have encouraging implications for immunotherapy and suggest that retardation of growth of an established tumor may ultimately be achieved by the induction of less than complete immunity to that tumor.

We concluded from the present experiments that parabiotic inhibition of tumor growth is an immunologic phenomenon. Studies are presently underway to further elucidate and quantitate the nature of this immunity.

REFERENCES

1. Attia, M., and Weiss, D.: Immunology of spontaneous mammary carcinomas in mice, Cancer Res. **26:** 1787, 1966.
2. Bunster, E., and Meyer, E. K.: An improved method of parabiosis, Anat. Rec. **57:** 339, 1933.
3. Falls, N. G., and Kirschenbaum, A.: Passive immunization of mice in parabiosis against a transplanted lymphosarcoma, Cancer Res. **13:** 741, 1953.
4. Fisher, J., and Hammond, W.: Parabiotic transfer of tumor specific immunity, Cancer **21:** 160, 1968.
5. Martinez, C., Smith, J., Shapiro, F., and Good, R.: Transfer of acquired immunological tolerance of skin homografts in mice joined in parabiosis, Proc. Soc. Exp. Biol. Med. **102:** 413, 1959.
6. Roseneau, W., and Morton, D. L.: Tumor specific inhibition of growth of MCA-induced sarcomas in vivo and in vitro by sensitized isologous lymphoid cells, J. Natl. Cancer. Inst. **36:** 825, 1966.
7. Rous, P.: Parabiosis as a test for circulating antibodies in cancer, J. Exp. Med. **11:** 810, 1909.
8. Sauerbruch, F., and Heyde, M.: Uber parabiose Kunstlichvereinigter warmbluter, Munchen. Med. Wochenschr. **55:** 153, 1908.
9. Sauerbruch, F., and Heyde, M.: Cited by Bunster and Meyer (1933).[2]
10. Takasugi, M., and Klein, E.: A microassay for cell-mediated immunity, Transplantation **9:** 219, 1970.
11. Takasugi, M., and Klein, E.: In vitro methods in cell-mediated immunity, New York and London, 1971, Academic Press, pp. 415-422.
12. Zaiman, H., Wilson, J., Rubel, J., and Stoney, J. R.: Studies on the nature of immunity to trichinella spiralis in parabiotic rats, Am. J. Hygiene **59:** 39, 1954.

Hernia presentation of cancer in the groin

Glenn W. Geelhoed, M.D., Roger C. Millar, M.D., *and* **Alfred S. Ketcham, M.D.,**
Bethesda, Md.

Seven patients with groin masses simulating hernias are presented who underwent operations planned for hernia repair but which led to cancer diagnoses. Other lesions simulating hernias that have been reported are reviewed. We would propose that malignant disease be considered a possible etiology in patients who present unexplained groin masses. Surgical exploration should be planned so that either diagnosis or definitive therapy can be carried out if malignancy is encountered. The surgeon should be prepared to deal with cancer if encountered in the groin or to be aware that re-excision of the operative site may be required at later definitive reoperation and to limit his exploration accordingly.

From the Surgery Branch, National Cancer Institute, National Institutes of Health, Bethesda, Md.

A SWELLING that appears in the groin near the inguinal or femoral canal regions usually signals one of the benign structural deformities that are common in these areas of weakness in the abdominal wall. Since most anatomic deformities in these areas often turn out to be hernias, the diagnosis of hernia is often presumed until a mass in these regions is proved to be otherwise. In most instances, the surgeon can predict the diagnosis of hernia after careful clinical examination. The prevalence of hernia at these sites should not lead the surgeon to exclude other possibilities, however. A mass masquerading as a hernia may signal malignant disease, and the operating surgeon should be alert for the possibility of encountering malignant disease in exploring masses at hernia sites.

At the Surgery Branch of the National Cancer Institute (NCI), we have seen seven patients whose groins have been explored with the presumptive diagnosis of hernia (Table I), but the operating surgeon was surprised by the encounter of malignant disease. The common features of this unusual cancer presentation have been reviewed to alert other physicians to consider all diagnostic possibilities when faced with a mass in the groin area that is presumed to be a hernia.

Accepted for publication Nov. 12, 1973.

Reprint requests: Dr. G. W. Geelhoed, 10N-116, National Cancer Institute, Bethesda, Md. 20014.

CASE REPORTS

Patient 1. V. W. (09-70-88-8) is a 38-year-old woman who noticed a painless right groin lump one month before she consulted her physician. She was referred to a surgeon who concurred in the diagnosis of incarcerated right femoral hernia. The groin was explored through a standard herniorrhaphy incision. Large matted lymph nodes were removed from the femoral triangle but no hernia was found. The diagnosis was changed following histologic examination to malignant melanoma metastatic from a primary in the anorectal mucosa. She was referred to the NCI where

Table I. *Summary of seven cancer patients with the initial diagnosis of groin hernia*

Patient	Age (yr.)	Sex	Duration of mass (mo.)	Preoperative diagnosis	Postoperative diagnosis
R. K.	62	F	1	Incarcerated left inguinal hernia	Metastatic melanoma—previously undiscovered L. calf primary melanoma
R. H.	48	M	1	Right inguinal hernia	Primary rhabdomyosarcoma in adductor longus
R. T.	33	M	3	Right inguinal hernia	Undifferentiated primary leiomyosarcoma
R. M.	60	M	2 (7 yr. after herniorrhaphy)	Recurrent right inguinal hernia	Primary undifferentiated sarcoma, type unclassified
V. W.	38	F	1	Incarcerated right femoral hernia	Metastatic melanoma—anorectal primary melanoma
J. M.	30	M	3	Incarcerated right femoral hernia	Primary leiomyosarcoma
J. M.	46	F	3	Left femoral hernia; persistent left inguinal neurofibrosarcoma	Metastatic neurofibrosarcoma; left femoral hernia

she underwent posterior exenteration and bilateral radical groin dissection three months after her "right femoral hernia" had appeared. At the time of the present follow-up study, she is twelve months postoperative.

Patient 2. R. K. (08-39-47) was a 62-year-old woman who noted a mass in the left groin associated with lower anterior abdominal pain for which she sought treatment at a University Hospital. She was admitted with the diagnosis of incarcerated inguinal hernia. After attempts to reduce the hernia failed, she underwent left groin exploration. No hernia was identified, but malignant melanoma was found in the inguinal lymph nodes. Postoperatively, she was re-examined and a bleeding mole was found on the posterior aspect of her left lower leg which was identified as the primary source of the metastatic melanoma. She was referred to the NCI, where wide local excision of the primary site with split-thickness skin graft coverage was performed. This was accompanied by radical inguinal and pelvic lymphadenectomy, including re-excision of the scar from the previously intended herniorrhaphy. Local control of the disease was achieved, but 18 months later the patient developed visceral and pulmonary metastases unresponsive to chemotherapy, and she died with widespread melanomatosis.

Patient 3. R. H. (08-39-30) was a 48-year-old man who developed right groin pain on straining one month before he noticed a lump in his right groin. He saw his physician, and he was referred to a surgeon; the surgeon agreed that the findings were compatible with an inguinal hernia. The right groin was explored through a standard inguinal hernia incision, and a mass of necrotic tumor was encountered. In obtaining a specimen of tumor, malignant cells were spilled in the surgical wound as the tumor drained. Frozen section diagnosis of a highly malignant sarcoma was obtained. The patient was referred to the NCI with the permanent section diagnosis of pleomorphic rhabdomyosarcoma originating in the head of the right adductor longus muscle. The patient underwent en bloc resection on the right lower quadrant abdominal wall encompassing the old herniorrhaphy incision. An in continuity resection of the pubis, adductor muscle compartment, and right orchiectomy were also performed. Six months later, the patient developed local recurrence of the sarcoma near the area where the inguinal incision had been. Along with this recurrence, pulmonary nodules representing metastatic sarcoma were demonstrated. His extensive disease did not respond to combined chemotherapy and radiation, and the patient died ten months following the surprising findings encountered at inguinal exploration.

Patient 4. J. M. (07-86-33) is a 30-year-old physician who discovered a soft, subcutaneous mass in the medial aspect of his right groin which caused some aching discomfort following the exertion of mowing his lawn. He consulted a general surgeon who admitted him to the hospital with the diagnosis of incarcerated femoral hernia. On reexamination in the hospital, it was felt that the hernia was reduced and elective groin exploration was undertaken several days later.

During the groin exploration under local anesthesia, a mass was removed that extended into the fossa ovalis. The mass was later diagnosed as leiomyosarcoma and the patient was referred to the NCI, where he underwent right radical groin dissection. Five years later, he is alive with no evidence of disease.

Patient 5. R. T. (09-31-30-5) is a 33-year-old man who was in good health until he noticed a small mass in his right groin three months before referral to the NCI. The lump appeared quite

Table II. *Review of thirteen cases of groin masses simulating hernias*

Author	*Date*	*Age (yr.)*	*Sex*	*Preoperative diagnosis*	*Postoperative diagnosis*
Salah[25]	1972	53	M	Strangulated inguinal hernia	Retroperitoneal hemorrhage, trauma
Phillips and Holmes[23]	1972	21	M	Strangulated inguinal hernia	Torsion infarction–ectopic cryptorchid
Brightmore[4]	1971	72	F	Strangulated inguinal hernia	Dermoid cyst–inguinal canal
Speed[28]	1972	72	M	Incarcerated inguinal hernia	Liposarcoma
Handmaker and Mehn[12]	1969	57	M	Incarcerated inguinal hernia	Spermatic cord hematoma–anticoagulation
Robertson[24]	1954	45	M	Incarcerated inguinal hernia	Hematoma–internal oblique muscle
Johnstone and Rintoul[16]	1970	50	F	Incarcerated inguinal hernia; recurrent inguinal hernia	Thrombophlebitis in a varix
Soudek[27]	1970	45	F	Inguinal hernia	Cyst–inguinal canal
Majewski[18]	1965	48	F	Inguinal hernia	Dermoid cyst–inguinal canal
Perrigard[22]	1947			Inguinal hernia	Supernumerary pectineus bursa
Manfredonia[20]	1943	36	M	Inguinal hernia	Preperitoneal lipoma
Bachhuber[1]	1943	48	F	Inguinal hernia	Pedunculated uterine fibroma
Stansfeld	1972	53	M	Strangulated femoral hernia	Lymph node infarction
		54	F	Femoral hernia	Lymph node infarction

abruptly after he had worked a 16-hour shift at heavy labor as a machinery operator. When he complained of some tenderness around this groin lump, his work-mates suggested to him that he had a hernia and should see his physician. His physician made the diagnosis of a right inguinal hernia and referred him to a surgeon who explored his right groin through a herniorrhaphy incision. A mass was encountered which on biopsy proved to be a leiomyosarcoma. At the NCI, he underwent a wide local excision of the groin scar and right radical groin dissection. He has subsequently done well with no further evidence of disease 18 months after his operation.

Patient 6. R. M. (08-73-74) was a 60-year-old man who underwent right inguinal herniorrhaphy in 1963. He was well until September, 1970, when a small knot appeared under the right inguinal hernia scar. He was seen by his physician who made the diagnosis of recurrent right inguinal hernia and explored the groin. A mass was encountered which was excised; no hernia was found. A diagnosis of malignancy was suspected but before a definitive diagnosis could be confirmed by another consultant, the mass recurred and the patient was referred to the NCI.

Physical examination on admission showed a firm 10 × 4 cm. subcutaneous mass in the right groin running along the previous hernia incision which was partially fixed to the inguinal ligament. After extensive preoperative evaluation, he underwent wide local excision of the right inguinal mass with abdominal wall resection. A bipedical flap from the chest and upper abdomen was mobilized to cover the defect which was created. Histologic diagnosis was undifferentiated sarcoma, type unclassified. Three months later, the sarcoma recurred beneath the graft covering the right inguinal region, and widespread metastatic sarcoma was found. Despite treatment with radiotherapy and chemotherapy, the patient succumbed to the sarcoma which had originated in his groin.

Patient 7. J. M. (09-18-36-2) is a 46-year-old woman with von Recklinghausen's disease. She had multiple neurofibromata scattered over her body, one of which gradually increased in size on her left anterior thigh over a three-year-period and the patient had noted tenderness in the area. This lesion was removed by excisional biopsy which yielded the diagnosis of malignant schwannoma. Three months later, a palpable left groin mass developed. She had had a femoral hernia on the right side repaired nine years before, and the mass in her left groin was thought to represent a left femoral hernia. She underwent a left groin exploration intended for hernia repair, but a mass was excised which was reported histologically to show metastatic neurosarcoma in one of three lymph nodes.

Postoperatively, a mass was still present in her left groin, and she was referred to the NCI for definitive therapy. She underwent groin exploration with a preoperative diagnosis of persistent malignant schwannoma metastatic to the left groin.

A superficial groin dissection was carried out. The specimen was entirely negative for neoplastic disease but a left femoral hernia was encountered and repaired. Through a separate incision, a deep groin dissection and radical lymphadenectomy was performed which revealed three of 11 pelvic lymph nodes involved with tumor. The patient's postoperative course was complicated by pulmo-

Table III. *Summary of reported round ligament abnormalities which presented as hernias*

Author	Date	No. of patients	Preoperative diagnosis	Postoperative diagnosis
Innocenti[14]	1948	1	Incarcerated inguinal hernia	Angioma—round ligament
Cullen	1896	1	Incarcerated inguinal hernia	Adenomyoma—round ligament
Moesgaard[21]	1943	1	Incarcerated inguinal hernia	Hemorrhagic cyst—round ligament
Martin[19]	1937	1	Inguinal hernia	Cyst—round ligament
Kershner and Shapiro[17]	1943	2	Incarcerated groin hernia	Endometrial cyst—round ligament
Jimenez and Miles[15]	1960	9	Inguinal hernia	Inguinal endometriosis
Von Hellens[13]	1951		Inguinal hernia	Inguinal endometriosis
Christopher[5]	1927	1	Inguinal hernia	Inguinal endometriosis
Dickinson[9]	1932	1	Inguinal hernia	Endometriosis—round ligament
Sanders[26]	1943	1	Inguinal hernia	Endometriosis—round ligament
Dormandy[10]	1956	3	Inguinal hernia	Endometriosis—round ligament
Daro and co-workers[7]	1954	1	Strangulated femoral hernia	Endometriosis—round ligament
Beck[3]	1936	1	Femoral hernia	Endometriosis—round ligament

nary embolism treated by anticoagulation and caval plication. Although she made an uneventful recovery following her embolic complications and on follow-up 12 months later showed no evidence of recurrence of her hernias or malignant disease, at 16 months postoperatively pulmonary metastases developed.

DISCUSSION

We wish to call attention to malignant disease in the differential diagnosis of masses simulating groin hernias. The diagnosis of femoral or inguinal hernia has been mistaken for a variety of lesions causing a mass in the groin area. A review of the literature reporting lesions which may simulate a groin hernia is listed in Tables II and III. All of the cases except one represent benign disease processes. Although Bailey[2] calls attention to enlarged lymph nodes in the differential diagnosis of inguinal and femoral hernias, only one case of malignant disease metastatic to lymph nodes simulating an inguinal hernia can be found in the literature.[21] As noted in our series of seven cases (Table I), cases 1 and 2 are patients with malignant melanoma metastatic to regional lymph nodes. Cases 3, 4, 5, and 6 are patients with primary soft tissue sarcomas in the groin area.

Patient 7 presents both interesting sides to the diagnosis of groin masses in relationship to malignant disease. She was first diagnosed as having a left femoral hernia based on her prior history of a previously repaired right femoral hernia. At groin exploration, metastatic schwannoma was found in matted left inguinal lymph nodes. When she presented to the NCI, the persistent left inguinal mass was diagnosed at metastatic tumor, but was found to be a femoral hernia which was not appreciated at the first exploration. This finding points out that hernias are still the most frequent structural abnormalities of the groin area even when such groin lumps develop in cancer patients.

The diagnosis of groin hernia is usually made by clinical examination and history. Patients present with the history of a mass in the groin area associated with pain. The appearance of a groin hernia may signal the presence of other physical problems which result in increased intra-abdominal pressure. As examples, chronic cough, constipation, and urinary obstruction are three such findings which may signal the onset of bronchogenic carcinoma, carcinoma of the colon, carcinoma of the prostate, or benign prostatic hypertrophy. These neoplasms arising elsewhere in the body can be reflected at the groin as genuine hernias secondary to the elevated intra-abdominal pressure. This was not the case in the series of patients presented above, none of whom had genuine inguinal or femoral hernias secondary to elevated intra-abdominal pressure from the presence of intra-abdominal visceral neoplasm. In none of the cases did abdominal visceral disease present at the hernia site either. The neoplasms encountered were either primary in the groin, or metastatic from the extremity or regional lymphatic drainage areas.

The important points in the diagnosis of a hernia are the location of the groin mass with respect to other anatomic structures, whether or not a tactile impulse is visible or palpable, the reducibility of the mass, and whether a hernia orifice can be palpated by the examining finger. Incarcerated or strangulated hernias which present as groin masses that are not reducible pose diagnostic problems. The differential diagnosis of this condition includes enlarging of the lymph nodes. Most of the lymph nodes in the superficial groin area lie either parallel and inferior to the inguinal ligament or in close proximity to the vessels. Femoral hernias generally present through the areolar tissue space and are easily confused with enlarged lymph nodes in that area. A mass which presents above the inguinal ligament or in the inguinal canal which does not have a tactile impulse and is not reducible should arouse suspicion. There will be confusion in many cases of groin masses as to the precise diagnosis preoperatively. These patients should be explored for the purpose of determining a diagnosis, and the possibility that malignant disease might be encountered should be entertained. When an irreducible mass is encountered in the groin with no tactile impulse or hernia orifice that can be appreciated, the surgeon is obligated to carefully examine the anatomic regions draining into that groin for occult inflammation or neoplasm.

Patient 6 poses the interesting problem of a mass appearing at the site of a previous herniorrhaphy simulating recurrent hernia. Careful examination with attention to the same criteria of reducibility, impulse, and orifice must be considered in the determination of recurrent hernia or a mass for which an etiology must be found.

In the event that a suspicious groin mass is encountered during exploration for inguinal hernia, the surgeon should establish the diagnosis without compromising definitive resection. If he is not prepared to perform definitive cancer extirpation, he should limit his dissection to excisional or minimal incisional biopsy with the awareness that later reoperation will have to encompass the field of his exploration. Subtotal resection as attempted in patient 3 compromised later definitive resection through unnecessary tumor contamination of tissue planes in the groin; thoughtless closure in patient 5 obligated much wider re-excision than would have been required for removal of the primary tumor. The greater mass of tissue resected requires primary wound closure under tension which might break down or graft coverage which might conceal recurrence.

REFERENCES

1. Bachhuber, C. A.: Pedunculated fibromyoma of the inguino-abdominal region, Am. J. Surg. **61:** 308, 1943.
2. Bailey, H.: Demonstrations of physical signs in clinical surgery, ed. 13, Baltimore, 1960, Williams & Wilkins Company, pp. 322-343.
3. Beck, W. C.: Endometrioma on the ligamentum rotundum uteri, Am. J. Surg. **31:** 105, 1936.
4. Brightmore, T.: Dermoid cyst of the inguinal canal simulating a strangulated inguinal hernia, Br. J. Clin. Prac. **25:** 191, 1971.
5. Christopher, F.: Inguinal endometriosis, Ann. Surg. **86:** 918, 1927.
6. Cronin, K., and Ellis, H.: Pus collection in hernia sacs an unusual complication of general peritonitis, Br. J. Surg. **46:** 364, 1959.
7. Daro, A., Capos, N., and Baserga, R.: Endometriosis of the round ligament, J. Int. Coll. Surg. **21:** 385, 1954.
8. Davies, J. D., and Stansfeld, A. G.: Spontaneous infarction of superficial lymph nodes, J. Clin. Pathol. **25:** 689, 1972.
9. Dickinson, A. M.: Endometriosis of the round ligament simulating hernia, Am. J. Obstet. Gynecol. **38:** 720, 1932.
10. Dormandy, T. L.: Inguinal endometriosis, Lancet **1:** 832, 1956.
11. Ficarra, B. J.: Hernia—masquerades of surgical disorders, Surg. Clin. North Am. **51:** 1401, 1971.

12. Handmaker, H., and Mehn, H.: Hemorrhage into spermatic cord and testicle simulating incarcerated inguinal hernia, Ill. Med. J. **135:** 697, 1969.
13. Hellens, A. von: Inguinal endometriosis diagnosed preoperatively as irreducible inguinal hernias: Case report, Ann. Chir. Gynaec. Fenn. **40:** 256, 1951.
14. Innocenti, M.: Angioma cavernoso del ligamento rotondo simulante un'ernia inguinale strozzata, Boll. e Mem. Soc. Tosco-umbra Chir. **9:** 43, 1948.
15. Jimenez, M., and Miles, R. M.: Inguinal endometriosis, Ann. Surg. **151:** 903, 1960.
16. Johnstone, J. M. S., and Rintoul, R. F.: Unusual cause of inguinal mass, Br. Med. J. **2:** 179, 1970.
17. Kershner, D., and Shapiro, A. L.: Multilocular serous cysts of the round ligament simulating incarcerated herniae, Ann. Surg. **117:** 216, 1943.
18. Majewski, W.: Niezwyke umiejscowienie torbieli skórzastej, Pol. Przegl. Chir. **37:** 1175, 1965.
19. Martin, W. S.: Case of cyst of round ligament simulating inguinal hernia, Mich. State Med. Soc. J. **36:** 572, 1937.
20. Manfredonia, M.: Lipoma preperitoneale simulante un á ernia inguinale obliqua esterna, Boll. Soc. Ital. di Med. e Ig. Trop. **2:** 76, 1943.
21. Moesgaard, J.: Tilfaelde af cyste i lig. rotundum uteri simulerende incarceration af inguinal hernie, Nord. Med. **25:** 244, 1945.
22. Perrigard, G. E.: Supernumerary bursa of pectineus muscle simulating hernia in inguinal region, Br. J. Surg. **34:** 314, 1947.
23. Phillips, N. B., and Holmes, T. W.: Torsion infarction in ectopic cryptorchidism: A rare entity occurring most commonly with spastic neuromuscular disease, SURGERY **71:** 335, 1972.
24. Robertson, B. M.: A case of haemorrhage into the internal oblique muscle simulating an incarcerated indirect inguinal hernia, Med. J. Aust. **2:** 674, 1954.
25. Salah, M. W.: Retroperitoneal haemorrhage simulating a strangulated inguinal hernia, Brit. Med. J. **4:** 403, 1972.
26. Sanders, R. L.: Endometriosis: Clinical and therapeutic considerations, SURGERY **13:** 224, 1943.
27. Soudek, V. K.: A cyst in the right inguinal canal simulating an inguinal hernia, Zentralbl. Gynaekol. **92:** 1429, 1970.
28. Speed, Terrell: Inguinal liposarcoma, Surg. Clin. North Am. **52:** 439, 1972.

Hemodynamics of coronary circulation during ventricular fibrillation

C. L. Sarin, M.D., Ch.M., F.R.C.S., *and* W. O. Nickel, M.D., F.A.C.S., *Detroit, Mich.*

Effects of electrically induced ventricular fibrillation on coronary circulation resistance were studied in 10 anesthetized dogs maintained on cardiopulmonary bypass. The aortic root was isolated and perfused by a separate pump at a pressure of 125 mm. Hg. On induction of ventricular fibrillation and on reversion to sinus rhythm there was no change in aortic root blood flow and pressure. It is concluded that induction of ventricular fibrillation does not alter the resistance in the coronary circulation.

From the Department of Surgery, Veterans Administration Hospital, Allen Park, Mich., and Wayne State University, School of Medicine, Detroit, Mich.

THE CYCLIC pattern of coronary blood flow is governed by the aortic pressure pulse and the impedance to the inflow resulting from physical compression of the coronary vessels by myocardial contraction.[5] Eighty to 90 percent of coronary inflow takes place during ventricular diastole. Ventricular fibrillation, being a continuous state of myocardial contraction, is frequently induced during clinical cardiac surgery. Does this state of continuous contraction increase the impedance to coronary blood flow at a constant aortic root pressure?

EXPERIMENTAL TECHNIQUE

Dogs weighing 18 to 29 kilograms were anesthetized with 10 mg. of hexobarbitol sodium per kilogram of body weight. An endotracheal tube was then inserted and anesthesia was maintained with 50 percent nitrous oxide diluted with oxygen and 0.25 to 0.5 percent Penthrane.

Supported by Research Funds of Veterans Administration Hospital.

Accepted for publication Nov. 26, 1973.

Reprint requests: C. L. Sarin, M.D., Department of Surgery, Veterans Administration Hospital, Allen Park, Mich. 48101.

The animal was then prepared for cardiopulmonary bypass. The chest was entered via the fourth right intercostal space and the pericardial sac was opened. Heparin sulfate (3 mg. per kilogram of body weight) was administered intravenously. Two No. 28 Bardic catheters were inserted into the superior and inferior venae cavae via the right atrial appendage. The left common femoral artery was exposed and a No. 16 to 18 Bardic catheter was inserted into the femoral artery for arterial return. The right brachiocephalic artery was isolated and a specially designed arterial return cannula was positioned into the root of the aorta via the right brachiocephalic trunk. A small polyethylene tube glued to the side of the cannula was used to record arterial pressure in the root of the aorta. A schematic diagram of the experimental model is shown in Fig. 1. A Rummell tourniquet was placed around the ascending aorta. A Bardic catheter was inserted into the left ventricle via the apex to vent the heart during cardiopulmonary bypass.

A pediatric Bentley oxygenator was primed with Ringer's lactate solution. The animal was placed on cardiopulmonary bypass at a flow of 80 ml. per kilogram of body weight. Right atrial pressure was maintained at 0 mm. Hg. Esophageal temperature was maintained at 37.5° C. When a steady state of circulation with cardiopulmonary bypass had been attained, the arterial return cannula in the root of the aorta was isolated from the rest of the systemic circulation by tightening the Rummell tourniquet. The aortic root perfusion flow was adjusted so as to continuously perfuse the aortic root at 125 mm. Hg pressure. The flow delivered by the precalibrated aortic pump was monitored by extracorporeal probe of an electromagnetic flowmeter.* The aortic root flow, the aortic root pressure, and the electrocardiogram (ECG) were recorded on an Electronics for Medicine Recorder throughout the procedure.

After a ten minute period of stabilization of the two circulations, ventricular fibrillation was electrically induced with a 4 to 6 volt alternating current (A.C.) delivered through electrodes attached to the surface of the heart. Ventricular fibrillation was continued for a period of 10 minutes, during which aortic root flow, arterial pressure, and ECG were continuously monitored. The heart was defibrillated at the end of this period by a direct current (D.C.) defibrillator. The above observations were continued for a period of 10 minutes.

RESULTS

Continuous records of aortic root blood flow (made with the use of an electromagnetic flowmeter and a calibrated perfusion pump), aortic root pressure and ECG were made with the animals on cardiopulmonary bypass. Initial records were made with the heart in sinus rhythm, followed by the heart in induced ventricular fibrillation and then on reversion to sinus rhythm (Fig. 2). From the data obtained on pressure and flow, resistance in coronary circulation was calculated by means of the formula:

*Statham Instruments, Calif.

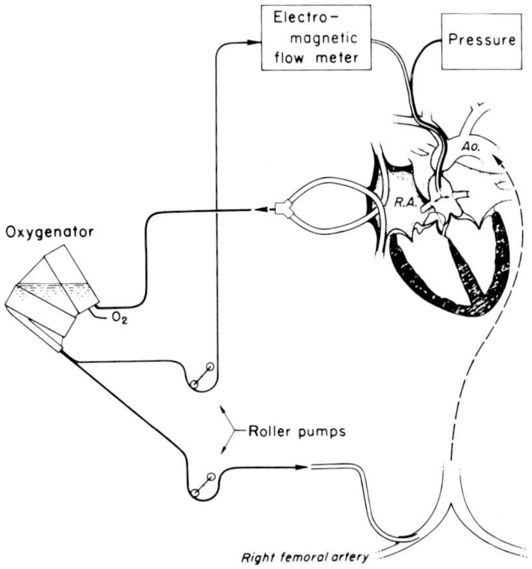

Fig. 1. Schematic diagram of the experimental model used in the present study. "Pressure" in this diagram means aortic root pressure measured by Statham transducer. For details see text.

$$\text{Resistance (PRU)} = \frac{\text{Mean arterial pressure} - \text{mean venous pressure}}{\text{Flow (ml./sec.)}}$$

As venous pressure was maintained at zero, this can be disregarded. Figures for the weight of the animals, aortic root flow, aortic root pressure, and coronary circulation resistance calculated in peripheral resistance units (PRU) are shown in Table I.

The blood flow required to attain an aortic root pressure of 125 mm. Hg varied from 220 to 350 ml. per minute with a mean flow of 292 ml. per minute ± 57.2 (S.D.) and a standard error (S.E.) of 18.29 ml. per minute. Coronary circulation resistance calculated from the data on flow and pressure ranged from 21.2 to 34.1 PRU with a mean of 26.7 ± 5.6 (S.D.) and S.E. of 1.8.

Once the desired arterial pressure was attained in the aortic root, blood flow required to maintain this pressure remained constant. After the induction of ventricular fibrillation the flow was maintained at the prefibrillation levels.

At a constant coronary artery flow any change in the coronary circulation resistance would have been reflected by changes

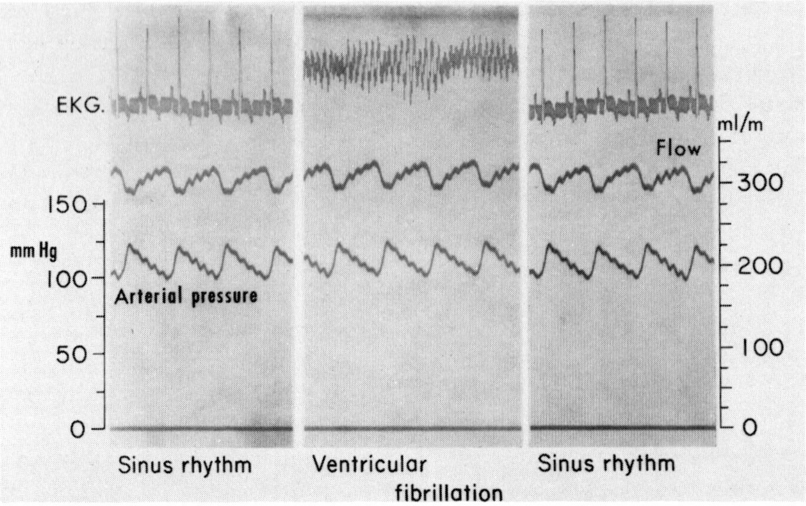

Fig. 2. The arterial pressure blood flow required to attain a mean pressure of 125 mm. Hg in the aortic root during sinus rhythm, during electrically induced ventricular fibrillation, and on reversion to sinus rhythm. Electrocardiographic tracings during three phases are also shown. (Paper speed, 25 mm. per second.)

Table I. *Coronary hemodynamics during ventricular fibrillation*

Dog No.	*Weight (Kg.)*	*Coronary blood flow* (ml./min.)*			*Pressure* (mm. Hg)*			*Resistance* (PRU)*		
		Sinus	*Fib.*	*Postfib.*	*Sinus*	*Fib.*	*Postfib.*	*Sinus*	*Fib.*	*Postfib.*
1	29	220	220	220	125	125	125	34.1	34.1	14.1
2	26	330	330	330	125	125	125	22.8	22.8	22.8
3	28	320	320	320	125	125	125	23.5	23.5	23.5
4	29	354	354	354	125	125	125	21.2	21.2	21.2
5	18	220	220	220	125	125	125	34.1	34.1	34.1
6	23	354	354	354	125	125	125	21.2	21.2	21.2
7	25	265	265	265	125	125	125	28.3	28.3	28.3
8	22	354	354	354	125	125	125	21.2	21.2	21.2
9	23	285	285	285	125	125	125	26.3	26.3	26.3
10	23	220	220	220	125	125	125	34.1	34.1	34.1
Mean		292.2						26.7		
S.D.		57.82						5.6		
S.E.		18.29						1.8		

*It is evident that these three parameters are not affected by induction of ventricular fibrillation or on reversion to sinus rhythm.

in aortic root pressure. Since that pressure remained unchanged on induction of ventricular fibrillation and on its reversion to normal sinus rhythm, we have shown that induction of ventricular fibrillation does not bring about any change in the resistance in the coronary circulation.

DISCUSSION

Cardiac standstill provides an ideal state for intracardiac maneuvers in open-heart surgery and is also helpful in coronary artery surgery. A quiet, nonbeating heart not only provides a still organ to work on but also prevents the accidental expulsion of air into the arterial system.

An ideal means to achieve cardiac standstill should be easily inducible, easily maintained, and quickly reversible; it should not damage the myocardial structure or impair its function. Achievement of cardiac asystole with the use of potassium citrate[4] or acetylcholine[3] has fallen into disrepute because it causes lasting myocardial damage. Prolonged anoxic arrest causes depression of myocardial function.[6] Senning[7] had introduced induced electrical fibrillation to attain cardiac standstill in experimental surgery and its use in clinical practice was introduced by Glenn and associates.[2] Since ventricular fibrillation provides a still heart, prevents air embolism, is easily induced, and can be instantaneously reversed, it has become the most acceptable method of achieving cardiac standstill during clinical cardiac surgery. However, one pays the price for cardiac standstill, since the oxygen requirements of fibrillating hearts are higher than those of empty beating hearts. As a result ischemia is less well tolerated in the fibrillating heart than in the empty beating heart.[10]

During cardiopulmonary bypass, coronary perfusion is dependent upon the mean pressure in the root of aorta which is a function of cardiac output and systemic resistance. However, when the aorta is opened, and we cannulate the coronary arteries individually, a separate pump is used to perfuse the coronary arteries. It has been shown that a linear correlation between coronary arterial perfusion pressure and flow exists. Optimal coronary perfusion as reflected in left ventricular function was achieved at a mean coronary perfusion pressure of 100 to 125 mm. Hg.[8] This pressure range seems to deliver adequate blood flow to prevent damage to the myocardial structure or function. When conducting coronary perfusion from a separate pump, only a narrow flow range permits perfusion in the physiologic range of pressure. Any undetected increase in coronary circulation resistance may reduce the flow, resulting in decrease in myocardial function, and a fall in resistance may result in an increased perfusion, which has been shown to damage the myocardium by subendocardial hemorrhage.[1] (Also, myocardial oxygen consumption is higher with rise in pressure.) Some surgeons avoid using the technique of ventricular fibrillation during operations, as this may offer increased resistance to coronary blood flow and thereby reduce the blood flow. Also they cannot see the ECG which may reveal the onset of myocardial anoxia during the operation.

Coronary blood flow has a cyclic pattern. Eighty to 90 percent of the coronary inflow takes place during diastole as myocardial contraction by physically compressing the coronary vessels impedes the coronary inflow. Though ventricular fibrillation is a state of continuous systole, it does not alter the resistance in coronary circulation as shown by the present study. It may be that only the coordinated ventricular contraction of systole compresses the coronary vessels and impedes the coronary inflow. During ventricular fibrillation, however, the myocardial muscle fibers are contracting out of phase with each other and therefore do not compress the coronary vessels. Whatever the subtle differences between systole and ventricular fibrillation may be, we have shown that under conditions of constant flow, coronary resistance occurred during ventricular fibrillation as compared to coronary blood flow with sinus rhythm. We suggest therefore that fibrillation is a safe way to produce cardiac standstill.

We would like to record our gratitude to Norman Thoms, M.D., for his help in editing this manuscript and to Mrs. R. Cunningham for secretarial help.

REFERENCES

1. Brown, A. H.: The effect of excessively high perfusion pressure on the histology, histochemistry, birefringence and function of the myocardium, J. Thorac. Cardiovasc. Surg. **58:** 655, 1969.
2. Glenn, W. W., Toole, A. L., Longo, E., Hume, M., and Gentsch, T. O.: Induced fibrillatory arrest in open heart surgery, N. Engl. J. Med. **262:** 852, 1960.
3. Lam, C. R., Graghegan, T., and Lepore, A.: Induced cardiac arrest for intracardiac surgical procedures, J. Thorac. Surg. **30:** 620, 1955.
4. Melrose, D. G., Dreyer, D. H., Bentall, H. H., and Baker, J. B. E.: Elective cardiac arrest, Lancet **2:** 21, 1955.
5. Rushmere, R. F.: Cardiovascular dynamics, ed. 3, Philadelphia, 1970, W. B. Saunders Company.
6. Sarin, C. L., Hall, R. W., and Ross, D. N.:

Effects of extracorporeal circulation on left ventricular function with and without anoxic arrest, J. Thorac. Cardiovasc. Surg. **56:** 395, 1968.
7. Senning, A.: Ventricular fibrillation during extracorporeal circulation used as a method to prevent air embolism and to facilitate intracardial operations, Acta Chir. Scand. **171** (Suppl.): 1-72, 1952.
8. Shaw, R. F., Mosher, P., and Ross, J.: Physiologic principles of coronary perfusion, J. Thorac. Cardiovasc. Surg. **44:** 608, 1962.
9. Sokol, D. M., Mundth, E. D., and Austen, W. G.: Optimal levels of coronary perfusion pressure during cardiopulmonary bypass, Surg. Forum **20:** 175, 1969.
10. Stoney, R. J., Zanger, L. C. C., and Roe, B. B.: Myocardial metabolism and ventricular fibrillation before and after induced ventricular fibrillation, SURGERY **52:** 37, 1962.

Alternatives for vascular access for hemodialysis: Experience with autogenous saphenous vein autografts and bovine heterografts

M. Haimov, M.D., L. Burrows, M.D., A. Baez, M.D., M. Neff, M.D., *and* **R. Slifkin, M.D.,**
New York, N. Y.

Alternatives to the standard arteriovenous fistula for hemodialysis, as applied to a group of 68 patients, are described. These included four proximal A-V fistulas, four brachiocephalic fistulas, and the use of 27 saphenous vein grafts and 40 bovine heterografts for fistulas in the forearm, arm, and upper leg. With the exception of the side-to-side brachiocephalic fistula and the loop vein or heterograft fistula, all other modalities were found acceptable. The serious ischemic complications that can follow construction of brachial artery fistulas are discussed.

From the Departments of Surgery and Medicine, Mount Sinai School of Medicine of the City University of New York, New York, N. Y.

For the patient requiring maintenance dialysis, a complication-free repeated access to the circulation is vital. The surgically created subcutaneous arteriovenous fistula (A-V fistula), originally described by Brescia and associates[1] has been the method of choice in our unit since 1968. Early and late results with this method in more than 200 patients have previously been reported.[4, 5] A group of patients exists, however, in whom a standard peripheral A-V fistula cannot be constructed. This article will deal with the alternatives applied to this select group of patients.

MATERIALS AND METHODS

Twenty-seven saphenous vein autografts and 40 modified bovine heterografts were used in the construction of subcutaneous A-V fistulas for hemodialysis in 60 patients; in four patients fistulas were constructed in the mid-forearm (Fig. 1, *A*); in four other patients, brachiocephalic fistulas were constructed at the elbow level. All surgical procedures were done with the use of local infiltration anesthesia and on an ambulatory basis, when applicable. The indication for an alternative access in all of these patients was the lack of arteries and/or veins which were patent and adequate in size in the distal forearm. Some of the patients exhibited extensive calcific obliterative arteriosclerosis involving medium-sized arteries with absent or weak peripheral pulses. Significant number of these patients were diabetic with end-stage renal disease. In two of them, even the brachial artery did not carry sufficient flow for hemodialysis, and the axillary artery was used as the outflow source (Fig. 2, *B*). In a second group of these patients, deficiency in the venous system was the predominant factor. In some, veins of adequate size were constitutionally absent, while in others the superficial veins were obliterated following repeated venapunctures in the predialysis period. In the remaining patients, both the arteries and veins were simultaneously deficient. Patients who have had multiple ac-

Accepted for publication Nov. 26, 1973.

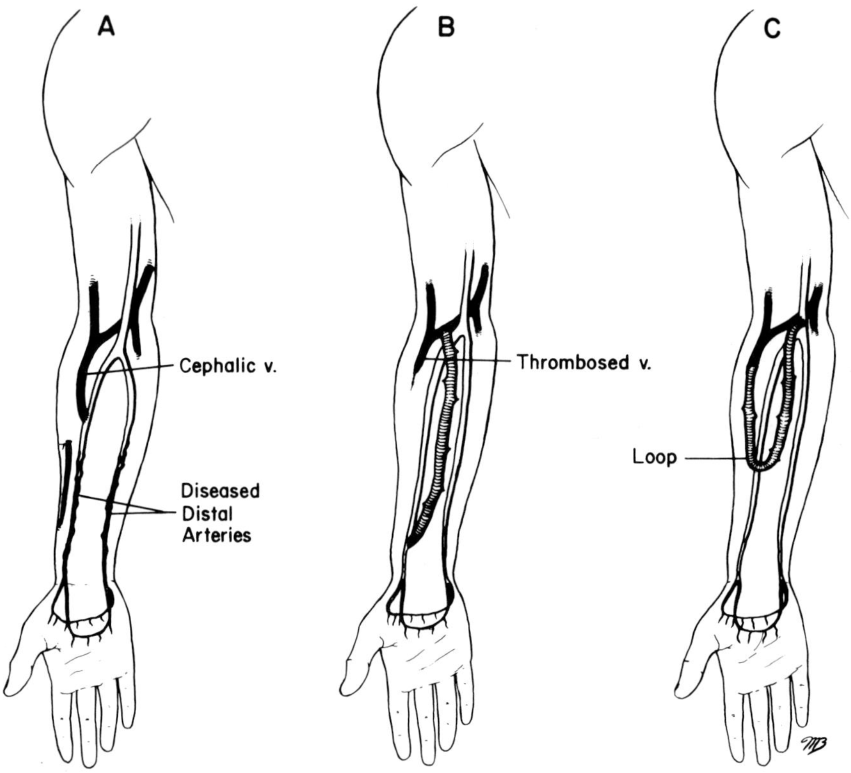

Fig. 1. *A,* Extensive arteriosclerotic process in the more distal portion of the radical or ulnar artery demonstrates the need for construction of an A-V fistula in the mid-forearm. *B,* "Straight" saphenous vein autograft. *C,* "Loop" saphenous vein autograft.

Table I. *A-V fistulas using autogenous saphenous vein grafts*

		No. of months on dialysis											
		3		*6*		*9*		*12*		*18*		*24–48*	
Type	*Total No.*	*No. open*	*%**	*No. open*	*%*	*No. open*	*%*	*No. open*	*%*	*No. open*	*%*	*No. open*	*%*
"Straight" forearm A-V fistulas	13	13	100	13	100	11	100	11	100	7	87.5	5	75
"Loop" forearm A-V fistulas	14	12	84	11	77	8	56	6	42	3	21	1	7

*Calculated for patients at risk.

cess procedures in the past constituted a major part of this last group.

RESULTS

In four patients, a proximal A-V fistula was constructed because of extensive arteriosclerotic process in the more distal portion of the radial or ulnar artery (Fig. 1, *A*). All these fistulas have remained open for a period of eight to 18 months. In four patients, A-V fistulas were done at the elbow level between the brachial artery and antecubital vein. In two of these patients, a side-to-side fistula was originally made; one of them developed severe vascular insufficiency necessitating narrowing and eventual closure of the fistula to alleviate symptoms. The second patient developed extensive swelling of the forearm with associated vascular insufficiency and in this patient also, the fistula eventually had to be closed. In the other two patients, in whom an end-to-side fistula was constructed

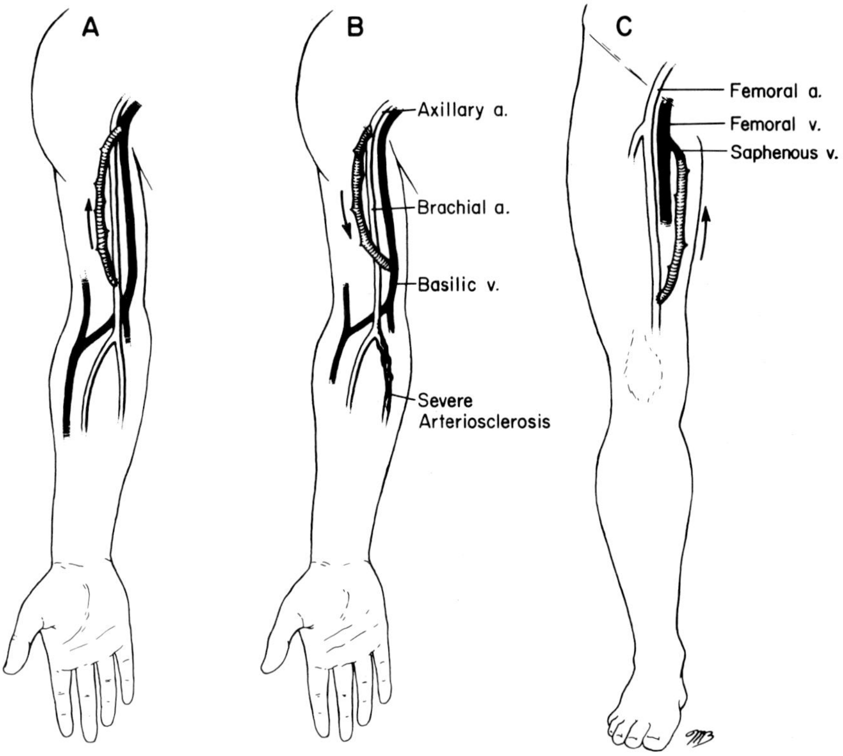

Fig. 2. *A,* A-V fistula between the brachial artery and the axillary vein. *B,* A-V fistula between the axillary artery and the brachial vein. *C,* A-V fistula between the femoral artery and a stump of the saphenous vein which had been excised previously.

Table II. *A-V fistulas using modified bovine heterografts*

Type	*No.*	*Open*	*Closed*	*Percent open**
"Loop" forearm A-V fistulas	4	0	4	0
"Straight" forearm A-V fistulas	20	16	4	80
"Straight" arm A-V fistulas	15	15	3	80
"Straight" leg A-V fistulas	1	0	1	0

*Follow-up period—three to 14 months.

(end of vein to side of artery), no neurovascular symptoms developed and these fistulas have been in use now for 12 and to 16 months.

The experience with autogenous saphenous vein grafts for A-V fistula is summarized in Table I. In 14 patients, a loop saphenous vein autograft was constructed in the upper extremity following the method originally described by May and co-workers[8] in 1969 (Fig. 1, *C*). Two of these grafts thrombosed within the first month following surgery; three grafts thrombosed within six months on hemodialysis; three additional grafts thrombosed within nine months resulting in a patency rate of 42 percent at the end of the first year of dialysis. As seen in Fig. 3, failure continued to plague this group of patients and only one patient has an open graft currently for more than two years. This patient also has had one episode of thrombosis, but the graft was successfully declotted. Thirteen patients had a straight saphenous vein autograft between the radial artery or ulnar artery and the brachial or antecubital vein (Fig. 1, *B*). This group of patients fared significantly better; one thrombosed after 18 and one after 19 months on dialysis, resulting in a patency rate at the end of one year of 100 percent and at the end of two years of 75 percent. In five of these patients, the grafts have now been in use of 26, 29, 30, 31, and 41 months.

The modified bovine heterograft* was used as a venous substitute 40 times in 33 patients (Table II). The smallest diameter graft available was used (7½ to 8 mm. diameter). All operations were done under local anesthesia with the use of standard vascular anastomotic technique and synthetic suture material. Anticoagulant agents were not used routinely. In four patients, a loop-type graft (Fig. 1, *C*) was placed in the forearm. Three of these grafts failed shortly after surgery. Thrombectomy was attempted in all three and was unsuccessful. No obvious technical factors were found to account for the failures. One graft remained open for a period of two months when it had to be removed because of graft infection which developed following accidental trauma to the subcutaneously placed graft.

Twenty heterografts were of the "straight" type (Fig. 1, *B*), and 16 of these have remained open for a period of three to 14 months. Four of these grafts have failed; the cause of failure was infection or unusually small arteries or veins and did not appear to be related to the nature of the graft per se.

Fifteen grafts were placed in the arm, 13 as a fistula between the brachial artery and the axillary vein (Fig. 2, *A*) and two as a fistula between the axillary artery and the brachial vein (Fig. 2, *B*). Three of these heterografts have failed, the causes of failure being false aneurysms in one, endophlebitis of the axillary vein and thrombosis in a second, and inadequate brachial artery flow in the third patient. Three patients of this group developed severe arterial insufficiency. In the first of these patients arterial insufficiency was present even before the graft was done; however, the fistula significantly worsened the ischemia, eventually leading to partial finger amputation. The amputation site did not heal, amputation of the hand at the wrist level was later required. In the second patient, who had had multiple access procedures in the forearm previously, massive small artery and vein thrombosis developed after an episode of ventricular fibrillation and cardiac arrest. Arterial and venous thrombectomy at the wrist level failed to restore adequate circulation and eventually a hand amputation wass required for this patient as well. In the third patient, the flow in the graft was measured directly with an electromagnetic flowmeter and was found to be 1,200 c.c. per minute. With the use of a Dacron cuff, the outflow of the fistula was narrowed until a flow of 400 c.c. per minute was recorded. There was complete symptomatic recovery and the ischemic symptoms disappeared. In one patient, in whom the arm heterograft failed as the result of an axillary vein endophlebitis, a second heterograft was placed in the lower extremity between the superficial femoral artery and a stump of the saphenous vein which has previously been excised (Fig. 2, *C*). Good flow was obtained in this graft, and it was used or dialysis for a period of two months, after which thrombosis occurred which on surgical exploration was found to be due to proximal ileofemoral thrombophlebitis. Thrombectomy was unsuccessful. There were two heterograft infections, both necessitating ligation of the graft and its removal. None of the patients with heterografts have developed aneurysms secondary to graft degeneration for the period of observation of three to 14 months on dialysis for a total of 301 dialysis months.

*Johnson and Johnson, Inc., New Brunswick, N. J.

DISCUSSION

The establishment of a successful access for hemodialysis will continue to challenge the vascular surgeon. Several factors contribute to the increasing number of "problem patients" referred to the surgeon. Maintenance dialysis has become an accepted method of treatment for patients with chronic renal failure, regardless of age or presence of other systemic diseases. The surgeon is therefore confronted with patients with advanced arteriosclerotic obliterative

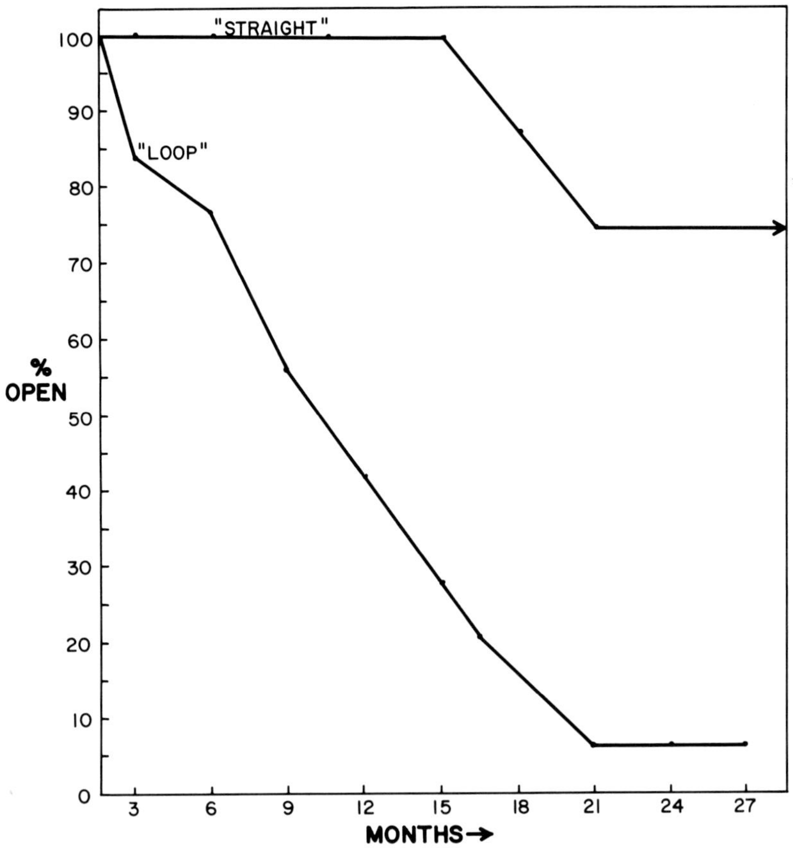

Fig. 3. Patency rate throughout the follow-up period for saphenous vein grafts used as A-V fistulas.

diseases. The second factor accounting for the increasing number of "problem patients" is that chronic dialysis is entering now its second decade and an increasing number of patients are being seen in whom all the conventional vascular access sites have been exhausted.

The standard peripheral A-V fistula remains the method of choice as vascular access for hemodialysis. The various methods used in these patients are all alternatives suggested in those cases, in which a standard A-V fistula cannot be constructed. If the distal radial artery or ulnar artery in the forearm are patent, the straight graft between this artery and the antecubital or deep brachial vein is the procedure of choice (Fig. 1, *B*). The autogenous saphenous vein or the modified bovine heterograft have been used successfully as a venous substitute, and both the short-term and long-term results appear satisfactory.

The arm fistula (Fig. 2, *A* and *B*) is reserved for patients in whom the arterial or venous circulation in the forearm is inadequate either because of obliterative arterial disease or following multiple previous shunt procedures. In some of these patients, a more proximal forearm procedure can be done (Fig. 1, *A*) or if the cephalic vein is superficial and prominent, a brachiocephalic fistula at the elbow level can be constructed. It is important that an end of vein–to–side of artery fistula be done at that level. The construction of a side–to–side fistula with the hope of superficial veins developing as the result of the retrograde pressure has been disappointing. The presence of competent valves prevents distal vein enlargement, and because of the back pressure, severe swelling develops causing marked patient discomfort without any additional pain.

Severe hand ischemia progressing to gangrene is a serious complication of A-V fistulas at the brachial or axillary artery level.[7] These patients are particularly prone to ischemia, since in many the very indication for this type of fistula is the absence of adequate arterial circulation to the forearm. If signs of ischemia develop following surgery, the flow in the graft would have to be measured and decreased to 400 to 500 c.c. per minute, which is adequate for dialysis purposes. Ideally, if facilities are available, the graft flow should be measured in each arm fistula. If the flow cannot be measured and the brachial pulse is not palpable at the end of the procedure, the anastomosis should be narrowed down to the point at which it can be palpated again.

The loop A-V fistula in the forearm (Fig. 1, *C*) with either autogenous saphenous vein or modified bovine heterograft has been found to be inferior to the straight variety for both the short-term and long-term patency. Although technical factors may play a role, the continuous drop in patency over the first two years of follow-up would indicate that a marked tendency to thrombosis is present in these fistulas (Fig. 3). We suspect that this may be the result of hemodynamic, rather than local obstructive factors.

Despite the fact that satisfactory experience with the modified bovine heterograft has been reported,[2, 6, 9, 10] one should be cautious in reaching the final verdict. In our own experience when the heterograft is used in peripheral vascular surgery it appears to be significantly inferior to the autogenous saphenous vein in the femoropopliteal position.[5] However, when used for an arteriovenous fistula, the high flow in the heterograft and the low peripheral resistance do create a situation in which the tendency to thrombosis is markedly decreased. If the long-term follow-up with the bovine heterograft proves satisfactory, it may become the prosthesis of choice for the purpose of vascular access instead of the saphenous vein. In this case use of the heterograft, in addition to simplifying the surgical procedure, will also preserve the saphenous vein for future use by either the cardiac or peripheral vascular surgeon.

REFERENCES

1. Brescia, M. J., Cimino, J. E., Appel, K., and Hurwich, B. J.: Chronic hemodialysis using venapuncture and a surgically created arteriovenous fistula, New Engl. J. Med. **275:** 1089, 1966.
2. Chinitz, J. L., Yokoyama, T., Bower, R., and Swartz, C.: Self-sealing prosthesis for arteriovenous fistula in arm, Trans. Am. Soc. Artif. Intern. Organs **18:** 452, 1972.
3. Haimov, M., and Jacobson, J. H.: Experience with the modified bovine arterial heterograft in peripheral vascular reconstruction and in vascular access for hemodialysis, Ann. Surg. In press.
4. Haimov, M., Singer, A., and Schupak, E.: Access to blood vessels for hemodialysis: Experience with 87 patients on chronic hemodialysis, SURGERY **69:** 884, 1971.
5. Haimov, M., Burrows, L., Casey, J. D., and Schupak, E.: Vascular access for hemodialysis —Experience with 214 patients: Special problems and causes for early and late failures, Proc. Eur. Dial. Transpl. Assoc. **9:** 173, 1973.
6. Keshishian, J. M., John, M., Smyth, N. P. D., Adkins, P. C., Camp, F., and Yahr, W. Z.: Clinical experience with the modified bovine arterial heterograft, Ann. Surg. **172:** 690, 1970.
7. Matolo, N., Kastagir, B., Stevens, L., Chrysanthakopoulos, S., Weaver, D., and Klinkman, H.: Neurovascular complications of brachial arteriovenous fistula, Am. J. Surg. **121:** 716, 1971.
8. May, J., Tiller, D., Johnson, J., Stewart, J., and Sheil, A. G. R.: Saphenous vein arteriovenous fistula in regular dialysis treatment, N. Engl. J. Med. **280:** 770, 1969.
9. Rosenberg, D. M. L., Glass, B. A., Rosenberg, N., Lewis, M. R., and Dale, W. A.: Experience with modified bovine carotid arteries in arterial surgery, SURGERY **68:** 1064, 1970.
10. Rosenberg, N.: The modified bovine arterial graft (editorial), Arch. Surg. **105:** 547, 1972.

Hemodynamic effects of femoral venous occlusion in the subhuman primate

Creighton B. Wright, M.D., Major, MC, USA, *and* **Robert W. Hobson, M.D., Lieutenant Colonel, MC, USA,** *Washington, D. C.*

Data from the baboon, an animal phylogenetically close to man, demonstrated that femoral venous occlusion significantly reduced femoral arterial flow while significantly increasing femoral venous pressure and femoral vascular resistance. Restoration of venous continuity returns extremity hemodynamics to normal. The return of femoral arterial flow and resistance to control level 72 hours following sustained venous occlusion correlates the critical clinical interval associated with vascular trauma. Following occlusion of the femoral vein, lumbar sympathectomy increased femoral arterial flow without further increasing femoral venous pressure. In the presence of major venous injuries of the lower extremity, venous repair is the treatment of choice. When venous reconstruction is not feasible and when the venous outflow is limited, the surgeon should be aware that sympathetic denervation may increase flow in the extremity.

From the Division of Surgery, Walter Reed Army Institute of Research, Walter Reed Army Medical Center, Washington, D. C.

Combined arterial and venous injuries of the lower extremity have occurred commonly in both military and civilian experience.[2, 3, 8, 10, 11, 17, 19-21, 23, 27] Despite significant improvement in arterial reconstructive techniques and a shorter interval from injury to treatment, amputation rates following injuries of the femoral and particularly popliteal vessels have remained high.[2, 3, 19-21, 27, 28] Concomitant venous trauma is associated with 30 to 63 percent of major injuries of the lower extremity.[2, 3, 19, 24, 27] The usual management of these wounds has included reconstruction of the artery and ligation of the vein. Hughes[17] and Spencer and Grewe[27] noted occasional severe venostasis and gangrene following ligation of major veins. Veins were repaired in Korea with satisfactory results; however, the number of cases was small and did not permit a conclusion as to the value of venous reconstruction in the lower extremities. Rich and associates,[24] Sullivan and co-workers,[28] and Cohen and colleagues,[3] have recently reported that acute venous insufficiency caused by ligation of major veins of the lower extremity has contributed to the persistently high amputation rate. These authors recommended that venous reconstruction be part of the management of combined injuries.

The hemodynamic sequelae of acute and chronic occlusion of the femoral vein and its branches as well as the hemodynamics of venous reconstruction have been studied in the dog.[1, 15, 30, 31] The resultant data sup-

Accepted for publication Dec. 10, 1973.

"In conducting the research described in this report, the investigators adhered to the 'Guide for Laboratory Animal Facilities and Care,' as promulgated by the Committee on the Guide for Laboratory Animal Facilities and Care of the Institute of Laboratory Animal Resources, National Academy of Sciences–National Research Council."

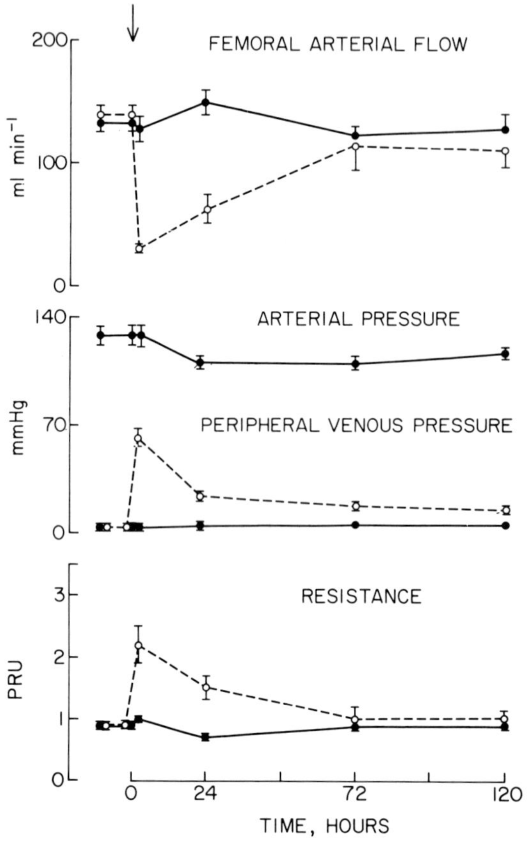

Fig. 1. The effects of femoral venous ligation on femoral hemodynamics are presented. Each point represents the mean ± S.E. of five experiments in five animals. Control, ●——●; femoral venous occlusion, O- - -O. The arrow indicates point of unilateral femoral vein ligation.

port the clinical recommendation for venous repair. Other studies in the dog have suggested that alpha-adrenergic blockade or sympathectomy may be alternate techniques for restoring arterial flow when ligation of major veins is unavoidable.[32-34]

Vascular anatomy of the canine hindlimb, particularly the veins, differs significantly from that in man. The present studies were designed to evaluate the hemodynamic effects of acute and chronic femoral venous occlusion in the subhuman primate, an animal phylogenetically closer to man than the dog. The effect of lumbar sympathectomy on the hemodynamic responses to femoral venous occlusion was evaluated.

MATERIALS AND METHODS

Eighteen adult baboons (*Papio anubis*) of either sex with a mean weight of 17 kilograms were immobilized with phencyclidine* (1.0 mg. per kilogram, given intramuscularly)and maintained under light anesthesia with intravenous supplements of pentobarbital. Femoral arterial blood flow was measured with an electromagnetic flowmeter† and flowmeter transducers‡ calibrated in vivo and in vitro with whole blood. Zero blood flow was recorded by temporarily occluding the femoral artery distal to the flow probe with a vascular clamp. Arterial and venous pressures were recorded with needles or catheters connected to tranducers§ which were calibrated with a mercury manometer at the start of each experiment. The data were collected simultaneously on a multichannel recorder.|| Resistance across the peripheral vascular bed was calculated from the arteriovenous pressure differential divided by flow and expressed in peripheral resistance units (PRU).

Three separate groups of animals were studied.

Group 1. Five animals had bilateral exposure of the femoral arteries and veins. Femoral arterial flow was measured on each side. Femoral arterial and peripheral venous (PVP) pressures were monitored. After a 30 minute recovery interval, base-line values were recorded and the femoral vein was doubly ligated unilaterally. Values were recorded for the subsequent one hour. The animals were reanesthetized 24, 72, and 120 hours following venous occlusion for repeat measurements of the same hemodynamic parameters.

Group 2. In these eight animals, a midline abdominal incision and unilateral exposure of the femoral vessels were performed. After a 30 minute recovery interval, femoral arterial flow and peripheral venous and

*Bio-Ceutic Laboratories, St. Joseph, Mo.
†Biotronex Laboratories, Silver Springs, Md.
‡In Vivo Metric Systems, Los Angeles, Calif.
§Statham, Hato Rey, Puerto Rico.
||Sanborn, Waltham, Mass.

arterial pressures were recorded. Femoral venous occlusion with a vascular clamp was carried out for 30 minutes and then the clamp was released. Subsequently, an ipsilateral lumbar sympathectomy was performed through the midline incision. A segment of the sympathetic chain, including at least three ganglia, was excised. After stabilization of the flow tracings, a repeat femoral venous occlusion of 30 minutes duration was performed.

Group 3. In these five animals, a midline abdominal incision and unilateral inguinal exposure of the femoral vessels was performed. Thirty minutes after completion of the operative procedure, base-line values were recorded and the femoral vein was occluded. After 30 minutes, an ipsilateral lumbar sympathectomy was performed. Hemodynamic parameters were monitored during continuous venous occlusion for an additional hour. At this time, the clamp on the femoral vein was released and observations were continued for 30 minutes. In a single additional animal, the skin of the thigh was circumferentially transected, and the same hemodynamic parameters were measured during femoral venous occlusion before and after sympathectomy.

Data are presented as the mean ± standard error and differences assessed for statistical significance by Student's t test for paired observations.[26]

RESULTS

Group 1. Base-line femoral arterial flows were 134 ± 7 ml. per minute and 142 ± 6 ml. per minute in the right and left hindlimbs, respectively. These values are not significantly different ($p > 0.1$). Arterial pressure was 129 ± 7 mm. Hg and venous pressure was 5 ± 1 mm. Hg. Peripheral resistance was 0.9 ± 0.1 PRU. Occlusion of the left femoral vein resulted in a significant ($p < 0.001$) reduction in flow to 32 ± 3 ml. per minute, while PVP increased significantly ($p < 0.001$) to 63 ± 5 mm. Hg and peripheral resistance increased to 2.2 ± 0.3 PRU ($p < 0.02$). Arterial pressure was unchanged. Contralateral arterial flow was not significantly ($p > 0.1$) different from the base-line values. At 24 hours, flow in the ligated extremity was 64 ± 12 ml. per minute, and this value was significantly ($p < 0.005$) below the control value. PVP remained significantly ($p < 0.01$) elevated at 25 ± 2 mm. Hg, and resistance was 1.5 ± 0.2 PRU in the ligated extremity and 0.7 ± 0.2 PRU ($p < 0.05$) in the control limb. At 72 hours, flow in the ligated extremity was 114 ± 21 ml. per minute, and this value was not significantly different ($p > 0.05$) from flow in the opposite limb. Arterial pressure was 109 ± 2 mm. Hg, PVP was 18 ± 1 mm. Hg, and resistance values were not significantly different ($p > 0.1$). Five days after ligation of the left femoral vein, flow was 109 ± 13 ml. per minute compared to a control value of 129 ± 12 ml. per minute. These values are not significantly different ($p > 0.05$). Arterial pressure was 118 ± 5 mm. Hg. PVP of 15 ± 3 mm. Hg was still significantly elevated ($p < 0.01$). Resistance of 1.0 ± 0.1 PRU was not significantly different ($p > 0.1$) from the control value. These data are presented in Fig. 1.

Group 2. Control femoral arterial flow was 107 ± 15 ml. per minute, arterial pressure was 123 ± 6 mm. Hg, peripheral venous pressure was 8 ± 1 mm. Hg, and peripheral resistance was 1.2 ± 0.1 PRU. Femoral venous occlusion produced a significant ($p < 0.001$) reduction in femoral arterial flow to 30 ± 5 ml. per minute, and this value was sustained throughout the 30 minute occlusion. Arterial pressure was unchanged. Peripheral venous pressure increased to 49 ± 3 mm. Hg ($p < 0.001$), and peripheral resistance increased significantly ($p < 0.01$) to 2.6 ± 0.3 PRU. Following release of the femoral venous occlusion, all values returned to control levels ($p > 0.1$). Following sympathectomy, flow increased ($p < 0.01$) gradually over the first 30 minutes to 203 ± 19 ml. per minute, while resistance decreased ($p < 0.001$) to 0.6 ± 0.1 PRU. Arterial and venous pressures were not sig-

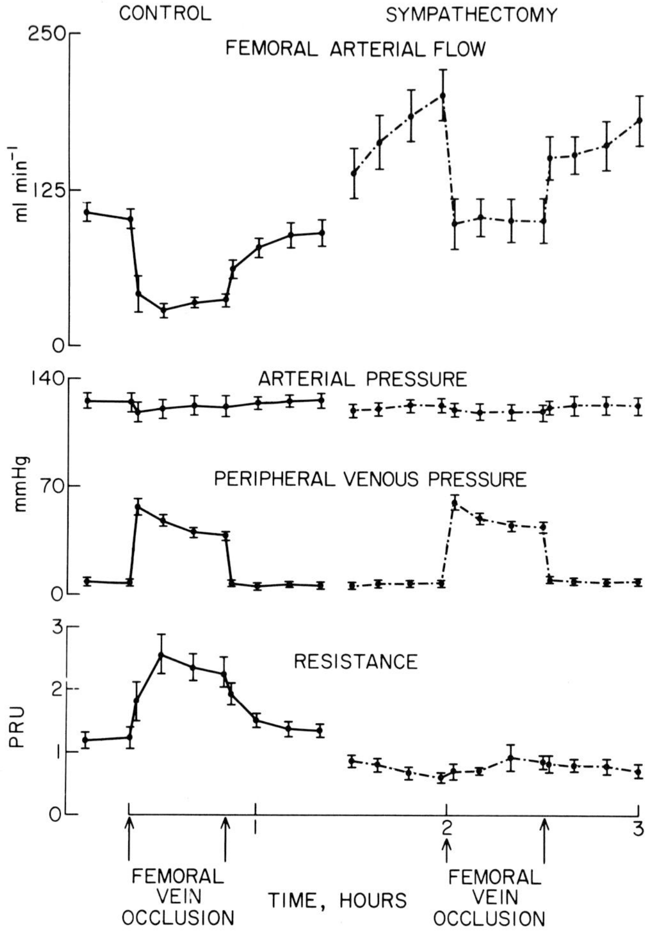

Fig. 2. The effects of femoral venous occlusion on femoral hemodynamics are presented before and after lumbar sympathectomy. Each point represents the mean ± S.E. of eight experiments in eight animals.

nificantly ($p > 0.1$) different from control values at 123 ± 5 mm. Hg, and 7 ± 2 mm. Hg, respectively. Femoral venous occlusion significantly reduced ($p < 0.001$) femoral arterial flow to 103 ± 19 ml. per minute. This value was not significantly different from control ($p > 0.1$). PVP increased significantly ($p < 0.001$) to 46 ± 3 mm. Hg. Resistance and arterial pressure were not significantly altered ($p > 0.1$). After 30 minutes of occlusion, the vascular clamp was removed. Femoral arterial flow increased significantly ($p < 0.001$) to 184 ± 21 ml. per minute while venous pressure decreased to 9 ± 1 mm. Hg and peripheral resistance remained 0.7 ± 0.1 PRU. Arterial pressure was 124 ± 6 mm. Hg. These data are presented in Fig. 2.

Group 3. Control flow was 114 ± 15 ml. per minute, arterial pressure was 131 ± 4 mm. Hg, and PVP was 8 ± 1 mm. Hg. Peripheral resistance was 1.2 ± 0.1 PRU. After venous occlusion, flow was reduced ($p < 0.005$) to 54 ± 9 ml. per minute, peripheral venous pressure was increased ($p < 0.005$) to 61 ± 5 mm. Hg with gradual reduction to 46 ± 4 mm. Hg after the 30 minute observation. Resistance was increased ($p < 0.05$) to a peak of 1.5 ± 0.2 PRU at the 30 minute observation. During continuous femoral venous occlusion, the effect of lumbar sympathectomy was an immedi-

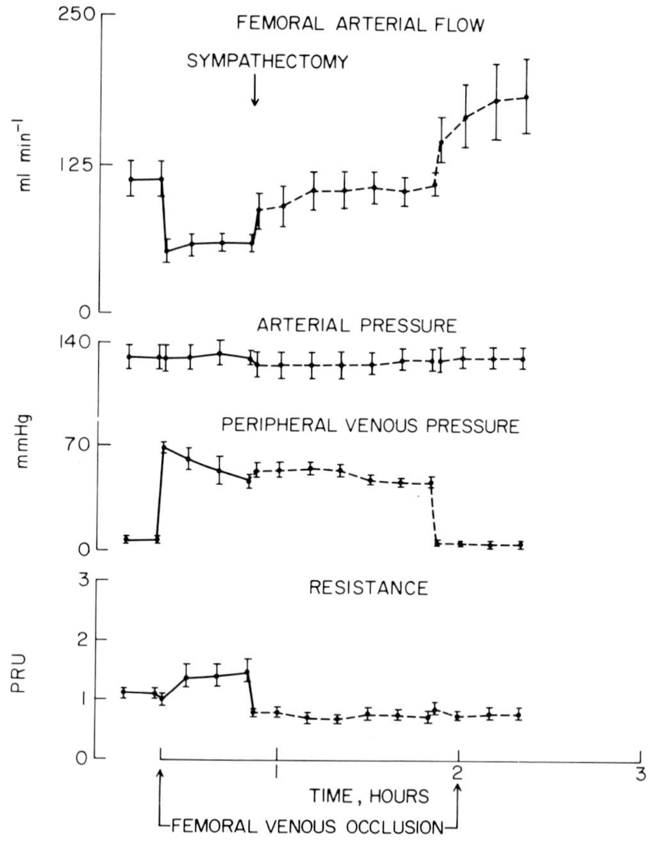

Fig. 3. The effects of lumbar sympathectomy on femoral hemodynamics are presented during sustained femoral venous occlusion. Each point represents the mean ± S.E. of five experiments in five animals.

ate increase in flow and the 60 minute flow was 115 ± 11 ml. per minute. This value was not significantly different ($p > 0.1$) from the base-line value. Venous pressure was 46 ± 1 mm. Hg ($p > 0.1$) and peripheral resistance was reduced ($p < 0.01$) to 0.7 ± 0.1. Arterial pressure was not significantly ($p > 0.1$) different at any point. Following release of the venous occlusion, arterial flow further increased ($p < 0.05$) to a maximum of 185 ± 32 ml. per minute. The venous pressure decreased to 6 ± 1 mm. Hg, while resistance and arterial pressure were unchanged. The data are reviewed in Fig. 3.

In the single separate study with division of the skin of the thigh, control flow was 130 ml. per minute. Femoral vein occlusion reduced flow to 65 ml. per minute. Following sympathectomy, base-line flow was 250 ml. per minute. Venous occlusion immediately reduced flow to 130 ml. per minute; however, at the 30 minute observation, flow was 175 ml. per minute. After release of the occlusion, flow increased to 230 ml. per minute. Distal venous pressure was increased to 35 mm. Hg during each occlusion (Fig. 4).

DISCUSSION

The data from the present study demonstrated that venous ligation in the lower extremity of the baboon was accompanied by a significant reduction in arterial flow as well as increases in femoral venous pressure and resistance. Although venous pressure was elevated throughout the period of observation, arterial flow and resistance re-

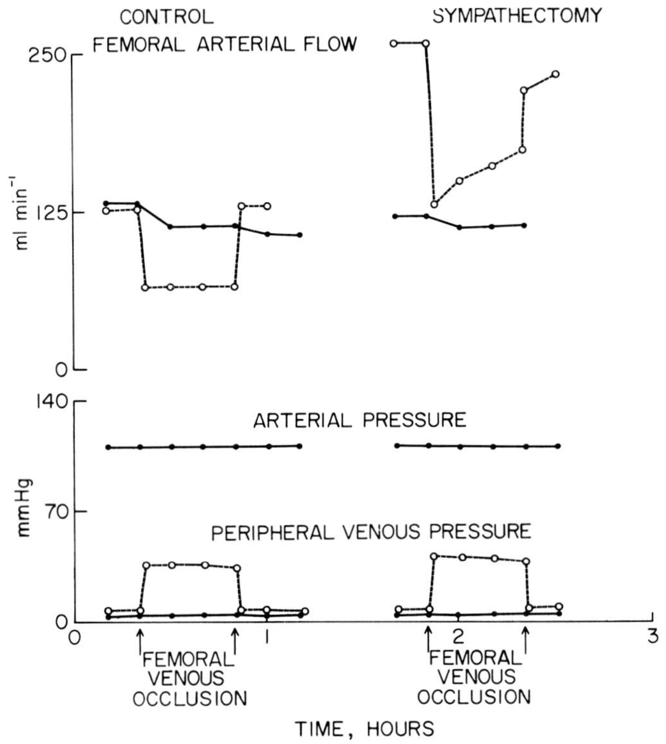

Fig. 4. The effects of femoral venous occlusion on femoral hemodynamics before and after sympathectomy in one animal with circumferential division of the skin of the thigh. Control, ●——●; femoral venous occlusion, ○- - -○.

turned to control levels 72 hours after femoral venous ligation. These data correlate the clinical observations of Cohen and associates[3] and Rich and colleagues[23] that the first 24 to 72 hours after vascular reconstruction are the most critical in determining patency and ultimate limb survival. The ischemic insult of venous occlusion may be in addition to that caused by hypovolemia, extensive soft tissue injury, and fractures. Although our study evaluates the influence of venous occlusion alone, we recognize that these combined factors may render the limb unsalvageable regardless of venous continuity.

Venous repair by lateral suture has been the most commonly recommended technique.[2, 17, 23, 24, 28] However controversy exists regarding venous reconstruction when grafts are required to bridge defects.[2, 11, 19, 24, 28] The reasons for this appear to be twofold: (1) technical considerations in completing and maintaining patency of the venous anastomosis and (2) fear of thromboembolism accompanying venous reconstruction.[4] The technical features for completion of the venous anastomosis and maintenance of high patency rates have been reviewed by several authors.[5, 12, 14, 16] Satisfactory results have been obtained both experimentally and clinically.[5, 9, 12, 14, 16, 18, 19, 22, 24, 28, 35] In general, autogenous sphenous vein has been the best venous substitute. Although the saphenous vein is acceptable for popliteal venous reconstruction, size discrepancy may limit its use in femoral venous reconstruction. However, previous investigations have shown that patency and hemodynamic improvement can be accomplished with even small grafts used in bypass or cross-over fashion.[6, 7, 13, 29] In these circumstances, distal venous pressure is reduced and arterial flow is improved significantly, although neither parameter returns entirely to normal levels.[29, 35] With regard to the problem of thromboembolism, Spencer and Grewe,[27] Rich and associates,[24] and Drapanas and colleagues[10] have reported a low incidence of thromboembolism following venous repair. In fact, the incidence of thromboembolism may be higher after venous ligation as compared with venous repair.[10, 11, 21, 23, 24] Reluctance to perform extremity venous reconstruction on the basis of these factors seems unwarranted by recent evidence.

Although our experimental data as well as a review of clinical reports lead to the recommendation for venous reconstruction, it is recognized that repair of the venous injury may not always be feasible. Previous studies in the dog[32-34] demonstrated that alpha-adrenergic blockade or lumbar sympathectomy increased femoral arterial flow in the presence of femoral venous occlusion. In this study, the results in Group 2 demonstrated the improvement in flow could be achieved following sympathectomy and during venous occlusion. In Group 3, sympathectomy performed in the presence of sustained venous occlusion also improved flow. These data confirm the effects of lumbar sympathectomy on improving femoral arterial flow while reducing peripheral resistance without creating additional significant increases in the femoral venous pressure. The mechanisms for these effects is uncertain; however, the elimination of sympathetic tonus of collateral veins, allowing for their passive dilation, may offer a possible explanation. The single additional experiment, with circumferential division of the skin of the thigh, demonstrated that following sympathectomy improvement of extremity flow occurred even with the femoral vein and cutaneous collateral vessels interrupted. Although not conclusive, this suggests the improvement in flow following sympathectomy is not entirely dependent on cutaneous venous channels.

The beneficial effects of sympathectomy on extremity blood flow are not permanent. Following a variable interval (two weeks to five years), blood flow and temperature return to pre-existing levels.[25] In the dog, femoral venous occlusion two weeks after unilateral sympathectomy produces similar responses in each extremity indicating a deterioration of effectiveness of the sympathectomy.[33] The improvement in extremity flow and temperature and the reduction of peripheral resistance are greatest during the first week after sympathectomy.[25] The hemodynamic effects of sympathectomy as demonstrated in the present study are maximally beneficial during the "critical" one to three days following femoral venous ligation. Following venous ligation when venous collateral channels develop, flow returns to normal as in the dog.[15] At that point, the effects of sympathetic denervation are no longer necessary. This has led us to recommend nonoperative sympathetic denervation, such as epidural anesthesia, when feasible, to transiently improve the hemodynamic situation.[32]

In clinical circumstances following major venous ligation when venous hypertension is evident and ischemic complications appear imminent, sympathetic denervation may be useful.

The technical assistance of PFC Robert Lamoy was greatly appreciated.

REFERENCES

1. Barcia, P. J., Nelson, T. G., and Whelan, T. J.: Importance of venous occlusion in arterial repair failure: An experimental study, Ann. Surg. **175:** 223, 1972.
2. Chandler, J. G., and Knapp, R. W.: Early definitive treatment of vascular injuries in the Vietnam conflict, J. A. M. A. **202:** 960, 1967.
3. Cohen, A., Baldwin, J. N., and Grant, R. N.: Problems in the management of battlefield vascular injuries, Am. J. Surg. **118:** 526, 1969.
4. Cook, F. W., and Haller, J. A.: Penetrating injuries of the subclavian vessels with associated venous complications, Ann. Surg. **155:** 370, 1962.
5. Dale, W. A.: Chronic iliofemoral venous occlusion including 7 cases of cross-over vein grafting, SURGERY **59:** 117, 1966.
6. Dale, W. A., and Scott, H. W.: Grafts of the venous system, SURGERY **53:** 52, 1963.
7. Dale, W. A., and Harris, J.: Cross-over vein grafts for iliac and femoral venous occlusion, Ann. Surg. **168:** 319, 1968.
8. De Bakey, M. E., and Simeone, F. A.: Battle injuries of the arteries in World War II, Ann. Surg. **123:** 534, 1946.
9. DeWeese, J. A., and Niguidula, F.: The replacement of short segments of veins with

functional autogenous vein grafts, Surg. Gynecol. Obstet. **110:** 303, 1960.

10. Drapanas, T., Hewitt, R. L., Weichert, R. F., and Smith, A. D.: Civilian vascular injuries: A critical appraisal of three decades of management, Ann. Surg. **172:** 351, 1970.
11. Gaspar, M. R., and Treiman, R. L.: The management of injuries to major veins, Am. J. Surg. **100:** 171, 1960.
12. Haimovici, H., Hoffert, P. W., Zinicola, N., and Steinman, C.: An experimental and clinical evaluation of grafts in the venous system, Surg. Gynecol. Obstet. **131:** 1173, 1970.
13. Hardin, C. A.: Bypass saphenous grafts for the relief of venous obstruction of the extremity, Surg. Gynecol. Obstet. **115:** 709, 1962.
14. Hobson, R. W., Croom, R. D., and Rich, N. M.: Influence of heparin and low molecular weight dextran on the patency of vein grafts in the venous system, Ann. Surg. **74:** 824, 1973.
15. Hobson, R. W., Howard, E. W., Wright, C. B., Collins, G. J., and Rich, N. M.: Hemodynamics of canine femoral venous ligation: Significance in combined arterial and venous injuries, Surgery **74:** 824, 1973.
16. Hobson, R. W., Wright, C. B., Rich, N. M., and Swan, K. G.: *In* Swan, K. G., editor: Evaluation of vein graft patency, venous surgery in the lower extremity, St. Louis, Mo., 1974, Warren H. Green, Inc.
17. Hughes, C. W.: Arterial repair during the Korean War, Ann. Surg. **147:** 555, 1958.
18. McLachlin, A. D., Carroll, S. E., Meads, G. E., and Amacher, A. L.: Valve replacement in the recanalized incompetent superficial femoral vein in dogs, Ann. Surg. **162:** 446, 1965.
19. McNamara, J. J., Brief, D. K., Beasley, W., and Wright, J. K.: Vascular injury in Vietnam combat casualties: Results of treatment at the 24th Evacuation Hospital, 1 July 1967 to 12 Aug. 1969, Ann. Surg. **178:** 143, 1973.
20. Morton, J. H., Southgate, W. A., and DeWeese, J. A.: Arterial injuries of the extremities, Surg. Gynecol. Obstet. **123:** 611, 1966.
21. Perry, M. O., Thal, E. R., and Shires, G. T.: Management of arterial injuries, Ann. Surg. **173:** 403, 1971.
22. Rich, N. M., and Sullivan, W. G.: Clinical recanalization of autogenous vein graft in the popliteal vein, J. Trauma **12:** 919, 1972.
23. Rich, N. M., Baugh, J. H., and Hughes, C. W.: Popliteal artery injuries in Vietnam, Am. J. Surg. **118:** 531, 1969.
24. Rich, N. M., Hughes, C. W., and Baugh, J. H.: Management of venous injuries, Ann. Surg. **171:** 724, 1970.
25. Simeone, F. A.: Intravascular pressure, vascular tone, and sympathectomy, Surgery **53:** 1, 1963.
26. Snedecor, G. W., and Cochran, W. G.: Statistical methods, 6th ed., Ames, Iowa, 1967, Iowa State University Press.
27. Spencer, F. C., and Grewe, R. V.: The management of arterial injuries in battle casualties, Ann. Surg. **141:** 304, 1955.
28. Sullivan, W. G., Thornton, F. H., Baker, L. H., LaPlante, E. S., and Cohen, A.: Early influence of popliteal vein repair in the treatment of popliteal vessel injuries, Am. J. Surg. **122:** 528, 1971.
29. Webster, J. H. H.: Blood-flow in established iliac venovenous grafts, Br. J. Surg. **53:** 725, 1966.
30. Wright, C. B., and Swan, K. G.: Hemodynamics of venous occlusion in the canine hindlimb, Surgery **73:** 141, 1973.
31. Wright, C. B., and Swan, K. G.: Hemodynamics of venous repair in the canine hindlimb, J. Thorac. Cardiovasc. Surg. **65:** 195, 1973.
32. Wright, C. B., Swan, K. G., Reynolds, D. G., and Nelson, T. G.: Venous occlusion in the canine hindlimb: Hemodynamic effects of adrenergic stimulation and blockade, Surgery **73:** 507, 1973.
33. Wright, C. B., Sayre, J. T., Casterline, P. F., and Swan, K. G.: Hemodynamic effects of sympathectomy on canine femoral venous occlusion, Surgery **74:** 405, 1973.
34. Wright, C. B., Casterline, P. F., Sayre, J. T., and Swan, K. G.: Management of venous ligation, *in:* Swan, K. G., editor: Venous surgery in the lower extremity, St. Louis, Mo., 1974, Warren H. Green, Inc.
35. Wright, C. B., Hobson, R. W., and Alix, E. C.: Results following reconstruction of the canine femoral vein, *in:* Swan, K. G., editor: Venous surgery in the lower extremity, St. Louis, Mo., 1974, Warren H. Green, Inc.

The effects of gastric exclusion operations on pancreatic exocrine secretion

John W. Thomas, M.D., M.S.,* *Lexington, Ky., and* **Edward E. Mason, M.D., Ph.D., F.A.C.S.,** *Iowa City, Iowa*

Three dogs with pancreatic fistulas were subjected in succession to two-thirds gastric bypass, antral exclusion, and two-thirds gastric resection. Three feeding experiments were done after each operation. Each consisted of a standard meal and collection of nine half-hour samples of pancreatic juice. The volume, bicarbonate, and protein content of each sample was determined. This experiment differed from previous experiments in that pancreatic juice was continuously replaced into the duodenum. Previously reported depressions in pancreatic secretion following gastric bypass and gastric resection were not seen in this experiment. The principle effect of the gastric exclusion operations was on the pattern of secretion rather than on the quantity of secretion. The effects of gastric bypass were a late rise in volume secretion and a 30 minute delay in peak protein secretion. However, delay in the peak protein secretion following gastric resection was 60 minutes; therefore, the impairment in mixing of food and pancreatic juice should not be as great after gastric bypass as after a comparable gastric resection.

From the Department of Surgery, University of Iowa, Iowa City, Iowa.

Bayliss and Starling[3] noted in 1902 that the activity of the pancreas is normally called into play by events occurring in the alimentary canal. Operations upon the gastrointestinal tract which alter its function might therefore be expected to alter the secretory activity of the pancreas. Division of the stomach with formation of a loop gastrojejunostomy results in afferent and efferent limbs of small bowel. Since the distal stomach segment is closed proximally the afferent limb of small bowel, duodenum and two thirds of the stomach are excluded from the main flow of gastrointestinal contents. A variety of such exclusion operations is possible depending on where the stomach is divided, whether a portion of the stomach is resected, the length of the afferent limb, and the type of gastrojejunostomy performed. This study was limited to three selected exclusion operations: two-thirds gastric bypass, antral exclusion, and two-thirds gastric resection.

Gastric exclusion operations have been studied utilizing dogs with Pavlov pouches.[17] Gastric bypass caused a depression of acid secretion following a standard meal. It was theorized that gastric bypass removed the antrum from the usual stimuli, yet retained the inhibitory effect of acid secreted by the bypassed segment. When the antral exclusion was produced, there was a steady rise in acid secretion which was attributed to an increase in gastrin secretion. When the an-

Accepted for publication Dec. 13, 1973.

This article is from a thesis submitted as partial fulfillment of the requirements for the Master of Science Degree in Surgery at the University of Iowa, May, 1973.

*Present address: Department of Surgery, Division of Cardiothoracic Surgery, University of Kentucky, Lexington, Ky. 40506.

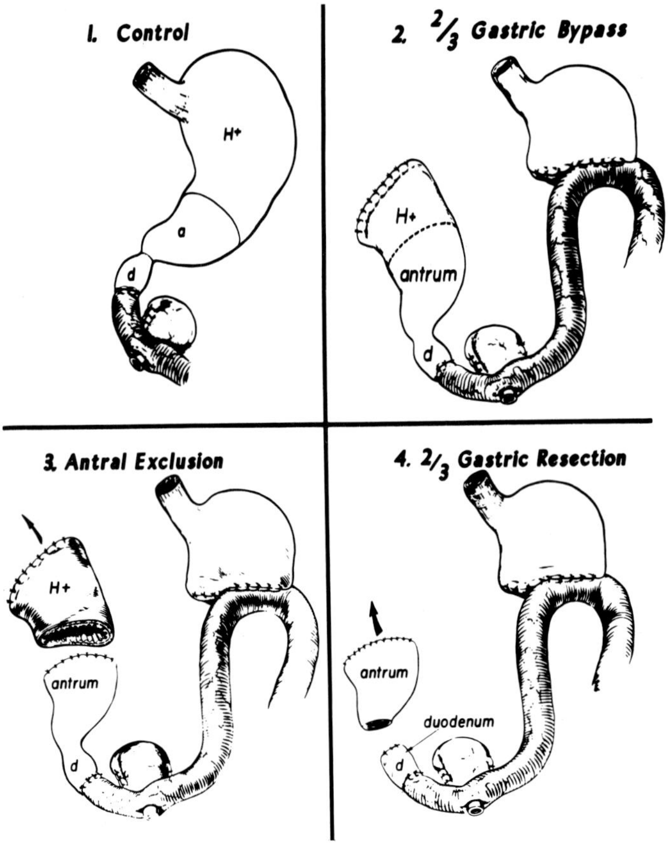

Fig. 1. The four operations which were performed in sequence on each dog.

trum was excised, the acid secretion fell to its lowest level.

One of the other effects of gastrin is that it is a stimulus for pancreatic enzyme secretion.[5, 19, 20] This fact led to the hypothesis that gastric bypass would cause a decrease in pancreatic enzyme secretion following a standard meal in the same manner that it had decreased Pavlov pouch acid secretion. In a prior study, gastric bypass resulted in a 40 percent decrease in pancreatic protein secretion.[18] The pancreatic secretory rate for protein was returned to normal by reconstruction of the stomach, but it was further depressed by transthoracic vagotomy. The reduction in pancreatic digestive enzyme secretion was thought to be due to reduced stimulation from gastrin or possibly less pancreozymin. Division of vagal branches in the wall of the transected stomach was not a factor.

The effect of antral exclusion upon pancreatic secretion has not previously been studied. Stomal ulceration follows antral exclusion, and this has been attributed to gastrin release because the antrum is not inhibited by hydrochloric acid. In dogs, subjected to various ulcerogenic treatments, a two-thirds gastric bypass provides more protection from stomal ulceration than a two-thirds gastric resection.[17]

Gastric resection with gastroenterostomy represents one extreme of the exclusion type of operation in which the excluded stomach segment is reduced to zero. Partial gastrectomy is generally considered to significantly diminish the pancreatic response to a standard meal.[2, 24, 26]

The results of earlier studies in our laboratory[17, 18] suggested a further experiment in which the sequence of gastric exclusion operations used in the Pavlov pouch experiment[17] would be repeated, but now pancreatic protein secretion rather than Pavlov pouch acid secretion would be measured. In most prior studies,[2, 18, 24, 26] the total pancreatic secretion has been removed and none replaced. The present experiment was designed to return pancreatic juice to the duodenum as precisely as possible so as to simulate what would occur in a patient or in an experimental animal without a pancreatic fistula.

MATERIALS AND METHODS

Three female mongrel dogs, each weighing 17.5 kilograms, were used in the experiment. Intravenous Nembutal (pentobarbital) was used as the anesthetic agent in an initial dose of 25 mg. per kilogram. The sequence of operations is shown in Fig. 1. At each operation, penicillin and streptomycin were given.

In the control operation, the dogs were prepared with a permanent pancreatic fistula similar to that described by Preshaw and Grossman[19] and modified by Stening.[25] This preparation allows pancreatic juice to flow into the duodenum between collections. The details of this operation are illustrated in Fig. 2. The accessory pancreatic duct was ligated and divided. The Gregory cannula and Thomas cannula were drawn through multiple layers of folded omentum. No sutures were used between the pancreatic pouch and the duodenum. This was done to lessen the likelihood of fistula formation.

In the two-thirds gastric bypass operation, the stomach was divided with an estimated two-thirds of the stomach distal to the resection line. The ligament of Treitz was taken down. A retrocolic antiperistaltic Hofmeister modification of the Billroth II operation was done. Approximately 4 cm. of the greater curvature side of the proximal stomach was used to form the gastrojejunostomy. The defect in the mesocolon was sutured around the stomach. The bypassed stomach segment was sutured to the parietal peritoneum.

In the antral exclusion operation, 50 mg. of Histalog (betazole) were given intramuscularly just prior to opening the bypassed segment of stomach along the greater curvature. The mucosa was gently washed with normal saline and covered with a single layer of fine mesh gauze. The gauze was then moistened with a saturated solution of Congo red.[14] The acid-secreting portion of the bypassed stomach was identified by a blue-black color change and was amputated. Random sections of the transected edges showed parietal cells in all three specimens, and some sections (dog 1 and dog 2) showed small areas of antral mucosa on the same sections.

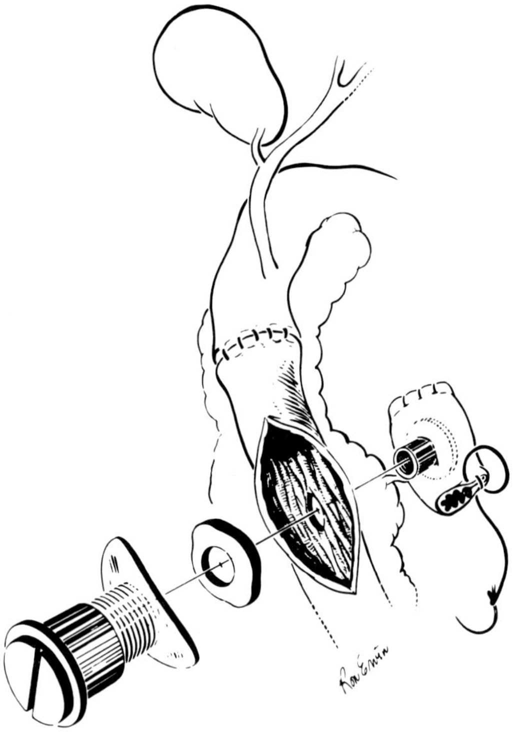

Fig. 2. The techniques used in constructing the pancreatic pouch and in placing the Gregory and Thomas cannula.

In the final stage, the duodenum was transected just distal to the pylorus and the antrum was excised, converting the preparation to a two-thirds gastric resection.

Following completion of the experiment, the dogs were killed. The gastrointestinal tract was examined for evidence of disease or parasites and none was found. The surgically constructed items were all intact. By using the weights of the various stomach

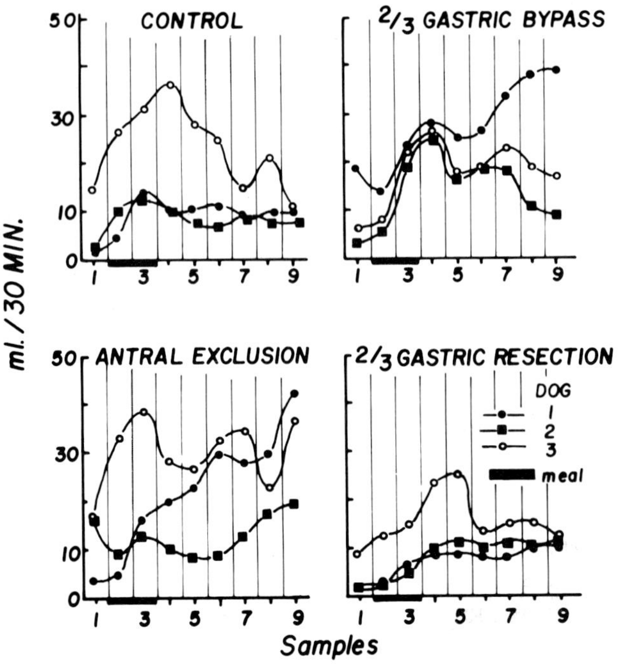

Fig. 3. Volume data. Each point represents the average from three feeding experiments.

segments, the percentage of the stomach which had been excluded in the gastric bypass and resected in subsequent operations was calculated. These percentages were 72.5, 81.0, and 79.3 for dogs 1, 2, and 3, respectively, and to the extent there was any atrophy from disuse, these represent minimal figures.

Before the feeding experiments began, and again after they were finished, each pancreatic pouch was tested for leaks. Methylene blue in normal saline was used at a pressure of 100 cm. of saline. No leaks were demonstrated. Several weeks were allowed between each operation and the subsequent feeding experiments. Several days were allowed between each run of the experiment. Each run of the experiment was done in the morning. Food was removed from the cage the previous evening, but water was never withheld. The Thomas cannula was extended by replacing the screw cap with the internal portion of another Thomas cannula. The catheter for intubating the Gregory cannula was prepared from a No. 16 Foley catheter with the tip cut off and a piece of No. 240 polyethylene tubing inserted into the lumen to maintain patency. A long piece of No. 160 polyethylene tubing for pancreatic juice replacement was taped along the Foley catheter. A No. 5 tracheostomy cuff was placed around both the Foley catheter and No. 160 polyethylene tubing. The Gregory and Thomas cannulas were sealed by inflating the Foley catheter and tracheostomy cuff balloons, respectively. Warm paraffin was molded over the Thomas cannula, squeezed tightly around the protruding tubes, and allowed to harden. The No. 160 polyethylene tubing was connected to a stopcock attached to a calibrated syringe and a reservoir for pancreatic juice. A pool of pancreatic juice was prepared for each dog and kept frozen at $-2°$ C. This was started by making a preliminary run and maintained with juice not used in the chemical analyses.

The standard meal consisted of 8 ounces of commercial canned animal food (Prescription Diet, revised), and was fed in six portions at equal intervals over the course of an hour. This eliminated the problem of regurgitation noted in previous dogs with small stomach pouches. Water was allowed as desired.

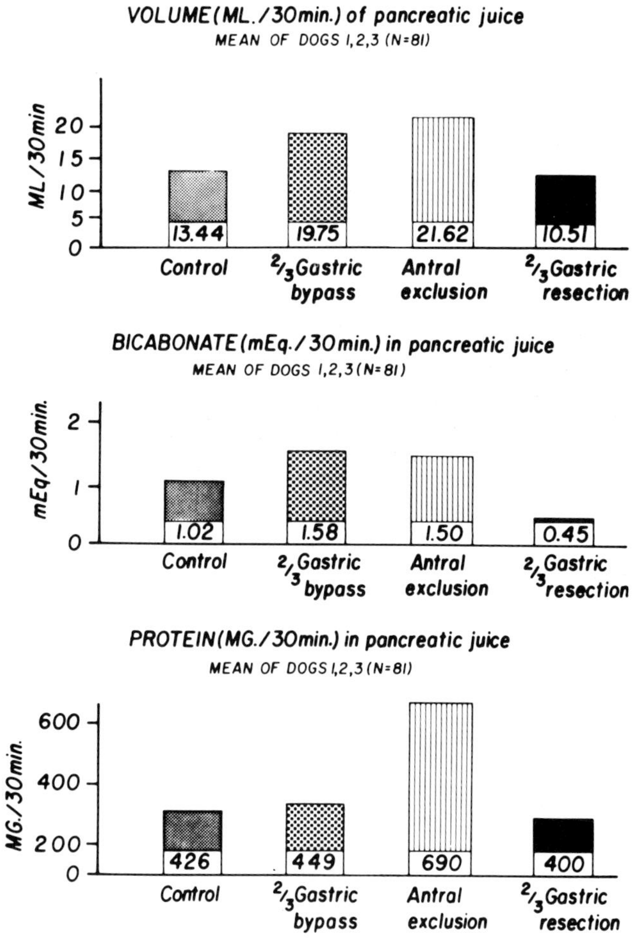

Fig. 4. Fluxes in pancreatic secretion with various gastric procedures. Shown alone are the averages for all pancreatic juice collected during the three experiments in the three dogs following each operation.

Each run of the feeding experiments consisted of collecting pancreatic juice for nine consecutive 30 minute periods. One sample was collected before, two during, and six following the standard meal. Three runs were made following each of the four operations performed. Pancreatic juice was replaced into the duodenum at five minute intervals. The replacement was begun with the use of pancreatic juice from the pool. When each sample was complete, the volume was recorded and an aliquot was kept for chemical analysis. The remainder was returned to the duodenum.

The determinations of bicarbonate and protein secretion were based on methods described by Preshaw and Grossman.[19] The bicarbonate determinations were made by adding excess 0.1N hydrochloric acid and back-titrating with 0.02N sodium hydroxide to the phenolphthalein end point. The protein determinations were made by diluting the juice 1:100 in quartz cuvettes and reading the optical density at 280 mμ. A standard curve using bovine serum albumin was plotted for each cuvette in order to eliminate cuvette error.

RESULTS

Volume showed a change in pattern (Fig. 3) but not a significant change in total volume of secretion between the different operations (Fig. 4). It was at the end of the experiment that the greatest difference

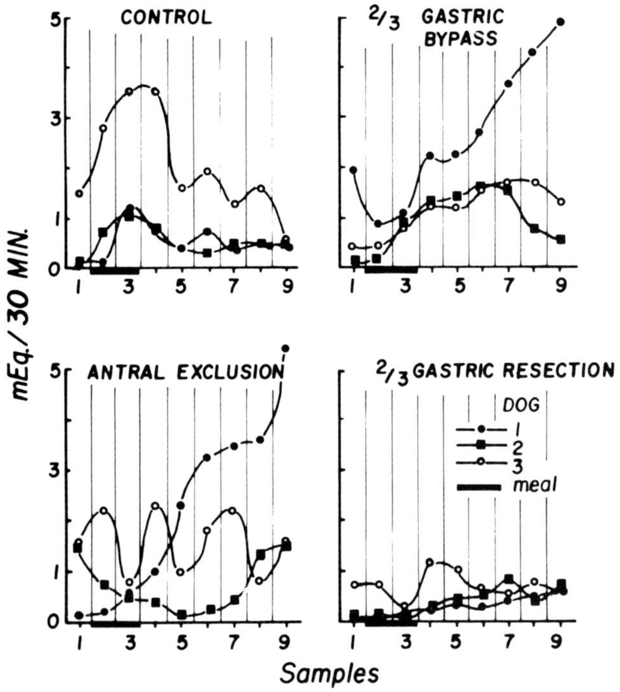

Fig. 5. Bicarbonate data. Same experiments as shown in Fig. 3.

in volume was noted and when both gastric bypass and antral exclusion caused high volumes in comparison to low volumes in the control experiments and after gastric resection.

There was less bicarbonate secretion after gastric resection and more after gastric bypass than in the control but none of these simple operative effects were significant at the 0.05 level (Fig. 5). The only significant differences were observed between control and antral exclusion and between control and gastric resection during the third collection period when interactions between operation and collection periods were examined. In both there was a decrease in bicarbonate secretion. Bicarbonate secretion was well sustained after gastric bypass at all times and in all three dogs.

Protein secretion (Fig. 6) was well sustained after each operation and, although there were no statistically significant differences in the total secretion or in the multiple comparisons between different time periods and operations, there does appear to be a consistent difference between the operations in terms of the time when peak protein secretion was reached.

DISCUSSION

From our earlier study of pancreatic pouch secretion we expected considerable variation in the data and this was found, as can be seen in Figs. 3, 4, 5, and 6. However, through the use of an experimental design which allows assignment of portions of the variation to the various simple effects of difference between animals, difference between operations, difference between times of sampling following a standard meal and the various interaction effects, it has been possible to detect, at a p value less than 0.05, a significant difference which should make a difference to the digestive function of such animals and probably to humans who might be subjected to such operations.

The findings in this experiment indicate that quantitative differences (Fig. 4) in the pancreatic response to a standard meal following gastric exclusion operations are not significant. The significant effect of gastric exclusion operations is on the *pattern* of the

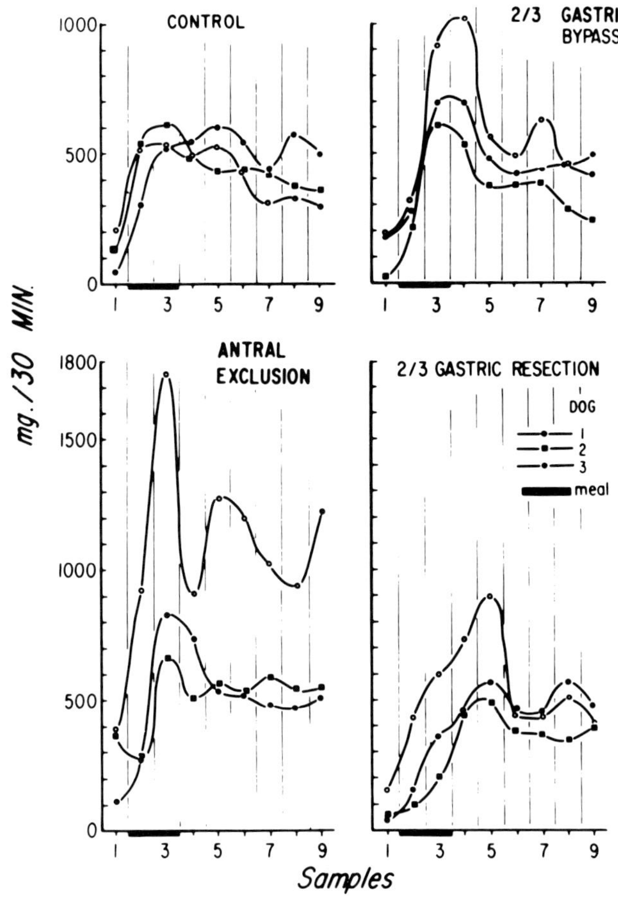

Fig. 6. Protein data.

pancreatic secretory response to a meal. Prior animal studies[2, 18, 24] did contain data pertinent to the effects of gastric exclusion operations upon the *pattern* of the pancreatic secretory response to a standard meal; however, this feature of the results was never emphasized. Human studies and animal studies in which pancreatic juice was replaced correlate well with the results of this experiment, both quantitatively and as regards secretory pattern.[1, 4, 6, 9, 11, 15, 21] Animal studies in which pancreatic juice was not replaced correlate well with the results of this experiment as regards secretory patterns, but not quantitatively.[2, 18, 24] Previously reported depressions in pancreatic secretion following gastric bypass and gastric resection were not seen in this experiment.

At least part of the explanation for the quantitative differences between this and other animal experiments may be that in this experiment a different standard feeding technique was used. Feeding of multiple small portions simulates human meal ingestion and is a more effective stimulus for pancreatic secretion in dogs with an intact stomach and duodenum than feeding a single portion of the same quantity of food.[21]

Another factor is that in this experiment pancreatic juice was returned to the duodenum while in the other experiments it was excluded. Gregory[7] wrote that: "If the normal response of the pancreas to a meal in the conscious dog is to be determined, it is essential to return continuously the pancreatic juice collected, and to the same region of the duodenum as that to which it would normally have been delivered." Replacing pancreatic juice could have eliminated falsely elevated control values for volume and bicarbonate. Volume and bicarbonate data obtained without pancreatic juice replacement[1, 2, 18, 21] are generally higher than comparable data obtained with pancreatic juice replacement, as in this experiment and others.[1, 4]

Excluding pancreatic juice from the duodenum in prior feeding experiments following gastric exclusion operations might have produced pancreatic secretory responses which were falsely depressed. The products of protein digestion are powerful stimuli for pancreatic enzyme secretion as well as volume and bicarbonate secretion.[27] Returning pancreatic juice probably increases digestion within the afferent limb. The intestinal phase of pancreatic secretion is due to stomach acid and digestion products releasing secretin and cholecystokinin-pancreozymin from the intestinal mucosa.[8] Recent reports[8, 10] indicate that secretin and cholecystokinin-pancreozymin have a potentiating effect on bicarbonate secretion and an additive effect on protein secretion.

Returning the pancreatic juice might elevate the pH in the duodenum but should have no effect on secretin release which depends on the rate of introduction of acid into the duodenum and is essentially independent of pH changes below 4.5.[8, 21] The replacement of pancreatic juice could conceivably release gastrin from the duodenal bulb[22, 28] and the antrum.[29] Gastrin is about 0.3 to 0.4 as potent a stimulus for pancreatic flow and enzyme secretion as cholecystokinin-pancreozymin.[8]

The ability of products of digestion to stimulate pancreatic enzyme secretion in normal patients has been studied by infusing the duodenum with various solutions and measuring duodenal enzyme levels.[6] The curves obtained in man with the use of an amino acid mixture approximates that obtained in dogs at the control stage in this experiment using a standard meal.

Postgastrectomy patients have been studied with the use of a long intestinal tube and a standard meal.[15] The curve for secretion of protein by the pancreas after Billroth II gastrectomy in our study is similar to the trypsin concentration curve obtained in man by collecting juice near the gastroenterostomy. Some differences between the curves would be expected, since a greater volume of pancreatic juice and a greater concentration of pancreatic enzymes can be obtained at the level of the ampulla of Vater than at levels further down.[12]

Data obtained during the control periods showed a constant pattern during the nine experiments. These secretory patterns are characterized by a late gradual decline in secretion. The control volume, bicarbonate, and protein peaks occurred during the second 30 minutes of feeding. Peak protein secretion after gastric exclusion operations occurred, after feeding started, as follows: two-thirds gastric bypass, 30 to 90 minutes; antral exclusion, 30 to 60 minutes; and two-thirds gastric resection, 90 to 120 minutes. A delay in peak protein secretion is considered to be a significant factor in malabsorption and especially when rapid gastric emptying and rapid intestinal passage occurs, as in some patients with Billroth II gastrectomy. This has been referred to as "pancreaticocibal asynchrony."[16]

The gastric bypass operation was designed with the intent of limiting food intake but allowing normal digestion of the food that is eaten. The effects of gastric bypass in these experiments were a late rise in volume secretion and a slight delay in peak protein secretion. Some impairment in mixing of food with the pancreatic juice might thus be predicted. However, the delay in peak protein secretion was not as great as that which occurred following gastric resection and therefore the impairment in mixing of food and pancreatic juice should not be as great after gastric bypass as after a comparable gastric resection. Furthermore, there was a decrease in the volume of secretion following gastric resection which was not seen following gastric bypass and this could be a factor in mixing.

Antral exclusion was used early in the history of duodenal ulcer surgery but was abandoned because of stomal ulceration. There was a delay in bicarbonate secretion following antral exclusion in these experiments which was not seen following gastric bypass. This could be a factor in the formation of stomal ulcers. There was also an elevated basal protein secretion after antral exclusion as compared to that secreted after gastric resection. This may be evidence of an elevated basal gastrin level after antral exclusion which is not present after gastric resection. In the gastric bypass operation, the antral release of gastrin may have been controlled by the acid-secreting portion of stomach excluded with the antrum. If it were not for the risk of stomal ulcer, antral exclusion might be considered the best procedure since pancreatic enzyme secretion occurred early and in high concentration following a meal.

If a surgeon were looking for an operation which would allow the pancreas to remain in a non-secretory state following a meal, as in patients with chronic relapsing pancreatitis, then antral exclusion would be the worst possible choice and neither gastric resection nor gastric bypass would be effective. Gastric resection has been used (without success) in the treatment of pancreatitis[23] on the thesis that there would be less stimulation of the pancreas because the antrum and duodenum were bypassed. These data serve to explain the error in the premise which probably led to failure of such operative treatment.

The size of the gastroenterostomy stoma influences the rate of emptying of the stomach and in these dogs the size was a measured 4 cm. which is twice as large as we currently use in obese patients subjected to gastric bypass. Our patients are limited both in the volume of food they can eat and in the rate at which they can ingest food. Dogs normally bolt their food but, since these animals were fed small amounts over an hour, the eating pattern approaches what is observed in patients with gastric bypass.

The rate of emptying of the stomach is a factor in digestion of food after a gastroenterostomy. In gastric resection and gastric bypass, optimum digestion is an objective which could be approximated by providing a stoma which would allow food to enter the intestine in synchrony with the secretion and passage of bile and pancreatic enzymes past the stoma. Such a perfect substitution for the normal regulatory action of the pyloric sphincter cannot be expected, but it is reassuring to find that both the quantity and pattern of protein (pancreatic digestive enzyme) secretion after gastric bypass is more nearly normal than after gastric resection. Gastric bypass can be used to limit the volume of food eaten without interfering with the digestion and absorption of what is eaten and weight loss can be produced without the risk of introducing malnutrition.

REFERENCES

1. Annis, D., and Hallenbeck, G. A.: Effect of excluding pancreatic juice from duodenum on secretory response of pancreas to a meal, Proc. Soc. Exp. Biol. Med. **77:** 383, 1951.
2. Annis, D., and Hallenbeck, G. A.: The effects of partial gastrectomy on canine external pancreatic secretion, SURGERY **31:** 517, 1952.
3. Bayliss, W. M., and Starling, E. H.: The mechanism of pancreatic secretion, J. Physiol. (Lond.) **28:** 325, 1902.
4. Cooke, A. R., Nahrwold, D. L., and Grossman, M. I.: Diversion of pancreatic juice on gastric and pancreatic response to a meal stimulus, Am. J. Physiol. **213:** 637, 1967.
5. Emas, S., Billings, A., and Grossman, M. I.: Effects of gastrin and pentagastrin on gastric and pancreatic secretions in dogs, Scand. J. Gastroenterol. **3:** 234, 1968.
6. Go, V. L. W., Hofmann, A. F., and Summerskill, W. H. J.: Pancreozymin bioassay in man based on pancreatic enzyme secretion: Potency of specific amino acids and other digestive products, J. Clin. Invest. **49:** 1588, 1970.
7. Gregory, R. A.: Secretory mechanisms of the gastrointestinal tract, London, 1962, Edward Arnold, Ltd., p. 134.
8. Grossman, M. I.: Control of pancreatic secretion, *in* Beck, I. T., and Sinclair, D. G., editors: The exocrine pancreas, Proceedings of a symposium held at Queen's University, Kingston, Ontario, June, 1969, London, 1971, J. & A. Churchill, Ltd.
9. Henriksen, F. W., and Rune, S. J.: Effect of vagotomy on the canine pancreatic secretion after feeding, Scand. J. Gastroenterol. **4:** 435, 1969.
10. Henriksen, F. W., and Worning, H.: The interaction of secretin and pancreozymin on the external pancreatic secretion in dogs, Acta Physiol. Scand. **70:** 241, 1967.
11. Henriksen, F. W., and Worning, H.: External pancreatic response to food and its relation to

the maximal secretory capacity in dogs, Gut **10:** 209, 1969.
12. Lenninger, S. G., White, T. T., and Magee, D. F.: Studies of pancreatic juice in the proximal loop after Billroth II gastrectomy, Surg. Gynecol. Obstet. **120:** 507, 1965.
13. Lindquist, E. F.: Design and analysis of experiments in psychology and education, Boston, 1953, Houghton Mifflin Company.
14. Lowicki, E., and Littlefield, J. B.: An experimental method of precisely defining the dimensions of the gastric antrum, Surg. Forum **12:** 308, 1961.
15. Lundh, G.: Intestinal digestion and absorption after gastrectomy, Acta Chir. Scand. Suppl., **231:** 1, 1958.
16. Lundh, G.: The mechanism of postgastrectomy malabsorption, Gastroenterology **42:** 637, 1962.
17. Mason, E. E., and Ito, C.: Gastric bypass in obesity, Surg. Clin. North Am. **47:** 1345, 1967.
18. Mason, E. E., and Ito, C.: Gastric bypass and pancreatic secretion, SURGERY **69:** 526, 1971.
19. Preshaw, R. M., and Grossman, M. I.: Stimulation of pancreatic secretion by extracts of the pyloric gland area of the stomach, Gastroenterology **48:** 36, 1965.
20. Preshaw, R. M., Cooke, A. R., and Grossman, M. I.: Sitmulation of pancreatic secretion by a humoral agent from the pyloric gland area of the stomach, Gastroenterology **49:** 617, 1965.
21. Preshaw, R. M., Cooke, A. R., and Grossman, M. I.: Quantitative aspects of response of canine pancreas to duodenal acidification, Am. J. Physiol. **210:** 629, 1966.
22. Richards, E. A., and Anderson, S.: Effect of antrectomy on gastric secretion following duodenal exclusion, Am. J. Dig. Dis. (New Series) **14:** 267, 1969.
23. Richman, A., and Colp, R.: Chronic relapsing pancreatitis: Treatment by subtotal gastrectomy and vagotomy, Ann. Surg. **131:** 145, 1950.
24. Richman, A., Lester, L. J., Hollander, F., and Dreiling, D. A.: The effect of subtotal gastrectomy upon external pancreatic secretion in dogs, Gastroenterology **26:** 210, 1954.
25. Stening, G. F.: A modification of a chronic pancreatic fistula in the dog, Br. J. Surg. **56:** 308, 1969.
26. Thistlethwaite, J. R.: The effect of banthine, vagotomy, and subtotal gastrectomy upon pancreatic secretion, Surg. Gynecol. Obstet. **93:** 616, 1951.
27. Wang, C. C., and Grossman, M. I.: Physiological determination of release of secretin and pancreozymin from intestine of dogs with transplanted pancreas, Am. J. Physiol. **164:** 527, 1951.
28. White, T. T., Stacher, G., and Tea, J. P. T.: Heidenhain pouch hypersecretion after intraduodenal injection of pancreatic juice, SURGERY **60:** 107, 1966.
29. Woodward, E. R., Fried, W., and Schapiro, H.: Further studies on the isolated gastric antrum, Gastroenterology **32:** 868, 1957.

Brief clinical report

Ascending aorta–bilateral femoral artery bypass for the totally occluded infrarenal abdominal aorta

Stephen L. Frantz, M.D., Martin J. Kaplitt, M.D., Arthur R. Beil, Jr., M.D., *and*
Harry L. Stein, M.D., *Manhasset, N. Y.*

This paper presents a safe and simple method of bypassing the abdominal aorta in those cases in which the infrarenal portion of the aorta is unusable for proximal grafting. When the aorta is judged to be inadequate, the abdominal incision is extended to a median sternotomy and the ascending thoracic aorta is used for the proximal anastomosis. A review of the literature reveals several alternate methods of bypassing the abdominal aorta. Our method offers several advantages including the simple and rapid exposure of the ascending thoracic aorta, the technical ease with which the proximal anastomosis can be performed, and the low morbidity rate associated with a median sternotomy.

From the Division of Thoracic and Cardiovascular Surgery and the Departments of Surgery and Radiology, North Shore University Hospital and Cornell University Medical College, Manhasset, N. Y.

THE STANDARD aortofemoral artery bypass graft is applicable in most cases of the totally occluded abdominal aorta. A bifurcation graft is usually interposed between the abdominal aorta and the femoral arteries. There are cases, however, in which the infrarenal abdominal aorta is either unsuitable or entirely unusable for proximal grafting. This can be due to dissection, severe atherosclerosis, arteritis, or, as in the present case, complete replacement of the aortic lumen by a solid fibrous cord. Several alternate methods of bypassing the abdominal aorta have been reported.[1-4] We have devised a relatively simple method for avoiding the severely diseased abdominal aorta, particularly in those cases in which this problem is discovered during the operative procedure.

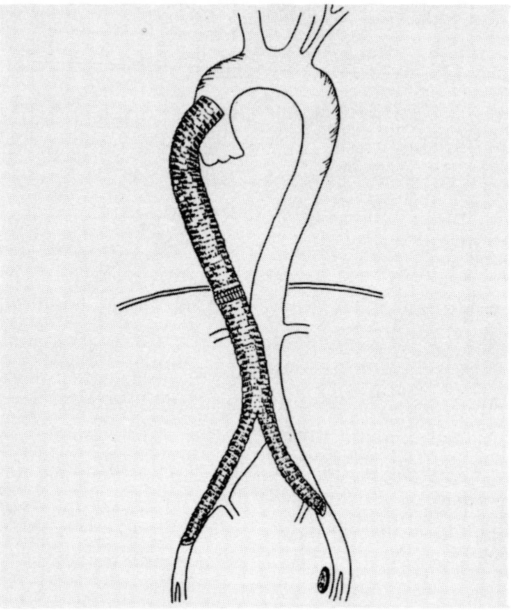

Fig. 1. A diagrammatic representation of the ascending aorta–bilateral femoral artery bypass.

Accepted for publication Dec. 10, 1973.

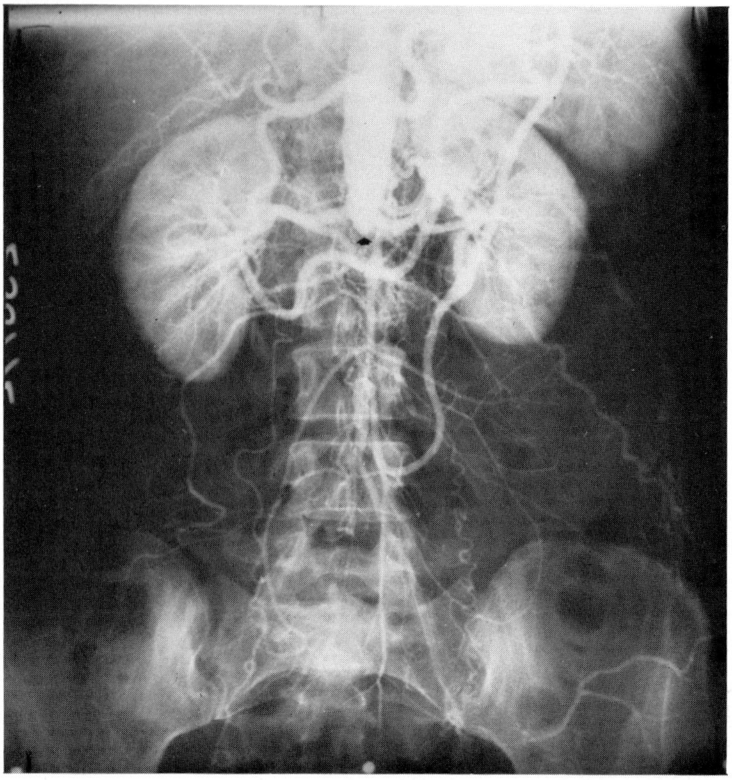

Fig. 2. Preoperative percutaneous right transaxillary abdominal aortogram and peripheral arteriogram. Frontal projection, abdominal study, reveals a complete occlusion of the abdominal aorta (arrow) just below the origin of the renal arteries. Note the large, well-developed middle-left colic artery (Arc of Riolan) with filling of patent inferior mesenteric artery and retrograde opacification of aortic bifurcation and a segment of left common iliac artery. Large systemic-systemic collaterals are also visualized.

OPERATIVE TECHNIQUE

The patient is placed in a supine position with the chest, abdomen, and both groins prepared for surgery. Preoperative arteriograms delineate the distal runoff, and both femoral areas are explored to ascertain the quality of the femoral arteries. When this examination is judged to be adequate, the operation is continued with an exploratory laparotomy through a midline abdominal approach. If the infrarenal abdominal aorta is found to be unusable, the midline incision is extended to a midsternal incision for exposure of the ascending thoracic aorta. A Dacron tube graft can be sutured end to end to the proximal limb of a bifurcation graft. The graft is then measured and the proximal limb of this newly fashioned graft is sutured end to side to the ascending thoracic aorta. The graft is brought subxiphoid through the gastrohepatic ligament, into the retroperitoneum, and sutured to the femoral arteries bilaterally (Fig. 1).

CASE REPORT

A 41-year-old non-diabetic mother of four children presented with a history of intermittent claudication upon walking less than one-half block. Past history included moderate hypertension for eight years and toxemia associated with her last three pregnancies. A hypertensive work-up in the past had been unrewarding. The claudication had progressed, with pain developing in hips and thighs upon minimal exertion. Additionally, she had developed paresthesias of the distal extremities. She stated that she was now unable to care for her children. Physical examination revealed a normally developed and well-nourished 41-year-old female

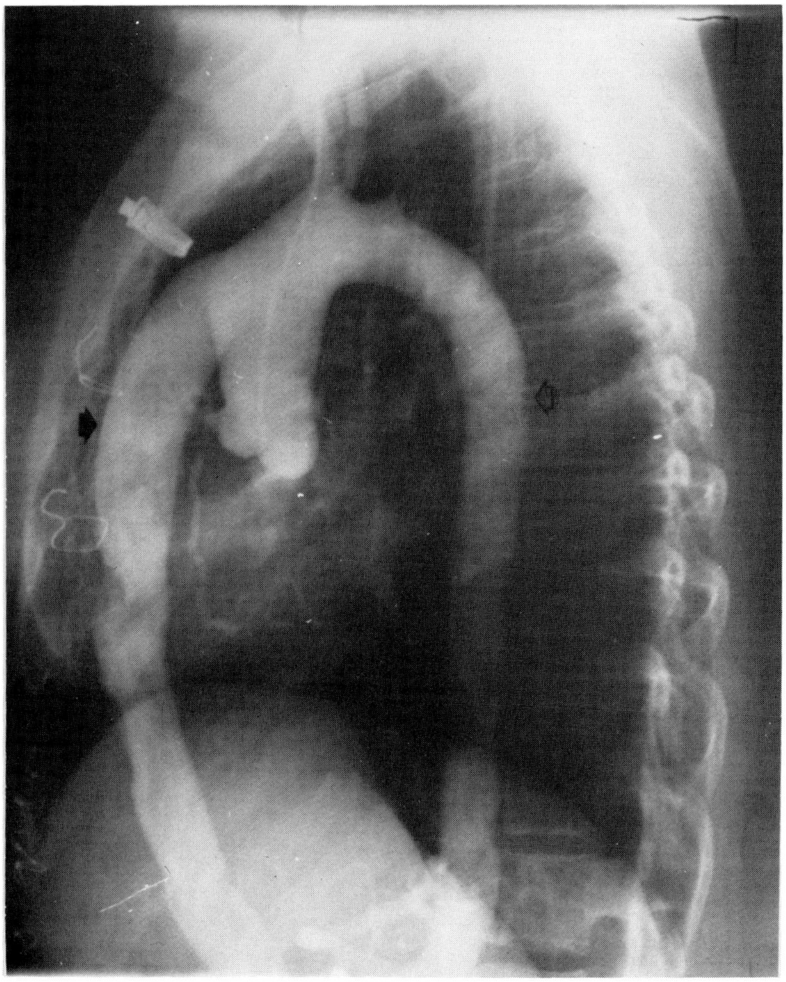

Fig. 3. Postoperative right transaxillary thoracic aortogram. Lateral projection reveals opacified, patent graft anteriorly (solid arrow), and normal descending thoracic aorta (open arrow). Note occlusion of left subclavian artery.

with no pulsations in the lower abdomen or in either leg. Pulses in the upper extremities were within normal limits. The results of laboratory tests and the appearance of routine chest x-ray films were within normal limits. An aortogram was performed through an axillary artery and the abdominal aorta was found to be completely obstructed below the level of the renal arteries (Fig. 2). The superior mesenteric artery was stenotic and filled from collateral sources. The femoral arteries were small, but patent with good runoff. At operation, femoral exploration confirmed the arteriographic findings. The abdominal aorta was found to be enveloped by a thick inflammatory reaction. When visualized, it was found to be a thick fibrous cord with no lumen and was completely unusable for grafting. The midline abdominal incision was extended to the chest with a sternal splitting incision. A graft was placed between the ascending thoracic aorta proximally and the femoral arteries distally. At the end of the procedure, the patient's extremities were warm with pulsations in both feet. An aortogram at four months showed a completely patent graft revascularizing the femoral arteries (Figs. 3, 4*A*, and 4*B*). At one year, the patient continues to be asymptomatic, with excellent pulses bilaterally.

DISCUSSION

The severely diseased abdominal aorta can present a perplexing problem to the vascular surgeon when he is attempting to perform

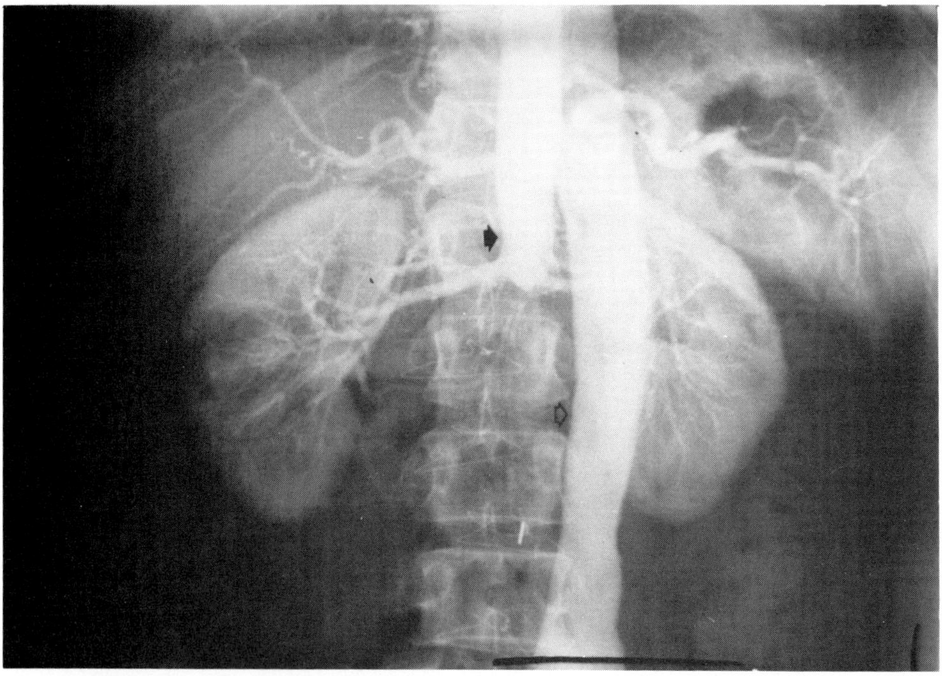

Fig. 4*A*. Postoperative right transaxillary abdominal aortogram and peripheral arteriogram. Frontal projection, abdominal study, reveals the occluded abdominal aorta (solid arrow) as previously visualized, and the patent graft to the left of the aorta (open arrow).

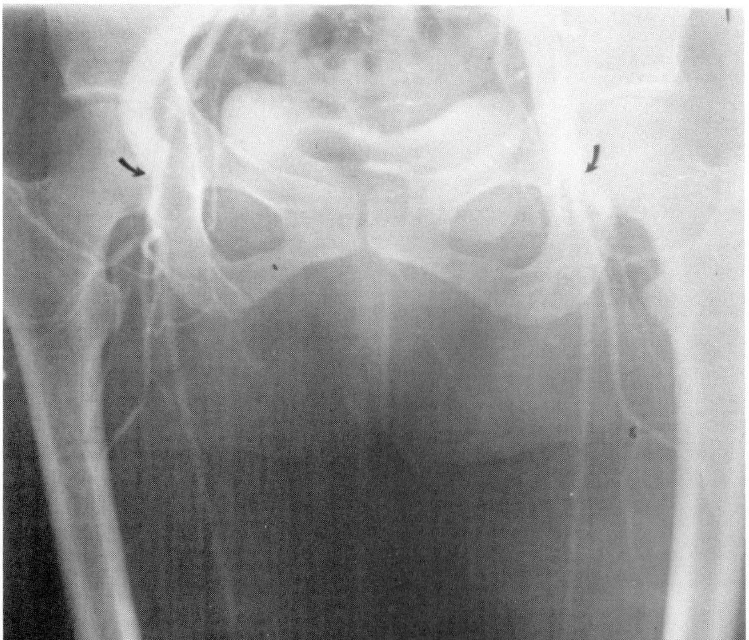

Fig. 4*B*. Postoperative right transaxillary abdominal aortogram and peripheral arteriogram. Frontal projection, film of pelvis and upper thighs, reveals the anastomoses of the limbs of the graft with each of the common femoral arteries (curved arrows). Note the good runoff into grossly normal proximal superficial femoral and profunda femoral arteries.

an aortofemoral bypass. In some patients, the abdominal aorta is totally unusable and an alternate approach must be found. In others, however, the indications for alternate methods are not as clear, but the aorta may be so severely diseased that the surgeon would appreciate a simple and safe alternative. A review of the literature reveals several methods of bypassing the abdominal aorta. In 1963, Blaisdell and Hall[1] described the axillofemoral bypass for lower extremity ischemia. This can be particularly useful in bypassing the abdominal cavity in cases of infection, but the late results have been very disappointing.[3] De Bakey[2] has described a bypass from the descending thoracic aorta to the distal abdominal aorta, and Nunn and Kamal[4] have reported a graft from the descending thoracic aorta to the femoral arteries. These operations can be accomplished only through a difficult exposure and could present a problem if the patient is not properly positioned prior to the beginning of the operation. Robinson and associates[5] presented a method of bypassing a recurrent dissecting aneurysm of the descending aorta by placing a tube graft between the ascending thoracic aorta and the distal abdominal aorta. Our method utilizes this concept in bypassing the highly diseased aorta. It offers several advantages over the other methods, including the simple and rapid exposure of the ascending thoracic aorta through a midsternal incision. A midline abdominal incision can easily be extended without any change in the patient's position and with extreme rapidity. After the pericardium is opened, the ascending thoracic aorta is completely exposed without any further dissection. The proximal anastomosis can be accomplished with technical ease since this portion of the aorta is an anterior structure and is usually less involved with the severe atherosclerotic changes often present in other portions of the arterial tree. The median sternotomy avoids the pleural cavities, is associated with a low morbidity, and can be closed safely and quickly. While other techniques are available for avoiding the dangers of a severely diseased abdominal aorta, it is our feeling that this technique adds an additional dimension to the surgical armamentarium available for peripheral vascular reconstruction.

REFERENCES

1. Blaisdell, F. W., and Hall, A. D.: Axillofemoral artery bypass for lower extremity ischemia, SURGERY **54:** 563, 1963.
2. De Bakey, M.: Basic concepts of surgery in arterial disease, N. Y. Acad. Med. **39:** 707, 1963.
3. Mannick, J. A., Williams, L. E., and Nasbet, D. C.: The late results of axillofemoral grafts, SURGERY **68:** 1038, 1970.
4. Nunn, D. B., and Kamal, M. A.: Bypass grafting from the thoracic aorta to femoral arteries for high aortoiliac occlusive disease, SURGERY **72:** 749, 1972.
5. Robinson G., Siegleman, S., and Attai, L.: Recurrent dissecting aneurysm of aorta, N. Y. J. Med. **72:** 2328, 1972.

Letters to the editors

No need for autoclavable information

To the Editors:

The communication by Burt Meyers (SURGERY 74: 794, 1973) suggesting that surgeons might benefit from autoclaved instruction sheets available at the table to carry them through an operation reminded me painfully of the late Dean Lewis.

I vividly remember a Friday noon clinic, in which, when a student failed to respond appropriately to a question on anatomy, Dr. Lewis stopped and said, "I was in ______ Hospital the other day, and the surgeon had an anatomy book open on a reading stand. The reading stand was painted white. They must have used it every day. It nearly made me vomit."

Dr. Meyers suggests that his aids may be useful to "an otherwise preoccupied surgeon." If a surgeon is preoccupied, i.e., occupied with other matters, he ought not be operating. The illustrations shown are taken from Woodward's paper on esophageal hiatus hernia in *Current Problems in Surgery,* December, 1970. I have reread this carefully. The texual operative description is painstakingly clear, there are innumerable details in the text which are not shown in the drawings. A surgeon who could not read this text through and understand the technique of the operation without reference at the operating table to diagrams is not ready to undertake the operation. I deplore this anti-intellectual, cookbook approach to surgery. This may be appropriate technique for assembling the children's toys the night before Christmas, but it could hardly be seriously proposed as appropriate to the operating room.

Mark M. Ravitch, M.D.
Surgeon-in-Chief and
Professor of Surgery
Department of Surgery
University of Pittsburgh
School of Medicine
Pittsburgh, Pa.

Reply

To the Editors:

I can see no point arguing with Dr. Ravitch about the qualifications of a surgeon, but I still feel that at times any surgeon might want printed information at the operating table. The illustration used with the article may have been a poor one, but the point is that the technique is available and all surgeons should know about it.

M. Bert Myers, M.D.
Department of Surgery
Veterans Administration Hospital
1601 Perdido St.
New Orleans, La.

Volume 75 Number 4

SURGERY

APRIL, 1974

Original communications

Specific tissue and tumor responses of chimpanzees following immunization against human melanoma

Maria O. Hornung, M.D., *and* **Edward T. Krementz, M.D.,** *New Orleans, La.*

Anti-human melanoma immunization of adult normal chimpanzees was expressed by a mononuclear cell infiltrate surrounding inoculated melanoma cells. This inflammatory response resulted in the formation of a small nodule (2 cm. by 1 cm.) which disappeared by day 12. Lymphocytes from these chimpanzees destroyed melanoma cells cultured from several sources but did not affect other types of cultured cells. The appearance of vitiligo in the hyperimmunized chimpanzees indicated that the general nature of the immunity was tissue specific. However, the vitiligo was not inflammatory whereas a strong inflammatory response to melanoma occurred in all immunized chimpanzees, along with the vitiligo. It is of general interest that a malignant tissue cell was the antigen responsible for an "autoimmune" type reaction.

From the Department of Surgery, Tulane University School of Medicine, New Orleans, La.

A CLOSE genetic relationship between chimpanzee and human species has been emphasized by recent analyses of amino acid sequences of certain proteins.[4] In these studies, identity was demonstrated for the fibrinopeptides, the alpha- and beta-globulin chain genes of both species. Near identity (132 of 133 residues examined) was found for carbonic anhydrases. Further, inter-species reassociation of non-repeating DNA polynucleotide sequences has been achieved experimentally.[8] From these data, one may presume that in many instances cellular recognition mechanisms of chimpanzee and man resemble those occurring within one species. This presumption might be exploited to study the immunology of human tumors. Among human tumors, malignant melanoma is generally considered to be antigenic in the host and there is some evidence

Supported by grants from the Cancer Association of Greater New Orleans, United States Public Health Service Research Grant No. 5 PO2 CA05837-12, and the J. Douglas Eustis Fund for Cancer Research.

Accepted for publication Jan. 29, 1974.

that spontaneous remission is associated with host cellular immunological reactivity.[2, 12, 13]

We therefore chose to implant human melanoma cell populations in normal chimpanzees and study their cellular responses, hoping the information gained might be useful in developing concepts applicable to the immunotherapy of human tumors. The control animals were non-immunized chimpanzees, a chimpanzee immunized with normal skin from one of the melanoma donors and a chimpanzee immunized with complete Freund's adjuvant (CFA) alone.

Our first objective was to produce in the chimpanzees a population of lymphocytes reactive to the target (melanoma or normal) cells. We attempted to do this by active immunization with the use of living cultured human cells in CFA, followed by repeated booster doses of cells alone. Following immunization, we implanted various melanoma cell populations intradermally in the breast area sought evidence for tumor growth, type of host cellular response, and ultimate fate of the melanoma population. We also examined the animals regularly for "autoimmune" type responses to their own normal melanocytes. In vitro tests for lymphocyte cytotoxicity employed mixed cell culture techniques and were monitored by time lapse photography.

We report here the results of experiments designed to answer the following questions: (1) Would human melanoma cells multiply significantly in normal (non-immunosuppressed) chimpanzees? (2) Was it possible to produce in the chimpanzees a population of lymphocytes reactive against the tumor cells? (3) Was the chimpanzee cellular reaction specific for only the individual immunizing melanoma or for all melanomas available for testing? (4) Was this reaction species specific? If so, the melanoma-immune lymphocytes would affect all human cell lines equally. As a corollary, immunization with normal human skin would cause the chimpanzees to produce lymphocytes cytotoxic for all human skin and melanoma cells. (5) What role did HL-A antigens play in the responses? Some melanoma cell lines carry HL-A antigens, others do not.[7] If the chimpanzees were recognizing only the HL-A antigens on the melanoma cells, then the lymphocytes from chimpanzees immunized against melanoma cells would respond in the same fashion to both melanoma and normal cells from that donor. Conversely, the chimpanzee immunized with normal skin cells would react to various test cell populations in a manner showing HL-A associated selectivity. (6) Also, was there any evidence that the reaction was tissue specific? If so, one could expect some effect on the normal melanocytes of chimpanzees immunized against malignant melanoma. Such an effect could be compared to the response by the same chimpanzee to implanted melanoma cell populations.

MATERIALS AND METHODS

Chimpanzees. These were adult males and females purchased and housed in the vivarium at Tulane Medical School. They weighed between 85 and 135 pounds. Medical histories showed they had never been immunized with human materials. They were cared for by veterinarians who were receiving advanced degrees in veterinary medicine. Care included routine physical examinations including chest x-ray films and hematological and clinical biochemical evaluations. The animals remained free of bacterial or parasitic diseases. Their sera were negative for Australian antigen.

Human cell types.

Melanoma. Human melanoma tissue was obtained during surgery. Tumor cells were harvested and cultured in Tc199 medium containing 15 percent fetal calf serum, 0.01 percent glutamine, penicillin (100 U. per milliliter), streptomycin (100 U. per milliliter), and fungizone (0.25 mg. per milliliter). At the third or fourth passage, cultures containing only melanoma cells (no fibroblasts) were selected for melanoma-immunizing procedures. Aliquots (3×10^6 melanoma cells per tube) were frozen at −170° C. for subsequent subculturing. Four melanoma cell lines (JC, BL, MG, and Ta) were available for use throughout the study. One of these

(BL) consistently produced melanin in culture. The other three either produced small amounts of melanin (MG) or were amelanotic (JC, Ta).

Normal skin. Normal skin cells were obtained from two of the melanoma donors (JC and Ta). These were cultured and grown as described above. Other normal skin fibroblasts (Al, Mt) were established in culture from human foreskin.

Carcinoma. Human colon carcinoma cells (Mu) were established in culture and used in one set of experiments.

HL-A typing. Lymphocytes from two of the melanoma donors (JC and Ta) were evaluated for HL-A antigens by the tissue typing laboratory at the University of California at Los Angeles.

The presence of HL-A antigens on melanoma cells and fibroblasts was determined by the method of McDonald and associates[10] with the use of monospecific HL-A antisera. One thousand melanoma cells in each well were treated with 5 γ of a 1:2 dilution of guinea pig complement. Subsequently 2 γ of the appropriate antiserum was added. The control animals contained cells with complement alone, cells with media alone, and cells with antiserum only. Rabbit antiserum prepared against human melanoma cells served as a positive control.

Immunization protocol. Cultured melanoma (or normal skin) cells grew as monolayers. At harvesting, the medium was poured off, and the monolayer rinsed gently three times in phosphate-buffered injectible saline (PBS). The cells were then removed by a rubber policeman, counted, and tested for viability by dye exclusion. After three more washings in PBS, they were gently mixed with an equal amount of CFA and inoculated intramuscularly in the deltoid muscle. An average inoculum contained 3×10^6 cells in a total volume of approximately 1 ml. This procedure was repeated three weeks later. Subsequently, booster injections containing 3×10^6 cells in PBS were inoculated intradermally in the breast area at monthly intervals. One chimpanzee received only CFA (two injections of 1 ml. each three weeks apart).

Chimpanzee lymphocytes. At each bleeding, the chimpanzees were plasmapheresed for 700 ml. of blood. Following return of the red cells and plasma, lymphocytes were separated from other cells by passage through nylon fiber columns. Viability was regularly better than 95 percent and the average yield of lymphocytes was 3×10^9 cells.

The chimpanzee lymphocytes were scanned for the presence of viral particles by the method of Beltran and Stuckey.[1] Briefly, at each plasmapheresis a cell pellet consisting of 0.2 ml. of packed washed lymphocytes was fixed in 1.5 percent glutaraldehyde in 0.067M cacodylate buffer (pH, 7.3) and postfixed in one percent O_sO_4. The sample was dehydrated, embedded in Maraglas, stained with lead citrate and uranyl acetate, and examined with a Phillips 300 microscope.

In vivo test for cellular response to melanoma. Melanoma cells were harvested as described above, and an inoculum containing 3×10^6 cells (without adjuvant) was injected intradermally into the shaved breast area and observed for signs of tumor growth inflammation, and induration. Microscopic examination of biopsied areas was the method used to detect tumor cell multiplication and the character of the cellular response.

Response to normal melanocytes was evaluated by examination of normally heavily pigmented areas of chimpanzee skin for evidence of vitiligo. Skin biopsies were examined after staining with differential stains (Fontana-Masson, PAS, hematoxylin and eosin.

In vitro test for specificity of chimpanzee cellular response to human melanoma. At approximately three-week intervals, the chimpanzees were bled and their lymphocytes were tested for cytotoxic activity against the immunizing cell line, other melanoma cell lines, normal skin fibroblasts of the melanoma donor, another melanoma donor, and two normal sources. One cell

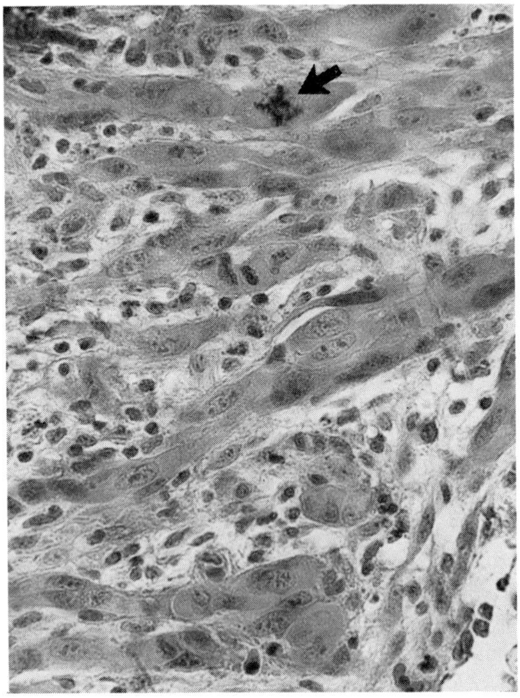

Fig. 1. Human melanoma cells growing in non-immunosuppressed chimpanzees. Arrow points to abnormal metastatic cell surrounded by lymphocytic infiltrate (×400).

line derived from carcinoma of the colon was available for one set of experiments.

The target cells were harvested, counted, and their viability was determined. For quantitative studies 1 or 2 × 10^5 viable melanoma (or other) cells were placed in small plastic bottles in 7 ml. of Tc^{199} containing 15 percent fetal calf serum and incubated at 37° C. In five percent CO_2 for approximately six hours to ensure cell attachment, verified microscopically. Occasionally longer periods of time (up to 18 hours) were required before all cells were attached to the plastic surface. Lymphocytes were then added in lymphocyte/target cell ratios of 10:1, 50:1, 200:1. Control animals received no lymphocytes. At 24, 48, and 72 hours three bottles of each cell mixture and three bottles of control target cells were rinsed free of lymphocytes, and the target cells were harvested and tested for viability by dye exclusion. A count was made of cells in each bottle and sensitization was estimated by comparing the number of viable target cells in the experimental and control cultures. Cell dispersion was usually nearly complete. Small clumps which occurred were never counted as more than three cells each. The paired t test for small samples was used to determine significant differences between experimental and control cultures.

RESULTS

In preliminary studies, melanoma cell populations (10^6 cells) were implanted in seven normal chimpanzees. There were no local reactions at the inoculation sites. Neither the serum nor lymphocytes of these chimpanzees gave evidence of anti-melanoma or anti-species immunity on subsequent testing by the methods described above.

Following immunization with melanoma cells in CFA, the implantation of melanoma cells resulted in a local reaction which appeared red and indurated at 48 hours. The induration was 22 to 25 mm. in diameter. The nodule increased in size to 10 mm. in height by day 6 and subsequently decreased, disappearing by day 13 to 14. This was a characteristic response which occurred in every immunized chimpanzee following the monthly booster shots with melanoma cells. Fig. 1 shows a biopsy of one of these nodules which contained multiplying melanoma cells surrounded by lymphocytes and histiocytes. In some sections, there was an occasional eosinophil. When a chimpanzee immunized against BL melanoma cells received implants of Ta melanoma cells in one breast area and Ta skin cells in the other breast area, the typical nodule described above appeared in the area receiving Ta melanoma, and there was no reaction at the site receiving Ta skin cells.

Electron microscopy of lymphocyte pellets taken at plasmapheresis (Fig. 2) indicated the absence of viral particles detectable by this procedure. Prior to immunization, the chimpanzee lymphocytes were innocuous to the melanoma cell cultures. The lymphocytes from one chimpanzee who received CFA alone did not damage melanoma cells

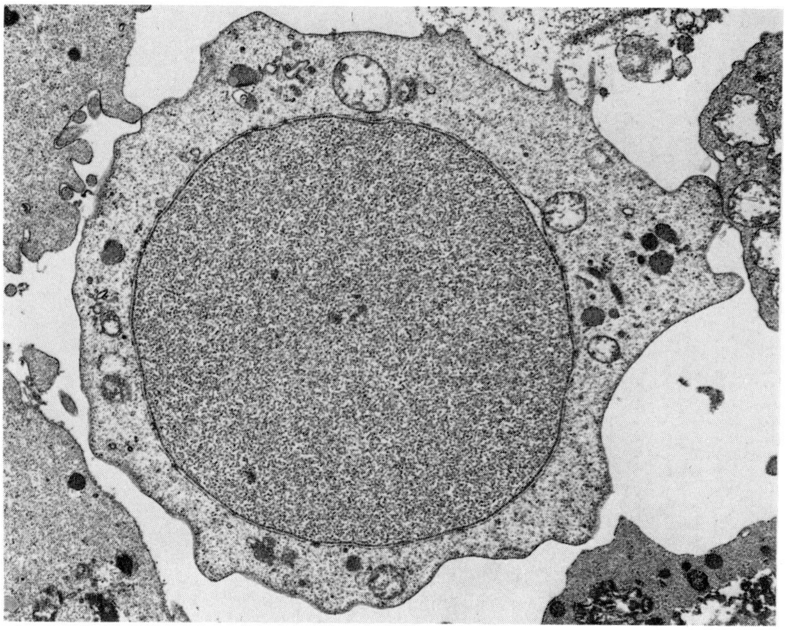

Fig. 2. Electron microscopic picture of typical chimpanzee lymphocyte used in mixed culture experiments. (×10,830.)

in culture. Also one culture of colon carcinoma cells (Mu) were unaffected by lymphocytes from chimpanzees immunized against melanoma cells. These three experiments were carried out at a lymphocyte/target cell ratio of 300:1. Higher lymphocyte numbers (500:1 or above) sometimes, but not always, had the effect of increasing the lag phase of growth. At lymphocyte/target cell ratios of 10:1, there was no effect by either immune or non-immune lymphocytes. Fig. 3 shows the time sequence and dose response curves of a typical experiment in which melanoma cell cultures were exposed to lymphocytes from non-immunized and immunized chimpanzees at two different cell ratios (50:1 and 200:1).

After 24 hours of culture there was no significant effect on the target cells by non-immune lymphocytes (200:1) or immune lymphocytes (50:1). There was some effect (52 percent cell reduction) by the immune lymphocytes at 200:1 ratio. At 48 hours, there was a highly significant ($P < 0.01$) reduction in target cell population by immune lymphocytes at both (50:1 and 200:1) cell ratios. This effect was a general one for all immunized chimpanzees and persisted throughout the test period (18 months) during which time the chimpanzees received monthly booster doses of melanoma cells without adjuvant. Under these experimental conditions, the affected target cell cultures did not become established but died out completely after a few days.

Table I. *Cross-reactions between cultured human melanomas demonstrated by immune chimpanzee lymphocytes*

*Chimpanzee lymphocytes added**	*Melanoma cell JC*	*Culture† BL*
None	114‡ ± 1	129 ± 6
Non-immune	151 ± 10	109 ± 10
Anti-JC	26§ ± 7	73§ ± 3
Anti-BL	66‖ ± 7	35§ ± 2

*10^5 melanoma cells placed in each culture.
†5×10^6 lymphocytes added to each melanoma culture.
‡Melanoma cell count after 48 hours growth ($\times 10^3 \pm$ S.E.).
§$P < 0.01$.
‖$P < 0.02$.

Table I presents one typical experiment in which lymphocytes from two immunized chimpanzees were compared for their respective activities against (1) the specific

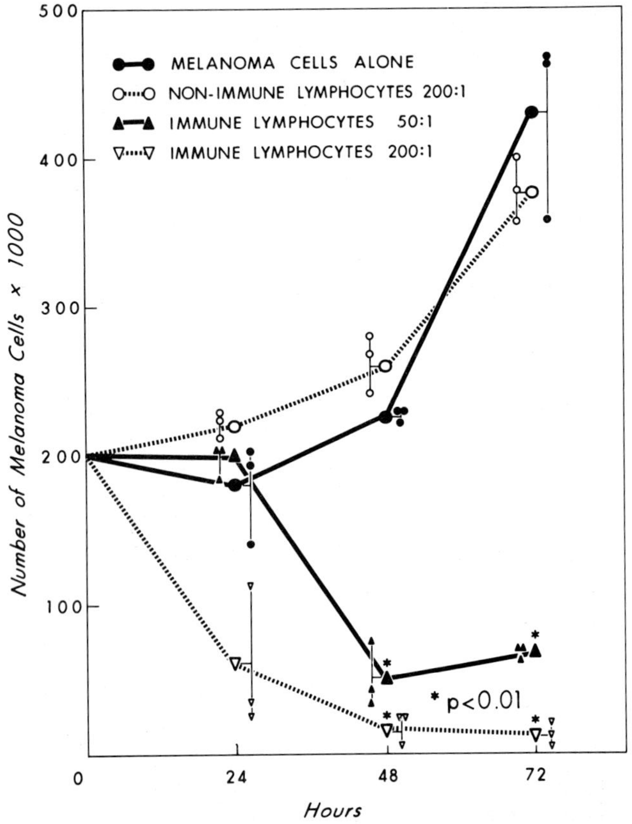

Fig. 3. Effect of immune chimpanzee lymphocytes on cultured human melanoma cells.

Table II. *Effect on cultured skin and melanoma cells by lymphocytes from chimpanzee immunized to Ta normal skin*

	Preimmunization		*Postimmunization*	
	*Control**	*Experiment†*	*Control*	*Experiment*
Ta skin	143‡ ± 13	109 ± 10	147 ± 22	62§ ± 11
Ta melanoma	180 ± 11	143 ± 28	96 ± 2	44§ ± 2
JC skin	116 ± 18	135 ± 9	136 ± 4	106 ± 25
JC melanoma	116 ± 5	97 ± 6	143 ± 23	73‖ ± 5
BL melanoma	138 ± 5	129 ± 6	158 ± 9	127 ± 6
MG melanoma	ND	ND	119 ± 3	123 ± 4
Al skin	ND	ND	128 ± 7	127 ± 10
Mt skin	ND	ND	147 ± 7	123 ± 4

*10^5 target cells.
†10^5 target cells plus 5×10^6 lymphocytes.
‡Target cell number after 48 hours growth ($\times 10^3 \pm$ S.E.).
§$P < 0.01$.
‖$P < 0.1$.

immunizing melanoma cell population and (2) a second melanoma cell population. In every instance, chimpanzees immunized against one melanoma cell population reacted to all other melanoma cells available for study. In the experiment illustrated here, JC was an amelanotic cell whereas BL produced large amounts of melanin. In each case the reaction against the immunizing melanoma (73 percent cell reduction at 48 hours) was greater than the reaction against the other melanoma (42 and 44 percent reduction, respectively), but this difference did not reach statistical significance.

The HL-A antigens of Ta were 7 and

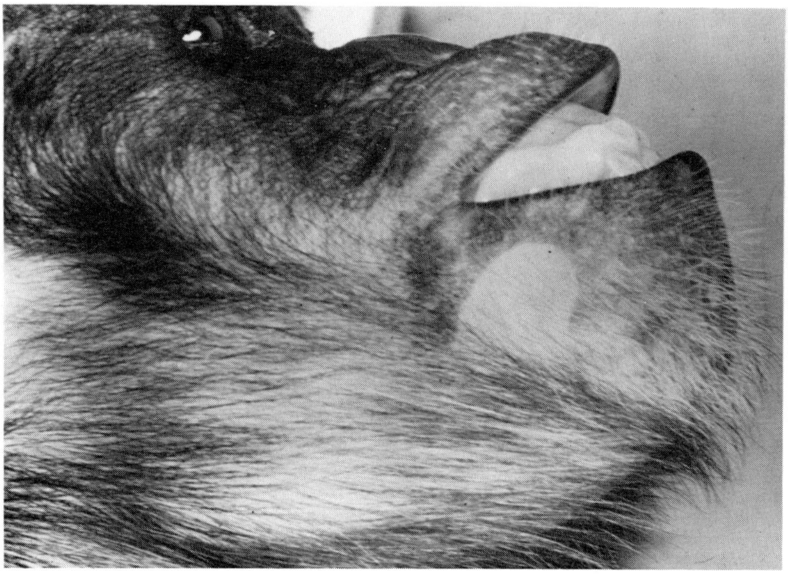

Fig. 4. Chimpanzee Zelda, showing depigmented skin area following eight months immunization with human melanoma (Ta).

W-12. Those of JC were 2, 3, 7, and 17. A chimpanzee immunized with Ta skin as described above produced lymphocytes which had a highly significant ($p < 0.01$) destructive effect on both Ta skin and Ta melanoma (Table II). There was no significant effect on JC skin cells but growth of JC melanoma was somewhat inhibited ($P < 0.1$). Both of these donors had HL-A 7. There was no effect on two other melanoma cell lines (BL and MG) nor on two other cell lines derived from normal donors (AL and Mt). The HL-A antigens of these latter four donors were not known.

Some facial areas of chimpanzee skin are highly pigmented and these were observed regularly for signs of auto-immune response to normal chimpanzee melanocytes. After six to eight months of the immunization protocol described above, all chimpanzees developed vitiligo in these pigmented areas. Figs. 4 and 5 demonstrate the depigmentation observed. Fig. 6, *A* illustrates the microscopic appearance of a biopsy of this vitiligo area at the juncture between the heavily pigmented and depigmented skin. The epidermis showed irregular hypopigmentation with reduction in the pigment of the basal layer. In some areas, the basal layer was heavily pigmented and the melanocytes

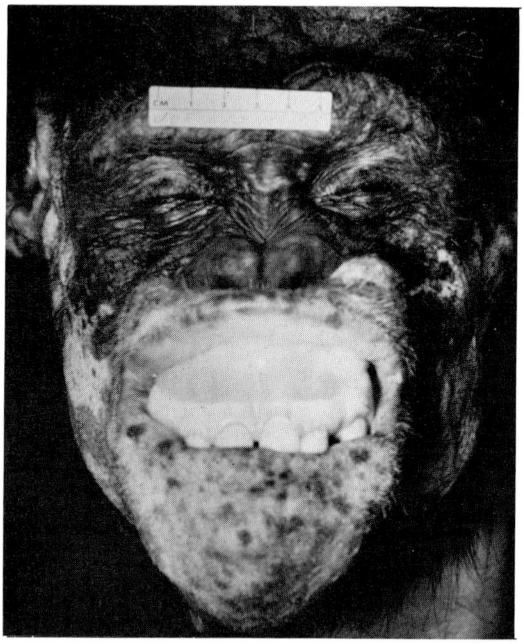

Fig. 5. Chimpanzee Joe showing piebald appearance of facial skin occurring after nine months continuous immunization with human melanoma (BL).

were hypertrophic. There was no significant thickening of the basement membrane. Many prominent pigmented dendritic cells were found in the reticular dermis in the perivascular spaces and about small cuta-

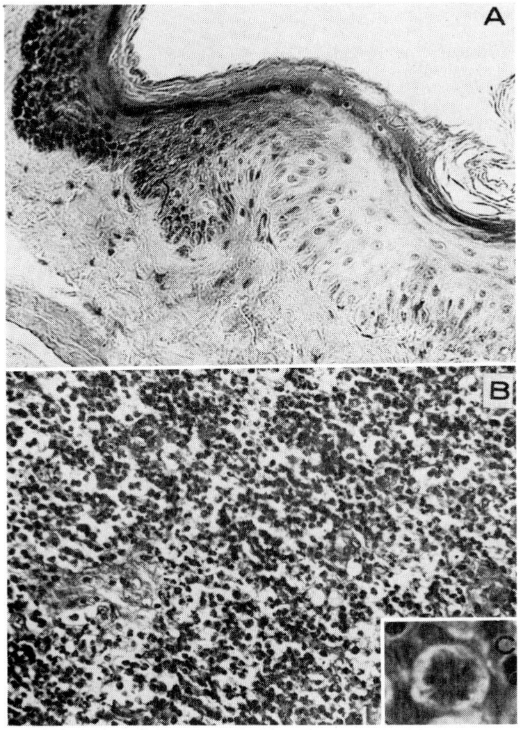

Fig. 6. Response of chimpanzee Joe to *(A)* his own pigmented skin (vitiligo), and *(B)* human melanoma cells (JC). This response consisted of masses of lymphocytes surrounding implanted growing melanoma cells, one of which is shown enlarged *(C)*. (Magnification: *A* and *B*, ×240; *C*, ×1,200.)

neous nerves. There was also evidence of dermal fibrosis. There was no evidence of mononuclear cell infiltration or inflammation. This same chimpanzee gave a strong inflammatory response (Fig. 6, *B*) to living malignant melanoma cells (Fig. 6, *C*) and his lymphocytes destroyed melanoma cells in culture.

DISCUSSION

The heterotransplantation of human melanoma has succeeded in several animal species immunosuppressed with radiation, drugs, and antilymphocyte globulin. Manuelidis[9] has transferred such tumors to the brains of non-immunosuppressed guinea pigs where they have been maintained for many years. Recently Visfeldt and colleagues[15] showed that human melanomas transplanted into nude (thymic aplastic) mice grew and maintained their human chromosome composition. In all of these studies, the normal animal response (hyperacute rejection) was abrogated and there was no lymphocytic or other mononuclear cell reaction characteristic of cellular immunity. We chose to study human melanomas in the chimpanzee in the hope of producing in this close relative of man a cellular immune response transferrable to man.

The lack of local reaction to the small inocula (10^6 cells) used in preliminary trials seemed to indicate: (1) that the animals were not making the hyperacute rejection response characteristic of anti-species immunity and (2) that the cells were probably moving or being carried away into the circulation. These animals made no immune response detectable by the procedures described above. CFA was added to the living cell inoculum to increase its antigenicity, and this occurred since subsequent tumor cell inocula always produced small nodules containing multiplying melanoma cells surrounded by lymphocytic infiltrates (Fig. 1). Further evidence against an anti-species type of reaction came from the fact that a chimpanzee immunized against BL tumor produced a nodule when injected with Ta tumor but no reaction to Ta skin cells inoculated at the same time.

The in vitro test system employed large numbers (1 to 2×10^5) of target cells because preliminary experiments showed that lower cell densities caused distortions in the growth curve (long lag phases) or occasional loss of the control cultures. Electron microscopy of the washed packed chimpanzee lymphocytes (Fig. 2) was chosen as our best available procedure to rule out the presence of infective viral particles. Since no virus was ever found and the chimpanzees remained healthy, it was assumed that viruses played no role in the test reaction.

In the test system, non-specific toxicity of the lymphocyte medium was ruled out by the fact that: (1) there was a dose-response relationship to the number of lymphocytes

(Fig. 3) and (2) such non-specific toxicity would probably be evidenced at 24 hours. Time lapse photography confirmed that the melanoma cells were being killed by highly active living lymphocytes which attacked them repeatedly, sticking to the tumor cells and pulling at the membranes until they burst. This process continued until the last tumor cell in the field was disrupted. Non-immune lymphocytes moved slowly to and away from the melanoma cells and did not stick to each other or inhibit the growth of the melanoma cell population which gradually filled the field being photographed.

The ability of immune lymphocytes to attack more than one melanoma cell population (Table I) was not unexpected since this finding had been reported for human lymphocytes from melanoma patients.[3, 6]

Immunization with melanoma cells regularly failed to produce an HL-A type response. Not only were donor skin fibroblasts unaffected but in one instance (Ta melanoma), donor lymphocytes (Ta) were available and the chimpanzee serum was not cytotoxic for Ta lymphocytes in the standard lymphocytotoxicity test, although this chimpanzee's lymphocytes killed Ta melanoma cells in culture. This chimpanzee and its melanoma donor (Ta) both had HL-A antigen 7. Ta also had HL-A W-12 but no others were found in either chimpanzee or Ta (human donor). Kersey, and associates[7] studied eight melanoma cell lines and found four of the eight had lost all donor HL-A antigens. Of the other four, only one retained all HL-A antigens present on the lymphocytes of the melanoma cell donor. Consequently our failure to produce anti–HL-A activity by immunization with melanoma cells could be explained by assuming that: (1) the melanoma cells had lost some or all HL-A antigens in culture, (2) the chimpanzee and its human donor shared major HL-A antigens, or (3) the melanoma antigen(s) competitively inhibited anti–HL-A responses.

Anti–HL-A responses are not easily induced in man or chimpanzee and in fact more prolonged immunization (four months) was required to produce an immune response to normal human fibroblasts derived from Ta skin.

When sensitization to Ta skin did occur, the lymphocytes from this chimpanzee destroyed both the fibroblasts and melanoma cells of the fibroblast donor (Ta). Table II shows that they also had an effect of some significance ($P < 0.1$) on the melanoma cells of JC who shared an HL-A antigen 7 with Ta. Cytotoxicity tests with monospecific HL-A antisera showed that JC melanoma cells carried JC antigens 3 and 7 but had lost HL-A 2. Monospecific antiserum for HL-A 17 (the fourth JC antigen) was not available. JC fibroblasts were unaffected, as were the other two (BL and Mg) melanoma cell lines and the other (Al and Mt) normal skin fibroblasts. Since 95 percent of cultured adult human fibroblasts carry the donor HL-A antigens,[7] the best explanation of these results appeared to be that the chimpanzee responded to the HL-A antigen 7 present on Ta fibroblasts and also on JC melanoma. The failure to damage JC fibroblasts was probably due to the greater hardiness of fibroblasts in culture as compared to melanoma cells or possibly JC fibroblasts had lost HL-A 7. This latter could not be determined since these fibroblasts gave unsatisfactory results in HL-A typing procedures.

The appearance of vitiligo (Figs. 4 and 5) in the hyperimmunized chimpanzees was of particular interest since this condition has been often associated with spontaneous remission of melanoma in human patients. In 1953, Summer[14] drew attention to these areas of skin depigmentation which occurred at the time of regression and were present four years later at which time the patient was still free of disease. Everson[2] also found that spontaneous regression of extensive metastatic melanoma was accompanied by "bone-white" depigmented areas. McPeak[11] has reported that successful intralymphatic therapy with immune lymphocytes produced vitiligo in the treated patient. All chimpanzees immunized against human melanoma eventually (six to eight months of hyperimmunization) developed vitiligo.

This fact allows the conclusion that the chimpanzee response to human melanoma was immunologically specific for normal melanocytes and was a tissue-specific response. However, the vitiligo was never inflammatory (Fig. 6, *A*) while the reaction to melanoma cells was always inflammatory (Fig. 6, *B*) so there was a marked difference between these two responses. The malignant tissue cell initiated an "autoimmune" type response to normal cells of the same tissue. This vitiligo did not appear to cause the chimpanzees any discomfort. In a recent review of human immunity to melanomas and neuroblastomas, Hellstrom and Hellstrom[5] concluded that "it may be that there is antigenic cross reactivity between neoplastic and normal cells of the same tissue. Even if this is true one must still remember that the reactions against these (melanoma) antigens gave delayed hypersensitivity in vivo (generally believed to be correlated with a tumor destructive ability) and led to tumor cell destruction in vitro, implying that the antigens involved did not at all appear as self to the organism and thus may be useful for tumor prevention and therapy."[5] These studies on chimpanzee response to melanoma support the Hellstrom hypothesis presented above and indicate that this close relative of man may prove to be a good model for certain human malignant and autoimmune diseases.

The authors wish to acknowledge the assistance of Dr. James C. Harkin, who performed the electron microscopy studies.

REFERENCES

1. Beltran, G., and Stuckey, W. L.: Nuclear lobulation and cytoplasmic fibrils in leukemic plasma cells, Am. J. Clin. Path. **58:** 159, 1972.
2. Everson, T. C.: Spontaneous regression of cancer, Ann. N. Y. Acad. Sci. **114:** 72, 1964.
3. Fossatti, G., Colnaghi, M., Della, P. G., Cascinelli, N., and Veronesi, U.: Cellular and humoral immunity against human melanoma, Int. J. Cancer **8:** 344, 1971.
4. Goodman, M., Barnabas, J., Matsuda, G., and Moore, G. W: Molecular evolution in the descent of man, Nature **233:** 604, 1971.
5. Hellstrom, K., and Hellstrom, I.: Immunity to neuroblastomas and melanomas, Ann. Rev. Med. **23:** 19, 1972.
6. Hellstrom, I., Hellstrom, K. E., Sjogren, H. O., and Warver, G. A.: Demonstration of cell mediated immunity to human neoplasms of various histological types, Int. J. Cancer **7:** 1, 1971.
7. Kersey, J. H., Yunis, E. J., Todaro, G. J., and Aaronson, S. A.: HL-A antigens of human tumor derived cell lines and viral transformed fibroblasts in culture, Proc. Soc. Exp. Biol. Med. **143:** 453, 1973.
8. Kohne, D. E.: Evolution of higher organism DNA, Q. Rev. Biophys. **3:** 327, 1970.
9. Manuelidis, E. E.: Heterologous transplantation of a tissue culture line of human melanoma, Yale J. Biol. Med. **43:** 307, 1971.
10. McDonald, J. C., Jacobbi, L., and Williams, R. W.: HL-A antigen studies with leukocyte cell lines, Transplantation **10:** 499, 1970.
11. McPeak, C. J.: Intralymphatic therapy with immune lymphocytes, Cancer **5:** 1126, 1971.
12. Oettgen, H. F., Old, L. J., and Boyse, E. A.: Human tumor immunology. Symposium on medical aspects of cancer, Med. Clin. North Am. **55:** 761, 1971.
13. Piessens, W. F.: Evidence for human cancer immunity, Cancer **26:** 1212, 1970.
14. Summer, W. C.: Spontaneous regression of melanoma, Cancer **6:** 1040, 1953.
15. Visfeldt, J., Povlsen, C. O., and Rygaard, J.: Chromosome analyses of human tumours following heterotransplantation to the mouse mutant "nude," Acta Pathol. Microbiol. Scand. (A). **80:** 169, 1972.

The interaction of glucagon and glucose on cardiorespiratory variables in the critically ill patient

Michael R. Drucker, M.D., Frank Pindyck, M.D., Robert S. Brown, M.D., David H. Elwyn, Ph.D., *and* **William C. Shoemaker, M.D.,** *New York, N. Y.*

The effect of glucagon on hemodynamic and oxygen transport was studied in 11 severely stressed surgical patients. When these responses were evaluated in relation to the patients' prior intravenous therapy, those patients who have received increased metabolic substrate (50 percent glucose) had, in general, greater and more consistent responses to glucagon infusion. It is suggested that exogenous glucose supplies the metabolic substrates necessary for the inotropic effect of glucagon. It is also suggested that the variability in response observed clinically with this hormone may be related to the carbohydrate availability. Since critically ill patients are frequently undernourished, therapeutic use of glucagon should be accompanied by adequate caloric intake.

From the Department of Surgery, Mount Sinai School of Medicine of the City University of New York, New York

THE CARDIAC effects of the pancreatic hormone glucagon were first described by Farah and Tuttle[6] in 1960; they observed a positive inotropic as well as chronotropic effect in various isolated heart preparations. Subsequently, numerous studies in laboratory animals[2, 8, 17, 27] and man[5, 13, 16, 24, 25, 37] have shown that glucagon can significantly increase myocardial contractility. It is well established that its effects are not altered by pretreatment with reserpine[2, 6, 8, 27] or beta blocking agents[8, 17] and are additive to the effects of digitalis preparations.[8, 25] Furthermore, it does not induce harmful arrhythmias despite its tendency to lower serum potassium levels.[5, 8, 13, 18, 24, 25, 37] Glucagon can inhibit gastrointestinal motility,[6, 33] but this undesirable side effect can easily be controlled with prochlorperazine.[18] Recently, reports of variability in its action, and at times lack of response, have cast doubt on the clinical usefulness of glucagon[11, 22, 23, 30, 31, 37, 38]; some of the factors involved have been reviewed by Glick.[7]

It is believed that the positive inotropic action of glucagon is mediated through its ability to activate the adenyl cyclase system, stimulating the formation of adenosine 3′-5′ monophosphate (cyclic AMP) from adenosine triphosphate (ATP).[14, 36] By activating various phosphokinases, cyclic AMP can produce multiple metabolic effects. In the heart, this includes the activation of phosphorylase, inactivation of glycogen synthetase, and increased incorporation of calcium.[20, 35] The subsequent increased availability of oxidative substrate in the form of glucose phosphate may partially explain the enhanced myocardial contractility following glucagon.

Since the action of glucagon is intimately related to glucose metabolism, possibly a relative deficiency of this nutrient could ac-

Accepted for publication Jan. 28, 1974.

Table I. *Summary of clinical data*

Patient	*Age (yr.)*	*Sex*	*Disease*	*Operation*	*Outcome*
F. L.	79	M	Chronic bronchitis and emphysema, sepsis, abdominal aortic aneurysm	None	Died
I. I.	76	M	Stab wound, left ventricle	Thoracotomy, suture, left ventricle	Survived
J. R.	90	M	Ruptured abdominal aortic aneurysm	Aneurysmectomy	Died
A. K.	80	M	Gastrointestinal bleeding	Suture ligation, gastric ulcer	Survived
H. S.	58	M	Cervical cord transection	None	Died
H. L.	79	M	Multiple fractures, cerebral concussion, sepsis	Reduction and internal fixation, left femur	Survived
J. S.	78	M	Ruptured abdominal aortic aneurysm	Aneurysmectomy	Died
H. G.	46	M	Stab wound, left ventricle	Thoracotomy, suture, left ventricle	Survived
J. S.	56	M	Carcinoma of stomach	Esophagogastrectomy	Survived
D. W.	70	M	Small bowel obstruction, sepsis	Lysis of adhesions	Died
D. H.	80	M	Carcinoma of colon, complete obstruction	Transverse colostomy	Survived

count for the variable effectiveness. In the unanesthetized dog, glucagon administration increased hepatic blood flow and hepatic glucose output: This hepatic response was markedly depressed if the dogs were glycogen depleted.[29]

The present clinical study was performed to determine whether adequate carbohydrate may be a limiting factor for the inotropic action of glucagon in severely stressed surgical patients. The cardiorespiratory changes produced by glucagon are compared with the responses to hypertonic glucose described by Pindyck and associates.[26]

METHODS

Clinical material. Eleven severely stressed surgical patients, in various degrees of shock were monitored in the surgical metabolic unit; twenty-three separate studies were performed on these eleven patients, who were all males, between the ages of 46 and 90 (mean age, 72). The relevant clinical data are summarized in Table I; there were a variety of complicated surgical problems including hemorrhage, sepsis, bowel obstruction, bowel infarction, and spinal cord transection. For purposes of this analysis, no attempt was made to separate patients into etiologic categories, but depending upon prior intravenous therapy, each patient was placed in either of two groups: Group I, patients maintained on conventional (five percent glucose) intravenous therapy for at least 24 hours prior to study; and Group II, patients who had received intravenously at least 2,000 calories as 50 percent glucose in the 24 hours prior to the study.

Hemodynamic measurements. Methods used in these studies have previously been reported in detail.[28] Briefly, either the brachial or subclavian vein was catheterized percutaneously with a large gauge polyethylene catheter and advanced sufficiently into the superior vena cava for direct measurement of the central venous pressure. The systemic arterial pressure was measured by catheterization of the axillary artery percutaneously; on rare occasion, radial artery cut-down was required. A No. 7 Fr.

Table II. *Hemodynamic and oxygen transport variables after glucagon (mean ± S.E.)*

	Group I (5% glucose)			*Group II (50% glucose)*		
	Control	*Glucagon*	*P value*	*Control*	*Glucagon*	*P value*
Heart rate (beats × min.$^{-1}$)	90.8 ± 6.2	94.6 ± 5.8	0.010	83.6 ± 5.0	86.5 ± 4.9	N.S.
Mean arterial pressure (mm. Hg)	81.5 ± 4.6	82.9 ± 4.7	N.S.*	87.7 ± 5.3	88.5 ± 6.4	N.S.
Cardiac index (L. × min.$^{-1}$ × M.$^{-2}$)	3.84 ± 0.50	4.45 ± 0.54	0.010	3.77 ± 0.31	5.13 ± 0.76	0.050
Stroke index (ml. × M.$^{-2}$)	45.2 ± 5.4	51.8 ± 6.3	0.050	47.0 ± 6.3	62.8 ± 5.7	0.025
Mean transit time (sec.)	25.3 ± 2.2	23.2 ± 2.2	0.100	25.0 ± 2.0	23.2 ± 2.1	0.025
Mean pulmonary artery pressure (cm. saline)	22.0 ± 2.5	20.6 ± 3.0	N.S.	27.9 ± 2.3	24.5 ± 1.8	0.100
Left atrial pressure (cm. saline)	5.6 ± 2.1	4.8 ± 2.5	N.S.	10.2 ± 0.9	8.7 ± 1.7	N.S.
Left stroke work index (Gm. × M. × M.$^{-2}$)	50.1 ± 6.8	52.2 ± 6.5	0.100	51.7 ± 95	73.6 ± 14.7	0.050
Right stroke work index (Gm. × M. × M.$^{-2}$)	13.0 ± 2.3	15.7 ± 2.7	N.S.	15.5 ± 1.4	20.2 ± 2.7	0.100
Total peripheral resistance (dyne × sec. × cm.$^{-5}$ × M.$^{-2}$)	1,760 ± 176	1,522 ± 187	0.050	1,908 ± 166	1,438 ± 197	0.005
Pulmonary vascular resistance (dyne × sec. × cm.$^{-5}$ × M.$^{-2}$)	380 ± 64	345 ± 88	N.S.	402 ± 70	332 ± 54	N.S.
Oxygen availability (ml. × min.$^{-1}$ × M.$^{-2}$)	491 ± 66	590 ± 81	0.005	535 ± 57	737 ± 127	N.S.
Oxygen extraction (%)	29.1 ± 2.7	31.8 ± 3.9	N.S.	25.8 ± 1.5	27.9 ± 3.1	N.S.
Oxygen consumption (ml. × min.$^{-1}$ × M.$^{-2}$)	132 ± 14	164 ± 18	0.005	139 ± 19	185 ± 24	0.050

*N.S. = not significant.

Swan-Ganz flow-directed catheter was introduced percutaneously and advanced into a distal pulmonary artery for measurement of pulmonary and precapillary wedge pressures; the pressure wave contour was used as a guide to placement of this catheter. The pressures were measured with microdot (MS5) transducers and continuously recorded. Cardiac output was measured by the Stewart-Hamilton dye dilution principle[12] with indocyanine green as the indicator. The dye was injected rapidly into the right atrium, and the dye concentration in arterial blood was measured by a Gilford photodensitometer. The dye curve and all pressures were simultaneously recorded on a Beckman multichannel dynagraph and, through electronic interfacing equipment, on magnetic tape. Cardiac output was calculated digitally from the area under the primary washout curve by a digital computer and a program which used an algorithm based on ratios of the log of digital values taken every 0.1 second in order to differentiate the dye recirculation from the primary washout curve. Stroke volume, mean transit time, systemic and pulmonary vascular resistance, and left and right stroke work were calculated according to standard formulas; all of the primary and derived caculations were performed by a digital computer programmed for this purpose. The measurements were divided by surface area and expressed as indexed values for purposes of comparison.

Oxygen transport. Mixed venous and systemic arterial blood samples were collected anaerobically in heparinized syringes and immediately analyzed for Po_2, Pco_2, and pH at 37° C. with an Instrumentation Laboratory (IL) gas analyzer and microblood pH assembly. Hemoglobin and oxygen saturation were measured with an IL 182 co-oximeter. Oxygen content was calculated from the oxygen saturation and the hemoglobin values. Oxygen extraction ratio was calculated as the arteriovenous content difference divided by the arterial oxygen content. Oxygen availability was calculated as the product of the arterial oxygen content

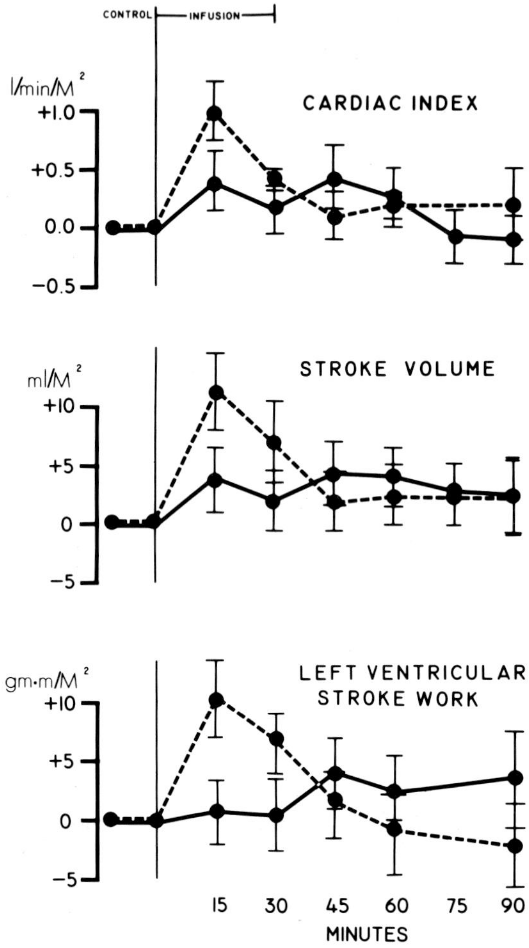

Fig. 1. Serial changes in cardiac index, stroke volume and left ventricular stroke work before, during, and after a 30 minute infusion of glucagon. Dots indicate mean values. Vertical bars represent standard errors of the mean. ——, Group I (5 percent glucose; - - - -, Group II (50 percent glucose).

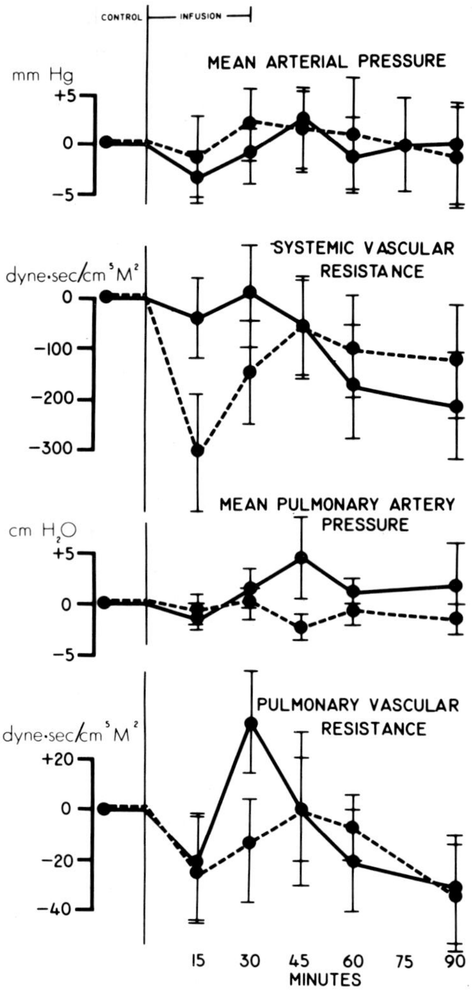

Fig. 2. Serial changes in arterial pressure, systemic vascular resistance, pulmonary artery pressure, and pulmonary vascular resistance before, during, and after a 30 minute infusion of glucagon. Dots indicate mean values. Vertical bars represent standard errors of the mean. ——, Group I (5 percent glucose); - - - -, Group II (50 percent glucose).

and the cardiac index. Oxygen consumption was calculated as the product of the arteriovenous oxygen content difference and the cardiac index. All measurements of cardiorespiratory function were obtained during relatively stable periods, when the patient did not exhibit anxiety or agitation.

Protocol. After suitable control measurements had demonstrated a reasonably steady state, 5 mg. of glucagon (Lilly), dissolved in the accompanying diluent and made up to a volume of 50 ml. with normal saline, was constantly infused over a 30 minute period with a Harvard pump. Hemodynamic and oxygen transport measurements were made at 15, 30, 45, 60, and 90 minutes following the beginning of this infusion. During the period of observation, no other active therapy was given.

RESULTS

The control and maximum hemodynamic and oxygen transport responses following glucagon infusion are listed in Table II. The sequential values expressed as changes from control values are illustrated in Figs. 1, 2, and 3.

The control serum glucose level in Group I averaged 166 mg. per 100 ml., while Group II had control levels of 251 mg. per 100 ml.; the latter value is consistent with the increased exogenous supply of glucose in Group II. Following glucagon infusion, the maximum increase in serum which occurred 45 minutes after onset of the infusion, averaged 120 mg. per 100 ml. (72 percent above control) in Group I and 68 mg. per 100 ml. (27 percent above control) in Group II.

Hemodynamic response. The chronotropic effects of glucagon were minimal in both groups; the increase in heart rate averaged 5.2 percent in Group I ($P < 0.05$) and 4.0 percent in Group II. However, the inotropic effects of glucagon infusion were appreciable in both groups. Although blood pressure was essentially unchanged, there were substantial increases in cardiac index, stroke volume, and stroke work with a reduction in both the systemic and pulmonary vascular resistances. The inotropic effect was greater and more consistent in Group II than in Group I. The less impressive hemodynamic effect in Group I was maximal 45 minutes after onset of the infusion; the response in Group II was greatest at the 15 minute period. Cardiac index increased 16 percent in Group I ($P < 0.01$) as compared to 31 percent in Group II ($P < 0.05$). Eight patients in Group I had increased flow and three had slight decreases in flow. By contrast, all of the Group II patients responded to glucagon infusion with increased cardiac output. Similarly, with respect to stroke work, Group I increased only 15 percent ($P < 0.10$); six of these patients had increases; two had slight decreases, and the values of two patients remained unchanged from control values. In Group II, the left stroke work increased 28 percent ($P < 0.05$); all but one of these patients responded. The changes in Group II were significantly different from the first group ($P < 0.05$). The maximum increase in stroke volume was 18 percent in Group I ($P < 0.05$) as compared to 31 percent in Group II ($P < 0.025$).

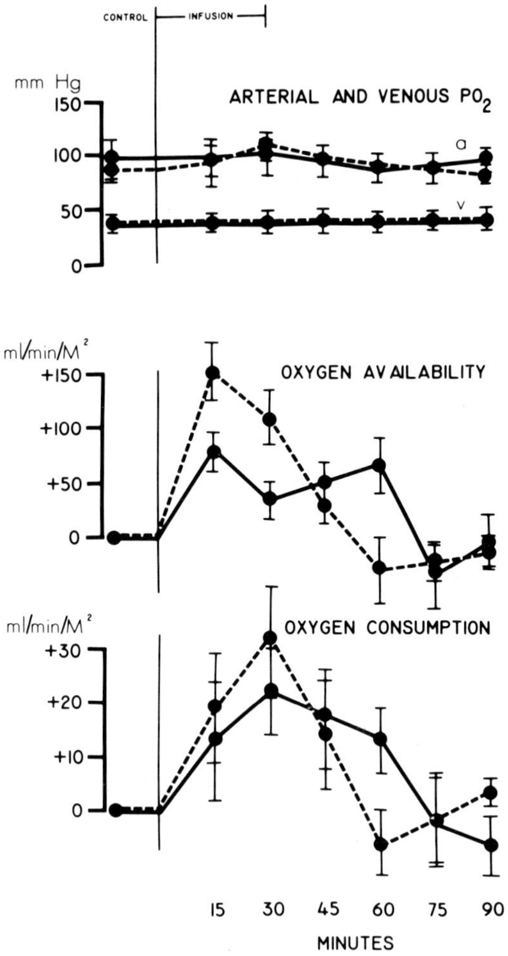

Fig. 3. Serial changes in arterial Po_2, oxygen availability and oxygen consumption before, during, and after a 30 minute infusion of glucagon. Dots indicate mean values. Vertical bars represent standard errors of the mean. ——, Group I (5 percent glucose); - - - -, Group II (50 percent glucose).

The systemic and pulmonary vascular resistance fell. There was an average decrease of 14 percent in systemic vascular resistance in Group I ($P < 0.05$); eight of the 11 patients in this group had decreases. Greater and more consistent responses were noted in Group II; the average decrease was 26 percent ($P < 0.005$) and all but one of these patients had decreased resistance.

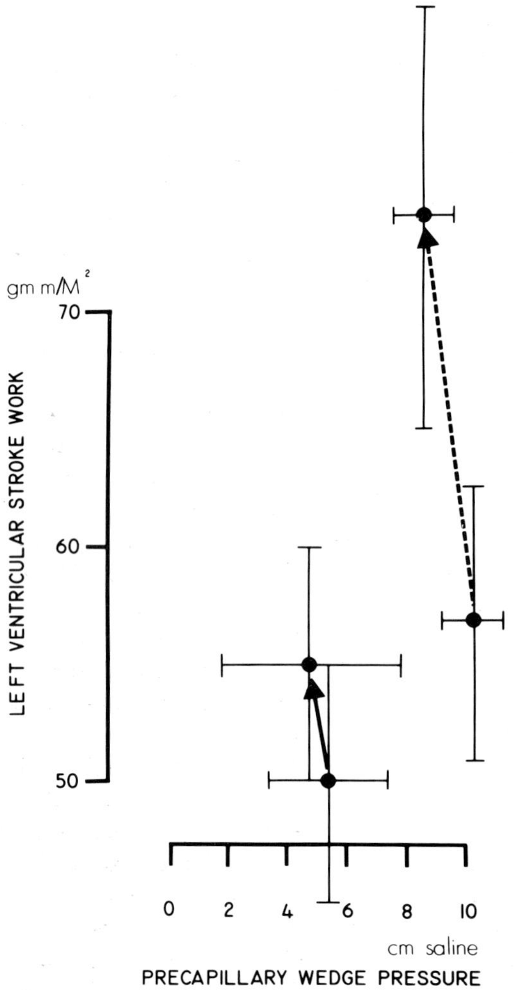

Fig. 4. Left ventricular stroke work values plotted against their corresponding precapillary wedge pressures prior to and at the maximum response following glucagon infusion in two groups of critically ill patients. ——, Group I (5 percent glucose); - - - -, Group II (50 percent glucose).

Ventricular function. Figure 4 represents left ventricular stroke work values plotted against their corresponding precapillary wedge pressures in the standard Starling curve for myocardial performance. Group II patients had slightly higher control filling pressures. Following glucagon administration there was a more pronounced improvement in ventricular function in Group II as compared with Group I. The precapillary wedge pressures tended to fall minimally in both groups after glucagon was given.

Oxygen transport. The oxygen extraction increased slightly in both groups. The increased oxygen availability in Group I was 23 percent; in Group II, it was 41 percent. The oxygen consumption rose 27 percent in Group I ($P < 0.05$) as compared to 37 percent in Group II ($P < 0.05$).

DISCUSSION

The data presented herein show that glucagon has significant hemodynamic and oxygen transport effects in critically ill patients who had been given approximate caloric replacement. That is, patients who had received 2,000 calories or more of 50 percent glucose in the preceding 24 hour period had greater and more consistent responses to glucagon infusion than those maintained on standard intravenous therapy. Although the energy requirements of the acutely stressed patient are variable and not precisely known, there is abundant evidence that additional caloric intake can improve wound healing[33] and cellular function.[3] Glucose loading of the anoxic myocardium can also improve myocardial contractility.[1] Recently, increased adenyl cyclase activity and myocardial contractility were demonstrated in animal hearts perfused with glucose solutions.[4]

The conventional Starling myocardial performance curve considers cardiac output, left ventricular stroke work, or some other measure of cardiac function plotted against the simultaneously measured inflow pressure. The experimental variable usually has been the addition or withdrawal of blood or plasma volume expanders, but the effects of a therapeutic agent may also be evaluated by its influence on the stroke work–inflow pressure relationship.

In the study by Pindyck and associates,[26] control studies indicated that comparable volumes added by the glucagon infusion did not appreciably affect cardiorespiratory variables. Both groups of the present series were given the same volume of diluent, namely 50 ml. of saline over a 30 minute period; this rate is equivalent to 2,400 ml. of fluid per day, which is the normal rate of fluid loss and therefore not an unreasonable rate of fluid replacement. No other fluids were given during the period of observation.

The Starling myocardial performance convention, which considers any pair of stroke work–inflow pressures, is an accepted convention for evaluating the response of a drug as well as that of blood withdrawal or fluid loading. The slopes of the function curves in the two groups appear very similar. This is consistent with the conclusion that glucagon in the depleted, critically ill patient produces a small, transient change, while glucagon together with adequate glucose produces a greater improvement in cardiac function as well as peripheral perfusion and oxygen transport. That the direction of the change is the same but the degree of change is different suggests that the responses of the two clinical groups were quantitatively, but not qualitatively, different.

The mean precapillary wedge pressure values of the two groups in the control period were different, but because of the variability within each group, the difference was not statistically significant. Moreover, the values of both groups were normal; i.e., wedge pressures up to 15 cm. H_2O in our hands, are considered to be within the normal range. After glucagon administration, the mean wedge pressures decreased slightly, but not significantly, in both groups, indicating that changes in myocardial performance were not due to changes in ventricular filling.

Although the hemodynamic and oxygen transport responses were greater in Group II patients, the hyperglycemic response to glucagon was more pronounced in Group I patients. This suggests that the inotropic effects of glucagon were direct effects of this agent on the heart and vasculature. Glucose and insulin effects on carbohydrate metabolism, cardiac hemodynamics, osmotic effects, and blood volume changes are considered in the communication by Pindyck and colleagues.[26]

The variability in inotropic action previously observed when the glucagon was used clinically may in part be explained by the data of the present study. The increased energy demands of acute illness may rapidly deplete the amount of available carbohydrate needed to maintain optimal cellular metabolism and therefore limit glucagon responses. It is possible that the additional parenteral carbohydrate load our Group II patients had received prior to glucagon infusion was sufficient to sustain or replenish carbohydrate stores and to provide greater amounts of glycogen upon which the enzyme systems could act. Moreover, evidence from carefully controlled experimental studies indicated that physiologic manifestations of glucagon may be absent or attenuated in depleted animals.[29] Repeated doses of glucagon have been observed to produce the phenomenon of tachyphylaxis in man[31] and experimental animals.[6] This also may be explained by rapid glycogenolysis and consequent depletion of carbohydrate stores.[29] When there is limited carbohydrate stores or increased demands of acute illness, oxidative substrates become less available for cellular function and myocardial contractility.

In severe *chronic* congestive heart failure both myocardial contractility and activation of adenyl cyclase following glucagon administration is limited. By contrast, the action of glucagon is preserved in both the normal and the *acutely* failing heart.[9, 10, 15] Possibly, the ability of the poorly functioning myocardium to store and mobilize adequate energy substrates is sufficiently depressed that the glucagon response is attenuated. The normal and acutely failing heart may still retain the ability to respond.

REFERENCES

1. Austen, W. G., Greenberg, J. J., and Piccinini, J. C.: Myocardial function and contractile force affected by glucose loading of the heart during anoxia, SURGERY **57:** 839, 1965.
2. Bower, M. G., Okude, S., Jolley, W. B., and Smith, L. L.: Hemodynamic effects of glucagon, Arch. Surg. **101:** 411, 1970.
3. Currer, P. W., Willmore, D. W., Mason, A. D., Newsome, T. W., Asch, M. J., and Pruitt, B. A.: Intracellular cation alterations following major trauma: Effect of supranormal caloric intake, J. Trauma **11:** 390, 1971.
4. Dhalla, N. S., Sulakhe, P. V., Khandelwal,

R. L., and Olson, R. E.: Adenyl cyclase activity in the perfused rat heart made to fail by substrate lack, Cardiovasc. Res. **6:** 344, 1972.
5. Eddy, J. D., O'Brien, E. T., and Singh, S. P.: Glucagon and hemodynamics of acute myocardial infarction, Br. Med. J. **4:** 663, 1969.
6. Farah, A., and Tuttle, R.: Studies on the pharmacology of glucagon, J. Pharmacol. Exp. Ther. **129:** 49, 1960.
7. Glick, G.: Glucagon: A perspective, Circulation **45:** 513, 1972.
8. Glick, G. G., Parmley, W. W., Weschsler, A. S., and Sonnenblick, E. H.: Glucagon: Its enhancement of cardiac performance in the cat and dog and persistence of its inotropic action despite beta-receptor blockade with propranolol, Circ. Res. **22:** 789, 1968.
9. Gold, H. K., Prindle, K. H., Levey, G. S., and Epstein, S. E.: Effects of experimental heart failure on the capacity of glucagon to augment myocardial contractility and activate adenyl cyclase, J. Clin. Invest. **49:** 999, 1970.
10. Goldstein, R. E., Skelton, C. L., Levey, G. S., Glancy, D. L., Beiser, G. D., and Epstein, S. E.: Effects of chronic heart failure on the capacity of glucagon to enhance contractility and adenyl cyclase activity on human papillary muscles, Circ. **44:** 638, 1971.
11. Greenberg, B. H., Tsakiris, A. G., Moffitt, E. A., and Frye, R. L.: The hemodynamic and metabolic effects of glucagon in patients with chronic valvular heart disease, Mayo Clin. Proc. **45:** 132, 1970.
12. Hamilton, W. F., Moore, J. W., Kinsman, J. M., and Spurling, R. G.: Studies on the circulation, Am. J. Physiol. **99:** 534, 1932.
13. Klein, S. W., Morch, J. E., and Mahon, W. A.: Cardiovascular effects of glucagon in man, Can. Med. Assoc. J. **98:** 1161, 1968.
14. Levey, G. S., and Epstein, S. E.: Activation of adenyl cyclase by glucagon in cat and human heart, Circ. Res. **24:** 151, 1969.
15. Levey, G. S., Prindle, K. H., Jr., and Epstein, S. E.: Effects of glucagon on adenyl cyclase activity in the left and right ventricles and liver in experimentally produced isolated right ventricular failure, J. Mol. Cell. Cardiol. **1:** 403, 1970.
16. Linhart, J. W., Barold, S. S., Cohen, L. S., Hildner, F. J., and Samet, P.: Cardiovascular effects of glucagon in man, Am. J. Cardiol. **22:** 706, 1968.
17. Lucchesi, B. R.: Cardiac actions of glucagon, Circ. Res. **22:** 777, 1968.
18. Lvoff, R., and Wilcken, D. E. L.: Glucagon in heart failure and in cardiogenic shock, Circulation **45:** 534, 1972.
19. McNamara, J. J., Mills, D., and Aaby, G. V.: Effect of hypertonic glucose on hemorrhagic shock in rabbits, Ann. Thorac. Surg. **9:** 116, 1970.
20. Major, P. W., and Kilpatrick, R.: Review: cyclic AMP and hormone action, J. Endocrinol. **52:** 593, 1972.
21. Moffat, J. G., King, J. A. C., and Drucker, W. R.: Tolerance to prolonged hypovolemic shock: Effect of infusion of an energy substrate, Surg. Forum **19:** 5, 1968.
22. Murtagh, J. G., Binnion, P. F., Lal, S., Hutchinson, K. J., and Fletcher, E.: Hemodynamic effects of glucagon, Br. Heart J. **32:** 307, 1970.
23. Nord, H. J., Fontanes, A. L., and Williams, J. F.: Treatment of congestive heart failure with glucagon, Ann. Intern. Med. **72:** 649, 1970.
24. Parmley, W. W., Glick, G., and Sonnenblick, E. H.: Cardiovascular effects of glucagon in man, New Engl. J. Med. **279:** 12, 1968.
25. Parmley, W. W., Matloff, J. M., and Sonnenblick, E. H.: Hemodynamic effects of glucagon in patients following prosthetic valve replacement, Circulation **390-400** (Suppl. 1): 163, 1969.
26. Pindyck, F., Drucker, M. R., Brown, R. S., and Shoemaker, W. C.: Cardiorespiratory effects of hypertonic glucose in the critically ill patient, SURGERY **75:** 11, 1974.
27. Regan, T. J., Lehan, P. H., Henneman, D. H., Behar, A., and Hellems, H. K.: Myocardial metabolic and contractile response to glucagon and epinephrine, J. Lab. Clin. Med. **63:** 638, 1964.
28. Shoemaker, W. C.: Cardiorespiratory patterns in complicated and uncomplicated septic shock, Ann. Surg. **174:** 119, 1971.
29. Shoemaker, W. C., and Van Itallie, T. B.: The hepatic response to glucagon in the unanesthetized dog, Endocrinology **66:** 260, 1960.
30. Siegel, J. H., Levine, M. J., McConn, R., and Del Guercio, L. R. M.: The effect of glucagon infusion on cardiovascular function in the critically ill, Surg. Gynecol. Obstet. **131:** 505, 1970.
31. Simianis, J., and Goldberg, L. I.: The effects of glucagon on sodium, potassium and urine excretion in patients in congestive heart failure, Am. Heart J. **81:** 202, 1971.
32. Sporn, J., and Necheles, H.: Effect of glucagon on GI motility, Am. J. Physiol. **187:** 634, 1956.
33. Steiger, E., Allen, T. R., Daly, J. M., Vars, H. M., and Dudrick, S. J.: Beneficial effects of immediate post-operative total parenteral nutrition, Surg. Forum **22:** 89, 1971.

34. Snedecor, G. W.: Statistical methods, ed. 5, Ames, Iowa, 1962, Iowa State University Press, p. 45.
35. Sutherland, E. W., and Robison, G. A.: The role of cyclic AMP in the control of carbohydrate metabolism, Diabetes **18:** 797, 1969.
36. Sutherland, E. W., Robison, G. A., and Butcher, R. W.: Some aspects of the biological role of adenosine 3′,5′-monophosphate (cyclic AMP), Circulation **37:** 279, 1968.
37. William, J. F., Jr., Childress, R. H., Chip, J. N., and Border, J. F.: Hemodynamic effects of glucagon in patients with heart disease, Circulation **39:** 38, 1969.
38. Vander Ark, C. R., and Reynolds, E. W., Jr.: Clinical evaluation of glucagon by continuous infusion in the treatment of low cardiac output states, Am. Heart J. **79:** 481, 1970.

Fatty acid absorption in jejunal autograft and allograft

William P. Stamford, M.D., *and* Mark A. Hardy, M.D., *Bronx, N. Y.*

Absorption studies of short and long chain fatty acids (lauric acid and oleic acid) were performed in jejunal Thiry-Vella loops, autografts and untreated allografts. Lauric acid absorption in jejunal allografts correlated well with progressive morphologic signs of rejection, thus suggesting its usefulness in predicting intestinal allograft rejection. Oleic acid was not absorbed in the absence of lymphatic regeneration. The first appearance of oleic acid absorption in autografts (two to four weeks) was related to regeneration of the lymphatic vessels as shown by lymphangiography. It is therefore suggested that oleic acid absorption may ultimately serve as a test of functional capacity of regenerating lymphatic vessels of intestinal allografts.

From the Transplantation Service, Department of Surgery, Albert Einstein College of Medicine, Bronx, N. Y.

IN ORDER to achieve successful clinical transplantation of the intestine, not only morphological but also functional survival must be accomplished. In the present study, we wish to report on the absorption of lauric and oleic acids by segmental jejunal autografts and allografts deprived of neural and lymphatic connections. In previous reports,[2, 7, 8] we described functional survival of intestinal allografts in relation to glucose and arabinose absorption, and this study extends our continuing interest in the correlation between morphologic and functional survival of intestinal allografts.

MATERIAL AND METHODS

Adult, unmatched, mongrel dogs weighing 20 to 25 kilograms were used in all experiments. They were maintained on a standard kennel diet and were not fed on the night prior to surgery and prior to each absorption study.

Operative procedure. Diabutal (0.5 ml. per kilogram) anesthesia was used with an endotracheal tube in place. An eight-inch segment of proximal jejunum was isolated as a Thiry-Vella loop in four dogs. The vascular, lymphatic, and neural connections to the isolated jejunal loop were carefully preserved. The remaining bowel was reanastomosed in an end-to-end fashion.

Autografts and allografts were performed by isolating an eight-inch segment of proximal jejunum with an intact vascular pedicle. In allografts in which the donors were killed, the dissection extended to the superior mesenteric vessels. The resected jejunal segment was perfused with cold (4° C.) balanced, lactated Ringer's solution containing heparin and lidocaine until the venous effluent was clear. Circulation to the graft was re-established by an end-to-end anastomosis

Accepted for publication Feb. 6, 1974.

Reprint requests: Dr. M. A. Hardy, Chief, Transplantation Service, Department of Surgery, Albert Einstein College of Medicine, 1300 Morris Park Ave., Bronx, N. Y. 10461.

of the superior mesenteric artery to the internal iliac artery and by an end-to-side anastomosis of the superior mesenteric vein to the common iliac vein. Following the vascular anastomosis, both stomas of the jejunal segment were exteriorized for future absorption studies and biopsies. This technique proved successful in 85 percent of allografts. In autografts, for which a segmental artery and vein were used, the patch-graft technique described by Taylor and associates[15] was employed. Four autografts were placed in the heterotopic position and four autografts were placed in a completely orthotopic position. The latter proved to be technically more difficult, and the success rate of the surgical procedure was only 50 percent. The appearance of the Thiry-Vella loops and autografts was assessed daily. Intraluminal punch biopsies were performed three times a week for morphological studies. Tissue was fixed in ten percent formalin, sectioned and stained with hematoxylin-eosin and Mowry's stains.

Absorption studies. Absorption studies were performed on the jejunal segments with uniformly labeled C^{14} lauric acid* and C^{14} oleic acid* on alternate days. After dose-response curves for each substance in the Thiry-Vella loops were determined, it was found that 20 μc of the labeled substance dissolved in 2.5 c.c. of buffered saline and 1 c.c. of ox bile gave consistently reproducible absorption curves for both lauric and oleic acids. After a control blood sample was obtained, 20 μc of the test substance at a pH of 7.5 was introduced into mechanically closed intestinal lumen. Peripheral blood samples were then obtained at 5, 10, 20, 30, 40, 60, 120, 180, and 240 minutes. Plasma fraction of the sample (0.5 c.c.) was then separated by Folch lipid extraction,[3] yielding a filtrate containing all lipids except the phospholipids, which in other experiments proved to be present only in insignificant amounts. After the evaporation of the solvents (two parts chloroform to one part methanol), the sediment was suspended in 10 c.c. of Omnifluor.* Radioactivity of each sample was then counted in duplicate on a Beckman liquid scintillation counter.

*New England Nuclear, Boston, Mass.

Lymphangiography. Lymphangiography was performed by injection of 0.5 to 1 c.c. of three percent Evans blue into the exposed intestinal submucosa, thus outlining a lymphatic channel in the grafted mesentery. This lymphatic channel was then dissected and cannulated with a No. 26 needle through which 5 c.c. of Diodrast was injected. Radiographs of the abdomen and chest were performed during the injection and at 30, 60, and 120 minutes after the injection.

RESULTS

Morphological graft survival.

Group I. This group consisted of four animals with Thiry-Vella loops. The intestinal segments were studied throughout the period of the experiment and manifested normal intestinal behavior in terms of clear intraluminal secretions and excellent peristalsis. Histological sections obtained at various intervals revealed normal intestinal mucosa. Three months after surgery, there was a minimal hypertrophy of the villi with an increase in the number of the mucin-secreting cells.

Group II. This group consisted of eight untreated animals with jejunal autografts. Four autografts were in an orthotopic position and four autografts were in the heterotopic position in the abdomen. The gross appearance of the graft stoma was the same as that in the control group. All autografts remained viable until the time of death. Histological sections revealed normal intestinal mucosa with a minimal decrease in the height of the villi. The mucin-secreting cells remained intact. There was mild dilatation of lymphatic channels in both Groups IIA and IIB.

Group III. This group consisted of six dogs receiving intraperitoneal heterotopic jejunal allografts. Donors and recipients were not matched for histocompatability transplantation antigens.

*New England Nuclear, Boston, Mass.

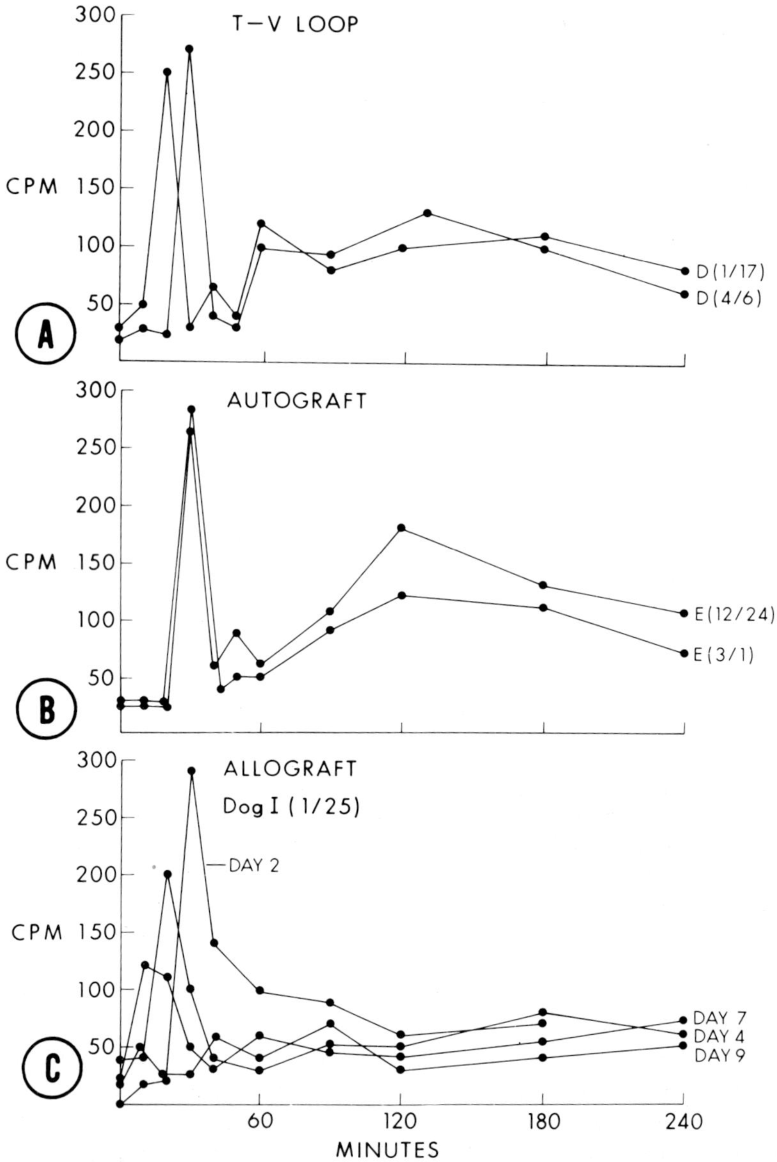

Fig. 1. C^{14} lauric acid absorption curves recorded as counts per minute (CPM) with each period of study lasting four hours. *A,* Absorption curves in a Thiry-Vella loop in one dog on two days three months apart. *B,* Absorption curves in an autograft in one dog on two days three months apart. The curves in *A* and *B* are similar in both the time of peak of absorption and the shape indicative of active absorption. *C,* Absorption curves in a non-immunosuppressed segmental jejunal allograft in one dog on days 2, 4, 7, and 9 as indicated. There is gradual decrease in the peak of lauric acid absorption from day 2 through 7, and the curve is almost flat on day 9 when gross rejection was apparent.

The rejection of the allografts occurred between days 5 and 9, and was heralded by edema and congestion of the mucosa of the stoma and by blood-stained secretions from the lumen of the allograft.

The histological rejection pattern was similar in all allografts studied and occurred at variable periods. In the first three to four days, there were few significant morphological changes except for dilated lacteals, occasional areas of hemorrhage, and mild edema. The initial histological changes con-

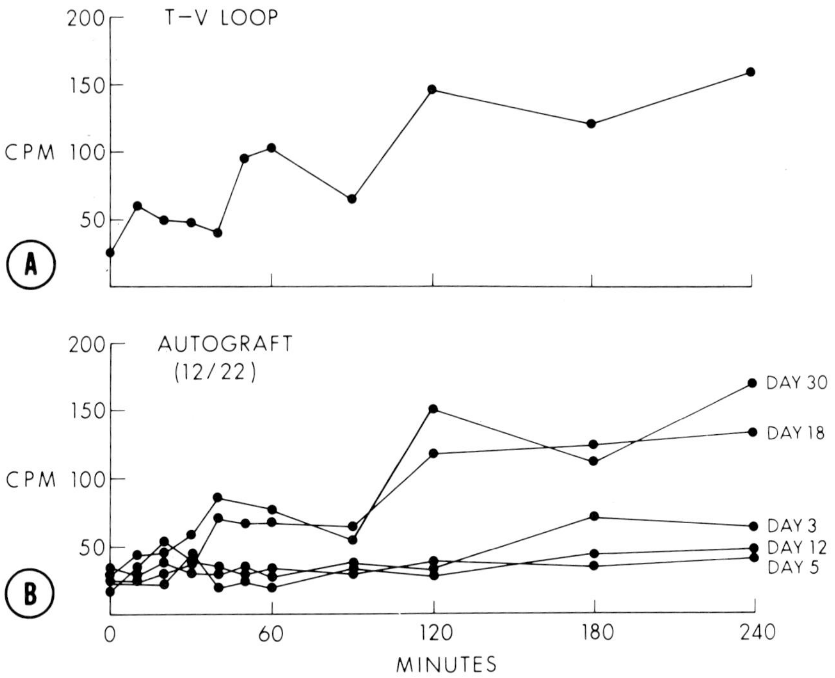

Fig. 2. C^{14} oleic acid absorption curves recorded as counts per minute (CPM) with each period of study lasting four hours. *A,* Absorption curve in a Thiry-Vella loop showing slow rise suggestive of both active and passive absorption which may partially depend on recirculating C^{14}-labeled products of oleic acid breakdown. *B,* Absorption curves on five different days in one autograft. On days 3, 5, and 12 the curves are almost flat. On days 18 and 30, there is a rise in oleic acid absorption. The magnitude and shape of the curves on days 18 and 30 approximate that found in *A*.

sisted of a cellular infiltration of the lamina propria by lymphocytes and plasma cells. At the same time, there was a flattening in the villi which then progressed to necrosis of the epithelial cells. The final event consisted of necrosis of the surface epithelium with marked infiltration of leukocytes into the submucosal layer. This was accompanied by fibrosis of the muscularis, mucosae.

Functional graft survival.

Lauric acid absorption. C^{14} lauric acid absorption curves in the Thiry-Vella loops and autografts (II) were quite similar, as illustrated in Fig. 1, *A* and *B*. The active absorption of lauric acid in these control groups served as the standard for all further lauric acid absorption studies in the jejunal allografts. The peak plasma levels were obtained at ten to twenty minutes in both Thiry-Vella loops and autografts which differed anatomically by the initial absence of lymphatic and neural connections in the autografts. The absorption curves were consistently reproducible in both groups over a three-month period of study. In Group III, consisting of segmental jejunal allografts in dogs receiving no immunosuppression, there was a gradual decrease in the peak absorption of lauric acid as illustrated in Fig. 1, *C* in one dog. The serial curves in the other five allografts showed similar decreases in peak absorption depending on the length of survival; when the allograft survived only five days, active absorption of lauric acid was demonstrated in the study at two days while the remaining curves (days 4 and 6) were flat. In two dogs peak absorption ($>$ 100 CPM) was present on days 2 and 5, and in the remaining two dogs, three separate studies (days 2, 4, and 7) demonstrated peak absorption of lauric acid. This correlated well with the appearance of progressive histological rejection.

Oleic acid absorption. C^{14} oleic acid was

actively absorbed in Thiry-Vella loops in which the lymphatic and neural connections were intact. The curves in Fig. 2, *A* and *B,* suggest a recirculating pattern rather than the prompt disappearance pattern seen with lauric acid. In autografts, oleic acid was not absorbed early in the experiment. In these animals, absorption of oleic acid began to appear two to three weeks after transplantation. Although all animals with autografts showed absorption of oleic acid four weeks after transplantation, the peaks of absorption were variable and not consistently reproducible in subsequent studies. In allografts, no oleic acid absorption was demonstrated.

Lymphangiography. Two dogs with Thiry-Vella loops were studied and showed prompt and excellent lymphatic drainage from the jejunal segment to the cisterna chyli.

The lymphangiography studies were done in Groups IIA and IIB in an attempt to correlate the regeneration of the lymphatic channels to the autograft with the fatty acid absorption studies. Six of the eight dogs had to be killed after the performance of this study. Lymphangiography was performed on separate dogs at two, four, six, and eight weeks after transplantation. Two studies were done at four weeks and two at six weeks. All animals studied demonstrated regeneration of the lymphatic connections four weeks after transplantation, where passage of the contrast material from the graft to the cisterna chyli was demonstrated. We did not demonstrate lymphatic regeneration at two weeks in one dog studied.

In Group III, in vitro injection roentgenographic studies of the graft lymphatic connections at autopsy, after allograft rejection, did not demonstrate any lymphatic connection between the allograft and the host lymphatic systems.

DISCUSSION

In previous studies,[8] we have reported on the direct correlation between C^{14} glucose absorption and morphological survival of heterotopic canine jejunal allografts in the neck. We and others[13] have performed similar studies on glucose absorption in intraperitoneal jejunal allografts, both untreated and immunosuppressed, again showing the very close and direct relationship between morphological and functional survival in relation to glucose absorption.

The present studies analyze the functional capability of jejunal autografts and allografts in relation to the absorption of short chain fatty acid (lauric acid) and long chain fatty acid (oleic acid). If, in the future, we are to expand clinical intestinal transplantation, then the methods of assessing graft survival by morphologic criteria by the use of repeat biopsies as suggested by Holmes and colleagues[9] are not only fraught with danger but also are impractical on a long-term basis. Tests of physiologic integrity and function of intestinal transplants that correlate with morphologic rejection must be developed. The changes in C^{14} lauric acid absorption described here in both autografts and allografts correlate closely with the histological appearance of the intestinal mucosa during progressive rejection.

Lauric acid absorption remained good and quite constant throughout the period of studies in the Thiry-Vella loops and autografts. The absorption of this substance did not appear to depend at all on lymphatic regeneration and neural connections. The observation of the gradual decrease in the peak of absorption of lauric acid in non-immunosuppressed allografts during progressive rejection is highly significant. Since in our experiments histological sections of the allografts were not available for study until termination of absorption studies, we were able to predict in almost every instance the prognosis of the allograft in terms of rejection on the basis of lauric acid absorption studies. This was confirmed by the impartial evaluation of coded histological sections.

Holmes and colleagues,[10] in their elegant morphologic studies, point out that careful histologic assessment, particularly the mitotic index and villus:crypt ratio, is superior to glucose absorption studies in predicting rejection. We have no doubt that daily histologic evaluation may be most accurate in predicting rejection and our own studies using pyrrhynophillic cell number per villus confirm this. However, this is not practical in a clinical situation, and our previous findings on glucose absorption and present studies of lauric acid absorption are simple to perform and correlate closely enough with histological rejection to offer a reliable predictive parameter of intestinal rejection. Westbroek and associates[17] have also reported on the usefulness of absorption studies in diagnosing rejection of intestinal allografts, as have Toledo-Pereyra and Najarian.[16] It is important that substances used for such absorption studies are actively transported by intestinal mucosa since those that are passively transported are of little value in evaluating the integrity of the allografted intestinal epithelium.

Oleic acid studies yielded the interesting preliminary observation that the presence of this substance in the circulating plasma appears to be determined to a major degree by the presence of intact lymphatic connections between the graft and the host. Oleic acid absorption curves in the Thiry-Vella loops were present after surgery and remained reproducible for a three-month period of study. In autografts, however, the first observations of oleic acid absorption were not made until two to three weeks after transplantation. Even at that time the absorption curves differed from dog to dog, although they were reproducible in the same experimental animal. This may be explained by minor differences in the length of the autografted segments and by small variations in the anatomical configuration of the venous drainage of the autografts in relation to portal circulation. The most likely explanation, however, is the difference in the rate of regeneration of the lymphatic vessels of the autograft. The lymphangiography studies showing the regeneration of lymphatic channels in the autografts at about four weeks suggest that detection of oleic acid absorption in the intestinal autografts depends to a major extent on the intact lymphatic communications between the graft and the host. Preliminary studies in immunosuppressed allografts confirm our findings in autografts that oleic acid absorption is closely related to the regeneration of lymphatic channels. This may perhaps serve as a test of lymphatic regeneration of intestinal allografts and help to determine the progressive reduction in dietary restrictions that patients receiving segmental intestinal allografts will undoubtedly need.

It is interesting to note that in the extensively described case of human intestinal transplantation by Olivier and colleagues,[14] and in the recent case described by Alican and associates,[1] no regeneration of lymphatic channels was noted at the end of the survival period of 26 days. However, regeneration appeared to be present at 76 days at autopsy in the patient with the longest surviving intestinal allograft reported by Fortner[4] between the second and the third week after transplantation, by Goott and associates[5] and by Kocandrle and colleagues,[12] and at 30 days in the heterotopic intestinal transplants by Grenier and co-workers.[6] The oleic acid absorption studies described here correlate well with the roentgenographic demonstration of lymphatic regeneration and may serve in the future as a test of the functional capacity of lymphatic regeneration in intestinal allografts.

We are grateful to Mrs. Dagmar Fabian and Mr. Felix Revera for their excellent technical assistance, to Dr. Robert Bases for his helpful advice on the use of radioactive isotopes, and to Dr. William A. Cook for his encouragement.

REFERENCES

1. Alican, F., Hardy, J. D., Cayirli, M., Varner, J. E., Moynihan, P. C., Turner, M. D., and Anas, P.: Intestinal transplantation: Laboratory experience and report of a clinical case, Am. J. Surg. **121:** 150, 1971.
2. Cohen, W. B., Hardy, M. A., Quint, J., and State, D.: Absorptive function in canine jejunal autografts and allografts SURGERY **65:** 440, 1969.
3. Folch, J., Lees, M., and Sloane-Stanley, G. H.: A simple method for the isolation and purification of total lipides from animal tissues, J. Biol. Chem. **226:** 497, 1957.
4. Fortner, J. G.: Clinical and experimental orthotopic intestinal allografting after massive intestinal resection, Biol. Gastroenterol. **5:** 438c, 1972.

5. Goott, B., Lillehei, R. C., and Miller, F. A.: Mesenteric lymphatic regeneration after autografts of small bowel in dogs, SURGERY **48:** 571, 1960.
6. Grenier, J. F., Doremieux, J., Wong, P., and Botescu, V.: Transplantations d'intestin grêle chez le chien: Enseignments tirés d'une statistique de 100 cas, Chirurgie (Mem. Acad. Chir.) **96:** 958, 1970.
7. Hardy, M. A., Quint, J., Cohen, W. B., and State, D.: C^{14} D-Glucose absorption in heterotopic jejunal allografts, Gastroenterology **54:** 1295, 1968.
8. Hardy, M. A., Quint, J., and State, D.: Effect of antilymphocyte serum and other immunosuppressive agents on canine jejunal allografts, Ann. Surg. **171:** 51, 1970.
9. Holmes, J. T., Klein, M. S., Winawer, S. J., and Fortner, J. G.: Morphological studies of rejection in canine jejunal allografts, Gastroenterology **61:** 693, 1971.
10. Holmes, J. T., Yeh, S. D. J., Winawer, S. J., Kawano, N., and Fortner, J. G.: Absorption studies in canine jejunal allografts, Ann. Surg. **174:** 101, 1971.
11. Holmes, J. T.: Small bowel transplantation: An experimental study, Ann. R. Coll. Surg. Engl. **52:** 165, 1973.
12. Kocandrle, V., Honttuin, E., and Prohasha, J. V.: Regeneration of the lymphatics after autotransplantation and homotransplantation of the entire small intestine, Surg. Gynecol. Obstet. **122:** 587, 1966.
13. Mach, K. M., Merkel, F. K., and Preston, F. W.: Glucose absorption from canine Thiry fistulas, autografts and allografts, Biol. Gastroenterol. **5:** 589c, 1972.
14. Olivier, C., Rettori, R., Olivier, Ch., Baur, O., and Roux, J.: Un cas de transplantation orthotopique du jejuno-ileon et des colons droit et transverse, Presse Med. **77:** 1275, 1969.
15. Taylor, R. M. R., Watson, J. W., Walker, F. C., and Watson, A. J.: Prolongation of survival of jejunal homografts in dogs treated with azathioprine, Br. J. Surg. **53:** 134, 1966.
16. Toledo-Pereyra, L. H., and Najarian, J. S.: Preservation of the small intestine for allotransplantation, Surg. Gynecol. Obstet. **137:** 445, 1973.
17. Westbroek, D. L., Van Stekelenburg, L., Rothengatter, C. Kort, W., Dikmen, M. E., de Vries, M. J., and MacDicken, I.: Orthotopic total small bowel allografting in the genetically controlled situation, Biol. Gastroenterol. **5:** 587c, 1972.

Experimental cancer immunotherapy using a neuraminidase-treated non-viable frozen tumor vaccine

Angelyn Rios *and* **Richard L. Simmons, M.D.,*** *Minneapolis, Minn.*

Firmly established tumors in syngeneic mice will regress if the host is challenged with living tumor cells which have been exposed to **Vibrio cholerae** neuraminidase (VCN) in vitro. The present study demonstrates that rapid freezing of the VCN-treated tumor challenge at –95° C. and storage at –70° C. does not interfere with its immunoregressive potency but does prevent regrowth of the tumor cells from the challenging vaccine. The clinical potential of this finding is discussed.

From the Department of Surgery, University of Minnesota, Minneapolis, Minn.

WE HAVE previously shown that total regression of a variety of firmly established syngeneic murine tumors could be induced by inoculation of living tumor cells treated in vitro with *Vibrio cholerae* neuraminidase (VCN).[16, 18, 22] Regression could not be induced with cells treated with inactivated VCN or cells incubated with VCN and an excess of sialic acid (a specific feedback inhibitor of VCN).[22] The regression is immunospecific and can only be induced with VCN-treated cells identical in type with the growing tumor.[22]

In designing a protocol of tumor immunotherapy which might have some potential clinical application, one would like to avoid the need for repeated operations to obtain autologous tumor tissue and prevent the growth of the tumor cells within the tumor vaccine, i.e., the production of a metastasis.

Supported by Grant No. CA 11605 from the United States Public Health Service and Grant No. IM-20A from the American Cancer Society.

Accepted for publication Jan. 29, 1974.

Reprint requests: R. L. Simmons, M.D., Box 185, Mayo Memorial Building, University of Minnesota, Minneapolis, Minn. 55455.

*John and Mary R. Markle Foundation Scholar in Academic Medicine.

The present experiments were designed to compare tumor regression induced by living fresh and non-viable stored VCN-treated tumor cells.

MATERIALS AND METHODS

Mice. C3H/HeJ female mice, age 8 to 16 weeks, were obtained from the Jackson Laboratories, Bar Harbor, Maine. The animals were housed in covered plastic cages, ten or less per cage, and provided with tap water and a standard laboratory diet (Purina Chow Checkers) ad libitum.

Tumors. Two different fibrosarcomas (MC-42, MC-43) were induced wth 0.5 mg. 3-α-methylcholanthrene (MCA) dissolved in 0.1 percent trioctanoin injected intramuscularly into the hind legs of C3H/HeJ female mice. The immunogenic characteristics of these tumors have been thoroughly investigated by Haywood and McKhann.[8] The tumors have been serially transplanted in syngeneic female mice without any evidence of antigen modification or deletion. In unimmunized C3H/HeJ female mice, an inoculum of 120 MC-42 cells, or 1280 MC-43 cells, will kill 50 percent of the recipients.[8] Spontaneous regression does not occur. The tumors are specific for the strain in which they arose, and they do not grow on mice of different H-2 histocompatibility types. Haywood and McKhann[8] have demonstrated that these tumors are weakly immunogenic, i.e., inoculation of the tumor followed by amputation leads to tumor-specific resistance against subsequent inoculation.[8] The MC-42 tumor, however, does not immunize against MC-43, or vice versa.

Sterile tumor cells for inoculation were prepared from tumors (0.5 to 1.0 cm. in diameter) growing in C3H/HeJ female mice approximately three weeks following subcutaneous transfer. Cells were pressed through a stainless steel screen (45 mesh) in medium 199 (M199) (Grand Island, N. Y.) without addition of trypsin. Cell clumps were then allowed to settle and the supernatant containing single cells in suspension was retained, and the cells were washed three times in M199 and counted in hemocytometers. Viability was determined by trypan blue exclusion.[5] The cells were then injected subcutaneously into the lateral posterior flank of recipient C3H/HeJ female mice. The mice were inspected daily to determine the day of the initial appearance of a palpable tumor. The largest diameter of the growing tumor was measured by calipers three times weekly, and the day of death was also recorded.

Neuraminidase. *Vibrio cholerae* neuroaminidase (VCN)* is said to contain 500 U. of enzyme per milliliter. (One unit of activity is defined as that quantity which will release 1 μg of N-acetylneuraminic acid from a glycoprotein substract in 15 minutes at 37° C., at a pH of 5.5.) VCN is inactivated by heating to 65° C. for 30 minutes.[24] A number of investigators[1, 6, 7, 14, 15, 17, 24] have demonstrated that sialic acid is released from cell surfaces of normal and malignant cells by VCN without affecting cell viability.

Mitomycin-C. Mitomycin-C† was incubated with tumor cells in a concentration of 25 μg per milliliter per 10^6 cells in the same incubation mixture with VCN or heat-inactivated VCN. We have previously demonstrated that the mitomycin-C has no adverse effect on the efficacy of VCN-treated cells to induce immunospecific regression of firmly established methylcholanthrene fibrosarcomas in C3H/HeJ mice.[19, 21] Mitomycin-C treatment of MC-42 or MC-43 tumor cells does not increase the uptake of trypan blue by such tumor cell suspensions but effectively prevents the growth of palpable tumors from the treated cells.[19, 21]

Technique of freezing and storage. Tumor cell suspensions were prepared as described above, and incubated with VCN, inactivated VCN, and/or mitomycin-C in the fresh state. After being washed, the cell suspensions were dispensed to ampules in 2.4 ml. volumes containing 12 × 10^6 cells (85 percent viable) and were frozen rapidly to −95° C. in a bath of acetone and Dry Ice. After being frozen, the ampules were stored at −70° C. and allowed to thaw at room temperature prior to use. Cells were used after various periods of frozen storage. Frozen cells did not grow into palpable tumors in any case.

Experimental protocol. The basic experimental design was to inoculate adult female C3H/HeJ mice (Jackson Laboratory, Bar Harbor, Maine) with fresh viable untreated tumor cells. Fifteen days thereafter, a series of challenging inocula of tumor cells were given, using either fresh viable or frozen tumor cells which had been incubated with VCN, heat-inactivated VCN, and/or mitomycin-C.

RESULTS

Comparative effect of fresh or frozen neuraminidase-treated MC-42 cells on the growth of established MC-42 tumors in C3H/HeJ mice. Untreated MC-42 cells (20,000) were injected into the subcutaneous tissue of the left flank of syngeneic C3H/HeJ mice on day 0. Fifteen days after inoculation, tumor-bearing mice were challenged with 10^6 fresh or frozen MC-42 tumor cells which had been exposed to VCN

*Behring Diagnostics, Somerville, N. J.

†Sigma Chemical Company, St. Louis, Mo.

Table I. *Comparative effect of fresh or frozen stored neuraminidase (VCN)-treated MC-42 cells on the growth of MC-42 tumors in C3H/HeJ mice*

Group No.	Cell viability*	Cell treatment†	Fraction 1° tumors regressing	Mean tumor diameter (d. 20) (cm. ± S.E.)	Mean day of death (± S.S.)‡
1	No challenge	—	0/16	1.89 ± 0.07	58.0 ± 1.5
2	Fresh	VCN + mitomycin C	3/24	1.06 ± 0.12§	60.9 ± 2.8
3	Fresh	Inactive VCN + mitomycin C	0/18	2.16 ± 0.09	47.5 ± 3.4
4	Fresh	Mitomycin C	0/16	1.88 ± 0.08	57.0 ± 1.6
5	Frozen-stored	VCN	4/24	1.30 ± 0.13§	59.7 ± 3.3
6	Frozen-stored	Inactive VCN	0/24	1.90 ± 0.08	61.8 ± 1.9
7	Frozen-stored	No treatment	0/16	2.21 ± 0.14	52.1 ± 2.7

*Cells frozen in acetone and Dry Ice bath (−95° C.) and stored at −70° C. for two to four weeks (six inocula).

†Challenging inocula consisted of six injections of 10^6 MC-42 cells. The first challenge was given 15 days after tumor inoculation with subsequent challenges at two-day intervals.

‡Does not include mice whose tumors totally regressed.

§$p \leq 0.05$ when compared to Groups 1, 3, 4, 6, and 7.

or heat-inactivated VCN (plus mitomycin-C). Subsequent challenges were given at two-day intervals for a total of six inoculations. Treatment of fresh or frozen tumor vaccine with heat-inactivated VCN and/or mitomycin had no effect on the growth of the primary tumor. In contrast, both fresh and frozen VCN-treated MC-42 cells strongly inhibited the growth of the tumor. All tumors showed temporary cessation of growth and seven of 48 tumors totally regressed and disappeared. All animals whose tumors regressed survived for an indefinite period. There was no difference between the effects of frozen or fresh VCN-treated cells (Table I).

Effect of storage time on the immunoregressive effect of frozen neuraminidase-treated MC-43 cells on the growth of established MC-43 tumors in C3H/HeJ mice. The experiments were repeated with the use of an immunodistinct (MC-43) methylcholanthrene-induced fibrosarcoma (Table II). MC-43 tumor cells (40,000) were implanted in the subcutaneous tissue of the left flank of syngeneic C3H/HeJ mice on day 0. Fifteen days thereafter mice were challenged with a series of six injections with MC-43 cells which were fresh or stored for various periods of time from 18 hours to 12 weeks (Table II). VCN-treated MC-43 tumor cells were capable of inducing the immunoregression of MC-43 tumors on C3H/HeJ mice, whether the tumor cells were fresh or had been stored frozen for 18 hours or 12 weeks. Tumor cells treated with heat-inactivated VCN and utilized in the fresh condition or after freezing for various intervals had no immunoregressive potency whatsoever (Table II).

DISCUSSION

Our previous experiments demonstrated that it was possible to severely inhibit the growth of firmly established methylcholanthrene fibrosarcomas by challenge of the tumor-bearing mice with living tumor cells which had been treated with VCN.[18, 22] Some tumors were permanently cured.[18, 22] Regression could not be induced with cells treated with heat-inactivated VCN, or cells incubated with VCN in an excess of competitive feedback inhibitor of the enzyme (sialic acid).[22] Regression induced by VCN-treated tumor cells was immunospecific and could be induced only by VCN-treated cells identical in type with the growing tumor.[22] We have subsequently demonstrated that the immunospecific regression of firmly established syngeneic transplantable tumors is not restricted to methylcholanthrene-induced tumors; the growth of mammary tumors in C3H/HeJ mice and B16 melanomas in C57 BL/6 mice will also be inhibited if their hosts are challenged with VCN-treated tumor cells of the same tumor line.[16] Similar

Table II. *Effect of stored neuraminidase (VCN)-treated MC-43 cells on the growth of MC-43 tumors in C3H/HeJ mice*

Group No.	*Period frozen**	*Cell treatment†*	*Fraction 1° tumors regressing*	*Mean tumor diameter (d. 30) (cm. ± S.E.)*	*Mean day of death (± S.E.)‡*
1	No challenge	—	0/10	1.79 ± 0.10	55.7 ± 3.5
2	Fresh	VCN + mitomycin C	0/10	0.47 ± 0.05§	69.9 ± 4.5
3	Fresh	Inactive VCN + mitomycin C	0/10	1.61 ± 0.06	59.1 ± 3.6
4	18 hr.	VCN	1/10	0.47 ± 0.06§	79.2 ± 4.6¶
5	18 hr.	Inactive VCN	0/10	1.60 ± 0.09	60.8 ± 4.8
6	2 wk.	VCN	0/10	0.45 ± 0.05§	82.2 ± 6.1¶
7	2 wk.	Inactive VCN	0/10	1.50 ± 0.09	62.7 ± 3.7
8	4 wk.	VCN	2/10	0.41 ± 0.07§	83.8 ± 5.2¶
9	4 wk.	Inactive VCN	0/10	1.56 ± 0.06	65.4 ± 2.7
10	12 wk.	VCN	1/10	0.42 ± 0.05§	85.6 ± 6.9¶
11	12 wk.	Inactive VCN	0/10	1.55 ± 0.08	60.5 ± 2.5

*Cells frozen in acetone and Dry Ice bath (–95° C.) and stored at –70° C.

†Challenging inocula consisted of six injections of 10^6 MC-43 cells. The first challenge was given 15 days after tumor inoculation with subsequent challenges at two-day intervals.

‡Does not include mice whose tumors totally regressed.

§$p \leq 0.05$ when compared to Groups 1, 3, 5, 7, 9, and 11.

¶$p \leq 0.05$ when compared to Groups 1, 2, 3, 5, 7, 9, and 11.

results have been obtained by Bekesi and Holland[2-4] (also personal communication) and by Kollmorgen and associates,[13] who have demonstrated the immunospecific regression of transplantable and spontaneous murine lymphomas and leukemias. We have also demonstrated that spontaneous mammary tumors can be made to regress by intralesional injections with VCN and BCG but not by BCG or VCN alone.[20]

To translate this immunotherapeutic potential to man will require either that the tumor itself be accessible to intratumor injection of VCN and BCG or that the tumor be excised, treated in vitro with VCN, and reinjected back into the patient. The regrowth of the tumor after reinjection into the patient can be prevented by treatment of the tumor cells in vitro with mitomycin-C, which does not interfere with the immunogenicity of the tumor challenge.[19] In order to avoid repeated operations to obtain fresh tumor, some technique of tumor storage had to be designed which would not interfere with the immunogenicity of the tumor cells. Tissue culture has been shown to reduce the immunogenicity of normal tissue as well as tumor cells and may not be suitable.[9-12, 23] The present experiments demonstrate that rapid freezing in acetone-Dry Ice at –95° C. will render the tumor vaccine non-viable without diminishing the immunoregressive potency of the VCN-treated tumor cells. Storage for 12 weeks also did not reduce immunoregressive effect.

If fresh viable tumor is not required for immunotherapy, greater flexibility in treatment protocols is possible. Relatively early tumors can be excised, treated with VCN, and stored pending recurrence of the tumor, or termination of a course of adjunctive chemotherapy or radiotherapy. Time can be allowed for the recovery of the patient from his surgical operation and recovery of his immune response from the surgical, radiotherapeutic, or chemotherapeutic insult. Further savings in money can be achieved in this method by avoiding the use of large doses of mitomycin-C which are required to insure that tumor regrowth of VCN-treated inocula will not occur since freezing appears to be capable of injuring tumor cells sufficiently to prevent their regrowth. Freezing, thus appears capable of interfering with tumor viability without interfering with the augmented immunogenicity of VCN-treated tumor cells.

REFERENCES

1. Bagshawe, K. D., and Currie, G. A.: Immunogenicity of L 1210 murine leukemia

cells after treatment with neuraminidase, Nature **218:** 1254, 1968.

2. Bekesi, J. G., St. Arneault, G., Walter L., and Holland, J. F.: Immunogenicity of leukemia L 1210 cells after neuraminidase treatment, J. Natl. Cancer Inst. **49:** 107, 1972.
3. Bekesi, J. G., Walter, L., and Holland, J. F.: Immunogenicity of neuraminidase-treated 6C3HED lymphoma in C3H/HeJ and C3H/f mice, Proc. Am. Assoc. Cancer Res. **13:** 113, 1972.
4. Bekesi, J. G., Walter, L., and Holland, J. R.: The fate of neuraminidase-treated leukemia L 1210 cells as an immunogen in nonimmunized mice, Proc. Am. Assoc. Cancer Res. **14:** 64, 1973.
5. Boyse, E. A., Old, L. H., and Chourorlinkow, I.: Cytotoxic test for demonstration of mouse antibody, *in:* Methods in medical research, Chicago, 1964, Yearbook Medical Publishers, p. 39.
6. Currie, G. A., and Bagshawe, K. D.: The role of sialic acid in antigenic expressions: Further studies of the Landschutz ascites tumour, Br. J. Cancer **23:** 843, 1968.
7. Currie, G. A., and Bagshawe, K. D.: Tumour-specific immunogenicity of methylcholanthrene-induced sarcoma cells after incubation in neuraminidase, Br. J. Cancer **23:** 141, 1969.
8. Haywood, G., and McKhann, C. F.: Antigenic specificities on murine sarcoma cells: Reciprocal relationship between normal transplantation antigens (H-2) and tumor-specific immunogenicity, J. Exp. Med. **133:** 1171, 1971.
9. Jacobs, B. B.: Growth of tumors in allogeneic hosts after organ culture explanation. II. Tumor-host interactions, J. Natl. Cancer Inst. **42:** 537, 1969.
10. Jacobs, B. B.: Altered host-allograft relationships for mouse tumors modified by prior passage in vitro and in vivo, J. Natl. Cancer Inst. **45:** 263, 1970.
11. Jacobs, B. B., and Huseby, R. A.: Growth of tumors in allogeneic hosts following organ culture explanation, Transplantation **5:** 410, 1967.
12. Jacobs, B. B., and Huseby, R. A.: Successful growth of tumor allografts following explanation: Effect of various culture conditions, Proc. Soc. Exp. Biol. Med. **127:** 957, 1968.
13. Kollmorgen, G. M., Erwin, D. N., Killion, J. J., Hoge, A. F., and Sansing, W. A.: Combination chemotherapy and immunotherapy of transplantable murine leukemia, Proc. Am. Assoc. Cancer Res. **14:** 69, 1973.
14. Ray, P. K., Gewurz, H., and Simmons, R. L.: Complement sensitivity of neuraminidase-treated lymphoid cells, Transplantation **12:** 327, 1971.
15. Ray, P. K., and Simmons, R. L.: Failure of neuraminidase to unmask allogenic antigens on cell surfaces, Proc. Soc. Exp. Biol. Med. **138:** 600, 1971.
16. Rios, A., and Simmons, R. L.: Immunospecific regression of various syngeneic mouse tumors in response to neuraminidase-treated tumor cells, J. Natl. Cancer Inst. **51:** 637, 1973.
17. Sanford, B. H., and Codington, J. F.: Further studies on the effect of neuraminidase on tumor cell transplantability, Tissue Antigens **1:** 153, 1971.
18. Simmons, R. L., and Rios, A.: Immunotherapy of cancer: Immunospecific rejection of tumors in recipients of neuraminidase-treated tumor cells plus BCG, Science **174:** 591, 1971.
19. Simmons, R. L., and Rios, A.: Immunospecific regression of methylcholanthrene fibrosarcomas with the use of neuraminidase. V. Quantitative aspects of the experimental immunotherapeutic model, Israel J. Med. Sci. **13:** 71, 1974.
20. Simmons, R. L., Rios, A., and Kersey, J. H.: Regression of spontaneous mammary carcinomas using direct injections of neuraminidase and BCG, J. Surg. Res. **12:** 57, 1972.
21. Simmons, R. L., Rios, A., Lundgren, G., and Ray, P. K.: Immunotherapy of methylcholanthrene fibrosarcoma using neuraminidase, Fed. Proc. **30:** 246, 1971.
22. Simmons, R. L., Rios, A., Lundgren, G., Ray, P. K., McKhann, C. F., and Haywood, G. R.: Immunospecific regression of methylcholanthrene fibrosarcoma using neuraminidase, SURGERY **70:** 38, 1971.
23. Summerlin, W. T., Broutbar, C., Faanes, R. B., Payne, R., Stutman, O., Hayflick, L., and Good, R. A.: Acceptance of phenotypically differing cultured skin in man and mice, Transplant. Proc. **V:** 707, 1973.
24. Woodruff, J. J., and Gesner, B. M.: The effect of neuraminidase on the fate of transfused lymphocytes, J. Exp. Med. **129:** 551, 1969.

The adequacy of myocardial oxygen delivery in acute normovolemic anemia

John Brazier, M.D., Norman Cooper, M.D., James V. Maloney, Jr., M.D., *and*
Gerald Buckberg, M.D., *Los Angeles, Calif.*

Subendocardial ischemia with patent coronary arteries is recognized increasingly as a cause of previously unexplained cardiac failure. Subendocardial muscle flow is diastolic, and subendocardial oxygen delivery is determined by oxygen content as well as coronary blood flow. Hemodilution (open-heart surgery, refusal of transfusion) reduces oxygen content by acutely lowering the hemoglobin levels; this study assesses its effects on the adequacy of myocardial oxygen delivery. In ten anesthetized dogs, we produced anemia by exchanging blood with a dextran solution while measuring aortic and left atrial blood pressure, cardiac output, coronary blood flow, and endocardial and epicardial EKG's. Myocardial blood flow distribution, aortic blood pressure, and cardiac output remained normal with hemoglobins ranging from 14 to 5 Gm. percent. Myocardial oxygen delivery was maintained by increasing coronary blood flow from 75 to 127 c.c. per 100 Gm. per minute. Coronary flow became redistributed away from subendocardial muscle ($P < 0.025$) and myocardial failure occurred with hemoglobins below 5 Gm. percent. Failure was associated with ischemic endocardial EKG's despite total left ventricular coronary blood flow increasing to 310 percent above control levels. We conclude that (1) oxygen delivery to the entire left ventricle remains adequate over a wide range of hemoglobin levels in normal hearts, and (2) subendocardial ischemia and cardiac failure occur when coronary blood flow becomes maldistributed and cannot compensate for decreased oxygen-carrying capacity of the blood. We would expect these adverse changes to occur at higher hemoglobin levels with valvular or ischemic heart disease, abnormal circulatory dynamics, or increased myocardial oxygen requirement.

From the Division of Thoracic Surgery, UCLA School of Medicine, Los Angeles, Calif.

ACUTE normovolemic anemia is frequently encountered in surgical practice as a result of hemodilution during cardiopulmonary bypass operations where religious beliefs prevent blood transfusion or as a consequence of resuscitation from hemorrhagic shock with non-hemoglobin–containing fluids. In normal hearts with acute normovolemic anemia, tissue oxygen delivery is maintained when cardiac output increases to compensate for the reduced oxygen-carrying capacity of the blood.

Pathologic studies, however, have shown that subendocardial ischemia and necrosis can occur in hearts of patients who were anemic.[16] High-output cardiac failure may be associated with anemia in these patients and their electrocardiograms frequently show ST and T wave changes consistent with subendocardial ischemia.[2, 12, 15]

This study was supported by Grants-in-Aid from the Wilbur May Foundation, Frank W. Clark Charities, and the United States Public Health Service.

Accepted for publication Jan. 7, 1974.

Reprint requests: Gerald Buckberg, M.D., Division of Thoracic Surgery, UCLA Medical Center, Los Angeles, Calif. 90024.

Subendocardial ischemia in the presence of patent coronary arteries is becoming recognized increasingly as a possible cause of previously unexplained myocardial failure.[8, 16, 21]

Subendocardial muscle is particularly vulnerable to ischemia because it must receive most or all of its flow during diastole. This is because systolic intramyocardial compressive forces are highest in the subendocardium and therefore prevent perfusion during ventricular contraction.[1, 3, 14] Our experimental studies have shown that subendocardial ischemia can be produced by varying the diastolic determinants of subendocardial flow and that the adequacy of that flow (i.e., how it meets oxygen demands) can be predicted from readily obtained pressure measurements at the bedside or in the cardiac catheterization laboratory.[4]

Oxygen delivery to the subendocardium, however, is determined by both coronary flow and the oxygen content of arterial blood. Normally, there is almost complete extraction of oxygen from coronary blood as it passes through the myocardium, so that coronary flow must increase if raised oxygen requirements are to be met adequately.[6, 13] This increased flow is achieved through coronary artery dilatation which lowers vascular resistance.[6]

Augmentation of coronary flow alone may not provide adequate myocardial oxygenation when the oxygen content of arterial blood is decreased because of reduced hemoglobin levels. In this experiment we studied how acute normovolemic anemia effects the distribution and adequacy of coronary blood flow in anesthetized dogs.

METHODS

Preparation. Ten mongrel dogs weighing 15 to 25 kilograms were anesthetized with 3 mg. per kilogram of morphine intramuscularly and 15 mg. per kilogram of chloralose intravenously. Ventilation was maintained by delivering 100% oxygen through an endotrachial tube with a positive pressure respirator. After bilateral thoracotomy, polyethelene catheters were placed into the left atrium, right atrium, and ascending aorta; the coronary sinus was cannulated through the right atrium. These catheters were connected to Statham P23DB pressure transducers and pressures were recorded on a Hewlett Packard multichannel recorder. Cardiac output was monitored by placing a Statham Electromagnetic Flow Transducer around the pulmonary artery. Zero flow was determined from the diastolic flow signal. Mean flow was electronically integrated.

Endocardial and epicardial electrocardiograms. A unipolar platinum electrode was placed into the left ventricular cavity from the carotid artery to record endocardial electrocardiograms and leads were sutured to the epicardium to record epicardial electrocardiograms.

Total and regional flow. Total and regional coronary flow was measured by determining the myocardial distribution of 8 to 10 μ microspheres labeled with ^{125}I, ^{141}Ce, ^{85}Sr, and ^{46}Sc injected into the left atrium and collecting a reference sample from a peripheral artery.[4, 7] After completion of the experiment, the dogs were killed, and the hearts were removed. The left ventricular free wall was divided into subepicardial, subendocardial, and mid-myocardial layers of approximately equal thickness. These tissue samples were counted with a Nuclear Chicago 512 Channel Pulse Height Analyzer. Total and regional flow were calculated from the equation:

$$F_h = C_h \cdot \frac{F_r}{C_r}$$

where F_h is the flow to the heart, F_r is the flow in the reference sample in cubic centimeters per minute, C_h is the counts in the heart, and C_r is the counts in the reference sample. Flows were expressed as cubic centimeters per 100 Gm. of heart per minute.

The pH and P_{CO_2} were measured by the Astrup method, venous oxygen contents were measured directly (Lex-O-Con, Lexington Instrument Corp.), and arterial oxygen content was calculated from the equation:

$$O_2 \text{ content} = 1.34 \times \text{hemoglobin (Gm. \%)} \times \%\ O_2 \text{ saturation} + 0.003 \times P_{O_2} \text{ (mm. Hg)}.$$

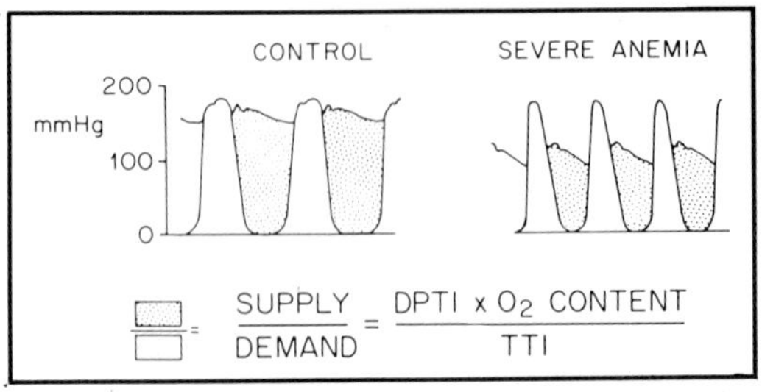

Fig. 1. Simultaneous tracings of aortic and left ventricular pressures during control (Hgb > 10 Gm. percent) and severe anemia (Hgb < 5 Gm. percent). The stippled area between the aortic and left ventricular pressure was used to calculate the diastolic pressure time index. The tension time index was calculated from the area between perpendicular lines from the beginning and end of aortic systole.

Oxygen saturation was measured with an American Optical Oximeter, hemoglobin was measured by the cyanohemoglobin method, and arterial Po_2 was measured by radiometer Po_2 electrodes.

Calculation of indices. Potential subendocardial flow was estimated from the diastolic pressure time index (DPTI). This index describes diastolic pressure time relationships and is obtained by planimetry of the area between the aortic and left ventricular pressure curves in diastole. In some experiments, mean left ventricular diastolic pressure was estimated from mean left atrial pressure. DPTI times heart rate is equal to DPTI per minute (mm. Hg × sec./min.) (Fig. 1). Potential oxygen delivery to the subendocardium was calculated from the expression: DPTI × O_2 content.

Myocardial oxygen demands were estimated from the tension time index (TTI) obtained by planimetry of the area beneath the left ventricular systolic pressure curve from the onset of ventricular contraction to the dicrotic notch.[20] TTI times heart rate is equal to the tension time index per minute (mm. Hg/sec./min.) (Fig. 1).

The following expression was used to express the supply/demand ratio:

$$\frac{\text{DPTI} \cdot O_2 \text{ content}}{\text{TTI}}$$

Procedure. After control measurements were obtained, the dogs were made isovolemically anemic by withdrawing blood from the femoral artery and simultaneously replacing equal volumes of 6% Dextran in 0.9N NaCl. The exchange of blood for Dextran was stopped intermittently and after stabilization had occurred for approximately 5 minutes, measurements of blood pressure, cardiac output and epicardial and endocardial electrocardiograms were made and microspheres were injected.

RESULTS

Oxygen delivery.

Control. During the control period (hemoglobin > 10 Gm. percent), blood oxygen content was 17.2 vol. percent. Mean total left ventricular blood flow was 82 c.c. per 100 Gm. per minute and left ventricular subendocardial muscle received 92 c.c. per 100 Gm. per minute. The endocardial to epicardial flow ratio was 1.13 to 1 (endocardial/epicardial = 1.13) (Fig. 2).

Moderate anemia (hemoglobin, 5 to 10 Gm. percent): With moderate anemia blood oxygen content was 10.7 vol. percent. Total left ventricular flow increased to 106 c.c. per 100 Gm. per minute, and left ventricular subendocardial flow increased to 116 c.c. per 100 Gm. per minute ($P < 0.05$). There was no significant change in distribution of flow through the left ventricular myocardium (endocardial/epicardial flow ratio of 1.07 to 1) (Fig. 2).

Severe anemia (hemoglobin, < 5 Gm. percent). When hemoglobin was reduced to below 5 Gm. percent, blood oxygen content was lowered to 4.9 vol. percent. Total left ventricular coronary flow increased further to 190 c.c. per 100 Gm. per minute and left ventricular subendocardial flow increased to 150 c.c. per 100 Gm. per minute ($P < 0.01$). However, this more severe form of anemia was associated with a redistribution of flow across the myocardial wall so that the proportion of the flow delivered to the subendocardium fell 35 percent; the endocardial/epicardial flow ratio fell to below 1.0 ($P < 0.01$) (Fig. 2).

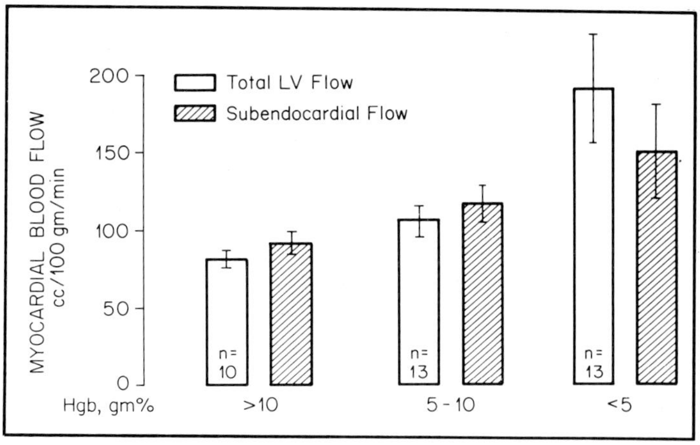

Fig. 2. Myocardial blood flow for the entire free wall of the left ventricle (total) and subendocardial muscle, during control (Hgb > 10 Gm. percent), moderate anemia (Hgb 5-10 Gm. percent), and severe anemia (Hgb < 5 Gm. percent). Note the proportion of total flow delivered to the subendocardium during severe anemia is significantly reduced.

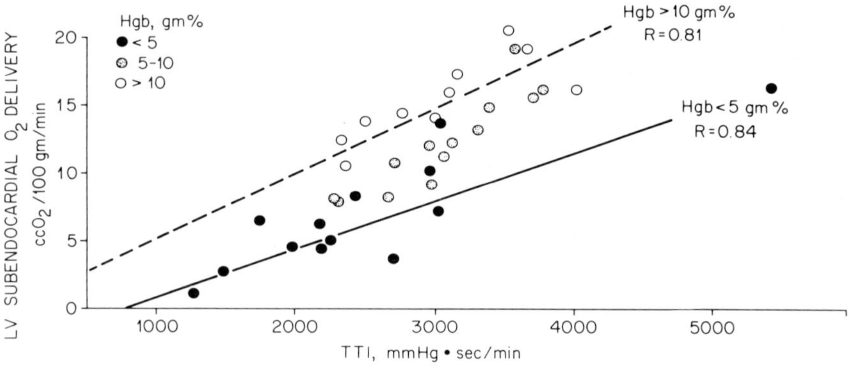

Fig. 3. Total and subendocardial oxygen delivery (flow in cubic centimeter per 100 grams per minute × oxygen content) is plotted against the tension time index (TTI). The broken line is the regression line for dogs with a normal coronary flow distribution (endocardial/epicardial > 1): $Y = 0.00421X + 2.606$; $R = 0.81$. The solid line represents the regression line for those animals with an altered flow distribution (endocardial/epicardial < 1): $Y = 0.00318X - 1.40$; $R = 0.84$. Note the significant reduction in oxygen delivery per unit of TTI when Hgb < 5 Gm. percent.

Oxygen delivery relative to demand. In all experiments, both total and subendocardial oxygen delivery (subendocardial flow times oxygen content) increased relative to myocardial oxygen demands as estimated from the tension time index (TTI) (Fig. 3). There was, however, a significant difference in the values for subendocardial oxygen delivery at any given level of demand when dogs with normal oxygen content were compared with those with severe anemia. When blood oxygen content was normal (control), subendocardial oxygen delivery per unit of demand was significantly higher than that seen when blood oxygen content was lowered with severe anemia. The lowest values for subendocardial oxygen delivery per unit of demand always occurred when coronary flow was redistributed away from the subendocardium.

Electrocardiograms. Under control conditions, the ST segments in both the epicardial and the left ventricular cavitary electrocardiograms were isoelectric, and flow was

Table I. *Values during control and anemic states**

	Arterial hemoglobin (Gm. %)	Oxygen content (vol. %)	Left ventricular flow	
			Total	Subendocardial
Control	12.7 ± 1.1	17.2 ± 2.1	82 ± 19	92 ± 21
Moderate anemia	7.6 ± 1.4	10.7§ ± 2.2	106.4§ ± 32.4	116.5§ ± 44.5
Severe anemia	3.4 ± 1.1	4.9§ ± 1.9	191 ± 127	150§ ± 109

*Values are mean ± S.D.
†DPTI = Diastolic pressure time index (mm. Hg·sec./min.)
‡TTI = Tension time index (mm. Hg·sec./min.).
§P < 0.05.

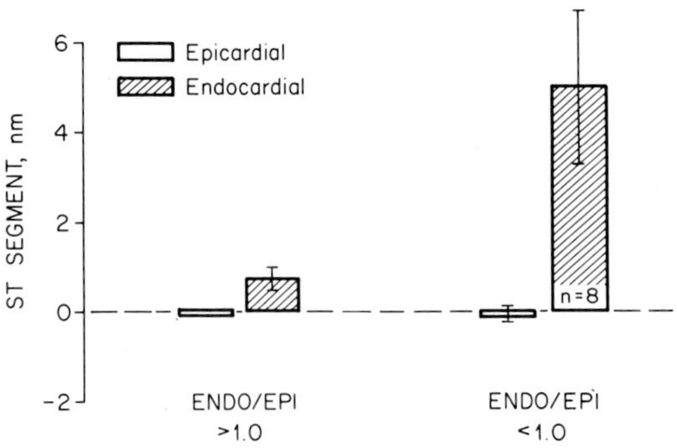

Fig. 4. The change in ST segment (from isoelectric) during control (Hgb > 10 Gm. percent) and with severe anemia (Hgb < 5 Gm. percent). Note: Although the ST segment of the epicardial lead remains isoelectric during control (endocardial/epicardial flow ratio > 1.0), with severe anemia (endocardial/epicardial < 1.0) the ST segment on the intracavitary lead becomes significantly elevated.

evenly distributed across the left ventricular myocardial wall. With moderate anemia (hemoglobin, 5 to 10 Gm. percent), coronary flow distribution remained relatively homogenous and no significant electrocardiographic changes were observed in either epicardial or endocardial electrocardiographic leads.

Conversely, with severe anemia (hemoglobin < 5 Gm. percent), the ST segment recorded from the intracavitary electrocardiogram was elevated 5 mm. above base line (P < 0.01) when coronary blood flow became redistributed away from the subendocardial region (endocardial/epicardial flow less than 1.0) (Fig. 4). While occasional changes in the epicardial electrocardiogram were seen, the mean value of the ST segment did not significantly differ from control values despite the marked alterations in myocardial flow distribution and endocardial ST changes.

Cardiac output. Systemic oxygen delivery was maintained by increasing cardiac output 20 percent above control values (P < 0.05) with moderate decreases in the oxygen content of arterial blood (hemoglobin, 5 to 10 Gm. percent). When hemoglobin was reduced further, cardiac output initially increased to 50 percent above control values (P < 0.05). This augmented output could not, however, be sustained when changes in myocardial flow distribution occurred (endocardial/epicardial < 1.0). We saw a progressive decline in both cardiac output and mean arterial pressure which was reversible only by reinfusion of shed blood.

Indices of supply and demand.

Pressure determinants of flow and the DPTI. With moderate anemia (hemoglobin, 5 to 10 Gm. percent), heart rate increased from a control value of 154 ± 35 beats per minute to 170 ± 20 beats per minute (P < 0.05). The diastolic pressure decreased significantly as the pulse pressure widened and peripheral vascular resistance fell. Consequently, the diastolic pressure time index decreased from 4,320 mm. Hg sec. per minute to 3,864 mm. Hg sec. per minute (P < 0.05).

With severe anemia, heart rate fell slightly but the systolic ejection period became prolonged so that the diastolic filling period of

Cardiac output: (%) control	Endocardial / Epicardial	DPTI† (c.c./100 Gm./min.)	TTI‡ (c.c./100 Gm./min.)	DPTI·O_2 content (vol. %·mm. Hg·sec./min.)	DPTI·O_2 content / TTI
—	1.13	4,320	3,039	74.7	24.9
	± 0.07	± 1,094	± 568	± 22.0	± 6.6
120§	1.07	3,864	3,063	41.3§	13.5§
± 23	± 0.14	± 768	± 483	± 11.5	± 4.1
150§	0.70§	2,441§	2,524	14.9§	4.7§
± 70	± 0.21	± 1,205	± 1,103	± 11.3	± 2.1

the coronary arteries was significantly shortened ($P < 0.01$). Of greater significance was a progressive lowering of both mean and diastolic arterial blood pressure so that the DPTI fell further to 2,473 mm. Hg sec. per minute ($P < 0.01$).

DPTI × oxygen content. Estimated potential subendocardial oxygen delivery (DPTI × oxygen content) decreased progressively as the oxygen content of arterial blood was lowered. With moderate anemia, DPTI × O_2 content fell 45 percent. DPTI fell only slightly (11 percent), but the O_2 content was reduced 37 percent. With severe anemia, both determinants of potential subendocardial oxygen delivery were reduced markedly. DPTI fell 57 percent and 0_2 content fell 73 percent. Consequently, the value DPTI × O_2 content was lowered 80 percent below the control value (Table I).

Oxygen requirements and the TTI: Myocardial oxygen requirements as estimated by the tension time index (TTI) did not change significantly with either moderate or severe anemia.

DPTI × O_2 content/TTI. Fig. 5 shows the relationship between subendocardial and subepicardial flow distribution and the supply to demand relationship estimated from the expression: DPTI × O_2 content/TTI. With moderate anemia, the mean value for DPTI × O_2 content/TTI fell 46 percent, but coronary flow remained evenly distributed across the left ventricular myocardium. Endocardial and epicardial electrocardiograms remained isoelectric. With

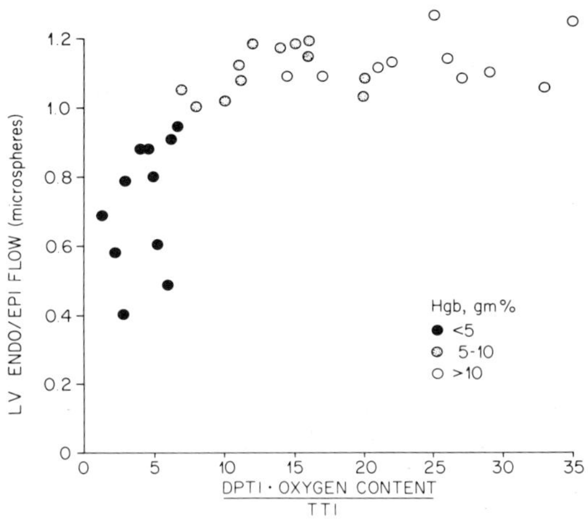

Fig. 5. Left ventricular myocardial flow distribution (endocardial to epicardial flow ratio) versus the supply (DPTI · O_2 content) to demand (TTI) ratio. Note altered flow distributions (endocardial/epicardial < 1) occur only when the supply/demand ratio is below a critical value.

severe anemia, the mean value for DPTI × O_2 content/TTI fell 87 percent and was below 10 in each instance. Fig. 5 shows that the proportion of total left ventricular flow delivered to the subendocardium became reduced when this ratio was less than 10. These changes in distribution of coronary flow were also associated with significant elevations of the endocardial ST segment and inability of the dog to maintain cardiac output and arterial blood pressure.

DISCUSSION

These studies demonstrate that oxygen delivery to both the left ventricle and the subendocardial muscle is adequately maintained over a wide range of hemoglobin levels in normal dogs with patent coronary arteries. Previous studies have shown that the coronary arteries dilate in order to insure the adequacy of oxygen delivery when the oxygen content of arterial blood is lowered; and that cardiac output increases to maintain systemic oxygen delivery.[6] Our findings confirm these observations and demonstrate that coronary blood flow is evenly distributed across the left ventricular myocardium both during control and with moderately severe anemia (hemoglobin as low as 5 Gm. percent). We could detect no electrocardiographic changes suggesting ischemia over this wide range of hemoglobin levels in these experiments. This augmented coronary blood flow resulted from reduction in coronary vascular resistance caused by both coronary vasodilatation and lowered blood viscosity.[6, 19]

With severe anemia, a further increase in both total and subsendocardial flow was observed. However, there was a significant reduction in the proportion of that flow delivered to the subendocardial region (endocardial/epicardial flow ratio < 1). The augmented levels of cardiac output could not be sustained, and a progressive fall in both systemic blood pressure and systemic blood flow occurred. The coronary and systemic hemodynamic changes were associated with a significant rise in the ST segment recorded from the intracavitary electrocardiogram. Wolferth and associates[22] have shown that this reflects injury in the subendocardial muscle and suggests that oxygen delivery is inadequate to meet simultaneous oxygen needs. Fig. 3 shows that the actual oxygen delivery per unit of demand was lowered when changes in coronary blood flow distribution and in intracavitary electrocardiograms were observed.

Evidence that the subendocardial muscle become ischemic when the proportion of total left ventricular coronary blood flow delivered to it is reduced can be marshalled from several sources. Hirshorn and Kaiser[10] and Monroe and associates[17] observed intracavitary electrocardiographic changes (ST elevation) when coronary blood flow became redistributed away from the inner shell of the left ventricle. Griggs and associates[9] have recently reported subendocardial anaerobic metabolism associated with alterations and redistribution of coronary flow. Previous experiments have demonstrated ischemia by histochemical techniques when the subendocardial muscle is underperfused relative to the subepicardium.[5] The present studies confirm this observation and demonstrate that the electrocardiographic changes occur when measured subendocardial delivery is reduced relative to simultaneous oxygen needs. These ECG abnormalities did not occur in control experiments, or if levels of anemia or coronary blood flow distribution remained homogenous, and regressed when flow distribution returned to normal. It is unlikely, therefore, that they were due to injury to the subendocardium by the electrodes. Epicardial electrocardiograms remain normal so that the ischemia seemed limited to the subendocardial muscle.

Under normal circumstances, the adequacy of coronary blood flow across all layers of the left ventricular myocardium is maintained by autoregulation. The coronary arteries dilate to increase flow as oxygen needs rise, the coronary driving pressure is lowered, or the oxygen content of arterial blood becomes reduced.[4, 6, 13] The subendocardial muscle, however, is more vulnerable to ischemia than other parts of the heart because it must receive most or all of its flow during diastole. Studies by Baird and associates[1] and Brandi[3] have demonstrated that intramyocardial compressive forces are highest in the subendocardial region and retard perfusion during systole. Despite this, coronary blood flow is normally evenly distributed across the left ventricular wall.[11, 18] In order for the subendocardium to receive the same amount of flow as the subepicardium it must have a lower vascular resistance. It is reasonable to assume, therefore, that the capacity of subendocardial vessels to vasodilate is more limited than that of vessels in other parts of the heart. Consequently, maximum coronary dilatation will, in all probability, occur first in the subendocardial region.

When maximum vasodilatation does occur, coronary blood flow to the subendocardium is determined by the coronary driving pressure (i.e., the difference between the coronary diastolic blood pressure and the opposition to flow offered by intramyocardial compressive forces or coronary sinus pressure, whichever is greater), and the duration of diastole. Oxygen delivery to the subendocardium, however, is determined both by the coronary blood flow and the oxygen content of arterial blood. Thus, with maximum vasodilatation oxygen delivery will fall if the coronary driving pressure is lowered, the diastolic filling period of the coronary arteries is shortened, or blood oxygen content is reduced. The subendocardium will become ischemic when the oxygen delivery fails to meet oxygen needs.

Our studies demonstrate that several of the determinants of subendocardial oxygen delivery (flow and oxygen content) are altered simultaneously with anemia. The oxygen content of arterial blood is progressively lowered as the anemia becomes more severe. The recognized reduction in peripheral vascular resistance is associated with a fall in the diastolic coronary blood pressure, and the associated tachycardia shortens the diastolic filling period of the coronary arteries. These determinants of flow are described by the diastolic time pressure index and changes in potential oxygen delivery described by the expression DPTI $\times$ O_2 content. In these studies, despite a marked reduction in the determinants of subendocardial oxygen delivery, we observed a preservation of the normally even distribution of flow across the myocardial wall with moderately severe levels of anemia (hemoglobins above 5 Gm. percent). The adequacy of subendocardial oxygen delivery was maintained by autoregulation (i.e., coronary vasodilatation). Although oxygen demands (TTI) did not change with progressive anemia in these studies, we observed that coronary blood flow was redistributed away from the subendocardial region and ischemia resulted when the hemoglobin level fell below 5 Gm. percent. This only occurred when the supply/demand ratio described by the expression DPTI $\times$ O_2 content/TTI fell below a critical value.

The clinical implication of these findings are that coronary blood flow remains adequately distributed over a wide range of hemoglobin levels in patients with normal hearts and patent coronary arteries. If however, there is an associated rise in myocardial oxygen requirements (i.e. hypertension, valvular heart disease, fever) or lowering of potential coronary blood supply (coronary artery disease) resulting in significant coronary vasodilatation at rest, the margin of safety in acute normovolemic anemia may become compromised.

SUMMARY

These studies show that in anesthetized dogs with normal coronary arteries, coronary blood flow remains normally distributed and myocardial oxygen delivery is adequately maintained with moderately severe levels of normovolemic anemia (hemoglobin above 5 Gm. percent). Redistribution of coronary blood flow and subendocardial ischemia occur when hemoglobin is reduced below 5 Gm. percent. Changes in flow distribution and the occurrence of electrocardiographic evidence of ischemia could be predicted from measurements of blood pressure and blood oxygen content that could be made at the bedside.

REFERENCES

1. Baird, R. J., Manktelow, R. T., Shah, P. A., and Ameli, F. M.: Intramyocardial pressure study of its regional variations and its relationship to intraventricular pressure, J. Thorac. Cardiovasc. Surg. **59:** 810, 1970.
2. Bhatia, M. L., Manchanda, S. C., and Roy, S. B.: Coronary hemodynamic studies in chronic severe anemia, Br. Heart J. **31:** 365, 1969.
3. Brandi, G., and McGregor, M.: Intramural pressure in the left ventricle of the dog, Cardiovasc. Res. **3:** 472, 1969.
4. Buckberg, G. D., Fixler, D. E., Archie, J. P., and Hoffman, J. I. E.: Experimental sub-

endocardial ischemia in dogs with normal coronary arteries, Circ. Res. **30:** 67, 1972.
5. Buckberg, G. D., Towers, B., Paglia, D. E., Mulder, D. G., and Maloney, J. V., Jr.: Subendocardial ischemia after cardiopulmonary bypass, J. Thorac. Cardiovasc. Surg. **64:** 669, 1972.
6. Case, R. B., Berglud, E., and Sarnoff, S. J.: Ventricular function: Changes in coronary resistance and ventricular function resulting from acutely induced anemia and the effect thereon of coronary stenosis, Am. J. Med. **18:** 397, 1955.
7. Domenich, R. J., Hoffman, J. I. E., Noble, M. I. M., Sanders, K. B., Henson, J. R., and Subijanto, S.: Total and regional cononary blood flow measured by radioactive microspheres in conscious and anesthetized dogs, Circ. Res. **25:** 581, 1969.
8. Friedberg, C. K., and Horn, H.: Acute myocardial infarction not due to coronary artery occlusion, J. A. M. A. **112:** 1675, 1939.
9. Griggs, D. M., Tihokoev, V. V., and Chi-Chen, C.: Transmural differences in ventricular tissue substrate levels due to coronary constriction, Am. J. Physiol. **222:** 705, 1972.
10. Hirshorn, S., and Kaiser, G. A.: The effect of changes in left ventricular and diastolic pressure on the distribution of coronary blood flow on the electrical activity of the heart, Curr. Top. Surg. Res. **2:** 463, 1970.
11. Hoffman, J. I. E., Buckberg, G. D., Fixler, D. E., and Archie, J. P.: Regional flow in the right and left ventricular free walls and septum during tachycardia, aortic constriction and arteriovenous fistulas, *in* Maseri, A., editor: Myocardial blood flow in man: Methods and significance in coronary disease, Torino, Italy, 1972, Minerva Medica.
12. Jones, H. L., Wetzel, F. E., and Black, B. K.: Sickle cell anemia with striking electrocardiographic abnormalities, and other unusual feature, with autopsy, Ann. Intern. Med. **29:** 928, 1948.
13. Katz, L. M., Feinberg, H.: The relation of cardiac effort to myocardial oxygen consumption and coronary flow, Circ. Res. **6:** 656, 1958.
14. Kirk, E. S., and Honig, C. R.: An experimental and theoretical analysis of myocardial tissue pressure, Am. J. Physiol. **207:** 361, 1964.
15. Master, A. M., and Jaffee, H. L.: Coronary insufficiency and myocardial necrosis due to acute hemorrhage, J. Mt. Sinai Hosp. **7:** 26, 1940.
15. Master, A. M., Dack, S., Horn, H., Friedman, B. J., and Field, L. E.: Acute coronary insufficiency due to acute hemorrhage: An analysis of one hundred and three cases, Circulation **1:** 1302, 1950.
17. Monroe, R. G., Bramble, W. J., LaFarge, C. G., Jumar, A. E., Stark, J., Sanders, G. L., Pharnphulkul, C., and Davies, M.: The anrep effect reconsidered, J. Clin. Invest. **51:** 2573, 1972.
18. Moir, T. W., and DeBra, D. W.: Effect of left ventricular hypertension, ischemia and vasoactive drugs on the myocardial distribution of coronary flow, Circ. Res. **21:** 65, 1967.
19. Murray, J. F., and Escobar, E.: Circulatory effects of blood viscosity: Comparison of methemoglobinemia and anemia, J. Appl. Physiol. **25:** 594, 1968.
20. Sarnoff, S. J., Braunwald, E., Welch, G. H.: Hemodynamic determinants of oxygen consumption of the heart with special reference to the tension time index, Am. J. Physiol. **192:** 148, 1958.
21. Tawes, R. L., Berry, C. L., Aberdeen, E., and Graham, G. R.: Myocardial ischemia in infants, Ann. Thorac. Surg. **8:** 383, 1969.
22. Wolferth, C. C., Bellet, S., Linezey, M. M., and Murphy, F. D.: Negative displacement of the RS-T segment in the electrocardiogram and its relationships to positive displacement; an experimental study, Am. Heart J. **29:** 220, 1945.

An experimental study of the antral gastrin mechanism

S. R. Friesen, M.D., Ph.D., I. Crosby, M.D., M. D. Boggan, M.D., E. Fiallos, M.D., J. M. Lees, M.D., D. B. Cudnik, M.D., J. Underwood, III, M.D., M. S. Peckler, M.D., C. C. Craig, M.D., R. H. Friesen, M.D., R. E. Bolinger, M.D., *Kansas City, Kan., and* J. E. McGuigan, M.D., *Gainesville, Fla.*

Over a period of four years, experiments were carried out in 120 dogs in which the gastric antral mucosa was subjected on a chronic basis to nine different environmental conditions in three general categories of influence: antral "stimulation," antral "inhibition," and "neutral" (neither antral stimulation nor inhibition). To substantiate the endocrine function of the antrum, the influence of the antral mucosal environment on antral gastrin release was measured directly by repeated serum gastrin concentrations and indirectly by gastric acid concentrations and the incidence of ulceration. The results show that the antrum of the dog is responsive to chronic experimental stimulation by distention and by alkaline secretions of the colon, duodenum, and gallbladder, as evidenced by significant elevations of serum gastrin concentrations ($p < 0.001$) and by an increase in the incidence of acid-peptic ulceration. When the antrum is in juxtaposition to acid-secreting gastric mucosa, no significant increases in serum gastrin content occur; furthermore, if the antral mucosa is chronically exposed to histamine-provoked acid hypersecretion, significant reductions in serum gastrin content are observed ($p = 0.025$), suggesting inhibition of antral gastrin release. The antral mucosa is dynamically responsive to experimental changes in its environment without evidence of fatigue within the observed experimental period of six months.

From the Departments of Surgery and Medicine, University of Kansas School of Medicine, Kansas City, Kan., and the Department of Medicine, Universtiy of Florida, Gainesville, Fla.

AN ENDOCRINE function of the gastric antrum was first postulated by Edkins[5] in 1905 when he speculated that foodstuffs in the stomach caused a release of a chemical substance from the antral portion of the stomach; he called this chemical substance "gastrin," which had the capacity to stimulate secretions from the stomach. Heidenhain[16] had already demonstrated that food placed in the main part of the stomach of dogs caused their miniature stomachs (denervated fundic pouches) to secrete gastric juice, but many years elapsed before Grossman and colleagues[14] in 1948, confirmed the physiologic existence of the "gastrin mechanism" by demonstrating a "humoral" transmission of the distention stimulus. This mechanical stimulus, as well as the alkaline stimulus, was demonstrated in an ingenious experiment by Dragstedt and associates[4] in 1951. These investigators showed that experimental hyperfunction of the gastric antrum could cause gastrojejunal ulcers in dogs in which the antrum

These investigations were supported by American Cancer Society Grants No. 67R1793, 1C-38D, and T-528, by National Institutes of Health Grants No. CA-03292-10 SGYA and AM 12711, and by the Agustin Morales-Tijerina Research Fund.

Accepted for publication Jan. 30, 1974.

was attached to the colon as a diverticulum. The ulcerogenic effect of this hyperfunctioning antrum was thought to be due to an increased release of the antral hormone gastrin which produced increased secretion of gastric acid.

An increased incidence of gastrojejunal stomal ulceration has also been reported when the gastric antrum is surgically excluded from the acid-secreting portion of the stomach[27]; under these circumstances, the retained, excluded antrum is considered to be free from the inhibiting effects of gastric acid secretions and is responsive to the alkaline stimulation by duodenal contents.

Although Edkins[5] had suggested that the gastric antrum was the source of gastrin, it was not until 1959 that Gregory and Tracy[11] extracted and prepared a substance from the antral mucosa which possessed the physiologic properties of gastrin. By 1963 and 1964, Anderson and associates[1] and Gregory and Tracy[12] had identified the structure of gastrin as a polypeptide with 17 amino acid residues, and gastrin was synthesized. In 1968, this led McGuigan,[19] using an immunofluorescent technique, to the first positive intracellular localization of gastrin in cells of the antral mucosal glands; others[25] have also identified the polypeptide-secreting gastrin cells (G cells) of the antral mucosa by cytochemical and electron microscopic methods. Furthermore, McGuigan[20] developed the immunochemical methods for the quantitative measurement of circulating gastrin in the serum, and the content of gastrin in tissues. These immunochemical techniques then made it possible to determine alterations in gastrin storage and release in clinical and experimental conditions.[7, 8, 22]

Reports of altered serum gastrin concentrations as related to antral function have been meager. Experimental studies of the antral gastrin mechanism have usually been designed as acute or short-term experiments, and conclusions from these experiments often have been based indirectly on gastric acid secretory responses.

Direct confirmation of the presumed enhanced antral gastrin release by measurement of serum gastrin concentrations in chronic experimental preparations has not been previously reported. It is the purpose of this study to substantiate the endocrine function of the antrum and to elucidate some of the influences upon it which may alter rates of gastrin release as measured directly in chronic experimental conditions.

MATERIALS AND METHODS

Method. Experimental preparations were designed to subject the gastric antral mucosa of the dog on a chronic basis to nine different environmental conditions, which may be further grouped into three general categories (Groups A, B, and C) of influence:

Group A ("hypergastrin" dogs). This group is composed of dogs in which the antral mucosa was primarily stimulated by available contact with the contents of the colon, duodenum or gallbladder.

Group B ("hypogastrin" dogs). In these dogs, the antrum was primarily in contact with the acid-secreting stomach or the acid-hypersecreting stomach.

Group C ("neutral" dogs). In this group of dogs, the antrum was neither experimentally stimulated nor inhibited (as outlined in Groups A and B above).

Over a period of four years, data were obtained from 120 dogs (beagles), in which studies were continued in individual dogs up to a maximum period of six months. All surgical procedures were performed aseptically while the animals were under anesthesia (intravenous sodium pentobarbital). The following were the procedural objectives: (1) to establish the experimental canine preparations as described below; (2) to surgically re-explore at monthly intervals for visual inspection of the gastrointestinal mucosa for ulceration and to obtain serial biopsies of antral mucosa and pancreas for special studies to be reported in the future; and, (3) to convert the antral preparation sequentially from one experimental Group and/or Type to another.

Peripheral venous blood (10 ml.) was obtained from each dog in the fasting, awake

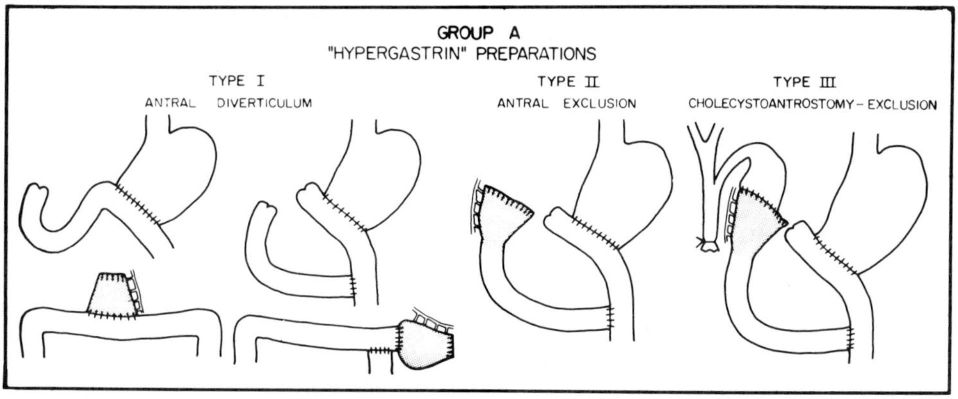

Fig. 1. Diagrammatic representation of the experimental preparations in Group A ("hypergastrin" dogs) in which the antral mucosa was primarily stimulated by available contact with the contents of the colon, duodenum or gallbladder, or by distention. In the Type I (antral diverticulum) preparations, the gastric antrum with its intact blood supply was anastomosed as a diverticulum to either the side or the end of the transverse colon. In the Type II (antral exclusion) preparations, the retained, excluded antrum was separated from the body of the stomach and remained in continuity with the duodenum. In the Type III (cholecystoantrostomy–antral exclusion) preparations, the retained, excluded antrum was anastomosed to the fundus of the gallbladder, and the distal common bile duct was ligated and divided. In those operations in which the gastrojejunostomy was fashioned by the Roux-en-Y technique, the isoperistaltic Roux limb was relatively long (16 to 20 inches) in order to minimize reflux of alkaline contents.

state for serum gastrin determinations prior to each operation, and at monthly intervals (weekly in Types VI and VII) and prior to the death of the dog. The blood was centrifuged for separation of the serum which was immediately frozen until radioimmunoassay measurements of gastrin were performed. The immunochemical assays for gastrin content of serum samples were done on coded (double-blind) specimens by McGuigan; in the weekly determinations in some of the experiments the immunochemical assays of serum gastrin were done by Bolinger. All data involving observations in several hundred operations and serum gastrin measurements were tabulated for determination of the mean of the basal serum gastrin concentrations, the mean of the maximal gastrin responses achieved in each of the dogs in each group, and the mean of the total serum gastrin concentrations in each experimental preparation. These data, analyzed by computer for statistical significances, were correlated with the experimental preparation which had been constructed and the incidence of ulceration and the gastric acid secretory response.

Experimental preparations.

Group A ("hypergastrin") preparations (Fig. 1).

TYPE I (ANTRAL DIVERTICULUM). This type describes operations in which the antrum was separated from the body of the stomach and the duodenum and was anastomosed with intact blood supply as a diverticulum to either the side or the end of the transverse colon. Gastrointestinal continuity was reestablished by gastrojejunostomy with or without duodenojejunostomy Roux-en-Y. The proximal end of the duodenal stump was closed.

TYPE II (ANTRAL EXCLUSION). These operations were those in which the antrum was separated from the body of the stomach and remained in continuity with the duodenum. Gastrointestinal continuity was restored by gastrojejunostomy Roux-en-Y. The proximal end of the antral stump was closed.

TYPE III (CHOLECYSTOANTROSTOMY WITH ANTRAL EXCLUSION). These operations were those in which the antrum was separated from the body of the stomach and remained in continuity with the duodenum (as in Type II). In addition, the antrum was anasto-

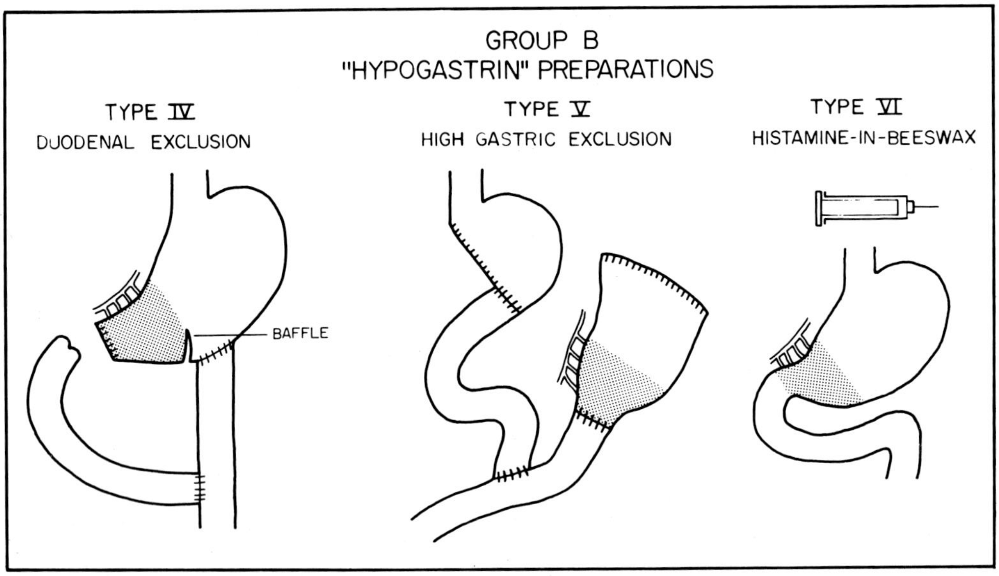

Fig. 2. Diagrammatic representation of the experimental preparations in Group B ("hypogastrin" dogs) in which the gastric antrum was primarily in contact with the acid-secreting stomach or the acid-hypersecreting stomach. In the Type IV (duodenal exclusion) preparations, the duodenum was excluded and the antrum was retained in contact with the acid-secreting body and fundus of the stomach. An intragastric baffle was constructed to prevent enteric contents from contact with the antral mucosa. In the Type V (high gastric exclusion) preparations, the stomach was divided high in the gastric body so that the antrum was left in continuity with a major portion of the acid-secreting body of the stomach; the duodenum was also excluded from the antrum. In the Type VI (histamine-in-beeswax) preparations, the antrum remained in situ so that the antral mucosa was primarily in contact with the acid-hypersecretion of the exocrine stomach produced by daily intramuscular injections of histamine imbedded in beeswax (30 mg. histamine base). In the Type IV and Type V operations, the isoperistaltic Roux limb leading from the gastrojejunostomy or the antrojejunostomy was relatively long (16 to 20 inches) in order to minimize reflux of alkaline contents.

mosed to the fundus of the gallbladder. Gastrointestinal continuity was restore by gastrojejunostomy Roux-en-Y. The distal common duct was divided and ligated.

Group B ("hypogastrin") preparations (Fig. 2).

TYPE IV (DUODENAL EXCLUSION). These operations were those in which the duodenum was divided immediately distal to the pylorus and was excluded by closure of both margins, with the antrum retained in contact with the acid-secreting body and fundus of the stomach. Gastrointestinal continuity was restored by gastrojejunostomy Roux-en-Y. An intragastric baffle (Fig. 2) was constructed by partial division and suture just distal to the gastrojejunostomy to prevent enteric contents from contact with the antral mucosa.

TYPE V (HIGH GASTRIC EXCLUSION). In these operations, the stomach was divided high in the gastric body so that the antrum was left in continuity with a major portion of the acid-secreting body of the stomach. In addition, the duodenum was divided and excluded from the antrum. Gastrointestinal continuity was restored by fundoduodenostomy and by antrojejunostomy Roux-en-Y.

TYPE VI (HISTAMINE-IN-BEESWAX). In these preparations, the dogs were given daily intramuscular injections of histamine imbedded in beeswax[14] (30 mg. histamine base) for periods up to 42 days. Blood was drawn at weekly intervals for serum gastrin determinations. The animals were killed when evidence of ulceration was obvious or at 42 days.

Group C ("neutral") preparations (Fig. 3).

TYPE VII (BEESWAX). In these prepara-

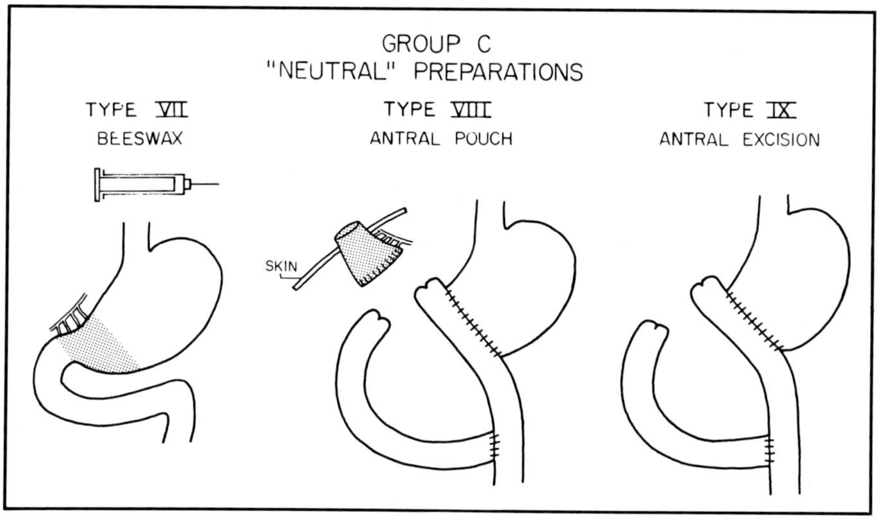

Fig. 3. Diagrammatic representation of the experimental preparations in Group C ("neutral" dogs) in which the gastric antrum was neither stimulated nor inhibited. In the Type VII (beeswax only) preparation, the antrum remained in situ in a homeostatic environment in which the dogs were given daily intramuscular injections of beeswax only (without histamine). In the Type VIII (antral pouch) preparations, the antrum was separated from both acid and extra-antral alkaline environments in conversion experiments by the construction of an innervated cutaneous antral pouch which was neither stimulated nor inhibited. In the Type IX (antral excision) preparations, the antrum was surgically excised during the course of conversion experiments, thus eliminating the prior antral environments in these dogs.

tions, the dogs were given daily intramuscular injections of beeswax only (without histamine) for 42 days. Blood was drawn at weekly intervals for serum gastrin determinations, and the animals were killed at 42 days.

TYPE VIII (ANTRAL POUCH). In these operations, the antrum was separated from both acid and extra-antral alkaline environments or the antrum was detached from its original environment in conversion experiments. The pyloric end of the antrum was sutured to the skin as a stoma and its proximal end was closed, thereby constructing an innervated antral pouch with intact blood supply. Gastrointestinal continuity was maintained by gastrojejunostomy Roux-en-Y.

TYPE IX (ANTRAL EXCISION). In these operations, the antrum was excised in conversion experiments. Gastrointestinal continuity was maintained by gastrojejunostomy Roux-en-Y.

In all operations in which a gastrojejunostomy or antrojejunostomy was constructed by the Roux-en-Y technique, the isoperistaltic Roux limb leading from the stomach or antrum was approximately 18 inches long in order to minimize reflux of alkaline contents.

Two dogs in each of Type I (antral diverticulum) and Type IV (duodenal exclusion) operations also had denervated fundic (Heidenhain) pouches constructed in order to monitor acid secretion of humoral origin. In Types VI (histamine-in-beeswax) and VII (beeswax) preparations, gastric acid concentration determinations by pH and titration were obtained by orogastric intubation.

RESULTS

In those dogs in Group A in which the antrum was excluded from the remainder of the stomach and stimulated by distention or by alkalinization—Types I (antral diverticulum), II (antral exclusion), and III (cholecystoantrostomy)—gastrin concentrations in the serum increased significantly over basal values (Table I) ($p < 0.001$). The serum gastrin levels in the dogs in Group A were also significantly greater ($p < 0.001$) than those in Group B, in which the antrum was in contact predominantly with gastric

Table I. *Effect of antral environment on serum gastrin and acid concentrations and incidence of ulceration**

Experimental preparation	*No. of dogs*	*Mean serum gastrin concentration (pg./ml.)*			*Incidence ulceration*†		*Mean gastric HCl (mEq./L.)*	
		Basal	*Total*	*Maximum*	*No.*	*%*	*Basal*	*Maximum*
Group A ("hypergastrin")	58	67 ± 7 (58)	307 ± 28‡ (139)	446 ± 56‡ (58)	27/58	47		
Type I (antral diverticulum)	32	53 ± 7 (32)	318 ± 45 (57)	385 ± 68 (32)	20/32	63	5	88
Type II (antral exclusion)	16	87 ± 18 (16)	301 ± 35 (50)	504 ± 75 (16)	3/16	19		
Type III (cholecystoantrostomy)	10	79 ± 16 (10)	295 ± 74 (32)	547 ± 212 (10)	4/10	40		
Group B ("hypogastrin")	43	43 ± 5 (43)	50 ± 4 (117)	75 ± 8 (43)	17/43	40		
Type IV (duodenal exclusion)	24	38 ± 6 (24)	52 ± 6 (64)	75 ± 11 (24)	6/24	25	5	12
Type V (high gastric exclusion)	9	42 ± 14 (9)	72 ± 15 (17)	101 ± 20 (9)	1/9	11		
Type VI (histamine-in-beeswax)	10	57 ± 12 (10)	35 ± 4§ (36)	50 ± 9 (10)	10/10	100	5	124
Group C ("neutral")	19	58 ± 9 (19)	65 ± 6 (44)	66 ± 6 (19)	0/19	0		
Type VII (beeswax)	5	56 ± 14 (5)	68 ± 5 (30)	92 ± 6 (5)	0/5	0	6	5
Type VIII (antral pouch)	9	49 ± 8 (9)	73 ± 16 (9)	73 ± 16 (9)	0/9	0		
Type IX (antral excision)	5	77 ± 8 (5)	27 ± 7‖ (5)	27 ± 7‖ (5)	0/5	0		

*In this table, *Total* refers to the mean of the serum gastrin concentrations measured throughout the experiments in each group; *Maximum* refers to the mean of the maximum serum gastrin levels achieved in each of the dogs in each group; ± no. refers to the standard error of the mean (S.E.M.), $\sqrt{\frac{\Sigma X^2}{N(N-I)}}$; number in parentheses refers to the number of determinations used for the determination of mean values.

†There is a significant difference in the incidence of ulceration between dogs of Group A (I, II, III, 47 percent) and dogs of Group B (IV and V, 21 percent) ($p < 0.02$).

‡Group A, total and maximum serum gastrin concentrations are significant elevations over Group A basal concentrations ($P < 0.001$) and over Groups B and C, total and maximum concentrations ($p < 0.001$).

§Group B, Type VI total serum gastrin concentration is a significant decrease from basal concentration ($p = 0.025$); there are no significant elevations of total over basal concentrations in Groups B and C ($p > 0.05$).

‖Group C, Type IX total serum gastrin concentration is a significant decrease from basal concentration ($p < 0.001$).

acid secretions, and were also greater ($p < 0.001$) than those in Group C, in which the antrum was neither stimulated nor inhibited experimentally (Table I). In Group A, the maximum serum gastrin concentrations occurred within the first three experimental months in 31 of the 32 dogs of Type I (antral diverticulum) and in eight of the ten dogs in Type III (cholecystoantrostomy), but in 15 of the 16 dogs in Type II (antral exclusion), the maximum serum gastrin concentrations were achieved later, i.e., in the last four months. There were no significant increases in the serum gastrin concentrations in Groups B and C over their basal values ($p > 0.05$). In dogs of Type VI of Group B, in which active acid-inhibition of the antrum was simulated by gastric hypersecretion of acid produced by daily administration of histamine-in-beeswax, there were no increases of serum gastrin levels, i.e., no individual values were greater than the initial levels. Furthermore, in these dogs the mean serum gastrin concentrations, determined at weekly intervals, were substantially lower ($p = 0.025$) than basal levels (Table I). The only

Table II. *Successive changes in serum gastrin concentrations (pg./ml.) with conversions of antral environments**

Dog No.	*Basal*	*"Hypogastrin" B-IV: Duodenal exclusion*	*"Hypergastrin" A-I: Antral diverticulum*	*"Neutral" C-VIII: Antral pouch*	*"Hypergastrin" A-I: Antral diverticulum*	*"Neutral" C-IX: Antral excision*
34	20 →		227 →	80		
59	70 →		125 →	70		
92	20 →		410 →	115		
36	40 →		33 →	20		
21	20 →	100 →	399 →	70		
56	70 →		230 →	20 →	210	
57	65 →		750 →	180 →	235	
37	67 →		740 →	50 →	650 →	26
69	65 →	100 →	422 →	52 →		22
40	110 →		367 →			28
47	80 →		500 →			27
43	65 →	80 →				32
Mean	58 →	91 →	382† →	73‡ →	365† →	27‡

*In this Table, the antral environment was changed by surgical conversion of one experimental preparation to others as indicated by arrows pointing to the right.

†Group A–Type I mean serum gastrin concentrations are significant elevations over their basal concentrations ($p < 0.01$).

‡Group C–Types VIII and IX mean serum gastrin concentrations are significant reductions from Group A–Type I mean serum gastrin concentrations ($p < 0.01$).

Table III. *Mean serum gastrin concentrations in dogs with and without ulceration**

Experimental preparation	*With ulceration†*				*Without ulceration†*			
	No. of dogs	*Mean serum gastrin concentrations (pg./ml.)*			*No. of dogs*	*Mean serum gastrin concentrations (pg./ml.)*		
		Basal	*Total*	*Maximum*		*Basal*	*Total*	*Maximum*
Group A ("hypergastrin")	27	70 ± 8 (27)	342 ± 52‡ (57)	497 ± 97‡ (27)	31	64 ± 11 (31)	282 ± 31‡ (82)	401 ± 62‡ (31)
Group B ("hypogastrin")	17	52 ± 9 (17)	47 ± 7 (52)	66 ± 15 (17)	26	37 ± 6 (26)	56 ± 7 (65)	80 ± 9 (26)
Group C ("neutral")	0	—	—	—	19	58 ± 9 (19)	65 ± 6 (44)	66 ± 6 (19)

*In this Table, *Total* refers to the mean of the serum gastrin concentrations measured throughout the experiments in each group; *Maximum* refers to the mean of the maximum serum gastrin levels achieved in each of the dogs in each group; ± number refers to the standard error of the mean (S.E.M.); number in parentheses refers to the number of determinations used for the determination of mean values.

†There is no significant difference in the attained serum gastrin concentrations between dogs with and without ulceration ($p > 0.05$).

‡The means of the total and maximal serum gastrin concentrations in Group A are significantly elevated over basal concentrations ($p < 0.001$).

other experimental circumstance after which uniform and significant decreases in serum gastrin concentrations occurred below basal levels was in dogs receiving antrectomy, i.e. Type IX ($p < 0.001$).

The results of serum gastrin responses in 12 dogs following surgical conversion of the antral environment from one experimental group to others are shown in Table II. There were resultant significant elevations of mean serum gastrin concentrations whenever the antrum was attached as a diverticulum to the colon ($p < 0.01$), and reductions in serum gastrin levels were produced when, as sequential procedures, the antrum was altered to construct the experimental conditions of Type VIII (antral pouch) and Type IX (antral excision) ($p < 0.01$).

As shown in Table III, there were no significant differences in the mean maximum serum gastrin concentrations which were observed between those dogs which developed ulceration and those which did not ($p > 0.05$). No dogs in Group C ("neutral" procedures) developed ulcers, but ulceration was present in 47 percent (27 of 58) of the dogs in Group A and 40 percent (17 of 43) of the dogs in Group B. As was anticipated, 100 percent (10 of 10) of the dogs of Type VI (histamine-in-beeswax) developed histamine-provoked ulcers; if this experimental group is excluded from Group B, the incidence of ulceration in Group B, Types IV (duodenal exclusion) and V (high gastric exclusion) is 21 percent; this incidence rate is significantly less than that observed in Group A ($p < 0.02$). The highest incidence of ulceration in the operated preparations occurred in Types I (antral diverticulum) and III (cholecystoantrostomy) dogs, being 63 and 40 percent respectively; in these types, it will be recalled, the increased and maximum serum gastrin responses were early, i.e., within the first three months. In Type II (antral exclusion) dogs, in which the incidence of ulceration was 19 percent, the majority of the maximum serum gastrin responses occurred in the third to sixth month of the experiments.

In the conversion experiments (see Table II), when 11 dogs with antral diverticula had developed stomal ulcers, nine were converted to Type C-VIII (antral pouch) preparations and two were converted to Type C-IX (antral excision) preparations, after which the ulcers healed. Three of the nine Type C-VIII dogs were then converted back to Type-A-I (antral diverticulum) preparations; these dogs then developed ulcerations, one with perforation. One of these three dogs with recurrent ulceration was then further converted by excision of the antral diverticulum to form the Type C-IX (antral excision) preparation and the ulcer healed.

Twenty of the 27 dogs with ulceration in Group A ("hypergastrin") preparation had serum gastrin levels over 200 pg. per milliliter; the four perforated ulcers in Group A dogs occurred in Type I (antral diverticulum) preparations and were associated with high serum gastrin levels ($>$ 400 pg. per milliliter). In the Group B experiments all ulcerations were associated with serum gastrin values under 220 pg. per milliliter (15 of 17 dogs had values under 100 pg. per milliliter). In Group B, two of the five perforations occurred in Type IV (duodenal exclusion) preparations, and three perforations occurred in Type VI (histamine-in-beeswax) experiments.

The measurement of concentration of gastric hydrochloric acid from the fundic pouches of the dogs in Type I (antral diverticulum) and Type IV (duodenal exclusion) reflected the serum gastrin concentrations in these dogs and confirms a humoral influence. The concentration of gastric hydrochloric acid in the dogs of Type VI (histamine-in-beeswax) was elevated directly upon stimulation by histamine, independently of serum gastrin concentrations.

DISCUSSION

There were significant and persistent increases in the gastrin content of the peripheral sera of dogs when the antrum was chronically stimulated by the presence of alkaline secretions or distention and also when the antrum was excluded from acid-secreting gastric mucosa. These findings are in accord with Edkins'[5] original identification of a humoral secretagogue originating from the gastric antrum. Such antra in Group A preparations were stimulated and non-inhibited. Homeostasis of gastrin release could not occur in these dogs because there was no opportunity for acid inhibition of the stimulated antrum.

No significant elevations of serum gastrin levels were detected in any of the experiments in which the antral mucosa was in juxtaposition with acid-secreting gastric mucosa. That active acid-inhibition of gastrin release does occur is suggested by the significant reductions of serum gastrin concentrations measured in the dogs of Type VI (histamine-in-beeswax) of Group B, in which acid hypersecretion was produced by chronic histamine-in-beeswax administration. There was no instance of increased serum gastrin content in any of the determinations, and it was noted that even the maximal gastrin responses in the five- to six-week period were lower than basal levels.

The lack of significant increases or decreases in serum gastrin concentrations in dogs of Type IV (duodenal exclusion) and Type V (high gastric exclusion) in Group B may be interpreted in a number of ways. It may be that the isoperistaltic Roux limb leading from the gastrojejunostomy or antrojejunostomy prevented reflux alkaline stimulation of the antrum, as was intended, in which case the normal gastric acid secretions were of insufficient concentration to depress serum gastrin content below normal levels. On the other hand, if reflux of alkaline intestinal secretions or antral distention did occur, such an expected stimulation of antral gastrin release either obliterated the effect of acid inhibition or was, in fact, inhibited by the normal gastric acids in contact with the antral mucosa, in which case homeostasis of gastrin release occurred because of the presence of acid inhibition. It is known from other experiments[6, 7] that the extremes of pH of either antral stimulation or inhibition exert greater changes in systemic serum gastrin concentrations in dogs than do moderate alterations of the pH of antral content.

These experimental observations tend to confirm Pavlov's[24] suggestion in 1910 that there is an autoregulation on the part of the stomach which participates in the control of the rate of secretion of gastric juice and that an accumulation or increase of acid within the stomach prevents further secretion of gastric acids. The acid-inhibiting effect of acid upon gastrin release from the antrum has been suggested also in acute experimental studies.[3, 7, 10, 17] Clinically, Yalow and Berson[28] have shown that, in patients who have pernicious anemia with gastric achlorhydria, the high serum gastrin values can be promptly and significantly reduced by placement of hydrochloric acid into the stomach. Whereas the serum gastrin values tend to be high in patients with pernicious anemia and achlorhydria[21] or with gastrin-producing tumors,[20] the content of gastrin in the serum of patients with gastric hypersecretion associated with duodenal ulcer is not elevated, but is rather within normal range.[22] The possibility of acid inhibition of gastrin release from the G cells of the antrum has been suggested also by cytochemical, immunofluorescent, and electron microscopic studies on the basis that, in patients with acid hypersecretory states, and with normal serum gastrin concentrations, the G cells of the antrum are increased in number and appear to be full of gastrin-containing cytoplasmic granules.[9, 26] These observations provide evidence to indicate that the gastrin cell of the antrum is a dynamic cell which is responsive to both stimulation and inhibition.

The capacity of the antrum to respond to sequential changes in the state of its chronic environment was clearly shown in the conversion experiments of Table II, in which both the concentration of gastrin in serum and the development and healing of stomal ulceration reflected the influence of the antral environment.

Antrectomy in the Type IX (antral excision) experiments significantly reduced (> 50 percent reduction) but did not eliminate the content of gastrin in the serum; in such situations, the remaining, albeit reduced, serum gastrin values are presumably accounted for by pancreatic[6, 13, 18] and/or intestinal[2, 23] release of gastrin.

All serum gastrin determinations were carried out on serum obtained in the dogs' fasting, awake state; serum gastrin response to feeding was not measured because of the chronic nature of the experiments and because the anticipated responses would have occurred only in those animals in which the antrum was in contact with food and nonexcluded.

Acid-peptic ulcerations occurred in dogs during these experiments as a result of several different pathophysiologic mechanisms. In Group A experiments, the ulcerations and the increased gastric acid concentrations occurred presumably as a result of the significant elevations of circulating gastrin when the antrum was stimulated. In Group B, Type IV (duodenal exclusion) and Type V (high gastric exclusion), the ulcerations developed secondary to the diversion of neutralizing alkaline secretions from the acid-bathed gastrojejunostomy. The high incidence of ulceration in Type VI (histamine-in-beeswax) preparations is due to the high gastric acid secretory response to histamine stimulation.

CONCLUSIONS

The antrum of the dog is responsive to chronic experimental stimulation by distention and by alkaline secretions of the colon, duodenum, and gallbladder, as evidenced by significant elevations of serum gastrin concentrations and by an increase in the incidence of acid-peptic ulceration. When the antrum is in juxtaposition to acid-secreting gastric mucosa, no significant increases in serum gastrin content occur. If the antral mucosa is chronically exposed to histamine-provoked acid hypersecretion, significant reductions in serum gastrin content are observed, suggesting inhibition of antral gastrin release. The antral mucosa is dynamically responsive to experimental changes in its environment without evidence of fatigue within the observed experimental period of six months.

REFERENCES

1. Anderson, J. C., Barton, M. A., Gregory, R. A., Hardy, P. M., Kenner, G. W., MacLeod, J. K., Preston, J., Sheppard, R. D., and Morley, J. S.: Synthesis of gastrin, Nature **204:** 933, 1964.
2. Berson, S. A., and Yalow, R. S.: Nature of immunoreactive gastrin extracted from tissues of gastrointestinal tract, Gastroenterology **60:** 215, 1971.
3. De La Rosa, C., Manzano, C. A., Woodward, E. R., and Dragstedt, L. R.: Effect of variations in antrum acidity on gastrin release, Arch. Surg. **93:** 286, 1966.
4. Dragstedt, L. R., Oberhelman, H. A., Jr., and Smith, C. A.: Experimental hyperfunction of the gastric antrum with ulcer formation, Ann. Surg. **134:** 332, 1951.
5. Edkins, J. S.: On the chemical mechanism of gastric secretion, Proc. R. Soc. Lond. **76:** 376, 1905.
6. Frazier, R., and Friesen, S. R.: Pancreatic and peripheral vein gastrin after antrectomy in the dog. Unpublished data.
7. Friesen, R. H., Frazier, R. L., Lukert, B. P., Bolinger, R. E., and Friesen, S. R.: Antral influence on pancreatic islet function in dogs, Surg. Forum **23:** 367, 1972.
8. Friesen, S. R., Bolinger, R. E., Pearse, A. G. E., and McGuigan, J. E.: Serum gastrin levels in malignant Zollinger-Ellison syndrome after total gastrectomy and hypophysectomy, Ann. Surg. **172:** 504, 1970.
9. Friesen, S. R., Schimke, R. N., and Pearse, A. G. E.: Genetic aspects of the Z-E syndrome: Prospective studies in two kindred; antral gastrin cell hyperplasia, Ann. Surg. **176:** 370, 1972.
10. Gillespie, I. E., and Grossman, M. I.: Effect of acid in pyloric pouch on response of fundic pouch to injected gastrin, Am. J. Physiol. **20:** 557, 1962.
11. Gregory, R. A., and Tracy, H. J.: The preparation and properties of gastrin, J. Physiol. **149:** 70, 1959.
12. Gregory, R. A., and Tracy, H. J.: Constitution and properties of two gastrins extracted from hog antral mucosa, J. Physiol. **169:** 18, 1963.
13. Greider, M. H., and McGuigan, J. E.: Cellular localization of gastrin in the human pancreas, Diabetes **20:** 389, 1971.
14. Grossman, M. I., Robertson, C. R., and Ivy, A. C.: Proof of a hormonal mechanism for gastric secretion: The humoral transmission of the distention stimulus, Am. J. Physiol. **153:** 1, 1948.
15. Hay, L. J., Varco, R. L., Code, C. F., and Wangensteen, O. H.: The experimental production of gastric and duodenal ulcers in laboratory animals by the intramuscular injection of histamine in beeswax, Surg. Gynecol. Obstet. **74:** 170, 1942.
16. Heidenhain, R.: Über der absonderung die Fundusdrüsen des Magens, Pflügers Arch. **19:** 148, 1879.
17. Jackson, B. M., Reeder, D. D., Searcy, J. R., Watson, L. C., Hirose, F. M., and Thompson, J. C.: Correlation of the surface pH histology and gastrin concentration of gastric mucosa, Ann. Surg. **176:** 727, 1972.
18. Lomsky, R., Langr, F., and Vortel, V.: Immunohistochemical demonstration of gastrin in mammalian islets of Langerhans, Nature **223:** 618, 1969.
19. McGuigan, J. E.: Gastric mucosal intracellular localization of gastrin by immunofluorescence, Gastroenterology **55:** 315, 1968.
20. McGuigan, J. E.: Immunochemical studies with synthetic human gastrin, Gastroenterology **54:** 1005, 1968.

21. McGuigan, J. E., and Trudeau, W. L.: Serum gastrin concentrations in pernicious anemia, N. Engl. J. Med. **282:** 358, 1970.
22. McGuigan, J. E., and Trudeau, W. L.: Gastrin release in normals and patients with duodenal ulcer, N. Engl. J. Med. **288:** 64, 1973.
23. Miller, J. H., Jackson, B. M., and Thompson, J. C.: Effect of total gastrectomy and partial evisceration on circulating gastrin concentration, Surg. Forum **21:** 295, 1970.
24. Pavlov, I. P.: The work of the digestive glands, translated by W. H. Thompson, London, 1910, Charles Griffin & Company.
25. Pearse, A. G. E., Coulling, I., Weavers, B., and Friesen, S. R.: The endocrine polypeptide cells of the human stomach, duodenum and jejunum, Gut **11:** 649, 1970.
26. Solcia, E., Capella, C., and Vassallo, G.: Endocrine cells of the stomach and pancreas in states of gastric hypersecretion, Rendie. R. Gastroenterol. **2:** 147, 1970.
27. Waddell, W. R.: Effects of antral exclusion on gastric secretion, J. Appl. Physiol. **9:** 222, 1956.
28. Yalow, R. S., and Berson, S. A.: Radioimmunoassay of gastrin, Gastroenterology **58:** 1, 1970.

Regional organ preservation program in the New England area

Sang In Cho, M.D., Robert P. DerHagopian, M.D., Robert S. Krane, M.D., *and* **Donald C. Nabseth, M.D.,** *Boston, Mass.*

A regional organ preservation laboratory for 13 transplant centers in the New England area has been established, and 107 kidneys were preserved during the period from July, 1972, to May, 1973. Ninety-three kidneys were transplanted and 14 kidneys were discarded because of multiple reasons. Among the 93 kidneys transplanted, 53 percent had immediate function, 44 percent had acute tubular necrosis (ATN), and three percent of the kidneys never functioned and were removed. Although the incidence of ATN in this series was higher than the incidence of ATN reported from individual centers, multiple advantages have been gained in the transplantation programs in this region by the utilization of organ preservation with pulsatile perfusion. Poor correlation between the initial flow rate on the pump and the final quality of the kidneys transplanted was demonstrated, but there was good correlation between the increase in flow observed during the period of preservation and the final quality of the kidneys.

From the Organ Preservation Laboratory, Interhospital Organ Bank; Department of Surgery, Tufts University Medical School; and the Veterans Administration Hospital, Boston, Mass.

THE CADAVER has become the main source of kidneys used for clinical renal transplantation in recent years. An increased number of cadaver kidneys has been made available for transplantation by applying the technique of pulsatile organ preservation. Two types of preservation are currently used for clinical organ preservation; one utilizes a solution similar to the intracellular fluid advocated by Collins and associates[6] and the other, advocated by Belzer and colleagues,[3] which consists of hypothermic unit, membrane oxygenator, and pulsatile pump using cryoprecipitated plasma.

This work was supported by the Interhospital Organ Bank, Inc., Contract No. V523P-3017.

Accepted for publication Jan. 29, 1974.

Reprint requests: to: S. I. Cho, M. D., Director, Organ Preservation Laboratory, Veterans Administration Hospital, 150 South Huntington Ave., Boston, Mass. 02130.

A regional organ preservation laboratory which employs the method of Belzer and Kountz[1] was established in July, 1972, as a part of the Interhospital Organ Bank. The majority of cadaver kidneys harvested in the New England area have been preserved in this laboratory. While the kidneys were being preserved, HL-A, phenotyping and cross-matching studies were performed at the tissue-typing laboratory of the Interhospital Organ Bank, and the potential recipients were selected for transplantation.

Such a regional organ preservation program has been found to be a reasonable approach in terms of increasing efficiency of organ preservation and maintaining strict control of the quality of preservation.[10, 13]

A total of 107 cadaver kidneys was preserved in an eleven-month period, and the experience derived from this group forms the basis for this report.

MATERIALS AND METHODS

From July, 1972, to May, 1973, 107 cadaver kidneys were preserved. These organs were harvested in the university and community hospitals located in the New England area by ten organ procurement physicians designated by the Interhospital Organ Bank and surgeons in the community hospitals. The locations of transplant centers, tissue-typing laboratory, and organ preservation laboratories are described in Fig. 1. The central preservation laboratory is located in the Veterans Administration Hospital, Boston, while the three satellite preservation laboratories are located at the University of Vermont Medical Center, Maine Medical Center, and Miriam Hospital, Providence, R. I. Some of the kidneys harvested outside of Boston were initially preserved in the satellite preservation laboratories and then transferred to the central laboratory in which further preservation was carried out until transplantation.

All the cadaver donors were treated with intravenous heparin and mannitol prior to nephrectomy. Lasix was given to the donor in certain instances. Twenty-seven percent of the cadaver donors were given 20 mg. of Regitine and 1 Gm. of Solu-medrol intravenously prior to nephrectomy.

The majority of the harvested organs were immediately perfused with cold Ringer's lactate solution, placed in sterile, plastic bags, and transferred to our perfusion laboratory in styrofoam boxes containing ice. When the HL-A typing and cross-matching studies were completed and the recipients selected, the majority of the preserved kidneys were again transferred to the recipient hospital in the same manner. Thirty-nine percent of the preserved kidneys were transported to recipient hospitals in the transport module which maintained pulsatile flow to the kidneys up to the time of transplantation.

The majority of the preserved kidneys were transplanted in the Boston area. Sixty-five percent of the preserved cadaver kidneys were harvested from heart-beating cadavers, and 35 percent of the kidneys were harvested from cadavers after cardiac arrest.

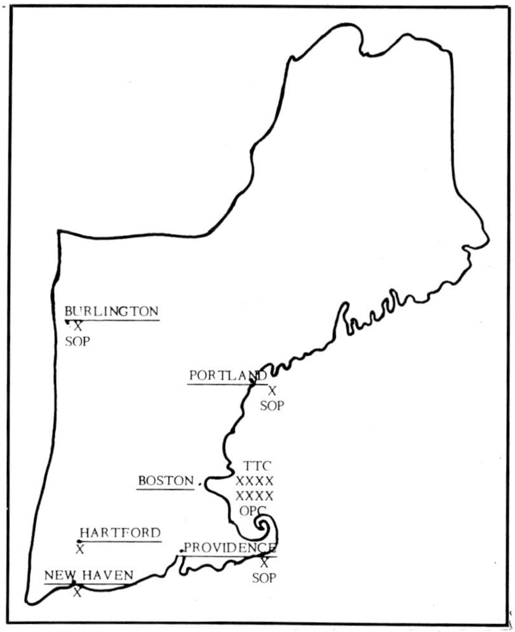

Fig. 1. Locations of transplant centers, tissue-typing laboratory, and organ preservation laboratories in the New England region. *X,* Transplant center; *TTC,* tissue typing center; *OPC,* organ preservation center; *SOP,* satellite organ preservation unit.

The perfusion unit consists of organ chambers, hypothermic unit, membrane oxygenator, pulsatile pump which uses cryoprecipitated plasma, and multiple monitoring units.[1] Organ preservation by continuous perfusion has been carried out with four perfusion units.* The consoles were located in the operating room suite of the hospital. The alarm systems were set to alert the technicians of important changes in the perfusion system.

Type-specific or AB human plasma was obtained from the Blood Bank as the single unit of fresh-frozen plasma. Because of the hypertonicity of bank plasma, 850 ml. of plasma were diluted with 135 ml. of distilled water and 15 ml. of 25 percent mannitol. This reconstituted plasma was kept frozen at −20° C. until the cadaver kidneys were

*Two Mox 100 and two Mox 100 TM, Waters Co., Rochester, Minn.

Table I. *Causes for discarded kidneys*

Causes	*No. of kidneys*
Poor flow	4
Multiple vessels	3
Extended warm ischemia time (75 min.)	2
Contused kidney	2
Contamination of plasma perfusate with ethylene glycol	2
Multiple intimal flaps of renal artery	1
Total	14

Table II. *Donor serum creatinine*

Group type	*No. of kidneys*	*Serum creatinine (Mean ± S.D.) (mg./100 ml.)*	*Range (mg./100 ml.)*
Immediate function	38	1.1 ± 0.3	0.6 – 2.3
ATN	31	1.0 ± 0.4	0.5 – 2.3

Table III. *Sources of donor kidneys*

Donor source	*No. of kidneys*	*Group type*			
		Immediate function		*ATN**	
		No.	*Percent*	*No.*	*Percent*
Heart-beating cadaver	50	32	64	18	36
Cadaver after cardiac arrest	27	10	37	17	63

*ATN of heart-beating versus cardiac arrest ($P < 0.05$).

available for preservation. When the kidneys were available, the reconstituted plasma was thawed quickly at 39° C. and 500,000 U. of penicillin G, 8 mg. of magnesium sulfate, 8 mg. of Decadron, 120 U. of crystal insulin, and 1 ml. of phenolsulfonphthalein dye were added to 1,000 c.c. of plasma. This preparation was filtered through a Millipore filter unit which contained a prefilter and 1.2, 0.45, and 0.22 μ Millipore filters.[4] Filtered plasma, 600 ml., was used for the priming of the pump. The Po_2 of plasma was maintained between 170 to 230 mm. Hg, and the pH of plasma was maintained in a physiological range with Co_2.[12]

When kidneys arrived in the perfusion laboratory, the renal artery was cannulated with an arterial cannula of appropriate size and connected to the arterial line of the pump. The initial perfusion systolic pressure was adjusted to 60 mm. Hg. When the systolic pressure fell, a single readjustment to 60 mm. Hg was made. The systolic rate was set at 60 per minute. The temperature of the perfusate was maintained at 7 to 9° C. Temperature, flow rate, perfusion pressure, and systolic rate were monitored continuously and the Po_2, Pco_2, and pH were checked every 12 hours.

RESULTS

In the group of 107 kidneys, 93 kidneys (87 percent) were transplanted at 12 transplant centers in the New England area. Fourteen kidneys (13 percent) were not transplanted because of multiple reasons and were discarded (Table I).

Transplanted kidneys were classified into three groups: immediate function, acute tubular necrosis (ATN), and non-function. In the immediate function group, the kidneys produced urine immediately, and patients did not require dialysis in the posttransplant period. In the ATN group, the patients were dialyzed in the immediate posttransplant period. In the nonfunction group, the kidneys never regained function and were removed.

Among the 93 kidneys that were transplanted, 49 kidneys (53 percent) displayed immediate function, 41 kidneys (44 percent) had ATN, and three kidneys (three percent) had non-function. The causes of transplant failures in these three kidneys were hyperacute rejection, rupture of the kidney, and renal arterial thrombosis.

In the remaining 90 kidneys, various aspects of donation and preservation were considered. Because of incomplete records in the early period of this series, all 90 of the organs were not able to be compared, and tables in this report reflect the number of organs with available data.

Donor serum creatinine was compared be-

Table IV. *Cold storage time*

Group type	*No. of kidneys*	*Preperfusion cold storage (Mean ± S.D.) (hr.)*	*Postperfusion cold storage (Mean ± S.D.) (hr.)*
Immediate function	49	2.2 ± 1.7	0.75 ± 0.78
ATN	41	2.5 ± 2.3	0.68 ± 0.61

Table V. *Flow rate*

Group type	*No. of kidneys*	*Initial flow[a] (Mean ± S.D.) (ml./min.)*	*Final flow* (Mean ± S.D.) (ml./min.)*
Immediate function	48	119 ± 54	191 ± 71
ATN	41	114 ± 47	156 ± 50

*Final flow rate: Immediate Function versus ATN ($P < 0.02$).

Table VI. *Perfusion time*

Total perfusion time (hr.)	*No. of kidneys*	*Immediate function*		*ATN*	
		No.	*Percent*	*No.*	*Percent*
1 – 15	31	15	48	16	52
16 – 30	59	34	58	25	42

tween the immediate function and ATN groups (Table II). There was no significant difference in the donor serum creatinine between these two groups. The majority of the cadaver donors maintained good urinary output, and their serum creatinine measured below 1.5 mg. percent. Although the acceptable upper limit of donor serum creatinine was 2.0 mg. percent in the majority of cases, it was increased to 3.0 mg. percent in a small number of selected cases.

Sixty-five percent of the kidneys were harvested from heart-beating cadavers, and 35 percent of the kidneys were harvested from cadavers after cardiac arrest. The incidence of ATN was compared in these two groups (Table III) and the difference (36 versus 63 percent) was statistically significant ($P < 0.05$).

The preperfusion and postperfusion cold storage time was compared between the immediate function and the ATN groups (Table IV). There was no significant difference in the cold storage time between these two groups.

Plasma flow rate during the perfusion period was compared between the immediate function and the ATN groups (Table V). Although the initial flow rates were similar in both groups, the final flow rates, following a period of continuous perfusion, were significantly greater in the group of kidneys having immediate function following transplantation ($P < 0.02$).

The mean perfusion time was 17.4 hours for the immediate function group and 17.6 hours for the ATN group. The perfusion time ranged between five and 30 hours. There was no statistical difference in the incidence of ATN whether the kidneys were preserved up to 15 hours or up to 30 hours (Table VI).

Twenty-five kidneys were harvested from cadaver donors who were treated with 20 mg. of Regitine and 1 Gm. of Solu-medrol administered intravenously just prior to nephrectomy, and 68 kidneys were harvested from cadavers without this treatment. The incidence of ATN in the former group was 52 percent, and the incidence of ATN in the latter group was 39 percent. This difference was not statistically significant.

Warm ischemia time was compared between the immediate function and ATN groups. The mean warm ischemia time was ten minutes in the immediate function group and 14 minutes in the ATN group. This difference was not statistically significant.

DISCUSSION

Although only approximately 50 percent of cadaver kidneys were preserved by continuous perfusion at the beginning of this program, the number of kidneys preserved by this method has steadily increased and at present almost all cadaver kidneys available to this region are preserved in this manner. It is felt that multiple advantages have been gained by the utilization of this type of preservation. All the recipients were better prepared for transplantation. Transplantation became a relatively elective procedure, and kidneys of poor quality were screened and discarded.

Since the beginning of the perfusion program in this region, the number of cadaver kidneys has increased 150 percent. Obviously other factors such as the development of the procurement physician program have been largely responsible for this increase. However, it is felt that the availability of the perfusion laboratory has enhanced the enthusiasm for kidney donation and procurement and has been at least partially responsible for the increase in the number of organs contributed to the Interhospital Organ Bank.

There was no significant difference in the preperfusion and postperfusion cold storage time between the immediate function and ATN groups. This finding indicates that transportation of preserved kidneys within the city can be carried out safely by simple hypothermia which eliminates some technical problems related to the transportation of kidneys on the pulsatile pump. It has also been shown to be possible to carry out interstate transportation of preserved kidneys by means of simple hypothermia.[9]

The over-all incidence of ATN in this series is higher than the incidence reported from other centers.[2, 10] Although the majority of kidneys in our series were harvested from cadavers with adequate renal function and two thirds of the kidneys were harvested from heart-beating cadavers, it has been a not uncommon experience to receive kidneys that were poorly flushed, mottled, and with poor initial flow (less than 50 ml. per minute). Some of these kidneys showed grossly bloody venous effluent when they were flushed again in the laboratory. This finding reflects the diversity of surgical techniques applied by many surgeons engaged in organ harvesting in our region, and it is felt to be at least partially responsible for the higher incidence of ATN. Because our regional program has preserved kidneys for thirteen transplant centers and one half of the kidneys were harvested from non-transplant hospitals, a higher incidence of ATN has been anticipated compared to the incidence of ATN reported from individual centers.

Thirty percent of the kidneys preserved in this laboratory contained multiple renal arteries which required separate cannulations. It is to be emphasized that kidneys with multiple arteries are best harvested by removal of a segment of the aorta which contains both renal arteries allowing easy cannulation for continuous perfusion and providing the Carrel patch for the arterial anastomosis.

Poor correlation frequently was observed between the initial flow rate of plasma at the beginning of perfusion and the subsequent function of the kidneys. There was a significant correlation, however, between the ultimate function of the kidneys and the increase in the flow rate during the period of preservation. In this study, the initial flow rates in both the ATN and immediate function groups were similar, but the final flow rates were significantly greater in the group of kidneys having immediate function following transplantation. Such an increase in flow was observed in the first two-hour period of preservation. This finding may be attributed to the fact that cadaveric donors in our series were not treated with "injectable Dibenzyline,"* and these cadaver kidneys had sustained initial vasospasm.[5, 11] To aid in the elimination of initial vasospasm, treatment of cadaveric donors with 100 mg. of Dibenzyline prior to nephrectomy has been started in this program.

There was no significant difference in the mean warm ischemia time between the immediate function and ATN groups. There was difficulty in determining the accurate warm ischemia time of kidneys derived from the donor whose nephrectomy was begun before cardiac arrest but the cardiac arrest developed during the nephrectomy. In this situation, the warm ischemia time was reported in various ways. This may be the reason for poor correlation between the inci-

*Phenoxybenzamine hydrochloride; Smith, Kline and French Laboratories, Philadelphia, Pa.

dence of ATN and the warm ischemia time in this series.

Several advantages of the Waters pump have been demonstrated in this laboratory. The transport module (Mox 100 TM) weighs 60 lb. and is 18 by 13½ by 22½ inches in size. Because of its small size, it can be carried in the technicians own automobile anywhere within the New England area. This fact has eliminated the cost necessary for a van required for the operation of the mobile preservation unit. The plastic perfusion chamber of this unit has been made disposable and interchangeable between the hospital console and the transport module. This has allowed us to interchange the perfusion unit without having to disturb the kidney or prepare a new batch of plasma, thereby lessening the danger of contamination of the plasma and making the transportation of the preserved kidneys easily carried out with the transport module.

The frequency of the mechanical failure of this pump has become somewhat a problem in this laboratory. In the past eleven-month period of operation, there have been two occasions of malfunctioning of the hypothermic unit which required replacement of the unit. The mechanical failure of the pulsatile pump was observed once every six months and required total replacement of the pump. On six occasions, there was leakage of plasma from the plastic perfusion chambers requiring repair or change of perfusion chambers. On one occasion, there was a small crack in the heat exchanger which allowed cross-circulation of antifreeze solution into the plasma. This last incident caused the loss of two kidneys.

A longer period of preservation of cadaver kidneys (up to 50 hours) has been attained with a preservation unit utilizing pulsatile perfusion than with a simple hypothermic method.[1] This finding may be related to better preservation of adenosine triphosphate (ATP) of the renal cortex accomplished with a preservation unit utilizing pulsatile perfusion as demonstrated by Collste and associates.[7] It may be possible to achieve even longer periods of kidney preservation by enhancing the intracellular synthesis of ATP of the renal cortex during the preservation period through supplying the energy substrates for ATP synthesis. There are evidences that the renal cortex consumes free fatty acid for the synthesis of ATP.[8] Further investigation is needed to explore this possibility of maintaining longer periods of organ preservation.

We would like to express our appreciation to all of the transplant centers in the following hospitals which have participated in the activity of the Interhospital Organ Bank: Beth Israel Hospital, Boston City Hospital, Children's Hospital, Hartford General Hospital, Lahey Clinic, Maine Medical Center, Massachusetts General Hospital, Miriam Hospital, New England Medical Center, Peter Bent Brigham Hospital, University Hospital, University of Vermont Medical Center, Veterans Administration Hospital, and Yale-New Haven Medical Center.

We would also like to thank Mr. James Bradley and Mr. Thomas Zolad for their technical assistance.

REFERENCES

1. Belzer, F. O., and Kountz, S. L.: Preservation and transplantation of human cadaver kidneys: A two-year experience, Ann. Surg. **172:** 394, 1970.
2. Belzer, F. O., Schweizer, R. T., Hoffman, R., and Kountz, S. L.: Preservation and transplantation of human cadaver kidneys, Transplantation **14:** 363, 1972.
3. Belzer, F. O., Ashby, B. S., and Dunphy, J. E.: 24-hour and 72-hour preservation of canine kidneys, Lancet **2:** 536, 1967.
4. Belzer, F. O., Ashby, B. S., Huang, J. S., and Dunphy, J. E.: Etiology of rising perfusion pressure in isolated organ perfusion, Ann. Surg. **168:** 382, 1968.
5. Belzer, F. O., Reed, T. W., Pride, J. P., Kountz, S. L., and Dunphy, J. E.: Cause of renal injury in kidneys obtained from cadaver donors, Surg. Gynecol. Obstet. **130:** 467, 1970.
6. Collins, G. M., Bravo-Sugarman, M., and Terasaki, P. I.: Kidney preservation for transportation, Lancet **II:** 1219, 1969.
7. Collste, H., Bergstrom, J., Hultman, E., and Melin, B.: ATP in the cortex of canine kidneys undergoing hypothermic storage, Life Sci. **10** (Part I): 1201, 1971.
8. Huang, J. S., Downes, G. L., and Belzer, F. O.: Utilization of fatty acids in perfused hypothermic dog kidneys, J. Lipid Res. **12:** 622, 1971.

9. Kaufman, H. M., Rodgers, R. E., Gross, B. M., Shreffler, B. M., Ivanovich, P., Merkel, F. K., Bergan, J. J., and Moore, T. C.: Human kidney preservation and shipping, Transplantation **15:** 465, 1973.
10. Moore, T. C., Berne, T. V., and English, T. S.: Use of a mobile transplant kidney preservation unit in a large metropolitan area, Am. J. Surg. **124:** 229, 1972.
11. Pryor, D. P., Keaveny, T. V., Reed, T. W., and Belzer, F. O.: Improved immediate function of experimental cadaver renal allografts by elimination of agonal vasospasm, Br. J. Surg. **58:** 184, 1971.
12. Santiago-Delpin, E. A., Moberg, A., Mozes, M., Campos, R., Mason, R., and Najarian, J. S.: Oxygen dynamics in a static membrane oxygenator for organ preservation, J. Surg. Res. **14:** 20, 1973.
13. Sterling, W. A., Pierce, J. C., Lee, H. M., Hume, D. M., Hutcher, N. E., and Mendez-Picon, G.: Renal preservation by hypothermic storage plus pulsatile perfusion, Surg. Gynecol. Obstet. **135:** 589, 1972.

The prevention and treatment of the persistent perineal sinus

William Silen, M.D., *and* **Donald J. Glotzer, M.D.,** *Boston, Mass.*

The perineal wound which closes and heals after proctectomy does so because the pelvic cavity is obliterated, mainly by downward descent of the peritoneal floor and to some extent by posterior movement of the urogenital structures bounding this space anteriorly. This process, in many instances, can be aided and hastened by primary closure with suction drainage. Acute and chronic sepsis within this cavity produces a thick-walled, rigid tract which precludes obliteration of the space with the resultant development of a chronic sinus. Under this circumstance, only adequate drainage, sometimes requiring excision of the coccyx and sacrum will suffice to marsupialize the wound and thus allow healing.

From the Departments of Surgery, Harvard Medical School and Beth Israel Hospital, Boston, Mass.

A PERSISTENT perineal sinus is a too frequent sequel of proctectomy for inflammatory disease of the colon, often seriously marring the excellent effects of operation on the patient's health and well-being. Despite the morbidity and anguish of this important complication, little light has been shed on its prevention or cure. The long list of diverse treatments for the established sinus including repeated curettage, the gamut of local and systemic antibacterial and antibiotic agents, local nitrogen mustard, and skin grafting attests to the lack of efficacy of any of these therapies.

A better understanding of the uncomplicated healing of the perineal wound after proctectomy will not only aid in the prevention of the persistent perineal sinus but will also serve to make more rational the therapy for this complication. Careful observation of patients undergoing excision of the rectum in which the perineal wound has been managed by a variety of methods, together with experience in the treatment of a number of persistent perineal sinuses, have led to the development of the concept of the mode of healing of these wounds presented in this communication. While it is recognized that for the most part only clinical observations can be produced to support them, we suggest that these principles represent nothing more than attention to the fundamental concepts of wound healing directly analogous to and apparently valid for a number of other surgical conditions.

HEALING OF THE UNCOMPLICATED PERINEAL WOUND

Excision of the rectum leaves a large space in the pelvic cavity bounded anteriorly in the female by the uterus, cervix, and vagina and in the male by the prostate, seminal vesicles, and bladder (Fig. 1). The posterior and lateral bony boundaries, the

Accepted for publication Jan. 8, 1974.

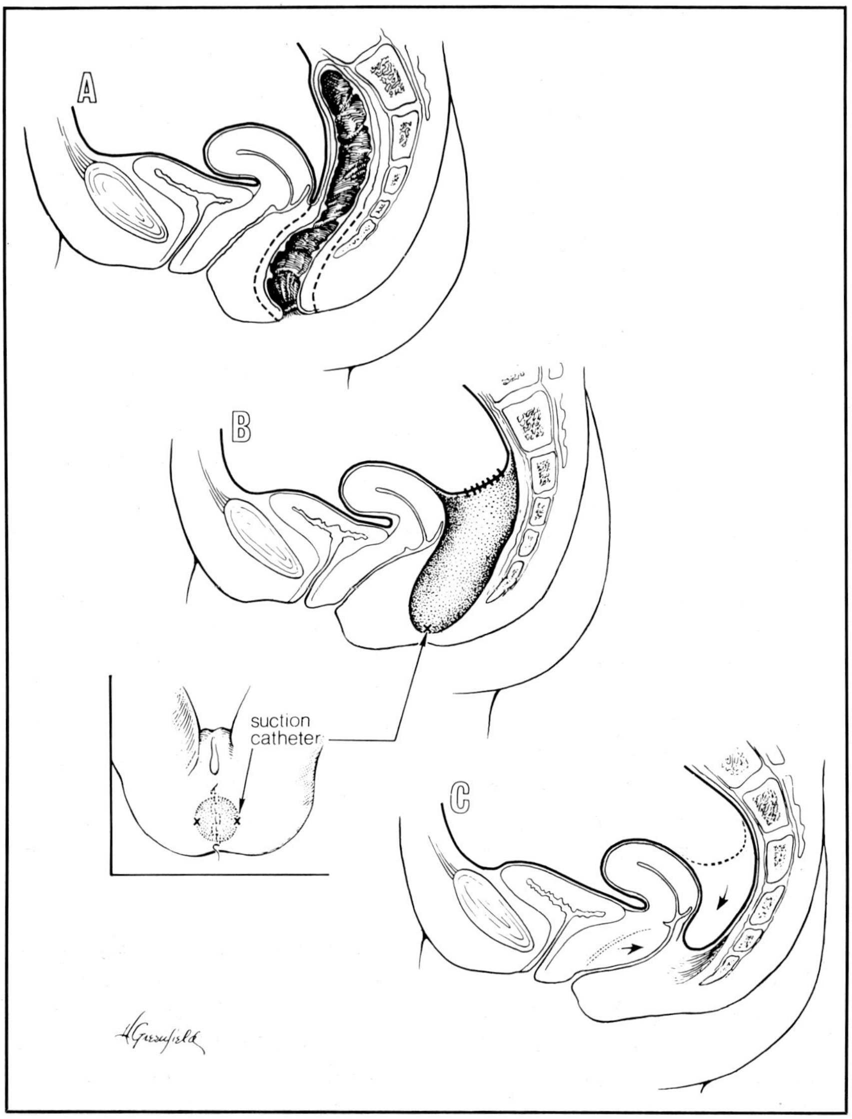

Fig. 1. *A,* Excision of the extraperitoneal rectum leaves a large space bounded by bony and relatively fixed soft tissue structures. *B,* The space is obliterated by shifting of the urogenital structures and, most importantly, by downward descent of the peritoneal floor. This process sometimes can be hastened by primary closure and suction catheters (inset).

ischia, sacrum, and coccyx, are particularly important since they are completely fixed and unyielding, thus tending to prevent apposition of the remaining soft tissue structures. Similarly, relatively little posterior displacement of the urogenital structures can occur since they are reasonably well anchored anteriorly to bony and muscular structures, even after division of the portions of the levator ani and urogenital diaphragm attached to the rectum. Moreover, the pelvic peritoneum is usually closed during proctectomy, preventing, to an extent, prolapse of the small intestine to fill the pelvic cavity. Thus, a large unoccupied space is present, rather analogous to the pleural space which remains after pneumonectomy.

How then does the large space left by removal of the rectum heal under uncomplicated conditions? If one takes the opportunity to observe an open perineal wound on a daily basis, it is clear that the *single most important factor in causing disappearance of the pelvic space is the descent of the pelvic peritoneal floor.* Any factor which interferes with this descent will contribute significantly to the development of a persistent perineal sinus.

Most surgeons deal with the perineal wound by closing the skin loosely about rubber drains placed in the pelvis below the previously closed pelvic peritoneum. The drains are removed after a period of time and the wound is left to "granulate in" during which time the patient usually has irrigations and/or sitz baths. A moment of reflection suggests that the notion that the large cavity comprising the true pelvic basin can close by growth of granulation tissue is probably preposterous. The space is obliterated rather by descent of the pelvic peritoneum, posterior displacement of the urogenital structures, and perhaps by upward shifting of the soft tissue of the buttock (Fig. 1). Only the outer portion of the wound below the level of the levators normally closes by a combination of cicatrization and epithelization of the granulating surfaces.

If, on the other hand, the perineal wound is managed by primary closure, the resultant cavity will fill with fluid just as the pleural space fills with fluid after pneumonectomy. So long as the fluid remains sterile and is not present for a period protracted enough to cause fibrosis and rigidity of the pelvic peritoneum at a high level, healing per primam will eventually occur. Thus, suction catheters placed below the pelvic floor are advantageous, not only for the removal of the fluid as usually proposed, but because they enhance and hasten the downward descent of the pelvic peritoneum.

Whatever the method, the outcome of the race between obliteration of the pelvic cavity and inevitable infection resulting from prolonged placement of the catheter or drains will determine whether primary healing, or abscess and persistent sinus is the result.

CAUSES OF PERSISTENT OR INFECTED PERINEAL SINUS

Infection or contamination of the perineal wound. If infection of the perineal wound occurs, the structures which normally slide over or descend to occupy the space previously taken by the rectum become fibrotic, thickened, and rigid. This morbid fibrotic process is similar to the thickening and fibrosis of the "peel" over a chronic empyema. The longer this obliteration of the pelvic cavity is delayed, the more rigid the walls of the cavity become, and the less likely the space is to close. Packing of the perineal wound for a prolonged period beginning immediately after resection will lead to sepsis with its attendant deleterious effects mentioned above. Although packing may be necessary because of otherwise uncontrollable hemorrhage, the consequences of packing should preclude its use as a routine method of management of the perineal wound. Jalan and associates[8] found that packing was the most significant identifiable factor favoring non-healing of perineal wounds.

Relationship to primary disease. There seems to be a general consensus that persistent perineal sinus is more common after proctectomy for inflammatory disease of the colon than after resection for carcinoma of the rectum[2, 6-9, 12, 14, 15] and also more frequent in Crohn's disease than in ulcerative colitis.[9] Although this contention cannot be completely verified by data currently available, a review of our personal cases tends to support this view. Solid and complete healing seldom occurred in less than five months and periods up to one year were not uncommon following proctectomy for inflammatory bowel disease, whereas after resection for carcinoma, healing regularly took place in six to eight weeks. Perineal sepsis in inflammatory disease of the colon may contribute to delayed healing as might the poor nutritional status of some of these patients.

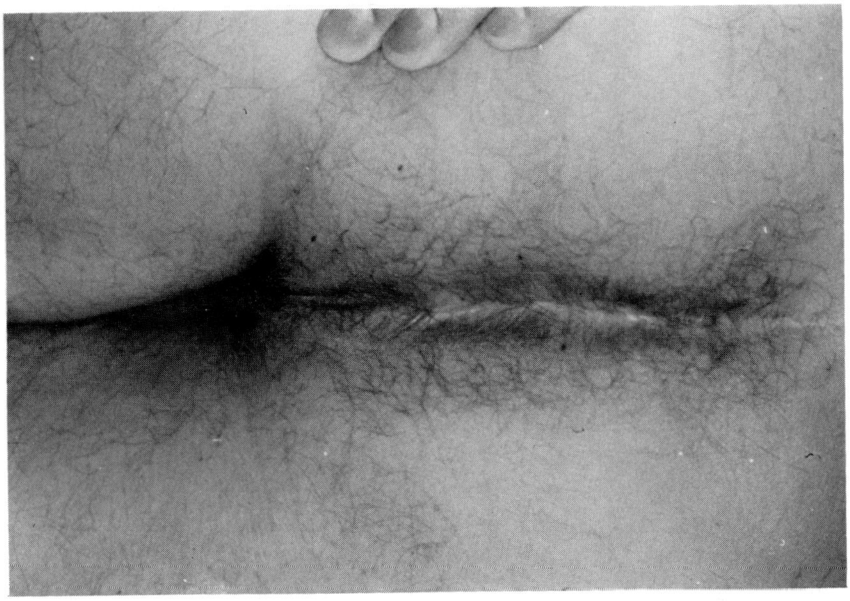

Fig. 2. Healed perineum in Case 1 after wide unroofing and coccygectomy.

However, delayed healing may even occur when the proctectomy is performed secondarily after subtotal abdominal colectomy at which time the patient has fully recovered and is in excellent nutritional condition.

It has been suggested that differences in technique and the state of the local tissue may account for the different rates of healing after proctectomy for cancer as opposed to that in inflammatory disease. The factors that have been emphasized are: (1) better drainage afforded by the wider resection for carcinoma[2, 6, 14]; (2) pararectal inflammation in inflammatory disease rendering the tissue remaining after proctectomy rigid and less apt to obliterate the space. This is particularly true of the peritoneum which is described as a fixed tent or diaphragm after closure[12, 14]; (3) removal of this proximal colon for inflammatory disease leaving less intestine to fill the abdomen with a lesser propensity for the small bowel to fall into the pelvic and obliterate the space.[14]

Corticosteroids. Although steroids have been implicated in the causation of persistent perineal sinus,[6, 12, 15] Jalan and coworkers,[8] in their rather careful analysis, found that the administration of steroids did not adversely affect the healing of the perineal wound. Unquestionably, steroids retard wound healing,[3, 4] particularly if the wound is open and granulating. However, it is doubtful that corticosteroids can be the overriding detrimental factor since many such wounds heal under steroid treatment, and the complication may develop in the absence of the use of these agents.

POOR HEALING AS A RESULT OF ACTIVE DISEASE

There is, thus, considerable doubt that there is a fundamental defect in healing in patients with inflammatory bowel disease which causes persistent perineal sinus. Nevertheless, activation of inflammatory disease of the intestine clearly appears to have a detrimental effect on the healing of the perineal wound. We have observed healed or nearly healed perineal wounds break down in the presence of reactivation of intestinal disease.

CASE REPORT

Case 1. H. C. (BIH No. 34-00-65), a 21-year-old dental student, underwent a total abdominal colectomy and ileostomy for granulomatous colitis in September, 1966. The proximal rectum was brought out as a mucous fistula since multiple perineal abscesses and fistulas were present. On May 8, 1967, an abdominal perineal excision of the rectum was performed, excising the fistulas and leaving the wound wide open. A persistent perinatal sinus developed and resisted all local maneuvers used to induce it to heal. An excision of the external skin and portions of the tract along with curettement of the sinus were carried out on Dec. 20, 1967, and again on Aug. 13, 1968, because of failure to heal. Both procedures were to no avail. On July 21, 1969, the sinus was excised and widely unroofed to the cephalic extent of the sinus, the latter being accomplished by adding a coccygectomy. The resultant huge wound granulated well and by February, 1970, the wound was virtually healed. However, the patient developed prestomal ileitis and a para-ileostomy abscess in March, 1970. The previous defect which had largely healed, quickly enlarged and the previously healthy granulations on the surface literally melted away leaving an indolent wound. On March 30, 1970, the ileostomy was revised by excising the diseased terminal ileum and relocating the ileostomy to the left lower quadrant. The patient recovered and has remained well since. The perineal wound quickly became healthy again and closed completely by May 29, 1970. It has remained solidly healed since that time (Fig. 2).

PREVENTION OF PERSISTENT PERINEAL SINUS

Open treatment. Contamination and subsequent infection arise most commonly from either operative disruption of the rectal wall during the pelvic dissection or from contamination of the perineal wound by pre-existent perianal sepsis. Every effort must be made to avoid either of these circumstances. Gentle and knowledgeable dissection of the pelvic colon will usually prevent entry into the rectum. Should perianal sepsis be present, occasionally this can be encompassed by the excision, especially if fistulas are close to the anal verge and can be excluded from the wound by inversion with the perianal purse-string suture. If larger fistulas are present, the various arborizations should be excised in continuity with the rectum and the wound should be left widely open for drainage.

Open perineal wounds must be examined by the surgeon at frequent intervals especially early in the postoperative period to make certain that no pockets have developed deep within the wound and also to assure that the external portions of the wound do not close prematurely. The surrounding skins should be shaved at each visit to prevent ingrown hairs. We have found, as did Hughes,[6] loose hair at the bottom of some persistent perineal sinuses, suggesting that these contributed to the persistence of the sinus.

Primary closure. If contamination or perirectal sepsis are absent, healing per primam can be expected in the majority of cases if the wound is closed. However, meticulous technique and absolute hemostasis are necessary. Suction catheters will never serve as a substitute for hemostasis and are not meant for the aspiration of uncontrolled bleeding. These suction catheters are brought through stab wounds in both ischiorectal fossae rather than through the wound itself (Fig. 1, inset). The catheters are irrigated daily under aseptic technique with bacitracin-neomycin solution,[5] and the volume of the cavity is calibrated by the amount of solution necessary to produce a slight sensation of distension. The space is usually obliterated in five to seven days as judged by this calibration and are removed. Our technique varies only in detail from the methods used successfully by others.[1, 7, 11] Altemeier[1] has recently reported extremely encouraging results with per primam healing in the vast majority of cases. Although primary closure may sometimes succeed after minimal contamination by the use of local and systemic antibiotic agents, in general, contamination is synonymous with infection and should dictate open treatment of the perineal wound.

TREATMENT OF PERSISTENT OR INFECTED PERINEAL SINUS

The persistent or infected perineal sinus may be defined as a perineal wound which has not healed by one year after operation. These sinuses invariably have two anatomical characteristics: (1) a narrow external opening and (2) a long tract lined by an extremely thick and unyielding fibrous "peel" covered by granulation tissue. In

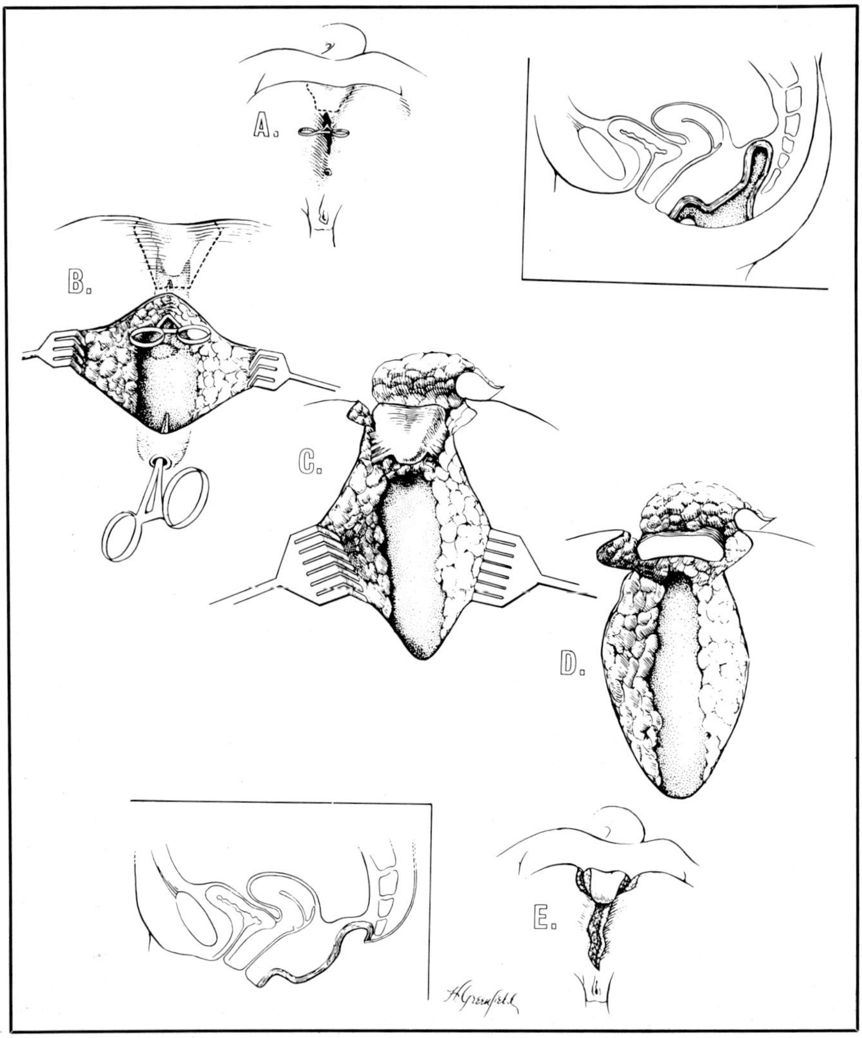

Fig. 3. Steps in unroofing operation for persistent perineal sinus. *A,* Partially open sinus tract which in inset to right is noted to have a narrow external opening and to extend cephalad beneath the coccyx and a portion of sacrum. *B,* A flap of skin and subcutaneous tissue over the coccyx is outlined and raised in *C.* In *D,* coccyx and portion of sacrum are removed and covered by the skin flap in *(E),* the rest being left wide open. The marsupialized defect is diagramed in lower inset. The flap is not always used, but was deemed advisable in this case because of the extreme proximal extent of the sinus.

some instances, if the tract is not too deep, an excision of skin and granulating lining of the tract in the narrow external portion in the shape of a cone with curettement of the more inaccessible portion may promote healing. However, the deeper and the more chronic the tract, the less likely is this approach to succeed. Under these circumstances, the presence of the immovable sacrum and coccyx is completely analogous of the chest wall (ribs, etc.) over a chronic empyema. Since the coccyx and lower two sacral segments may be removed without fear of disturbance of bladder or sexual function, the space problem in the perineal wound can be most directly and surely solved by resection of varying portions of the coccyx and sacrum sufficient to allow complete access to the apex of the cavity (Fig. 3). With careful and frequent attention to the details of wound management, healing will ensue gradually by means of contraction and with ingrowth of epithelium from the buttocks to the depths of the cavity. Skin grafting[16] may hasten closure of such a large wound, but is unnecessary in most instances. It is the unroofing of the cavity and not the skin grafts which is of primary importance. Moreover, skin grafting may prevent some of the contraction which takes place after unroofing of the cavity and hence may cause a deeper internatal cleft than if the wound is allowed to heal by secondary intention.

ADDITIONAL ILLUSTRATIVE CASES

Case 2. D. L. M. (BIH No. 30-04-14), a 23-year-old woman, had a subtotal colectomy and ileostomy for ulcerative colitis at the age of 12. Proctectomy was carried out one year later and was complicated by perineal sepsis. For the ensuing eight years, the patient had at least six curettements of the perineal sinus and three injections of nitrogen mustard at another institution without relief. Each injection of nitrogen mustard was followed by prostration and high fever for which she was transported to this hospital. Every conceivable combination of antibiotic agents was to no avail. During these eight years, the patient became addicted to narcotics and was then victim of persistent and recurrent pyoderma gangrenosum involving not only the perineum but also the extremities and abdominal wall. Continual sepsis and foul, purulent drainage were present. Repeated physical and x-ray examination of the ileostomy showed no evidence of recurrent inflammatory disease nor did microscopic study of the repeated curettements show retained fragments of rectal mucosa.

In August, 1970, the pelvic cavity was unroofed by excision of the coccyx and lower two segments of the sacrum. The overhanging edges of skin and gluteal muscle were excised to produce a completely marsupialized wound. The extremely rigid walls of the pocket in some areas were as much as one inch thick. The wound progressively healed and was closed completely by July, 1972. The pyoderma cleared and the patient voluntarily discontinued narcotics which at one point were being consumed at the rate of 6 mg. of dilaudid every two hours. The patient married and entered nursing school.

Case 3. A. L. (BIH No. 44-58-78), a 38-year-old man, underwent a two-stage colectomy and ileostomy for ulcerative colitis, the second stage having been carried out in January, 1971, at another hospital. Infection of the perineal wound developed and in the ensuing year the patient had repeated episodes of fever. Six attempts to cure the persistent sinus by curettement and drainage of the wound had failed. The patient lost 25 pounds and was almost totally bedridden at the time he was first seen at this institution. It was observed that whenever the patient stood, purulent drainage literally poured from his perineal wound.

On Oct. 31, 1971, the coccyx and lower two segments of sacrum were excised to produce a completely marsupialized wound. The walls of the cavity were more than one inch in thickness just anterior to the coccyx and sacrum. Following operation, the wound granulated cleanly and healing was complete in October, 1972. The patient has gained 65 pounds since the unroofing operation. He is again gainfully employed and scores below 80 for 18 holes of golf!

Comment. In each of the examples above, prior to the unroofing operation the patients were treated by a variety of methods without success. In some cases, internists prescribed prolonged courses of multiple antibiotics without an understanding of the pathogenesis of the lesion. The specific type of organism at this stage of the disease is almost inconsequential compared to the mechanical factors characteristic of the chronic sinus. The rationale for the introduction by surgeons of nitrogen mustard is totally unclear and would not appear to be based on sound principles of wound healing. Multiple curettements through a tiny external orifice can be compared to an attempt to decorticate a chronic empyema through a tube tract. Although chronic empyema can be cured by decortication, excision of perineal sinuses can be accomplished only in their external portions since such an attempt in the cephalad portion is fraught with danger to normal anatomical structures and the intestine lying in the pelvic cavity. The only sound method of unroofing such a cavity is to remove the rigid bony structure from behind so that the cavity is completely marsupialized and healing can occur by secondary intention.

DISCUSSION

We believe that descent of the pelvic peritoneum, shifting of the urogenital structures, and perhaps upward movement of soft tissue of the buttocks normally obliterate the pelvic cavity resulting from excision of the rectum. Although delayed healing is not infrequently observed after excisions for inflammatory bowel disease and uncommon after those for carcinomas of the rectum, mystical factors regarding wound healing need not be invoked to explain this phenomenon. The persistent sinus remains persistent because of its thick, uncollapsible, fibrotic wall. Its incidence can be decreased by avoidance of contamination, provision of wide-open drainage and careful wound care if managed open, and by primary closure in selected cases. Stubborn, established cases can be cured by wide unroofing of the cavity which frequently requires excision of the coccyx and portions of the sacrum. Treatment with occult therapies not based on sound principles of wound healing can only be deplored.

REFERENCES

1. Altemeier, W.: Presentation at annual meeting of Society for Surgery of the Alimentary Tract, New York, May, 1973.
2. Bacon, H. E., and Nuguid, T. P.: Problem of persistent perineal sinus following removal of the rectum for ulcerative colitis, Dis. Colon Rectum **5:** 370, 1962.
3. Ehrlich, H. P., and Hunt, T. K.: Effects of cortisone and vitamin A on wound healing, Ann. Surg. **167:** 324, 1968.
4. Ehrlich, H. P., and Hunt, T. K.: The effects of cortisone and anabolic steroids on the tensile strength of healing wounds, Ann. Surg. **170:** 203, 1969.
5. Glotzer, D. J., Goodman, W. S., and Geronimus, L. H.: Topical antibiotic prophylaxis in contaminated wounds, Arch. Surg. **100:** 589, 1970.
6. Hughes, E. S. R.: Surgery in ulcerative colitis, Med. J. Aust. **1:** 743, 1964.
7. Hulten, L., Kewenter, J., Knutsson, U., and Olbe, L.: Primary closure of perineal wound after proctocolectomy or rectal excision, Acta Chir. Scand. **137:** 467, 1971.
8. Jalan, K. N., Smith, A. N., Ruckley, C. V., et al.: Perineal wound healing in ulcerative colitis, Br. J. Surg. **56:** 749, 1969.
9. Lockhart-Mummery, H. E., and Morson, B. C.: Crohn's disease (regional enteritis) of the large intestine and its distinction from ulcerative colitis, Gut **1:** 87, 1960.
10. Miles, A., Miles, E. M., and Burke, J.: The value and duration of defense reactions of the skin to the primary lodgement of bacteria, Br. J. Exp. Pathol. **38:** 79, 1957.
11. Oates, G. D., and Williams, J. A.: Primary closure of the perineal wound in excision of the rectum, Proc. R. Soc. Med. (Suppl.) **63:** 128, 1970.
12. Van Prohaska, J., and Siderius, N. J.: Surgical aspects of acute and chronic ulcerative colitis, Surg. Clin. N. Am. **42:** 1245, 1962.
13. Stephens, F. O., Dunphy, J. E., and Hunt, T. K.: Effect of delayed administration of corticosteroids on wound contraction, Ann. Surg. **173:** 214, 1971.
14. Tolstedt, G. E., Bell, J. W., and Harkins, H. N.: Chronic perineal sinus following total colectomy for ulcerative colitis, Am. J. Surg. **101:** 50, 1961.
15. Watts, J. Mck., DeDombal, F. T., and Goligher, J. C.: Long-term complications and prognosis following major surgery for ulcerative colitis, Br. J. Surg. **53:** 1014, 1966.
16. Wise, L., Efrom, G., Glotzer, D. J., and Turnbull, R. B., Jr.: Symposium: Ulcerative colitis and Crohn's disease, Contemp. Surg. **2:** 84, 1973.

Delayed presentation of carotid intimal tear following blunt craniocervical trauma

Michael M. Crissey, M.D., *and* **Eugene F. Bernstein, M.D., Ph.D.,** *La Jolla, Calif.*

Blunt craniocervical trauma may produce carotid artery stenosis and occlusion with delayed and unusual clinical manifestations. This condition is illustrated by two patients with traumatic intimal tears, presenting with transient neurologic deficit or asymptomatic bruits several months or years after injury. Such injuries usually follow cranial trauma which stretches the carotid artery by sudden extension and counter-rotation of the head or by direct blunt trauma to the carotid bifurcation. The hallmark of such blunt carotid artery injury is the delayed onset of symptoms, which usually result from an intimal flap and subsequent embolic phenomena. While the symptoms are generally those of carotid insufficiency, a diagnosis of cervical carotid trauma is seldom made clinically because the entity is easily confused with intracranial injury. Aggressive angiographic evaluation and recent improvements in the safety of carotid artery surgery should improve the otherwise poor prognosis for those patients correctly diagnosed in whom operation is properly timed and performed.

From the Department of Surgery, University of California, San Diego, School of Medicine, La Jolla, Calif.

CAROTID ARTERY stenosis or occlusion following non-penetrating cervical or cerebral trauma is an uncommon, although well-described, condition. The most common pathophysiologic mechanism is an intimal tear with subsequent thrombosis. Such injury involves the extracranial internal carotid artery or the carotid bifurcation in approximately 85 percent of cases,[18, 21] and symptoms usually occur a few hours or several days following trauma. The longest previously reported delay from injury to the onset of symptoms was two weeks.[4] Only one case of traumatic intimal tear presenting as an asymptomatic bruit has been reported.[13] We have encountered two patients with delayed and unusual clinical presentations which illustrate the variable pathologic nature of the injury.

Accepted for publication Jan. 7, 1974.

CASE REPORTS

Case 1. C. S., is a 44-year-old black female admitted in January, 1972, with recurrent abdominal pain diagnosed as chronic pancreatitis. On routine physical examination, a left carotid bruit was noted. She had been evaluated two years previously for episodic dizzy spells usually lasting 5 to 15 minutes, occasionally associated with falling, but without loss of consciousness. No mention was made of either the presence or absence of a bruit at that time. Evaluation included electrocardiogram, electroencephalogram, and skull films, all of which were normal. No diagnosis was made. In 1957, she had been involved in an automobile accident in which she sustained injuries to her head and a fracture of her left leg. Despite repeated careful inquiry, she was unable to recall any more recent traumatic episodes of any kind.

Physical examination was marked only by mild hypertension and the carotid bruit. Carotid pulses were full and equal, and neurologic and cardiovascular exams were normal.

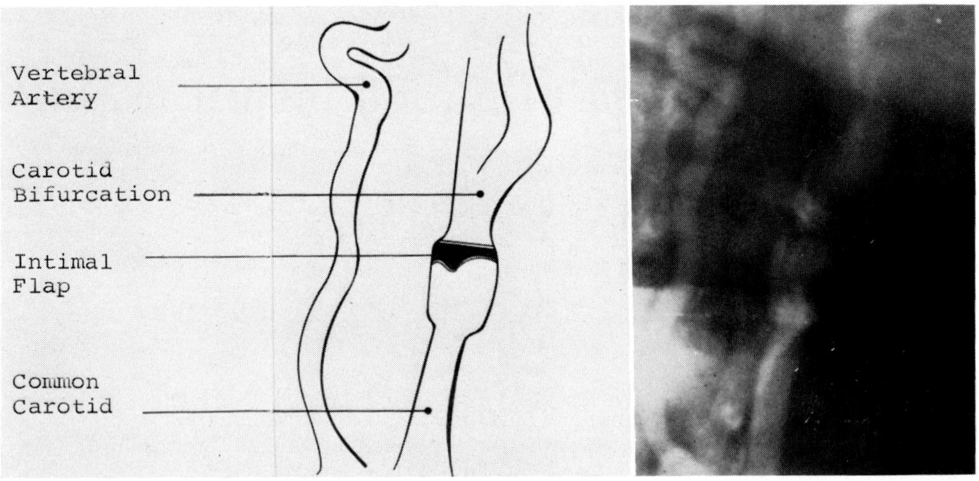

Fig. 1. Diaphragmlike lesion almost completely occluding the common carotid artery about 1 cm. below the bifurcation. Note proximal dilatation and faint distal concentration of contrast.

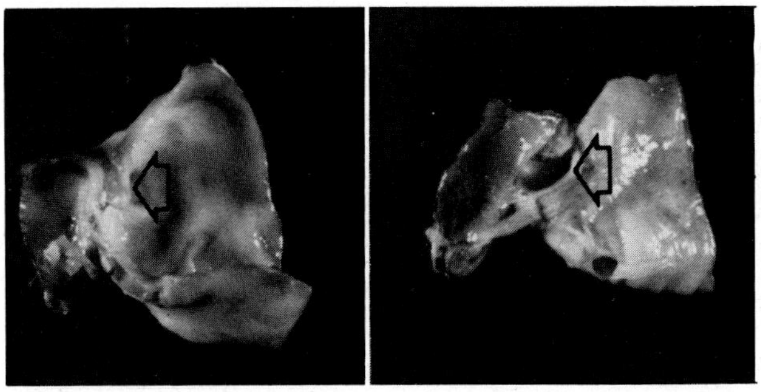

Fig. 2. Resected cylindrical fragment of intima and media about 2 cm. in length, containing the circumferential intimal flap with its markedly narrowed orifice *(arrow)*. Specimen has been opened longitudinally with distal end to the right.

A four-vessel cerebral arteriogram (Fig. 1) revealed a diaphragmlike lesion almost completely occluding the left common carotid artery, 1 cm. proximal to the bifurcation. Fibromuscular dysplasia of the left vertebral artery was suggested by these films, but no angiographic signs of atherosclerosis were identified.

At operation, the distal common carotid was enlarged and thickened, and the adventitia appeared fibrotic. The internal and external carotid arteries and the carotid bifurcation area were normal. Upon incising the thickened common carotid vessel, a fibrotic web was encountered, confluent with the distal intima, with a lumen of 3 to 4 mm. The luminal edge appeared thickened and rolled. A plane of dissection was developed between the intima and normal adventitia and carried 1.5 cm. cephalad. The intima was excised circumferentially, and the web was removed en bloc (Fig. 2). The proximal and distal intima was then tacked down with No. 6-0 sutures. A postoperative arteriogram revealed no residual obstruction. The postoperative course was uncomplicated, and the bruit disappeared. However, her episodes of dizziness have persisted.

Pathologic examination of the specimen revealed intima and elastic media. There were no changes suggesting cystic medial necrosis or atherosclerosis (Figs. 3 and 4).

Comment. Operative correction of this patient's carotid lesion was not undertaken in the hope that it would relieve her symptoms, but rather on the basis that the stenotic lesion was likely to cause more serious future symptomatic difficulty.

Pathologic examination of the specimen demonstrated its traumatic origin. However, the only history of trauma was 15 years prior to discovery of the bruit. This is a unique mode of presentation of this lesion, the location and character of which were also unusual.

Case 2. S. T. is a 31-year-old white man in-

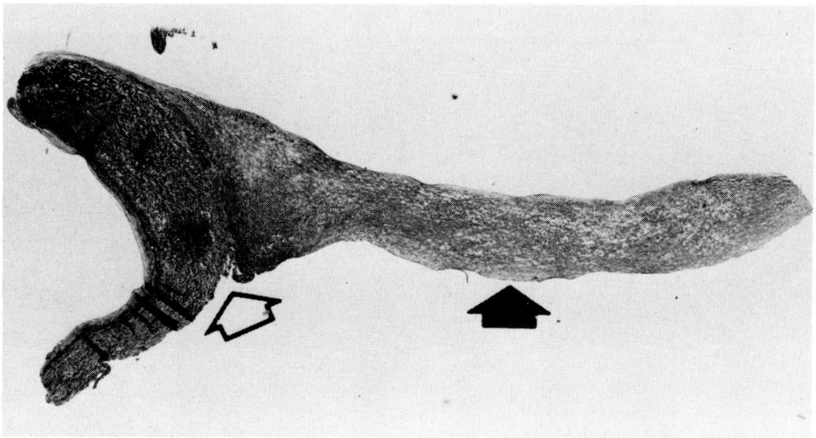

Fig. 3. Low-power photomicrograph of intimal flap *(solid arrow)* and vessel wall in longitudinal hemisection. Note point of intimal separation at junction of flap and media *(open arrow)*.

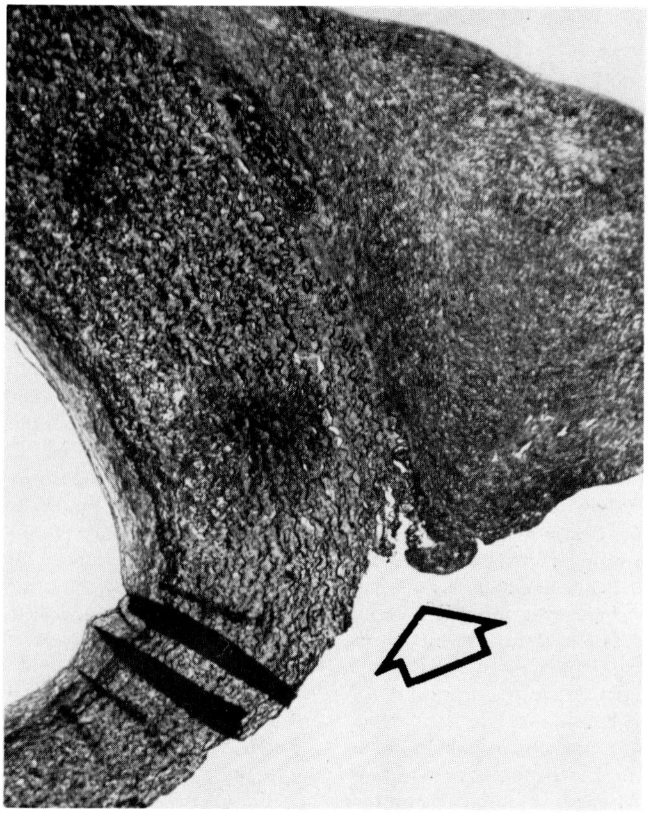

Fig. 4. Higher magnification of area of intimal separation *(arrow)*. Flap and lumen to the right.

volved in a motorcycle accident in January, 1971. He was rendered transiently unconscious and awoke with complete loss of vision in his left eye, diagnosed as optic nerve injury. Physical examination at that time revealed numbness, facial abrasions, and edema of the left cheek and eye. The left pupil reacted consensually but not directly. Extra-ocular movements were normal, as were the findings of the remainder of the neurologic examination. There was no sign of neck trauma. No mention of carotid pulses or bruits was made. X-ray films revealed a left frontal skull fracture

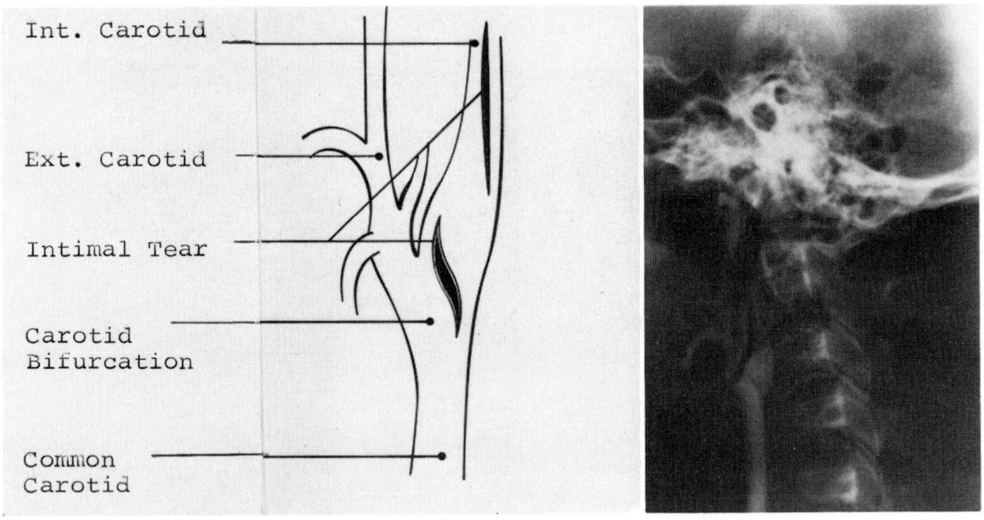

Fig. 5. Linear filling defect is present at the origin of the internal carotid artery. It appears discontinuous but can be seen to extend well up into the internal carotid, markedly compromising flow. The internal carotid was completely occluded just distal to the ophthalmic branch.

extending into the orbit not involving the optic foramen, a non-displaced left zygomatic fracture.

The patient was discharged and did well except for the persistence of blindness in the left eye, until November, 1971, when he was admitted with right hemiparesis, hypalgesia, and dysarthria of sudden onset. There was no history of dizziness or headache and no disturbance of consciousness. Eye examination revealed optic atrophy on the left. Carotid pulses were 2+ bilaterally without bruits. His symptoms cleared in less than 24 hours and a diagnosis of transient ischemic attack was made. A brain scan revealed decreased flow to the left hemisphere. Cervical and cerebral angiography revealed a localized occlusion of the left internal carotid just distal to the ophthalmic branch with collateral filling from the right side. In addition, an irregular linear filling defect was present at the origin of the left internal carotid artery extending distally 1 to 2 cm. (Fig. 5).

Because of the history of cerebral trauma, carotid obstruction, and the transient nature of the ischemic episode, exploration of the left carotid artery was undertaken to search for and attempt to eliminate a focus for the future generation of cerebral emboli. At operation the vessel appeared normal externally but on opening the artery a small amount of tissue approximately 2 mm. in diameter was seen, partially obstructing the origin of the internal caroid artery. In addition, a 3 mm. transverse intimal tear was present at the entrance to the external carotid artery, and a similar tear was present just distal to the mound of tissue in the internal carotid. The mound was felt to represent a platelet thrombus resulting from turbulent flow in the area of the intimal tears, and it was excised. No repair of the small tears seemed possible or advisable, as they were quite superficial, not completely through the intima, and the distal thrombosis would not be relieved. The immediate postoperative course was uneventful. However, six months later the patient experienced several episodes of light-headedness, once associated with tingling of his right side.

Pathologic examination of the specimen revealed the presence of some elastic media as well as intima, and a moderate amount of organized atherosclerotic material (Fig. 6).

Comment. The nature of the lesions in this patient's carotid bifurcation indicated that they were most certainly traumatic in origin, despite the lack of history of direct neck trauma. The cerebral occlusion may have resulted at the time of initial injury as a result of the skull fracture or may have been secondary to an embolus which originated at the carotid bifurcation. Pathologic examination of the resected carotid tissue idicates that it may have represented a small intimal flap altered by thrombosis. Again the length of delay in presentation of this lesion is unusual, as is the character of the lesion.

DISCUSSION

Carotid artery occlusion resulting from non-penetrating head and/or neck injury was first reported by Verneil in 1872,[18] and approximately 100 cases have been reported.[1, 3-5, 7, 8, 10-14, 17-21] associated with various etiologic mechanisms, including

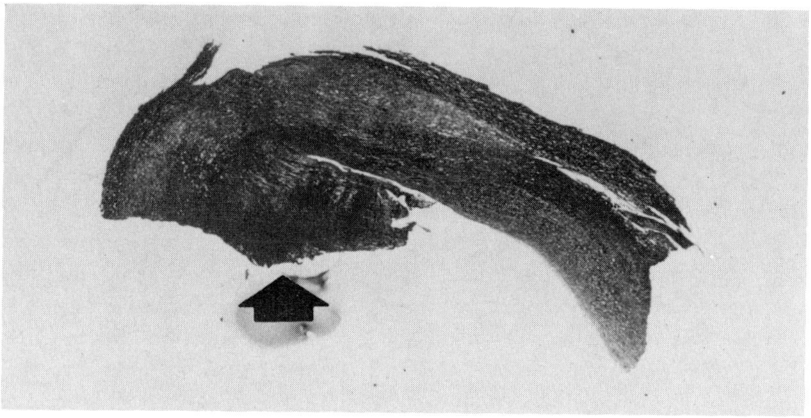

Fig. 6. Fragment of tissue excised from the origin of the internal carotid artery in Case 2. The intimal specimen includes a mound of organized thrombus *(arrow)*. Elastic media is seen superiorly.

spasm,[5] contusion, thrombosis, intramural hematoma,[19] mural fibrosis,[19] aneurysm,[1, 11] and an intimal tear. The latter is by far the most common pathologic finding. Yamada and associates,[19] in reviewing 52 cases, found an intimal tear in 62 percent of the cases in which the pathology was known. This figure may represent an underestimate, since more recent reports frequently mention the presence of a tear. Intimal tear is less common in thrombosis of peripheral arteries following blunt trauma and, when present, is frequently associated with fracture of a long bone of the extremity.[6] Circumferential tears, as seen in patient 1, occur less often than partial tears.

Four types of craniocervical injury may produce traumatic thrombosis of the carotid artery:

Type 1. A direct blow to the anteromedial neck is the mechanism in about 50 percent of cases. It is frequently seen in older patients with significant atherosclerosis in the region of the bifurcation and is associated with a fracture of the atherosclerotic plaque. Thrombosis of the carotid bifurcation is common after direct trauma, presumably because the bifurcation is the most common site of atherosclerotic plaques.[19]

Type 2. A blow to the side of the head, resulting in hyperextension and rotation of the head away from the side of the flow and lateral flexion of the neck, carries the carotid artery upward and backward on the side of the blow and stretches it across the transverse process of the third cervical vertebra or the bony mass of the first and second cervical vertebrae. This results in rupture of the intima and media at the level of the third cervical vertebra with preservation of the more elastic adventitia. This injury is less likely to occur in older individuals in whom the carotid artery has become elongated and tortuous and can withstand such extreme extension without fracture.[3, 8, 12]

Type 3. Blunt intra-oral trauma has been reported as a cause of carotid artery injury.[14]

Type 4. Basal or skull fractures may cause thrombosis of the intrapetrous portion of the internal carotid artery.[20]

The site of thrombosis is usually in the area of the carotid bifurcation or just above it in the first 1 to 3 cm. of the internal carotid artery.[21] Complete common carotid occlusion is rare, occurring only three times in the 52 cases of carotid injury presented by Yamada and associates.[19] McGough and associates[13] recently described the first case of common carotid stenosis without occlusion secondary to intimal tear presenting as an asymptomatic bruit, which is similar to case 1 in this report.

Fifty percent of patients with carotid artery injuries have no sign of cervical trauma. Seventy-five percent have an admission diagnosis of cerebral trauma, and only 37 percent have a diagnosis of cervical region injury. An admission diagnosis of carotid artery injury is rarely made (about six percent).[19]

Symptoms of carotid arterial injury are generally those of carotid insufficiency—either as transient ischemic attacks (TIA) or frank stroke. In addition, physical signs of trauma, such as hematoma in the lateral neck, are reported with some frequency. Horner's syndrome may also be present.[10] The hallmark of this entity is a delay in onset of symptoms. Only ten percent of patients will be symptomatic on admission. The majority will develop symptoms in the first 24 hours, but 17 percent do not develop symptoms until at least 24 hours after trauma.

The reason for the delay in symptoms is still speculative. The intimal tear must occur at the time of injury. In most cases, a thrombus probably develops at the site of the intimal damage shortly after injury, and symptoms are prevented by an adequate collateral circulation. Later, however, symptomatic embolization occurs.[4, 8]

The prognosis for these injuries is relatively poor. A mortality rate of 40 percent has been reported and only 11 percent of patients in the series studied by Yamada and associates returned to gainful employment.[19] Improvement in prognosis may follow earlier recognition of the cause of the patient's neurologic deficit and appropriate surgical management. In recent years, carotid artery surgery has been employed for atherosclerotic disease with increasing safety and success. Mortality rates are low with good functional results in properly selected patients. Patency rates in the range of 98 percent and operative mortality rates of approximately one percent have been reported from several institutions for patients with TIA's.[2, 15, 16] Furthermore, a substantial number of patients have undergone surgery for asymptomatic bruits with a mortality rate approaching zero.

A recent report by Towne and coworkers[17] stresses a non-operative approach to patients with acute carotid occlusion following blunt trauma. Of three patients approached surgically, two died and one patient survived with mild hemiparesis and aphasia. A fourth patient treated with heparin and dextran recovered completely. We also advocate a non-operative approach for patients with established stroke on the basis of traumatic carotid occlusion, unless the diagnosis is made within four to six hours of the onset of symptoms or symptoms are fluctuating in nature. Improvement in prognosis for carotid artery injury must come from earlier diagnosis, so that such lesions may be treated shortly after the onset of symptoms, when emergency surgical management might be appropriate. A higher index of suspicion of carotid injury should be exercised and careful inspection, palpation, and auscultation of the neck should be carried out in all cases of face, head, or neck trauma. Later application of carotid artery reconstruction also should be considered for those patients who present with TIA's (patient 2) or in the unusual patient who presents with an asymptomatic bruit (patient 1).

REFERENCES

1. Calcaterra, T. C., and Holt, G. P.: Carotid artery injury, Laryngoscope **82:** 321, 1972.
2. DeWeese, J. A., Rob, C. G., Satran, R., Morris, F. H., Lipchik, E. O., Zehl, D. N., and Long, J. M.: Surgical treatment for occlusive disease of the carotid artery, Ann. Surg. **168:** 85, 1968.
3. Fleming, J. F. R., and Petric, D.: Traumatic thrombosis of the internal carotid artery with delayed hemiplegia, Can. J. Surg. **11:** 166, 1968.
4. Gurdjian, E. S., Hardy, W. G., and Thomas, L. M.: Closed cervical cranial trauma associated with involvement of carotid and vertebral arteries, J. Neurosurg. **20:** 418, 1963.
5. Gurdjian, E. S., Blaise, A., Renato, W. S., and Thomas, L. M.: Spasm of the extracranial internal carotid artery resulting from blunt trauma demonstrated by angiography, J. Neurosurg. **35:** 742, 1971.
6. Hare, R. R., and Gaspar, M. R.: The intimal flap, Arch. Surg. **102:** 552, 1971.
7. Horner, T. G., Maroon, J. C., and Campbell, R. L.: Traumatic occlusion of the internal carotid secondary to closed craniocervical in-

jury, J. Indiana Med. Assoc. **63:** 136, 1970.

8. Hughes, J. T., and Brownell, B.: Traumatic thrombosis of the internal carotid artery in the neck, J. Neurol. Neurosurg. Psychat. **31:** 307, 1968.
9. Javid, H., Ostermiller, W. E., Heughesh, J. W., Dye, W. S., Hunter, J. A., Najafi, H., and Julian, C.: Carotid endarterectomy for asymptomatic patients, Arch. Surg. **102:** 389, 1971.
10. Jernigan, W. R., and Gardner, W. C.: Carotid artery injuries due to closed cervical trauma, J. Trauma **11:** 429, 1971.
11. Little, J. M., and May, J.: Civilian arterial injuries, Med. J. Aust. **1:** 841, 1972.
12. Little, J. M., May, J., Vanderfield, G. K., and Lamond, S.: Traumatic thrombosis of the internal carotid artery, Lancet **2:** 926, 1969.
13. McGough, E. C., Helfrich, L. R., and Hughes, R. K.: Traumatic intimal prolapse of the common carotid artery, Am. J. Surg. **123:** 724, 1972.
14. Pitner, S .E.: Carotid thrombosis due to intraoral trauma, New Engl. J. Med. **274:** 764, 1966.
15. Thompson, J. E., Austin, D. J., and Patman, R. D.: Carotid endarterectomy for cerebrovascular insufficiency, Ann. Srug. **172:** 663, 1970.
16. Thompson, J. E., Kartchner, M. M., Austin, D. J., Wheeler, C. G., and Patman, R. D.: Carotid endarterectomy for cerebrovascular insufficiency (stroke): follow-up of 359 cases, Ann. Surg. **163:** 751, 1966.
17. Towne, J. B., Neis, D. D., and Smith, J. W.: Thrombosis of the internal carotid artery following blunt cervical trauma, Arch. Surg. **104:** 565, 1972.
18. Verneil, M.: Contusions multiples, délire violent, hémiplégic à droit, signes de compressoin cérébrale, Bull. Acad. Nat. Med. (Paris) **36:** 46, 1872.
19. Yamada, S., Kindt, G. W., and Youmans, J. R.: Carotid artery occlusion due to nonpenetrating injury, J. Trauma **7:** 333, 1967.
20. Yashon, D., Johnson, A. B., II, and Jane, J. A.: Bilateral internal carotid artery occlusion secondary to closed head injuries, J. Neurol. Neurosurg. Psychiat. **27:** 547, 1964.
21. Zilkha, A.: Traumatic occlusion of the internal carotid artery, Radiology **97:** 543, 1970.

Transvenous adrenal destruction: Clinical trials in patients with metastatic malignancy

C. E. Zimmerman, M.D., H. Eisenberg, M.D., R. Spark, M.D., *and* C. B. Rosoff, M.D., *Boston, Mass.*

Transvenous adrenal destruction, produced by retrograde venous extravasation of a mixture of contrast medium and nitrogen mustard, was studied in six patients with metastatic malignancy. The procedure is one of low morbidity in patients with marked debilitation from their primary disease. In four or five patients in whom the procedure was technically satisfactory, adrenal function was absent at six weeks, as measured by beta 1-24 ACTH (Cortrosyn) stimulation tests. Profound depression of adrenal function in these patients can last at least as long as six months.

From the Departments of Surgery, Radiology, and Medicine, Beth Israel Hospital, Harvard Medical School, Boston, Mass.

Adrenalectomy can offer patients with metastatic carcinoma of the breast prolonged remissions from the disabling symptoms of their disease.[8] The response rate is not uniform, however, and the inability to predict with full accuracy the results of the operation often leaves the attending physician reluctant to recommend major surgery to a patient perhaps already debilitated and with a poor ultimate prognosis. The venous architecture of the adrenal gland is delicate, and since the introduction of adrenal venography, occasional reports have documented accidental gland infarction occurring during diagnostic studies.[1, 3, 5, 6] Infarction almost uniformly occurred in glands involved in a pathologic process,[1, 5, 6] and loss of function on occasion appeared to be permanent.[3] The purposeful destruction of adrenal function via this transvenous route appeared to hold potential for therapy in patients with metastatic malignancy of the breast. Acting upon the original suggestion of one of the authors (CBR), Zimmerman and associates[11] demonstrated that canine adrenal glands could be totally infarcted via transvenous extravasation of a mixture of nitrogen mustard and contrast medium. This report summarizes the clinical experience with this procedure in six patients with metastatic malignancy. It should be stressed at the beginning that since the purpose of this study was to demonstrate that retrograde venous extravasation could achieve long-term suppression of adrenal function, with minimal morbidity, patients were selected on the basis of advanced disease alone, rather than on potential for clinical response.

STUDIES AND METHOD

All patients in this study had proved metastatic malignancy (five breast cancers, one prostate cancer), which had become resistant to various forms of chemotherapy and radiotherapy. Functional adrenal in-

Accepted for publication Dec. 28, 1973.

Reprint requests: Clarence E. Zimmerman, M.D., c/o Beth Israel Hospital, 330 Brookline Ave., Boston, Mass. 02215.

tegrity was assessed before and after the procedure by determination of base-line levels of plasma cortisol as well as response of plasma cortisol to an intramuscular injection of beta 1-24 ACTH (Cortrosyn) (Fig. 1 and Table I). Base-line plasma cortisol value was determined between 8:00 and 10:00 A.M. Repeat plasma cortisol determination 30 minutes after the injection of beta 1-24 ACTH was obtained to assess the ability of the adrenal to respond to its trophic hormone. Plasma cortisol was determined by the competitive protein-binding method of Murphy.[9] Patients selected for transvenous adrenal destruction were brought to the X-ray Department fasting from the previous midnight and were given small doses of intramuscular Valium (5 to 10 mg.) on the morning of the procedure. Under local anesthesia, a catheter was guided via percutaneous femoral vein puncture into the orifice of the right adrenal vein. After adrenal venograms documented the position of the catheter, it was wedged into position, and the patient was given a supplement of intravenous morphine (2 to 3 mg.) and 250 μg of beta 1-24 ACTH prior to the retrograde injection. Under fluoroscopic control, forceful retrograde injection was repeated until a small bleb of extravascular contrast material (Renograffin 76) was seen within the adrenal parenchyma. A mixture of this contrast material and nitrogen mustard, the latter calculated to deliver 0.1 mg. per kilogram of body weight per adrenal gland, was prepared in a total volume of 10 to 20 c.c., depending upon the estimated size of the adrenal gland. This solution was extravasated through the previous venous rent into the gland, until the adrenal capsule was completely filled with contrast material, or a rupture of the capsule was produced. The procedure was then repeated on the opposite side. Patients were kept fasting for the rest of the day and were given medication for nausea and pain as necessary. Following the extravasation, patients were maintained on physiologic replacement doses of cortisone or prednisone as well as fludrocortisone as noted in the individual case reports. On the day before a repeat ACTH test, the only glucocorticoid administered was a physiologic dose of dexamethasone. This was done to ensure accurate estimation of endogenous production of corticosteroids in the base-line state as well as after provocation with ACTH. Patients were followed with repeated beta 1-24 ACTH stimulation tests postoperatively, and clinical and radiologic evaluation of tumor response was recorded.

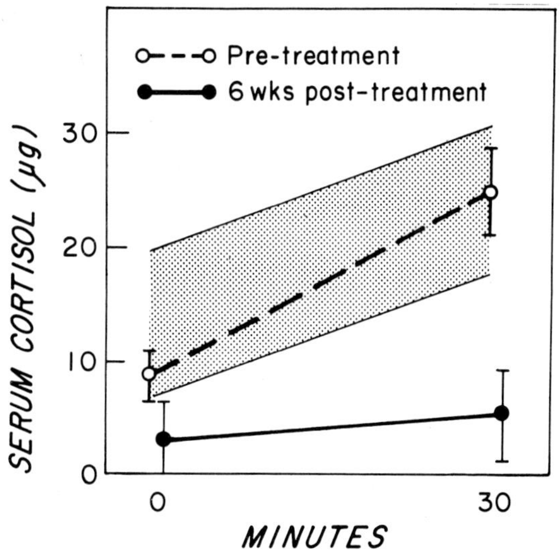

Fig. 1. Mean values (± 1 S.D.) for base-line serum cortisol values and thirty-minute response levels after 250 μg beta 1-24 ACTH, measured before and six weeks after transvenous adrenal destruction. The shaded area indicates the normal range of response.

CASE REPORTS

Case 1. A. B. (No. 44-90-27), a 69-year-old woman, underwent right radical mastectomy and radiation in 1969 with six of 22 nodes positive. In August, 1970, she developed chest wall and pulmonary metastases. The skin metastases responded to local irradiation and diethystilbesterol, 15 mg. daily. In April of 1971, she underwent modified left radical mastectomy for a new malignancy, 13 of 19 nodes positive. Diethylstilbesterol was replaced by prednisone 15 mg. a day. In May of 1971, skin lesions recurred, and thoracentesis demonstrated a malignant pleural effusion. Nitrogen mustard was instilled. In August, 1971, she was begun on 5-fluorouracil, with some improvement, and later Halotestin, 30 mg. a day, was given. The pulmonary effusion recurred in November of 1971, with left lower leg

Table I. *Individual base-line serum cortisol values and the thirty-minute response levels after the intramuscular injection of 250 μg beta 1-24 ACTH, measured before and after transvenous adrenal destruction*

	Pretreatment		Post treatment					
			6 wk.		10 wk.		30 wk.	
Patient	Base line	Beta 1-24 ACTH response	Base line	Beta 1-24 ACTH response	Base line	Beta 1-24 ACTH response	Base line	Beta 1-24 ACTH response
A. B.*	10.0†	20.5	10.5	12.0				
E. S.	16.5	40	0.5	1.5	0.0	6.5	0.5	5.5
H. N.	6.0	22.5	0.0	1.0	1.0	7.0		
A. C.	1.0	11.0	0.0	1.5			0.0	2.0
J. B.	2.5	13.5	1.0	3.5				
G. D.	16.0	40.0	5.0	11.0				

*Technically unsatisfactory.
†Serum cortisol (μg).

edema, thought to be secondary to retroperitoneal venous obstruction, a right pleural effusion, and a swollen right arm with extensive bilateral chest wall metastases. Chest x-ray films showed bilateral pulmonary metastases and multiple osteoblastic lesions. Liver chemistries were abnormal, and the liver was enlarged. On Dec. 17, 1971, the patient underwent transvenous adrenal destruction. Extravasation on the right side proved very difficult, and was not deemed to be technically satisfactory. She had one day of mild nausea, but otherwise did well. However, she never demonstrated any subjective or objective evidence of response. She was discharged on prednisone, 5 mg. a day. In March of 1972 she was started on the Cooper regimen of multiple drug therapy, with some hepatic evidence of response. The patient died of Lysteria meningitis on Aug. 4, 1972. At autopsy, the right adrenal gland demonstrated a thin cortex, but the over-all architecture was preserved. The left gland was infarcted with a fibrotic capsule and scant cortical rim, containing lysed red blood cells, fibrin, and prominent cholesterol clefts. Capillary ingrowths into the organizing hemorrhage were seen (Fig. 2, A). A tiny fragment of glandular tissue was found at the periphery of the lower pole (Fig. 2, B).

Case 2. E. S. (No. 31-03-11), a 60-year-old woman, underwent left radical mastectomy and irradiation with three of 21 axillary nodes positive in 1961. In October, 1970, chest wall recurrence was treated successfully with 3,000 rads. In July of 1971, chest wall lesions reappeared. Diethylstilbesterol administration was without effect. On Feb. 8, 1972, a technically satisfactory transvenous adrenal destruction was performed. Known disease was limited to the chest wall with massive swelling of the left arm. The patient tolerated the procedure well, incurring 24 hours of nausea and vomiting but with rapid recovery. White count rose briefly from 5,000 to 11,000, but she had an afebrile course. There was rapid disappearance of much of the swelling in her left arm immediately following the procedure. She was maintained postoperatively on prednisone (7.5 mg. a day) and Florinef (0.05 mg. daily). The patient did not demonstrate any objective signs of remission in her skin recurrences, and in June, 1972, she underwent transphenoidal radiofrequency hypophysectomy. At this time she had in addition sclerotic lesions noted in the eleventh thoracic vertebra, the pelvis, and right femur. She had no clinical response to the hypophysectomy, which appeared to be complete. The patient was still alive in October, 1973, undergoing multiple drug therapy.

Case 3. H. N. (No. 37-04-55), a 61-year-old man, was found in January, 1971, to have carcinoma of the prostate with widespread regional lymph node and multi-focal bone metastases. The patient underwent bilateral orchietomies. He was placed on Decadron (2 mg. twice a day). He developed a myelopthisic anemia with extreme fatigue and inability to continue work. Repeated transfusions maintained a hematocrit of around 30. Acid phosphatase was 81.6 with a prostatic fraction of 70.4. The patient was admitted in June, 1972, for hypophysectomy in an effort to control his anemia, but an unusual sella turcica made this procedure inadvisable, and on June 21, 1972, he underwent a technically satisfactory transvenous adrenal destruction. The patient had a very benign postprocedure course, with one day of mild nausea, no fever, and very slight leukocytosis. The patient was discharged on prednisone (7.5 mg. a day) and did well with regard to his anemia and bone pain, never requiring a subsequent transfusion, holding a hematocrit in the range of 31 to 33. Within one week of the procedure, acid phosphatase had fallen to 5.1 sigma units with a prostatic fraction of 3.8. Four months

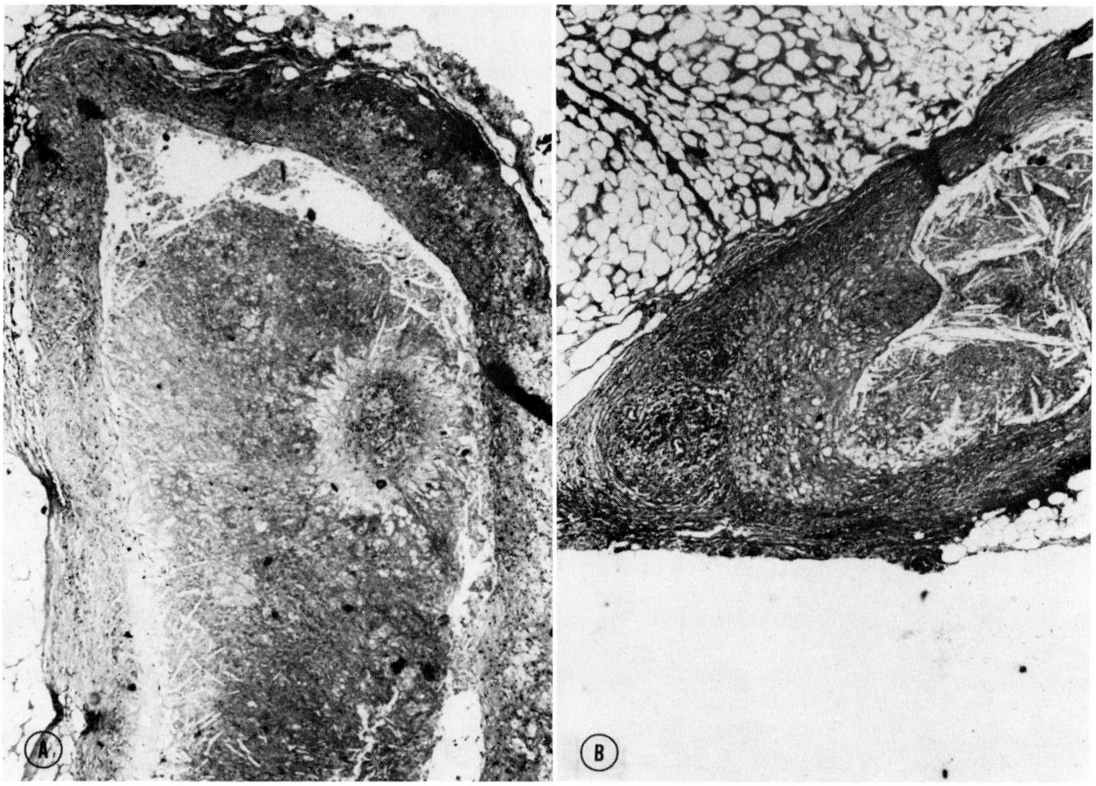

Fig. 2. *A*, Autopsy specimen of left adrenal gland from Patient A. B., removed eight months following transvenous adrenal destruction. Full-thickness cortical necrosis exists throughout, with organizing hemorrhage and prominent cholesterol clefts in the medulla. *B*, Lower pole of the same adrenal gland from Patient A. B. The small rounded nodule at the tip of the pole, on magnification, is a fragment of viable adrenal cortex. It is estimated that this represents less than 5% of the original functioning tissue in this gland. (Hematoxylin and eosin stain.)

later, the acid phosphatase level was 4.2 with an 0.28 prostatic fraction. He returned to full-time work for five months until two weeks prior to his final admission in December, 1972. At this time, he entered in hypercalcemic crisis. Efforts to decrease serum calciums were unsuccessful, and the patient died on Jan. 3, 1973. Postpermission was refused.

Case 4. A. C. (No. 38-19-08), a 52-year-old woman, underwent left radical mastectomy and irradiation in March, 1969. In October, 1971, a lytic lesion in the skull was irradiated. In August, 1972, she developed a pathologic fracture in the left ninth rib and a lesion in the right pelvis. Both areas were irradiated. Diethystilbesterol and Halotestin were unsuccessful in alleviating persistent bone pain. In November, 1972, new lesions were found in the calvarium, pelvis, and left femur, and in the second and fourth lumbar vertebrae, with severe lower back pain radiating to the left leg. She was at this time largely bedridden and unable to work. On November 9, 1972, the patient underwent a technically satisfactory transvenous adrenal destruction, followed by a benign course with two days of mild nausea and vomiting, a mild elevation in her white count, and marked improvement in her lower back and left leg pain. This symptomatic improvement lasted for six months, during which she was fully mobile, although x-ray films failed to show healing of her lumbar spine and pelvic metastases. In June, 1973, she re-entered with complaints of new bone pain in the left ribs and groin, and left arm swelling. At this time, she was given radiation therapy to her ribs and pelvis.

Case 5. J. B. (No. 30-78-05), a 69-year-old woman, underwent left radical mastectomy and radiotherapy. In 1968, metastatic disease to the fourth lumbar vertebra was treated by local irradiation and diethystilbesterol (5 mg. three times a day) with a good clinical response. In 1969, the patient had a left pleural effusion. In 1970, recurrent severe back pain and metastatic involvement of the second and third lumbar vertebrae was treated with local irradiation, with little response. A transphenoidal radiofrequency hypophysectomy was performed for intractable pain in 1971, without relief, but postoperative hormonal evaluation suggested that the hypophysectomy was incomplete. Since late 1971, the patient had difficulty in walking secondary to lower back pain radiating to both legs, frequent nausea, vomiting, and dypsnea. In March, 1972, a lytic lesion was seen in the skull and in the fifth lumbar vertebra. For over one year, the patient had been on cortisone. On November 14, 1972, the patient underwent a technically satisfactory transvenous adrenal destruction. She tolerated the procedure well, with nausea and vomiting for 48 hours after the procedure. She had no temperature elevations but did experience a brief leukocytosis. This depressed patient achieved no relief from her lower back pain. Over the next two months, she was readmitted twice for similar persistent back pain and general deterioration. An attempt to begin a multi-drug therapy course was halted because of leukopenia. She died in late January, 1973 at a chronic care hospital.

Case 6. G. D. (No. 39-55-30), a 55-year-old woman, underwent left radical mastectomy and irradiation in October, 1969. A chest wall recurrence was noted in April, 1971. She received additional radiation to her left chest wall, but after initial improvement, the skin lesions recurred. Estrogen therapy induced local flare-up, and combination chemotherapy was employed from January, 1972, until March, 1973, when the initial improvement disappeared. Halotestin was briefly tried with poor effect. A bone scan immediately prior to transvenous adrenal destruction suggested metastases in the sixth and seventh thoracic vertebrae and the right iliac crest. On April 5, 1973, the patient underwent technically satisfactory transvenous adrenal destruction, which she tolerated very well, suffering only one day of mild nausea and vomiting. Although her prominent left arm edema decreased for two weeks immediately following destruction, it slowly reaccumulated, and there has been no evidence of regression of the multiple nodules on her chest wall.

DISCUSSION

In both the preliminary canine experiments and this study, an effort was made to employ a solution for extravasation which would cause reproducible local tissue destruction. The known toxicity of extravasated constrast material is related to its marked degree of hypertonicity in relation to intracellular osmolarity and to its ability to induce widespread small vessel thrombosis. Cytotoxity of nitrogen mustard, mediated by its action on formed nucleic acids, is also direct and locally effective. Total mustard dosage, however, was only 50 percent of that usually given in systemic therapy. The infusion of beta 1-24 ACTH immediately before extravasation was given in an effort to stimulate the cortical cells to maximum metabolic activity and thus enhance their ischemic vulnerability. While technical problems did prevent adequate extravasation in the right adrenal gland of the patient in Case 1, bilateral catheterization of the adrenal veins, in experienced hands, is possible for between 90 and 95 percent of individuals. Failure rate will largely be determined by those in whom the right adrenal drainage is into a hepatic vein. However, adrenal atrophy, induced by prolonged steroid therapy, does make successful catheterization and extravasation more tedious.

These patients initially treated have included cases of metastatic carcinoma of the breast that are less amenable to hormonal manipulation: three patients with post-irradiation chest wall recurrences and five patients seen over one year after the diagnosis of metastatic breast carcinoma, all representing failures of drug therapy and radiotherapy.[4] While the two clinical responses seen in this series (Cases 3 and 4), are gratifying, they are in no way predictive of results that might be expected in the general population of patients with metastatic malignancy. Transvenous adrenal destruction was accomplished with satisfactorily low morbidity and is a procedure that is well tolerated by patients whose general debilitation would make major surgery formidable. Pain from the extravasation was characterized by most patients as moderate to severe, but lasting a short period of time. A period of 24 to 36 hours of nausea was common, but most patients were able to take clear liquids on the following day and had returned to normal diets by 48 hours. Such an interval of nausea is common after parenteral therapy with nitrogen mustard and may represent systemic absorption or the effects of drug which leaked back around the catheter into the vena cava. Paralytic ileus, while anticipated, was not seen. A transient leukocytosis was noted on the day after surgery, but no significant fevers or evidence of retroperitoneal bleeding, the major potential hazard, was noted. The pain had considerably lessened by the evening of the procedure, and pain medication was required only occasionally as early as the following day. Most patients not otherwise hampered by their disease could with reason be planned for discharge in four days.

While Fig. 1 demonstrates the dramatic drop in mean response to beta 1-24 ACTH stimulation after treatment, Table I is more informative of the true response patterns. If the first patient, in whom the procedure was technically unsatisfactory, is eliminated, it can be seen that four of five patients had little or no demonstrable adrenal function at six weeks after treatment. One of these (A. C.), has continued to show essentially no adrenal function at 30 weeks after treatment, while two others have had slight but demonstrable return of some adrenal function by the beta 1-24 ACTH stimulation test. Patients exhibiting flat stimulation tests at six weeks, without clinical responses, are probably doubtful candidates for surgical hormonal ablation. In this respect, patient E. S. did fail to respond to hypophysectomy after failure to respond to a transvenous adrenal destruction that appeared complete at six weeks. The clinical significance for remission of such slight returns of adrenal function as appeared at ten weeks in patients E. S. and H. N. is not clear and would require larger patient populations of more favorable prognosis. Such small glandular remnants as were found at autopsy in patient A. B. (Fig. 2) might result in detectable hormone levels on stimulation without affecting the malignancy at low basal outputs. Patient H. N.'s clinical and objective response was unaffected by the degree of functional recovery recorded. The profound and long-lasting reduction in adrenal function that technically satisfactory transvenous destruction is capable of achieving also raises the possibility of the use of this technique in pathologic conditions of the gland, such as the adrenal hyperplasia of the ectopic ACTH syndrome or Cushings' disease, in which exquisite sensitivity to venous infarction has already been documented.[5] Adrenal destruction in the management of widespread metastatic carcinoma of the prostate can induce objective remissions, although the duration of response in general is shorter than for patients with metastatic carcinoma of the breast.[2, 7, 10] This transience favors the use of the procedure with the least morbidity that is still effective. Transvenous adrenal destruction deserves further trial in this group.

REFERENCES

1. Bookstein, J. J., Conn, J., and Reuter, S. R.: Intra-adrenal hemorrhage as a complication of adrenal venography in primary aldosteronism, Radiology **90:** 778, 1968.
2. Butler, W. S., III, Grayhack, J. T., Ransom, C. I., and Scott, W. W.: Metabolic studies on the bilateral adrenalectomy patient, J. Urol. **70:** 657, 1953.
3. Eagan, R. T., and Page, M. I.: Adrenal insufficiency following bilateral adrenal venography, J. A. M. A. **215:** 115, 1971.
4. Eckles, N. E.: Sequence of therapy for metastatic breast cancer, in breast cancer, early and late, Chicago, Ill., 1970, Year Book Medical Publishers, p. 395.
5. Fellerman, H., Dalakos, T. G., and Streeten, D. H. P.: Remission of Cushing's syndrome after unilateral adrenal phlebography, Ann. Intern. Med. **73:** 585, 1970
6. Fisher, C. E., Turner, F. A., and Horton, R.: Remission of primary hyperaldosteronism after adrenal venography, New Eng. J. Med. **285:** 334, 1971.
7. Harrison, J. H., Thorn, G. W., and Jenkins, D.: Total adrenalectomy for reactivated carcinoma of the prostate, New Engl. J. Med. **248:** 86, 1953
8. Moore, F. D., Woodrow, S. I., Aliapoulios, M. A., and Wilson, R. E.: Carcinoma of the breast, New Engl. J. Med. **277:** 460, 1967.

9. Murphy, B. E. P.: Some studies of the protein binding of steroids and their application to the routine micro and ultramicro measurement of various steroids in body fluids by competitive protein-binding radioassay, J. Clin. Endocrinol. Metab. **27:** 973, 1967.
10. Murphy, G. P., Reynosos, G., Schooness, R., Gailani, S., Bourke, R., Kenny, G. M., Mirand, E. A., and Schalch, D. S.: Hypophysectomy and adrenalectomy for disseminated prostatic carcinoma, J. Urol. **105:** 817, 1971.
11. Zimmerman, C. E., Kettyle, W. M., Eisenberg, H. R., Spark, R., Rosoff, C. B., and Cohen, R. B.: Transvenous adrenalectomy, J. Surg. Res. **12:** 124, 1972.

Venoarterial bypass with a membrane oxygenator: Successful respiratory support in a woman following pulmonary hemorrhage secondary to renal failure

E. Lawrence Hanson, M.D.,* Philip A. Drinker, Ph.D., Hillary F. Don, M.D., Stephen H. Van Devanter, M.D., Jacques Bonnet-Eymard, M.D., *and* **Francis D. Moore, M.D.,** *Boston, Mass.*

A young woman, whose respiratory function was acutely compromised by pulmonary hemorrhage associated with glomerulonephritis in a transplanted kidney, was supported for 90 hours by using venoarterial bypass with a membrane oxygenator. This support permitted access to the airway for lavage and suction and made it possible to decrease the tidal volume, peak inspiratory pressure, and inspired oxygen concentration. The course of the patient on bypass illustrates the effects of relieving the lung of a large portion of its flow, and oxygenating the blood extracorporeally. The immediate increase in arterial oxygen content with the initiation of bypass may be due to several factors, acting singly or in combination: retrograde perfusion in the aorta by the oxygenator; an improved ventilation-perfusion relationship; or simply the increased oxygen content of the venous blood entering the lungs resulting from improved oxygenation of the lower body. The latter effect was documented and appears to have been the predominant mechanism in the improved oxygenation seen in this case. This experience also demonstrates recovery of the lungs following an acute episode of pulmonary hemorrhage. Once the cause of bleeding had been eliminated, systemic heparinzation necessary for bypass caused no further bleeding from the lungs and the lesion proved reversible.

From the Departments of Surgery, Anesthesia, and Division of Bioengineering, Harvard Medical School, Peter Bent Brigham Hospital, Boston, Mass.

A TYPE OF reversible pulmonary lesion is presented as an example of the acute, often lethal, respiratory diseases in which extracorporeal oxygenation can extend the limits of treatment and lead to long-term survival. The documentation of the course and response to treatment provide a basis to discuss the rationale for venoarterial pumping with oxygenation and its use in patients with pulmonary insufficiency.

This study was supported in part by a special fellowship from the National Heart and Lung Institute (ELH) and through background investigations under grants from the National Science Foundation, The John A. Hartford Foundation, Inc., the National Heart and Lung Institute, and a contract with the United States Army Medical Research and Development Command.

Accepted for publication Jan. 29, 1974.

*Present address: Upstate Medical Center, 750 E. Adams St., Syracuse, N. Y. 13210.

CASE REPORT

A 33-year-old woman was hospitalized with the chief complaints of hematuria and malaise, nine months following renal isografting from her identical twin. During the first week after her admission, biopsy specimen showed a recurrence of glomerulonephritis involving the transplanted kidney. This, together with progressive hemoptysis, presented a picture similar to that described by Goodpasture[3] in 1919.

Oxygen tensions in the arterial blood (Pa_{O_2})

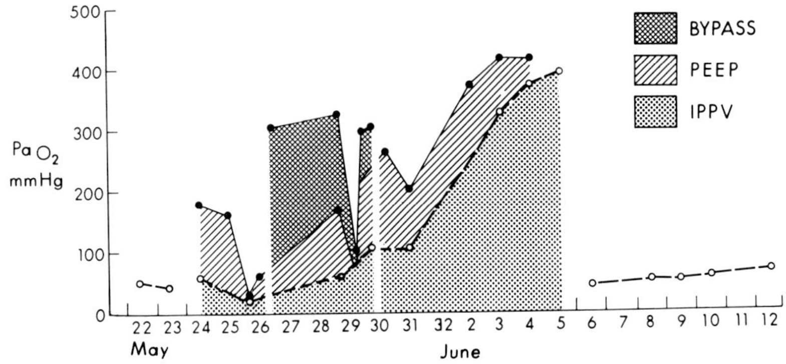

Fig. 1. Po_2 of arterial blood sampled from the left radial artery in test periods during the course of bypass showing the additive effects of PEEP and venoarterial bypass to IPPV. F_IO_2 was 1.0 for all samples except May 22-23 and June 6-12 when it was 0.21, and the patient was breathing without ventilator.

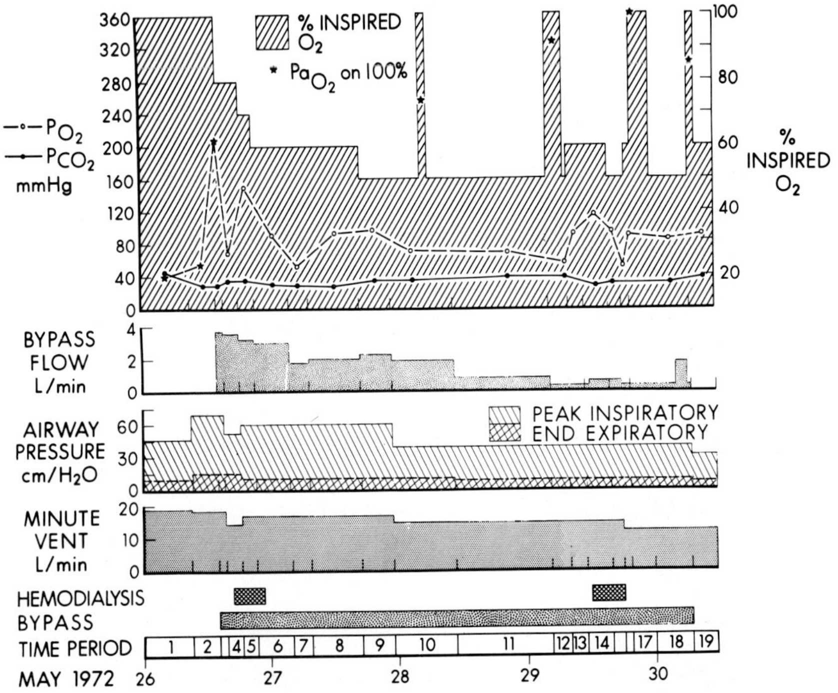

Fig. 2. Summary of the course of bypass illustrating the relationships of Pa_{O_2} and Pa_{CO_2} to changes in percent of inspired O_2 ventilation. Bypass flow is represented as the mean value for the fluctuations during the time period. The values of Pa_{O_2} during the tests at $F_IO_2 = 1$ are shown separately. The time Periods 1-19 were defined either as periods of relative stability, in which cases mean values are given, or to show isolated events.

before bypass are summarized in Fig. 1. At the start of mechanical ventilation (indicated by IPPV), the Pa_{O_2} on 100 percent oxygen ranged from 43 to 60 mm. Hg, increasing to 180 mm. Hg with the application of 5 cm. H_2O (PEEP). Over the next two days she had intermittent minor episodes of hemoptysis and finally, while being dialyzed, bled massively from the lungs. Removal of the kidneys stopped the bleeding immediately, but gas exchange continued to deteriorate.*

Post-operatively, during the first eight hours

*The details of this case prior to emergency nephrectomy will be reported elsewhere. Carpenter, C. B., et al.: In preparation.

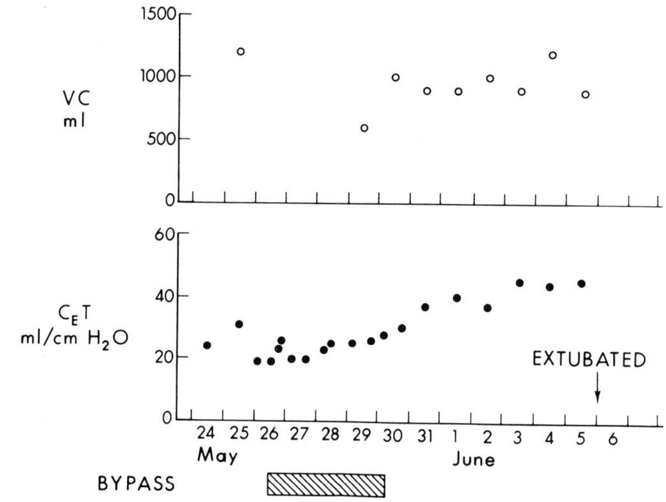

Fig. 3. Vital capacity (VC) and effective compliance of the total respiratory system before, during, and after bypass. Effective compliance is calculated as the ratio of tidal volume in milliliters to (PIP-PEEP), cm. H_2O.

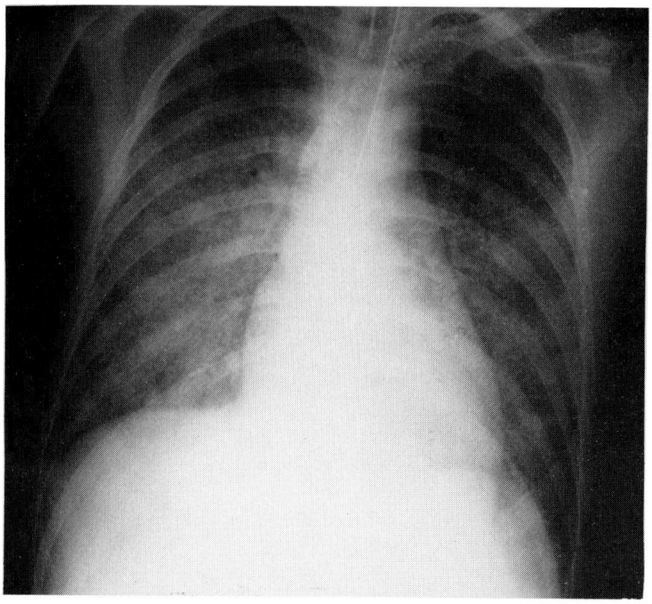

Fig. 4. Chest x-ray film taken the day bypass was started, showing the venous cannula with the tip in the inferior vena cava. Use of the right jugular would be preferred because it is more direct, but prior use of this site made the left-sided cannulation necessary, and it presented no problem.

(Fig. 2, Period 1), the mean blood pressure in the radial artery was 54 mm. Hg, the pulse 140 per minute; norepinephrine was infused at 4 to 8 μg per minute to support the circulation, while a total of 2 L. of blood was given. During this time, the Pa_{O_2} ranged from 31 to 45 mm. Hg at an F_IO_2 of 1.0, the Pa_{CO_2} ranged from 32 to 55 mm. Hg, and the pH ranged from 7.13 to 7.44. Severe peripheral cyanosis and hypotension indicated not only hypoxia but extreme circulation compromise. Suctioning of the airway through the endotracheal tube was hazardous because of immediate onset of cardiac arrhythmias which followed even brief interruption of mechanical ventilation.

With volume replacement, norepinephrine could be discontiued, and for the following five hours (Period 2) the mean blood pressure remained

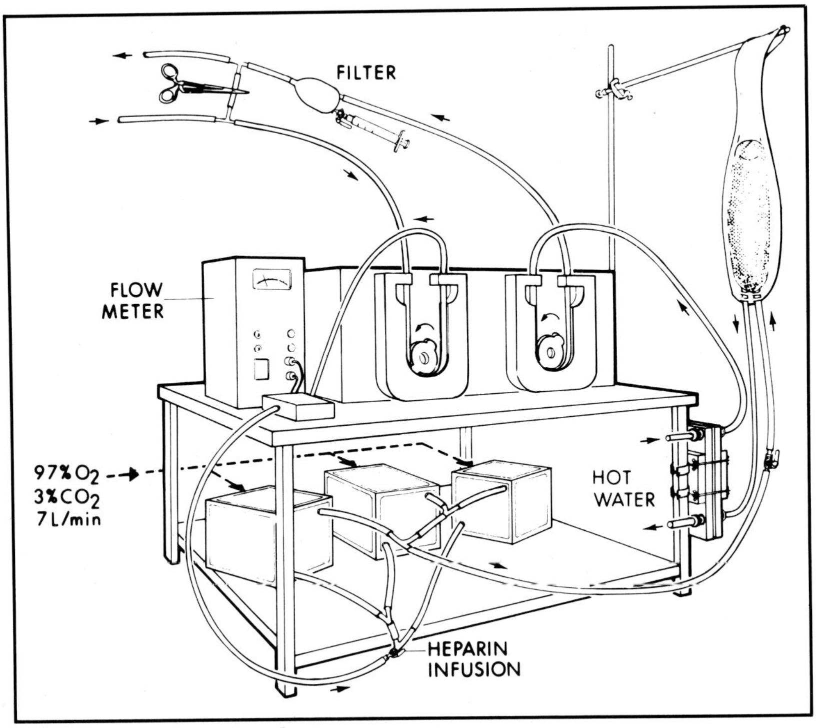

Fig. 5. Bypass circuit used in the perfusion. See text for details.

between 60 and 70 mm. Hg, and the pulse rate was 110 per minute. In spite of the improved hemodynamic status, respiratory condition continued to deteriorate. The tidal volume was raised to 1,100 ml. at a rate of 17 per minute and the PEEP was raised to 15 cm. H_2O, giving a PIP of 70 cm. H_2O. Effective compliance (Fig. 3) had fallen to 19 ml. per cm. H_2O. The Pa_{O_2} increased only minimally and ranged between 46 and 66 mm. Hg. Pa_{CO_2} ranged between 25 and 40 mm. Hg, and the pH ranged between 7.38 and 7.50. With these indications of the continuing severity of cardiopulmonary failure, the decision to proceed with bypass was affirmed, and the procedure was started 13 hours after the emergency nephrectomy.

Following heparin administration (200 units per kilogram, given intravenously) the venous cannula was inserted via the internal jugular vein into the inferior vena cava just below the right atrium (Fig. 4). The arterial cannulas were inserted proximally and distally into the left femoral artery in the groin, with provision for flow regulation in the distal cannula to maintain normal perfusion in the leg.

Three 3 M.[2] membrane lungs* were used in parallel in the circuit shown in Fig. 5. Oxygen with three percent CO_2 flowed into each oxygenator at 7 L. per minute. Blood from the patient was pumped through the oxygenators, collected in a collapsible reservoir, and returned through a heat exchanger* and filter† with the use of a second pump. Blood flow was monitored with an electromagnetic flowmeter.‡ The arterial pump was used throughout bypass, but the venous pump was required only for blood flows greater than 2 L. per minute.

The tubing was silicone rubber§ (3/8 inch internal diameter) connected by polycarbonate fittings|| and pumping chambers were of silicone tubing¶ with an internal diameter of 1/2 inch. The system was primed, after an initial saline rinse, with 1 L. of whole blood, 1 L. of normal saline, and 75 Gm. of salt-poor albumin.

When bypass was initiated, the flow was increased to the maximum obtainable, 4 L. per min-

*Lande-Edwards, Edwards Laboratories, Santa Ana, Calif.

*Travenol, Morton Grove, Ill.

†Johnson & Johnson, New Brunswick, N. J.

‡Statham Instruments, Oxnard, Calif.

§Dow Corning Corporation, Midland, Mich.

||Bentley Laboratories, Norwalk, Conn.; Cobe Laboratories, Lakewood, Colo.

¶Recently we have changed over to PVC tubing because of the observation that silicone tubing fatigues on the internal surface by sloughing, whereas in PVC, fatigue cracks start at the outside and are visible. (Hyans, T: Personal communication, Edwards Laboratories, Santa Ana, Calif.)

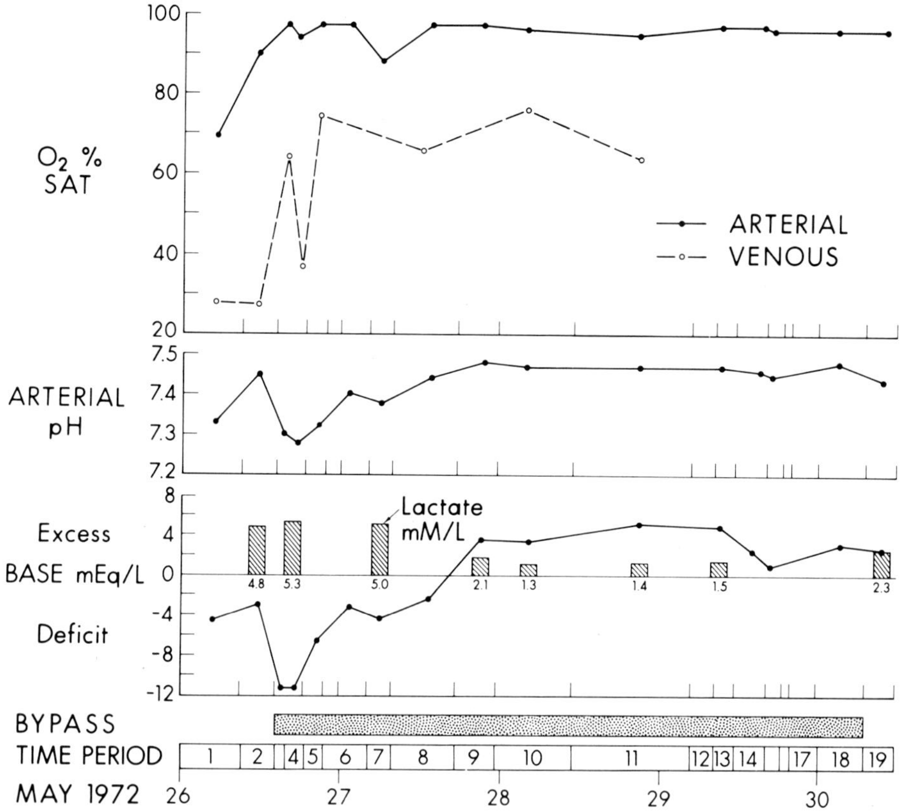

Fig. 6. The response to venoarterial bypass with oxygenation, of venous and arterial saturation, pH, base excess, and lactate are shown. The venous saturation is seen to be very dependent upon the lung ventilation (Period 4) as well as on the bypass flow.

ute (75 to 80 per cent of the estimated cardiac output). The patient's temperature was reduced from the prebypass level, 102.4° F., and was maintained at 97° F.

Over the first 30 minutes, the Pa_{O_2} (left radial artery) rose from 66 to 304 mm. Hg. Mean values for this time period are shown in Fig. 2, Period 3. This improvement in oxygenation made it possible to decrease the F_IO_2, but an attempt to decrease the tidal volume, thereby lowering the PIP, caused a marked fall in Pa_{O_2} (Fig. 2, Period 4). With increase in tidal volume, the Pa_{O_2} again rose, Period 5. The arterial and venous saturations in Fig. 6 indicate the return of A-V oxygen difference to normal. Except for the episode of inadequate ventilation during Period 4, the normal A-V O_2 difference was maintained.

During the initial seven to eight hours (Periods 3 to 5 in Fig. 2) improvement was rapid. The F_IO_2 was lowered from 1.0 to 0.7, and the PEEP was lowered from 15 to 10 cm. H_2O. It is of interest to note that even after 39 hours of bypass, the momentary reduction of PEEP from 8 cm. H_2O to 0 decreased Pa_{O_2} from 324 to 100 mm. Hg ($F_IO_2 = 1.0$) (Fig. 1).

Hemodialysis which had been carried out immediately prior to nephrectomy was repeated during this time with the use of hypertonic solution to expedite the removal of water. The forearm arteriovenous shunt had ceased to function, and the dialyzer was attached to sampling ports of the bypass circuit. This dialysis probably contributed to the rise of Pa_{O_2} noted during Period 5, which allowed a further decrease in F_IO_2 to 0.6.

With the initiation of bypass, mean arterial pressure rose from 75 to 100 mm. Hg. Volume shifts, when they occurred, were immediately reflected in the systolic pressure, while it was primarily the diastolic pressure which varied with changes in bypass flow rate.

Subsequent to this initial phase of rapid improvement, more gradual progress was seen over the next 54 hours (Periods 6 to 11, Fig. 2). During Period 7, failure of the venous pump caused the flow rate to fall from 3.0 to 1.2 L. per minute, at its lowest point. At this time, the Pa_{O_2} fell from 116 to a low of 37 mm. Hg. While the pump was being replaced, edema of the face was noted and the chest x-ray film indicated increased pulmonary water (Fig. 7). Five hundred

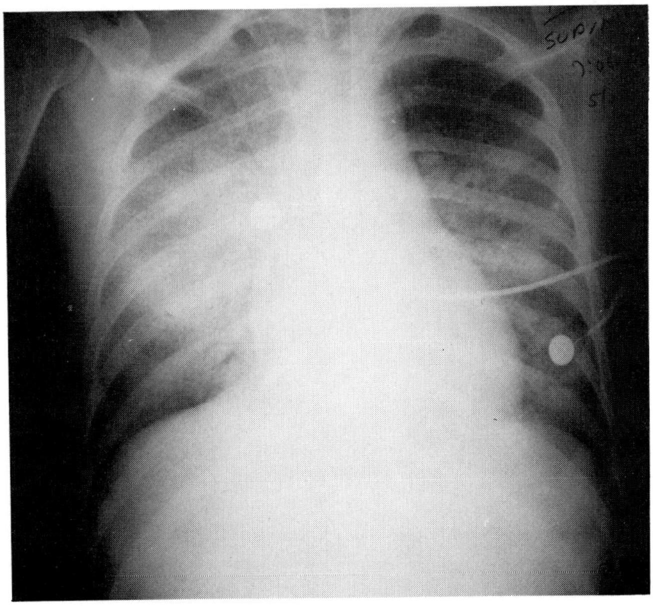

Fig. 7. Chest film taken when the venous pump was non-functional (Period 7) and the Pa_{O_2} had fallen, indicating the increased pulmonary interstitial fluid volume.

milliliters of blood were rapidly removed, and subsequently, with pumping capability regained, only a minimal increase in flow was necessary to restore the Pa_{O_2}. The blood removed was centrifuged and the packed cells reinfused. This plasmapheresis was continued intermittently throughout the bypass with a total of 3,500 ml. of whole blood removed and the cells replaced (Fig. 8).

Effective compliance (C_ET) of the total respiratory system increased from 19 to 25 ml. per centimeter of H_2O during the first seven hours of bypass (Fig. 3). This value fell transiently to 20 ml. per centimeter of H_2O the next day, associated with the episode of pulmonary edema. Vital capacity (Fig. 3) was 1,200 ml., 24 hours prior to bypass; when it could be next measured, on the third day of bypass, it was 600 ml.

Treatment applied to the lungs during bypass consisted of chest physiotherapy, turning the patient from side to side each hour, injecting saline (75 ml.) into the trachea, aspirating the material from the endotracheal tube, and postural drainage by lowering the head of the bed for 15 minutes each hour.

At the start of Period 10, with a further reduction in tidal volume and minute ventilation, the Pa_{O_2} remained at approximately 80 mm. Hg, while pH and base excess were normal. The lactate levels fell from the high values, 5 mM. per liter, associated with inadequate oxygen transport, to nearly normal levels of 1.4 mM. per liter (Fig. 6).

After 62 hours of bypass, the patient's cyanosis had cleared, and she was sufficiently improved to decrease the bypass flow to token levels. At this time, it is likely that bypass could have been terminated, but it was considered preferable to maintain the option of reinstituting pulmonary support if necessary for another day. Hemodialysis was repeated in this final phase (Periods 14 and 15) during which time the bypass flow was increased to permit adequate flow for the dialyzer.

Immediately prior to decannulation, with zero flow, Pa_{O_2} was 301 mm. Hg with an F_IO_2 of 1.0 and a PEEP of 8 cm. H_2O. The removal of PEEP caused a drop in Pa_{O_2} to 103 mm. Hg. At this time, the vital capacity was 1,000 ml., maximum inspiratory pressure achieved by the patient was –60 cm. H_2O, and effective total compliance was 29 ml. per centimeter of H_2O.

Throughout the entire 90 hour period, the patient was responsive and was able to communicate rationally after the first day. There was never any evidence of a neurologic deficit during or after bypass.

Cumulative fluid balance over the 90 hours of bypass is shown in Fig. 8 as the total fluid added and that removed by plasmapheresis and for samples. Fluid removed by the hypertonic dialysis could not be measured but was estimated at 2,000 ml. for each six hours of dialysis. Water loss through the membranes could account for an additional 1,000 ml. per day. The summary of known fluids administered and removed shows a balance in this anephric patient amounting to not

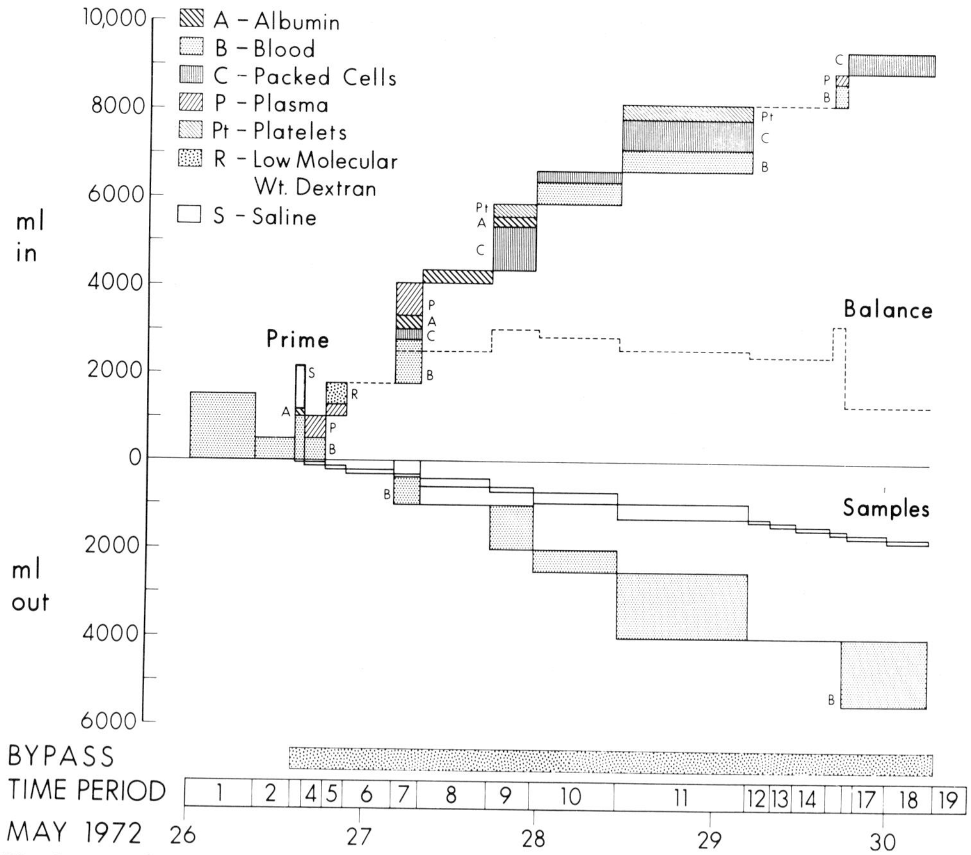

Fig. 8. The fluid balance is shown as measured intake and output with the difference represented by the dotted line. This balance does not include additional estimated losses (see text).

more than 450 ml. per 24 hours for the four days. The additional losses which can only be estimated would place her in a negative balance.

The average heparin dose given by continuous infusion was 25 U. per kilogram per hour and was regulated by using activated clotting times measured every 20 to 40 minutes.*

A fall in the platelet count from 350,000 to 10,500 per cubic millimeter during the first 24 hours on bypass was associated with bleeding from the surgical incisions and prompted platelet infusions; however, no pulmonary bleeding was seen. The platelet count remained at 20,000 per cubic millimeter for the remainder of the bypass. By the fourth day after bypass, the platelet count was 117,500 and by the tenth day it was 180,000. Blood-tinged gastric aspirate was noted early in the patient's course and was managed by instilling antacid into the stomach.

*The activated clotting time is a modification of Hattersley's[4] method using diatomite (Cellite Johns Mansville) in a test tube with 1 c.c. of whole blood, maintained at room temperature, and tipped every 30 seconds until a clot is observed. Normal, 90 seconds; anticoagulation for bypass, five to seven minutes.

Plasma hemoglobin levels, first measured after three hours of bypass, started at 30 mg. per 100 ml. and fell during the 90 hour period to 2 mg. per 100 ml., probably reflecting an initial loading caused by the prebypass transfusion.

Following the extracorporeal support, there was a period of six days during which the patient required continued mechanical ventilation. Periodic test of Pa_{O_2} on 100 percent oxygen showed improvement both with and without PEEP (Fig. 1). PEEP was maintained because it appeared to be of therapeutic benefit, maintaining the patency of terminal airways. After five days, PEEP was discontinued, and on the sixth day, the patient was extubated when she had shown stable gas exchange for periods of spontaneous ventilation. The Pa_{O_2} ($F_IO_2 = 1.0$) was 392 mm. Hg, vital capacity was 900 ml., and C_ET was 45 ml. per centimeter of H_2O (Fig. 3). Following extubation, she made further recovery of pulmonary function so that on the thirteenth day after bypass, her Pa_{O_2} on air was 71 mm. Hg. She was discharged from the hospital 11 days later, and she is currently being maintained in a chronic dialysis program.

DISCUSSION

Galletti[2] has described venoarterial pumping as a constant phlebotomy with continuous arterial infusion of oxygenated blood. This concise statement provides the basis for an intuitive understanding of the mechanics as well as the effects of partial heart lung bypass. The use of phlebotomy to relieve the effects of an excessive volume in the pulmonary circulation has been a common practice. Arterial infusion is a somewhat more controversial subject, but it appears to be of potential benefit by improving both perfusion and arterial oxygenation as demonstrated by the response of this patient to the start of bypass. The mechanism of this response, however, has not been explained. Why should the oxygen content of blood sampled from a radial artery be increased by perfusion of oxygenated blood into the femoral artery? Several mechanisms can be suggested: (1) retrograde flow of the oxygenator-return up the aorta, mixing with left ventricular output; (2) an improved relationship between ventilation and perfusion ($\dot{V}_A/\dot{Q}$) in the lung, for example by decreased pulmonary interstitial fluid volume; (3) increased pulmonary artery oxygen content caused by improved oxygenation of the lower body.

Considering the first of the three possibilities listed above, it seems reasonable that if cardiac output were sufficiently limited, the oxygenator flow could contribute to the perfusion of the upper extremities. Studies by Dow and associates[1] in animals and, more recently, by Hill and colleagues[5] suggest that only when bypass flow exceeds 70 percent of the cardiac output is mixing likely to occur in the arch of the aorta. Considering the broad A-V gradient before bypass was started (Fig. 6), which together with the patient's low blood pressure, is indicative of an extremely low cardiac output, it is quite likely that some of the initial rise in Pa_{O_2} was due to oxygenator flow in the aorta. This may well have been a transient effect until cardiac function improved on bypass.

Changes in ($\dot{V}_A/\dot{Q}$) and pulmonary shunt ($\dot{Q}_S/\dot{Q}_T$) cannot be documented without sampling from the left side of the heart because of the possibility of mixing in the aorta. In a patient treated a few months after this case,* who was in intractable heart failure following cardiac surgery, it was possible to determine shunt while on bypass because there was an indwelling left atrial catheter. In that case, a reduction in $\dot{Q}_S/\dot{Q}_T$ was seen immediately after the patient went on bypass. After 24 hours, however, with the onset of uncontrolled pulmonary hemorrhage (due to underlying gram-negative septicemia) the shunt increased to over 90 percent, and it was not possible to oxygenate the patient. Evidently if the lungs are sufficiently damaged, improvement in $\dot{V}_A/\dot{Q}$ is unlikely to occur and adequate support with partial bypass is difficult to achieve.[5] As with aortic mixing, it is possible that in this woman, some of the initial improvement in systemic oxygenation was due to an improved $\dot{V}_A/\dot{Q}$.

The final possibility, increased venous O_2 content, is documented in this patient, and may well have been the predominant factor in her initial improvement. By presenting the lungs with venous blood containing more oxygen, a higher O_2 content in the arterial blood would be expected, even if the gas transferred by the lungs did not increase.

The decision to intervene with bypass in this patient was based upon the clinical judgment that conventional modes of support had proved inadequate, and that death was imminent. The blood lactate levels, obtained by later analysis, were consistent with hemodynamic data and blood gases in showing a serious deficiency in O_2 transport and cardiac function. Although maximal ventilation during the prebypass period produced a slight increase in Pa_{O_2}, the $P\bar{v}_{O_2}$ remained low, indicating that she could not compensate for the insufficient oxygen supply by increasing her cardiac output.

*Don, H. F., Drinker, P. A., Hanson, E. L., et al.: The mechanisms of improvement in arterial oxygen during partial cardiopulmonary support: A case report. In press, J. A. M. A.

Following the initiation of bypass, arterial and venous oxygen saturations rose and the A-V oxygen difference narrowed. The pH and calculated base deficit dropped indicating elimination of acid metabolites from areas previously poorly perfused, presumably skin and muscle. This took longer than expected, but related temporally to the time required to restore pinkness and warmth to the extremities. It is probably fortunate that this "wash out" was gradual, since rapid mobilization of the total acid load could be detrimental.

Lavage, positioning of the patient, and removal of plasma were carried out during the bypass. The lavage and positioning were responsible for the removal of blood and material which had collected during hemorrhage. Possibly the most important effect of the bypass was that it allowed aggressive therapy to be undertaken, whereas previously the patient could not tolerate even short periods disconnected from the ventilator.

The decreased Pa_{O_2} which accompanied the temporary loss of the venous pump appeared to be associated with an increased volume of fluid in the lungs which was reflected in the chest x-ray film. In animal experiments, the same change has been observed and is associated with a rise in pulmonary arterial pressure. Its reversal with the collection of blood in the reservoir justified the removal of plasma in this case and suggests that the benefit derived may relate to a decrease in pulmonary blood volume.

The course of this patient also indicates that recent pulmonary hemorrhage is not an absolute contradiction to a bypass procedure. Thirteen hours after the lung had been hemorrhaging uncontrollably, heparin was used safely once the factors responsible for hemorrhage had been stopped.

The authors would like to acknowledge the work of the following members of the Bioengineering Division: Eleanor LaCava, Christian Stetz, and John L. Lehr, Ph.D.; the Staff Physicians: Karen Kagey, M.D., Richard E. Wilson, M.D., Jan Dmochowski, M.D., and Gordon Vineyard, M.D. We would also like to acknowledge the work of: Mrs. Helen Kordis and members of the Nursing Staff of the Bartlett Unit and Intensive Care Unit; the following Resident Physicians: Dwight Geha, M.D., Kathryn McGoldrick, M.D., and Alan R. Baker, M.D.; members of the Respiratory Therapy Team who functioned as assistant pump technicians; and the staff of the Surgical Research Laboratories directed by Miss Margaret R. Ball.

REFERENCES

1. Dow, J. W., Dickson, J. F., and Hamer, A. J.: Experimental evaluation of venoarterial pumping: A proposed technique for circulatory support, Dis. Chest **38:** 323, 1960.
2. Galletti, P. M.: Experimental heart-lung bypass and assisted circulation, Progr. Cardiovasc. Res. **11:** 312, 1969.
3. Goodpasture, E. W.: The significance of certain pulmonary lesions in relation to the etiology of influenza, Am. J. Med. Sci. **158:** 863, 1919.
4. Hattersley, P. G.: Activated coagulation time of whole blood, J. A. M. A. **196:** 150, 1966.
5. Hill, J. D., O'Brien, T. G., Murray, J. J., et al.: Prolonged extracorporeal oxygenation for acute post-traumatic respiratory failure (shock-lung syndrome): Use of the Bramson membrane lung, New Engl. J. Med. **286:** 629, 1972.

Ultrapore filter–induced thrombocytopenia*

Alfred S. Gervin, Major, MC, USA, Kenneth Mason, B.S., *Washington, D. C.,*
Tom Limbird, B.S., *and* **Donald Silver, M.D.,** *Durham, N. C.*

A new method for the production of acute thrombocytopenia in canines is presented. The passage of blood through ultrapore filters placed in the limbs of arteriovenous fistulas decreases platelet counts 95 percent and white blood cell counts 50 percent in four hours. Hematocrits are unaffected by this procedure. Pretreatment with aspirin (25 mg. per kilogram twice daily for five days) reduces the absolute degree of thrombocytopenia achieved (95 percent vs. 80 percent). Platelet counts in both groups return to normal values within 48 hours. Potential mechanisms for the removal of platelets by ultrapore filters are discussed and potential clinical applications are suggested.

From the Division of Surgery, Walter Reed Army Institute of Research, Walter Reed Army Medical Center, Washington, D. C., and the Department of Surgery, Duke University Medical Center, Durham, N. C.

EXPERIMENTAL thrombocytopenia may be produced by whole body irradiation,[8] antiplatelet antisera,[24] bone marrow suppression with antimetabolic drugs,[33] infusion of thromboplastic suspensions to produce intravascular coagulation,[1] adsorption to activated charcoal[11] or selective platelet plasmaphoresis.[21] These methods are time-consuming, complex and often alter the biochemistry and/or physiology of the experimental animal.

In 1969, a new method for the creation of thrombocytopenia in animals was introduced.[16] This procedure was based upon the observations of Hellem[15] that platelets have a marked affinity for glass beads. The method, consisting of the continuous passage of blood through columns of glass beads which had been inserted between the limbs of an arteriovenous (A-V) fistula, produced significant decreases in platelet counts in three to four hours. The thrombocytopenia thus produced was associated with minimal alterations in the physiologic state of the experimental animal. However, the commercial unavailability and difficulty in preparation of these specialized columns preclude widespread acceptance of this technique.

Recent observations on the effects of ultrapore filtration on platelets in fresh blood[14] suggest that commercially available ultrapore filters might be used to produce experimental thrombocytopenia.

METHODS

Healthy mongrel dogs of either sex, weighing 24 ± 2 kilograms, were anesthetized with intravenous pentobarbital (30 mg. per kilo-

Accepted for publication Dec. 13, 1973.

*"In conducting the research described in this report, the investigators adhered to the 'Guide for Laboratory Animal Facilities and Care,' as promulgated by the Committee on the Guide for Laboratory Animal Facilities and Care of the Institute of Laboratory Animal Resources, National Academy of Sciences—National Research Council."

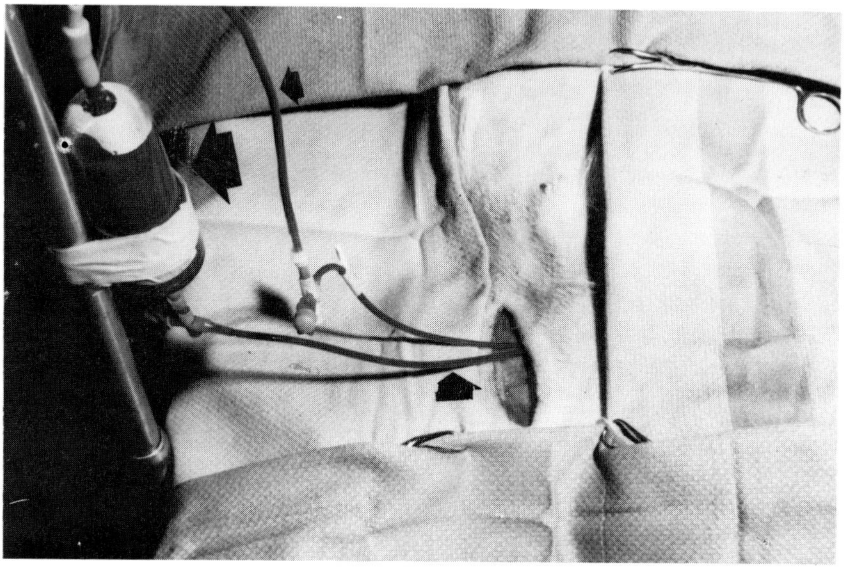

Fig. 1. The Dacron wool filter in position between the femoral artery and femoral vein. Small arrow identifies the femoral arterial cannula; medium arrow identifies the femoral venous cannula and large arrow identifies the Dacron wool filter. Head of the animal is to the top of the illustration.

gram). The femoral artery and vein were exposed and cannulated with No. 14 gauge catheters which were connected with silicone rubber tubing to form an A-V fistula. An initial dose of heparin* (100 U. per kilogram, given intravenously) was administered and supplemented with a second dose (50 U. per kilogram, given intravenously) given two hours after the onset of filtration. At the conclusion of the experiment, protamine sulfate (30 mg. per kilogram, given intravenously) was administered. Animals were randomly placed in one of four groups:

Group 1. Dacron wool filters,† primed with normal saline, were connected to the A-V fistula in ten dogs (Fig. 1). Blood flowed from the artery through the filter and back to the vein. Flow rates were determined by the cardiovascular status of the animals. Filters were changed hourly for four hours. The approximate time for filter change was 30 seconds. Hematocrits, platelet counts,[5] and white blood cell counts[4] were obtained before filtration, after administration of heparin, and at 1, 2, 3, 4, 24, and 48 hours. At the conclusion of four hours of filtration, whole blood clotting times,[18] partial thromboplastin times,[17] and thrombin times[27] were performed to determine the adequacy of heparinization. Filters were then removed, the A-V fistula was repaired, and protamine sulfate was administered.

Group 2. Eight control dogs underwent similar heparinization, creation of an A-V fistula, and neutralization of heparin. Dacron wool filters from which the filter elements had been removed were placed in the A-V fistula and changed hourly for four hours. Platelet counts, white blood cell counts, hematocritis, and coagulation studies were obtained as in Group 1.

Group 3. Eight animals were treated with aspirin (25 mg. per kilogram orally twice daily) for 5 days. A-V fistulae were then created and filters were inserted as in Group 1. Platelet counts, white blood cell counts, hematocrits, and coagulation studies were obtained as in Group 1.

Group 4. Four control animals were treated with aspirin as in Group 3. These animals underwent sham filtration as in

*Bovine Intestinal Heparin, 1,000 units/c.c., Upjohn Co., Kalamazoo, Mich. 49001.

†Swank, IL200, Pioneer Filters, Beaverton, Ore. 97005.

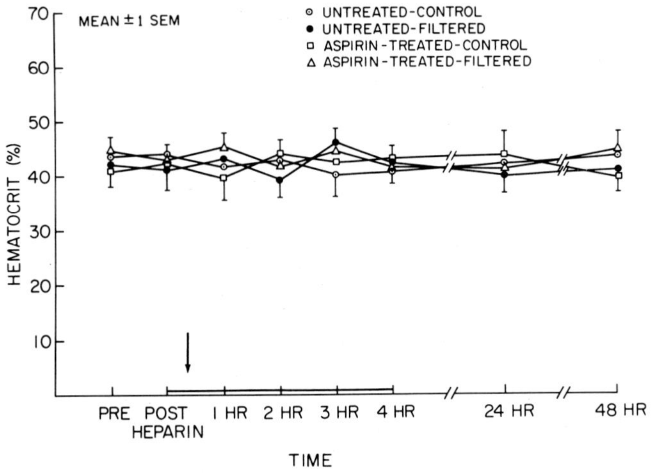

Fig. 2. Effect of ultrapore filtration on hematocrit. Arrow marks the onset of filtration. No changes occur.

Table I. *Statistical analysis*

	Group 1 vs. Group 2	*Group 3 vs. Group 4*	*Group 1 vs. Group 3*
Platelet count			
Preheparinization	NS	NS	NS
Postheparinization	NS	NS	NS
1 hr.	$p < 0.025$	$p < 0.05$	NS
2 hr.	$p < 0.001$	$p < 0.025$	NS
3 hr.	$p < 0.001$	$p < 0.001$	NS
4 hr.	$p < 0.001$	$p < 0.001$	NS
White blood cell count			
Preheparinization	NS	NS	NS
Postheparinization	NS	NS	NS
1 hr.	$p < 0.05$	$p < 0.05$	NS
2 hr.	$p < 0.05$	$p < 0.025$	NS
3 hr.	$p < 0.001$	$p < 0.025$	NS
4 hr.	$p < 0.001$	$p < 0.025$	NS

Group 2. The data are presented as mean values; standard errors of the mean were determined. The data were subjected to Student's nonpaired t test for statistical analysis.

RESULTS

The results are presented in Figs. 2, 3, and 4. All groups maintained constant hematocrits for the duration of the experiment (Fig. 2). As shown in Fig. 3, platelet counts decreased approximately 50 percent in all groups following administration of heparin. In the control groups, platelet counts returned to normal within three hours. In the filtered groups (Groups 1 and 3), platelet counts continued to decline. In Group 1, platelet counts decreased to 20 percent of control values following two hours, and 5 percent of control values following four hours of filtration. In Group 3 (aspirin treated), platelet counts decreased to 35 percent of control values after two hours and to 20 percent after four hours of filtration. Mean platelet counts after four hours of filtration were $15 \pm 5 \times 10^3$ per cubic millimeter in Group 1, $310 \pm 5 \times 10^3$ per cubic millimeter in Group 2, $60 \pm 1.5 \times 10^3$ per cubic millimeter in Group 3, and $295 \pm 6 \times 10^3$ per cubic millimeter in Group 4. In Groups 1 and 3, platelet counts returned to approximately 50 percent of control values after 24

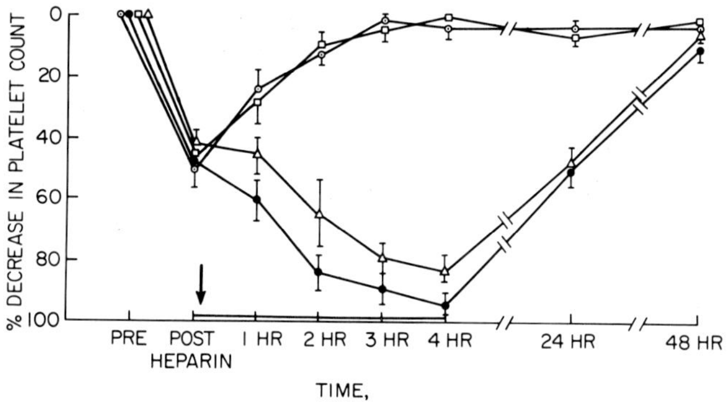

Fig. 3. The effect on the platelet count of passage of blood through Dacron wool filters. Arrow marks the onset of filtration. All platelet counts decrease following heparin administration. Values of control animals return to normal within two hours. Platelet counts decrease to five percent of original values in nontreated animals and 20 percent of original values in ASA-treated animals after four hours of filtration. Symbols: ⊙, Untreated control; ●, untreated, filtered; □, aspirin-treated control; △, aspirin-treated, filtered.

hours; at 48 hours the values had returned to prefiltration levels in all groups. Six days after filtration, a thrombocytosis of approximately twice control level was noted in several animals tested in each group.

In control animals, white blood cell counts were unchanged at one to four hours and at 24 hours (Fig. 4). Groups 1 and 3 displayed decreases in white blood cell counts of 43 and 28 percent, respectively, at one hour and 66 and 55 percent, respectively, at two hours. After two hours of filtration, white blood counts remained unchanged at approximately 50 percent of control values.

All animals were adequately anticoagulated as documented by whole blood clotting times of greater than 60 minutes, partial thromboplastin times greater than four times control times, and infinite thrombin times after four hours of filtration.

Statistical analyses are presented in Table I.

DISCUSSION

A new method for the production of experimental thrombocytopenia in animals is presented. This method, utilizing commercially available ultrapore filters, is inexpensive, convenient and effective. The versatility of the method permits a broad range of thrombocytopenia to be achieved; a desired degree of platelet reduction can be effected by simple variation of the filtration time.

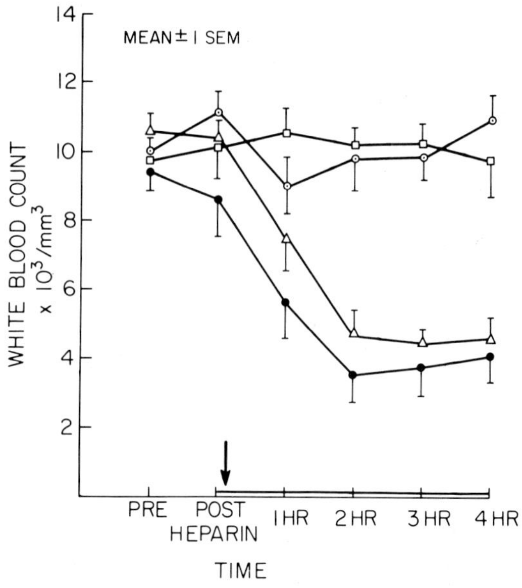

Fig. 4. The effect of ultrapore filtration on white blood counts. Arrow marks the onset of filtration. White blood counts in experimental groups decrease to 50% of control values in 2 hours—then remain unchanged. Symbols: ⊙, Untreated control; ●, untreated, filtered; □, aspirin-treated control; △, aspirin-treated, filtered. Each value is the mean ± S.E.M.

The expunction of platelets and white blood cells by Dacron wool filters is well known.[14, 25, 34] It is proposed that Dacron wool filters selectively remove platelets either by passively trapping the particles within the interstices of the filter or by providing a foreign surface to which the particles might adhere. The effective filtration size of the Dacron wool filter is reported to be approximately 10 to 15 μ[32]; particles smaller than 10 μ should pass through the filter undisturbed while larger particles should be readily retained. Since the canine platelet (1 to 3 μ)[30] is significantly smaller than the effective element size of the Dacron wool filter, the platelet must undergo some alteration of size or physiologic process if it is to be retained within the filter. Transient contact between the Dacron wool filter and the platelet could cause release of platelet procoagulants (adenosine diphosphate, platelet factor 3, serotonin, thrombin), which would then initiate the clumping of individual platelets. Platelet aggregates thus formed might have diameters in excess of 10 μ and be retained within the filter on a critical size basis.

Platelets actively adhere to many foreign substances[15, 20, 22, 28, 38] Dacron wool offers an appropriate surface to which healthy platelets could actively stick. The active adherence of one platelet might then initiate a series of platelet agglutinations on the filter similar to those observed in the early stages of hemostasis.[10] In this situation, the retention of platelets within the filter would depend upon the adhesiveness of the individual platelet or upon the ability of the platelet to release its procoagulant factors. Medications known to reduce platelet adhesiveness or block secondary platelet release would decrease the attraction of the platelet for the element and prevent the formation of platelet aggregates. Platelets would then pass unimpeded through the filter and the over-all effectiveness of the filter in producing thrombocytopenia would thus be reduced.

A further explanation for the removal of platelets during filtration might involve volume or size changes of the platelets during passage through the filter. Individual platelets could swell or change configuration so that their dimensions would be adequate for passive retention by the filter.

In this study, pretreatment with aspirin (an inhibitor of the platelet release phenomenon)[23, 36, 39] decreased the absolute levels of thrombocytopenia achieved after four hours of filtration (95 vs. 80 percent). However, these values were not significantly different ($p > 0.05$ but < 0.1). This suggests that the release of procoagulants by platelets with the formation of platelet aggregates is not a major mechanism of platelet removal by the filter. As aspirin does not inhibit the adhesion of platelets to foreign bodies,[13] one may assume that the adherence of individual platelets to the filter element may significantly contribute to the retention of platelets by the filter. Inspection of blood smears obtained during all phases of filtration revealed no significant changes in platelet dimensions.

The decrease in platelet counts following heparin infusion is an idiosyncracy of the canine species.[6, 12] In this series, all animals demonstrated a decrease in platelet count of approximately 50 percent in response to intravenously administered bovine intestinal heparin. Platelet counts in control animals returned to normal values within two hours. No animal manifested a further decrease in platelet count in response to the supplemental dose of heparin given at two hours. Because of species variation, caution must be exercised whenever applying data obtained from the experimental animals to the human. It is now known that many similarities and differences exist between the platelets of the human and those of the canine.[3, 9, 29, 35] The platelets of both species are similar quantitatively[7] and morphologically.[30] Differences occur, however, in the in vitro function of these platelets when aggregating agents are added to platelet-rich plasma. Canine and human platelets both respond with similar primary aggregation (measured by the turbidometric method of Born and Cross[2]) when aggregating agents, adenosine diphosphate (ADP) or epinephrine (EP), are employed. After primary aggregation, however, the canine platelet may undergo rapid deaggregation. The secondary wave of platelet aggregation occurs in both species in response to epinephrine but is more frequent in the human. Eighty percent of humans, but only 50 percent of canines, manifest secondary aggregation with ADP; epinephrine produces secondary aggregation in 80 percent of humans but only in 17 percent of canines. Higher concentrations of both agents are required (ADP, 0.25 to 10 vs. 5 to 10 μM; epinephrine, 0.005 to 10 vs. 100 μM) to produce this effect in the canine.[19] The secondary aggregation of the canine platelet often proceeds slowly and the aggregates formed undergo spontaneous deaggregation.

The platelets of both species aggregate when placed under glass slides and subjected to ADP, thrombin, and purified collagen. However, only human platelets aggregate in this situation with epinephrine, norepinephrine, or serotonin.

The preincubation of platelets with adenosine monophosphate (AMP) inhibits ADP aggregation in both species, although to a lesser extent in the canine.[31]

These findings suggest that, although the platelets of the human and the canine are not identical in all respects, sufficient similarities exist such that the data obtained from the canine model may well be applicable to the human. Reports of reduction of platelet number following the passage of fresh human blood through ultrapore filters[14, 22, 25] further strengthen the suggestion that similar mechanisms may exist in the human situation. Thus, this method may have promise as a therapeutic modality in patients in whom the reduction of elevated platelet counts (with increased probability of cerebral vascular accidents or intravascular thrombosis) or the reduction of elevated white blood cell counts is desired. The greatest degree of absolute thrombocytopenia can be achieved if aspirin or other platelet inhibiting medications[26, 37] are avoided.

A new method for the acute production of thrombocytopenia in animals is presented. The method is inexpensive, uncomplicated, and effective in decreasing platelet counts. The techniques for the use of this method are described and potential clinical applications are suggested.

REFERENCES

1. Adelson, E., Rheingold, J. J., Parker, O.: Platelet and fibrinogen sequestration, Blood **15:** 596, 1960.
2. Born, G. V., and Cross, M. J.: Aggregation of blood platelets, J. Physiol. **168:** 178, 1963.
3. Born, G. V., and Cross, M. J.: Effect of adenosine diphosphate on concentration of platelets in the blood, Nature **197:** 974, 1963.
4. Berkson, J., Magath, T., and Burn, J.: Error of estimate of blood cell counts as made with the hemocytometer, Am. J. Physiol. **128:** 309, 1940.
5. Brecher, G., and Cronkite, E. P.: Morphology and enumeration of human blood platelets, J. Appl. Physiol. **3:** 365, 1950.
6. Copley, A. L., and Robb, T. P.: Effect of heparin *in vivo* on the platelet count of mice and dogs, Am. J. Clin. Pathol. **12:** 416, 1942.
7. Copley, A. L., and Robb, T. P.: Studies on platelets. I. The method of Vilarino and imentel and a new direct method of counting blood platelets, Am. J. Clin. Pathol. **12:** 362, 1942.
8. Cronkite, E. P.: Induction of thrombocytopenia in mammals by ionizing radiation, *in* Blood coagulation, hemorrhage and thrombosis, New York, 1964, Grune & Stratton, Inc., p. 62.
9. Cuthbertson, W. F., and Mills, D. C.: Some factors influencing platelet clumping, J. Physiol. **169:** 9, 1963.
10. Deykin, D.: Thrombogenesis, New Engl. J. Med. **276:** 622, 1967.
11. Dutton, R. C., Dedrick, R. L., and Bull, B. S.: A simple technique for experimental production of acute platelet deficiency, Thromb. Diath. Haemorrh. **21:** 367, 1969.
12. Fidler, C., and Jacques, L. B.: Effect of commercial heparin on platelet counts, J. Lab. Clin. Med. **33:** 1410, 1948.
13. George, J. N.: Direct assessment of platelet adhesion to glass, Blood **40:** 862, 1973.
14. Gervin, A. S., Limbird, T. J., Pucket, C. L., and Silver, D.: The effects of ultrapore hemofiltration on the coagulation and fibrinolytic mechanisms in fresh and stored blood, Arch. Surg. **106:** 33, 1973.
15. Hellem, A.: The adhesiveness of human platelets in vitro, Scand. J. Clin. Lab. Invest. **12:** 1, 1960.
16. Kraytman, M.: A simple method for the

induction of acute thrombocytopenia, J. Lab. Clin. Med. **73:** 350, 1969.

17. Langdell, R., Wagner, R., Brinkhous, K.: Determination of partial thromboplastin time, *in:* Blood coagulation, hemorrhage and thrombosis, New York, 1964, Grune & Stratton, Inc., p. 103.
18. Lee, R. I., and White, P. D.: A clinical study of coagulation time of blood, Am. J. Med. Sci. **145:** 495, 1913.
19. MacMillan, M. R., and Sim, A. K.: Comparative study of platelet aggregation in man and laboratory animals, Thromb. Diath. Haemorrh. **24:** 385, 1970.
20. Mason, R. G.: Simple test for quantitation of platelet adhesion to glass, Thromb. Diath. Haemorr. **25:** 21, 1971.
21. Matter, A. J., Hartman, J. R., DeMarsh, Q. B., and Finch, C. A.: A study of thrombopoesis in induced acute thrombocytopenia, Blood **15:** 174, 1960.
22. Moolten, D.: Adhesiveness of blood platelets in thromboembolism, Am. J. Clin. Pathol. **19:** 701, 1949.
23. O'Brien, J. R.: Effect of salicylates on human platelets, Lancet **1:** 779, 1968.
24. Odell, T. T., McDonald, T. P., and Detwiler, T. C.: Stimulation of platelet production by serum of platelet-depleted rats, Proc. Soc. Exp. Biol. **108:** 428, 1961.
25. Osborn, J. J., Swank, R. L., Hill, J. D., et al.: Clinical use of Dacron wool filters during perfusion for open-heart surgery, J. Thorac. Cardiovasc. Surg. **69:** 575, 1970.
26. Packham, M. A., and Mustard, J.: Platelet reactions, Semin. Hematol. **8:** 30, 1971.
27. Peder, J., and Brecher, G.: Thrombin time, *in:* Blood coagulation, hemorrhage and thrombosis, New York, 1964, Grune & Stratton, Inc., p. 333.
28. Salzman, E. W.: A measure of platelet adhesiveness, J. Lab. Clin. Med. **62:** 724, 1963.
29. Salzman, E. W., Chambers, D. A., and Nevi, L. L.: Possible mechanisms of aggregation of blood platelets by adenosine diphosphate, Nature **210:** 167, 196.
30. Schalm, O. W.: Veterinary hematology, Philadelphia, 1965, Lea & Febiger, Publishers, pp. 193, 210.
31. Sinakos, Z., and Coen, J. P.: Platelet aggregation in mammalians: A comparative study, Thromb. Diath. Haemorrh. **17:** 99, 1967.
32. Solis, R. T., and Gibbs, M.: Filtration of microaggregates in stored blood, Transfusion **12:** 240, 1972.
33. Spector, B.: *In vivo* transfer of a thrombopoetic factor, Proc. Soc. Exp. Biol. **108:** 146, 1961.
34. Swank, R. L.: Alteration of blood on storage: Measurement of ageing of platelets and leukocytes and their removal filtration, New Engl. J. Med. **265:** 728, 1961.
35. Tocantins, L. M.: The mammalian platelet in health and disease, Medicine **17:** 155, 1938.
36. Weiss, H.: Effect of salicylates on hemostatic properties of man, J. Clin. Invest. **47:** 2164, 1968.
37. Weiss, H.: Pharmacology of platelet inhibition, *in* Spaet, T., editor: Progress in hemostasis and thrombosis, New York, 1972, Grune & Stratton, Inc., pp. 199-221.
38. Wright, H.: Adhesiveness of platelets in normal subjects, J. Pathol. Anat. **53:** 255, 1941.
39. Zucker, M. B., and Peterson, J.: Inhibition of adenosine diphosphate-induced secondary aggregation and other platelet functions by acetylsalicylic acid ingestion, Proc. Soc. Exp. Biol. **127:** 547, 1968.

Chronic salt-loading of donor and recipient in renal transplantation

Sherman Jay Silber, M.D., *Melbourne, Australia*

Chronic salt-loading is known to protect rats from glycerol-induced hemaglobinuric renal failure. Experiments with transplantation in salt-drinking and H_2O-drinking rats demonstrated that chronic salt-loading of both donor and recipient are necessary to protect against acute tubular necrosis from transplant ischemia time. Plasma volume expansion at the last minute will not provide this protection from renal failure. It appears, however, that a kidney so protected and given glycerol cannot tolerate the added ischemic insult of a transplant. Chronic increase in salt intake, insofar as it does not produce dangerous hypertension, may be useful for patients undergoing elective major renal vascular procedures.

From the Section of Urology, Department of Surgery, University of Michigan Medical Center, Ann Arbor, Mich.

UNTIL RECENTLY, there was very poor understanding of the pathophysiology or prevention of acute renal failure. Severe acute tubular necrosis can be produced in normal rats by injecting 50 percent glycerol to induce hemoglobinuria. However, in rats chronically receiving one percent NaCl instead of tap water, glycerol produces a much milder renal failure which completely clears within 24 hours.[3] This salt protection is *not* due to blood volume expansion, since transfusing the water-drinking rats to a comparable blood volume as the salt-drinking rats just prior to glycerol injection has no protective effect.

Plasma renin activity has been shown to be elevated in the oliguric phase of acute renal failure.[2] It is speculated, therefore, that renin plays a potent role in the development of acute renal failure, and that chronic saline loading protects against it by depleting the body of renin.

Accepted for publication July 18, 1973.

Current address: Department of Surgery, University of Melbourne, Melbourne, Australia.

Oken's group has shown through elaborate micropuncture studies that in acute renal failure, there is an almost complete cessation of glomerular filtration.[4, 8, 9] The majority of surface nephrons are initially collapsed, and no tubular obstruction or disruption was noted in studies of the early recovery phase.[5] In short, they found that acute tubular necrosis was not really a tubular entity at all, but rather resulted from renal ischemia and a protracted afferent arteriolar constriction with resultant loss of glomerular filtration. In chronic salt-drinking rats, the cessation of glomerular filtration (GFR) after glycerol injection was transient, and GFR returned to 75 percent of normal value within 12 hours.[7]

In humans, similarly, Hollenberg and associates[1] have shown through xenon washout studies that acute tubular necrosis results from decreased renal cortical perfusion and sustained preglomerular vasoconstriction, producing a cessation in glomerular filtration.[1]

With this improved understanding of acute

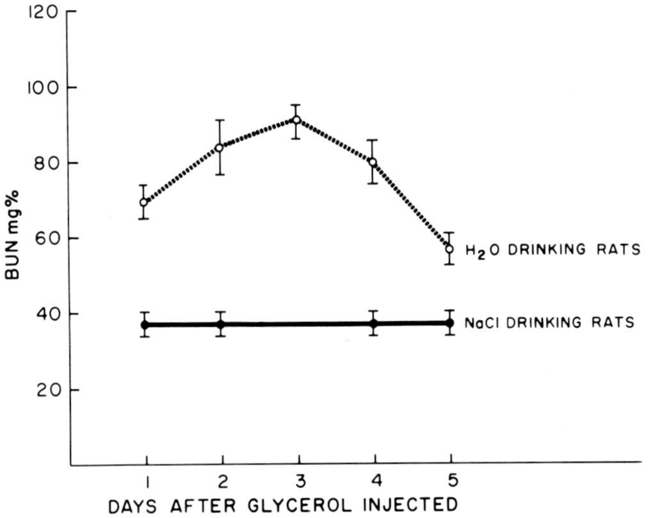

Fig. 1. Glycerol given but no transplant: H_2O-drinking rats all developed renal failure after glycerol injection, but NaCl-drinking rats were protected.

renal failure and its experimental prevention, we have been interested in determining the following:

In renal transplantation, is it more important to chronically salt load the donor or the recipient; or are they of equal importance? The answer to this question will be of considerable theoretical importance because it will tell us whether saline loading protects the kidney from renal failure through some *intrinsic* intrarenal mechanism, or whether it protects the kidney by way of an *extrinsic* effect upon the host.

Can a kidney challenged with glycerol but protected from acute failure by salt-loading tolerate the added insult of a transplant ischemia time and function in a suitably protected host?

METHOD

Isogeneic female Lewis rats weighing approximately 250 Gm. each were divided into two groups, one of which received tap water only to drink, and the other one percent NaCl. They were kept in the laboratory under these conditions for two months before any studies were carried out. A standard rat chow was provided (Na = 200 mEq. per kilogram; K = 185 mEq. per kilogram. The method of Silber and Crudup[6] was used for all transplants and has been described previously.

The animals were subdivided into the following experimental groups of five each.

Controls. A group of salt-drinking and H_2O-drinking rats were each injected with 50 percent glycerol I.M., 10 ml. per kilogram and followed daily for 5 days for BUN levels. They were then sacrificed and the kidneys examined histologically.

Transplantation with glycerol.

Group 1. A group of salt-drinking rats had glycerol injected as described, and one hour later their kidneys were transplanted into H_2O-drinking rats whose own kidneys were then removed.

Group 2. A group of H_2O-drinking rats had glycerol injected, and one hour later their kidneys were transplanted into NaCl-drinking rats whose own kidneys were then removed.

Group 3. A group of NaCl-drinking rats had glycerol injected, and one hour later their kidneys were transplanted into other NaCl-drinking rats whose own kidneys were then removed.

Ischemia times for rats in Groups 1, 2, and 3 were less than 45 minutes, and previous studies have shown minimal renal failure to occur postoperatively.[9]

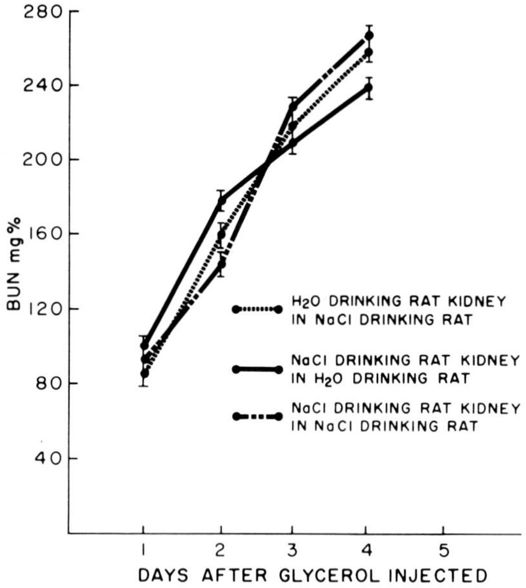

Fig. 2. Transplant one hour after donor was given glycerol: Kidneys from glycerol-injected rat donors, with or without salt protection, developed severe failure.

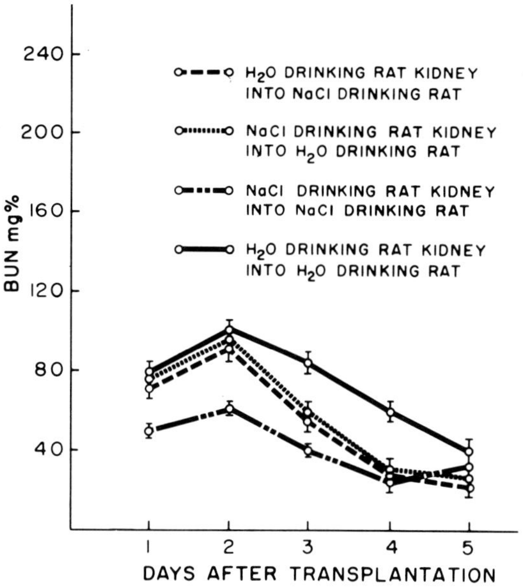

Fig. 3. No glycerol given: Only kidneys from NaCl-drinking donors and transplanted into NaCl-drinking recipients had maximal protection from ischemic renal failure.

Transplantation without glycerol. Without any glycerol injection one group of NaCl-drinking rats underwent bilateral nephrectomy and received kidney transplants from H_2O-drinking rats, and the other from rats that were also NaCl-drinkers. One group of H_2O-drinking rats similarly received kidneys from NaCl-drinking rats, and the other from rats that were also H_2O-drinkers. The ischemia time was intentionally standardized at 1½ hours in these rats.

All animals were followed with daily BUN till death or 5 days post transplant.

RESULTS

As Fig. 1 demonstrates, after glycerol injection, the blood urea nitrogen (BUN) level rose rapidly in H_2O-drinking rats but hardly changed in the salt-drinkers ($p < 0.001$). As in Fig. 2, regardless of whether donor or recipient rats were chronically salt-loaded, glycerol-induced renal failure in the transplanted kidney could not be prevented. In fact, the kidneys of the salt-protected donors, which would not have developed renal failure if left alone, did so after transplantation, regardless of whether or not the recipient too was salt-protected.

As in Fig. 3, without glycerol injection, ischemia from the transplantation caused mild renal failure in the salt-drinking rats who received kidneys from H_2O-drinkers and in H_2O-drinking rats who received kidneys from NaCl-drinking donors. The most sustained rise in the postoperative BUN level was seen when kidneys from H_2O-drinkers were transplanted into other H_2O-drinkers. Only the NaCl-drinking recipients who received kidneys from other NaCl-drinking donors had a normal postoperative BUN ($p < 0.01$).

Fig. 4 demonstrates the typical *histologic* picture of acute tubular necrosis seen in glycerol-injected rats, whether salt-protected or not.

DISCUSSION

These studies demonstrate that chronic salt-loading protects against acute renal failure in the rat by a combination of an intrinsic effect on the kidney and an extrinsic effect on the host. Only salt-loaded rats

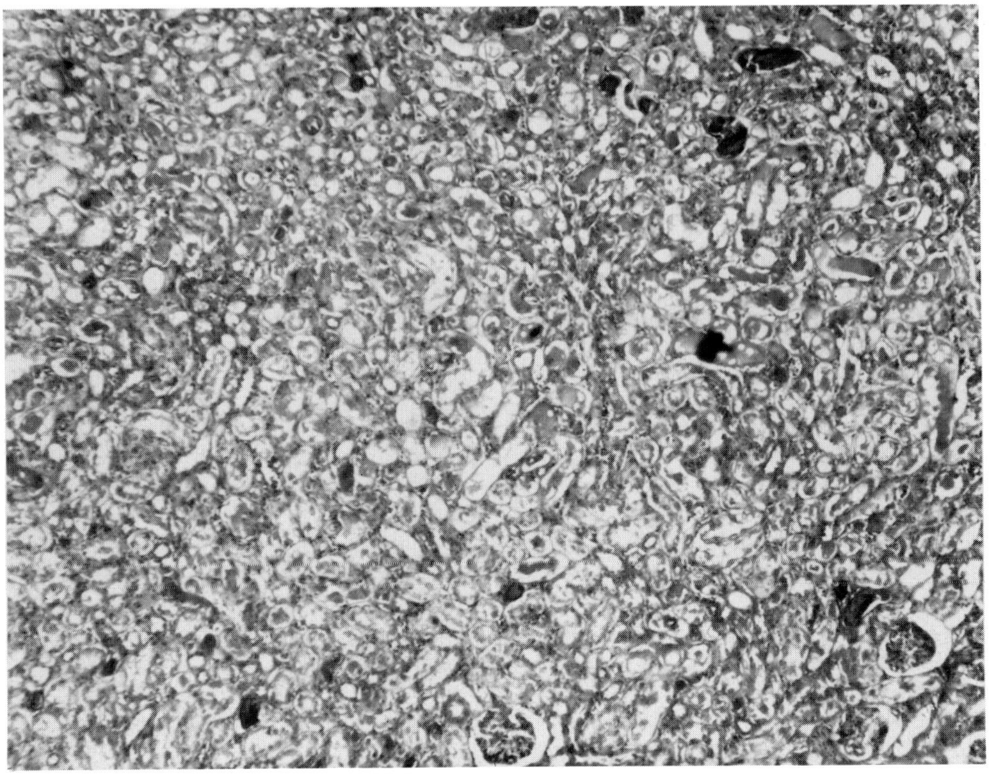

Fig. 4. Histology of glycerol-injected rat kidneys.

which received kidneys from other salt-loaded rats were fully protected from the ischemic time encountered in the transplantation process. If any human correlation can be made, it seems clear that last-minute plasma volume expansion in the dehydrated transplant recipient-to-be is not likely to prevent acute tubular necrosis. Many dialysis patients are intentionally dehydrated to allow better blood pressure control. It might be wise to start increasing their sodium intake several weeks to a month prior to the expected transplant, if acute tubular necrosis is to be avoided. In addition, in related transplants, though the problem is much less frequent, it might be wise to increase the salt intake of the donor a month in advance.

We cannot rule out the possibility of successfully transplanting a kidney already in acute tubular necrosis. However, we can see that even in a salt-protected rat injected with glycerol, which otherwise would have been protected from renal failure, the added insult of transplantation into another salt-protected host produced severe renal failure. Again, if any clinical correlation can be inferred, a severely ischemic kidney may not tolerate the added insult of a transplant procedure, whether or not the host is adequately salt-loaded.

It is ironic that patients undergoing renal revascularization procedures often are salt-depleted to help control their hypertension. If a difficult procedure is contemplated, with a prolonged ischemia time, it would be wise to increase salt intake as much as is safely possible for a month before the operation.

REFERENCES

1. Hollenberg, N. K., Adams, D. F., Oken, D. E., et al.: Acute renal failure due to nephroxins, N. Engl. J. Med. **282:** 1329, 1970.
2. Kokot, F., and Kuska, J.: Plasma renin activity in acute renal insufficiency, Nephron **131:** 115, 1969.
3. McDonald, F. D., Thiel, G., Wilson, D. R., et al.: The prevention of acute renal failure

in the rat by long-term saline loading: A possible role of the renin angiotensin axis, Proc. Soc. Exp. Biol. Med. **131:** 610, 1969.
4. Oken, D. E., Arce, M. L., and Wilson, D. R.: Glycerol-induced hemoglobinuric acute renal failure in the rat. I. Micropuncture study of the development of oliguria, J. Clin. Invest. **45:** 724, 1966.
5. Oken, D. E., DiBona, G. F., and McDonald, F. D.: Micropuncture studies of the recovery phase of myohemoglobinuric acute renal failure in the rat, J. Clin. Invest. **49:** 730, 1970.
6. Silber, S. J., and Crudup, J.: Kidney transplantation in inbred rats, Am. J. Surg. **125:** 551, 1973.
7. Thiel, G., McDonald, F. D., and Oken, D. E.: Micropuncture studies of the basis for protection of renin-depleted rats from glycerol-induced acute renal failure, Nephron **7:** 67, 1970.
8. Wilson, D. R., Thiel, G., Arce, M. L., et al.: Glycerol-induced hemoglobinuric acute renal failure in the rat. III. Micropuncture study of the effects of mannitol and isotonic saline on individual nephron function, Nephron **4:** 337, 1967.
9. Wilson, D. R., Thiel, G., Arce, M. L., et al.: The role of the concentration mechanism in the development of acute renal failure, Nephron **6:** 128, 1969.

Hazards of surgical treatment due to microorganisms in the bile

M. R. B. Keighley, D. M. Lister, S. I. Jacobs, *and* G. R. Giles, *Leeds, England*

The occurrence of microorganisms in the bile at the time of operation has been recorded from 150 cases. Positive cultures were invariably present in patients requiring emergency cholecystectomy and in 90 percent of patients with stones in the common bile duct who were jaundiced at the time of operation. The incidence of infected bile in subjects undergoing elective surgery for cholelithiasis, but who were not jaundiced was only 17 percent. The importance of these bacteria as a cause of postoperative morbidity was also studied. Wound sepsis was twice as common when surgery was undertaken in the presence of bacteria in the bile. Infective complications were doubled when the common bile duct was explored as a result of microorganisms isolated in the T tube after operation. In addition to local sepsis, bacteremia, caused by organisms previously cultured from the bile, was an additional hazard in ten patients after operation. This occurred most often after cholangiography. There were three cases presenting with endotoxic shock, two of which accounted for the only deaths in this study.

From the University Department of Surgery and Microbiology, Leeds (St. James') University Hospital, Leeds, England

For many years, biliary tract operations have been known to be attended by a high incidence of infective sequelae.[2, 9, 20] The relationship of microorganisms in the biliary tract to postoperative infection has not been extensively studied.[14, 22] The purpose of this report is to assess the clinical and pathological significance of bacteria in the bile among patients requiring surgical treatment. The incidence of these organisms and their relationship to postoperative morbidity is recorded from 150 consecutive patients requiring biliary tract surgery.

MATERIALS AND METHODS

During the course of this prospective study, samples of bile were obtained at operation from the gallbladder and common bile duct. Later, cultures were also taken from the gallbladder wall, liver, and duodenum. To identify the presence of bacteria in the bile after operation, samples were collected from the T tube on the fifth postoperative day. It has been routine practice to decompress the biliary tract with a T tube in every patient requiring choledochotomy.

Species were submitted for immediate aerobic and anaerobic culture. Samples were inoculated at 37° C. for 48 hours on blood agar and McConkey plates. Anaerobiosis was obtained by flushing with hydrogen in the presence of a cold catalyst. Quantitative results were obtained by inoculating culture plates with serial dilutions of bile in thioglycollate broth. Bacteria were identified by colonial and biochemical tests. In a small number of cases with positive bile cultures and *E. coli* bacteremia, colicine

Accepted for publication July 24, 1973.

Table I. *Incidence of bacteria in the biliary tract at operation*

Clinical situation	No. of cases	Positive bile cultures No.	Positive bile cultures Percent
Emergency cholecystectomy	11	11	100
Elective operations	139	38	27
a) Jaundiced patients	30	20	67
Malignant obstruction	12	4	25
Calculous disease	18	16	90
b) Remainder	109	18	17
Total No. of cases	150	49	33

Table II. *Organisms from the T tube drainage after choledochotomy and their relation to positive bile cultures at operation*

Procedure and findings	No.	Organisms in the bile: At operation No.	At operation Percent	From the T tube drainage No.	From the T tube drainage Percent
Procedure:					
Choledochotomy with T tube drainage	41	23	56	31	75
Findings:					
Same organisms at both sites		18		18	58
Identical cultures				11	36
Additional organisms in the T tube				7	22
Different organisms at both sites		5		5	16
Sterile bile at operation		—		8	26

and serological typing were also used for precise identification of the particular microorganism.

Clinical infection occurring during the postoperative period was confirmed by bacteriological study. Routine blood cultures were also taken on the fifth postoperative day, within 24 hours of T tube cholangiography, and in any patient with an unexplained pyrexia after operation.

RESULTS

Organisms in the biliary tract. The overall incidence of positive cultures in the bile at operation was 33 percent (Table I). Where acute cholecystectomy for suspected perforation of the gall bladder was indicated, the biliary tract was always infected. There was a much higher incidence of organisms in the bile among jaundiced patients requiring elective operation (67 percent) than in the remainder (17 percent). In the former group, pathogens were much more common in the presence of calculi (90 percent) than in patients with malignant obstruction (25 percent).

Exploration of the common bile duct with T tube drainage was performed in 41 patients. In 23 of these cases, positive cultures were obtained at operation. By the fifth postoperative day, however, as many as 31 bile samples had become infected (Table II). Despite the incidence of bacteria at operation in these patients, there were only 11 cases (36 percent) in which identical organisms were found in the T tube.

Quantitative studies have confirmed the pathological significance of positive bile cultures. Bacterial counts have all been between 10^5 and 10^9 organisms per milliliter, except in three early cases where error occurred from dilution when samples were taken after operative cholangiography. When organisms were cultured from multiple sites, those bacteria found in the bile were also isolated throughout the biliary tract. This work is the subject of a separate report.

Infective postoperative complications. In-

Table III. *Complications in relation to infected bile at operation*

Infective complications	*No. of patients*	*Percent with sterile bile (101 cases)*	*Percent with positive bile cultures (49 cases)*
Total No.	65	41	49 (83)*
Complications:			
Wound sepsis	32	18	36 (90)
Respiratory infection	29	23	12 (66)
Urinary infection	13	8	10 (80)
Bacteremia	19	6	6 (100)

*Numbers in parentheses refer to percentage of infective complications resulting from the same organism as found in the bile.

Table IV. *Complications after choledochotomy with T tube drainage*

Infective complications (%)	*Choledochotomy with T tube drainage (%) (41 patients)*	*Remainder (%) (101 patients)*
Overall: 43	64	35
Wound sepsis	40	15
Respiratory infection	10	18
Urinary infection	4	9
Bacteremia	17	2

Table VA. *The importance of bacteria in the T tube in the occurrence of infective complications*

		Postoperative infection due to the same organism in the bile	
Bacteria in the bile	*No.*	*No.*	*Percent*
At operation	23	12	46
From the T tube	31	26	100

fective complications occurred in as many as 65 patients (43 percent). These were only marginally more common when surgery was performed in the presence of biliary tract organisms (Table III). When postoperative infection occurred, however, microorganisms in the bile were responsible for the majority of these sequelae. Infected bile at the time of surgery was certainly related to a high incidence of wound sepsis after operation.

Table IV shows that infective complications were nearly twice as common after choledochotomy with T tube drainage. Exploration of the common bile duct was attended by a high incidence of wound sepsis and bacteremia. Organisms cultured from the bile at the time of operation were responsible for postoperative infection in only half of these patients. Cultures from the T tube, however, were far more important in the etiology of infective sequelae (Tables VA and VB). Sepsis in the postoperative period occurred only in the presence of bacteria in the T tube. In the instances in which the contents of the T tube were sterile, these events did not occur.

Positive blood cultures were obtained in ten patients after surgery or direct radiology on the biliary tract. There were seven cases of bacteremia attending choledochotomy. In each case, identical cultures were obtained from the T tube and in many of these patients sterile bile had been found at operation (Table VI).

T tube cholangiography performed at a time when the bile was infected was considered to be responsible for five of the seven cases of bacteremia after choledochotomy. Positive cultures from the bloodstream were isolated within 24 hours of cholangiography in these cases. Severe septicemia and fatal endotoxic shock occurred in two patients with bacterbilia who underwent transhepatic cholangiography. In each case, these events were unquestionably the result of organisms isolated in the bile. There was one case in which operative cholangiography performed

Table VB

Bacteria in the T tube	No.	Infective complications		No infection	
		No.	Percent	No.	Percent
Organisms found	31	26	84	5	16
No organisms found	10	—	—	10	100

Table VI. *Cases of bacteremia in relation to surgical treatment*

Blood cultures	Bile from T tube	Bile at operation	Cholangiography	Clinical findings	Mortality
1. *E. coli**	*E. coli*	Sterile	After T tube cholangiography	Endotoxic shock and renal failure	—
2. *Klebsiella aerogenes*	*Klebsiella aerogenes*	*E. coli*	After T tube cholangiography	Rigors	—
3. *E. coli*	*E. coli*	Sterile	After T tube cholangiography	No symptoms	—
4. *E. coli*	*E. coli* *Streptococcus faecalis*	Sterile	After T tube cholangiography	Rigors	—
5. *E. coli*	*E. coli*	*E. coli*	After T tube cholangiography	No symptoms	—
6. *Pseudomonas pyocyanea*	*Pseudomonas pyocyanea*	*Pseudomonas pyocyanea*	No relation to cholangiography	Rigors	—
7. *E. coli*†*	*E. coli*	Sterile	No relation to cholangiography	Endotoxic shock and renal failure	Died
8. *Klebsiella aerogenes*	No drainage†	*Klebsiella aerogenes*	After operative cholangiography	Febrile	—
9. *E. coli*†*	*E. coli*	*E. coli*	After transhepatic cholangiography	Endotoxic shock and renal failure	Died
10. "Coli"	No drainage†	"Coli"	After transhepatic cholangiography	Febrile	—

*Cases where colicine and serotyping was used to identify the organism.

†Exploration of the common bile duct with T tube drainage not performed.

in the presence of infected bile was thought to be responsible for positive blood cultures in the early postoperative period.

Bacteremia presented as endotoxic shock in three patients. In each case, this was complicated by renal failure, from which two patients died. There were no other deaths in this survey.

DISCUSSION

This study has demonstrated the hazards of surgery performed in the presence of microorganisms in the bile. Wound sepsis is particularly common in these patients. The association between infective bile and local complications in the wound has also been reported elsewhere.[14] Patients who are particularly prone to these sequelae during elective surgery are those who are jaundiced at the time of operation. Bacteria appear to be much more commonly found in the bile when jaundice is due to stones rather than malignant obstruction.[9, 18]

When exploration of the common bile duct is also necessary, infective complications are at least twice as common. This is not only due to a higher incidence of bacteria in the bile at the time of operation. In our experience, local and distant infection after choledochotomy is directly related to the incidence of bacteria in the T tube after surgery. Organisms isolated in the bile at the time of operation were responsible for only a third of patients with infected T tube bile. Despite a closed drainage system, therefore, it is possible that bacteria may occur as a result of outside contamination. It is conceivable that the T tube, as a foreign body, acts as a means of potentiating infection from organisms which would not normally multiply in the presence of free drainage. The role of latent L forms in the bile under these circumstances is being investigated. When bile which has been sterile at the time of operation later becomes infected following T tube decompression, this usually has occurred by the fourth postoperative day. Once bacteria become established in the T tube, the bile remains infected throughout the period of drainage.

The majority of infective complications consisted of wound sepsis and respiratory infection, but there were ten cases of bacteremia occurring in relation to surgical treatment. It is significant that identical cultures were isolated from the bile and the bloodstream in every patient with proven bacteremia. Colicine and serotyping has confirmed that the same organism was present in both sites in three patients with *E. coli* septicemia. There was a close correlation between positive blood cultures and cholangiography. It is conceivable that any form of cholangiography performed in patients with infected bile may be complicated by bacteremia or even fatal endotoxic shock.[13]

Local wound sepsis is probably due to contamination by infected bile, particularly when drains and T tubes are used through the abdominal incision. Distant infection on the other hand is almost certainly the result of bacteremia following ascending biliary infection. Asymptomatic bacteremia has been demonstrated on at least two occasions during this study. Evidence that bloodstream spread can occur from the biliary tract has been shown both anatomically and by cholangiovenous reflux at cholangiography.[7, 10] There were two patients with *E. coli* urinary tract infections after surgery which were shown to be of biliary origin on the basis of serotyping. It is not unreasonable to assume that these events are the result of transient bacteremia from infected bile.

It could be argued that these sequelae would be reduced if routine T tube drainage were not used. It has been shown elsewhere that the incidence of infective complications and the duration of hospital stay is reduced when direct suture of the common bile duct is undertaken.[5] The use of routine transduodenal exploration has been advocated by others for the same reason.[4, 11] On the other hand, the dangers of pancreatitis after this procedure appear to be considerable.[12]

It has been argued that routine antibiotic therapy might effectively sterilize the bile prior to surgical treatment, thereby reducing the incidence of local and distant infection. The value of various agents as a prophylaxis against these events has been studied.[1, 3, 15, 17] There are many who advise antibiotic cover routinely before transhepatic cholangiography in jaundiced patients[16, 21] and the avoidance of this procedure, if an antecedent history of cholangitis is obtained.[6] We have shown that the hazards of systemic infection are particularly common in patients with biliary obstruction. It is in these high-risk cases, however, that the biliary excretion of antibiotics is probably ineffective.[18] From a group of 30 patients in whom tetracycline (100 mg., given intramuscularly four hours before operation) was randomly allocated, the incidence of bacterbilia was not reduced.

Although this is the subject of further study, present evidence suggests that routine antibiotic cover does not sterilize the bile, particularly in the presence of obstruction. These agents, therefore, probably do not protect against local infective complications, even though they may play a part in preventing bacteremia in the presence of adequate serum antibiotic concentrations.

We wish to thank the following for their cooperation in this study: D. B. Feather, N. G. Graham, W. G. Harris, D. Pratt, and G. Wilson.

REFERENCES

1. Ancocella, G., Mattiussi, R., Nichols, F. B., Pallanza, R., and Fenconi, L. T.: Biliary ex-

cretion of antibiotics in man, Gut **9:** 536, 1968.

2. Bartlett, M. K., and Quinby, W. C.: Surgery of the biliary tract: Mortality and complications of cholecystectomy and choledochostomy for chronic cholecystitis, New Engl. J. Med. **254:** 155, 1956.
3. Bevan, P. G., and Williams, S. J. D.: Rifamide in acute cholecystitis, Br. Med. J. **III:** 284, 1971.
4. Carter, A. E.: Kocher's periampullary approach for common bile duct calculi, Br. J. Surg. **60:** 117, 1973.
5. Collins, P. G., Redwood, C. R. M., and Wynne-Jones, G. Primary closure of the common bile duct, Br. J. Surg. **47:** 661, 1960.
6. Dodd, G. R.: Percutaneous transhepatic cholangiography, Surg. Clin. N. Am. **47:** 1095, 1967.
7. Edlund, Y. A., and Hanzon, V.: Demonstration of the close relationship between bile capillaries and sinusoids walls, Acta Anat. **17:** 105, 1953.
8. Edlund, Y. A., Mollstedt, B. O., and Ouchterlony, O.: Bacteriological investigation of the biliary system and liver in biliary tract disease correlated to clinical data and micro structure of the gall bladder and liver, Acta Chir. Scand. **116:** 461, 1958.
9. Hight, D., Lingley, J. R., and Hurtubise, F.: An evaluation of operative cholangiography as a guide to common duct exploration, Ann. Surg. **150:** 1086, 1959.
10. Hultborn, A., Jacobson, B., and Rosengren, B.: Cholangio-venous reflux during cholangiography—an experimental and clinical study, Acta. Chir. Scand. **123:** 111, 1962.
11. Hunter, R. R.: Choledochometry and transduodenal sphincterotomy, Ann. R. Coll. Surg. Engl. **51:** 250, 1972.
12. Keighley, M. R. B., and Graham, N. G.: The aetiology and prevention of pancreatitis following biliary tract operations, Br. J. Surg. **60:** 149, 1973.
13. Keighley, M. R. B., Wilson, G., and Kelly, J. P.: Fatal endotoxic shock of biliary tract origin complicating trans-hepatic cholangiography, Br. Med. J. **3:** 147, 1973.
14. Larmi, T. K. I., Fock, G., and Yuopio, P.: Occurrence and antibiotic sensitivity of aerobic bacteria in the bile and their role in postoperative inflammatory complications in biliary tract diseases, Acta Chir. Scand. **117:** 379, 1958.
15. Mortimer, P. R., Mackie, D. B., and Haynes, S.: Ampicillin levels in human bile in the presence of biliary tract disease, Br. Med. J. **III:** 88, 1969.
16. Ritchie, G. W., Jackson, D. C., and Eaglesham, H.: Percutaneous transhepatic cholangiography—experience with 54 cases, Can. Med. Assoc. J. **100:** 110, 1969.
17. Sales, J. E. L., Sutcliffe, M., and O'Grady, F.: Cephalexin levels in human bile in the presence of biliary tract disease, Br. Med. J. **II:** 441, 1972.
18. Scott, A. J.: Bacteria and diseases of the biliary tract, Gut **12:** 487, 1971.
19. Scott, A. J., and Khan, G. A.: Origin of bacteria in bile duct bile, Lancet **II:** 790, 1967.
20. Swedburg, J.: Routine cholangiography at operation for gall stones, Acta Chir. Scand. **103:** 175, 1952.
21. Turner, F. W., and Costopoulos, L. B.: Percutaneous transhepatic cholangiography: A study of 115 cases, Can. Med. Assoc. J. **99:** 513, 1968.
22. Waton, J. R.: The role of bacterial infection in acute cholecystitis—a prospective clinical study, Milit. Med. **134:** 416, 1969.

Venous drainage of the ischemic kidney

Richard Brodman, M.D., William W. Pfaff, M.D., Birdwell Finlayson, M.D., *and*
Raymond L. Hackett, M.D., *Gainesville, Fla.*

Following 90 minutes of renal ischemia, gravity-drained venous blood is reduced in quantity, dilution by extravascular fluid is lessened and fluid is retained in the kidney. Venous potassium content is elevated to 14 to 20 mEq. per liter and reflects interstitial concentrations. Volume alterations may represent initiation of an immediate edematous response to this form of injury. Potassium concentrations of the observed range are sufficient to induce smooth muscle contraction and may play a role in post-ischemia malperfusion.

From the Departments of Surgery and Pathology, University of Florida College of Medicine, Gainesville, Fla.

In the intact, normally perfused animal, the renal venous blood differs little in non-gaseous constituents from arterial blood. In contrast, venous electrolyte concentrations are significantly altered with cessation of arterial inflow. Studying the gravity-drained venous effluent of the resected kidney, Swann and associates[3, 4] noted dilution of the cellular elements, lesser concentrations of protein, and increased levels of potassium, chloride, phosphate, and urea. On the basis of his investigations, he concluded that the source of this hyperkalemic, hypoproteinemic fluid was the interstitial space. When the concentrations of the vascular fluid were known, the gravity-drained venous blood could be analyzed to gain information as to the constituents of the interstitial space under a variety of circumstances. This model with modifications has been used in this study to reveal alterations in venous effluent composition following renal ischemia.

This work was supported in part by the John A. Hartford Foundation, Inc.

Accepted for publication Jan. 29, 1974.

Address all correspondence to: W. W. Pfaff, M.D., Department of Surgery, University of Florida, Gainesville, Fla. 32610.

MATERIALS AND METHODS

Fasted male and female mongrel dogs, weighing 15 to 25 kilograms, were anesthetized with sodium pentobarbital (30 mg. per kilogram), and a femoral artery cannula was advanced into the abdominal aorta. The animal was placed in a prone position and through extraperitoneal flank incisions, the right and left kidneys were freed of surrounding attachments including complete dissection of the main renal artery and vein. Following a 30 minute period for stabilization, the left renal artery was doubly clamped for 90 minutes in five animals. In five other animals, the left renal artery and vein were occluded. During the period of left renal ischemia, the right renal hilar structures were doubly clamped and the kidney was immediately excised, rapidly weighed, placed on a wire platform, and suspended over a beaker containing 500 U.

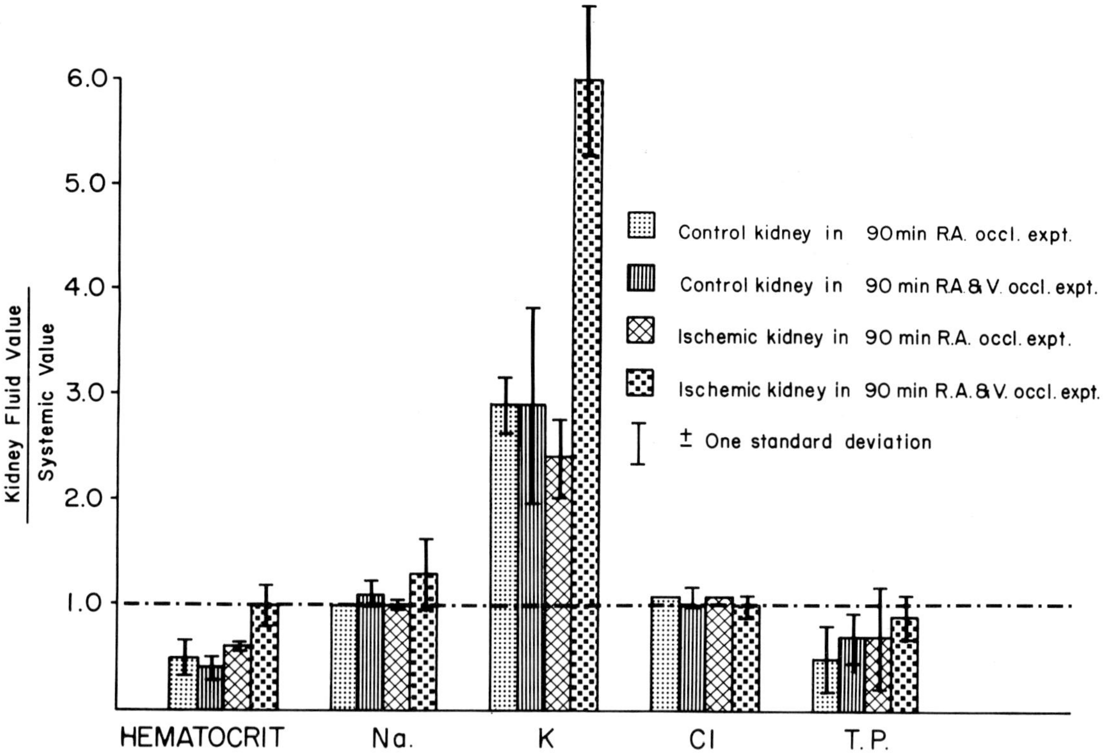

Fig. 1. Relative composition of kidney fluid.

Table I. *Kidney weight plus kidney fluid volume*

	90 minutes of occlusion of left renal artery		*90 minutes of occlusion of left renal artery and vein*	
	Left kidney (Mean)	*Right kidney (Mean)*	*Left kidney (Mean)*	*Right kidney (Mean)*
Weight of distended kidney (Gm.)	63.1 44–88*	62.4 34–94	63.2 48–80	62.7 49–76
Weight of drained kidney (Gm.)	55.8 36–79	44.8 28–61	55.6 ± 4.7†	46.6 ± 3.3
Volume of kidney fluid (c.c.)	8.4 2–14	17.8 4–30	6.3 ± 0.8	15.8 ± 2.0
Kidney fluid (c.c./100 Gm. of kidney)	12.1 ± 2.6	28.4 ± 2.4	9.9 ± 1.0	24.9 ± 1.4

*Ranges are rounded to 2 significant figures.

†Standard deviation given in instances when P < 0.01.

of heparin in 0.5 ml. The renal vein was incised and allowed to drain for five minutes. This differs from Swann's protocol in which drainage was maintained for 15 minutes. The kidney was then reweighed, stripped of its capsule and perihilar fat, and weighed again. The left kidney was handled in a similar manner after 90 minutes of ischemia without resuming perfusion of the organ. Venous fluid was analyzed for volume, hematocrit, total protein, sodium, potassium, and chloride.

In describing the venous effluent, Swann's[3] nomenclature is utilized. "Kidney fluid" is the total volume collected by gravity drainage; "diluting fluid" is that portion of the kidney fluid identified by dilution of the cellular elements and assumed to reflect vol-

Table II. *Volume and composition of diluting fluid*

	90 minutes of occlusion of left renal artery		90 minutes of occlusion of left renal artery and vein	
	Left kidney	*Right kidney*	*Left kidney*	*Right kidney*
Volume				
Diluting fluid (c.c./100 Gm. of kidney)	4.3	15	0	13.9
Composition				
Na (mEq./L.)	150	140	—	166
K (mEq./L.)	15.6	20	—	14.5
Cl (mEq./L.)	141	138	—	134
T.P. (Gm. %)	2.9	0.7	—	3.1

umes added from extravascular compartments as determined by change in the concentration of the formed elements.

RESULTS

Initial renal weights revealed no significant difference between right and left kidneys (Table I). Following drainage of the venous tree, the volume collected was greater from the right kidneys (control) when compared to the left kidneys that had been occluded for 90 minutes ($P < 0.01$).

Kidney fluid drained from the right kidney ranged from 24.9 to 28.5 percent of the distended kidney weight. Following arterial occlusion, the drained fluid varied from 8.2 to 22.1 percent of the distended weight and differed from individual controlled kidneys ($P < 0.01$). After occlusion of the artery *and* vein for 90 minutes, the kidney fluid weight was 7.2 to 13 percent of the distended kidney mass ($P < 0.001$).

The composition of drained kidney fluid relative to arterial blood values are presented in Fig. 1. The kidney fluid hematocrit in control kidneys averaged 43 percent of systemic values and differs from Swann's value (63 percent). Control kidney effluent potassium concentration was 2.9 times systemic concentrations, whereas the ratio in Swann's[3] experiment was 1.8 and again reflects greater dilution by non-cellular fluid in our study.

Following pedicle occlusion, higher elevation of potassium levels was noted. The ratio to systemic values was 6.0, and the absolute values ranged from 15.6 to 21.1 mEq. per liter with a mean value of 20.5 mEq. per liter. When compared with control values, there is a highly significant change in potassium concentration ($P < 0.001$).

Composition of diluting fluid (Table II), the cell-free additive to the vascular compartment, was computed by identifying the plasma component with the use of hematocrit reduction and subtracting the calculated plasma volume from the observed total volume of drainage. It was then possible to estimate the concentrations of the constituents of the interstitial fluid that had entered the vascular compartment.[3] There is no recorded diluting fluid from kidneys in which artery and vein were occluded, as no net dilution of the formed elements was recorded. In control kidneys, the diluting fluid potassium was fourfold systemic arterial levels (Fig. 2). A slightly lower level was calculated from data derived from ischemic kidneys.

Red blood cell potassium concentrations were similar in all experiments, eliminating this potential source of plasma potassium hyperconcentration. In addition, there was no significant variation in red cell mean corpuscular volume or in the degree of hemolysis in the specimens.

DISCUSSION

The volume of gravity-drained venous effluent is reduced following 90 minutes of arterial occlusion. Escape into the intact venous channel during occlusion did not occur, as control and experimental kidney weights were identical. Rather, there was

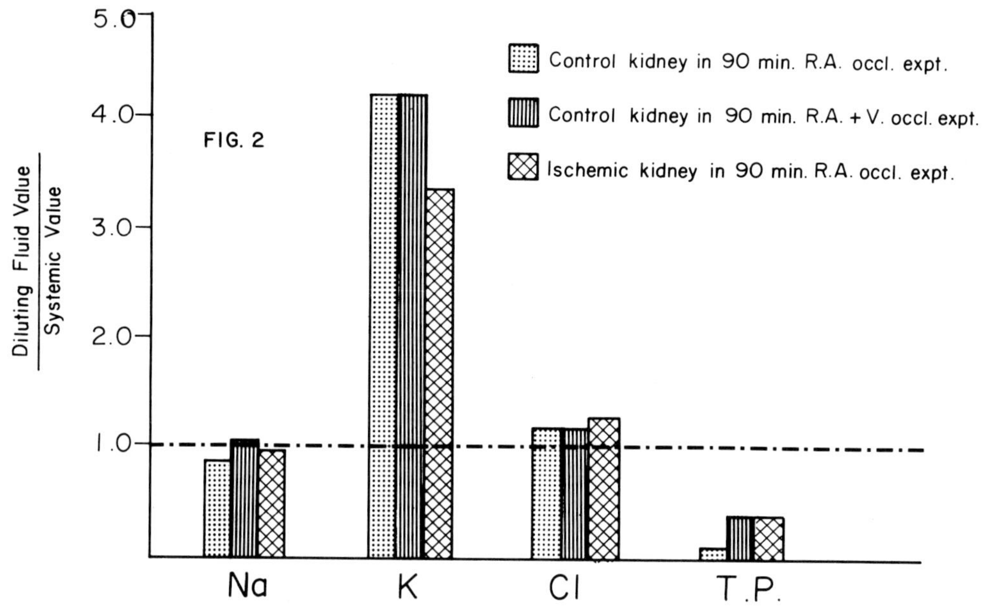

Fig. 2. Relative composition of diluting fluid.

retention of both formed elements (35 percent reduction in efflux), plasma, and diluting fluid. The effluent collected after occlusion of artery and vein differed, in that there was no reduction of the hematocrit and thus no net fluid shift into the vascular compartment. When compared to control kidneys, there again was intra-renal retention.

These experiments do not distinguish between retention in intravascular or extravascular sites, but they, however, point out the very early development of impedance to emptying of the kidney.

Potassium concentrations were elevated when kidneys were simply removed and drained, attained similar levels following renal artery occlusion, but were significantly higher when the artery and vein were clamped for 90 minutes. We have no evidence to dispute Swann's[3, 4] thesis that interstitial fluid potassium concentrations might be identical with those of "diluting fluid." The concept of the kidney as a turgid organ seems feasible, favoring passive displacement of extravascular fluid into the capillary bed once vascular hydrodynamic forces have been arrested by occlusion of the arterial supply. The similarities of potassium concentration in immediately drained and prolonged ischemic kidneys further supports the thought that venous potassium elevations are predominantly the result of mechanical phenomena rather than sustained anoxia.

After occlusion of the renal artery and vein for 90 minutes, potassium content of the venous effluent was higher than that of controlled kidneys and after arterial occlusion but was similar to the potassium concentration of diluting fluid, the presumed interstitial value. As the duration of vascular arrest was identical, the differences must be attributed to the effect of disallowing venous drainage into the vena cava during the period of ischemia. The entry of increased amounts of potassium into the vascular compartment can be viewed as a dialysis phenomenon. When the entire pedicle is occluded and hydrodynamic pressure is maintained, passive vascular dilatation should provide maximum surface area for electrolyte migration, allowing equilibration between the vascular and perivascular compartments.

The principal responses to renal ischemia observed in these experiments have practical import. First, pedicle occlusion for 90 minutes resulted in fluid retention when compared to minimally ischemic control kidneys. Though the pattern, distribution and many potential causes of retention are not within the scope of this study, the observation suggests that renal edema as commonly observed after anoxic injury may be initiated immediately and that preventive measures should therefore be instituted promptly on recognition of an actual or potential ischemic episode.

Increased potassium concentrations in the venous tree reflect similar or higher concentrations in the perivascular interstitial space. There was immediate rise in venous concentrations in Swann's[3] experiments and a similar one in our own control experiments. Thus potassium liberation is in part an acute response. Prolongation of pedicle occlusion results in further elevation to mean intravascular levels of 20 mEq. per liter. These alterations may greatly change the state of contractility of the vascular bed. The effect of increased potassium levels on smooth muscle is biphasic.[1, 2] With modest elevations, vascular dilatation has been observed. With further increase to 12 to 18 mEq. per liter, smooth muscle contraction ensues, with reduction in flow and increased vascular resistance. The observed venous concentrations of potassium following 90 minutes of pedicle occlusion represent net minimal perivascular concentrations and are in a range that one might expect to produce vascular smooth muscle contraction. A mechanism is thereby established wherein renal blood flow following an ischemic insult might be compromised by potassium-mediated vascular contraction, sufficient to induce postrelease malperfusion.

REFERENCES

1. Emmanuel, D. A., Fleishman, M., and Haddy, F. J.: Effect of potassium on small and large blood vessels of the dog forelimb, Am. J. Physiol. **197:** 637, 1959.
2. Levowitz, B. S., Kamil, N., Goldson, H., Rashkin, A., and LaGuerre, J.: Vascular responses to the potassium ion, Surg. Gynecol. Obstet. **129:** 979, 1969.
3. Swann, H. G.: The functional distention of the kidney, Tex. Rep. Biol. Med. **18:** 566, 1960.
4. Swann, H. G., Valdivia, L., Ormsby, A. A., and Witt, W. T.: Nature of fluids which functionally distend the kidney, J. Exp. Med. **104:** 25, 1958.

The blood supply of experimental liver metastases. IV. Changes in vascularity with increasing tumor growth

Norman B. Ackerman, M.D., Ph.D., *Kansas City, Mo.*

Vascularity of solitary Walker tumors implanted within the liver was studied in Holtzmann rats. Changes in arterial and portal vascularity were documented in tumors ranging in size from < 1 mm. to 33 mm. in diameter. Colored silicone rubber solutions were injected into the arterial and portal circulations in each animal, and specimens were studied under a stereomicroscope. The very smallest tumors (< 1 mm. in diameter) appeared as a blank space without any newly developed circulation. Tumors slightly larger, 1 to 2 mm. in diameter, induced the development of new vessels which encircled the tumor. These vessels were derived from either the arterial or portal circulation, or from both, which were mixing freely. All moderate-sized tumors, which were 3 to 7 mm. in diameter, had well-developed arterial circulations. Massive tumors, ranging from 7 by 8 mm. to 33 by 33 mm. in size, developed a wide variety of vascular patterns. These ranged, in a random fashion, from predominantly arterial to predominantly portal, as well as a combination of both vascular systems. Over-all vascularity varied from sparse to well developed. It is concluded that the pattern of vascularity of liver metastases is at least in part dependent on the size and growth of the tumors and that this vascularity is a continually changing phenomenon.

From the Department of Surgery, Menorah Medical Center and School of Medicine, University of Missouri, Kanas City, Kansas City, Mo.

It has been generally accepted as the result of data from both experimental and clinical studies, that metastatic tumors in the liver derive their blood supply predominantly from the hepatic artery system. The portal system seems to play a relatively minor role in feeding large, well-established tumors. However, arteriograms performed on patients with liver metastases demonstrate a wide range of vascular patterns in the area of these metastases. Most of these clinical series include studies performed on patients with all stages of tumor growths, from those barely recognizable on x-ray films to the most massive tumors which have replaced large portions of normal liver.

Accepted for publication Feb. 11, 1974.

It has been our feeling that tumor vascularity within the liver is not a simple matter of a constant development of arterial blood supply keeping pace with tumor growth. We have previously demonstrated an interplay between arterial and portal circulation under some circumstances in experimental tumors of moderate size.[1, 7] The present studies are an attempt to document changes in vascularity that occur as these tumors grow from an extremely small size, barely recognizable on gross examination, to a massively enlarged size.

MATERIALS AND METHODS

These experiments were performed on Holtzmann rats weighing approximately 200

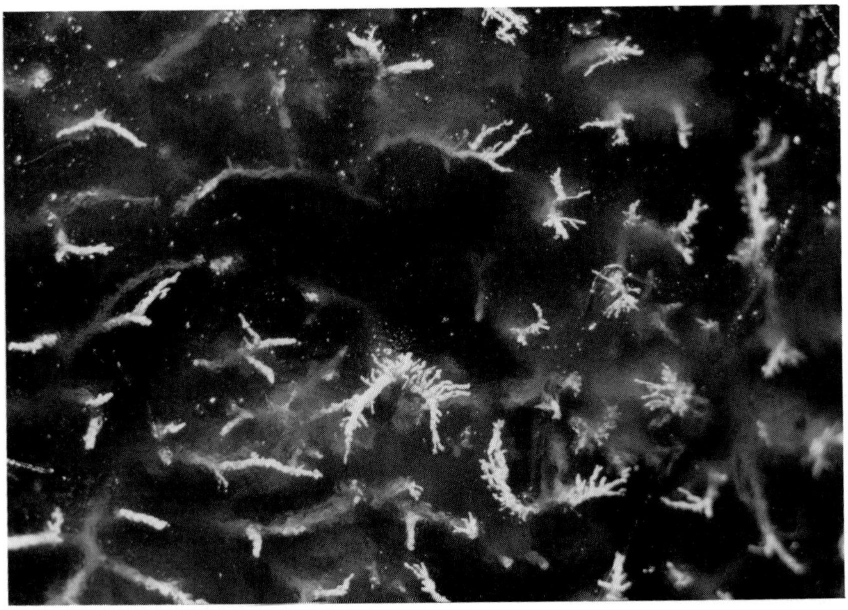

Fig. 1. Tumor less than 1 mm. in diameter appearing as blank space without newly developed circulation. (Original magnification ×17.)

Table I. *Vascularity of small tumors*

Tumor size (mm.)	Origin of circulation: Arte-rial	Origin of circulation: Por-tal	Description
<1	0	0	—
<1	0	0	—
<1	?+	0	Very early
1	+	0	Early
1	0	+	Early
1	+	0	Developed
1 – 2	+	0	Well developed
1 × 3	0	+	Developed
2	+	+	Developed, mixed
2	+	0	Very well developed

to 250 Gm. Solitary Walker-256 carcinosarcoma tumors were implanted within the left lateral lobe of the liver, with the use of a technique described in earlier reports.[7] Tumor "take" was 100 percent.

Tumor vascularity was studied in 26 animals with tumors ranging in size from less than 1 mm. to 33 mm. in diameter. Tumor size was controlled both by the size of the implant and the length of time between implant and death. The animals were studied as early as three days after implantation and as long as 17 days after. The animals were divided into three arbitrary groups; ten had small tumors, ranging in size from less than 1 mm. to 2 mm. in diameter, six animals had moderate-sized tumors, from 3 to 7 mm. in diameter, and ten animals had massive sized tumors from 7 by 8 mm. to 33 by 33 mm. in size. Tumors of a moderate size had been studied more extensively in an earlier report.[7]

Tumor vascularity was demonstrated by the perfusion of a silicone rubber solution (Microfil*) into the arterial and portal circulation. A polyethylene tube (size PE 90) was positioned in the abdominal aorta cranially, with the tip of the tube reaching just below the takeoff of the celiac artery. The aorta was occluded above the celiac artery, and arterial branches to the gastrointestinal tract were also occluded. A similar plastic tube was also placed within the portal vein. Both of these catheters were connected to syringes containing the silicone rubber solution. For arterial perfusion, Microfil MV-118 (red) was used, and MV-112 (white) was injected into the portal side. Injections

*Canton Bio-Medical Products, Swarthmore, Pa.

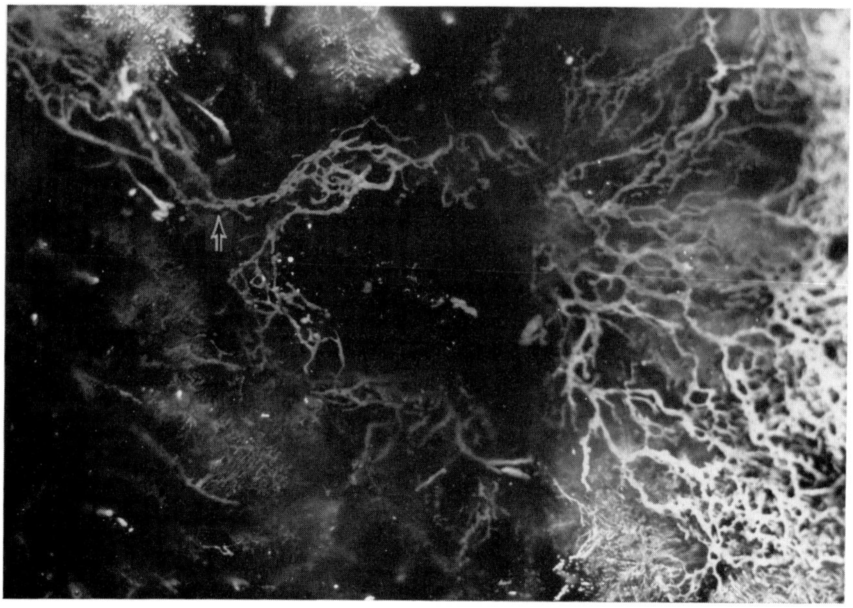

Fig. 2. Tumor 1 mm. in diameter with encircling vessel derived from arteriole *(arrow)*. (Original magnification ×17.)

were carried out manually, without manometric control which was found to be unnecessary in previous experiences. The injections were terminated when the vasculature of the liver seemed to be filled and the solutions were draining freely from the hepatic vein circulation.

Curing of the silicone rubber and clearing of the tissues was carried out as described previously.[7] The clearing procedure consisted of immersion in increasing concentrations of ethyl alcohol from 25 to 100 percent, and finally in a solution of methyl salicylate. The specimens were then examined and photographed under the stereomicroscope.

RESULTS

Small tumors (Table I). The ten smallest tumors demonstrated an interesting variety of patterns. After silicone rubber injection, the very smallest tumors appeared as a blank space without any newly developed circulation, surrounded by normal liver vasculature (Fig. 1). Since tumor "take" was 100 percent, it is assumed that these cancers were viable and were receiving nourishment by diffusion from the surrounding normal circulation. One of these small tumors, measuring less than 1 mm. in diameter, appeared to have a new arteriole growing in its vicinity, but it was not encircling the tumor.

As the tumors reached the size of 1 mm. in diameter, new vessel formation could easily be demonstrated. An arterial circulation varying from that which can be described as "early" to "well developed" was apparent in several animals. In its earliest stage, this consisted of a single vessel encircling the new tumor (Fig. 2). Two other animals had the same pattern of vasculature, but the vessels were clearly derived from the portal circulation (Fig. 3). One additional animal had newly formed vessels obviously

Table II. *Vascularity of moderate-sized tumors*

Tumor size (mm.)	*Origin of circulation*		*Description*
	Arterial	*Portal*	
3	+	0	Very well developed
4	+	0	Very well developed
4	+	0	Very well developed
4	+	0	Very well developed
5	+	0	Very well developed
7	+	0	Very well developed

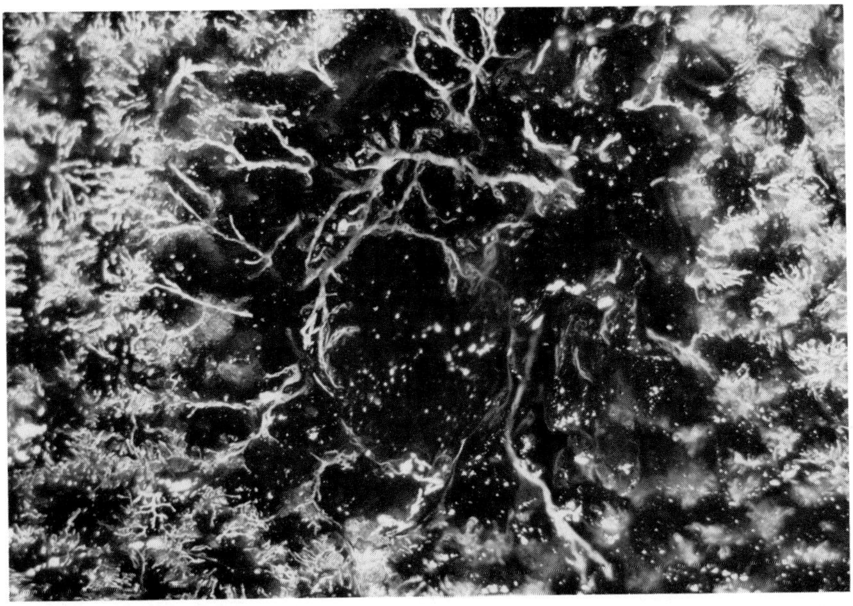

Fig. 3. Tumor 1 mm. in diameter with encircling vessel derived from portal vessels. (Original magnification ×17.)

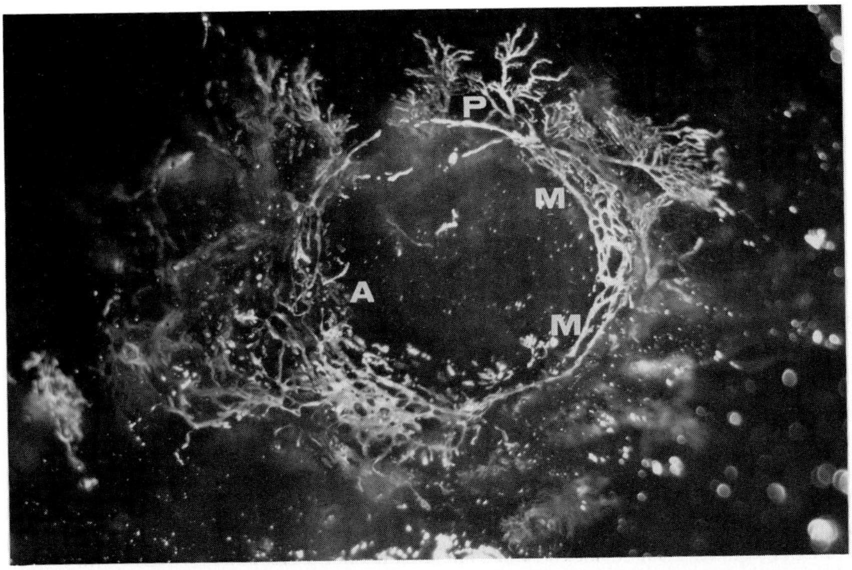

Fig. 4. Tumor 2 mm. in diameter with encircling vessels derived from both arterial and portal circulations, and freely mixing. A = arterial. P = portal. M = mixed. (Original magnification ×17.)

derived from both arterial and portal elements with free mixing of the two colored solutions (Fig. 4). Thus, the early developed circulation in these tumors consisted of either arterial or portal elements, or both.

Moderate-sized tumors (Table II). Tumors ranging from 3 to 7 mm. in diameter all had well-developed arterial circulations (Fig. 5). These vessels appeared similar to those described in an earlier report from this laboratory.[7] Portal vessels were seen close to the growing edge of the tumor, and in past studies, occasionally, small areas of the tumor plexus were fed directly from the portal

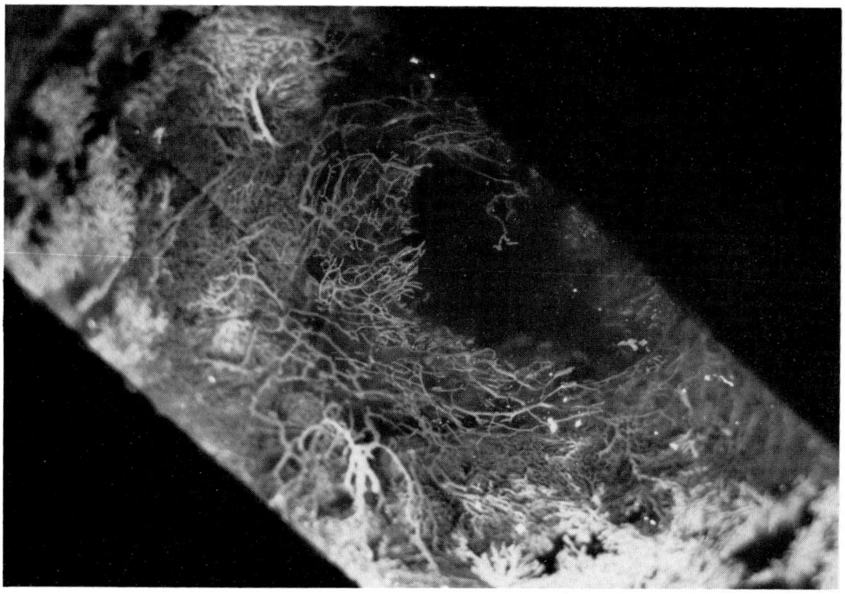

Fig. 5. Cut section of tumor 4 mm. in diameter. Well developed vascular plexus derived from arterial circulation. (Original magnification ×17.)

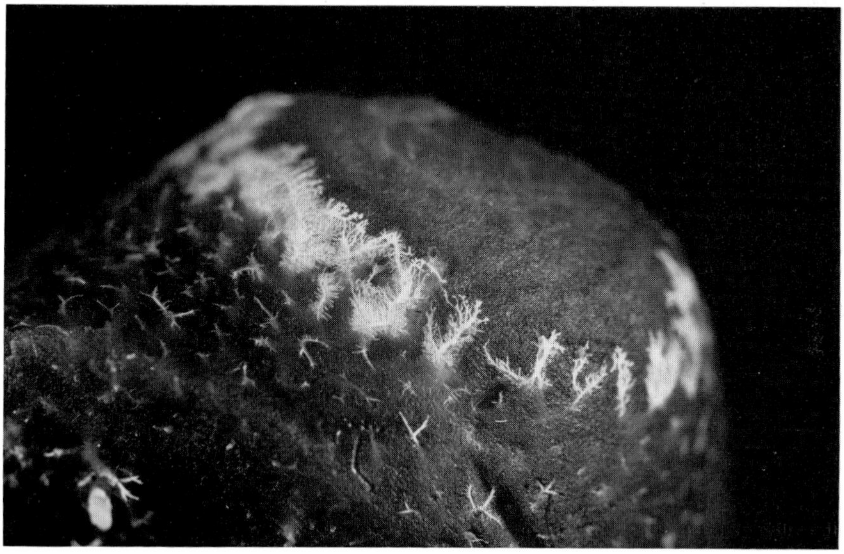

Fig. 6. Tumor 12 × 13 mm. with vasculature in periphery derived solely from portal circulation. (Original magnification ×6.)

circulation. In the present experiments, the tumor vessels appeared to be entirely arterial. These vessels were similar to those described by other authors, with tortuosity, irregularity of the lumen diameter, and a disorderly pattern compared to that of the normal liver vessels.

Massive tumors (Table III). The ten largest tumors, ranging from 7 by 8 mm. to 33 by 33 mm. in size, demonstrated a wide variety of patterns and a great variability in extent of vascularity. Several of the tumors appeared to have little or no arterial circulation, with portal vessels vary-

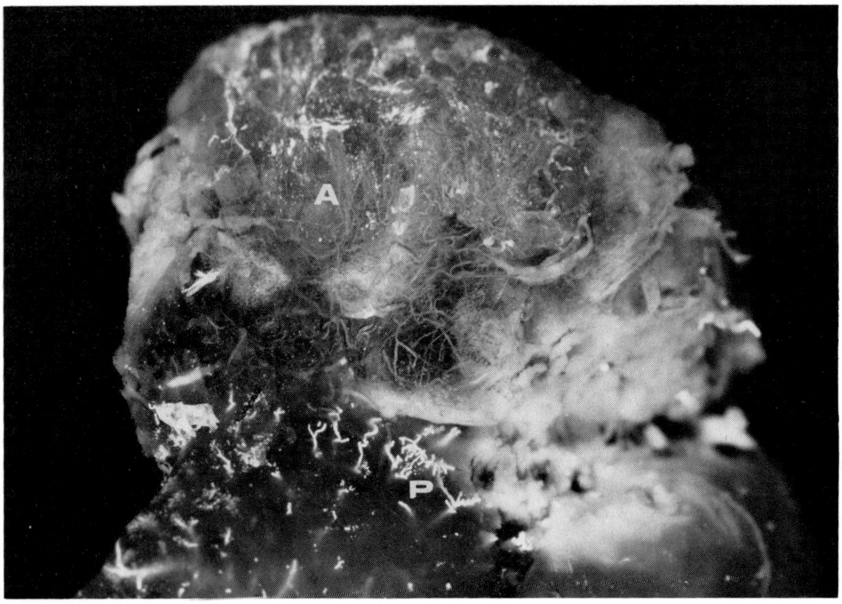

Fig. 7. Tumor 12 × 13 mm. with vasculature derived predominantly from arterial circulation. *A,* arterial; *P,* portal. (Original magnification ×6.)

Table III. *Vascularity of massive-sized tumors*

Tumor size (mm.)	Origin of circulation: Arterial	Origin of circulation: Portal	Description
7 × 8	0	+	Sparse
11 × 12	0	+	Sparse
12 × 13	0	+	Well developed, orderly
12 × 13	+	±	Well developed
15 × 16	±	±	Very sparse
17 × 17	+	±	Well developed
25 × 25	+	+	Well developed
27 × 28	±	±	Sparse
27 × 29	±	+	Sparse in areas
33 × 33	+	+	Sparse in areas

ing from sparse to well developed (Fig. 6). Others had a predominantly arterial circulation, which also varied from sparse to well developed (Fig. 7). Several animals had tumors with both arterial and portal elements combined to varying degrees (Fig. 8). One tumor had a very well-developed blood supply consisting of elements from both circulations, and the largest tumor had a similar pattern, but some areas of the tumor were relatively avascular. Most of the tumors had avascular areas, particularly in the central portion. The variability of vascular patterns of these tumors was similar to that described in arteriographic studies in humans.

DISCUSSION

For many years, there have been discrepancies in the literature regarding the extent of vascularity of cancers. Although the overabundance of new vessels formed in the area of new cancers has been well recognized for many years, others have noted the scarcity of vascularity in regions of other tumors. A great variability in the vascular pattern has been noted in arteriographic studies, beginning with some of the earliest work by Bierman and associates[3] and continuing to the present time. Bosniak and Phanthumachinda[4] reported that patients with metastatic cancer in the liver generally had avascular or poorly vascular lesions without obvious "tumor vessels." Healey,[5] using vinyl acetate cast studies on autopsy specimens, described three types of vascular patterns. Two of these types, generalized subcapsular infiltration and nodular infiltration, had a decreased vascularity. The third

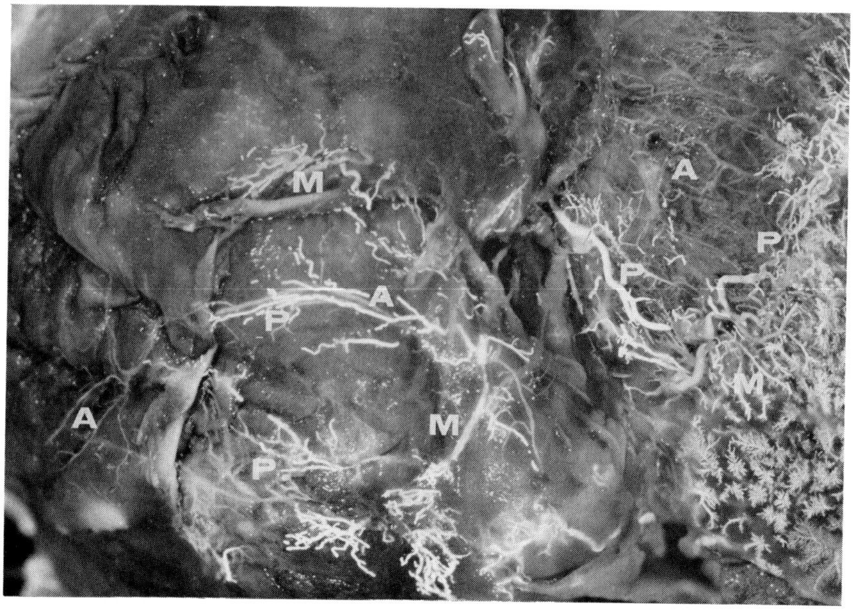

Fig. 8. Tumor 25 × 25 mm. with vasculature derived from both arterial and portal circulations. *A*, arterial; *P*, portal; *M*, mixed. (Original magnification ×3.)

type appeared to have a normal arterial vascularity. It should be emphasized, however, that most of these studies on human subjects dealt with liver metastases in the late stages of the disease with tumors of generally large and massive size.

There may be several factors influencing the degree of vascularity of liver metastases. The possibility that the anatomic site of the primary cancer may be an important factor in determining the type of blood supply to the metastases has been discussed by Healey.[5] He noted that primary tumors which were located in an organ which drained into the portal system tended to produce metastases in the liver with a more developed vascularity. Cancers originating in extraportal areas appeared to develop less vascular liver metastases. There were, however, exceptions, and mixed patterns were observed. Assa[2] discussed the relationship of the age of tumor in the donor before transplanting as a factor in determining vascularity of the tumor in the host. In studies with rabbit tumors, "older" tumors produced a decreased vascularity in liver implants in comparison to the vascularity produced by "younger" tumors.

The effects of size or age of the metastatic tumor itself on vascularity have not been studied in any detail. Kido[6] used aortography to study the growth and changes in vascularity of Walker tumors in rat livers. In his study, the smallest tumors observed on the x-ray films already had a well-developed vasculature, but these tumors were reported to be at least 4 mm. in diameter. Large tumors had developed the typical tumor plexus pattern, and some avascularity was noted.

At this point, a word should be said about the various techniques used to study this problem. Arteriography or aortography are techniques most readily available for studying vascularity in both animal and human subjects. However, one is unable to observe simultaneously the appearance of the portal circulation in these studies. Furthermore, these are relatively gross studies, and individual capillary components of the tumor circulation are probably not seen as clearly as in the silicone rubber preparation. The silicone rubber has the disadvantage of being limited to autopsy specimens or experiments on animals to be killed. However, resolution appears to be greater with this technique.

With aortography, Kido[6] was unable to recognize tumors less than 4 mm. in diameter, while in the present study done with the use of silicone rubber, tumors 1 mm. or less in diameter were clearly identified. Vinyl acetate has the same disadvantages as silicone rubber and is considerably less useful since the plastic is unable to penetrate into the smaller vessels and capillaries.

The present studies with silicone rubber show that tumor vascularity in the liver is a continually changing phenomenon. The smallest or earliest tumors appeared to exist initially without their own blood supply and probably depend on diffusion from surrounding vessels for nourishment. As the tumors continue to grow, angiogenesis occurs with a blood supply consisting of vessels developed from surrounding arterial or portal components. In some instances, both arterial and portal components coexist and connect with each other. As the tumors reach a larger size, the arterial role becomes predominant, and portal vessels are generally displaced and obliterated. However, in occasional tumors, there may be a small portal component in the well-developed tumor plexus, and portal vessels may play an important role in feeding the growing edges of the tumor as they penetrate into the surrounding liver. With further growth to large and massive size, angiogenesis appears unable to keep up with the destruction and displacement of these tumor vessels. A breakdown of the well-organized pattern occurs with development of irregular, poorly organized arterial or portal vessels. The extent of vascularity appears to be randomized with some areas having a hypervascular circulation and other areas having a sparse, avascular pattern. A mixed arterial and portal circulation may occur in these tumors.

It is impossible to correlate the findings in these experimental studies directly with the vascularity which occurs with increasing size in human tumors. Similarities which might account for the various findings described in arteriographic studies in patients are apparent, however. At the minimum, it is probably safe to conclude that there is a variability in the vascularity of metastatic tumors in the liver, caused, at least in part, by size and growth of the tumor.

REFERENCES

1. Ackerman, N. B., Lien, W. M., and Silverman, N. A.: The blood supply of experimental liver metastases. III. The effects of acute ligation of the hepatic artery or portal vein, SURGERY **71:** 636, 1972.
2. Assa, J.: Differential patterns of vasculature to liver tumours, Br. J. Cancer **24:** 360, 1970.
3. Bierman, H. R., Byron, R. L., Jr., Kelley, K. H., and Grady, A: Studies on the blood supply of tumors in man. III. Vascular patterns of the liver by hepatic arteriography in vivo, J. Natl. Cancer Instit. **12:** 107, 1951.
4. Bosniak, M. A., and Phanthumachinda, P.: Value of arteriography in the study of hepatic disease, Am. J. Surg. **112:** 348, 1966.
5. Healey, J. E., Jr.: Vascular patterns in human metastatic liver tumors, Surg. Gynecol. Obstet. **120:** 1187, 1955.
6. Kido, C.: Hepatic angiography of experimental transplantable tumor, Invest. Radiol **5:** 341, 1970.
7. Lien, W. M., and Ackerman, N. B.: The blood supply of experimental liver metastases. II. A microcirculatory study of the normal and tumor vessels of the liver with the use of perfused silicone rubber, SURGERY **68:** 334, 1970.

Beta-islet cell tumors of the pancreas: Results of a study on 1,067 cases

Paride Stefanini, M.D.,* Manlio Carboni, M.D., F.I.C.S., Neri Patrassi, M.D., F.I.C.S.,
and **Antonio Basoli, M.D.,** *Rome, Italy*

The results of an international investigation and a review of the existing literature on beta-islet cell tumors are reported. Of the 1,067 well-documented cases of insulinoma, 12 were from the personal experience of the authors. Common clinical aspects and the diagnostic investigations primarily used are described, with details of arteriography. Treatment was investigated in particular on the basis of the cases gathered. Medical treatment, indications, effects of various drugs, surgical treatment, incidence of operations, death rate, complications, and postoperative results are reported.

From the Second Surgical Clinic and Surgical Anatomy of The University of Rome Medical School

MORE THAN 20 years have passed since Howard and colleagues[18] published a review of 398 cases in the then-existing literature on tumors of the pancreas causing hypogylcemia. These data were updated by Moss and Rhoads[30] in 1960 with 549 cases of insulinoma. Since then works published on this disease, which still arouses considerable interest, have been even more numerous. During the past ten years findings in 12 patients with tumors of the pancreas which resulted in hypoglycemia have been recorded at the Second Surgical Clinic of the University of Rome.

These observations prompted us to conduct research on these extremely rare tumors, which are now being recorded more frequently. We extensively reviewed the literature and conducted an international investigation. Two questionnaires were sent to authors who have been most interested in this topic. Since our study is based on data supplied by the authors who were so kind as to complete our questionnaires, we cannot present 1,067 cases fully documented. In fact, some authors were not inclined to spend much time investigating insulinomas that they were not directly concerned with. As a result, the cases reported by physicians lack documentation with reference to surgical treatment. Moreover, some patients died before operation, others did not undergo operation, and still other cases were identified only at postmortem examination. For these reasons these cases could not be included in the tables concerning surgical treatment. Consequently, we selected those cases which were well documented from the diagnosis and treatment viewpoint or those cases which presented a special interest or a specific aspect. The complete list of cases is given in Table I to show the origins of the series collected. This study was particu-

Accepted for publication Jan. 23, 1973.

Reprint requests: Paride Stefanini, M.D., Second Surgical Clinic of the University of Rome Medical School, Policlinico Umberto I, 00161, Rome, Italy.

*President of the International College of Surgeons.

Table I. *Results of international inquiry into cases of beta-islet cell tumors*

The 47 Italian authors yielded 94 cases:	
Amasio, 1	Martinoli, 1
Austoni,* 6	Marcozzi, 1
Badini, 1	Mauri-Paolini, 1
Barbarino, 1	Michetti, 1
Beretta-Anguissola, 2	Monti, 3
Biancalana, 5	Montorsi, 1
Borghetti, 1	Nicora, 2
Bracco, 1	Pellegrini, 1
Chini, 1	Perrino, 1
Ciuffini, 1	Poli, 2
Coeli, 1	Possati, 6
Confalonieri, 1	Puglionisi, 2
Conti, 1	Quercio, 1
Crepaldi, 2	Rossini, 1
Crucitti, 1	Selli, 1
Galli, 1	Serra, 1
Gatti, 1	Stefanini, 12
Giardina, 2	Tonelli, 6
Goffrini, 2	Tuscano, 1
Legnani, 1	Vecchi, 1
Macchini, 1	Vecchioni, 1
Malan, 6	Vidili, 1
Marinaccio, 2	Zaccarini, 1
Marinoni, 3	
The 82 authors from other countries yielded 831 cases:	
Alfidi, 7	Mallinson, 2
Assan, 20	Mandache, 5
Blomquist, 8	Marks, 50
Bloodworth, 7	McGarity, 7
Bodner, 7	McGovern, 7
Bories-Azeau, 5	Mentouri, 2
Bozer, 1	Miller, 13
Child, 24	Molnar, 9
Creutzfeldt, 14	Murate, 2
De Peyster, 15	Murray-Lyon, 1
Delkonen, 6	Napalkov, 5
Dunn, 11	Niedner, 6
Enderlin, 1	Olsson,† 13
Falkmer, 1	Passaro, 8
Floquet, 8	Piroska, 2
Fonkalsrud, 10	Polak, 4
Fraser, 4	Porter, 47
Frawley, 15	Priestley, 154
Frederick, 1	Raia, 2
Fuchsig, 11	Raptis, 6
Ghnassia, 2	Reilly, 1
Govaerts, 2	Ribet, 4
Gulzow, 3	Ritchie, 12
Gurturk, 1	Rogers, 17
Heger, 5	Roux, 3
Hepp, 10	Sadoff, 3
Hess, 5	Saegesser, 11
Huguet, 17	Sato, 10
Iliescu, 1	Shamiyeh, 2
Juvara, 11	Singleton, 12
Kennedy, 9	Starr, 1
Kokkarakis, 1	Stoianovick, 2

*Austoni's cases were operated on by Cevese.

†Olsson's eight cases were operated on by Blomquist.

Table I. *Cont'd*

Kozakov, 1	Strotges, 1
Kugelberg, 13	Ton-That-Tung, 9
Kuo, 3	Toulet, 1
Lambert, 2	Urca, 6
Landor, 2	Zahnd, 15
Leger, 24	Zenker, 28
Lortat-Jacob, 4	White, 22
Magaldi, 1	Wolfe, 12
Mainetti, 4	Zollinger, 15
Review of the literature yielded 142 cases:	
Cady,[5] 1	Legre et al.,[22] 1
Clarke et al.,[7] 15	Mengoli and Le Quesne,[28] 3
De Gennes et al.,[8] 4	Olivier et al.,[33] 1
Deuil and Tugaye,[9] 5	Roth et al.,[37] 2
Epstein et al.,[10] 2	Salti and Walker,[38] 10
Gall,[12] 4	Scheinin and Tala,[39] 3
Grözinger,[16] 10	Schlicke and Berghan,[40] 3
Hartsuck and Brooks,[17] 16	Tompkins et al.,[45] 10
Irmer et al.,[19] 22	Warren,[50] 24
Koutras and White,[21] 8	Williams et al.,[52] 8

Authors who employed medical treatment:

Andreani, Austoni, Bodner, Bories Azeau, Child and Harrison, Creutzfeldt and Frerichs, De Peyster, Enderlin, Floquet, Fonkalsrud, Fraser and Kaufmann, Frawley, Fuchsig and Fritschs, Giardina, Goffrini, Gulzow, Hartsuck, Hepp, Hess, Irmer, Kennedy, Kokkarakis, Leger, Lortat Jacob, Mandache, Marinoni, Marks, Mercadier, Michetti, Miller, Murray Lyon, Nicora, Nieschlag, Passaro, Piroska, Porter, Raptis, Ribet, Ritchie, Roth, Sandoff, Salti, Schliche, Stanley, Toulet, Zahnd, Zenker, Zollinger, White, Williams, Wolfe

larly concerned with diagnosis and therapy, which continue to pose significant problems. The results of the investigation, and of our experience with beta-islet cell tumors of the pancreas, are reported in this paper.

CLINICAL MANIFESTATIONS AND DIAGNOSIS

Of the 1,067 patients with beta-islet cell tumors, 430 (40.3 percent) were male and 637 (59.7 percent) were female; the average age was 45½ years—68 percent of the patients with insulinomas were between 30 and 60 years of age; the oldest was 82 and the youngest was four. Hypoglycemia-inducing tumors of the pancreas in childhood are not rare. Apart from our investigation, we found over 30 cases documented by operation, most of which involved patients under two years of age.[3, 13, 15, 34, 41, 46, 47, 49]

The clinical manifestations of insulinomas are due to hypoglycemia and include neuropsychiatric, cardiovascular, and gastrointestinal symptoms. Neuropsychiatric symptoms, including loss of consciousness, sluggishness, confusion, asthenia, deep coma, dizziness, disturbances of vision, and epilepsy, were present in 981 patients (92 percent). Various types of irreversible damage to the central nervous system occurred in 6.8 percent of the cases. Temporary paralysis after a severe attack of hypoglycemia occurred in 4.5 percent of the cases. Cardiovascular symptoms, including palpitation, tachycardia, precordial pain, and arterial hypertension, were found in 180 patients. Gastroenterologic symptoms presented less frequently (93 patients); these usually included hunger, vomiting, and, occasionally, epigastric pain.

We do not have complete data on obesity since only a few authors indicated its presence; however, 19 of the authors found it in 68 of 144 patients.

The difficulty in correctly interpreting the symptoms explains why diagnosis often is not made until many years after the onset of clinical disturbances. Diagnosis of insulinoma was arrived at in 34 percent of the cases within one year, in 46 percent within one to five years, and in 20 percent after five years. The most frequent diagnoses made prior to identification of hyperinsulinism were psychiatric and neurologic, particularly epilepsy. Of the 162 cases reported by Breidhal, Abe,[1] White, Huguet, Floquet, and in our cases, the first diagnosis was epilepsy in 46 cases and a psychodepressive syndrome in 11.

The diagnosis of hypoglycemia-inducing islet cell tumors requires biochemical, radiologic, and radioisotopic investigations. Determination of the blood sugar levels, obviously done by all the authors consulted, is useful when associated with plasma insulin levels. Of the authors consulted, 64 specified that the diagnostic workup should include insulin level determinations. The existence of hypoglycemia of other origin (extrapancreatic neoplasms, hypopituitarism, hyperadrenalism, drugs, liver disease, glycogenesis, anomalies of childhood, gastric resection, or prediabetes) should be excluded. For such reasons it is necessary to utilize dynamic tests, the more important of which are summarized in Table II. Correct utilization and interpretation of tests are described in many works on the subject.[6, 8, 9, 12, 17, 19, 39, 45] Other tests used include the arginine (Austoni, Crepaldi, Raptis, Sato), lysine, and L-phenylalanine (Poli, Confalonieri, and Carnevali). Laurent, in a review of the literature, found that the epinephrine test used in 77 cases was helpful. This method has now been abandoned since newer tests give more gratifying results. Sixteen authors indicated that they still use the insulin-tolerance test, but this is not very helpful in diagnosing insulinomas. X-ray diagnosis of insulinomas is still looked upon with scepticism.

Table II. *Principal diagnostic tests and positive results (149 authors)*

Method	Authors using the test		Positive results
	No.	%	(%)
Prolonged fasting test	109	73	95
Tolbutamide tolerance test	101	68	80
Glucagon test	39	26	72
Glucose tolerance test	82	55	60
L-Leucine tolerance test	43	29	50

Selective arteriography is very helpful in localizing the tumor and is therefore an invaluable support for the surgeon at operation in that he already knows where the tumor is located; the main surgical difficulty lies in the localization of this tumor. The size of the tumor does not necessarily aid in locating it. Arteriography can show a tumor as small as 0.5 cm. Epstein and associates,[10] on the contrary, reported on 11 patients with tumors larger than 1 to 2 cm. where arteriography was negative. Consequently, the degree of vascularization of the tumor seems as important as size for angiographic diagnosis. Yet, in only 20 percent of the cases is vacularization represented by dilated sinusoids capable of a stable and intense opaqueness. Tumors with capillary structure are

Table III. *Results with arteriography and scintigraphy according to site of tumor (149 authors)*

Arteriography used by 67% of authors			*Scintigraphy used by 24% of authors*		
Author	*Total No. of investigations*	*Positive tests*	*Author*	*Total No. of investigations*	*Positive tests*
Alfidi	7	6	Austoni	4	2
Creutzfeldt	10	6	Bodner	5	0
Heger	5	4	Hartsuck	3	1
Hernandez	5	2	Hess	2	0
Hess	4	3	Leger	7	1
Mercadier	3	3	McGarity	3	1
Molnar	8	6	Napalkov	5	2
Olsson	9	8	Stefanini	5	0
Sato	10	8	Wolfe	2	1
Zenker	17	10	Zenker	10	3
Altri	92	56	Altri	35	4
Total	170	112 (65.9%)	Total	81	15 (18%)

less opaque and, therefore, not very helpful. For this reason, often it is easier to demonstrate by angiography the hepatic metastases of carcinomas than the primary lesion. The site is also important in detecting a tumor. Olsson found, in 11 cases where angiography was negative, that seven tumors were of the tail, two were of the body, and two were of the head of the pancreas. Bookstein and Oberman[4] reported four cases of large insulinomas of the tail of the pancreas in which angiography was negative. Since tumors of the tail are more difficult to trace, Olsson advised injecting the splenic artery if, upon initial examination, arteriography has been negative. Table III shows the results of research regarding selective arteriography and pancreatic scanning.

While Alfidi, Olsson, and Sato reported high percentages of success (81 percent), White and Zollinger maintained that arteriography is of little help. White, in particular, recounted that good angiograms made on 10 of his patients would not reveal the tumor. Instead, in a case of insular hyperplasia, arteriography gave a false-positive image which resulted in resection of the head of the pancreas as the initial operation. Furthermore, in two cases the angiography was complicated by an intimal dissection in the hepatic artery. In two other cases, plaques were dripped off at the femoral puncture site and, in a final case, a hematoma occurred adjacent to the hepatic artery.

As for pancreatic scanning, nearly all the authors consulted reported that it is of significant value in only a limited number of cases and only when the tumor is large and therefore easily located upon operation. Austoni, Napalkov, and Zenker have had considerable success with pancreatic scanning but White reported 15 cases in which scintigraphy was negative and Zollinger indicated that scans have been uninformative in all his cases in which they were performed. In our experience, pancreatic scanning has always been incapable of localizing the tumor. Moreover, in one case of insular hyperplasia, we experienced a false-positive image. In Table IV symptoms and diagnostic investigations of our series of 12 cases are reported.

MEDICAL TREATMENT

Medical treatment is only palliative; it is not curative. The only curative treatment for beta-islet cell tumors of the pancreas is surgical excision. Yet, medical treatment is effective in suppressing symptoms of hypoglycemia for several years. Results of our study indicate that 15 percent of patients with beta-islet cell tumors were treated medically. Usually this treatment is employed in those patients with inoperable

Table IV. *Symptoms and diagnosis of 12 personal cases*

Case No.	*Year*	*Age*	*Sex*	*Principal symptoms*	*Obesity*	*Previous diagnosis*	*EEG*	*Previous admission*	*Fasting*	*Tolbutamide*
1	1964	22	♀	Neuropsychic and gastrointestinal (2 yr.)	No	Epilepsy	3	2	+	±
2	1966	30	♂	Neuropsychic (4 yr.)	Yes	Epilepsy	2	—	+	+
3	1967	62	♀	Neuropsychic and gastrointestinal (7 yr.)	No	Epilepsy	5	3	+	+
4	1968	56	♂	Neuropsychic (12 yr.)	Yes	Epilepsy	8	8	+	+
5	1968	31	♀	Neuropsychic and cardiovascular (4 mo.)	No	—	—	1	+	+
6	1969	52	♀	Neuropsychic and gastrointestinal (1 yr.)	No	Epilepsy	1	—	+	+
7	1969	36	♂	Neuropsychic (3 yr.)	No	—	1	2	+	±
8	1970	37	♂	Neuropsychic and gastrointestinal (5 yr.)	Yes	Epilepsy	2	5	+	+
9	1970	41	♀	Neuropsychic (20 yr.)	No	Cerebral neoplasm	3	2	+	+
10	1971	63	♀	Neuropsychic (4 yr.)	Yes	—	—	1	+	∓
11	1971	67	♀	Neuropsychic and cardiovascular (3 yr.)	Yes	Neurosis	—	2	+	±
12	1971	42	♀	Neuropsychic (2 yr.)	No	—	1	1	+	+

islet cell carcinoma, patients who are unable to undergo operation, where surgical treatment is refused, or after surgical attempts at correction have been unsuccessful.

The drugs most commonly used in the medical treatment of islet cell tumors are diazoxide, corticosteroids, and Streptozotocin. Harrison and Child treated 16 patients with diazoxide for periods of three months to four and one half years with relief from hypoglycemic symptoms in 15 cases; Creutzfeldt and Frericks registered nine satisfactory results and four fair results in 13 patients treated over periods of one to three weeks to three months; Zenker reported five good results in six patients over periods of six weeks to five months. Marks treated all cases of insular carcinomas with diazoxide and reported one patient with insular carcinoma and hepatic metastases who survived for over eight years. De Gennes and group[8] noted in one patient that hepatic metastases regressed after the administration of diazoxide. On the contrary, the results achieved in the series of Sadoff, White, Gulzow, and Hartsuck and Brooks[17] were unsatisfactory.

Of the 55 cases documented, 24 received diuretics in association with diazoxide. The use of diuretics, which considerably increases hyperglycemia determined by diazoxide, did not provide significant results: the use of diuretics produced favorable results in 50 percent of the cases whereas without diuretics the results were favorable in 51 percent of the cases.

The complications encountered as a result of diazoxide therapy include hypotension, edema, nausea, shock, and hirsutism, as reported by Austoni, Creutzfeldt, Hess, Mandache, Piroska, Raptis, Irmer and colleagues,[19] and Zahnd. In particular, Creutzfeldt and Frericks report that of their 13 patients treated with diazoxide, five suffered nausea and occasional anorexia, three peripheral edema, three granulocytopenia, two sinus tachycardia, one severe hirsutism, and three others had normalization of hypertension.

Until a few years ago, corticosteroids were the drugs most frequently used but their use has recently been limited, as shown in our study. Hess, Lortat-Jacob, Mandache, Marks, Murray-Lyon, Piroska, and Zollinger maintain that in their experience the action of corticosteroids is insufficient and only transient. Moreover, with this treatment, obesity is aggravated and signs of hyperadrenalism appear.

Streptozotocin given intravenously or by catheterization of the celiac axis is principally indicated for patients with metastases. The three cases reported by Sadoff showed improvement of symptoms as did those reported by Marks, Kennedy, and Gulzow. Zollinger accomplished the disappearance of hypoglycemia in one case; in another case of diffuse metastases treated with Streptozotocin the patient died from sepsis. Stanley and Nieschslag and colleagues[32] have noted a reduction of heptic metastases after the administration of Streptozotocin. White, on the other hand, treated two patients with this drug and noted no significant improvement. Streptozotocin was used postoperatively by Toulet in a patient who submitted to an exploratory laparotomy for insular carcinoma with hepatic metastases. Piroska noted in one case toxic manifestations such as adynamia, vomiting, cyanosis, collapse, and tachycardia without improvement of the hypoglycemia. Streptozotocin presents a greater reliability when injected through the celiac axis (Stanley), yet toxicity increases and may cause kidney and hepatic damages (Sadoff).

It is not possible to correlate the toxic effects with the dosage of Streptozotocin utilized. Streptozotocin, an antibiotic, is a *Streptomyces achromogenes* derivative which inhibits the biosynthesis of insulin and, if applied in large doses, is very active against the beta cells. Child, Gulzow, Kennedy, Marks, Murray-Lyon, Nieschlas, Piroska, Sadoff, Stanley, and White have all used this drug but do not report any correlation between doses and side effects. The cases studied up to now number approximately 30 and every author uses a different dose.

Other drugs used with success, but in limited amounts, have been glucagon-zinc,[9, 37] zinc,[50] glucagon,[40] alloxan (Porter), and glucagon and azotic mustard (Fonkalsrud). Antimitotic substances were used by Leger and by Cady[5]; radiant therapy was used in only one patient by Blomquist. All the authors agree that medical measures are helpful in emergency treatment and in preoperative preparation, which includes proper diet and the administration of low doses of corticoids to maintain normal levels of blood sugar.

SURGICAL TREATMENT

Surgical management of beta-islet cell tumors still presents some very complex problems. Surgery is curative in most patients with insulinomas, but in many others it is unsuccessful. The persistence of hypoglycemia is generally caused by failure to detect the insulinoma or to completely excise it.

When the insulinoma is found, the choice of surgical procedure is based upon the site, number, volume, nature, and enucleability of the tumor.

One controversial point is the treatment of tumors of the body and tail of the pancreas. Of 132 authors whose orientation was deduced from the investigation data, 58 systematically performed distal resection in body and tail insulinomas. The other 74 authors performed enucleation or resection according to the pathologic findings.

When the tumor cannot be located, the procedure of choice is still under discussion. Until a few years ago blind distal resection was advised. Choice of this procedure was supported by the conviction that most insulinomas were located in the body and tail of the pancreas. In reality, occult tumors are often found in the head of the pancreas. In a review of 261 cases of occult insulinomas found at first or subsequent operations or at autopsy, 141 were located in the head, 53 in the body, and 26 in the tail of the pancreas. The remaining 31 were never located. Blind distal resection was performed in 172 cases at the first intervention and in 69 cases at the second intervention. Tumor was found in the resected specimen in 89 cases.

Our experience with occult insulinomas involves four patients, two of whom (cases 1 and 9) underwent blind distal resection. Only at reintervention was the insulinoma traced to the head of the pancreas. In one patient (case 5) a blind distal resection was performed without locating the tumor and, unfortunately, the patient refused a subsequent operation. In another patient (case 10) blind distal resection was performed and the insulinoma was found in the resected specimen. In one patient (case 11) who underwent blind resection, palpating once again the head of the pancreas, a small insulinoma arising in the uncinate process was found.

These findings are easily explained, considering that tumors of the head and of the uncinate process are often deeply situated in the parenchyma, while those of the body and tail are generally more superficial. Furthermore, the head of the pancreas is difficult to explore because of its thickness and anatomical position.

Based on these considerations, Flynn and McDonald,[11] Fonkalsrud, and Miller proposed, as an alternative to blind distal resection, blind pancreaticoduodenectomy.

De Peyster, Hartsuck and Brooks,[17] McGarity, Molnar, Rogers, Williams and associates,[52] and White recommended instead a progressive resection of the pancreas, beginning with the tail, which may require removal of 90 to 95 percent of the pancreas. The pancreatic tissue, progressively resected, must be histologically examined.

Mengoli and Le Quesne[28] advised that, when the tumor is not located, pancreatic resection should not be performed; rather, the pancreas should be re-examined after a year or two when presumably the tumor will have increased in size.

Often the only pancreatic disorder recognizable in blind resected specimens is a diffuse insular hyperplasia. The results of our study show that the incidence of insular hyperplasia was 6.5 percent, with 70 histologically documented cases. The symptoms and laboratory findings in these cases were the same as in those with insulinomas. In our experience we observed five patients with hyperplasia, of whom four submitted to a blind distal resection and one to a blind subtotal pancreatectomy.

The accompanying tables and figures summarize the results of our investigation into the surgical treatment of insulinoma. Table V summarizes the various types of

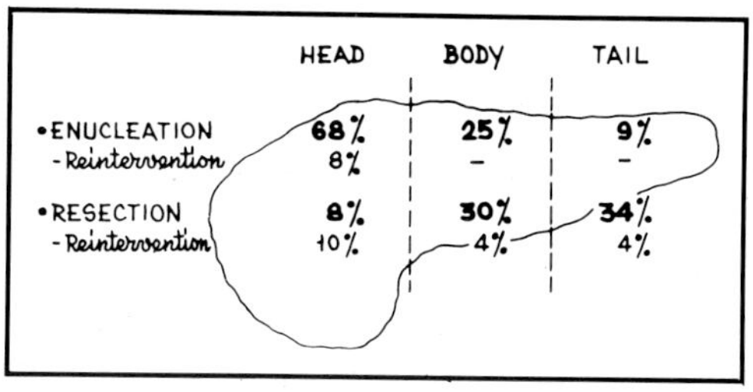

Fig. 1. Incidence of various interventions in relation to the site of the tumor (1,012 cases completely documented).

Table V. *Incidence of various types of intervention in 1,012 cases*

	Intervention		*Reintervention*	
	No. of cases	%	*No. of cases*	%
Enucleation	506	50	60	6
Distal resection	415	41	93	9.2
Pancreatoduodenectomy	15	1.5	24	2.4
Subtotal resection	20	2	37	3.7
Total resection	12	1.2	25	2.5
Exploratory laparotomy	44	4.3	—	—

operations and their incidence percentage. The reinterventions performed totaled 239 in 168 patients (23 percent).

The incidence of the various types of operation in relation to the site of the tumor is reported in Fig. 1. In the majority of tumors of the head of the pancreas, enucleation has been chosen; in insulinomas of the tail, pancreatic resection has been preferred. The percentages of tumors found at first operation and at successive ones are reported in Fig. 2. In the 17 percent of cases where the tumor was not found at operation, we included those cases in which only autopsy revealed the presence of an insulinoma, those where age and general conditions prevented further operations, and those in which the patients refused reintervention.

The difficulty encountered in finding the tumor at operation caused various authors to experiment with new techniques or to apply methods used for other diseases. Leger and Doublet have successfully used intraoperative pancreaticography and Monti used

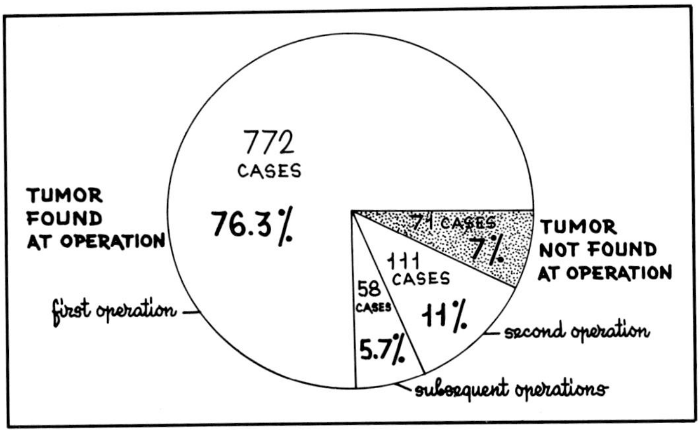

Fig. 2. Possibility of removing beta-islet cell tumors of the pancreas at operation.

Table VI. *Blood glucose and plasma insulin levels during operation*

Authors	*No. of cases*	*Results*
Bismuth	1	Good
Cevese	—	Good
De Peyster	—	Doubtful
Hartsuck	3	Good
Gentzen	1	Doubtful
Landor	2	Good
Leger	3	Good
McGarity	2	Good
McMillan	1	Good
Monti	3	Good
Scheinin	1	Doubtful
Schnelle	6	Good
Stefanini	3	Good
White	—	Good

cholangiography. Keaveny and co-workers[20] tried a method already used to distinguish other endocrine tumors, mainly parathyroids. Injection of toluidine blue into the splenic and gastroduodenal arteries may visualize an occult insulinoma. Nevertheless, the most useful test seems to be the measurement of serial blood glucose during operation (Table VI). This was proposed in 1951 by McMillan and Scheibe[26] and was based on the finding of "hyperglycemia on the rebound" which occur within the first 30 minutes of complete removal of the tumor.

De Peyster, although favoring this test, pointed out that there may be false-positive results in cases of diffuse adenomatoses submitted to subtotal resection or false-negative results when the hyperglycemia is late in appearing.

Table VII. *Pathologic findings in 951 completely documented cases*

	No. of cases	*Percent*
Topography:		
Head	305	32
Body	285	30
Tail	323	34
Uncinate	29	3
Ectopic	9	1
Number:		
Single	789	83
Multiple	123	13
Multiple endocrine adenomatosis	39	4
Parathyroid	16	1.5
Pituitary	10	1
Adrenal cortex	10	1
Thyroid	3	0.5
Size:		
< 0.5 cm.	47	5
0.5-1 cm.	323	34
1-5 cm.	504	53
> 5 cm.	77	8
Nature:		
Benign	798	84
Malignant	153	16
Metastases	47	5

Table VII reports the pathologic findings in 951 cases of insulinoma. Insulinomas are located in nearly equal percentages over the entire pancreas; for the most part they have a volume between 1 and 5 cm.; metastases were present in one third of the malignant tumors. Moreover, 10 percent of these insulinomas were multiple: 44 percent of the cases revealed two or three and 56 percent from four to a maximum of eight. To these cases which were certified at operation

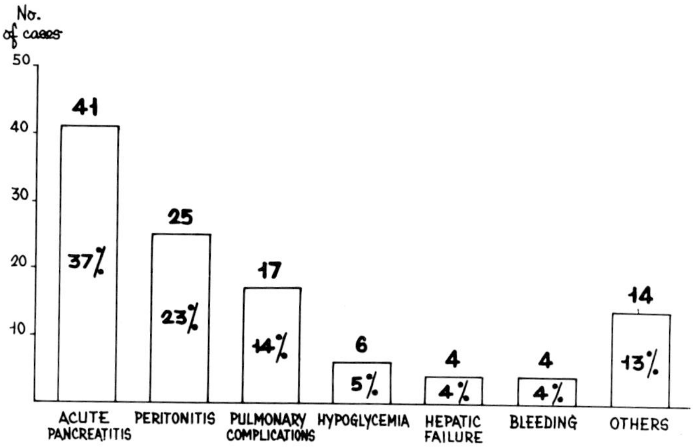

Fig. 3. Operative deaths (111 cases).

numerous other cases are added which have not been demonstrated: these include patients who, having undergone surgical removal of a tumor, present a persistence or recurrence of hypoglycemic crises.

RESULTS

The mortality rate in surgical treatment of beta-islet cell tumors was 11 percent—nearly three times as much in reinterventions (18 percent) as in first interventions (6.7 percent) (Table VIII). Nearly all the operative deaths that occur in larger procedures are due to acute pancreatitis or peritonitis. Deaths caused by peritonitis (22 cases) and acute pancreatitis (2 cases) occurred after pancreaticoduodenectomies and total pancreatectomies. Of 13 patients who had subtotal pancreatectomy, 10 died of acute pancreatitis. There is no question that acute pancreatitis occurs in the procedures including a higher risk for the pancreas integrity. Conversely, peritonitis occurs in procedures such as total pancreatectomy or pancreaticoduodenectomy where respectively two and three anastomsis are performed. The most frequent causes of death are summarized in Fig. 3. The high incidence of deaths for respiratory diseases can be easily explained if one considers the number of obese patients.

Postoperative complications may be general or specific after pancreatic surgery (Table IX). Those with enucleation have a frequency of 8 percent and primarily involve suppuration, bronchopneumonia, thrombophilia, and embolisms. As for specific complications, in patients undergoing distal resection pancreatic fistulas arise less often (4.5 percent) than after enucleation (12 percent of the cases). Urca advised the prevention of such complications through the use of pancreaticogastric anastomosis, which contacts the breach of the pancreas by a small opening in the posterior wall of the stomach. In only two cases, one of Mandache and one of Child, did the pancreatic fistula cause the death of the patient.

The pancreatic pseudocysts were nearly always caused by enucleation. White, in order to prevent fistulas and pseudocysts, advised performing a Roux-Y pancreaticojejunostomy after resection as well as after

Table VIII. *Death rate in relation to various interventions (1,012 cases completely documented)*

	Intervention		*Reintervention*	
	No. of cases	*%*	*No. of cases*	*%*
Enucleation	29	5.7	6	10
Distal resection	23	5.5	11	11.8
Pancreatoduodenectomy	4	26.6	8	33.3
Subtotal pancreatectomy	4	20	9	24.3
Total pancreatectomy	3	25	9	36
Exploratory laparotomy	5	11.3	—	—
Total	68	6.7	43	18
	111 (11%)			

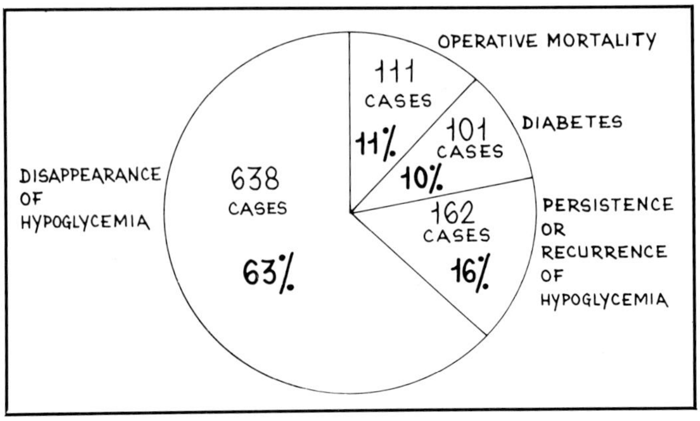

Fig. 4. Long-term results in 1,012 completely documented cases.

Table IX. *Incidence of postoperative complications in 882 completely documented cases in relation to different interventions*

		Fistulas		*Pseudocysts*		*Acute pancreatitis*		*Other complications*	
	No.	*No.*	*%*	*No.*	*%*	*No.*	*%*	*No.*	*%*
Enucleation	428	51	12	28	6.5	5	1.2	34	8
Distal resection	335	16	4.5	1	—	11	3.4	20	6
Pancreaticoduodenectomy	61	—	—	—	—	7	12	5	8
Other types of operation	58	—	—	—	—	—	—	9	15

local excision. Merkel,[29] however, reported that he used this technique in many patients without the presence of pseudocysts or fistulas.

Acute pancreatitis complicated the postoperative course of 12 percent of those patients submitted to pancreaticoduodenectomy; however, it sometimes occurred in other procedures and more often in distal resection than in enucleation.

Postoperative hyperglycemia was reported in many cases. When it occurs it is not a complication; when it is lacking one may suspect an incomplete treatment, as happened in two of our cases. This hyperglycemia is transient, lasting a maximum of 15 to 20 days. It remains between 200 and 300 mg. per 100 ml. and is accompanied by glycosuria and sometimes requires the use of insulin. Conversely, a persistent hyperglycemia pertains to subtotal and total pancreatectomy yet it is also present after minor operations. In the series collected (Fig. 4) from our investigations it recurred in 10 percent of the cases. The high incidence of cases (16 percent) with persistence or recurrence of hypoglycemia is to be emphasized. In many cases (6.8 percent) unsatisfactory results were due to nonresectable carcinomas or to multiple endocrine adenomatosis but the greater part (9.2 percent) consisted of unfound insulinomas and tumors in which inadequate resection had been performed.

In Table X we present our experience* which includes 10 adenomas, one carcinoma, and one case of unfound insulinoma. Eight were single, two were multiple, and one presented with multiple polyendocrine adenomatosis involving the adrenal cortex and the parathyroid. Three of these tumors were in the head, three in the body, four in the tail, and one in the uncinate process of the pancreas.

*In September, 1973, we observed another patient with an insulinoma of the tail. A corpocaudal resection was performed, and the patient is free of symptoms at 3 months.

Table X. *Surgical treatment and results (personal cases)*

Case No.	No., size, and site	Type of operation	Mortality rate	Complications	Long-term results
1	Single adenoma, 0.5 × 1 cm., head	Blind distal resection; enucleation	—	—	Hypoglycemia; cure at 2 yr.
2	Single adenoma, 1 × 1 cm., tail	Enucleation	—	Pseudocyst	Cure at 1 yr.
3	Multiple adenomas, 1.5 × 1 cm., body and tail	Corpocaudal pancreatectomy	—	Retroperitoneal abscess	Cure at 1 yr.
4	Multiple endocrine adenomatosis 1 × 0.5 cm., body, 1 × 2 cm., head	Corpocaudal pancreatectomy, enucleation	—	—	Cure at 6 mo.
5	Not found	Blind distal resection	—	—	Hypoglycemia
6	Single adenoma, 2.5 × 1.5 cm., tail	Corpocaudal pancreatectomy	—	—	Cure at 2 yr.
7	Single adenoma, 1.5 × 1 cm., body	Corpocaudal pancreatectomy	—	—	Cure at 1 yr.
8	Multiple adenomas, 2 × 3 cm., and 1 × 0.5 cm., body	Enucleation; blind distal resection	Died on day 3 from acute postoperative pancreatitis	—	Hypoglycemia
9	Carcinoma, 2 × 1.5 cm., body	Corpocaudal pancreatectomy; splenectomy	—	—	Cure at 9 mo.
10	Single adenoma, 0.5 × 1 cm., head	Blind distal resection; enucleation	Died on day 6 from massive intestinal infarction	—	Hypoglycemia
11	Single adenoma, 2 × 2 cm., tail	Blind distal resection; splenectomy	—	—	Cure at 6 mo.
12	Single adenoma, 1.5 × 1 cm., uncinate p.	Enucleation; blind distal resection	—	Pseudocyst	Cure at 6 mo.

*Adrenal cortex, parathyroid.

CONCLUSIONS

The following conclusions are drawn from the series collected in our investigations and personal experience.

1. The diagnosis of insulinomas is easily made when a tumor is suspected.

2. The real difficulty lies in locating the insulinoma rather than in technical surgical details. Of considerable help in this regard is the use of selective arteriography.

3. In occult tumors, rather than the classic blind distal resection, other procedures are presently advised. The most valuable one seems to be progressive resection from left to right with the extent being guided by pathologic examination of the successive portions of the pancreas removed and by the intraoperative blood sugar levels.

4. The operative mortality rate is elevated mainly in reinterventions and therefore every effort must be used to localize and remove the tumor at the first operation.

5. Fistulas and pseudocysts represent the most frequent complications.

6. The late results are good in cases where the insulinoma is found, less favorable when the insulinoma is not found.

We are greatly indebted to all those authors who sent up their personal communications and to all those who collaborated with their valuable information.

REFERENCES*

1. Abe, M., Iyanaga, T., and Yano, M.: Spontaneous hypoglycemia in Japan, Brain Nerve (Tokyo) **15:** 651, 1963.
2. Baum, S., Roy, R., Finkelstein, A. K., and Blakemore, W. S.: Clinical application of selective celiac and superior mesenteric arteriography, Radiology **84:** 279, 1965.
3. Bernheim, M., Francois, R., Sacrez, R., Mallet-Guy, P., Feroldi, J., Germain, D., Sherrer, M., Ruiton-Ugliengo, M., and Pra-

*References included in this paper concern only the authors from whom we did not receive direct information in our inquiry.

don, M.: Hypoclicémie par adenome pancréatique chez une fillette de 8 ans; intervention; guérison, Pediatrie **16:** 339, 1961.
4. Bookstein, J. J., and Oberman, H. A.: Appraisal of selective angiography in localizing islet cell tumours of the pancreas, Radiology **86:** 682, 1966.
5. Cady, B.: Palliative management of advanced carcinoma of the gastrointestinal tract, Surg. Clin. North Am. **51:** 761, 1971.
6. Carboni, M., Simi, M., and Patrassi, N.: Diagnosis and treatment of functioning beta-insular tumours and hyperplasias, Surg. Italy **3:** 206, 1971.
7. Clarke, M., Crofford, O. B., Graves, H. A., and Scott, H. W.: Functioning beta-islet cell tumours of the pancreas, Ann. Surg. **175:** 964, 1972.
8. De Gennes, J. L., Jungers, P., Saltiel, H., Mercadier, M., and De Court, J.: Sur les méthodes de diagnostic des hypoglycémies par adenome langerhansien, Presse Med. **33:** 1735, 1963.
9. Deuil, R., and Tugaye, A.: The diagnosis of hypoglycemia caused by malignant tumours, Presse Med. **75:** 2178, 1967.
10. Epstein, H. Y., Abrams, R. H., Beranbaum, E. R., and Locaho, S. A.: Angiographic localization of insulinomas, high reported success rate and two additional cases, Ann. Surg. **169:** 349, 1969.
11. Flynn, P. J., and McDonald, L. C.: Surgical treatment of the occult islet-cell tumour, Am. Surg. **25:** 843, 1959.
12. Gall, F.: Endokrine Pankreastumoren. Diagnostik und chirurgische Behandlung, Munch. Med. Wochenschr. **111:** 682, 1969.
13. Galli, T., and Pasini, G.: Malattia ipoglicemica infantile da adenoma insulare del pancreas, Clin. Pediat. **38:** 290, 1956.
14. Gray, R. K., Rosch, J., and Grollman, J. H.: Arteriography and diagnosis of islet-cell tumours, Radiology **97:** 39, 1970.
15. Gross, R. E.: The surgery of infancy and childhood, Philadelphia and London, 1953, W. B. Saunders Company, Firenze, 1956, S.E.S., p. 716.
16. Grözinger, K. H.: Klinik der endokrinen Pankreasgeschwülste. Med. Welt **44:** 2611, 1967.
17. Hartsuck, J. M., and Brooks, J. R.: Functioning beta islet-cell tumours. Preoperative tests and surgical approach, Am. J. Surg. **117:** 541, 1969.
18. Howard, J. M., Moss, H., and Rhoads, J. E.: Collective review: Hyperinsulinism and islet cell tumours of the pancreas. With 398 recorded tumours, Surg. Gynecol. Obstet. **90:** 417, 1950.
19. Irmer, W., Daweke, H., and Wedel, J.: Zur Diagnostik und Therapîe der Inselzelleadenome, Dtsch. Med. Wochenschr. **94:** 1, 1969.
20. Keaveny, T. V., Tawes, R., and Belzer, F. O.: A new method for intraoperative individuation of insulinomas, Br. J. Surg. **58:** 233, 1971.
21. Koutras, P., and White, R. R.: Insulin-secreting tumours of the pancreas. A diagnostic and therapeutic challenge, Surg. Clin. North Am. **52:** 299, 1972.
22. Legre, J., Guien, C., Clement, J. P., and Pietri, H.: Von Hippel-Lindau disease, cancer of the head of pancreas, hypoglycemic islet cell adenoma. Comparison of tumour radiologic aspects of angiomatous nature revealed by selective arteriography, Presse Med. **76:** 1911, 1968.
23. Lenarduzzi, G., Romani, S., and Zacchi, C.: La stimolazione farmacologica della funzione esocrina nella contrastografia opaca del pancreas, Radiol. Med. (Torino) **54:** 97, 1968.
24. Madsen, B.: Demonstration of pancreatic insuloma by angiography, Br. J. Radiol. **39:** 488, 1966.
25. McConnell, F., Thompson, A. G., and Kiss, J.: Selective celiac and superior mesenteric angiography, Can. J. Surg. **9:** 15, 1966.
26. McMillan, F. L., and Scheibe, J. R.: Islet-cell tumour of the pancreas, Am. J. Surg. **82:** 759, 1951.
27. Meaney, T. F., and Buonocore, E.: Arteriographic manifestations of pancreatic neoplasm, Am. J. Roentgenol. Radium Ther. Nucl. Med. **95:** 720, 1965.
28. Mengoli, L., and Le Quesne, L. P.: Blind pancreatic resection for suspected insulinoma: A review of the problem, Br. J. Surg. **54:** 749, 1967.
29. Merkel, F.: Quoted by White, *in* Karlie, H., and White, T.: Pancreatic beta islet cell tumors and hyperplasia: Experience in 14 Seattle hospitals, Ann. Surg. **175:** 326, 1972.
30. Moss, N. H., and Rhoads, J. E.: Hyperinsulinism and islet-cell tumours of the pancreas, *in* Howard, J. M., and Jordan, G. L., editors: Surgical diseases of the pancreas, Philadelphia, 1960, J. B. Lippincott Company, p. 321.
31. Nebesar, R. A., and Pollard, J. J.: A critical evaluation of selective celiac and superior mesenteric angiography in the diagnosis of pancreatic diseases, particularly malignant tumour: Facts and "artefacts," Radiology **89:** 1017, 1967.
32. Nieschlag, E., Wombacher, H., Kroeger, F. J., and Habighorst, L. V.: Therapie eines metastasierenden Inselzelltumours mit Streptozotocin, Acta Endocrinol. **67:** 405, 1971.

33. Olivier, C., Helemon, Epfelbaum, R., Toumieux, Favre, Rettori, R., and Baer, O.: Adenome langerhansien hypoglycemiant. L'image arteriographique, Presse Med. **45:** 2313, 1966.
34. Robinson, M. J.: Islet-cell adenoma in the new born report of two patients, Pediatrics **48:** 232, 1971.
35. Rochet, E., Gilly, R., and Dumas, B.: Hypoglycémie néonatale par adénome langerhansien, Bull. Féd. Soc. Gynécol. Obstet. franç. **13:** 314, 1961.
36. Rosch, J., and Bret, J.: Arteriography of the pancreas, Am. J. Roentgenol. **94:** 182, 1965.
37. Roth, J., Thier, S., and Segal, S.: Zinc glucagon in the management of refractory hypoglycemia due to insulin-producing tumors, N. Engl. J. Med. **274:** 493, 1966.
38. Salti, I. G., and Walker, T. M.: Islet-cell tumors of the pancreas, Arch. Surg. **85:** 238, 1962.
39. Scheinin, T. M., and Tala, E.: Diagnosis and treatment of pancreatic islet-cell adenomas, Acta Chir. Scand. **132:** 590, 1966.
40. Schlicke, C. P., and Berghan, R.: Hypoglycemia due to islet-cell tumour of the pancreas, Ann. Surg. **36:** 646, 1970.
41. Schwartz, J. F.: Islet-cell adenomatosis and adenoma in an infant, J. Pediatr. **79:** 232, 1971.
42. Smith, M. J., Hall, R., Stabler, J., and Hacking, P.: Successful localization of a pancreatic islet-cell adenoma by selective celiac angiography, Proc. R. Soc. Med. **63:** 337, 1970.
43. Smrcka, J., Bret, J., Hauer, J., and Polomis, V.: Arteriographic demonstration and successful removal of metastatic islet-cell tumors in liver, Diabetes **16:** 598, 1967.
44. Stefanini, P., and Ermini, M.: L'iperinsulinismo, Atti XXI Congr. Soc. Int. Chir. Philadelphia, 1965, p. 201.
45. Tompkins, R. K., Hardacre, J. M., Tzagournis, M., and Greider, M.: Definitive diagnosis of insulin-secreting tumors of the pancreas, Surg. Gynecol. Obstet. **125:** 1069, 1967.
46. Thompson, S., and Wech, K. J.: Surgery of the pancreas, *in* Benson, C. D.: Editor: Pediatric surgery, Chicago, 1962, Year Book Medical Publishers Inc., vol. 1, p. 629.
47. Underwood, L. E., and Jacob, N. M.: Familial endocrine adenomatosis, Am. J. Dis. Child. **106:** 218, 1963.
48. Vourinen, P., and Wegelius, N.: Angiography of the celiac area, Duodecimo **82:** 102, 1966.
49. Yacovac, W. C.: Beta-cell nesidioblastosis in idiopathic hypoglycemia of infancy, J. Pediatr. **79:** 226, 1971.
50. Warren, K. W.: Islet-cell tumors and hyperinsulinism, Surg. Clin. North Am. **42:** 709, 1962.
51. Wenz, W.: Selektive Arteriographie der Oberbauchorgane, Dtsch. Med. Wochenschr. **90:** 643, 1965.
52. Williams, C., Jr., Bryson, G. H., and Hume, D. H.: Islet-cell tumors and hypoglycemia, Ann. Surg. **169:** 757, 1969.

Brief clinical reports

The crossover femoropopliteal bypass

M. Haimov, M.D., *New York, N. Y.*

The crossover femoropopliteal bypass is suggested as a useful alternative in patients with unilateral iliofemoral occlusive disease, in whom groin dissection on the affected side is undesirable because of extensive scarring or infection. Two patients, in whom the procedure was successfully applied, are presented in brief.

From the Department of Surgery, Division of Vascular Surgery, Mount Sinai School of Medicine, City University of New York, New York, N. Y.

THE FEMOROFEMORAL bypass has been used successfully in patients with unilateral aorto-iliac obstructive disease.[5, 7] A modification, the crossover femoropopliteal bypass, has been found useful in a select group of patients. The indications and advantages of the procedure are illustrated in the following brief case reports.

CASE REPORTS

Case 1. A 42-year-old Caucasian male was admitted to the hospital with a six-month history of intermittent claudication of the left thigh and calf. The claudication was incapacitating and prevented the patient from continuing his occupation, which involved considerable physical exertion. On examination, the main findings were in the lower extremities. All the peripheral pulses were palpable in the right lower extremity, but there were no palpable pulses on the left. The left foot was cold, but sensation was normal and there were no signs of impending gangrene. Aortogram revealed an isolated left common and external iliac artery obstruction, with reconstitution of the common femoral artery and a second superficial femoral artery block with good distal "run-off." An unilateral aortofemoral bypass using 9½ mm. Dacron graft was performed through an extraperitoneal approach. The intraoperative and postoperative course up to the eighth postoperative day were uneventful. No prophylactic antibiotic agents were used. On the eighth day following surgery, the patient developed shaking chills with a rise in temperature to 104° F. Repeated blood cultures were sterile. Culture from a sinus which developed in the groin incision grew *Staphylococcus aureus,* coag. negative, and Streptococcus hemolytics. The patient was treated with intravenous antibiotics and local antibiotic drip to the groin sinus. Although the sinus in the groin did heal with this regimen, the systemic infection was not brought under control. After three weeks of persistent pyrexia, the patient underwent a second operation. A crossover femoropopliteal bypass (Fig. 1) was performed, through an uninfected area with the use of the reversed autogenous saphenous vein. After closure of all the incisions, the patient was redraped and the infected Dacron graft was removed, ligating the common femoral artery. A large abscess was found retroperitoneally above the inguinal ligament which was drained. The patient's temperature postoperatively returned to normal. All operative incisions healed primarily. Eight months following surgery, there are excellent pedal pulses in the left lower extremity and the patient is asymptomatic.

Comment. The crossover femoropopliteal bypass in this case allowed simultaneous ligation of the common femoral artery proximal to the deep femoral artery, removal of the infected aortofemoral Dacron prosthesis, and the preservation

Accepted for publication Jan. 14, 1974.

of the viability and function of the extremity. Other alternative solutions which may have been applicable were: obturator bypass through an uninfected plane[3, 6]; axillary popliteal bypass[1, 4]; or simple ligation of the femoral artery with removal of the prosthesis. All of these seemed to offer a more difficult, riskier, and less definitive solution for this gravely ill patient.

Case No. 2. A 65-year-old diabetic patient was admitted to the hospital with severe rest pain of the left foot. An unilateral Dacron aortofemoral bypass had been performed three years prior to this admission on the same side. The patient had been asymptomatic up to three weeks prior to admission, when he developed severe claudication and rest pain in the left foot and calf. Significant facts from the past history included diabetes of more than 15 years' duration and two episodes of myocardial infarctions in the last four years. On physical examination, the main findings were in the left lower extremity: the left foot was cold with the coldness extending to the mid-calf. There were no palpable peripheral pulses below the femoral pulse on the left. All pulses were present on the right. A translumbar aortogram showed complete occlusion of the left common iliac and external iliac arteries, with a patent Dacron aortofemoral bypass and open left deep femoral artery. The superficial femoral artery was occluded through its entire length. There was reconstitution of the popliteal artery above and below the knee with poor runoff caused by one vessel which was also occluded in the lower third of the leg.* In spite of the poor runoff, because of the severe rest pain and impending gangrene, a femoropopliteal bypass was performed. During surgery, extensive scarring was encountered in the area of the anastomosis of the Dacron graft to the femoral artery. Therefore, a crossover femoropopliteal bypass (Fig. 1) was performed by using the autogenous saphenous vein. Postoperatively, good popliteal pulse was palpable. The foot warmed up and the rest pain disappeared. Pedal pulses, however, have not appeared during the period of hospitalization and the subsequent one-year follow-up period. The bypass, however, has remained patent, the rest pain has disappeared, and the patient is free of symptoms on moderate exertion.

Comment. By refraining from further dissection in a previously operated groin, several potential complications were avoided: (1) injury to the anastomotic line or to the deep femoral artery which was the single outflow of the graft; (2) exposure of the Dacron prosthesis with its inherent danger of infection; (3) anastomosis of a vein to Dacron prosthesis which many consider undesirable.

*The right iliac and femoral arteries were patent.

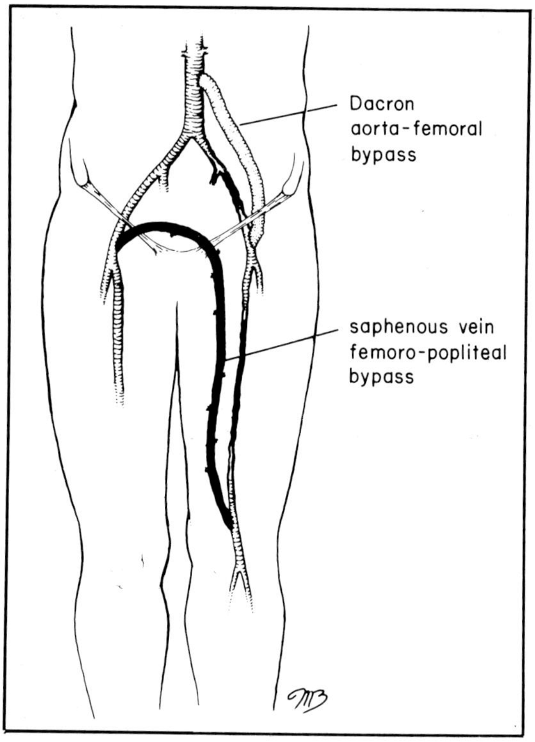

Fig. 1. Crossover femoropopliteal bypass performed with autogenous saphenous vein.

DISCUSSION

The femorofemoral bypass has been used by many with excellent immediate and long-term results.[2, 4, 5, 7] Although originally suggested as an alternative to the aortofemoral bypass in the poor-risk patient, its long-term results seem to be equally as good. Some surgeons have used it as the operation of choice in unilateral iliac artery obstruction, instead of the aortofemoral bypass, regardless of the general condition of the patient.[2] The crossover femoropopliteal bypass is a useful modification of this operation in patients in whom the groin on the affected side is either actually or potentially infected or is densely scarred from previous surgical procedures. It greatly simplifies the surgical approach to these difficult reconstructive problems and can be a limb-saving and occasionally life-saving procedure.

REFERENCES

1. Blaisdeal, F. W., and Hall, A. D.: Axillofemoral artery bypass for lower extremity ischemia, SURGERY **54:** 563, 1963.
2. Brief, D. K., Alpert, J., and Parsonnet, V.: Crossover femorofemoral grafts, Arch. Surg. **105:** 889, 1972.
3. DePalma, R. G., and Hubay, C. A.: Arterial bypass via the obturator foramen, Am. J. Surg. **115:** 323, 1968.
4. Mannick, J. A., William, L. E., and Nabseth, D. C.: The late results of axillofemoral grafts, SURGERY **68:** 1038, 1970.
5. Parsonnet, V., Alpert, J., and Brief, D. K.: Femorofemoral and axillofemoral grafts: Compromise or preference, SURGERY **67:** 26, 1970.
6. Shaw, R. E., and Baue, A. E.: Management of sepsis complicating arterial reconstructive Surgery, SURGERY **53:** 75, 1963.
7. Vetto, R. M.: The Femorofemoral shunt: An appraisal, Am. J. Surg. **112:** 162, 1966.

Inferior vena caval obstruction caused by expansion of an abdominal aortic aneurysm: Report of a case and review of the literature

Richard L. Snider, M.D., John M. Porter, M.D., *and* **Larry R. Eidemiller, M.D.,**
Portland, Ore.

Lateral vena caval displacement without caval obstruction occurs in a great majority of patients with expanding abdominal aortic aneurysms. In the patient described in this report, caval displacement was prevented by preexisting dense fibrous adhesions which may have resulted from previous aneurysmal leaks. Symptomatic vena caval obstruction occurred between the expanding aneurysm and the lateral adhesions. To our knowledge, this represents the first angiographically proved case of vena caval obstruction caused by aortic aneurysmal expansion.

From the Vascular Surgical Service, Department of Surgery, University of Oregon Medical School, Portland, Ore.

COMPLETE OCCLUSION of the inferior vena cava by an expanding abdominal aortic aneurysm is a rare clinical finding. Only a few such cases have been reported in the literature, and none have been documented angiographically. We recently treated a patient with a ruptured abdominal aortic aneurysm who had sustained complete symptomatic vena caval occlusion by aneurysmal expansion two weeks earlier. To our knowledge, this represents the first fully documented case of vena caval occlusion by an expanding aortic aneurysm. Our experience with the management of this patient and a review of the literature forms the basis for this report.

CASE REPORT

A 57-year-old unemployed male laborer entered our emergency room complaining of severe epigastric and mid-back pain and shortness of breath of 12 hours' duration. Two and one-half weeks prior to admission, he had noted the onset of sharp epigastric pain unrelated to meals. Several days later, he had developed painful swelling and a bluish discoloration of both legs. The leg swelling progressively increased until he was able to walk only with considerable difficulty. The epigastric pain subsided until 12 hours before admission. He gave no history of previous lower extremity claudication, venous disease, or edema.

Physical examination revealed an apical heart rate of 160 beats per minute and an unobtainable peripheral blood pressure. Although pale and diaphoretic, the patient was alert and oriented. Abdominal examination revealed an 8 by 6 cm. tender, pulsatile, epigastric mass. The lower extremities were massively edematous and cyanotic up to the inguinal ligaments.

The patient was immediately given a large intravenous volume of Ringer's lactate and albumin, and within ten minutes his blood pressure returned to 120/70. At that time arm pulses were easily palpable, but no lower extremity pulses could be felt. Laboratory results included a hematocrit of 43 percent, a leukocyte count of 27,000, a blood urea nitrogen (BUN) value of 72 mg. percent, normal urinalysis, normal serum electrolytes and arterial gases. An electrocardiogram showed only sinus tachycardia.

Accepted for publication Feb. 11, 1974.

Reprint requests: Dr. John M. Porter, Department of Surgery, University of Oregon Medical School, 3181 S.W. Sam Jackson Park Road, Portland, Ore. 97201.

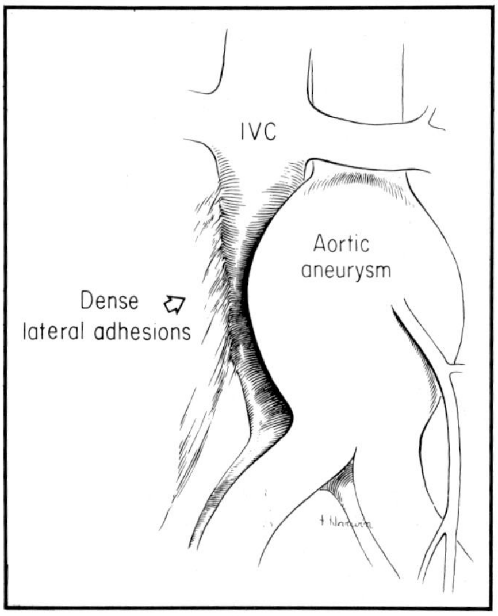

Fig. 1. Diagrammatic representation of the findings at surgery indicating the firm fixation of the vena cava to the retroperitoneum.

The patient was taken immediately to surgery with the diagnosis of ruptured abdominal aortic aneurysm and bilateral lower extremity venous occlusion. He was found to have a large ruptured abdominal aortic aneurysm with approximately 1,000 ml. of blood free both retroperitoneally and intraperitoneally. The inferior vena cava was surrounded by dense adhesions which extended from the renal veins to the caval bifurcation and fixed the cava firmly to the retroperitoneal tissues and to the aneurysm. The neck of the aneurysm and the iliac arteries were clamped, and the aneurysm was opened. The aneurysm had expanded laterally and had obliterated the caval lumen by compression of the medial caval wall against the lateral caval wall which was fixed by surrounding adhesions (Fig. 1). No bleeding occurred from the cava and the area of compression was densely fibrotic. Clots could be palpated in the iliac veins.

The aneurysm was replaced with a woven bifurcation Dacron prosthesis anastomosed proximally to the infrarenal aorta and distally to the femoral arteries. The patient's legs were elevated postoperatively, and within several days, the leg edema had completely resolved. Normal arterial pulses were easily palpated in both legs. Phlebograms were obtained postoperatively both above and below the site of caval obstruction (Figs. 2*A* and 2*B*). The patient was anticoagulated with warfarin and was discharged on the nineteenth postoperative day with elastic support stockings. He has done well postoperatively and, on his last clinic visit, was noted to have good arterial pulses in his legs and no leg edema.

DISCUSSION

In this case, the phlebograms depict clearly the complete interruption of the inferior vena cava at the site of the aneurysm and confirm the findings at operation. A review of the literature shows that there are four possible cases of inferior vena cava obstruction caused by an abdominal aortic aneurysm. In 1911, Pleasants[4] reviewed inferior vena caval obstruction and was able to find two probable cases of caval obstruction caused by abdominal aortic aneurysms reported in the British literature, although the available information was incomplete. He had no cases of aneurysmal obstruction of his own. In 1951, Herschowitz and Bagg[2] reported one case of a 70-year-old man who died of exsanguination from rupture of an abdominal aortic aneurysm into the third part of the duodenum. The patient had presented with "pitting edema" of both legs and autopsy showed that the aneurysm was "pressing on the inferior vena cava." Tein Eyck and Wellman[6] in 1959 reported a case of an abdominal aortic aneurysm that was infected with a strain of Salmonella. The patient developed massive edema of his legs and venous distention over his lower abdomen. Autopsy showed him to have died from rupture of the aneurysm into the duodenum and retroperitoneally. The aneurysm was pressing on the inferior vena cava and both iliac veins were thrombosed. The authors point out that the iliac vein thrombosis may have been caused by prolonged, contiguous sepsis alone.

Several authors[1, 5] have described aortocaval fistulas secondary to rupture of an abdominal aortic aneurysm into the adjacent vena cava. These patients usually present with edema of the lower extremities and venous distention over the lower abdomen, apparently representing functional vena caval obstruction caused by the high venous pressure at the arteriovenous fistula. Uniformly, these patients have not demonstrated anatomic caval interruption, and successful repair of the fistula and aneurysm has relieved the venous obstruction.

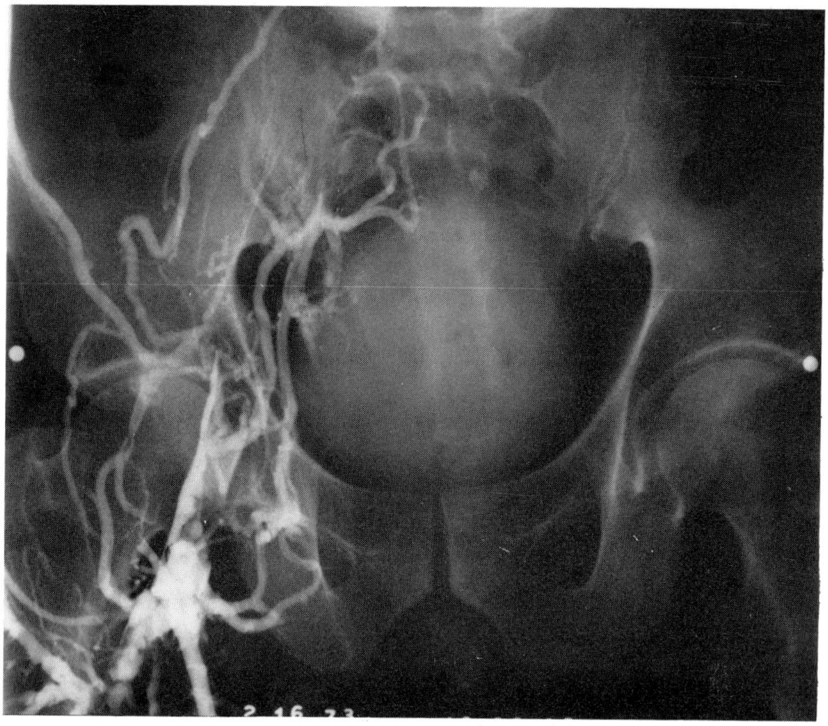

Fig. 2A. Postoperative phlebogram following peripheral injection showing occlusion of the right iliac venous system.

Our patient sustained complete occlusion of the inferior vena cava, presumably caused by aneurysmal expansion, two weeks prior to presentation with aneurysmal rupture. The abundant fibrosis at the site of caval occlusion suggests that the caval compression was of long standing and that the event two weeks before rupture represented the final total occlusion of a stenotic area. The dense fibrous adhesions found lateral to the inferior vena cava prevented lateral caval displacement as aneurysmal expansion occurred. The cause of the lateral caval adhesions in this patient is unknown but may represent a reaction to one or more prior retroperitoneal aneurysmal leaks, although the patient recalled no episodes of abdominal pain before two weeks prior to rupture of the aneurysm.

With the addition of this case, one may speculate that the inferior vena cava may respond in one of three ways to an abdominal aortic aneurysm. In a great majority of cases, without lateral caval fibrosis, aneurysmal

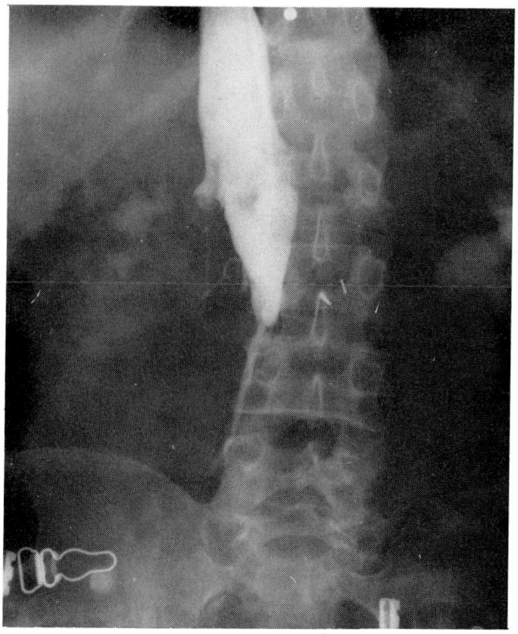

Fig. 2B. Postoperative phlebogram following vena cava injection showing occlusion of the inferior vena cava distal to the renal veins.

expansion causes lateral caval displacement without obstruction. Rarely, the cava may become fibrotically adherent to the aneurysm as a result of either aneurysmal leak or, possibly, atheromatous erosion. Further leak or erosion at this local area of caval adhesion may result in an aortocaval fistula. Finally, as shown by this patient, lateral caval fibrosis may trap the cava and result in caval occlusion by aneurysmal expansion.

REFERENCES

1. Beall, A. C., Cooley, D. A., Morris, G. C., and De Bakey, M. E.: Perforation of arteriosclerotic aneurysms into inferior vena cava, Arch Surg. **86:** 809, 1963.
2. Herschowitz, B. I., and Bagg, L.: Aneurysm of the abdominal aorta with a report of four unusual cases, Gastroenterology **18:** 361, 1951.
3. Missal, M. E., Robinson, J. A., and Tatum, R. W.: Inferior vena cava obstruction: Clinical manifestations, diagnostic methods and related problems, Ann. Intern. Med. **62:** 133, 1965.
4. Pleasants, J. H.: Obstruction of the inferior vena cava with a report of 18 cases, Johns Hopkins Hosp. Rep. **16:** 363, 1911.
5. Reckless, J. P. D., McColl, I., and Taylor, G. W.: Aortocaval fistulae: An uncommon complication of abdominal aortic aneurysms, Br. J. Surg. **59:** 461, 1972.
6. Tein Eyck, F. W., and Wellman, W. E.: Salmonellosis associated with abdominal aortic aneurysm and edema of the lower extremities. A case report, Postgrad. Med. **26:** 334, 1959.

Pinhole colonic perforation in breech-born infants

Å. Andersson, M.D., P.-Å. Hofer, M.D., D. E. W. Holmlund, M.D., *and* **H. Wendel, M.D.,**
Umeå, Sweden

A premature infant, second of twins, was born in assisted breech presentation with a pinhole perforation at the right colonic flexure. Similar colonic perforations have been reported earlier in breech-born infants. The genesis of this type of intestinal perforation is discussed. It is assumed that external compression of the cervical ring during delivery in assisted breech presentation can cause a rapid pressure rise inside the colonic flexures. In model studies in rabbits and in a postmortem specimen it is shown that a pinhole perforation of the intestinal wall occurs when the pressure inside the lumen increases rapidly.

From the Departments of Surgery, Pathology II, and Pediatrics, University Hospital of Umeå, Sweden.

ZILLNER[13] described in 1881 a diagonal slit in the sigmoid colon of newborns and assumed that the lesion was due to traction of the sigmoid colon during delivery. The aim of the present report is to describe another type of colonic perforation which also may be due to the delivery trauma.

CASE REPORT

A female infant (F. L.), second of twins, was born four weeks before term in assisted breech presentation. The delivery was uneventful and occurred five minutes after the birth of the first twin. The condition of the child was good. She weighed 1,580 grams and measured 42.5 cm. Umbilical artery catheterization was performed immediately to facilitate repeated analysis of arterial blood. After 14 hours the lumen of the catheter was occluded. An attempt to remove and replace the catheter caused blanching of the right leg. This blanching immediately disappeared when the catheter was withdrawn.

The patient needed parenteral nutrition and therefore the arterial catheter was replaced by an umbilical venous catheter. This was removed on the third day after birth. At this time it was noted that the abdomen was tympanitic and distended. An x-ray film of the abdomen showed free gas in the peritoneal cavity. Laparotomy was performed immediately. In the peritoneal cavity amounts of meconium were found. At the hepatic flexure there was an area of the colonic wall which was covered with fibrin. When these had been carefully removed it was possible, although with difficulty, to identify a *pinhole* perforation of the colonic wall. Ileocecal resection was performed. The postoperative period was uneventful and the patient was discharged in good health.

HISTOPATHOLOGIC EXAMINATION

The excised part of the bowel was fixed in a 10 percent solution of formalin and cut into 18 slices. All were dehydrated and embedded in paraffin. The sections, taken at numerous levels, were stained with hematoxylin and eosin and with van Gieson's stain.

The region which had been clinically observed to be slightly changed revealed upon

Accepted for publication Oct. 29, 1973.

Reprint requests: Dan E. W. Holmlund, M.D., Department of Surgery, University Hospital of Umeå, S-901 85 Umeå 6, Sweden.

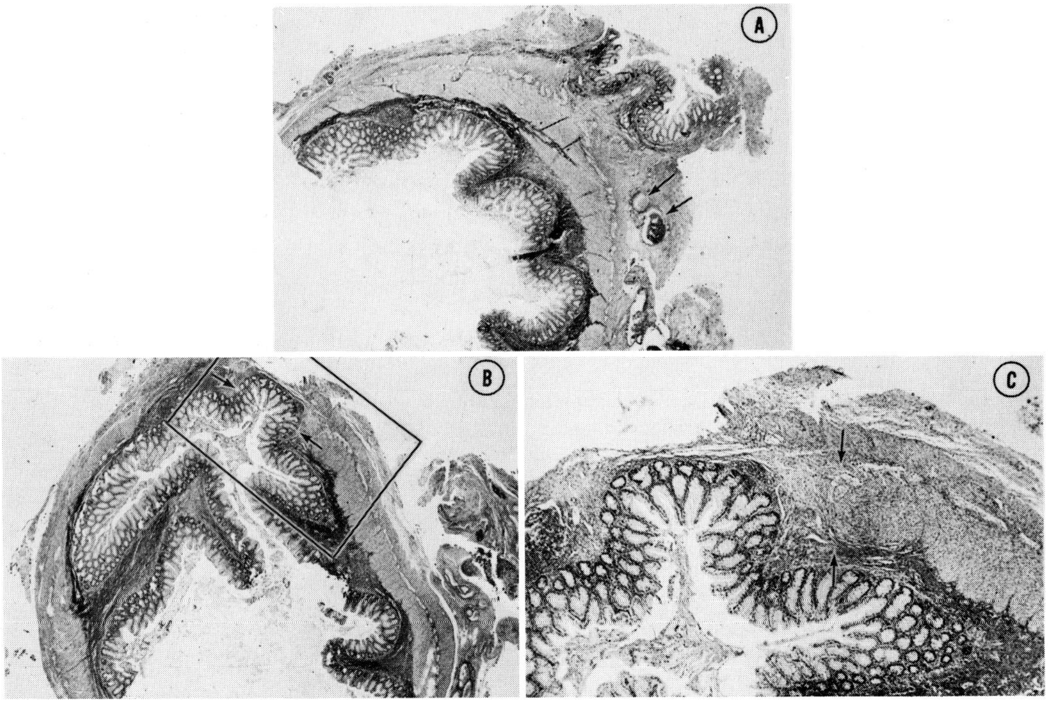

Fig. 1. *A,* Low-power photomicrograph of the wall of the large intestine close to the hepatic flexure, showing parts of the broken diverticulum (upper right corner). A few medium-sized blood vessels are seen outside the muscular coats not far from the diverticulum (arrows). (van Gieson's stain; ×8.) *B,* Another low-power photomicrograph of the colonic wall showing the inner opening of the diverticulum (between arrows). The diverticulum seems to run through the intestinal wall at an angle almost perpendicular to that of the plane of sectioning. (van Gieson's stain; ×8.) *C,* Enlargement of the area outlined in *B.* The circular muscular coat terminates (between the arrows) close to the inner opening of the diverticulum. (van Gieson's stain; ×20.)

histopathologic examination, a small diverticulum or diverticulum-like lesion, pushing through all the layers of the wall and coated with colonic mucosa (Fig. 1). The tip of this diverticulum was perforated. The diverticulum was not located right next to the mesentery but some fairly large blood vessels were seen near it. In the colonic wall, immediately next to the diverticulum, a slight inflammatory reaction was observed and there were newly formed blood vessels, granulocytes, and histiocytes. A very small part of the surface was covered with fibrin.

DISCUSSION

During the last few years many authors have reported intestinal perforations in newborn infants in connection with exchange transfusions[4-6] and after infusions into the umbilical vein.[9] Recently, in addition, colonic perforation has been observed following catheterization of the umbilical artery.[2] In all these cases the perforation had occurred in an area where an infarction apparently had weakened the intestinal wall. In these cases the infarction could be secondary to a disturbed circulation related to the catheterization.

In the present case there was no obvious infarction; there is, therefore, reason to analyze whether such a perforation may be caused by another mechanism than a locally disturbed circulation.

Nienhuis[8] described the case of a patient

with a similar perforation. This was also a twin, breech-born (weight at birth 2,500 grams). Twenty-four hours after delivery the child was operated on and a *pinhole* perforation was found in the right colonic flexure. Adjacent tissue was judged to be normal and the rupture was closed with silk sutures. The postoperative course was uneventful.

Anderson[1] reported the case of a premature infant (weight at birth 1,600 grams), also breech-born, who died eight hours after birth of respiratory insufficiency. At postmortem examination a very small but covered perforation was found in the left colonic flexure and a great deal of meconium in the peritoneal cavity. Levin and Isaacson[7] reported the case of an infant in whom meconium peritonitis was discovered during laparotomy but it had not been possible to localize the perforation during the operation. The child died within 24 hours and at postmortem examination a very small perforation was discovered in the right colonic flexure. Skiles[12] reported a case of meconium peritonitis in which the perforation had healed spontaneously. Rickham[11] and Rehbein and Wolfram[10] described similar cases in which it was not possible to find a perforation when exploration of the abdomen was carried out and where it was therefore assumed that there had been spontaneous healing. Anderson[1] presumed that colonic perforations of this type were due to a congenital defect in the muscular coats of the colonic wall. It is probable, however, that there is also another factor involved, i.e., a considerable pressure rise in the colonic lumen when a perforation occurs.

In studies of rabbits it has been shown that a *pinhole* perforation appears even in a normal intestinal wall if there is a rapid increase in pressure in the lumen.[3] These perforations always occurred near the mesentery and in the vicinity of relatively large vessels, i.e., in the parts of the intestinal wall where there are no muscular coats.

In a postmortem specimen we have also been able to show in the course of repeated experiments that if the pressure inside a colonic section is quickly increased a *pinhole* perforation occurs in the wall.

When a child is breech-born it is often desirable to finish the delivery as quickly as possible, especially if the infant is the second of twins. If the extraction is not accompanied by a simultaneous uterine contraction the abdomen of the infant may be compressed by the cervical ring and the contents of the abdominal cavity may then be violently pressed up against the thorax. A rapid rise in pressure may then occur in the colonic flexures, especially if both the incoming and outgoing part of the bowel are compressed. We think that this may be a possible explanation of the occurrence of the perforation in our case. This type of perforation of the colonic wall may be more common than was previously believed. Most of these early perforations would seem to heal spontaneously but leave behind them peritoneal adherences. Incidents of mechanical ileus in children who have not undergone laparotomy may sometimes be due to such adherences.

REFERENCES

1. Anderson, G. S.: Spontaneous perforation of the fetal colon, Am. J. Dis. Child. **103:** 166, 1962.
2. Andersson, Å, Hofer, P.-Å., Holmlund, D. E. W., and Wendel, H.: Colonic perforation secondary to thrombo-embolus from an umbilical artery catheter, Acta Pediatr. Scand. **63:** 155, 1974.
3. Bergman, F. O., Borgström, S. J. H., and Holmlund, D. E. W.: Synthetic absorbable surgical suture material (PGA), Acta Chir. Scand. **137:** 193, 1970.
4. Castor, W. R.: Spontaneous perforation of the bowel in the newborn following exchange transfusion, Can. Med. Assoc. J. **99:** 934, 1968.
5. Corkery, J. J., Dubowitz, V., Lister, J., and Moosa, A.: Colonic perforation after exchange transfusion, Br. Med. J. **4:** 345, 1968.
6. Friedman, A. B., Abellera, R. M., Lidsky, I., and Lubert, M.: Perforation of the colon after exchange transfusion in the newborn, N. Engl. J. Med. **282:** 796, 1970.
7. Levin, S. E., and Isaacson, C.: Spontaneous

perforation of the colon in the newborn infant, Arch. Dis. Child. **35:** 378, 1960.
8. Nienhuis, L. I.: Colon perforation in the newborn, Am. Surg. **29:** 835, 1963.
9. Orme, R. I. E., and Eades, S.: Perforation of the bowel in the newborn as a complication of exchange transfusion, Br. Med. J. **4:** 349, 1968.
10. Rehbein, F., and Wolfram, J.: Meconium peritonitis, Chirurg **30:** 149, 1959.
11. Rickham, P. P.: Peritonitis in the neonatal, Arch. Dis. Child. **30:** 23, 1955.
12. Skiles, J. H.: Prenatal rupture of the intestinal wall with subsequent dystonia, J. A. M. A. **90:** 1618, 1928.
13. Zillner, E.: Ruptura flexurae sigmoidis neonati inter partum, Virchows Arch. Pathol. Anat. **96:** 1999, 1881.

Amyloidoma (a solitary nodule of the lung)

João Batista Marchesini, M.D., Albano de Almeida Chaves Luis, M.D., *and*
Marco Aurelio Cravo, M.D., *Curitiba, Parana, Brazil*

A pulmonary solitary nodule, discovered in a 37-year-old woman, was removed surgically. It was a solitary amyloidoma of the left upper lobe. The clinical and pathological features of this disease were analyzed and the importance in the differential diagnosis among other pulmonary tumors is discussed.

From the Departments of Surgery, Pathology, and Medicine, Parana University Medical School and the Casa de Saude São Vicente, Curitiba, Parana, Brazil

AMYLOIDOSIS is an uncommon clinical entity, but when localized in a single organ as a tumor-like mass, it is very rare.[1-6] Amyloidoma is a localized deposit of amyloid material very similar to a tumor and, when found in the lung, is considered in the differential diagnosis with other pulmonary solitary nodules.

The first case report was published in 1877 by Lesser,[1] and by 1966, only seven cases were reported. Wichert,[5] in 1969, did a review of the literature and found only 30 cases. In 1970, Skagseth and Normann published a report of one more case.[4]

Our case has stimulated us to do the present report which adds one more to the medical literature. It is our intention to focus on the importance of the differential diagnosis and to record the interesting features of the tissue pathology.

CASE REPORT

An asymptomatic 37-year-old black woman from Curitiba, Parana, Brazil, was found during a routine chest x-ray to have a pulmonary nodule in the upper lobe of the left lung (Figs. 1, 2, and 3). She did not smoke or drink alcohol, never experienced weight loss, chest pain, cough, hemoptysis, or other respiratory symptoms. Twelve years prior to this admission, she had pneumonia which was successfully treated, and two years ago, she had a spiking fever which was interpreted as a virus infection. The physical examination showed a well-nourished female with a blood pressure of 140/80, a regular pulse (80 per minute), a

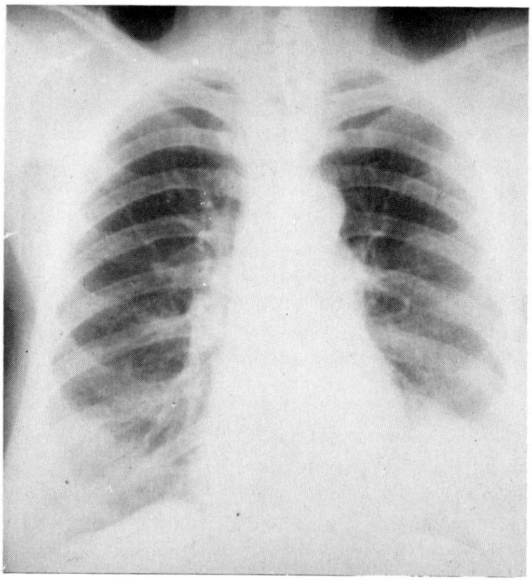

Fig. 1. Chest x-ray film. Anterior view showing a mass in the upper lobe of the left lung.

Accepted for publication Dec. 28, 1973.

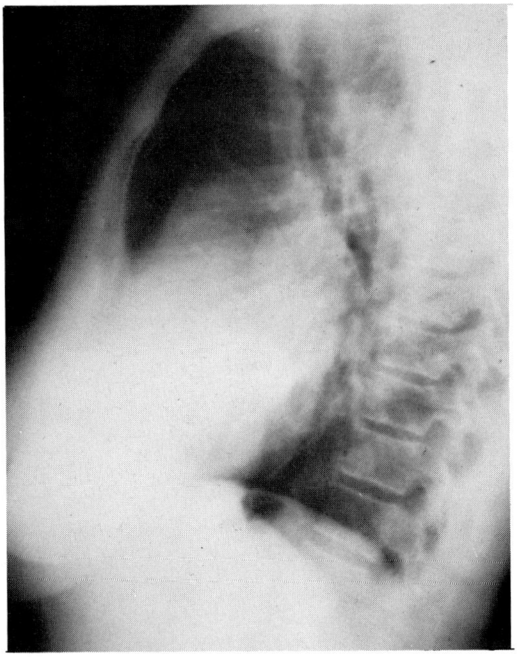

Fig. 2. Lateral view of the left chest showing a round mass overlying the heart shadow.

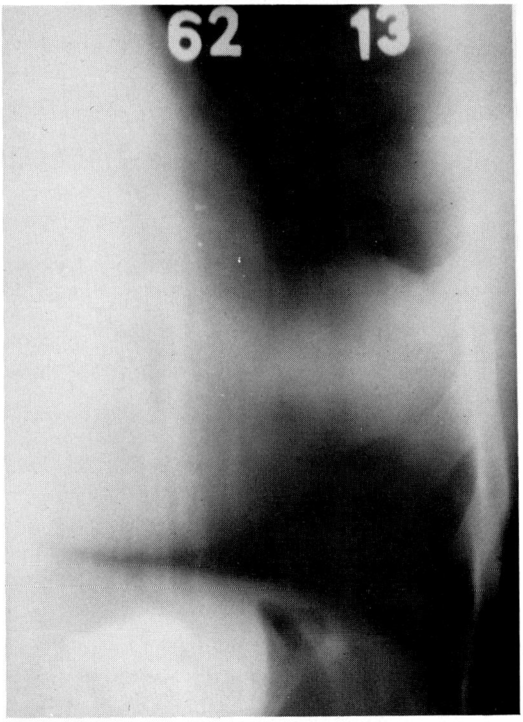

Fig. 3. Tomogram showing a round 5 cm. mass in the lingular segments.

temperature of 98° F., and a respiration rate of 16 per minute. The examination of the head and neck was not remarkable. The breath sounds were diminished in the anterolateral aspect of the left chest. Some moist rales were heard diffusely in both lungs which disappeared when the patient coughed. The examination of the breast, precordium, abdomen, and limbs was unremarkable. Laboratory studies were made. A chest x-ray film and tomograms showed a round (5 cm.) mass in the lingular segments of the upper lobe of the left lung. No hilar mass or satellite lesion was seen. Fluoroscopy of the chest demonstrated a normally moving diaphragm. The sputum examination was negative for malignant cells and for acid-fast bacilli, as well as for fungi. The patient was non-reactive on the P.P.D. test. A bronchoscopy showed a reddish area in the left main stem bronchus where the biopsy was taken. The tissue pathology report as well as bronchial washing examination were within normal limits. The ventilatory tests showed a vital capacity of 2,475 ml. (95 percent), M.V.V., 51,360 ml. per minute, and F.E.V./ls was 1.865 ml., calling attention to a ventilatory insufficiency of an obstructive type. The erythrocyte count was normal (5.2 million), the hematocrit was 40 percent, and the hemoglobin was 14 Gm. percent. The leukocyte count showed 4,700 leukocytes per cubic millimeter with a normal differential count. The blood urea was 32 mg. percent, and the creatinine 0.78 mg. percent. Fasting blood sugar was 85 mg. percent, and urinalysis was normal. The bone marrow was also examined and was normal as well. The electrocardiogram had a normal tracing.

An effort was made to determine if the lung mass was a primary or secondary lesion before starting surgical exploration. A thorough physical examination ruled out tumors of the breast, thyroid, neck masses, or other suspicious lesions. The results of an intravenous pyelogram, and upper gastrointestinal x-ray film and a barium enema were unremarkable. The patient was taken to the operating room. While the patient was under general anesthesia with selective endotracheal intubation with Carlens tube, a left thoracotomy was performed in the fifth rib bed which was resected. When the chest cavity was explored, a firm whitish, nonadherent, 5 cm. mass was found in the upper lobe, involving both lingular segments. A left upper lobectomy was performed. The chest cavity was drained and closed in layers in a routine manner. The recovery was uneventful. The chest tube was removed in 48 hours, the skin sutures in nine days, and the patient was discharged in two weeks.

Pathologic examination: the gross specimen was a 19 by 11 by 3 cm. upper lobe of the left

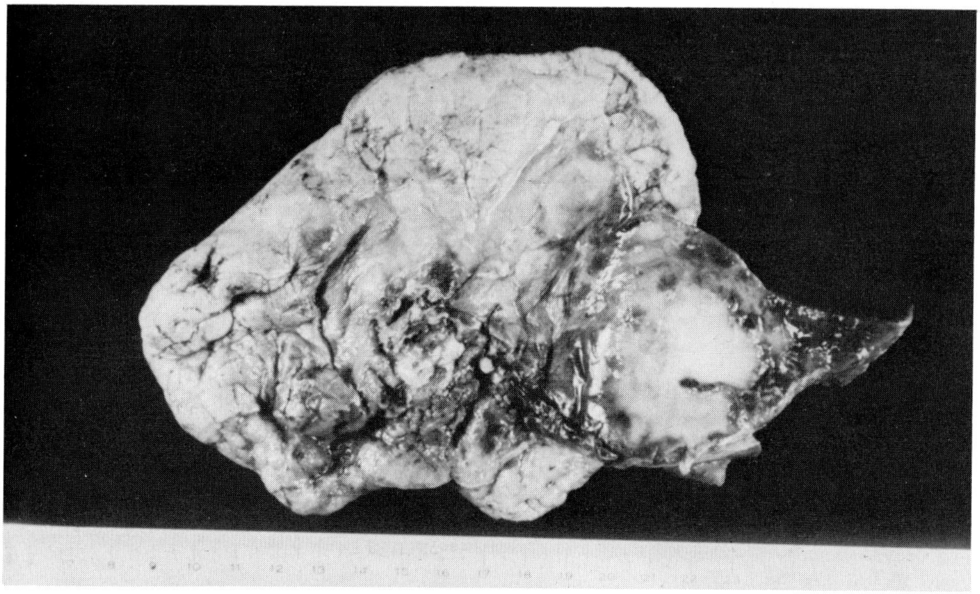

Fig. 4. Gross specimen with a view of the lingular mass.

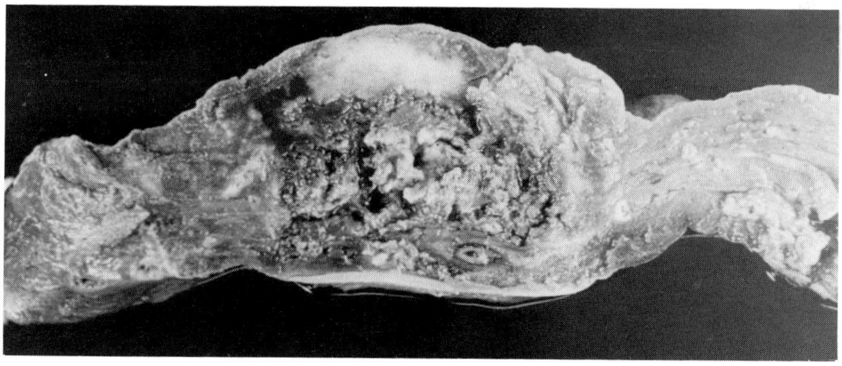

Fig. 5. Cross-section view showing a whitish round tumor with a necrotic center.

lung, with a 3 by 5 cm. round, firm, whitish mass which when cut showed a firm external wall surrounding an irregular cavity full of clotted blood and friable material. The rest of the specimen showed minimal crepitation (Figs. 4, 5, 6, and 7).

The microscopic examination of selected segments of the tumor surface showed part of the lung parenchyma somewhat preserved, intermingled with a large amount of an amorphous and hyaline eosinophilic material surrounding mostly the blood vessels occluding the lumen. Several groups of multinucleated giant cells were seen phagocyting this substance. The histologic pattern indicated the diagnosis of an amyloid tumor. Special stains with Congo red, crystal violet and periodic acid–Schiff were positive. Under poralized light and Congo red stain a birefringent green light was obtained. Adjacent to this lesion in the subpleural space, there was more of this amyloid deposit. The center of the mass contained necrotic and amorphous material as well as blood clots. An amyloid tumor was diagnosed.

DISCUSSION

An asymptomatic solitary pulmonary nodule when diagnosed in a routine chest x-ray film is usually considered to be one of the most common diseases, i.e., benign or malignant neoplasms, granulomatous lesions, abscess, or lymphomas. Since the beginning, the gross aspects of this tumor showed a different feature from those diseases men-

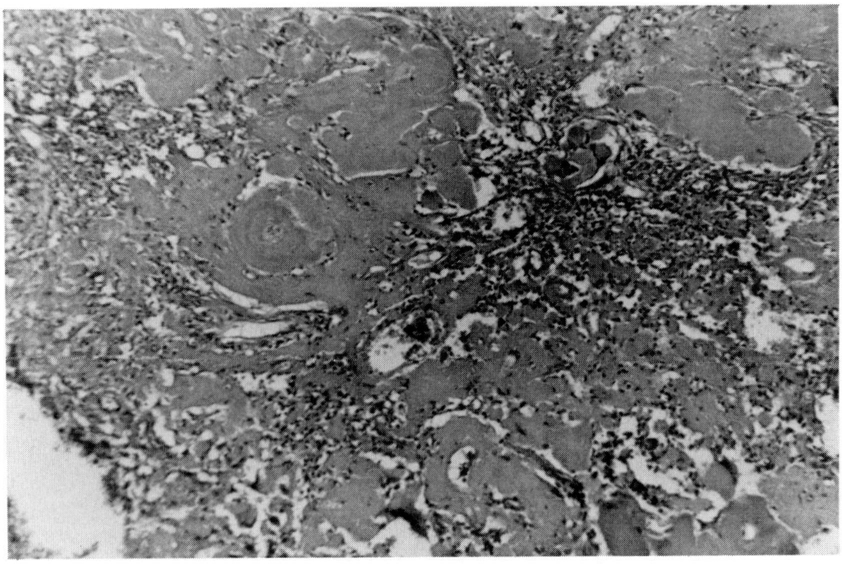

Fig. 6. Amyloid deposits in lung parenchyma surrounding blood vessels with small cells infiltrated. (Hematoxylin and eosin. Original magnification ×40.)

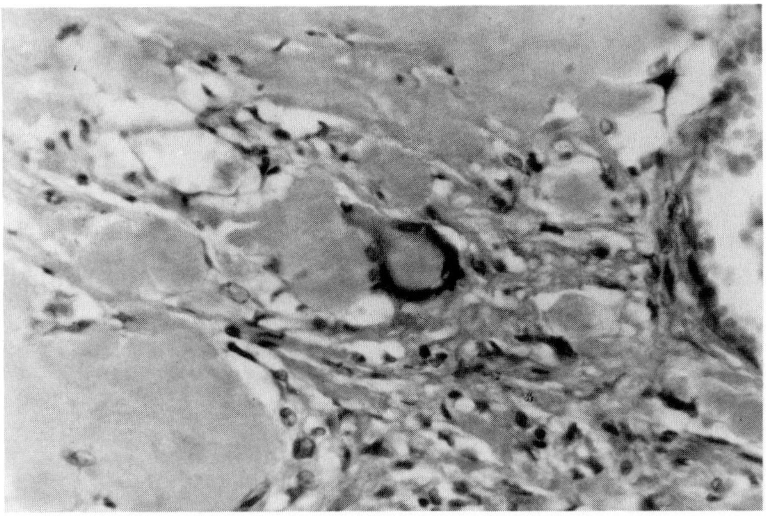

Fig. 7. Multinucleated giant cell phagocyting amyloid material. (Hematoxylin and eosin. Original magnification ×45.)

tioned above. It looked like an abscess but without a clear-cut exudate and had a firm and whitish wall. It resembled a malignant tumor with excavation but with somewhat different features. It did not have any caseous material suggestive of tuberculous granuloma and was not homogeneous enough to suggest other types of granulomas. The characteristics observed would not fit other solid lesions. Only the microscopic examination revealed the final diagnosis. In order to determine if the tumor was a systemic involvement or a localized lesion, we continued the investigation during the patient's hospitalization. Biopsies secured from the gums and from the rectum were negative. Serum

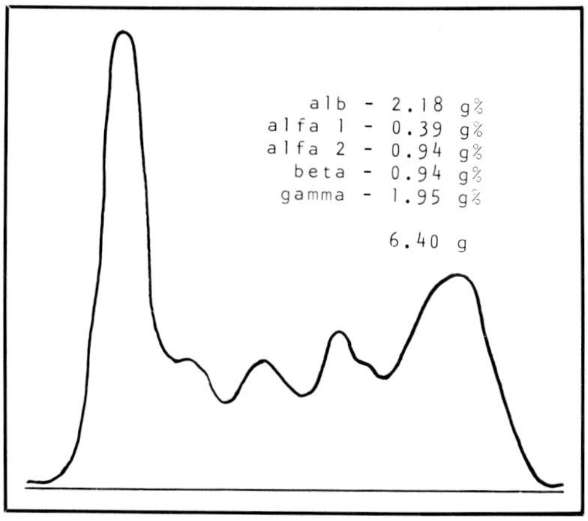

Fig. 8. Protein electrophoresis showing a normal gamma globulin.

protein electrophoresis did not present any hyper–gamma globulinemia and urinary electrophoresis showed no proteins (Fig. 8). There was no sign of systemic amyloidosis or other chronic disease to justify a diagnosis of systemic disease. Amyloidosis is a disease of uncertain etiology manifested by deposits, in different tissues, of a whitish and amorphous material composed of protein and sulfate-containing polysaccharide believed to be chondroitin sulfuric acid.[2] It may be primary or secondary. The primary type has an unknown etiology. The secondary one follows chronic diseases or degenerative processes.[2] According to Christensen,[4] amyloidosis may be classified as follows: (1) primary systemic; (2) secondary systemic; (3) amyloidosis associated with myelomatosis; (4) familial; (5) localized amyloid deposits; and (6) senescent.

Our case corresponds to a localized amyloid deposit which presents itself as a tumor called amyloidoma.

The lungs are involved in 30 percent of the cases of primary systemic amyloidosis and ten percent of the secondary forms.[4] However, localized amyloid deposits in the lung are rare,[1-6] and only about 30 cases have been reported.

Our patient has been followed for 14 months. Chest x-ray taken every three months showed no other lung mass. The patient is currently asymptomatic.

The authors are grateful to Dr. William S. Blakemore for his advice and review of this paper. Dr. Marchesini is indebted to Dr. William S. Blakemore, Professor and Chairman of the Department of Surgery, The Graduate Hospital of The University of Pennsylvania, Philadelphia, Pa., for training in surgery and to Mr. Jack Lloyd Griffith, F.R.C.S., Consultant Thoracic Surgeon, Hawkmoore Chest Hospital, Devon, England, for his thoracic surgical training.

REFERENCES

1. Chandhuri, M. R., and Parker, D. J.: A solitary amyloid nodule of the lung, Thorax **25:** 382, 1970.
2. Craver, W. L.: Solitary amyloid tumor of the lung, J. Thorac. Cardiovasc. Surg. **49:** 860, 1965.
3. Hayes, W. T., and Bernhardt, H.: Solitary amyloid mass of the lung, Cancer **24:** 820, 1969.
4. Skagseth, E., and Normann, T.: Localized amyloid tumor of the lung, Scand. J. Cardiovasc. Surg. **4:** 135, 1970.
5. Wichert, P. V.: Lungenrundherde als Symptom einer primaren Amyloidose, Thoraxchir. Vasc. Chir. **17:** 113, 1969.
6. Zundel, W. E., and Prior, A. P.: An amyloid lung, Thorax **26:** 357, 1971.

Editorials

A single step

George D. Zuidema, M.D., *Baltimore, Md.*

From the Department of Surgery, The Johns Hopkins Hospital, Baltimore, Md.

THERE IS AN ancient Chinese proverb which states:

> The tree that needs two arms to span its girth begins with the tiniest shoot. . . .Yon tower nine storeys high rose from a low mound of earth. . . . A journey of a thousand miles begins with a single step.[1]

American medicine finds itself in an unique position. On the one hand, it is capable of offering care of the highest quality available anywhere in the world; while on the other hand, there is considerable public dissatisfaction with what society perceives as its many inadequacies. There are undoubtedly aspects of medical practice which are uneven, and we are better at some things than others. I am convinced, however, that our profession is deeply sincere in its wish to see a uniform level of high-quality care available to the people of this country. The achievement of this objective will not be easy. There is now substantial public interest in accomplishing uniformity through legislation. There is no guarantee, however, that a plan devised by the Congress would be successful in solving our health-care problems in the most effective way. We cannot escape the harsh reality that our system will require changes and that we, as a profession, need to be involved in a creative and constructive way. This editorial addresses itself to only one aspect of the problems, but it is a beginning.

The American Board of Surgery was established and chartered in 1937 for the purpose of certifying surgeons who had met reasonable educational requirements and were found to be qualified to be responsible for the surgical care of patients. There are now a total of ten Surgical Boards, and these had, by 1972, certified some 48,000 specialists. The profile of surgical manpower in the United States was recently examined by Moore and associates.[2] Dr. Moore and his colleagues pointed out that the total number of persons performing surgery is approximately 93,000. Of this number, some 48,000 are Board-certified specialists, 20,600 are non–Board-certified practitioners, 16,000 are interns and residents in training, and nearly 10,000 are general practitioners who include the practice of surgery in their work.

The problem of surgical manpower is complicated in many ways, including a maldistribution of surgical specialists, variations in criteria established by hospital credential committees for clinical practice, and lack of uniformity of hospital accreditation. These factors obviously interact, and each will require attention if the delivery of surgical care is ever to be made of more uniform quality and accessibility. Nonetheless, there is a very real difference between the number of people practicing surgery and those whose credentials have been evaluated and have been certified by one or more of the surgical Boards. This is an important discrepancy, for apparently the lack of Board certification has not impaired, to any significant degree, the practice of those who lack these credentials. It has been estimated that approximately 40 percent of the operations per-

Accepted for publication Feb. 11, 1974.

Table I. *American Board of Surgery, Part I Examinations*

	Percent failed at first examination			Percent failed at reexamination			
	U. S. and Canadian graduates	Foreign graduates	Total	U. S. and Canadian graduates	Foreign graduates	Total	Grand total all candidates (percent failed)
1968	14.7	42.5	24.9	51	45	47	29
1969	13.8	47.6	26.1	53	68	63	34
1970	12.6	46.2	24.8	57	65	62	33
1971	13.8	53.4	30.1	57	76	70	41
1972	14.0	55.2	29.9	55	73	68	41
Five year average: 1968-1972	13.8	49.3	27.2	55	68	64	36

Table II. *American Board of Surgery, Part II Examinations: Calendar year 1972*

	No. of exams	No. failed	Percent failed	No. passed and certified
First examinations	883	195	22.1	688
Reexaminations	247	109	44.1	138
Part II totals	1,130	304	26.9	826

formed in this country are done by non-certified and general practitioner surgeons.

Together the ten surgical specialty Boards have shown a 90 percent increase in the output of specialists over the last 21 years, for an average increase of 4.5 percent per year. The maximum growth has actually taken place during the last six to ten years. These ten Boards have certified an average of 2,759 individuals a year during the last five years. Despite these dramatic increases in the number of certified surgeons, the problem of who is performing surgery continues to grow, for those who fail the certifying examination enter practice and join the staffs of hospitals as "Board-eligible" surgeons. By sitting for reexamination by the Board, general surgeons may remain in this category for up to ten years after completion of their training. The American Board of Surgery states that a candidate is not admissible to examination until "he has successfully fulfilled the requirements of the Board, . . . all his credentials have been considered and deemed acceptable, and his formal application has been approved." Despite this clear statement on the subject, the problem of "Board eligibility" as claimed by individuals and accepted by hospital credential committees remains.

The significance and scope of this problem can best be appreciated when it is considered in the light of the failure rates of the Part I and Part II examinations of the American Board of Surgery (Tables I and II).

These data show very clearly the high failure rates for both Part I and Part II examinations. It should also be noted that during the period 1968 to 1972, the total numbers of candidates examined rose from 1,122 to 1,505, indicating an absolute, as well as a relative increase in the failures.

The high failure rate has been a cause for concern for several reasons. First of all, it indicates that by virtue of either inadequate background or lack of proper educational setting, large numbers of surgeons fail to meet standards of competence. Furthermore, our system does not limit the practice of surgery to those of demonstrated competence. The tragedy, of course, is that the surgical candidates who fail the examination have invested four or more years of their lives in surgical training. Their careers will undoubtedly be limited when the day comes that the privilege to practice will depend on certification of competence. Our present system is geared to continue this practice and, therefore, perpetuate the problem indefinitely.

The American Board of Surgery could take a major step toward the solution of this problem by screening residents for competence at an early point in their training. The establishment of an in-service, qualifying examination would permit only limited numbers to proceed on into the final years of training. Such an examination could be offered during the second year of basic surgical education, and successful completion could be required before a candidate could enter the later years of an approved program. Successful candidates would be likely to perform much better on the final certifying examinations; and unsuccessful candidates could seek other career opportunities and be spared two or more years of surgical residency with little likelihood of achieving ultimate success. If any benefit has been gained by careful evaluation of surgeons' credentials and if the Board examinations have had any salutatory effect, patients could not help but profit from such change in our system.

At present, the Boards of Orthopedics, Ophthalmology, Anesthesiology, Otolaryngology, Neurosurgery, Plastic Surgery, and Obstetrics and Gynecology offer in-service examinations. All but the Orthopedic and Neurosurgery examinations are voluntary, however. Examinations of this kind are of help in demonstrating areas of weakness to both program directors and residents. To be effective in screening candidates and maintaining quality, however, a mandatory examination is necessary. Furthermore, successful completion of the test should be required for entrance into the final years of residency. Although one hesitates before suggesting the addition of one more hurdle in the form of a new examination, I cannot help but feel that patients, residents, and program directors will all benefit. Action of this kind would be an important first step toward solving the dilemma of who is permitted to perform surgery. The long-range implications are clear.

The proposal outlined above would do much toward correcting one inadequacy in our system. Obviously, taken alone, it would fall short of the kind of changes which need to be made. Other problems need to be addressed, and each will require careful study and thoughtful planning if we are to reach workable solutions. We have a group of Committees, Boards, and Agencies, sponsored by our professional organizations, which have the authority to effect change in most of the problem areas. It is vitally important that we, as a profession, begin to work through these voluntary organizations to correct these needs. It may seem like "a journey of a thousand miles," but it is now time to take a first step.

REFERENCES

1. Giles, L., translator: Sayings of Lao-Tzu, London, 1906, J. Murray, Publishers.
2. Moore, F. D., Boyden, C. M., Sabiston, D., Warren, R., Peterson, O. L., Zeppa, R, Heer, D., and Murthy, N.: The production, attrition, and biologic life-time of surgeons in relation to the population of the United States, Ann. Surg. **176:** 457, 1972.

Magnification and coronary artery surgery

William W. L. Glenn, M.D., *New Haven, Conn.*

From the Section of Cardiothoracic Surgery, Department of Surgery, Yale University School of Medicine, New Haven, Conn.

ONE OF THE strangest boasts ever made by sensible men is that they are able to do coronary artery anastomosis on 1.0 to 3.0 mm. diameter vessels "without optical assistance." During the past several years, a number of articles on coronary artery surgery have carried this phrase, or its equivalent, in their titles. In the present issue of the annual supplement to *Circulation* on Cardiovascular Surgery two such articles appear.[1, 2]

What in the name of common sense is the reason for not using a magnifier to assist in making these delicate anastomoses? It does not have to be a binocular scope, as suggested by Jacobson and used so effectively by Greene; but there is no conceivable reason why it should not be a simple magnifying lens worn as glasses, as advocated and practiced by Spencer. Cecil Drinker introduced the magnifying loupe to those of us working in his laboratory in Boston cannulating lymphatic vessels. I could not then imagine, nor can I now, carrying out anastomoses on vessels no larger than the thoracic duct without the benefit of the magnifying loupe. The technique for using the loupe is simple and can be mastered in only a few operations.

Accepted for publication Nov. 7, 1973.

I recall a few years ago having a prominent cardiac surgeon, approaching age 45, who was performing an aortic valve replacement, turn to me and say: "For a couple of years the lighting in this operating room was very poor and was getting worse—until my OR nurse suggested I get glasses."

Let us stop this nonsense about doing fine vascular work "without optical assistance." Who knows, maybe the long-term patency rate of coronary bypass grafts can be improved.

REFERENCES

1. Loop, F. D., Spampinato, N., Siegel, W., et al.: Internal mammary artery grafts without optical assistance: Clinical and angiographic analysis of 175 consecutive cases, Circulation **48** (Suppl. 3): 162, 1973.
2. Suzuki, A., Kay, E. B., and Hardy, J. D.: Direct anastomosis of the bilateral internal mammary artery to the distal coronary artery, without a magnifier, for severe diffuse coronary atherosclerosis, Circulation **48** (Suppl. 3): 190, 1973.
3. Jacobson, J. H., and Suarez, E. L.: Microsurgery in anastomosis of small vessels, Surg. Forum **11**: 243, 1960.
4. Green, G. E., Stertzer, S. H., and Rappert, E. H.: Coronary artery bypass graft, Ann. Thorac. Surg. **5**: 443, 1968.
5. Spencer, F. C.: Binocular loop (microtelescopes) for coronary artery surgery, J. Thorac. Cardiovasc. Surg. **62**: 163, 1971.

Letters to the editors

The young surgeon's dilemma

To the Editors:

I enjoyed Dr. Drew's account (SURGERY 74: 634, 1973) of the young surgeon's dilemma, academic surgery versus private practice, particularly since I was in a comparable quandry seven years ago. Having since then completed several years in both academia and in private practice, I might be considered as a young surgeon with perhaps a solution to the dilemma. I regret to state that the dilemma persists. Dr. Drew has succintly pointed out the extreme roles of academic surgery and private practice but neglected to emphasize several basic positive and negative points indigenous to both types of surgical practice. In academia, *time* is the priceless commodity. For the aggressive, driving academic surgeon, this means freedom for research, writing, reading, or just plain thinking. For others, however, time in academia can be turned toward personal pleasures, unending meetings, or sundry other activities that will assuredly *not* lead to fame or glory. Academia also offers *security,* an attraction to those concerned with their abilities to earn a livelihood, and independence, a blessing to those familiar with the enslaving "feeder" of private practice. Dr. Drew states that "the better surgeon operates." There is no doubt in my mind but that the academic surgeon operates too little and the private practitioner too much.

I have concluded that the choice of academic or private practice should be secondary to the realization by the young surgeon of a *commitment* to whichever practice of surgery he selects. This means the best *care* he can provide or arrange to have provided regardless of economic motivating factors or the lack thereof. Self-dedication to surgery will bring practice to the academician and academics to the practitioner. The gap might then be closed.

Herbert Dardik, M.D.
1555 Center Ave.
Fort Lee, N. J.

Reply

To the Editors:

I appreciated Dr. Dardik's comments on my editorial and as I began reading his letter I was encouraged that he might indeed have the solution to the dilemma. His point that "*time* is the priceless commodity" in academic surgery is precisely why I have chosen this course, at least for the present. Many, including Dr. Dardik, have made the observation that academic surgeons operate too little, and I for one will be looking for an academic position that allows for a certain number of private referrals. If the trend is away from such arrangements, I think it is a great mistake.

Though I understand the feelings behind the statements in his last paragraph, they strike me as nebulous and idealistic and not a specific solution at all, just as I offered no specific solution in my editorial. In order to "bring practice to the academician and academics to the practitioner," there must be a tangible mutual respect. The academician must discard his condescending manner, and the private practitioner should change his defensive posture. They need to get to know each other and each other's patients better.

John A. Drews, M.D.
Department of Surgery
Harbor General Hospital
Torrance, Calif. 90509

Volume 75 *Number* 5

SURGERY

MAY, 1974

Original communications

Morphology of the connective tissue grown in response to implanted silicone rubber: A light and electron microscopic study

Pablo Hernández-Jáuregui, V.M.D., Carlos Esperanza-García, M.D., *and* **Amador González-Angulo, M.D.,** *Mexico City, Mexico*

Silicone rubber cylinders were implanted into the subcutaneous tissue of 20 mongrel dogs. The fibrous connective tissue that grew in response to these implants had the same morphology as that of the cylinders used and they were allowed to reach maturity. They were studied with the light microscope after 2, 3, and 4 weeks, 6 months, and 1, 2, and 3 years. The minimum time required for the maturation of the cylinders was four weeks. At that time the conduits were composed of an inner layer made up of a lining of mesothelial-like cells arranged in several rows. These cells were identified as histiocytes with the electron microscope. The inner surface of the conduits was regarded as elements of the reticuloendothelial system with phagocytic functions. This becomes an advantage when such a conduit is used as a prosthesis where there is danger of infection. This layer of histiocytes also provides a favorable milieu for the migration or proliferation of those cells that normally cover conduits.

From Departmento de Investigación Científica and Hospital General, Centro Médico Nacional, Instituto Mexicano del Seguro Social, México City, México

Silicone rubber, when used for prostheses, does not produce any adverse tissue reaction[1, 3, 7] but several workers, when replacing pacemakers covered with silicone rubber, have observed the formation of a mold consisting of fibrocollagen tissues surrounding the pacemakers. This mold has a glistening, smooth, white, inner surface in close contact with the silicone rubber. When observed via the light microscope, an epithelial-like tissue layer is seen lining the inner

Accepted for publication June 30, 1973.

Reprint requests: P. Hernández-Jáuregui, V.M.D., Apartado Postal 73-032, México 73, D. F.

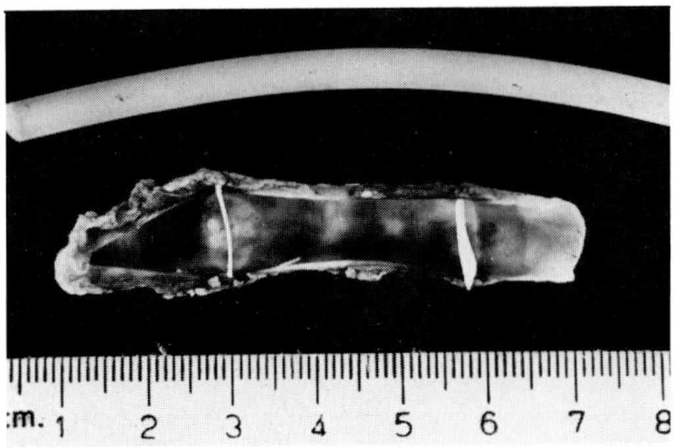

Fig. 1. Cylinder of connective tissue grown in the subcutaneous tissue of a dog in response to silicone rubber molds. The tissue has had three years of maturation.

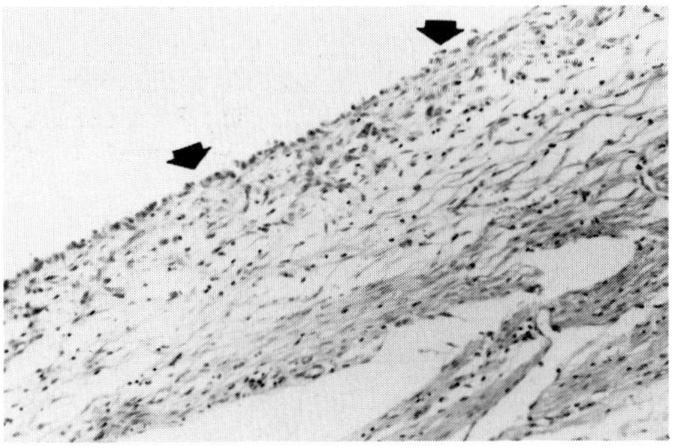

Fig. 2. Photomicrograph of a conduit of connective tissue grown in response to silicone rubber molds, of two weeks' maturation. The inner surface of the cylinder is composed of a simple layer of mesothelial-like cells (arrows). There are fibroblasts with collagen fibers underneath. (Hematoxylin and eosin; ×200.)

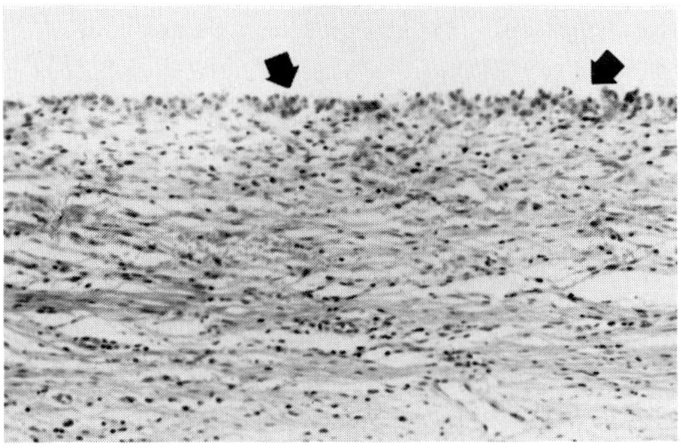

Fig. 3. Photomicrograph of a conduit of connective tissue grown in the subcutaneous tissue of a dog in response to silicone rubber molds, of three weeks' maturation. The number of mesothelial cells is increased (arrows). Well-organized connective tissue is seen beneath the mesothelial layer. (Hematoxylin and eosin; ×200.)

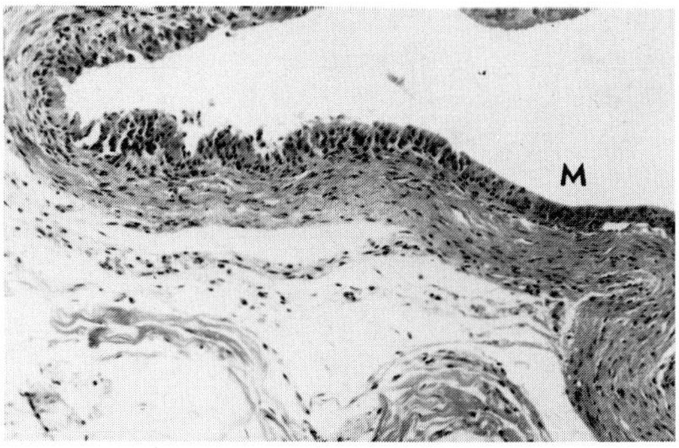

Fig. 4. Photomicrograph of a conduit of connective tissue grown in response to silicone rubber molds, of three weeks maturation. The stratified mesothelial layer *(M)* is well organized. (Hematoxylin and eosin; ×200.)

surface of the mold.[4, 9] The outer surface is composed of connective tissue firmly attached to the adjacent subcutaneous tissue, from which it can be separated by careful dissection.

Padula and associates[9] and Geha and associates[4] implanted silicone rubber molds of tubular and vascular forms into the subcutaneous tissue of dogs and obtained molds of connective tissue with a morphology similar to that of the silicone rubber. They used the connective tissue as valvular and vascular prostheses with good results. The histologic features of the connective tissue and the inner lining of the tube were, however, not described in detail. The purpose of the present study is to describe this tissue at various periods of maturation as seen with both light and electron microscopy, thereby arriving at a precise identification of the cell and fiber elements lining these newly formed conduits.

MATERIAL AND METHODS

Twenty mongrel dogs were conditioned for surgery for two weeks. An incision was made in the abdominal region and the subcutaneous tissue was exposed. A solid cylinder of silicone rubber, 3 by 1.5 cm., was implanted into the subcutaneous tissue of each dog. The connective tissue response to the implant was allowed to reach maturity, and then removed after 1, 2, 3, and 4 weeks, 6 months, and 1, 2, and 3 years. The tissues were dissected and immediately fixed in buffered 10 percent formalin for 24 hours and sections were conventionally treated for light microscopy studies. In all cases the following stains were used: hematoxylin and eosin, Masson's trichrome, Verhoeff's elastic fibers, and Gomori's reticulum.

Samples for electron microscopy were obtained from five dogs that had four weeks of connective tissue growth in response to the silicone rubber. The tissue was trimmed into small pieces and immediately fixed in a solution of 3 percent glutaraldehyde phosphate, buffered,[11] for one and a half hours, and post-fixed in a solution of 1 percent osmium tetroxide Millonig for one hour.[6] Samples were dehydrated in ethanol and embedded in araldite.[5] Sections 2 μ thick were cut on a Porter Blum MT-2 ultramicrotome and stained with Paragon for identification of suitable areas containing the cells of the inner surface of the connective tissue cylinder. Thin sections in the range of 800 Å, obtained with the same ultramicrotome, were stained with uranil acetate[12] and lead citrate[10] and observed with a Philips EM-300 electron microscope.

RESULTS

Two weeks' maturation. Grossly, the cylinders of tissue were soft and flexible; the inner surface was smooth and glistening (Fig. 1).

The light microscope revealed that the specimens were composed of connective tissue with areas of edema, lymphocytic and monocytic cell infiltrates, and hemorrhage. Two different layers of cells were observed. The inner layer was composed of polyhedric cells, irregularly oriented, and arranged in a single row. From this point on we will refer to this cell layer as the mesothelial layer. The cytoplasm of mesothelial cells was scarce and eosinophilic; the nuclei were ovoid with coarse chromatin. The second layer, or sub-

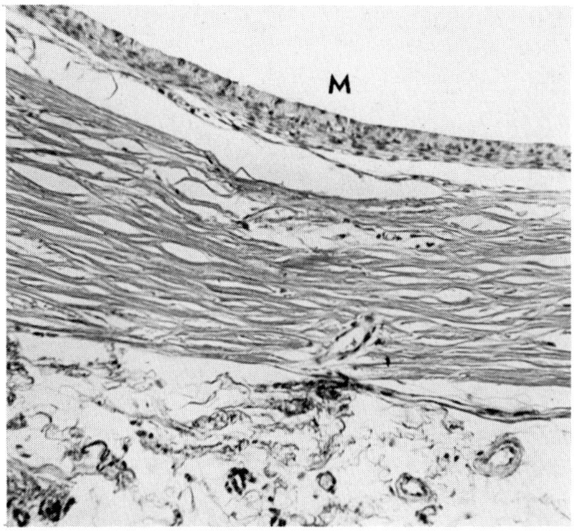

Fig. 5. Photomicrograph of a conduit grown in the subcutaneous tissue of a dog in response to silicone rubber molds, of three years' maturation. The cellularity in the mesothelial *(M)* and submesothelial layers is decreased. The fibroconnective tissue is hyalinized and has few blood vessels. (Hematoxylin and eosin; ×400.)

mesothelial tissue, was composed of fibroblasts, collagen, and reticular fibers. In this stage of maturation there was dissociation of fibers due to edema (Fig. 2).

Three weeks' maturation. The tissue was grossly more firm than after two weeks. The inner surface of the cylinder was also smooth and glistening. The number of mesothelial cells had increased and were arranged in two to three rows (Fig. 3). The reticular and collagen fibers evidenced with the special stains gave support to the mesothelial cells. The submesothelial tissue showed a definite increase in both reticular and collagen fibers that were arranged in a curly and whorly pattern. Blood vessels were numerous. At this stage of maturation fine bundles of elastic fibers were first seen.

Four weeks' maturation. The tissue was even more firm in consistency than previously; the inner surface was smooth, glistening, and white. The mesothelial cells were numerous and appeared as a stratified layer. Numerous collagen and reticular fibers beneath the mesothelial cell layer formed thick bundles of fibrous tissue, where clear-cut

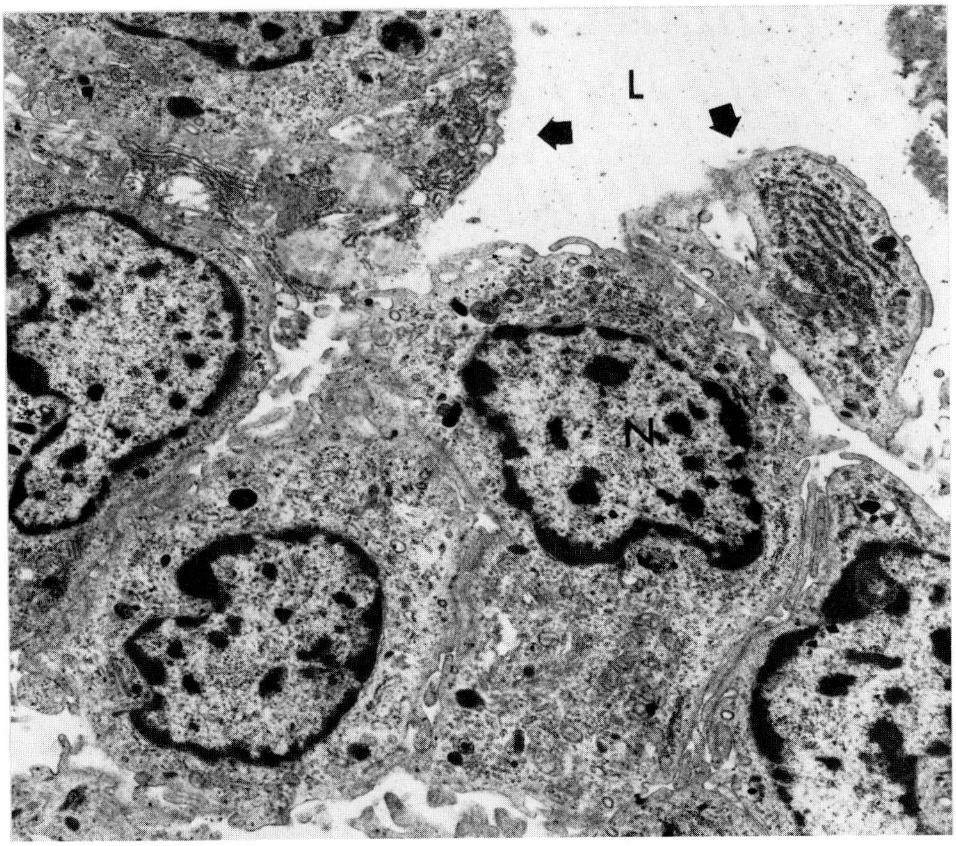

Fig. 6. Electron micrograph of the mesothelial layer of a conduit grown in response to silicone rubber molds of four weeks' maturation. A group of histiocytes is forming the mesothelium. The nuclei *(N)* are ovoid, indented, and polarized to one side of the cytoplasm. Mitochondria, vesicles, and smooth and rough endoplasmic reticulum are seen. Fragments of cytoplasm (arrow) of incomplete cells are present in the lumen *(L)* of the conduit (×15,000.)

elastic fibers were identified. At this stage of maturation, the mesothelial cells and connective tissue beneath the mesothelium were well organized and appeared to exhibit the minimum amount of time required for the organization of the tissue grown in response to silicone rubber (Fig. 4). Cylinders of tissue obtained at six months' maturation were quite similar to those obtained at one month.

One, two, and three years' maturation. Grossly, the cylinders of tissue obtained at one, two, and three years were quite firm in consistency. The inner surface was still smooth and glistening. The histologic pattern was similar and they will be described together. The deeper cells of the mesothelium were fusiform in shape and were identified as fibroblasts. The lining, more superficial, mesothelial cells were polyhedric and similar to those described previously. A large number of elastic fibers appeared between the cells. The submesothelial connective tissue was thick and hyalinized, it had few fibroblasts, and the blood vessels were also scarce. No elastic or reticular fibers were present (Fig. 5).

Electron microscopy. When the inner lining of the silicone rubber connective tissue mold was observed with the electron microscope, the so-called mesothelial layer appeared to be a lining made up of polyhedric cells identified as histiocytes. There were two to three rows of cells in close contact with neighboring cells with apposing cytoplasmic membranes with digitiform processes of their cytoplasms. There were no basement mem-

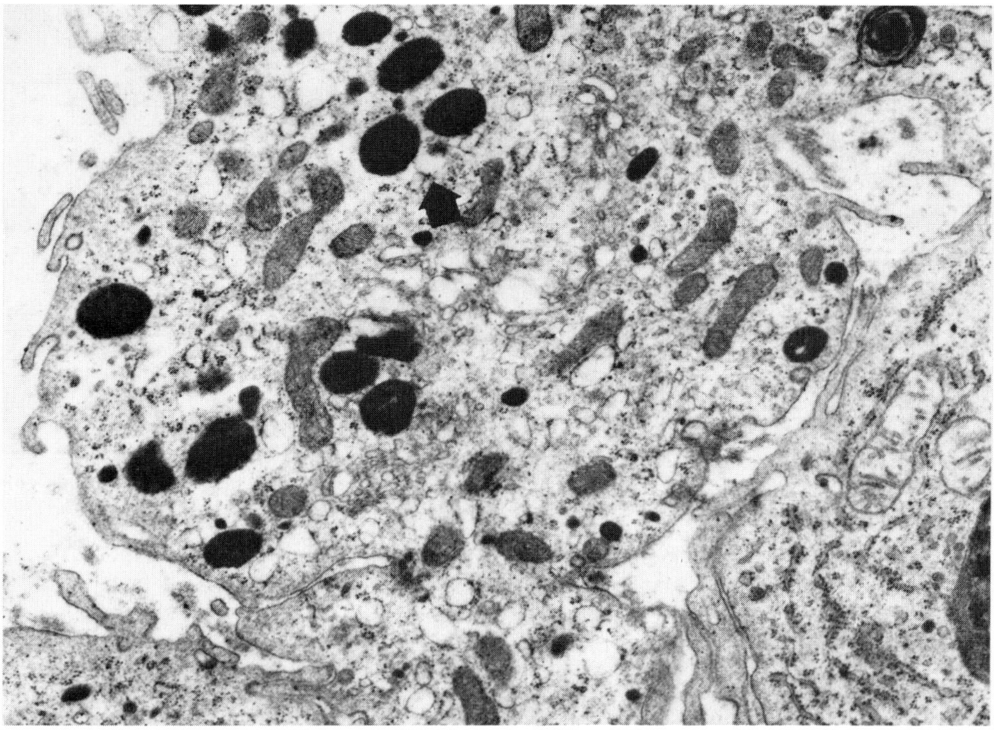

Fig. 7. Electron micrograph of the cytoplasm of a histiocyte. Note the large number of lysosomes (arrows). (×40,000.)

branes surrounding these cells. The nuclei were irregularly ovoid and oriented toward one side of the cytoplasm. The chromatin was found at the periphery of the nuclear membrane. The nucleoli were localized in the center of the nucleus and had low electron density. There were occasional lipid droplets within the cytoplasm.

The rough endoplasmic reticulum was scattered throughout the cytoplasm and in places it was quite prominent. The smooth endoplasmic reticulum had a similar distribution (Fig. 6). The majority of the cells had numerous lysosomes, myelin figures, and autophagic vacuoles (Figs. 7 and 8). The mitochondria were elongated and had transverse cristae. Numerous small vesicles, irregularly distributed along the cytoplasm, were usually found. The Golgi apparatus was prominent and located near the nucleus. Although the lumen of the cylinder was lined along most of its length with the cytoplasm of these histiocyte-type cells, there were areas where collagen and reticular fibers as well as fragments of cytoplasm of necrotic cells were seen. These were presumably dead histiocytes. Large numbers of collagen fibers and cells with the morphology of fibrocytes were observed deep in the tissue mold.

Long-term studies of the specimens revealed that they had the same appearance as those studied at two months. The illustrations for these reproduced rather poorly, but they are available.

DISCUSSION

The cylinders of connective tissue grown in response to silicone rubber molds had a well-conformed and defined shape, were flexible and elastic, and were therefore regarded as fully mature at the end of the fourth week. This observation is in keeping with the findings of Padula and Geha.

Few changes had taken place in the cylinders as much as six months after the molds were implanted. After a year, the vascularization and fibroblastic response decreased. At the same time the fibrous connective tissue

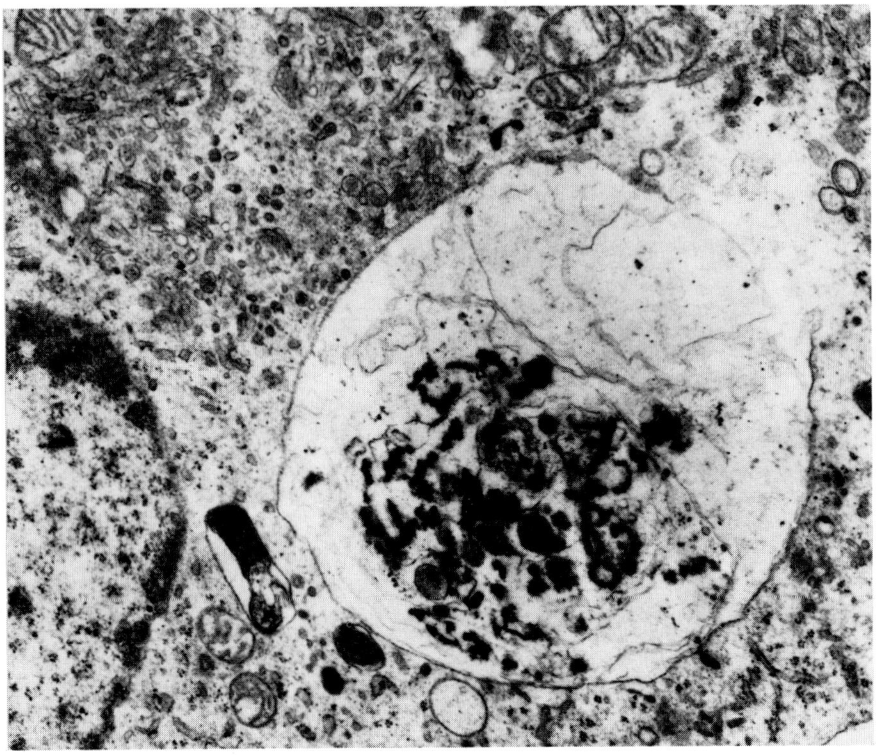

Fig. 8. Electron micrograph of the cytoplasm of a histiocyte. A cytosegrosome containing vesicles and cellular debris is present within the cytoplasm. (×40,000.)

became hyalinized, with disappearance of reticular and elastic fibers. Thus it seems reasonable to think that, should this newly formed conduit be utilized as a prosthesis, it must be used at a time when it is more vascularized, and when the connective tissue is less hyalinized, and therefore more extensible and flexible.

The lining mesothelial cells had been identified as histiocytes according to their morphology at the ultrastructural level.[2] The same cells seen with the light microscope had, indeed, the appearance of an epithelium as Padula had previously described. However, since no epithelial cell elements are normally present in the connective tissue, these lining cells should be regarded as mesenchymal in origin at the light microscope level. When observed with the electron microscope the rough inner surface is seen to be composed of histiocytes without junctional complexes but rather with cell membranes apposing each other with only occasional collagen fibers in between.

This capacity of the mesenchymal tissue to give rise to specialized connective tissue cells has long been seen with the use of Dacron prostheses where endothelial cells cover the inner surface of the Dacron hubs used to replace large blood vessels.[8]

Unpublished observations made in our laboratory indicate that when silicone rubber–produced cylinders are to replace a segment of esophagus, there is formation of a layer of epithelial cells lining the inner surface of the cylinder. In the present study the inner surface of the cylinder was composed of one to two rows of histiocytes. This cell has the potential ability to undergo changes according to functional needs. In this respect it may be regarded as a cell element of the reticular endothelial system with phagocytic functions. The findings of numerous lysosome and autophagic vacuoles within histiocytes by electron microscopy is indicative of the phagocytic capacity of these cells. This represents an advantage of utmost importance in keeping the tissue free from infection when the conduit is placed in organs where this complication is quick to occur. In addition, this layer of histiocytes provides a favorable milieu for the migration or proliferation of those cells that normally cover inner surfaces of conduits, whether blood vessels or other hollow tracts.

The elastic fibers began to appear during the third week of maturation of tissue grown in response to silicone rubber. This connective tissue, at this age of maturation, can be a suitable experimental mold for the study of the genesis of elastic fibers.

REFERENCES

1. Braly, S.: Use of silicones in plastic surgery, Arch. Otolaryng. **78:** 669, 1963.
2. Carr, I.: The fine structure of the mammalian lymphoreticular system, *in* Bourne, G. H., Danielli, J. F., and Jeon, K. W., editors: International review of cytology, New York, 1970, Academic Press, Inc., vol. 27, pp. 283.
3. Cronin, T. D., and Gerow, F. J.: Augmentation mammaplasty: A new natural feel prosthesis. Proc. III Int. Cong. Plast. Surg., Excerpta Medica Int. Cong. Serv. No. **66:** 41, 1963.
4. Geha, S. A., Salaymeth, T. M., Davis, L. G., and Bane, E. A.: Replacement of the aortic valve with molded autogenous grafts grown in response to implanted Silastic, J. Thorac. Cardiovasc. Surg. **60:** 661, 1970.
5. Glauert, A. M., and Glauert, R. H.: Araldite as an embedding medium for electron microscopy, J. Biophys. Biochem. Cytol. **4:** 191, 1958.
6. Millonig, G.: Further observations on a phosphate buffer for osmium solutions in fixation, *in* Breese, S. S., Jr., editor: Fifth International Congress for Electron Microscopy, New York, 1962, Academic Press, Inc., vol. 2, p. 8.
7. Mullison, E. Q.: Silicones as artificial internal tissue and organ subsitutes, Ann. N. Y. Acad. Sci. **120:** 540, 1964.
8. O'Neal, R. M., Jordan, G. L., Rabin, E. R., De Bakey, M. E., and Halpert, B.: Cells grown on isolated intravascular Dacron hub. An electron microscopic study, Exp. Mol. Pathol. **3:** 403, 1964.
9. Padula, T. R., Zeok, V. J., Pupi, A. P., and Camishion, C. R.: Replacement of the venae cavae with autogenous grafts grown in response to implanted Silastic, Surg. Forum **20:** 135, 1969.
10. Reynolds, E.: The use of lead citrate at high pH as an electron opaque stain in electron microscopy, J. Cell Biol. **17:** 208, 1963.
11. Sabatini, D. D., Bensch, K., and Barnett, R. J.: Cytochemistry and electron microscopy. The preservation of cellular ultrastructure and enzymatic activity by aldehyde fixation, J. Cell Biol. **17:** 19, 1963.
12. Watson, M. L.: Staining of tissue sections for electron microscopy with heavy metals, J. Biophys. Biochem. Cytol. **4:** 475, 1958.

The protection of the skin of fracture patients immobilized in plaster of Paris

Cyril Boroda, M.B.B.S., M.R.C.S., *and* **George L. Mouzas, M.D., F.I.C.S.,** *London, England*

A clinical evaluation of Betadine (povidone-iodine) aerosol in protecting the skin of patients encased in plaster of Paris casts was carried out in a controlled clinical trial with photographic assessment. The comparison with a control group and a group treated with a silicone cream showed that the aerosol gave significantly better results than either of the other groups ($P < 0.001$), with benefit in 95 percent of the patients compared with 10 percent for the dimethicone cream group and 3 percent for the control group.

From the Accident and Emergency Department, North Middlesex Hospital, London, England

When patients with limb fractures are encased in a plaster of Paris cast, apart from the unavoidable difficulties inherent in immobilization they also suffer from a variety of minor complications and discomforts which should be avoidable.

We have been struck by the frequent annoyance caused to such patients by the pruritus which frequently develops beneath the plaster and the odor which may be a source of considerable social embarrassment. A further cosmetic problem arises when the plaster cast is removed, revealing the all too common dry scaly skin which is resented by female and male patients alike.

These three problems stem from the same cause, namely, the overgrowth of normal skin bacteria, yeasts, and fungi. These organisms which are shed with exfoliated dead skin under normal conditions are prevented from so doing by the plaster and overgrowth of the skin flora results.

We have, therefore, tried various methods of avoiding these side effects of immobilization and, having experienced some success with a silicone cream, dimethicone cream BPC, and a germicidal aerosol, Betadine (povidone-iodine) aerosol, it was decided to carry out a comparative study in fracture patients comparing three groups of patients, one treated with the aqueous povidone-iodine aerosol, one with the silicone cream, and a third control group.

The rationale for the use of silicones was based on the various reports of their efficacy in skin protection and care[1]; dimethicone cream was chosen since it also contains cetrimide and chlorocresol, which could be expected to exert an additional antibacterial activity.

Povidone-iodine has been shown to be an effective germicidal agent by numerous investigations since the early reports[3] and has been previously used for skin protection under similar circumstances.[2]

MATERIAL AND METHODS

Patients were selected randomly from those attending the fracture clinic with limb fractures. The two treated groups received either

Accepted for publication Aug. 6, 1973.

Reprint requests: George L. Mouzas, M.D., F.R.C.S., Consultant Surgeon, West Hill Hospital, Dartford, Kent, England.

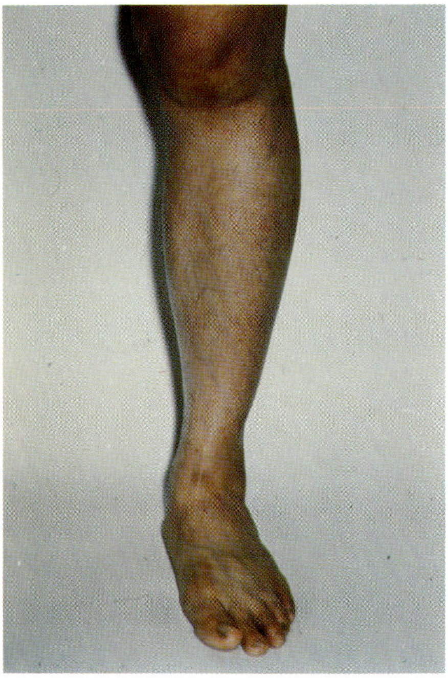

Fig. 1. A typical Betadine aerosol–treated patient.

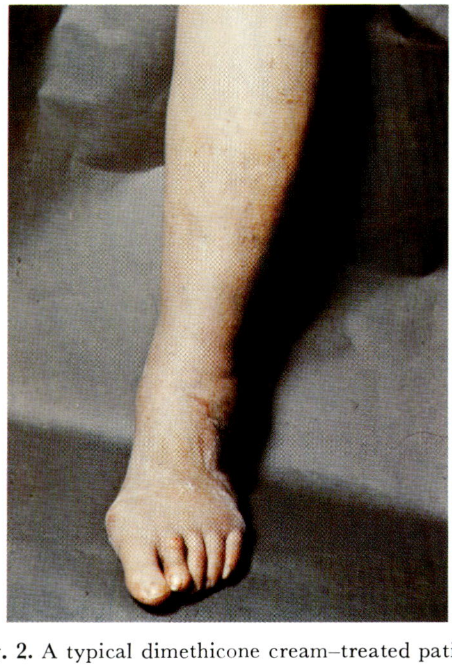

Fig. 2. A typical dimethicone cream–treated patient.

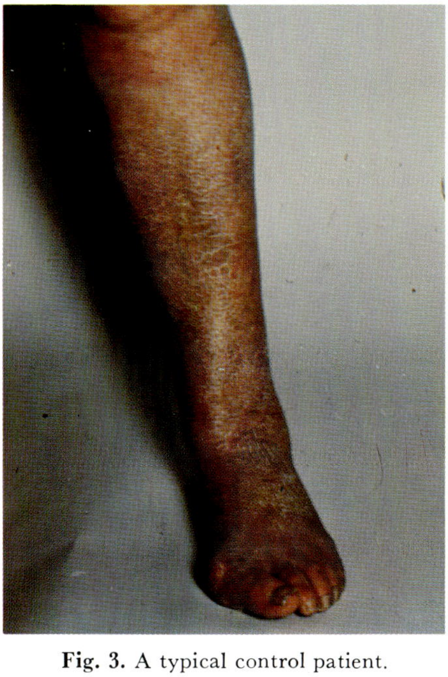

Fig. 3. A typical control patient.

the povidone-iodine aerosol, sprayed on generously as a uniform layer which was allowed to dry on the skin before application of the plaster of Paris cast, or the dimethicone cream, which was uniformly applied manually. The control group had no special skin preparation before the plaster was applied. The results were recorded when the plaster was removed by two independent observers having no knowledge of the previous skin treatment, if any. The skin condition was assessed with regard to its healthiness or otherwise, whether it was smooth or scaly, and the presence of odor. Additionally, a number of patients were photographed at the same time for a comparative and objective permanent record. Whether or not the patient developed irritation beneath the plaster was noted during clinical attendance.

RESULTS

The results are shown in Table I. Due to various factors, for example, failure to attend for follow-up, transfer, and so on, 40 patients treated with povidone-iodine, 20 treated with dimethicone cream, and 30 controls were assessed. As can be seen, the vast majority of patients (95 per cent) in the povidone-iodine group were found to have smooth skin with no scaling or irritation. In contrast, virtually all the control patients (97 per cent) had skin which was scaly and rough and had given rise to irritation and odor. The dimethicone group showed an intermediate result between these extremes with some protective action, but with the skin somewhat scaly, in 90 per cent of the patients. The over-all results were recorded as good, fair, or poor, the grading being based on the skin condition as previously detailed. These results are recorded in Table I.

The statistical analysis of the results using the χ^2 test gave the following results: the povidone-iodine–treated patients showed a highly significant advantage over the control group of patients ($P < 0.001$) and the dimethicone cream–treated group of patients ($P < 0.001$). There was no significant difference between the control group and the dimethicone group ($0.3 < P < 0.5$). The

Table I

	No. of patients	*Over-all assessment*		
		Good	*Fair*	*Poor*
Povidone-iodine	40	38	1	1
Dimethicone cream	20	2	8	10
Control group	30	1	6	23

groups were comparable in age range, the controls having a range of 5 to 69 (mean 50) years, the dimethicone group 10 to 68 (mean 41), and the povidone-iodine group 14 to 83 (mean 44). The sex ratio was also similar in the three groups, the percentage of male patients being 41, 49 and 40, respectively.

The distribution of upper and lower limb fractures in the three treatment groups were, respectively, 19:21, 10:10, and 14:16. The duration of immobilization in plaster was similar for the three groups, with a mean of five weeks for upper limb fractures and 12 weeks for lower limb fractures. The three groups, therefore, were entirely comparable.

DISCUSSION

The common occurrence of pruritus in patients who are encased in plaster of Paris casts is due to an overgrowth of the normal skin bacteria, as well as yeasts and fungi beneath the plaster. It results from occlusion by the plaster, which prevents the normal loss of exfoliated dead skin, and this situation favors overgrowth of the skin flora. This is accompanied by the dry, scaly condition of the skin normally seen when a plaster is removed. In contrast to the untreated group, those patients treated with Betadine aerosol showed a remarkable difference in appearance (Figs. 1 to 3). The skin was soft and of normal appearance, unlike the rough, scaly appearance of the control group. This group was also free of any skin irritation while the plaster was worn, and no complications or side-effects developed. Although the dimethicone-treated group also showed some advantages over the untreated group, these were not nearly as marked. This clinical difference is borne out statistically, with no significant advantage of the silicone cream compared with the untreated group, and with the povidone-iodine group showing a highly significant advantage over both the silicone cream and the control. It seems, therefore, that the bactericidal and fungicidal effects of povidone-iodine are of considerable practical benefit when applied to the skin before immobilization of a limb in a plaster of Paris cast, resulting not only in greater comfort to the patient, but a greatly improved cosmetic appearance of the skin when the plaster is removed.

Thanks are due to Sister P. Taylor, Senior Nursing Officer, Accident Department, North Middlesex Hospital, London, for her help in supervising the trials and to Napp Laboratories, Ltd., an affiliate of the Purdue Frederick Co., New York.

REFERENCES

1. Hughes, J. P. W., and Wigley, G. S.: Br. Med. J. **2:** 153, 1962.
2. Levine, S.: The effect of povidone-iodine in controlling skin flora beneath occlusive dressings, J. Am. Podiatr. Assoc. **60:** 486, 1970.
3. Shelanski, H. A., and Shelanski, M. V.: PVP-iodine: History, toxicity and therapeutic uses, J. Int. Coll. Surg. **25:** 727, 1956.

Inhibited platelet adhesion: A non-thrombogenic characteristic of a heparin-coated surface

H. Lagergren, M.D., P. Olsson, M.D., *and* **J. Swedenborg, M.D.,** *Stockholm, Sweden*

The thrombogenicity of plastic surfaces with a stable bound heparin layer was tested in dogs. The method for preparing the heparinized surface is described. The accumulation of ^{51}Cr-labeled platelets on specially designed arteriovenous shunts was used as a measure of platelet adhesion. The experiments were made on both fibrinogen-depleted and normal dogs. Non-treated shunts were occluded after a 30 minute test period in both groups of animals. Heparinized shunts remained open and the accumulation of platelets was less than ten percent of that on non-treated surfaces. Systemic heparinization did not markedly influence the adhesion of platelets on the shunts and untreated shunts were not kept open unless very large concentrations were used (> 5 I.U. per milliliter of plasma). It is concluded that the heparinized surface is non-thrombogenic, mainly because it prevents platelet adhesion. Systemic heparinzation does not have a similar effect.

From the Surgical Research Laboratory, Thoracic Clinics, Karolinska sjukhuset, Stockholm 60, Sweden

THE INCREASED use of non-biologic materials in contact with blood, e.g., in extracorporeal circulation, hemodialysis, and implantation of vascular grafts, has stimulated the development of new non-thrombogenic artificial surfaces. Several materials have been evaluated and the non-thrombogenic properties have been improved by different methods.[8] One such method is binding of heparin to the surface. The major problem with this procedure is the continuous release of heparin from the surface.[14] A promising solution to this problem has been achieved by the cross-linking of heparin with glutar aldehyde.[21]

The primary event in arterial thrombosis or thrombosis at a foreign surface is believed to be the adherence of platelets.[28, 31] These platelets subsequently release adenosine diphosphate (ADP), which presumably causes aggregation of platelets to the already adhered ones.[17] Initiation of plasma coagulation is then caused by release of platelet factor 3.[16] Fibrin deposition might thus be a secondary phenomenon in thrombosis at a foreign surface. This fact is also supported clinically since patients with an elevated platelet adhesiveness have a high incidence of occlusion of synthetic vascular grafts.[13]

The present study was undertaken to evaluate the non-thrombogenic properties of a plastic surface with a stable bound heparin layer in vivo. Particular attention was devoted to its capacity to prevent platelet adhesion, but the effect of systemic heparinization upon the adhesion of platelets was also investigated. In order to isolate the effect of platelets, some of the experiments were performed on fibrinogen-depleted dogs.

This study was supported by Grants No. B73-14x-3188-03A and K71-17x-3361-01 from the Swedish Medical Research Council and grants from the National Association against Heart and Chest Diseases and from the Torsten and Ragnar Söderbergs Foundation.

Accepted for publication Dec. 17, 1973.

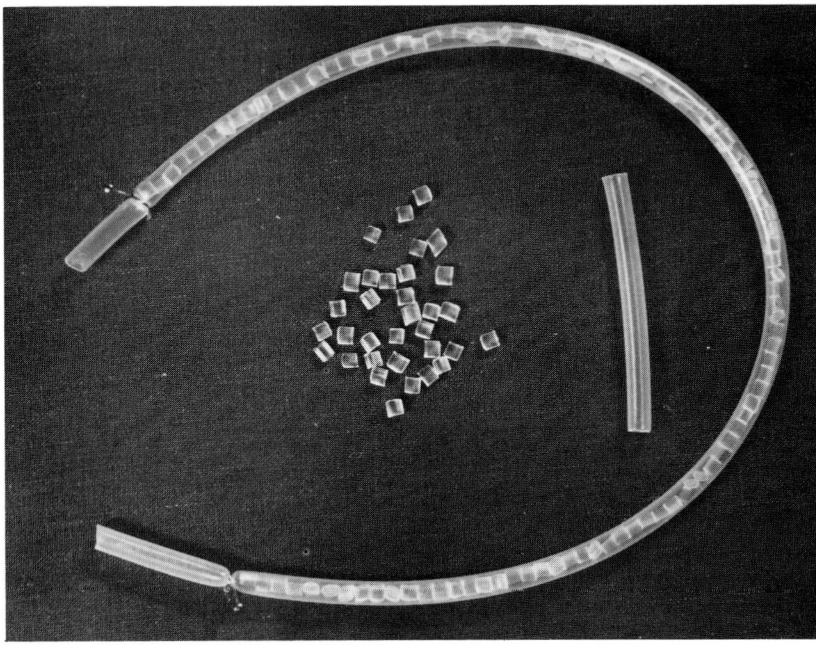

Fig. 1. An arteriovenous shunt used in the experiments.

METHODS

Preparation of arteriovenous shunts. A polyethylene tube (Portex PP 350) with a 3 mm. inner diameter was cut into lengths of 250 mm. and filled with small cubes of polypropylene which were positioned by a tightening ligature at both ends of the tube (Fig. 1). The inner surface area of the designed shunts was about 4.6 cm.^{2} and the flow of saline was about 40 ml. per minute at a pressure equal to 100 mm. Hg.

The heparin-treatment of the plastic material was carried out by a three-stage procedure.* The shunts were first placed in a circulating 0.5 mM. solution of the cationic surfactant cetylamine hydrochloride at a temperature of 90° C. for 30 minutes so that good flow through the inside of the shunts was assured. At this temperature, the lipophilic hydrocarbon chains of the surfactant penetrated into the plastic, thus providing the surface with positively charged ionic groups.[21]

In the second stage, the surfactant-containing shunts were placed in a flowing solution of heparin* (10 I.U. of heparin per milliliter 0.9 percent NaCl, pH 3.6) at 75° C. for 90 minutes. At this temperature, which is somewhat lower than that in the first stage, heparin is ionically bound to the amine groups in the surface. In the final stage, the heparin-bearing surface is stabilized by cross-linking in a one percent glutardialdehyde solution of 55° C. for ten minutes and then rinsed with 0.9 percent NaCl.

Labeling of platelets. The labeling of platelets was made essentially according to Aas and Gardner[1] as modified by Abrahamsen.[2, 3] Blood (150 ml.) was collected into a Fenwal TA-6 bag† containing 20 ml. of acid-citrate-dextrose (ACD) solution. The ACD solution had the following composition: sodium tricitrate 2 H_2O, 2.4 percent; citric acid, 1.5 percent; glucose, 2.5 percent. This solution has a lower pH than ordinary ACD solution and buffers the dogs' plasma to pH 6.1 to 6.3. A low pH results in better survival of the retransfused platelets.[4, 24] The

*Patents and patent applications are owned by Aminkemi A.B., 161 20 Bromma, Sweden.

*Vitrum, Stockholm, Sweden.

†Fenwal Laboratories, Morton Grove, Ill., U. S. A.

Table I. *Platelets × 10^3 per square millimeter on the surface of heparinized shunts before systemic heparinization**

Non-defibrinogenated dogs: 9 heparin-treated shunts tested in 4 dogs ($\bar{x}$ ± S.D.)	Defibrinogenated dogs: Heparin-treated shunts: 10 shunts tested in 4 dogs ($\bar{x}$ ± S.D.)	Defibrinogenated dogs: Non-treated shunts: 11 shunts tested in 4 dogs ($\bar{x}$ ± S.D.)
32.4 ± 18.1	24.4 ± 10.3	682 ± 220
	$p < 0.001$ (heparin-treated vs. non-treated)	
N.S. (non-defibrinogenated vs. defibrinogenated heparin-treated)		

*The statistical evaluation was made with the use of Student's t test.

Table II. *Initial heparin concentration in plasma and half-life time of four dogs with normal plasma fibrinogen and four defibrinogenated dogs*

Non-defibrinogenated animals			Debrinogenated animals		
Dose of heparin (I.U./Kg. b.w.)	Initial concentration of heparin (I.U./ml. plasma)	Half-life time (min.)	Dose of heparin (I.U./Kg. b.w.)	Initial concentration of heparin (I.U./ml. plasma)	Half-life time (min.)
400	9.5	50	400	11.6	81
400	9.1	50	400	11.2	63
400	8.6	49	400	13.0	48
800	13.5	129	800	26.0	58

TA-6 bag was centrifuged at 190 × g for 20 minutes and the resulting supernatant, which consisted of platelet-rich plasma (PRP), was transferred into a Fenwal transfer pack (TA-3). The latter was then centrifuged at 1,200 × g for 20 minutes, and the platelet-poor plasma (PPP) thus obtained was transferred into another transfer bag. The platelet button was then resuspended in Ringer's solution to which sodium tricitrate (three percent) and glucose (five percent) were added. After resuspension 250 μ Cu of ^{51}Cr as sodium bichromate was added. The platelets were incubated with ^{51}Cr for two hours at room temperature, when 0.5 ml. of ten percent ascorbic acid was added to oxidize excess chromate. All the PPP except 10 ml. was then added and after mixing, the bag was once again centrifuged for 20 min. at 1,200 × g. The supernatant was discarded and the remaining 10 ml. of PPP were used to resuspend the labeled platelets which were retransfused to the dogs. The labeling procedure was performed on the day before the actual experiments. Platelet counts were made in Buerker chambers according to Kristensson.[20] The ^{51}Cr activity was measured in a Packard well type scintillation counter.

Chemical methods. Fibrinogen was measured according to Bergström and associates.[6] The heparin level of plasma was kindly measured at AB Kabi Stockholm by Dr. Miller-Andersson.

The heparin assay was based on the principle of inactivation of activated factor X by heparin and its co-factor as described by Biggs and associates[7] and Yin and colleagues.[34] All components in the test system were purified proteins of human origin.

Experimental procedure. The series consisted of eight animals. Four of the animals were defribrinogenated by daily intravenous injections of Defibrase* in doses of 0.1 ml. per kilogram of body weight for two consecutive days before the experiment. On the experimental day, the dogs received a third dose of Defibrase. Anesthesia was induced and maintained with sodium pentothal. They were endotracheally intubated and ventilated with a volume controlled respirator. The femoral arteries and veins were carefully dissected on both sides and ligated distally.

*Pentapharm AG, Basel Switzerland.

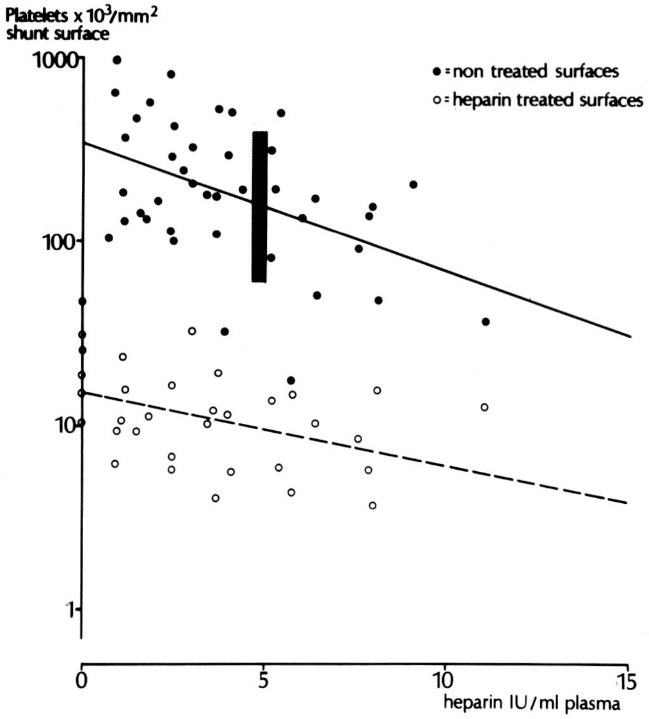

Fig. 2. Non-defibrinogenated dogs. Platelets per square millimeter of shunt surface plotted against heparin level of plasma in dogs with normal plasma fibrinogen levels. A semi-logarithmic plot is used. The bar on the line for non-treated surfaces represents the heparin level below which 90 percent of the shunts were occluded.

The arteriovenous shunts were then inserted, usually a treated shunt on one side and a non-treated on the other. The shunts were left in place for 30 minutes and then exchanged. After removal, the shunts were carefully rinsed with 20 ml. of saline and their ^{51}Cr activity was determined. Blood samples for determinations of platelet count, fibrinogen, heparin activity, and ^{51}Cr activity were taken through a catheter inserted into one carotid artery. The number of platelets per shunt was calculated by multiplying the ratio of platelet count of blood and ^{51}Cr activity of blood with the ^{51}Cr activity of the shunts. The number of platelets per square millimeter was then calculated by dividing this figure with the total shunt area.

RESULTS

Non-defibrinogenated animals.

Before systemic heparinization. As expected the non-treated arteriovenous shunts were closed by fibrin clots shortly after their insertion. It was not possible to flush them open after the 30 minute test period. The ^{51}Cr activity of these shunts was not determined since it would represent both surface-adhered and fibrin-trapped platelets.

The heparin-treated shunts remained patent during the thirty minutes. Their uptake of ^{51}Cr was measured after removal and gentle flushing with saline. This activity corresponded to $32.4 \times 10^3 \pm 18.1 \times 10^3$ platelets per square millimeter shunt surface (Table I).

After systemic heparinization. Systemic heparinization of the animals with 400 or 800 I.U. per kilogram resulted in the heparin levels shown in Table II. The heparin level of plasma then declined exponentially. Systemic heparinization initially prevented closure of the non-treated shunts. However, with declining heparin concentrations, they again ceased functioning during the 30 minute test period. It was found that

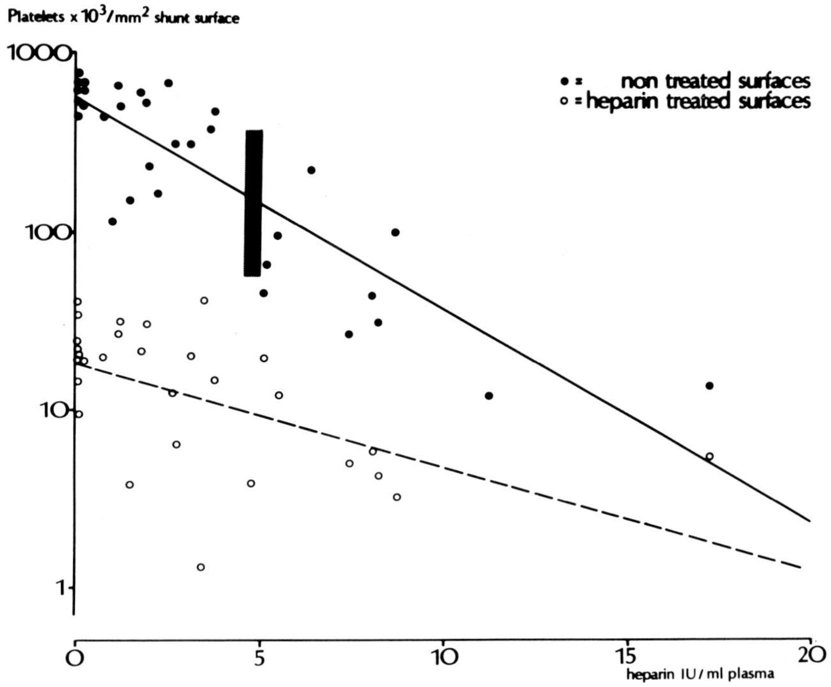

Fig. 3. Defibrinogenated dogs. Platelets per square millimeter of shunt surface plotted against heparin level of plasma in defibrinogenated dogs. A semilogarithmic plot is used. The bar crossing the line for the non-treated surfaces represents the heparin level below which 90 percent of the shunts were occluded.

90 percent of the non-treated shunts were closed when the plasma heparin level was below 5 I.U. per milliliter. The obliterating material, however, was easily removed by gentle flushing. The ^{51}Cr uptake on the shunt surface was correlated to the heparin level of plasma. This correlation proved to be negative (r = –0.46), i.e., the more heparin in plasma, the less uptake of ^{51}Cr on the surface (Fig. 2).

The heparin-treated shunts of course remained patent during heparinization as they did before. The uptake of ^{51}Cr on heparin-treated shunts was less than one tenth of that on non-treated shunts, irrespective of the heparin level in plasma. Also here, there was a weak negative correlation between ^{51}Cr activity and heparin level of plasma (r = –0.40) (Fig. 2).

Defibrinogenated animals.

Before systemic heparinization. On the experimental day, all the animals had no measurable amounts of plasma fibrinogen. The mean platelet count was 372 × 10^3 per cubic millimeter before defibrinogenation and 295 × 10^3 after. This difference is not statistically significant (Table III).

Despite defibrinogenation, all non-treated shunts were occluded when taken out after 30 minutes. In contrast to the non-treated shunts in the non-defibrinogenated animals, it was, however, possible to flush them with saline after removal. The uptake of ^{51}Cr activity in the non-treated shunts corresponded to 682 × 10^3 ± 220 × 10^3 platelets per square millimeter of shunt surface.

The heparin-treated shunts remained patent and their ^{51}Cr activity corresponded to 24.4 × 10^3 ± 10.3 × 10^3 platelets per square millimeter. Thus, the platelet accumulation on heparin-treated shunts was the same whether the animals were defibrinogenated or not (Table I).

After systemic heparinization. Systemic heparinization of the animals resulted in slightly higher heparin levels and slower de-

Table III. *Platelet counts and fibrinogen levels of four Defibrase-treated dogs before and after defibrinogenation and of four non-defibrinogenated dogs at the beginning of experiments*

Defibrinase-treated dogs (N = 4)				*Non-defibrinogenated dogs (N = 4)*
Before defibrinogenation		*After defibrinogenation*		
Platelet count (× $10^3/\mu l$ $\bar{x}$ ± S.D.)	*Fibrinogen concentration (g/100 ml. $\bar{x}$ ± S.D.)*	*Platelet count (× $10^3/\mu l$ $\bar{x}$ ± S.D.)*	*Fibrinogen concentration (g/100 ml. $\bar{x}$ ± S.D.)*	*(× $10^3/\mu l$ $\bar{x}$ ± S.D.)*
372 ± 117	0.28 ± 0.06	295 ± 113	0 ± 0	405 ± 191

cay than in the dogs with normal plasma fibrinogen levels (Table II).

Immediately after heparinization, the non-treated shunts remained open during the test period but became occluded with declining heparin levels. As in the case of non-defibrinogenated dogs, 90 percent of the shunts were closed when the plasma heparin level was below 5 I.U. per milliliter of plasma. There was a negative correlation between uptake of ^{51}Cr and plasma heparin level ($r = -0.84$) (Fig. 3).

The uptake of ^{51}Cr on heparin-treated shunts, which before systemic heparinization was only four percent of that of non-treated shunts, was somewhat more diminished by systemic heparinization. There was a weak negative correlation between ^{51}Cr uptake and heparin level ($r = -0.58$). This correlation was not as marked as for the non-treated shunts (Fig. 3). The regression lines for ^{51}Cr uptake versus heparin level for the treated shunts were almost the same in both defibrinogenated and non-defibrinogenated dogs.

DISCUSSION

The designed arteriovenous shunts have a resistance to blood flow which is the same or slightly higher than the femoral vascular bed of the anesthetized dog. The granules (alt. cubes) create a considerable surface of foreign material so that accumulation of platelets easily can be detected.

Some animals were defibrinogenated in order to elucidate, as far as possible, the interaction between the artificial surfaces and platelets without interference of clot formation. Defibrase-defibrinogenated animals have earlier been used for similar purposes.[11, 26] The snake venom enzyme Defibrase digests fibrinogen by splitting of fibrinopeptide A, but because of continuous synthesis, unmeasurable amounts of fibrinogen are very probably present in the circulation. The hemostatic function of platelets from Defibrase defibrinogenated dogs seems, however, to be largely unaffected.[26] Neither does the ^{51}Cr labeling seem to alter the function of the platelets.[9] The defibrinogenated dog with labeled platelets thus provides good possibilities for studying the reaction of platelets at artificial surfaces.

Non-treated shunts were obliterated in both defibrinogenated and normal animals. In the defibrinogenated animals, the shunts were easily flushed open since the platelet plug was not reinforced by fibrin. Both the adhesion of platelets to glass in in vitro test systems[15, 18] and aggregation induced by ADP[11] are impaired by lack of fibrinogen. In the present study, however, the adhesivity of the platelets after fibrinogen depletion was still sufficient to cause obliteration of the untreated shunts.

Systemic heparinization of the animals resulted in a decrease in the uptake of platelets on the surface of both non-treated and heparinized shunts. However, with declining levels of plasma heparin, the accumulation of platelets increased, and at levels below 5 I.U. per milliliter, the non-treated shunts became obliterated. The results were the same whether the animals were defibrinogenated or not. No distinction could be observed between the regression lines for heparin concentration versus platelet accumulation in the two groups. Thus, the effect of heparin on platelet adhesion did not seem to be affected by the presence of fibrinogen.

Conflicting reports about the effect of heparin on platelet adhesion and aggregation exist. Inhibition of adhesion at various concentrations of heparin have been reported[22, 30] while other authors have been unable to find any such effect.[25, 27] It has also been reported that heparin induces platelet aggregation.[10, 12] The postulation has also been made that heparin inhibits the release of ADP from platelets.[25] This finding might explain the gradual decline in platelet accumulation on the untreated shunts with increasing heparin levels in the blood, since inhibited release would inhibit ADP-induced aggregation to already adhered platelets. The results of the present study certainly show that if there is any effect of heparin in vivo on the platelets, the adhesivity is lowered. Like Salzman,[30] we conclude that this effect is weak and lacks clinical importance as much larger doses than those used in patients are required to obtain a significant effect.

It has been reported that heparin coating of plastic surfaces increases platelet adhesion.[32] The nature and degree of such effects might well, however, depend on the manufacturing procedure, the purity and stability of the heparin layer, etc. In the present study, the accumulation of platelets on heparin-treated surfaces was less than ten percent of that on untreated ones. This is in accordance with the findings of Jacobsson and Schlossman,[19] who found a diminished platelet adhesion from whole blood on vascular catheters heparinized with the same method as in the present study. Rembaum and associates,[27] using polyurethane heparin complexes, estimated the number of platelets per surface area by scanning electron microscopy. They obtained slightly lower values than ours but had much larger flows through their shunts.

There can be various and multiple reasons for the ability of the heparin surfaces to decrease platelet accumulation. One explanation is that the heparin coating renders the surface negatively charged and thereby repels the likewise negatively charged platelets.[33] Another explanation may be that some plasma protein preventing adhesion of platelets is attached to the heparin surface. Evidence of deposition of different plasma components on heparin surfaces and other surfaces have been put forward.[5, 29] However, the decreased platelet accumulation on heparin surfaces may not be due to a reduced adhesion of platelets to it, but to a reduced aggregation of circulating platelets on already adhered platelets. A third possible explanation to the decreased platelet accumulation on heparin surfaces may thus be attributed to the inhibitory effect of heparin on the platelet release reaction as described above.

The heparin coating of polypropylene and polyethylene according to the method used in the present study, results in a surface with markedly reduced thrombogenic properties, which is due to an inhibition of platelet adhesion.

REFERENCES

1. Aas, K. A., and Gardner, F. H.: Survival of blood platelets labeled with chromium^{51}, J. Clin. Invest. **37:** 1257, 1958.
2. Abrahamsen, A. F.: The effect of EDTA and ACD on the recovery and survival of Cr^{51} labelled blood platelets, Scand. J. Haemat. **2:** 53, 1965.
3. Abrahamsen, A. F.: A modification of the technique for Cr^{51}-labelling of blood platelets giving increased circulating platelet radioactivity, Scand. J. Haemat. **5:** 53, 1968.
4. Aster, R. H.: The anticoagulants of choice for platelet transfusions, Transfusion **6:** 32, 1966.
5. Baier, R. E., and Dutton, R. C.: Initial events in interactions of blood with a foreign surface, J. Biomed. Mater. Res. **3:** 191, 1969.
6. Bergström, K., Blombäck, B., and Kleen, G.: Studies on the plasma fibrinolytic activity in a case of liver cirrhosis, Acta Med. Scand. **168:** 291, 1960.
7. Biggs, R., Denson, K. W. E., and Akman, N., et al.: Antithrombin III, anti factor X, and heparin co-factor, Br. J. Haematol. **19:** 305, 1970.
8. Bruck, S. D.: Polymeric materials: Current

status of biocompatibility, Biomat. Med. Dev. Art. Org. **1:** 79, 1973.

9. Busch, C., and Olson, S.: Density distribution of ^{51}Cr-labelled platelets within the circulating dog platelet population, Thromb. Res. **3:** 1, 1973.
10. Copley, A. L., and Robb, T. P.: The effect of heparin on the platelet count in dogs and mice, Am. J. Physiol. **133:** 248, 1941.
11. Egberg, N., and Johnsson, H.: Platelet aggregation induced by ADP and thrombin in reptilase defibrinated dogs, Thromb. Res. **1:** 95, 1972.
12. Eika, C.: On the mechanism of platelet aggregation induced by heparin, protamine and polybrene, Scand. J. Haemat. **9:** 248, 1972.
13. Evans, G., and Mustard, F.: Platelet-surface reaction and thrombosis, SURGERY **64:** 273, 1968.
14. Falb, R. D., Takahaschi, M. T., Grode, G. A., and Leininger, R. I.: Studies on the stability and protein adsorption characteristics of heparinized polymer surfaces by radioisotope labeling techniques, J. Biomed. Mater. Res. **1:** 239, 1967.
15. Gugler, E., and Luscher, E. F.: Platelet function in congenital afibrinogenemia, Thromb. Diath. Haemorrh. **14:** 361, 1965.
16. Hardisty, R. M., and Hutton, R. A.: Bleeding tendency associated with a "new" abnormality of platelet behaviour, Lancet **1:** 983, 1967.
17. Holmsen, H., Day, H., and Stormorken, H.: The blood platelet release reaction, Scand. J. Haemat. **8:** 1, 1969.
18. Inceman, S., Caen, J., and Bernard, J.: Aggregation, adhesion, and viscous metamorphosis of platelets in congenital fibrinogen deficiencies, J. Lab. Clin. Med. **68:** 21, 1966.
19. Jacobsson, B., and Schlossman, D.: Thrombogenic properties of heparinized vascular catheters, Acta Radiol. (Diagn.) (Stockh.) **14:** 569, 1973.
20. Kristensson, A.: A new method for the direct counting of the so-called blood platelets in man, Acta Med. Scand. **57:** 301, 1922.
21. Lagergren, H. R., and Eriksson, J. C.: Plastics with a stable surface monolayer of cross-linked heparin: Preparation and evaluation, Trans. Am. Soc. Artif. Intern. Organs **17:** 10, 1971.
22. Lindsay, R. M., Prentice. C. R. M., Ferguson, D., Muir, W. M., and McNicol, G. P.: A method for the measurement of platelet adhesiveness by use of dialysis membranes in a test-cell, Br. J. Haematol. **24:** 377, 1973.
23. Miller-Andersson, M.: Personal communication.
24. Morrison, S., and Baldini, G.: Antigenic relationship between blood platelets and vascular endothelium, Blood **33:** 46, 1969.
25. O'Brien, J. R., Shoobridge, S. M., and Finch, W. J.: Comparison of the effect of heparin and citrate on platelet aggregation, J. Clin. Pathol. **22:** 28, 1969.
26. Olsson, P., and Johnsson, H.: Interference of acetyl salicylic acid, heparin and fibrinogen degradation products in haemostasis of reptilase-defibrinogenated dogs, Thromb. Res. **1:** 135, 1972.
27. Rembaum, A., Yen, S. P. S., Ingram, M., Newton, J. F., and Hu, C. L.: Platelet adhesion to heparin-bonded and heparin-free surfaces, Biomat. Med. Dev. Art. Org. **1:** 99, 1973.
28. Rodman, N. F., and Mason, R. G.: Compatibilty of blood with foreign surfaces, Thromb. Diath. Haemorrh. **40:** 145, 1970.
29. Rodman, N. F., and Mason, R. G.: Blood-foreign surface interaction, Thromb. Diath. Haemorrh. **42:** 61, 1970.
30. Salzman, E. W.: The limitations of heparin therapy after arterial reconstruction, SURGERY **57:** 131, 1965.
31. Salzman, E. W.: Role of platelets in blood-surface interactions, Fed. Proc. **30:** 1503, 1971.
32. Salzman, E. W., Merrill, E. W., Binder, A., Wolf, C. F. W., Ashford, T. P., and Austen, W. G.: Protein-platelet interaction on heparinized surfaces, J. Biomed. Mater. Res. **3:** 69, 1969.
33. Sawyer, P. N., and Srinivasan, S.: Metallic and plastic prosthetic devices as vascular wall substitutes: Biophysical criteria and methods for evaluation, J. Biomed. Mater. Res. **1:** 83, 1967.
34. Yin, E. T., Wessler, S., and Butler, J. V.: Plasma heparin: A unique practical submicrogram-sensitive assay, J. Lab. Clin. Med. **81:** 29, 1973.

A simplified kidney preservation system: Further development and results of extended perfusion

I. R. Hardie, G. J. A. Clunie, Glenda Balderson, J. F. Leditschke, *and* **I. J. Leslie,**
Brisbane, Queensland, Australia

Preliminary results with a greatly simplified continuous perfusion system indicated that satisfactory preservations of canine kidneys could be achieved in a small circuit from which much of the complexity required for pH, temperature, and pulse pressure control in conventional systems had been eliminated. Further development has been undertaken to simplify the pump control unit and to compare materials suitable for construction of the definitive circuit. Reliability of mechanical components and of preservation quality have been studied in a series of 48 hour perfusions of canine kidneys, with the use of both cryoprecipitated plasma and a five percent albumin solution as perfusates. Perfusions were carried out at both very low (0.5° C.) and low (5° C.) temperatures, since the operating temperature of the circuit, when immersed in chipped ice for simplified temperature control, depended on the material used in its construction. A total of 2,424 hours of perfusion was carried out, and no mechanical failure occurred; all components functioned efficiently and reliably. Plasma proved to be unsuitable at these low temperatures; only two of six dogs survived after 48 hours perfusion at 0.5° C. and six of nine survived at 5° C. All kidneys perfused with albumin at both temperatures survived, with maximum serum creatinines of 6.3 and 4.9 mg. percent, respectively, demonstrating that this solution is the more satisfactory of the two perfusates for this system.

From the Department of Surgery, University of Queensland, Brisbane, Australia.

INITIAL RESULTS with a simplified kidney perfusion system[8] indicated that this perfusion circuit provided 24-hour preservation comparable in quality to that of the the larger, more complex conventional circuits. The further development of this system forms the basis of the present report. Simplification of the solenoid control unit for the pneumatic pump has been achieved, suitable materials for the construction of the production unit were evaluated, and reliability of the unit was confirmed by a series of 48 hour perfusions of canine kidneys with the use of both cryoprecipitated plasma and a synthetic perfusate containing five percent albumin.

This project was supported by grants from the National Health and Medical Research Council, the Australian Kidney Foundation, and the Mayne Bequest Fund of the University of Queensland.

Accepted for publication Jan. 29, 1974.

Reprint requests: Dr. I. R. Hardie, Department of Surgery, Princess Alexandra Hospital, Ipswich Road, Woolloongabba, Brisbane, Q., Australia.

MATERIALS AND METHODS

Development of pump control unit. The final phase of operation to be simplified was the pump control function. The previous control unit required 240 v. A.C. power supply and utilized relatively large solenoid and constant pressure valves. For portability, a 12 v. D.C. power supply was selected, and provision was made for several alternative power sources, including a self-contained re-

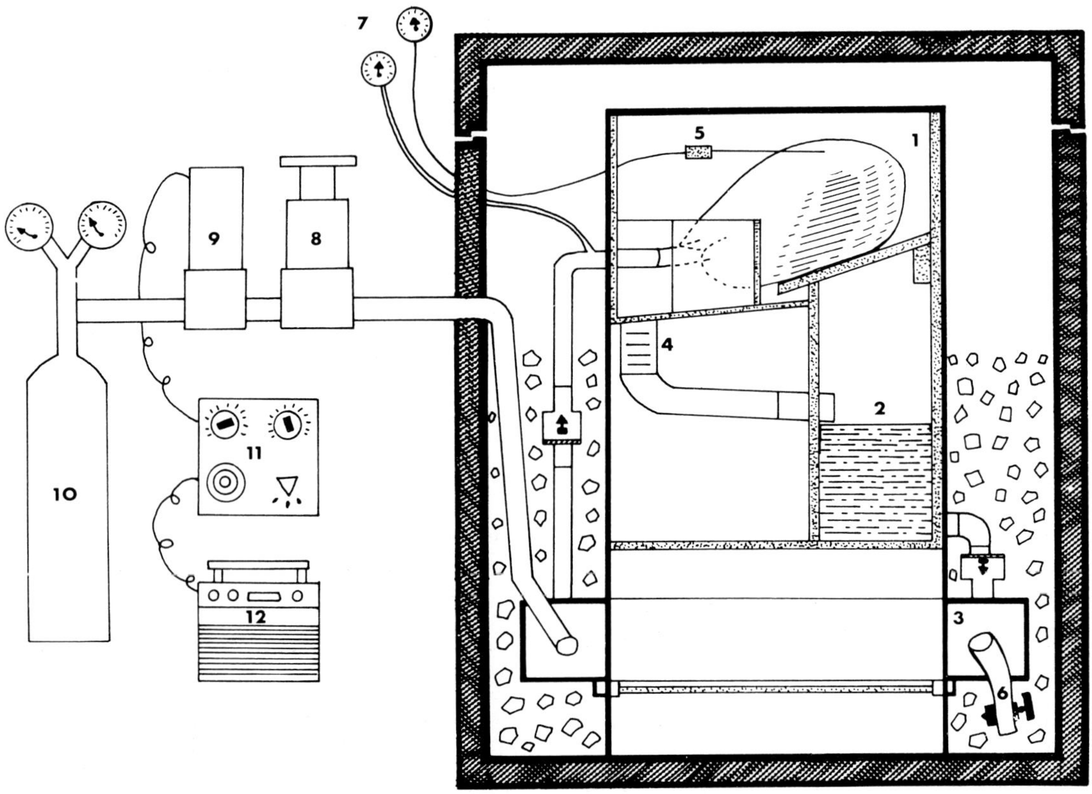

Fig. 1. Diagram of simplified kidney preservation system showing perfusion circuit (*1,* organ chamber; *2,* reservoir; *3,* oxygenator/pneumatic pump) immersed in ice, perfusate flow monitor *(4),* thermistor needle probe *(5),* pump air outlet constriction to control pulse wave form *(6),* arterial pressure and temperature monitors *(7),* constant pressure *(8),* and solenoid *(9)* values to control air release to drive pump, compressed air cylinder *(10),* control unit governing solenoid valve function *(11),* and portable 12 v. power source for control unit *(12).*

chargeable battery for use away from other sources, and 240/12 v. battery charger for local hospital storage. The rechargeable batteries use a semi-solid paste electrolyte/acid preparation which would be suitable for air transport.

Suitable electrical circuitry has been developed to provide a variable pulse frequency and an independently variable pulse duration; switched controls were used to ensure accurate selection of the required function. An alarm circuit provides an audible "pip" with each pulse and a continuous high pitched tone in the event of a decline in the voltage from the power source. The control unit measures 10 by 10 by 5 cm. and provides sufficient power output to operate a small (5 by 5 by 9 cm.) self-exhausting solenoid valve,* to the distal side of which is coupled a constant pressure valve of similar size.†

Evaluation of construction materials. The organ chamber and reservoir of the experimental circuit were made of polypropylene, and it is possible that toxins may have been leached out of this material,[1] thus accounting for some variability in results of preservation.[8] Furthermore, the acrylic non-return valves which were in use could not be autoclaved and so represented a double source of further potential contamination. New valves were therefore developed by using stainless

*Type UK3, Goyen Controls, Ltd., 151 Ipswich Rd., Woolloongabba, Brisbane, Q., Australia. (Goyen Controls [America] is a subsidiary.)

†Midget Regulating Valve, Type R125, Goyen Controls, Ltd.

Table I. *Perfusates used for continuous perfusion preservation of canine kidneys*

*Basic solution**			*Additives†*		
Plasma			Glucose	(50%)	5 ml.
1.5 L. pooled plasma, freeze-thaw-filter, osmolarity adjusted to 300 mOsm./L. with mannitol			Hydrocortisone		100 mg.
			Insulin		80 U.
			$MgSO_4$	(50%)	2 ml.
			H_3PO_4 (0.5M) to pH 7.5		
Albumin					
Saline	(0.9%)	500 ml.	Albumin	(25%)	200 ml.
Glucose	(5%)	100 ml.	$MgSO_4$	(50%)	2 ml.
Sucrose	(10.3%)	200 ml.	Hydrocortisone		100 mg.
K_2HPO_4	(200 mM)	75 ml.	Insulin		80 U.
			KOH (1N) to pH		7.5

*The plasma was stored frozen, after two cycles of freeze-thaw-filter, and thawed at 1° C. 48 hours before use.
†The additives were added to each solution immediately prior to use.

steel and a design similar to that of the former valves. Later, a stainless steel prototype circuit was constructed, providing an easily sterilized, non-toxic unit. Immersion of this unit in chipped ice for simplified temperature control resulted in a perfusion temperature rather lower than that provided by the polypropylene circuit, and some difficulties were encountered at this very low temperature, as will be discussed later. A polycarbonate plastic circuit was therefore constructed in order to utilize the advantages of reduced thermal conductivity, transparency, and lighter weight offered by this non-toxic, autoclavable material.[14]

Perfusion experiments. For reasons of economy, the perfusion experiments were performed in pairs, the perfusate being used without intervening filtration for consecutive 24 hour and, later, 48 hour periods on kidneys from two dogs. Nephrectomy and reimplantation were carried out under mannitol-induced diuretic conditions, as previously described.[5] After removal, the kidneys were cooled rapidly by immersion in iced saline slush and were then flushed until the effluent was clear with about 50 ml. of cold Ringer's lactate solution containing procaine (1.0 Gm. per liter) and heparin (500 U. per liter) and buffered to pH 7.4 before being weighed and placed on the perfusion circuit (Fig. 1). Thereafter, the temperature was maintained by immersion of the circuit in chipped ice, the actual operating range depending on the material used in the construction of the circuit. Renal cortical temperature, monitored by a thermistor needle probe, was in the range 4 to 5° C. in both plastic units and 0.5 to 1.0 C. in the stainless steel unit. Air pressure to the oxygenator/pump was set to maintain a renal systolic perfusion pressure of 60 mm. Hg. The rate of flow of effluent down the venous line was monitored regularly, together with the systolic and diastolic pressures and the perfusate arterial and venous pH, Po_2, and Pco_2 (measured at 37° C.).

Table II. *Final compositions of the perfusates used for continuous perfusion of canine kidneys*

	Cryo-precipitated plasma	*Albumin (5%)*
Sodium (mEq./L.)	146	108
Potassium (mEq./L.)	5.0	33
Magnesium (mEq./L.)	7.7	8.0
Chloride (mEq./L.)	75	77
Osmolarity (mOsm/L.)	295	310
pH	7.5	7.5
Glucose (mg./100 ml.)	300	860
Free fatty acid (mEq./L.)	1.0	2.5

After the period of perfusion, the kidneys were reweighed and reimplanted in the pelvis with the use of standard techniques, with immediate contralateral nephrectomy. Renal function was followed by daily estimations of the serum creatinine level. Animals becoming uremic were killed, while survivors

Table III. *Results of 24 hour perfusions with albumin solution at 4 to 5° C. in polypropylene circuit using two types of non-return valve*

	Maximum serum creatinine (mg./100 ml.)					
	A		B		Total	
Valves	*No.*	*Mean (S.D.)*	*No.*	*Mean (S.D.)*	*No.*	*Mean (S.D.)*
Acrylic	9	2.7 (1.0)	9	1.9 (0.9)	18	2.3 (1.0)
Stainless steel	6	2.7 (1.0)	5	2.4 (0.8)	11	2.6 (0.9)

Table IV. *Results of 48 hour perfusions at 0.5 to 1° C.*

Perfusate	*No. of dogs*	*No. of survivors*	*No. of uremic deaths*	*Maximum serum creatinine (mg./100 ml.)*
Plasma	6	2	4	5.0
				11.5
Albumin	5	5	0	Mean, 6.3 (S.D., 1.2)

were followed for at least four weeks. Sections taken from kidneys at autopsy were examined by light microscopy, with hematoxylin and eosin and Picro-Mallory stains.

Two perfusates were studied and compared (Table I). Cryoprecipitated pooled canine plasma was prepared by a modification of the method described by Belzer and associates,[2] subjecting it to an additional cycle of cold thawing, 48 hours ice storage, cold filtration, and refreezing in order to eliminate a further cryoprecipitate which became apparent with storage at 0° C., and substituting a phosphate buffer for the plasma bicarbonate buffer system by titrating with 0.5M phosphoric acid during the early stages of perfusion.[8] The second perfusate was a synthetic albumin solution similar to that described by Claes and colleagues.[4] The final compositions of the perfusates are shown in Table II.

Three groups of experiments were carried out. Technical failures were excluded from analysis when an obvious technical error was identified. Statistical analyses were carried out with the use of the Student's t test.

Group I. Perfusion with stainless steel valves. Twenty-four hour perfusions were carried out in the polypropylene circuit at 4° C., using either acrylic or stainless steel valves. For this experiment, only the albumin perfusate was used, in order to achieve accurate comparison between the two sets of valves within a single variant of the perfusate.

Group II. Perfusion at very low temperature. Forty-eight hour perfusions were carried out at 0.5 to 1.0° C. in the stainless steel circuit incorporating the new valves, with the use of either cryoprecipitated plasma or the albumin solution as perfusate.

Group III. Perfusion at low temperature. A further series of 48 hour perfusions was subsequently carried out at 4 to 5° C., the operating temperature provided by the polycarbonate circuit immersed in ice, with the use of the same perfusates.

RESULTS

Group I. Perfusion with stainless steel valves. The results of the 24 hour perfusions to test the stainless steel valves are summarized in Table III. The first and second kidneys from each consecutively perfused experimental pair have been grouped into Series A and Series B, respectively, before being combined to show the total result for the whole group. The only uremic deaths were due to technical failures caused by arterial and venous thrombosis, either alone or in combination, which complicated the postoperative course in three of the animals in Series A and one in Series B with acrylic valves. In two of these, one from each series, stable creatinine levels had been reached before this secondary rise characteristic of

Table V. *Perfusion characteristics of kidneys perfused for 48 hours at 0.5 to 1° C.*

Perfusate	No.	Diastolic pressure: Stable	Diastolic pressure: Increased No.	Diastolic pressure: Increased Mean (%)	Flow increase: Mean (%)	Flow increase: S.D.	Weight increase: No.	Weight increase: Mean % (S.D.)
Plasma								
Surivors	2	0	2	60	8	—	2	10.5 (—)
Nonsurvivors	4	0	4	85 (S.D., 47.0)	8.8	—	4	28.8 (13.4)
Albumin	5	1	4	60 (S.D., 25.8)	114.4	63.8	5	22.9 (12.2)

Table VI. *Results of 48 hour perfusions at 4 to 5° C.*

Perfusate	No. of dogs	No. of survivors	No. of uremic deaths	Maximum serum creatinine (mg./100) Mean	Maximum serum creatinine (mg./100) S.D.
Plasma	9	6	3	7.4	1.1
Albumin	8	8	0	4.9	1.7

the onset of thrombosis, and these levels have therefore been included, whereas the other two were excluded from further study. No vascular thrombosis occurred in either series in the stainless steel valve group. There were no technical failures due to circuit malfunction.

The rise in serum creatinine in Series B was almost always less than in Series A, but full analysis showed no significant difference between the two series with either type of valve. The comparison of the valves was therefore based on the total number of perfusions performed in each group, and again no significant difference was demonstrated between the results with the two types of valve.

Group II. Perfusion at very low temperature (0.5° C. to 1.0° C.). The results of the 48 hour perfusions at 0.5° C. to 1.0° C. are summarized in Table IV. Seventeen perfusions were performed, but six were technically unsatisfactory because of vascular thrombosis (one in each group), intussusception (one in the albumin group), leaking ureteroneocystostomy (one in the plasma group), or incorrect cannulation of the renal artery resulting in perfusion of only one major branch of the artery (one in each group), and were excluded from analysis. In both groups, there was no significant difference in maximum serum creatinine between the first and second kidneys in the pairs of perfusions and so all experiments in each group were combined for analysis.

Only two of the six kidneys perfused with plasma had life-sustaining function after reimplantation, and in these animals the serum creatinine rose to peaks of 5.0 mg. percent on day 1 and 11.5 mg. percent on day 5, respectively. The other four failed to support life, and the animals rapidly became uremic and died. Autopsy revealed a uniformly black kidney in each case, with all anastomoses intact and patent, and histologic examination showed extensive cortical necrosis. Details of the behavior of these kidneys during perfusion are summarized in Table V. The diastolic pressure rose progressively in every kidney perfused with plasma, while the perfusate flow rate increased only marginally and actually decreased in one kidney, which subsequently failed to support life. Every kidney increased in weight during perfusion, and most were frankly edematous at reimplantation. These features were more marked in the four which did not support life after reimplantation, but statistical comparison with the survivors is not possible with only two animals in the latter group.

In contrast, there were no uremic deaths in the group perfused with the albumin solution, and the mean maximum serum creatinine was 6.3 (S.D., 1.2) mg. percent.

Table VII. *Perfusion characteristics of kidneys perfused for 48 hours at 4 to 5° C.*

Perfusate	*No.*	*Diastolic pressure*		*Flow increase*		*Weight increase*		
		Stable	*Increased*	*Mean (%)*	*S.D.*	*No.*	*Mean (%)*	*S.D.*
Plasma								
Survivors	6	5	1 (50%)	66.7	12.5	3	3.0	2.4
Nonsurvivors	3	3	0	35.0	14.1	1	7.8	—
Albumin	7	7	0	79.6	22.1	6	13.5	10.9

Creatinine levels had returned to less than 2.0 mg. percent within ten days in all these animals and remained normal thereafter. Diastolic pressures during perfusion were more stable in this group and tended to rise less, while the flow showed a substantial increase of 114 percent (S.D., 64), which was significantly greater than in the plasma group ($p < 0.01$). However, all kidneys showed increases in weight which were not significantly different from the increases in the plasma group.

These animals were killed at intervals ranging from one to seven months after reimplantation and histologic examination of the kidneys revealed minimal changes.

Group III. Perfusion at low temperature (4 to 5° C.). The results of the 48 hour perfusions at 4 to 5° C. are summarized in Table VI. Nineteen experiments were performed, from which two technical failures were excluded, one with vascular thrombosis from the plasma group and one with air embolism from the albumin group. This was the only occurrence of this complication in all groups and was due to a clamp being inadvertently left on the venous line after recording the flow rate, causing accumulation of perfusate in the organ chamber until the reservoir level fell below the outlet and allowed air into the line. Awareness of this possible complication has helped to avoid any recurrence.

In the plasma group, there were three uremic deaths, all these kidneys appeared non-viable at autopsy, with histologic evidence of diffuse cortical necrosis. The remaining six in this group survived, the serum creatinine rising to a mean maximum of 7.4 mg. percent (S.D., 1.1). In the albumin group all eight survived, with no uremic deaths, and the mean maximum serum creatinine in this group was 4.9 mg. percent (S.D., 1.7), which was significantly lower ($p < 0.01$) than in the survivors of the plasma group. Once again, no significant difference was found between the first and second kidneys in the pairs of perfusions. Serum creatinine levels had fallen to less than 2.0 mg. percent between 18 days in the plasma group survivors and within ten days in the albumin group. Thereafter, all animals maintained normal creatinine levels for periods ranging from one to six months, at which time the animals were killed. These kidneys were macroscopically normal and showed minimal histologic change.

In all kidneys, the diastolic pressure remained stable throughout perfusion, while the flow rate increased during the first 12 hours and thereafter remained stable (Table VII). The flow increase was 79.6 percent (S.D., 22.1) in the albumin group, but rather less at 66.7 percent (S.D., 12.5) in the survivors of the plasma group, and this difference was not statistically significant. However, in the non-survivors of the plasma group, the flow increased by only 35.0 percent (S.D., 14.0), which was significantly less than the increase in both the survivors of the plasma group ($p < 0.02$) and the albumin group ($p < 0.01$).

Weight changes were variable in the plasma group, two of the survivors losing five and two percent of their original weight, while the other four gained less than five percent. One of the non-survivors lost 14 percent, while another gained 7.8 percent, and the weight of the remaining one was unchanged. Seven of the eight in the albumin group gained weight, but the extent varied greatly (mean, 13.5 percent, S.D., 10.9), and the eighth lost four percent of its original weight. Thus, there appeared to be no consistent relationship between weight change during perfusion and the ultimate function of the kidney.

DISCUSSION

The simplifications incorporated in every phase of the operation of this kidney perfusion system have resulted in the development of a small, simple, lightweight machine, the reliability of which is clearly demonstrated by the experiments described in this report. A total of 29 twenty-four hour and 36 forty-eight hour perfusions were carried out, and during these 2,424 hours of operation, no mechanical failure developed.

The pneumatic pump/oxygenator has provided flow rates up to 40 ml. per minute through the larger canine kidneys, at 60 mm. Hg systolic pressure, with peak flow rates ranging from 0.2 to 1.0 ml. per gram per minute. Separate observations on a small group of kidneys which were not reimplanted indicate that the pump can provide much greater flow rates if the pulse rate and/or duration or systolic pressure are increased. Oxygenation has been satisfactory at all times. The Po_2 of the arterial perfusate was always in the range 200 to 210 mm. Hg (at 37° C.), while the arteriovenous Po_2 difference never exceeded 80 mm. Hg, thus confirming the effectiveness of the pump/oxygenator.

The membrane oxygenators (Travenol 5M0321) have each been used for at least 288 hours of perfusion (three pairs of 48-hours) in order to test their reliability and for reasons of economy. After each use, they were thoroughly cleansed by flushing and then resterilized by exposure to ethylene oxide. No membrane failure was recorded, even with this extreme usage, and safe, reliable operation is therefore to be expected in clinical use, where the oxygenator is a disposable item.

Ice immersion has provided reproducible and stable temperature control. The ice supply has required only infrequent replenishment, although the interval depends to some extent on the ambient temperature.

The stainless steel valves proved mechanically sound and achieved the desired ease of sterilization. One valve which was thoroughly flushed with water after each use and then autoclaved without being taken apart, was found after 20 perfusions of 48 hours to be as clean inside as the other valve which had been disassembled for cleaning on each occasion. As a result of this, together with the demonstration that the change to these valves did not adversely effect preservation, the stainless steel valves were adopted for permanent use in the circuit.

The pH control by the phosphate buffer in each perfusate has been reliable. The pH remains stable over 96 hours of perfusion, thus eliminating the need for repeated pH estimations, improving the reliability, and effecting further simplification of operation additional to that already achieved by the elimination of a carbon dioxide supply and flow control.

The results of preservation of canine kidneys in this simplified perfusion system indicate a satisfactory quality of preservation. The results of 24 hour perfusions with cryoprecipitated plasma were reported previously,[8] and the maximum serum creatinine of 2.2 mg. percent (S.D., 1.0) was not significantly different from the over-all mean maximum serum creatinine for the 29 kidneys perfused for 24 hours with albumin in the present series. The two perfusates appear equally satisfactory for periods up to 24 hours, but the albumin is preferred because of its greater simplicity of preparation.

With both perfusates, the 24 hour results are comparable to those reported in the conventional perfusion systems. The albumin results compare favorably with those of Collste,[9] who reported a creatine peak of 3.6 mg. percent, and are considerably better than those Cooperman and associates[10] obtained with a 1.6 percent albumin solution, while Johnson and associates[12] reported a maximum creatine of 2.5 mg. percent with a similar solution utilizing a plasma protein fraction to provide colloid osmotic pressure. The plasma results are not significantly different from the peak level of 1.4 mg. percent reported by Woods and colleagues[19] with the Waters Mox-100 machine, and the peak of 1.5 mg. percent reported by Scott and associates[18] with the Belzer LI-400 machine.

The disappointing feature, however, was the realization that the over-all results of 24 hour perfusions, with a maximum serum creatinine after reimplantation of 2.4 mg. percent for all kidneys and both perfusates, are no better than the results of 24 hour preservation of similar kidneys by simple hypothermic storage in iced saline slush after initial flushing with the Collins C3 solution.[5-7] Since continuous perfusion represents a method of metabolic maintenance, it would be expected to provide preservation of superior quality to that of hypothermia alone, since the latter is based solely on metabolic inhibition. This provided a further reason, in addition to the aim of confirming the reliability of the system, for extending the preservation time to 48 hours, at which period hypothermia after C3 flush fails to provide consistently satisfactory preservation.[6, 9, 11, 15]

The major difference between this and the conventional perfusion systems is the operating temperature. It seems that, even with refined preparation, cryoprecipitated plasma is not as effective a perfusate at 5° C. as it is at 8 to 10° C. in the conventional units. The reason for this is not entirely clear but may be related in part to inhibition of the cellular membrane ATPase system below 10° C. leading to inability to consume available substrates to maintain cellular homeostasis,[13] and in part to the difficulties of clearing the plasma completely of all lipoid particles insoluble at this very low temperature.[3, 8] Similarly, the albumin results, while satisfactory on the whole, are not as good as would have been expected in view of the report by Claes and colleagues[4] that 72 hour perfusions of a small group of canine kidneys at 8° C. with a similar solution gave a mean maximum serum creatinine of 4.3 mg. percent. Once again, the probable inhibition of the membrane ATPase at 5° C. may provide a partial explanation.

The improvement produced by perfusion with an oxygenated solution over the results of simple hypothermic ischemic preservation indicates that the oxygenation is allowing the satisfaction of some metabolic need, even at the very low temperature employed in this experiment, thus leading to better maintenance of cellular viability. In this regard, it is interesting to note that the arteriovenous oxygen difference of 80 mm. Hg represents an oxygen extraction by the kidneys perfused at low temperatures in this experiment which is nearly double the 35 to 45 mm. Hg arteriovenous oxygen difference reported by Santiago-Delpin and associates[17] for kidneys perfused at 10° C. on the Mox-100 and LI-400 machines, with similar arterial Po_2 of 200 mm. Hg. It is apparent that further investigation is needed to define the metabolic pathways active at such low temperatures.

The results of the 48-hour perfusions were clearly dependent on the temperature at which the organs were perfused. At very low temperatures in the range 0 to 1° C. cryoprecipitated plasma proved to be unsuitable, with poor perfusion characteristics as evidenced by the rising diastolic pressure, the poor flow rates, and the poor survival rates after reimplantation. In the range 4 to 5° C., the plasma gave much better perfusion, but preservation was still of inconsistent quality.

On the other hand, the five percent albumin solution used in this experiment was superior at both temperature ranges and maintained life-supporting function in every instance. Preservation was essentially the same at both temperatures, the trend toward better results at the higher temperature not reaching statistical significance ($t = 1.545$: $p < 0.20$). The greater simplicity of preparation of the albumin solution, in addition to its clearly superior quality of preservation, establishes this solution as the optimal perfusate, in the present state of our knowledge, for use in the simplified kidney perfusion system.

The development of the perfusion technology has now reached a satisfactory level. Further advances in the quality of preservation may come from the use of improved perfusates. The development of such solutions depends on the elucidation of many as yet unknown aspects of the low temperature biochemistry and physiology of the kidney, from which it may be possible to deduce the optimal substrate composition of solutions for hypothermic perfusion at the very low operating temperatures of the simplified system. Of further interest is the recent finding by Sachs and colleagues[16] that results of simple hypothermic preservation could be greatly improved by using a hyperosmolar solution for the initial flush. Work at present in progress in our laboratory indicates that similar improvement in continuous perfusion preservation can be obtained when plasma is rendered hyperosmolar, results at 5° C. being equal to and perhaps better than those with standard albumin. Further experiments are planned to confirm this finding and extend it to the albumin solution in order to define the optimal osmolarity.

In the meantime, this simplified perfusion system is now being used with the albumin perfusate for the preservation of human cadaveric kidneys and commercial production is planned for the near future.

We wish to acknowledge the part played by Dr. Geoffrey Collins, now of the University of California, San Diego, in the initial development of the circuit, and the technical assistance of Mrs. Lizzie Hamlyn, Mr. Ron Hill, B.Sc., Mr. Del Sizemore, and Miss Dorothy Mackay, S.R.N.

REFERENCES

1. Atkins, R. C., Robinson, W. A., and Eiseman, B.: Cytotoxins released from plastic perfusion apparatus, Lancet **2:** 1014, 1968.
2. Belzer, F. O., Ashby, B. S., and Dunphy, J. E.: 24 and 72 hour preservation of canine kidneys, Lancet **2:** 536, 1967.
3. Belzer, F. O., Ashby, B. S., Huang, J. S., and Dunphy, J. E.: Etiology of rising perfusion pressure in isolated organ perfusion, Ann. Surg. **168:** 382, 1968.
4. Claes, G., Aurrell, M., Blohmé, I., and Pettersson, S.: Experimental and clinical results of continuous hypothermic albumin perfusion, Proc. Eur. Dial. Transplant Assoc. **9:** 484, 1972.
5. Collins, G. M., Bravo-Shugarman, M., and Terasaki, P. I.: Kidney preservation for transportation: 3. Initial perfusion and 30 hour ice storage, Lancet **2:** 1219, 1969.
6. Collins, G. M., Bravo-Shugarman, M., Terasaki, P. I., Braf, Z., Sheil, A. G. R., and Williams, G.: Kidney preservation for transportation: 4. Eight-thousand-mile international air transport, Aust. N. Z. J. Surg. **40:** 195, 1970.
7. Collins, G. M., Hartley, L. C. J., and Clunie, G. J. A.: Kidney preservation for transportation. Experimental analysis of optimal perfusate composition, Br. J. Surg. **59:** 187, 1972.
8. Collins, G. M., Hardie, I. R., and Clunie, G. J. A.: A simplified kidney preservation system. Development and initial results, Med. J. Aust. **1:** 59, 1973.
9. Collste, H.: Preservation of kidneys for transplanation. Experimental studies, Acta Chir. Scand. Suppl. **425:** 1, 1972.
10. Cooperman, A. M., Woods, J. E., Holley, K. E., and McIlrath, D. C.: Twenty-four hour perfusion and storage of canine kidneys with albumin and electrolyte solutions, Mayo Clin. Proc. **46:** 193, 1971.
11. Liu, W. P., Humphries, A. L., Jr., Russell, R., Stoddard, L. D., and Moretz, W. H.: 48-hour storage of canine kidneys after brief perfusion with Collins' solution, Ann. Surg. **173:** 748, 1971.
12. Johnson, R. W. G., Anderson, M., Flear, C. T. G., Murray, S. G. H., Taylor, R. M. R., and Swinney, J.: Evaluation of a new perfusion solution for kidney preservation, Transplantation **13:** 270, 1972.
13. Martin, D. R., Scott, D. F., Downes, G. L., and Belzer, F. O.: Primary cause of unsuccessful liver and heart preservation: Cold sensitivity of the ATPase system, Ann. Surg. **175:** 111, 1972.
14. Morgan, D. F., and Wendle, B. C.: Polycarbonates, *in* Modern plastics encyclopaedia, New York, 1968, McGraw-Hill, p. 217.
15. Panijayanond, P., Cho, S. I., Ulrich, F., and Nabseth, D. C.: Enhancement of renal preservation of furosemide, SURGERY **73:** 368, 1973.
16. Sachs, S. A., Petritsch, P. H., and Kaufman, J. J.: Canine kidney preservation using a new perfusate, Lancet **1:** 1024, 1973.
17. Santiago-Delpin, E. A., Moberg, A. W., Moses, M. F., Campos, R. A., Mason, R. V., and Najarian, J. S.: Comparative analysis of perfusion and non-perfusion methods for renal preservation, SURGERY **72:** 793, 1972.
18. Scott, D. F., Stephens, F. O., Keaveny, T. V., Kountz, S. L., and Belzer, F. O.: Evaluation of preservation of cadaver kidneys, Transplantation **11:** 90, 1971.
19. Woods, J. E., Holley, K. E., and DiPasquale, J. A.: Comparison of methods of 24-hour preservation of dog kidneys using the same perfusate, Transplantation **11:** 295, 1971.

Thymidine incorporation in esophageal wounds of zinc-deficient rats

R. A. MacMahon, M.S.(Colo.), F.R.C.S.(Edin.), F.R.A.C.S., L. J. Cussen, F.R.C.P.A., F. T. McDermott, F.R.C.S.(Eng.), F.R.A.C.S., *and* B. E. James, M.Sc., *Melbourne, Australia*

The relationship between zinc-deficiency, impaired wound healing, and DNA synthesis has been investigated by means of autoradiographic studies, performed with tritiated thymidine, of esophageal epithelial wounds of the rat. Zinc-deficient and pair-fed control rats were examined following pulse injection of tritiated thymidine three days after wounding. No significant differences were found in the pattern or frequency of labeling in the wound edges or in the total number of cells of the basal epithelial layer.

From the Departments of Paediatrics and Surgery, Monash University, Melbourne, Australia

ZINC-DEFICIENCY has been shown to impair wound healing in rats,[3, 8, 11, 13] and some workers[1, 4, 6] have suggested that it is at least a contributing factor in the poor wound healing observed in some human patients. The most marked effects of zinc deficiency occur in the renewing epithelial cell populations of skin and esophageal mucosa, and it is possible that these effects may be caused by reduced synthesis of DNA and decreased cell proliferation in these tissues. Results favoring this hypothesis have been obtained in rat liver,[12, 19] embryonic rat tissues,[18] wounded rat skin,[2, 17] and suckling rat brain,[14] but contrary evidence has been obtained showing that there is no significant impairment of DNA synthesis in rat liver,[20] kidney,[20] spleen,[20] testes,[5, 20] or skin[10] after several weeks of zinc deprivation.

This paper is a report of a study of the incorporation of tritiated thymidine by the basal layer of esophageal mucosa following longitudinal wounds of the esophagus in zinc-deficient and pair-fed control rats.

Accepted for publication Feb. 11, 1974.

MATERIALS AND METHODS

Male Hooded Wistar rats, age six weeks and weighing approximately 100 Gm. were made zinc-deficient over a period of four weeks by feeding them on a synthetic diet,[3] based on egg albumin, sucrose, and peanut oil, containing less than 1 μg of zinc per gram but able to meet all other known nutrient requirements of the animals. Control rats were pair-fed the same diet with 40 μg of added zinc per gram: Each day the control rats were fed an amount of food equal to the mean food intake of the deficient group on the previous day. Both groups of rats were housed in plastic and glass cages similar to the design proposed by McCosker,[7] and great care was taken to prevent zinc contamination.

The rats were wounded by making a transverse supraclavicular incision in the neck and gently mobilizing the esophagus behind the trachea. A longitudinal incision was made through all coats of the anterolateral side of the esophagus, and the incision was closed with three or four interrupted No. 6-0 Mersilene sutures through all coats.

Table I. *Effects of dietary regime*

Group	*No. of rats*	*Mean weight at operation (% of original weight)*	*Mean plasma zinc level at death (μg/100 ml.)*	*Mean erythrocyte zinc level at death (μg/100 ml.)*
Zinc-deficient	7	91.6	86.0	1193
Pair-fed controls	9	135.4	157.0	1188
U		0	1	30.5
p		< 0.001	< 0.001	> 0.05

Table II. *Data from autoradiography*

Group	*No. of rats*	*No. of wound edges*	*Mean No. of basal cells in section*	*Mean No. of labeled basal cells in 300 cell wound edge*	*Labeling index* (%)*
Zinc-deficient	7	14	924	52.3	17.4
Pair-fed controls	9	18	959	59.7	19.9
U			31	106	106
p			> 0.05	> 0.05	> 0.05

*Percentage of labeled cells in 300 basal cells adjacent to the wound edge.

On the third postoperative day, each animal received an intraperitoneal injection of 1 μCi of tritiated thymidine (Amersham thymidine-6-T (n), 5.0 Ci per millimole) per gram of body weight, and 75 minutes later blood was taken by cardiac puncture into zinc-free heparinized syringes and the animal was killed.

The esophagus was excised and immediately fixed in ten percent neutral buffered formol saline. Autoradiographs of 5 μ transverse paraffin sections, prepared by the dipping technique using Kodak nuclear track emulsion NTB2, were exposed for 12 days and then the sections were stained with hematoxylin and eosin. The criterion for labeling was five or more grains per cell.

Because preliminary assessment of the pattern of labeling showed that, although there was sporadic labeling of basal cells throughout the whole circumference of the esophagus, the area of most intense labeling was generally within 300 cells of the wound edge, the numbers of labeled and unlabeled basal cells were counted in successive blocks of 20 cells for the first 300 cells from the wound edge. In addition, the total number of cells in the basal layer of the epithelium was counted for each section.

Plasma and erythrocyte zinc levels were determined by atomic absorption spectrophotometry.[3]

The significance of differences between the zinc-deficient and pair-fed control rats was assessed by the Mann-Whitney U test.[15]

RESULTS

The data in Table I indicate the effectiveness of the dietary regime. During the four weeks that they received the low-zinc diet, the depleted rats gradually lost weight whereas the pair-fed control animals continued to grow so that the difference in weight between these two groups at the time of operation was significant at the 0.1 per cent level. Analysis of blood collected on the third postoperative day showed that the plasma zinc level of the zinc-deficient rats was significantly lower ($p < 0.001$) than that of the controls, but the erythrocyte zinc levels, as noted previously,[3] were not significantly changed by deprivation of zinc for this duration.

Table II shows the results for basal cell labeling in the wound edges. There was no significant difference between the two groups of animals in the total number of basal layer cells in each esophageal section,

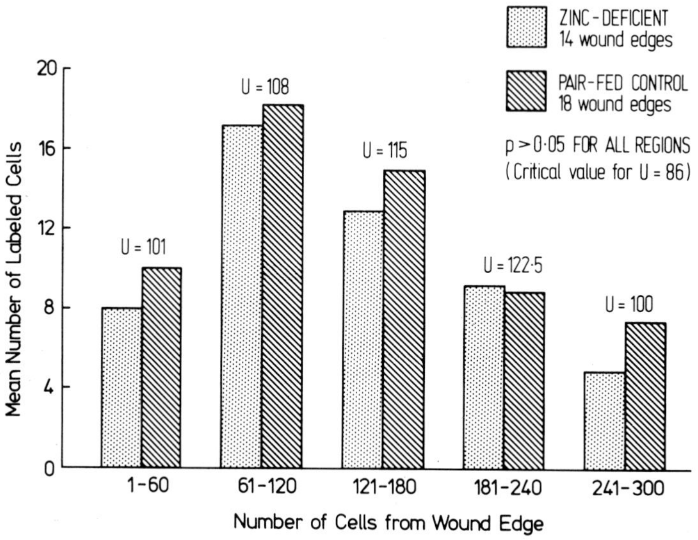

Fig. 1. Distribution of labeled basal cells.

and while the total number of labeled cells in the first 300 cells of the wound edge was lower in the depleted animals than in the control animals, the difference was not significant at the five percent level.

The distribution of labeled basal cells with the first 300 cells of the wound edge is shown in Fig. 1, where the data obtained by counting the number of labeled cells per block of 20 basal cells has, for clarity and ease of presentation, been recorded as the number of labeled cells per 60 basal cells. The pattern of labeling is qualitatively similar between the two groups of rats, and although there is a tendency toward decreased labeling in the zinc-deficient group, the differences between this group and the pair-fed control group are not significant for any area of the wound edge.

DISCUSSION

This investigation has shown that, while the total number of cells in the basal layer of esophageal epithelium and the percentage and distribution of labeled cells in the wound edges is decreased in zinc-deficient rats, the differences do not attain significance.

Hsu and Hsu[2] have studied the incorporation of tritiated thymidine into epithelial wounds in zinc-deficient rats and reported that the labeling index in cutaneous wounds of the back of zinc-depleted rats was lower than in control animals on days 2, 4, and 6 after wounding. The difference between groups on day 2 was least, being approximately three percent, but the difference increased to approximately nine and ten percent on days 4 and 6, respectively. Statistical evidence as to the significance of these differences was not presented. Our results, obtained three days after operation, show a difference in labeling index along the wound edge of 2.5 percent between the zinc-depelted and control rats, but this difference was not significant at the five percent level (Table II).

Hsu and Hsu[2] also expressed the opinion that, in unwounded epithelium, there appeared to be fewer cells in the zinc-deficient animals per unit of histological section when compared with sections from zinc-supplemented animals. In sections of wounded esophagus, we found fewer basal cells in zinc-deficient rats than in controls, but the difference was not significant.

Stephan and Hsu[17] used scintillation counting of DNA extracted from skin to study the short-term effects of zinc deficiency on radioactive thymidine incorporation into skin DNA of wounded rats. They found that the specific activity of skin DNA was significantly reduced in zinc-deficient rats at one hour after wounding but not at four hours after wounding; however, it was not made clear whether the skin analyzed came from an area adjacent to the wound or from another area.

Slater and associates[16] have shown that DNA polymerase from both bacterial and animal cells contains zinc and have suggested that zinc plays a functional role in the activity of this enzyme. While it might therefore be expected that restriction of dietary zinc intake would decrease DNA synthesis, this situation may not be encountered, since not all zinc-dependent enzymes are similarly susceptible to dietary zinc deprivation and different tissues reveal different activities for the same enzyme.[9]

Although this study has demonstrated no significant difference in thymidine incorporation in esophageal epithelial wounds, this finding does not preclude the possibility that the observed finding of impaired healing in zinc deficiency[3, 8, 11, 13] is consequent to a decreased rate of cellular proliferation.

REFERENCES

1. Henzel, J. H., De Weese, M. S., and Pories, W. J.: Significance of magnesium and zinc metabolism in the surgical patient. II. Zinc, Arch. Surg. **95:** 991, 1967.
2. Hsu, T. H. S., and Hsu, J. M.: Zinc deficiency and epithelial wound repair: An autoradiographic study of ^{3}H-thymidine incorporation, Proc. Soc. Exp. Biol. Med. **140:** 157, 1972.
3. James, B. E.: Zinc depletion: Its effects in the rat and its detection in man (M.Sc. thesis), Monash University, 1971.
4. Larson, D. L., Maxwell, R., Abston, S., and Dobrkovsky, M.: Zinc deficiency in burned children, Plast. Reconstr. Surg. **46:** 13, 1970.
5. Macapinlac, M. P., Pearson, W. N., Barney, G. H., and Darby, W. J.: Protein and nucleic acid metabolism in the testes of zinc-deficient rats, J. Nutr. **95:** 569, 1968.
6. MacMahon, R. A., Parker, M. LeM., and McKinnon, M. C.: Zinc treatment in malabsorption, Med. J. Aust. **2:** 210, 1968.
7. McCosker, P. J.: Design of cages for work with copper-deficient rats, Br. J. Nutr. **21:** 231, 1967.
8. Oberleas, D., Seymour, J. K., Lenaghan, R., Hovanesian, J., Wilson, R. F., and Prasad, A. S.: Effect of zinc deficiency on wound-healing in rats, Am. J. Surg. **121:** 566, 1971.
9. Prasad, A. S., and Oberleas, D.: Changes in activities of zinc-dependent enzymes in zinc-deficient tissues of rats, J. Appl. Physiol. **31:** 842, 1971.
10. Rao, V. H., and Bose, S. M.: Effect of zinc deficiency on the formation of collagen and nucleic acids in the albino rat skins and granulomas, Leather Sci. **18:** 211, 1971.
11. Sandstead, H. H., and Shephard, G. H.: The effect of zinc deficiency on the tensile strength of healing surgical incisions in the integument of the rat, Proc. Soc. Exp. Biol. Med. **128:** 687, 1968.
12. Sandstead, H. H., and Rinaldi, R. A.: Impairment of deoxyribonucleic acid synthesis by dietary zinc deficiency in the rat, J. Cell Physiol. **73:** 81, 1969.
13. Sandstead, H. H., Lanier, V. C., Jr., Shephard, G. H., and Gillespie, D. D.: Zinc and wound healing: Effects of zinc deficiency and zinc supplementation, Am. J. Clin. Nutr. **23:** 514, 1970.
14. Sandstead, H. H., Gillespie, D. D., and Brady, R. N.: Zinc-deficiency: Effect on brain of the suckling rat, Pediat. Res. **6:** 119, 1972.
15. Siegel, S.: Nonparametric statistics for the behavioral sciences, McGraw-Hill Book Company, Inc., New York, 1956, p. 116.
16. Slater, J. P., Mildvan, A. S., and Loeb, L. A.: Zinc in DNA polymerases, Biochem. Biophys. Res. Comm. **44:** 37, 1971.
17. Stephan, J. K., and Hsu, J. M.: Effect of zinc deficiency and wounding on DNA synthesis in rat skin, J. Nutr. **103:** 548, 1973.
18. Swenerton, H., Shrader, R., and Hurley, L. S.: Zinc-deficient embryos: Reduced thymidine incorporation, Science **166:** 1014, 1969.
19. Williams, R. B., Mills, C. F., Quarterman, J., and Dalgarno, A. C.: The effect of zinc deficiency on the in vivo incorporation of P into rat liver nucleotides, Biochem. J. **95:** 29p, 1965.
20. Williams, R. B., and Chesters, J. K.: The effects of early zinc deficiency on DNA and protein synthesis in the rat, Br. J. Nutr. **24:** 1053, 1970.

Spontaneous perforation of the extrahepatic bile ducts and bile peritonitis in infancy

John R. Lilly, M.D.,* William H. Weintraub, M.D., *and* R. Peter Altman, M.D.
Washington, D. C.

Spontaneous perforation of the extrahepatic bile duct is an uncommonly encountered condition in infancy but is second only to biliary atresia as a cause of surgical jaundice in the newborn period. The clinical features of extrahepatic bile duct perforation are characteristic of the condition and permit early diagnosis. Operative treatment is mandatory and simple drainage of the area of perforation is sufficient in most instances. Intestinal anastomoses to the perforation or "sac" under the misconception of a ruptured choledochal cyst are generally lethal. Properly treated, the majority of infants with bile duct perforation survive without sequelae. There is inferential evidence that spontaneous perforation of the extrahepatic bile ducts and choledochal cyst may be different manifestations of a common developmental fault in ductal embryogenesis.

From the Departments of Surgery, Children's Hospital National Medical Center and George Washington University Medical Center, Washington, D. C.

It is well recognized that, in children, congenital malformation of the extrahepatic bile ducts presents as a choledochal cyst or cystic dilatations of the common duct.[29, 37, 48] What has not been appreciated is that, with the exception of biliary atresia, the usual manifestation of common duct anomalies in infants is bile peritonitis consequent to spontaneous perforation of the extrahepatic biliary tree. Although not a common problem in the newborn infant, perforation of the extrahepatic bile duct is encountered with sufficient frequency to warrant recognition of its typical diagnostic features and to justify a reasonable plan of management. Currently, surgical recommendations for this lesion include simple peritoneal drainage,[13] operative closure of the perforation,[47] T tube drainage,[18] and Roux-en-Y intestinal anastomosis.[15] The purpose of this communication is to describe the characteristic findings of bile duct perforation in infancy, outline effective guidelines for surgical management, and present evidence indicating that spontaneous perforation of the extrahepatic bile duct and choledochal cyst are most likely different manifestations of a common developmental error in ductal embryogenesis. These conclusions are based on recent experiences with two infants with bile peritonitis at the Children's Hospital National Medical Center as well as on a study of other reported cases.

HISTORY

Spontaneous perforation of the biliary tract with bile peritonitis was first reported by Dijkstra[19] from the Netherlands in 1932 (Table I). He described the autopsy of a three-

Accepted for publication Feb. 11, 1974.

*Present address: Chief, Division of Pediatric Surgery, Department of Surgery, University of Colorado Medical Center, Denver, Colo.

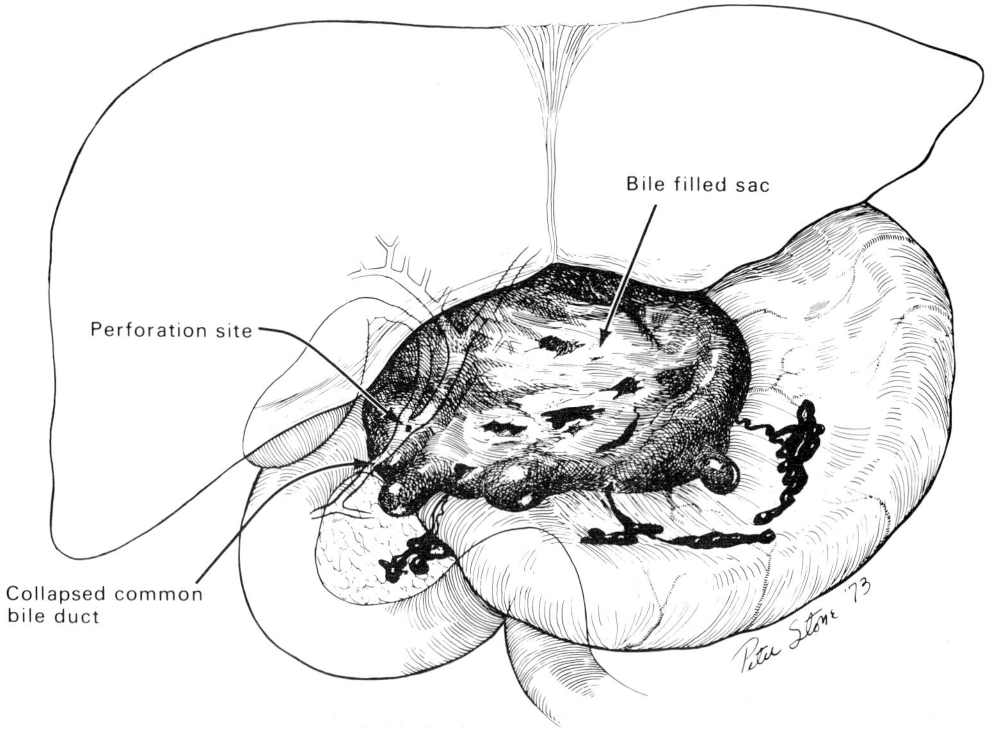

Fig. 1. Artist's depiction of the typical operative findings as seen in Case 1. The "sac" could be misinterpreted as a choledochal cyst.

month-old infant who died after five weeks of jaundice and progressive abdominal distension. Other than massive bilious ascites and a small perforation at the junction of the cystic and common ducts, the autopsy findings were unremarkable. In 1936, Caulfield[13] described two cases of common duct perforation in infancy. The first, a seven-week-old infant, was found to have extensive bile peritonitis at operation. Because of a severe inflammatory reaction in the porta hepatis, further exploration was abandoned and simple drainage of the portal area was done. The child survived and was well years later. Caulfield's second case was a ten-week-old infant who died without surgery after three weeks of jaundice and abdominal distension. At autopsy, there was a large amount of free bile and a false sac was found near the porta hepatis. The sac communicated with a tiny perforation at the junction of the common duct and cystic ducts. Since these first reports, numerous other cases have been described. Over fifty instances of spontaneous perforation of the extrahepatic bile duct have been reported during the past twenty years (Table I).

CASE REPORTS

Case 1. E. H. was a four-week-old female with low-grade fever, jaundice, and acholic stools of one week's duration. She appeared healthy except for moderate abdominal distension. White blood count (WBC) was 17,000; total bilirubin was 6 mg. percent (2.5, direct). Serum glutamic oxaloacetic transaminase (SGOT) and alkaline phosphatase levels were normal. Chest x-ray film showed right lower lobe pneumonia and *Klebsiella aerobacter* were cultured from the sputum. During the treatment of pneumonia, she developed abdominal tenderness and increasing distension. Surgery was performed fourteen days after admission. There was 200 ml. of bile-colored fluid in the peritoneal cavity which also cultured *Klebsiella aerobacter.* A loculated collection of thick, dark green fluid within a fibrinous sac was in the portahepatis (Fig. 1). A catheter cholecystogram demonstrated extravasation through a perforation in the common duct without flow into the duodenum (Fig. 2). Biopsy of the wall of the mass demonstrated inflammatory tissue. The catheter

Table I. *History*

Author	*Country*	*Date*	*Age (wk.)*	*Procedure*	*Comment**
Dijkstra[19]	Netherlands	1932	17	None	Died; "sac" present
Caulfield[13]	U.S.A.	1936	7	Simple drainage	Recovered
Caulfield[13]	U.S.A.	1936	12	None	Died; inspissated bile at autopsy; sac
Hindmarsch[30]	—	1947	22 mo.	Simple drainage	Recovered
Brautigam[9]	—	1949	4	Simple drainage	Died; "stenosis" of CBD at autopsy
Snyder et al.[47]	U.S.A.	1952	7	T tube drainage	"Gallstones"; CBD perforation sutured; recovered; sac
Byrne and Bottomley[10]	U.S.A.	1953	3	Simple drainage	Recovered
Lahary[34]	France	1954	14 mo.	None	Died; sac
Masson et al.[36]	U.S.A.	1954	7	T tube drainage	Perforation sutured; recovered
Masson et al.[36]	U.S.A.	1954	30 mo.	Cholecystoduodenostomy	Recovered; "stenosis" CBD
Von Krebs[54]	—	1954	13	None	Died; "stone" distal CBD, pancreatic necrosis
Coffey and Oweida[15]	U.S.A.	1955	3	Choledochojejunostomy	Died
Davies and Smith[18]	England	1955	7	T tube drainage	CBD "stones"; recovered
Davies and Smith[18]	England	1955	11	Choledochoduodenostomy	"Stenosis" CBD; recovered
Davies and Smith[18]	England	1955	8	Perforation sutured	Recovered; sac
Pettersson[41]	Denmark	1955	8	Perforation sutured	Recovered; sac
Pettersson[41]	Denmark	1955	7	T tube drainage	Bacterial peritonitis; recovered; sac
Pettersson[41]	Denmark	1955	2	Simple drainage	Bacterial peritonitis; died
Pettersson[41]	Denmark	1955	9	Perforation sutured	"Stone" in sac; recovered
Walker[56]	U.S.A.	1957	14	None	Died; CBD "stone"; bacterial cholangitis
Blumenstock et al.[4]	—	1957	15	Simple drainage	CBD "stones"; recovered
Eisnerova et al.[20]	Czechoslovakia	1958	21	Simple drainage	Inspissated bile; recovered
Von Simon and Schorr[55]	Germany	1958	3	Simple drainage	Bacterial peritonitis; recovered
Funder[24]	—	1958	12	T tube drainage	Perforation sutured; recovered
Assuied[2]	France	1958	11	Cholecystostomy	Died; sac
Volna[53]	—	1958	12	Cholecystectomy	Recovered; sac
Petit[42]	—	1959	8	Perforation sutured	Recovered
Gertz[25]	Denmark	1959	17	Choledochoduodenostomy	CBD "stone"; sac
Pouyanne et al.[43]	France	1959	4	Resection of sac	Died
Talalak[49]	Germany	1959	2	Cholecystectomy	
Talalak[49]	Germany	1959	5	Cholecystectomy	Died
Wright and Worsley[57]	U.S.A.	1959	1	T tube drainage	CBD "stone"; recovered
Ericsson and Rudhe[21]	Norway	1960	12	Hepaticoduodenostomy	CBD "stenosis"; "gallstones"; recovered
Partridge[39]	England	1960	15	Simple drainage	Partial excision of sac; recovered
Borde[6]	France	1960	7	Simple drainage	Bacterial peritonitis; recovered; sac
Toussaint[51]	Germany	1961	7	Simple drainage	Recovered
Gobbi and Perazzo[28]	Italy	1961	8	Hepaticocholedochostomy	
Johnston[32]	England	1961	6	Perforation sutured	Cholecystostomy drainage; recovered; sac
Oates[38]	Ireland	1961	8	Cholecystostomy	Sphincterotomy; recovered; sac
Toussaint[51]	Germany	1963	3	Simple drainage	CBD "stone"; recovered; sac
Colver[16]	U.S.A.	1964	7	Perforation sutured	CBD "stone"; cholecystostomy drainage; recovered

*CBD, Common bile duct.

Table I.—*Cont'd*

Author	*Country*	*Date*	*Age (wk.)*	*Procedure*	*Comment*
Caldera et al.[11]	France	1964	10	Sac excised	Bacterial peritonitis; recovered
Caldera et al.[11]	France	1965	17	Simple drainage	"Stones" removed at second operation; recovered; sac
Lees and Mitchell[35]	England	1965	16	Simple drainage	Recovered; sac
Lees and Mitchell[35]	England	1965	20 mo.	Cholecystoduodenostomy	
Hyde[31]	U.S.A.	1965	3	Simple drainage	Cholecystostomy drainage; recovered
Hyde[31]	U.S.A.	1965	21	Simple drainage	Cholecystostomy drainage; recovered
Segni et al.[45]	Italy	1965	10	Hepaticocholedochostomy	Died; sac
Fabrice[22]	France	1966	10	Hepaticojejunostomy	"Stenosis" common hepatic duct; cholecystectomy; recovered; sac
Van de Stadt[52]	Netherlands	1966	9	Simple drainage	Cholecystostomy drainage; recovered; sac
Danelatos-Athanassiadis et al.[17]	Greece	1970	6	T tube drainage	Recovered
Danelatos-Athanassiadis et al.[17]	Greece	1970	12	T tube drainage	Inspissated bile; recovered; sac
Kobayashi et al.[33]	Japan	1970	12	Simple drainage	Recovered; sac

was left in the gallbladder, and soft rubber drains were placed adjacent to the perforation site. The patient was fasted and started on intravenous hyperalimentation. Over the next two weeks, studies through the indwelling cholecystostomy catheter showed a persistent bile leak and obstruction of the distal common duct. Because of these findings and continued sepsis, it was decided that the patient should undergo a second exploratory operation. After an extraordinarily difficult dissection in the inflamed porta hepatis, the small perforation at the junction of the cystic duct and common duct was located and closed with fine silk sutures. The cholecystostomy tube was left indwelling, and multiple drains were left in the area of perforation. Postoperatively, a small bowel fistula developed and sepsis continued. Terminally, disseminated intravascular coagulopathy occurred, and the infant died eighteen days after her second operation.

Case 2. E. F. was an eight-week-old female with vomiting, light-colored, watery stools, and dark urine for five days. She was irritable, mildly jaundiced, and the abdomen was slightly tender. WBC was 11,500; total bilirubin was 7.4 mg. per-cent (4.4 direct). Lactic dehydrogenase (LDH), SGOT, and alkaline phosphatase were normal. A Rose Bengal I^{131} study demonstrated normal liver uptake (Fig. 3*A*). Twenty-four hours later, there was isotope activity in the free peritoneal cavity (Fig. 3*B*). At operation, 150 ml. of sterile, bile-stained fluid was found, and there were dense, fibrinous green adhesions forming a saclike structure in the porta hepatis. A catheter cholangiogram showed a leak at the junction of the common and cystic ducts and a miniscus sign in the distal common duct (Fig. 4). Dissection into the inflammatory tissue in the portal triad was not undertaken. The catheter was left in the gallbladder and soft rubber drains were inserted near the area of perforation. Postoperatively, the patient was fasted and started on total parenteral nutrition. Inadvertent removal of the abdominal drains at nine days was followed by progressive abdominal distension. At surgery to replace the drains, 650 ml. of bile had reaccumulated. Over the next week, her jaundice resolved, and bile drainage diminished and finally ceased. A tube cholecystogram at this time showed disappearance of the miniscus sign and a completely normal extrahepatic biliary tree with contrast passing freely into the duodenum. The drains and cholecystostomy tube were removed, and the patient is well one year later.

DISCUSSION

The most common developmental anomaly responsible for surgical jaundice in the early months of life is biliary atresia. For reasons that are unclear, there is a widely held view that choledochal cyst is also a common cause of surgical jaundice in infancy. In fact, manifestations of choledochal cyst are extremely rare in the neonatal pe-

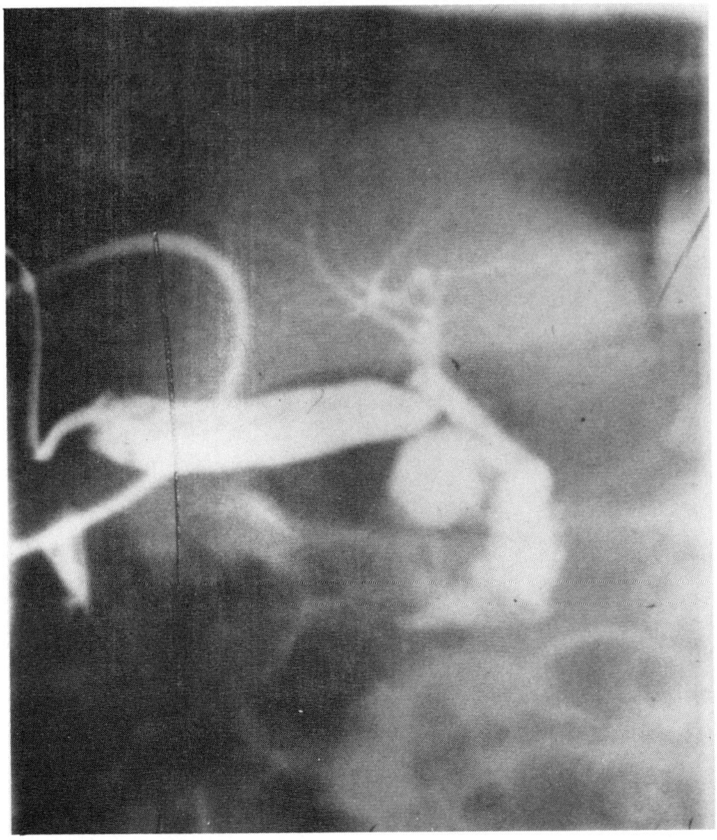

Fig. 2. Operative cholangiogram in Case 1 demonstrate ductal perforation near junction of common and cystic duct. There is partial encapsulation of contrast material in the porta hepatis and no flow into the intestine.

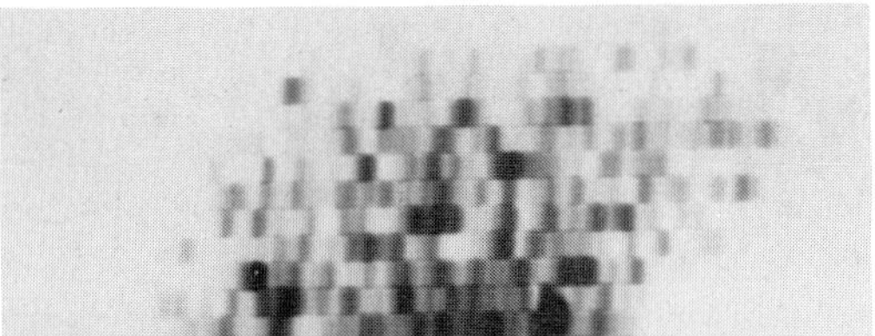

Fig. 3*A*. One-hour Rose Bengal I^{131} scan in Case 2 showing uptake in the liver.

riod,[1] and there are only scattered case reports of operation in the first few months of life.[3, 5, 7, 23, 26, 46, 58] Spontaneous perforation of the extrahepatic duct, on the other hand, occurs almost exclusively in the neonate.[44] During the past twenty years, over fifty documented cases have been reported and yet this lesion has been discussed either sketchily[37] or not at all[29, 48] in standard tests of pediatric surgery.

The inflammatory sac found in many infants with spontaneous perforation of the common duct has resulted in pernicious and at times disastrous diagnostic confusion with true cases of choledochal cyst. The operative findings may be misinterpreted as a "ruptured choledochal cyst" and so reported.[14] Such case reports are misleading as to the true incidence of the two conditions, but more importantly, the error has led to crucial mistakes in operative management. The flimsy sacs in these infants are comprised of inflammatory tissue only and primary intestinal anastomosis to them have been, for the most part, lethal.[14, 15, 28, 45, 49] Moreover, simple drainage of an erroneously di-

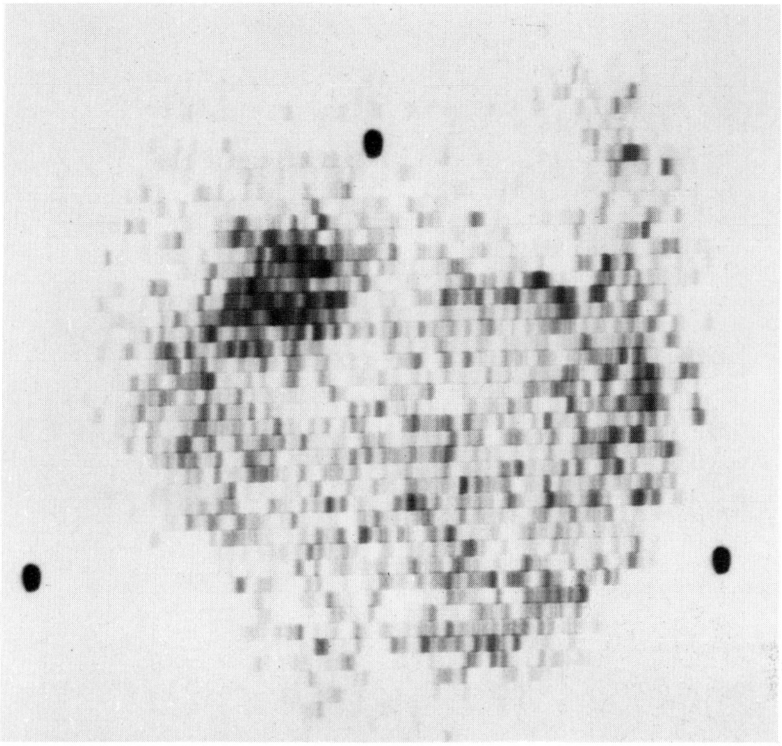

Fig. 3*B*. Twenty-four hours later, scan shows isotope free in the peritoneal cavity. There is a significant amount of the isotope under the left hemidiaphragm.

agnosed ruptured choledochal cyst has resulted in cure,[13, 14] a highly unlikely eventuality in a true choledochal cyst.

The pathogenesis of spontaneous perforation of the extrahepatic bile ducts is unknown. Distal common duct obstruction has been indicted in some cases where common duct stenosis or obstructing stones and sludge have been found. Ductal stenosis, however, has been a subjective surgical impression which in the small infant is difficult to evaluate. Furthermore, proximal common duct or gallbladder dilatation have not been observed, and liver biopsies have not demonstrated bile stasis[12, 14, 16] as might be expected if obstruction was severe enough to cause perforation. In addition, it is unclear if stones or sludge are a result of rather than a cause of perforation. The temporarily defunctionalized common duct distal to the perforation leads to bile stagnation and thus sludge or calculi within this portion[27] might be anticipated. The miniscus sign typical of a biliary calculus in our second case (Fig. 4) disappeared after spontaneous healing of the perforation. This would not have been predicted if the stone had been primarily responsible for the perforation.

A more attractive theory of the pathogenesis of spontaneous perforation of the common duct in infancy is that of a localized embryogenic mural malformation of the common duct. The location of the perforation in almost all instances to the area of union of cystic and common ducts suggests this junctional site may be particularly vulnerable to errors in development. This general concept is identical to that advanced for the pathogenesis of choledochal cysts.[8, 14, 29] Why in some instances the developmental error should lead to choledochal cyst formation and in others to perforation is speculative. A small circumscribed area of weakness may have a greater likelihood to rupture; whereas, more extensive common duct involvement might permit gradual dilatation and evolution to a choledochal cyst.

The reason for the temporal confinement

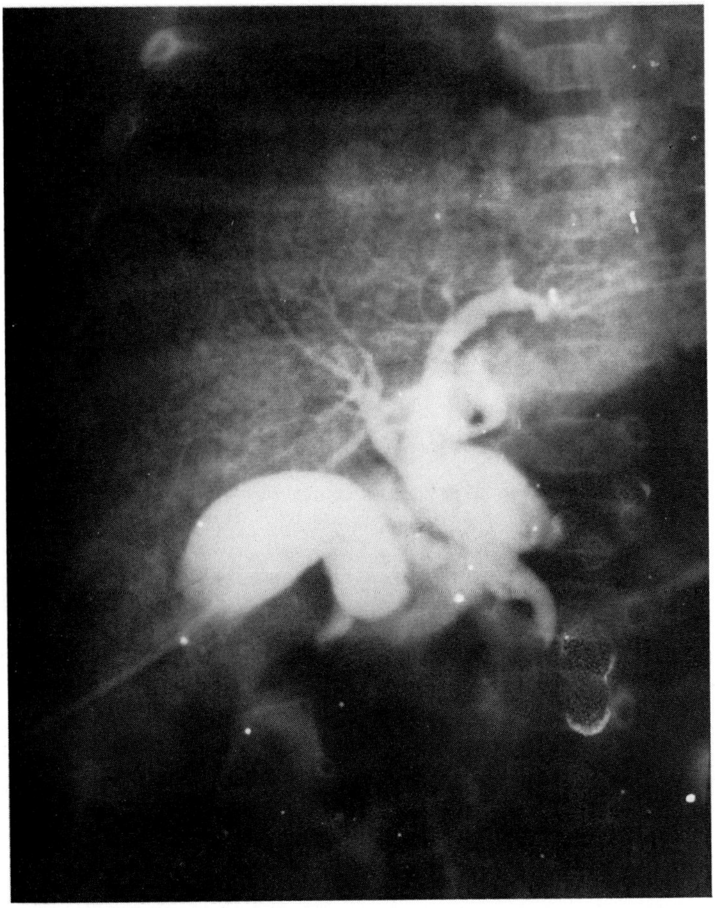

Fig. 4. Operative cholangiogram in Case 2. Again there is extravasation of contrast material into a fairly well-defined sac. Note appearance of miniscus sign suggesting a calculus obstruction of distal common bile duct.

of ductal perforation to infancy is unexplained. There have been no reported cases of bile peritonitis in the first days of life and only rarely has perforation occurred beyond twenty weeks of age. Most perforations have occurred when the infant was between the first and third month of life (Table I).

The presenting symptoms, diagnostic features, and early course described in our two case illustrations are faithful replicas of the typical clinical syndrome reported by most authors. In the first few weeks of life, the infants are normal. At varying periods thereafter, an indolent picture of irritability, failure to thrive, ascites, and mild jaundice develops. Except for elevated bilirubin, tests of liver function are usually normal, a feature which helps differentiate the condition from neonatal hepatitis. Definitive preoperative diagnosis may be made by intravenous cholangiogram[33] or, as in our second case by I^{131} Rose Bengal liver scan (Figs. 3*A* and 3*B*). Presence of the isotope in the free peritoneal cavity provides striking confirmatory evidence of bile extravasation.

The treatment of spontaneous perforation of the common duct in infants is surgical. A uniformly fatal outcome has followed expectant management.[13, 19, 34, 54, 56] Furthermore, once the diagnosis is made, early operation is indicated since delay may result in secondary infection. The general experience in the management of spontaneous perforation of the common duct indicates that a conservative surgical approach is fully justified. Spontaneous closure of the leak and subsequent cure has followed simple drainage of the perforation in most instances (Table I). More complicated procedures such as T tube drainage, common duct exploration and dilatation, suture repair, or intestinal anastomoses are unnecessary and probably foolhardy. The porta hepatis is involved in an acute inflammatory process making surgical identification of the individual structures difficult and technically hazardous.

We have found the most expeditious surgical approach to include an early operative cholecystogram. This permits precise identification of the common duct pathology. Surgical dissection in the inflamed portal triad is not undertaken. Multiple soft rubber drains are left in the area of perforation, and the abdomen is closed. We have also found it advantageous to leave the gallbladder catheter in place for postoperative studies. This small technical maneuver has given us a mechanism to assess the rate of healing of the perforation and the resolution of any distal common duct obstruction. The time necessary for spontaneous healing is variable. In our second case, closure of the leak was demonstrated at 25 days by tube cholangiogram. Inadvertent removal of the drains at nine days in this patient led to prompt reaccumulation of bile requiring operative reestablishment of drainage. Subsequently, a normal tube cholecystogram permitted permanent and safe removal of all drains including the cholecystostomy catheter.

Adjunctive treatment during the postoperative period in these infants should include the systemic administration of antibiotic drugs. The presence of partial common duct obstruction in many patients makes for special liability to the risk of ascending cholangitis, a hazard which persists until adequate biliary drainage is reestablished.

We also believe that ductal repair is facilitated by eliminating the intermittent stimulus to bile flow from ingestion of standard infant formulas. Consequently, caloric intake during early convalescenec should be provided by formulas free of fat or by parenteral hyperalimentation. In our patients, we elected to place the alimentary tract completely at rest and rely on parenteral nutrition.[40] Although it is known that a possible effect of prolonged hyperalimentation is cholestatic jaundice, an extended course seems necessary before this complication occurs.[50] We used a relatively brief period of fasting and total hyperalimentation (two weeks). Cholestatic jaundice did not occur.

In a preponderant number of infants with extrahepatic ductal perforation, the bile peritonitis at surgery will be sterile. Infrequently, secondary bacterial infection has been encountered.[6, 11, 41, 55, 56] In these cases, the infection may be a consequence of ascending cholangitis and spillage of infected bile through the ductal perforation. This appeared to be the course of events in our first case. The persistent septic course following the initial surgery prompted reoperation after two weeks to provide better drainage. In retrospect, the second operation was probably premature in that a longer period of observation might have resulted in spontaneous closure of the perforation. The second procedure unquestionably contributed to the infant's death. The exceptionally dense adhesions in the area of perforation led to inadvertent opening of the adjacent intestine and subsequent formation of a small bowel fistula.

The over-all experience with spontaneous perforation of the extrahepatic ducts in infancy indicates that the majority of these patients will survive. It would be expected that the prognosis might be improved further with prompt diagnosis and judicious surgical management. The lesion appears to be self-limiting and the sole error in ductal development. Thus, residual biliary tract disease or other sequelae would not be anticipated and have not been reported.

REFERENCES

1. Alaonso-Lej, F., Rever, W., and Pessagno, D.: Congenital choledochal cyst, Int. Abst. Surg. **108:** 1, 1959.
2. Assuied, D. R.: Les péritonites aigues neonatales, Dactylogr. 115 (Thèse Med.) Paris, 1958.

3. Attar, S., and Obeid, S.: Congenital cyst of the common bile duct; A review of the literature and a report of two cases, Ann. Surg. **142:** 289, 1955.
4. Blumenstock, D. A., Mithoefer, J., and Santulli, T. V.: Acute pancreatitis in children, Pediatrics **19:** 1002, 1957.
5. Bummelkamp, R., and Verboon, C. H.: Congenital cyst of the common bile duct in a newborn infant, Arch. Chir. Neerl. **1:** 113, 1949.
6. Borde, J., Bedouelle, J., and Carlioz, H.: Les péritonites neo-natales (à propos de 74 observations), Ann. Chir. Infant. **1:** 150, 1960.
7. Borde, J., and Cotoni, A.: Choleperitoine et perforation des voies biliaries chez le nourrisson, Ann. Chir. Infant. **7:** 387, 1966.
8. Bottger, H.: Zur atiologie der choledochuszysten, Zentralbl. Allg. Pathol. **87:** 407, 1951.
9. Brautigam, H.: Beitrag zur klinik und atiologie der galligen peritonitis, Zbl. Kinderheilk. **44:** 1239, 1949.
10. Byrne, J. J., and Bottomley, G. T.: Bile peritonitis in infancy, Am. J. Dis. Child. **85:** 694, 1973.
11. Caldera, R., Cayroche, P., and Borde, J.: Choleperitoine du nourrisson par perforation des voies biliaires, Sem. Hôpitaux **40:** 659, 1960.
12. Carter, R. F., and Saypol, G. M.: Symposium: Surgery for jaundice in infants and children, N. Y. State J. Med. **50:** 2945, 1950.
13. Caulfield, E.: Bile peritonitis in infancy, Am. J. Dis. Child. **52:** 1348, 1936.
14. Chen, W. J., Chang, C., and Hung, W.: Congenital choledochal cyst: With observations on rupture of the cyst and intrahepatic ductal dilatation, J. Pediatr. Surg. **8:** 529, 1973.
15. Coffey, R., and Oweida, L.: Unusual problems in biliary tract surgery, Am. J. Gastroenterol. **24:** 5, 1955.
16. Colver, H. D.: Perforation of the biliary tract due to gallstones in infancy. An established clinical entity, Ann. Surg. **2:** 226, 1964.
17. Danelotos-Athanassiadis, C., Tsakagiannis, E., Karpouzas, I., Mousatos, G., and Katerelos, C.: Bile peritonitis in infancy, Helv. Paediatr. Acta **6:** 655, 1970.
18. Davies, P. A., and Smith, A. E.: Bile peritonitis in infancy, Arch. Dis. Child. **30:** 174, 1955.
19. Dijkstra, C. H.: Graluistorting in de buikholte bij een zuigeling, Maandschr. Kindergeneeskd. **1:** 409, 1932.
20. Eisnerova, L. A., Piskacowa, A. and Zeman, L.: Biliarni peritonitida. Pozdni komplikace hermolytickeho onemocnemi novorozence, Cesk. Pediátr. **13:** 732, 1958.
21. Ericsson, N. O., and Rudhe, M.: Spontaneous perforation of the bile ducts in infants, Acta Chir. Scand. **48:** 439, 1960.
22. Fabrice, Ch.: *In* Prevat, J., and Babut, J.: Spontaneous perforation of the biliary tract in infancy, Progr. Pediatr. Surg. **3:** 187, 1971.
23. Fonkalsrud, E. W., and Boles, E. T., Jr.: Choledochal cysts in infancy and childhood, Surg. Gynecol. Obstet. **121:** 733, 1965.
24. Funder: *In* Prevat, J., and Babut, J.: Spontaneous perforation of the biliary tract in infancy, Progr. Pediatr. Surg. **3:** 187, 1971.
25. Gertz, T. C.: Spontaneous perforation of the common bile ducts. Report of a case, Arch. Surg. **78:** 7, 1959.
26. Gilliland, M., Holloway, C., and Lange, J.: Congenital choledochus cyst, J. Pediatr. **37:** 387, 1950.
27. Glenn, F.: Obstruction of the common bile duct, Surg. Gynecol. Obstet. **132:** 25, 1971.
28. Gobbi, U., and Perazzo, G.: Perforatione spontanea dell'epatico commune in lattante. 28 Congres It. di Pediat. (Torino) **3:** 128, 1961.
29. Gross, R. E., editor: The surgery of infancy and childhood, Philadelphia, 1953, W. B. Saunders Co.
30. Hindmarsch, F. D.: Bile peritonitis in infancy, Br. Med. J. **2:** 131, 1947.
31. Hyde, G. A.: Spontaneous perforation of bile ducts in early infancy, Pediatrics **35:** 453, 1965.
32. Johnston, J. H.: Spontaneous perforation of the common bile ducts in infancy, Br. J. Surg. **48:** 532, 1961.
33. Kobayashi, A., Obe, Y., and Akiyama, H.: Idiopathic acute bile peritonitis in infancy: Report of a case, Helv. Paediatr. Acta **25:** 59, 1970.
34. Lahary, J.: Dilatation pseudokystique de choledoque et choleperitoine chez un enfant de 14 mois, Dactylogr. 35 (Thèse Med.) Paris, 1954.
35. Lees, W., and Mitchell, J. E.: Bile peritonitis in infancy, Arch. Dis. Child. **41:** 188, 1966.
36. Masson, L. B., Bidbury, J. B., and Culang, S.: Rupture of the extrahepatic bile from non-penetrating trauma, Ann. Surg. **140:** 324, 1954.
37. Mustard, W. T., Ravitch, M. M., Snyder, W. H., Jr., Welch, K. J., and Benson, C., editors: Pediatric Surgery, ed. 2, Vol. 2, Chicago, 1969, Year Book Medical Publishers.
38. Oates, G. D.: Perforated empyema of the gallbladder in an infant, Br. J. Surg. **48:** 686, 1961.
39. Partridge, J.: Pseudocholedocus cyst, Br. Med. J. **2:** 36, 1960.
40. Peden, V. H., Witzleben, C. L., and Skelton,

M. A.: Total parenteral nutrition, J. Pediatr. **78:** 180, 1971.

41. Pettersson, G.: Spontaneous perforation of the common bile duct in infants, Acta Chir. Scand. **110:** 192, 1955.
42. Petit, P.: *In* Prévot, J., and Babut, J.: Spontaneous perforation of the biliary tract in infancy, Prog. Pediatr. Surg. **3:** 187, 1971.
43. Pouyanne, L., Moulies, J., Lasserre, J., et al.: Un eas de cholepéritoine en kyste de l'arrière cavite des epiploons chez un nouveau-né, Arch. Fr. Pediatr. **6:** 836, 1959.
44. Prevat, J., and Babut, J.: Spontaneous perforations of the biliary tract in infancy, Progr. Pediatr. Surg. **3:** 187, 1971.
45. Segni, G., Romano, C., and Grossi-Bianchi, M. L.: La perforazione spontanea della via biliaru nel primo trimestre di vita, Minerva Pediatr. **17:** 1736, 1965.
46. Shallow, T. A., Eger, S. A., and Wagner, F. B., Jr.: Congenital cystic dilatation of the common bile duct: Case report and review of the literature, Ann. Surg. **117:** 355, 1943.
47. Snyder, W. H., Chaffin, L., and Dettinger, L.: Cholelithiasis and perforation of the gallbladder in an infant with recovery, J. A. M. A. **149:** 1645, 1952.
48. Swenson, O., editor: Pediatric surgery, ed. 3, New York, 1968, Appleton-Century-Crofts.
49. Talalak, W. A.: Die perforation der gallenwege im sauglingsalter, Langenbecks Arch. Klin. Chir. **76:** 451, 1959.
50. Touloukian, R. J., and Downing, S. E.: Cholestasis associated with long-term parenteral hyperalimentation, Arch. Surg. **106:** 58, 1973.
51. Toussaint, W.: Spontane gallengangs perforation beim saugling; zugleich ein beitrag zur gallensekretion, Maandschr. Kinderheilk. **109:** 331, 1961.
52. Van de Stadt, F.: Spontaneous bile duct perforation in an infant, Arch. Chir. Neerl. **21:** 321. 1969.
53. Volná, G.: *In* Prévot, J., and Babut, J.: Spontaneous perforation of the biliary tract in infancy, Progr. Pediatr. Surg. **3:** 187, 1971.
54. Von Krebs, H.: Zur pathogenese der cholelithiasis mit pankreasbeteiligung im fruhen kindesalter, Maandschr. Kinderheilk. **102:** 327, 1954.
55. Von Simon, H., and Schorr, R.: Zur spontanperforation des ductus choledochus beim jungen saugling, Arch. Kinderheilk. **156:** 256, 1958.
56. Walker: *In* Prévot, J., and Babut, J.: Spontaneous perforation of the biliary tract in infancy, Progr. Pediatr. Surg. **1:** 197, 1971.
57. Wright, J. P., and Worsley, H. E.: A case of rupture of the hepatic duct in a newborn infant, Arch. Dis. Child. **175:** 277, 1959.
58. Wrightson, P.: Congenital cystic dilatation of the common bile duct, Austr. N. Z. J. Surg. **23:** 110, 1953.

A simple esophageal bypass operation by the high gastric division

Hiroshi Akiyama, M.D., *and* **Mamoru Hiyama, M.D.,** *Tokyo, Japan*

The simplest esophageal bypass operation using the divided distal stomach was performed on eleven patients with non-resectable malignancies (mostly carcinomas) of the esophagus. High division of the stomach is performed, and the large distal stomach is brought up to the neck through a retrosternal tunnel and anastomosed to the divided cervical esophagus. The small proximal stomach is anastomosed to the jejunum with the use of the Billroth II procedure as the standard technique. The divided distal end of the cervical esophagus is usually primarily closed but sometimes prepared as an esophagostomy for further investigation of the non-resectable tumor. The proximal stomach can also be anastomosed by using the Roux-en-Y technique or prepared as a cardiostomy for external drainage. A combination of these techniques is preferred, depending on the condition of the patient. All eleven patients survived the operation and were able to ingest a regular diet orally. Average blood loss during operation was about 200 ml., and the operation can be performed without blood transfusion and with ease because of the minimal surgical risks.

From the Department of Surgery, Toranomon Hospital, Tokyo, Japan

DESPITE THE numerous discussions of resectable carcinoma of the esophagus and its reconstructive methods, the greater part of cases are still left as being non-resectable, far advanced carcinomas. As a result, in esophageal surgery, a bypass procedure is very frequently needed and plays an important role in the palliative method.

Most patients with advanced carcinoma of the esophagus are usually emaciated and may not tolerate a major surgical procedure. Subsequently, a bypass operation itself should be done with minimal risk. Herewith, the technique of an esophageal bypass operation using the divided distal stomach with a retrosternal route is devised and reported. We believe this form of esophageal bypass surgery to be easier and simpler to perform.

Accepted for publication Feb. 11, 1974.

Non-resectable, malignant esophageal lesions with almost complete obstruction or with anticipated complete obstruction present adequate indications for this operation. The esophageal carcinoma with tracheoesophageal fistula is one of the strongest indicators for this procedure. Non-resectable carcinomas with marked invasion into the surrounding tissues can frequently be recognized by abnormalities of the "esophageal axis."[3]

Patients whose swallowing function has been disturbed by recurrent laryngeal nerve paralysis as the result of malignant invasion are not adequate candidates for this bypass operation. Also, those patients in advanced stages having distant metastases or marked cachexia and poor appetite are poor candidates. The general physical condition of prospective candidates should be at least as good as, for example, one able to tolerate a regu-

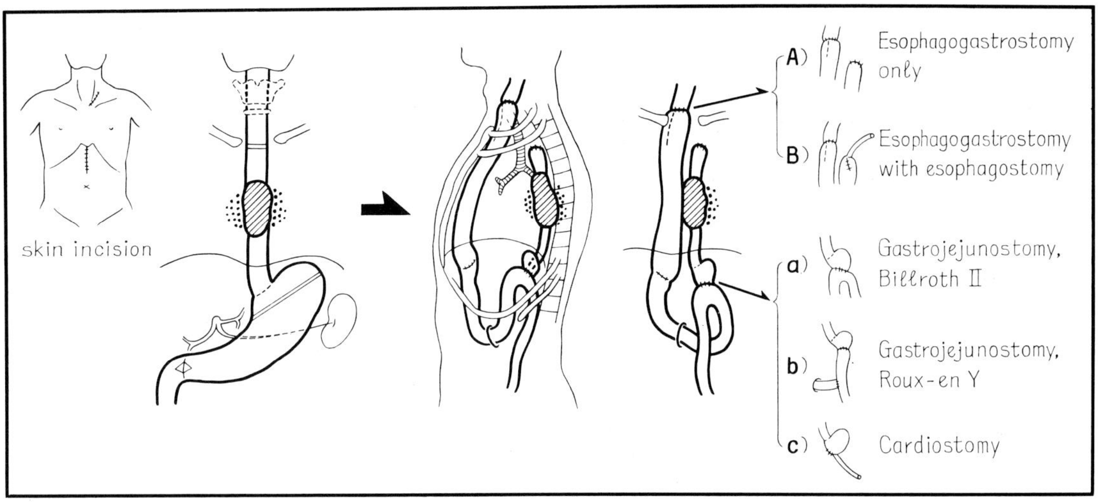

Fig. 1. Schema of the esophageal bypass operation.

lar gastrectomy. This procedure can also be applied to some benign strictures of the esophagus.

TECHNIQUE

Laparotomy is performed by a rather small upper median incision. The adequacy of performing this procedure should be reconsidered after a thorough investigation into the degree of intra-abdominal metastases.

First, the gastrocolic ligament is divided, preserving the right gastroepiploic vessels and severing the left gastroepiploic vessels. The short gastric vessels are divided along the greater curvature of the stomach; only a couple of short gastric vessels are left intact at the cardia. The right gastric artery is preserved. During lymph node dissection around the common hepatic artery, celiac axis, upper part of the lesser curvature of the stomach, and the bilateral pericardia, the left gastric artery is severed at its roots. Even in this palliative bypass operation, intra-abdominal lymph node dissection of this extent should be done if the nodes are found to be positive for cancer and not fixed to the surrounding tissue. This procedure is mandatory when the second-stage operation for resection of the primary tumor is expected. Otherwise, the left gastric artery can be severed at the higher level of the lesser curvature. Then the stomach is transected close to the cardia so that only a small portion of the fornix is left for gastrojejunostomy. At this time, the stomach is divided into two parts: (1) the small proximal and (2) the large distal (Fig. 1). Both cut ends of the stomach are closed in two layers, and a Heineke-Mukulicz pyloroplasty procedure is performed. Thus, the divided distal stomach is assured to be long enough to reach up to the neck (Fig. 2).

The small, oblique incision is placed on the left side of the neck along the anterior border of the sternocleidomastoid muscle, exposing the cervical esophagus; care is taken not to damage the recurrent laryngeal nerve. A tape is placed around the cervical esophagus, which is then pulled out and freed to some extent by finger dissection along the esophagus in the superior mediastinum. The cervical esophagus is then severed as low as possible, and the proximal end of the esophagus is placed aside for future esophagogastrostomy. The distal end of the esophagus is closed or prepared for esophagostomy. Both the sternohyoid and sternothyroid muscles are divided in order to widen the superior aperature of the anterior mediastinum.

The retrosternal tunnel is created by inserting a flat malleable intestinal retractor with a hole in one side (Fig. 3), along the posterior surface of the sternum through the abdominal incision. After this is done, a tape is passed through the tunnel with its

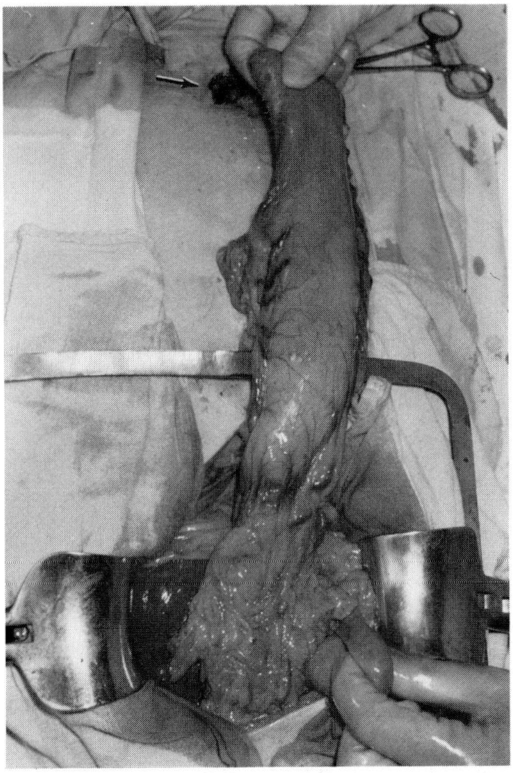

Fig. 2. Divided distal stomach is long enough to reach up to the cervical esophagus (Arrow).

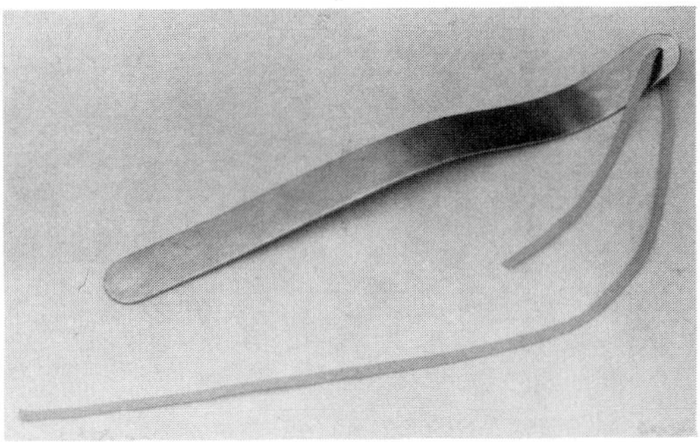

Fig. 3. Flat malleable intestinal retractor with a hole in one side for creating the retrosternal tunnel.

anchorage through the hole on the retractor. The distal stomach is then elevated to the neck through the retrosternal tunnel by pulling up on the tape previously connected to the distal stomach. The anastomosis is completed between the divided cervical esophagus and the proximal end of the distal stomach in two layers in the neck.[1] The esophageal bypass route is then accomplished.

MANAGEMENT OF THE PROXIMAL END OF THE EXCLUDED ESOPHAGUS

As routine procedure, the proximal end of the excluded esophagus with tumor is closed in two layers and pushed back into the posterior mediastinum (Fig. 1, technique A). In this fashion, the patient is quite comfortable since there is no fistula in his neck. When there is a necessity for further follow-up of the tumor or when the esophageal obliteration is complete and there is a fear of remaining abscess, a small rubber tube is inserted into the thoracic esophagus as an esophagostomy (Fig. 1, technique B). The tube is either pulled out of the skin or passed through behind the trachea and then pulled out of the skin on the other side of the neck. Later, contrast media can be injected through the tube for subsequent follow-up of the primary esophageal lesion.

MANAGEMENT OF THE PROXIMAL STOMACH

The divided, small proximal stomach should be externally drained or anastomosed to the small intestine to allow for drainage from the tumor and the rest of the esophagus. The routine anastomosis is accomplished through a retrocolic Billroth II procedure (Fig. 1, technique a). The anastomosis should be small in size since it is only to be used for drainage from the excluded esophagus. If the bypass procedure is done in patients with a tracheoesophageal fistula, the Roux-en-Y type gastrojejunostomy is preferred in order to prevent regurgitation (Fig. 1, technique b); also a simple cardiostomy[2] for complete external drainage (Fig. 1, technique c) is the appropriate technique for preventing regurgitation.

Any combination of techniques A, B and a, b, c may be used based on the over-all physical condition of the patient. The standard procedure involves the use of the A and

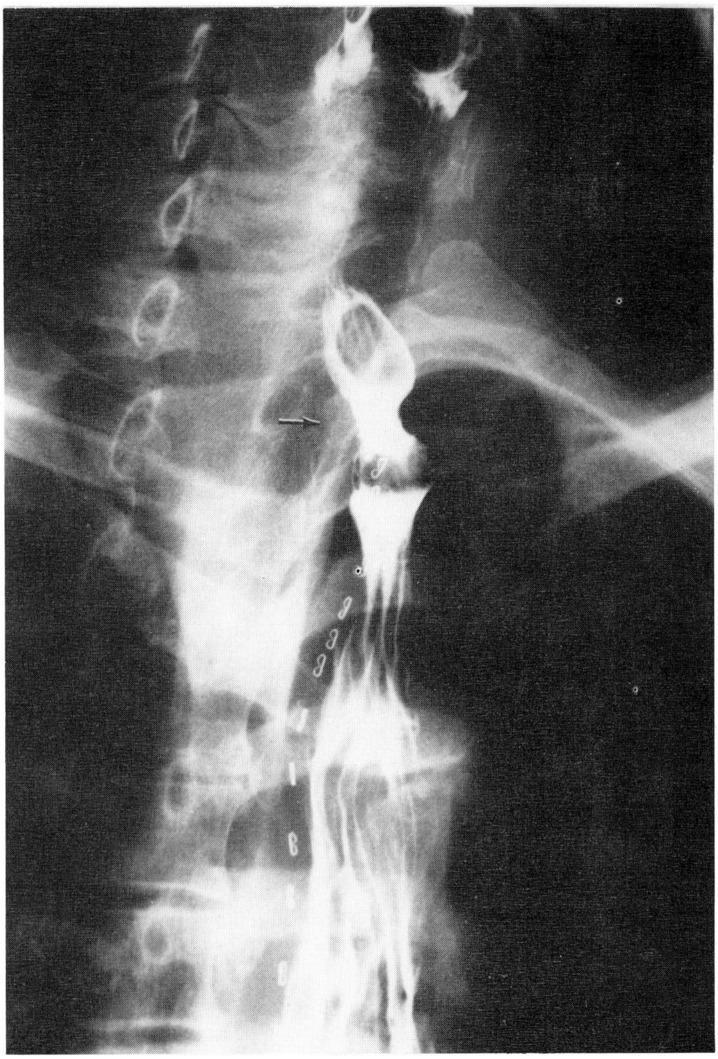

Fig. 4*A*. Postoperative x-ray of the well-functioning bypassed esophagus in the standard fashion (Case 8, Table I). Arrow shows cervical esophagogastrostomy on postoperative x-ray film of Case 8 (Table I).

a combination. This is the most simple form of bypass and also the one that is most comfortable for the patient.

RESULTS

Esophageal bypass operations which use the divided stomach have been performed on eleven cases since 1972 (Table I). It is only a palliative procedure; therefore, long-term survival is, of course, not expected. However, all patients survived the operation, resumed oral ingestion on the ninth postoperative day, and were able to have a soft-to-solid regular diet without difficulty.

Blood loss during operation was between 44 and 372 ml., with an average of 225 ml. Blood transfusion was not necessary in most cases.

Figs. 4*A*, 4*B*, and 4*C* are the postoperative x-ray films of an esophagus bypassed in our standard technique. Fig. 5 is a photograph of a 77-year-old man with cardiac complications who underwent the same operation (Case 3, Table I). He tolerated the operation

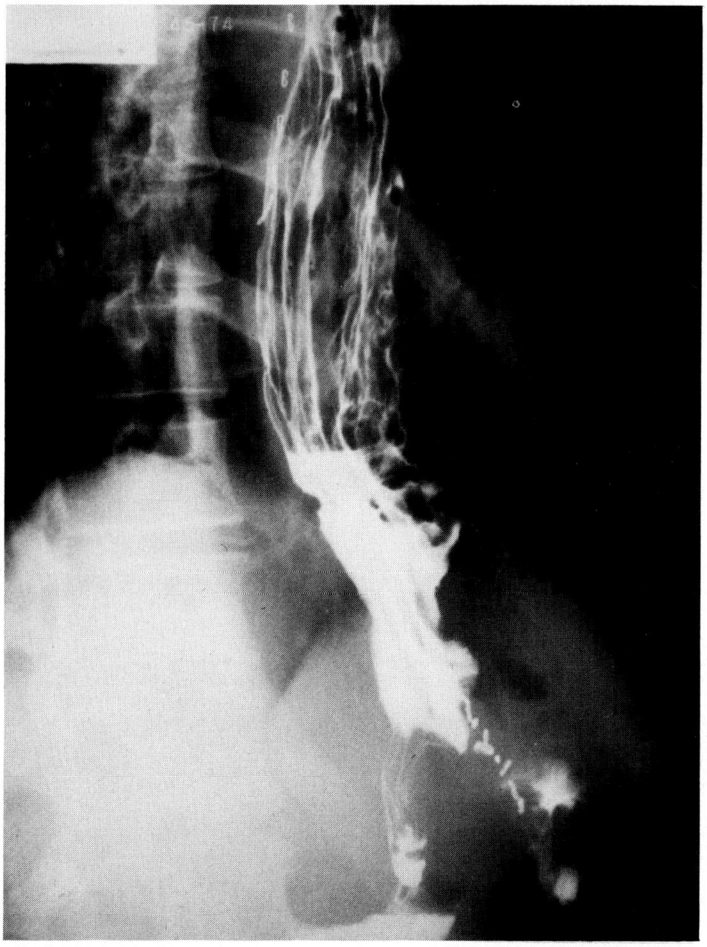

Fig. 4*B*. Retrosternal distal stomach used as the esophageal bypass is shown in postoperative x-ray film of Case 8 (Table I).

Table I. *Eleven cases of esophageal bypass operation by the high gastric division*

Case No.	*Patient*	*Age (yr.)*	*Sex*	*Location of lesion**	*Length of defect in x-ray (cm.)*	*Complication*
1	T. S.	55	M	U	15.0	TEF†
2	T. O.	65	F	M	7.0	DM
3	I. Y.	77	M	L	9.0	Cardiac
4	Y. S.	45	M	M	10.5	TEF
5	M. H.	60	M	L	5.0	—
6	G. O.	63	M	M	11.8	—
7	H. K.	65	F	L	7.0	Hypertension
8	D. K.	49	M	M	10.0	—
9	F. U.	61	F	L	9.0	—
10	S. D.	75	M	M	8.5	—
11	S. S.	64	M	U	9.0	—

*U, Upper third of the thoracic esophagus; M, middle third of the thoracic esophagus; L, lower third of the thoracic esophagus.

†Tracheoesophageal fistula.

‡A, Esophagogastrostomy only; B, esophagogastrostomy with esophagostomy; a, gastrojejunostomy, Billroth II; b, gastrojejunostomy

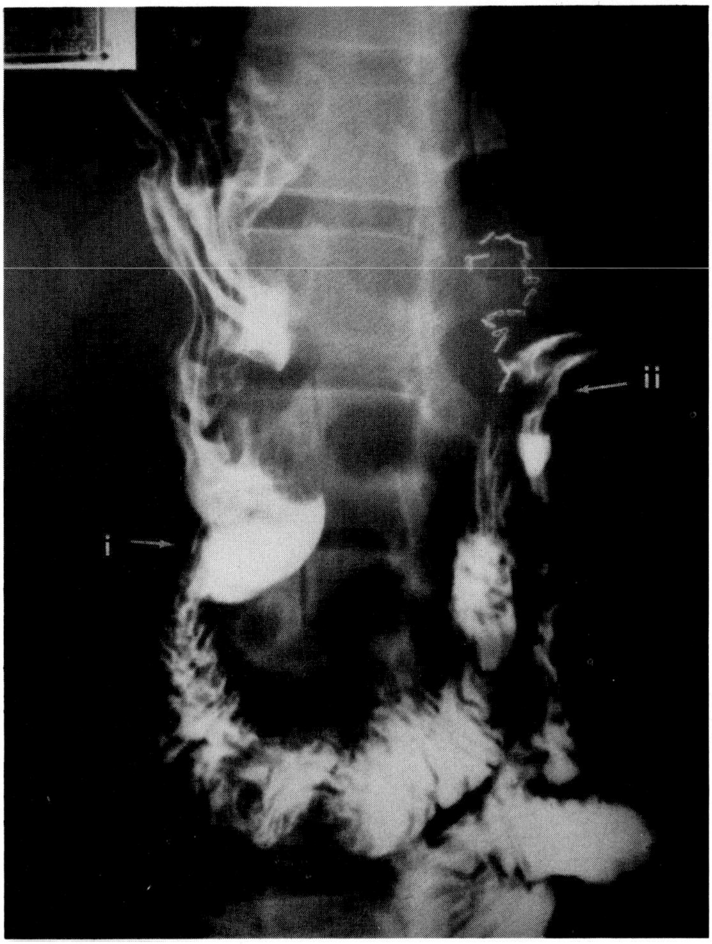

Fig. 4*C*. Arrow *i* shows pyloric region, and arrow *ii* shows Billroth II gastrojejunostomy in the x-ray film taken of the esophagus of Case 8 after operation (Table I).

Radiation (^{60}Co) (rads.)	*Blood loss during operation (ml.)*	*Blood transfusion (ml.)*	*Management of proximal end of excluded esophagus‡*	*Management of proximal stomach‡*	*Results*
12,000	339	600	B	c	Survived 1 yr., 2 mo.
3,600	100	0	A	a	Survived 3 mo.
5,000	245	200	A	a	Survived 11 mo.
900	250	0	A	b	Survived 3 mo.
—	319	0	B	a	1 yr., alive
7,400	330	0	B	a	9 mo., alive
2,700	160	0	A	a	4 mo., alive
5,580	156	0	A	a	5 mo., alive
360	372	0	A	a	Survived 3 mo.
4,650	44	0	A	a	2 mo., alive
—	162	0	B	a	2 mo., alive

Roux-en-Y; C, cardiostomy. (See Fig. 1 for diagrams of techniques.)

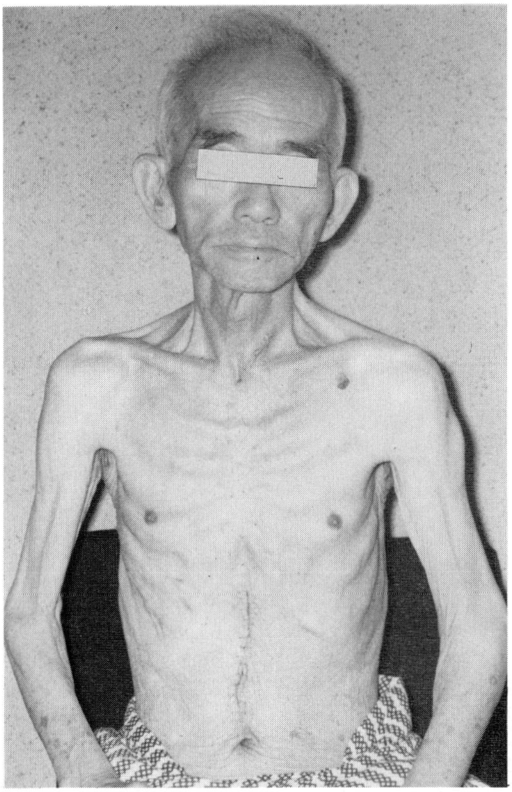

Fig. 5. Photograph of a 77-year-old male patient who underwent the esophageal bypass operation in the standard fashion (Case 3, Table I). Note very small skin incisions in the neck and abdomen.

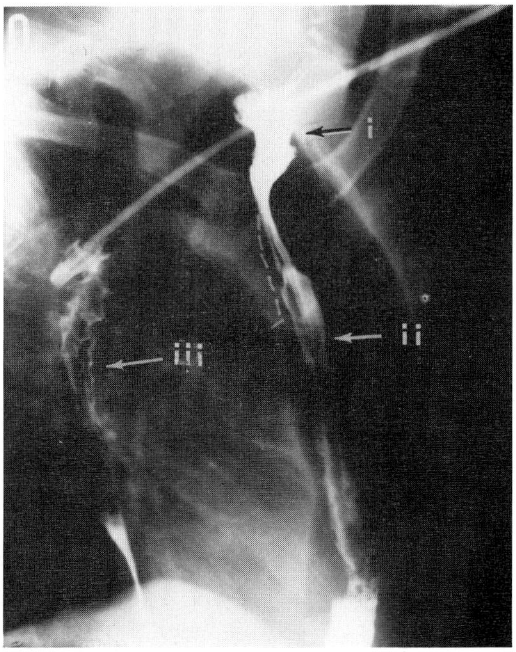

Fig. 6. Postoperative x-ray film of Case 1 (Table I). Arrows *i* and *ii* show cervical esophagogastrostomy and retrosternal distal stomach for bypass, respectively. Proximal end of the excluded esophagus is prepared as esophagostomy by inserting a tube. Subsequent follow-up of the primary tumor (arrow *iii*) is available.

well and enjoyed regular diet until his death. Postoperative x-ray film of the patient operated upon using the combination of B and c is shown in Fig. 6.

DISCUSSION

In cases of advanced, non-resectable esophageal lesions, the bypass operation is very useful and far more convenient than ordinary gastrostomy, if operative success can be reasonably assured. Of considerable import is the fact that this kind of operation can be performed with a minimum of surgical risks. We attribute this to the simplicity of our method. Bypass procedures have been one of the prime concerns among surgeons since very early in the history of esophageal surgery. The efforts of the past are shown in the paper by Yudin.[13] Many of the bypass procedures during the early period consisted of presternal skin tubes. Kirschner[8] used the stomach presternally as a bypass and anastomosed the abdominal esophagus with jejunum in Roux-en-Y fashion. The Roux-en-Y loop itself was used as an esophageal bypass by Herzen.[7] Currently, the colon is most frequently used for esophageal reconstruction or bypass.[6, 12] Most surgeons are concerned with whether the organ to be used will be able to reach the cervical esophagus. This is the reason that the colon has been the most popular esophageal substitution. However, the procedure of esophageal substitution by means of the colon is fairly complicated, and it involves many anastomoses. In this respect, the stomach is a more convenient organ for esophageal substitution, if it is properly used. It has been shown that the stomach can reach to the hypopharynx,[4, 5, 9, 10] provided the whole stomach is used and is brought up through the posterior mediastinum. In the early period, Kirschner[8] used the whole stomach presternally for the purpose of bypass. Ong[11] recently used this method and re-evaluated Kirschner's method of bypass procedure.

Our method has shown that use of the whole stomach is not necessary for bypass; rather, it has demonstrated that the distal stomach after high gastric transection is long enough to reach the cervical esophagus through a retrosternal route. The greatest advantage of our procedure is that, in leaving the proximal portion of the stomach, whether by gastrojejunostomy or cardiostomy, a drainage procedure from the excluded esophagus can become very easy.

A small gastrojejunostomy by the Billroth II method is especially simple. By combining the available ways of management of the divided distal end of the cervical esophagus and the drainage method of the proximal stomach, we can choose the suitable operative method, the choice of which is dependent upon the patient's prognosis, presence of tracheoesophageal fistula, necessity of follow-up, and other factors. Surgical risk is minimal.

REFERENCES

1. Akiyama, H.: Esophageal anastomosis, Arch. Surg. **107:** 512, 1973.
2. Akiyama, H., and Sato, Y.: Cardiostomy for malignant tracheoesophageal fistula, J. Abd. Surg. **13:** 144, 1971.
3. Akiyama, H., Kogure, T., and Itai, Y.: The esophageal axis and its relationship to the resectability of carcinoma of the esophagus, Ann. Surg. **176:** 30, 1972.
4. Akiyama, H., Sato, Y., and Takahashi, F.: Immediate pharyngogastrostomy following total esophagectomy by blunt dissection, Jap. J. Surg. **1:** 225, 1971.
5. Balasegaram, M.: Replacement of hypopharynx and esophagus, Am. J. Surg. **115:** 279, 1968.
6. Chrysospathis, P.: The large bowel as substitute for the esophagus, Pacific Med. Surg. **75:** 141, 1967.
7. Herzen, P.: Eine Modifikation der Roux'schen Ösophagojejuno-gastrostomie, Zentralbl. Chir. **35:** 219, 1908.
8. Kirschner: Ein neues Verfahren der Oesophagoplastik, Arch. Klin. Chir. **114:** 606, 1920.
9. LeQuesne, L. P., and Ranger, D.: Pharyngolaryngectomy with immediate pharyngogastric anastomosis, Br. J. Surg. **53:** 105, 1966.
10. Ong, G. B.: Carcinoma of the hypopharynx and cervical esophagus, *in* Smith, R., editor: Progress in clinical surgery, ser. 3, London, 1969, J. & A. Churchill, Ltd.
11. Ong, G. B.: The Kirschner operation—a forgotten procedure, Br. J. Surg. **60:** 221, 1973.
12. Petrov, B. A.: Retrosternal artificial esophagus created from colon, SURGERY **55:** 520, 1964.
13. Yudin, S. S.: The surgical construction of 80 cases of artificial esophagus, Surg. Gynecol. Obstet. **78:** 561, 1944.

Surgical treatment of abdominal angina: Review of 25 patients

George J. Reul, Jr., M.D., Don C. Wukasch, M.D., Frank M. Sandiford, M.D., Luigi Chiarillo, M.D., Grady L. Hallman, M.D., *and* Denton A. Cooley, M.D., *Houston, Texas*

Abdominal angina is a rare symptom that resembles angina pectoris which is associated with coronary artery disease. Over a nine-year period, 25 patients who ranged in age from 19 to 72 years underwent mesenteric revascularization for symptoms of abdominal angina. In most cases, postprandial abdominal pain and loss of weight combined with arteriographic findings of occlusive lesions of at least two of the three major visceral arteries—that is, the celiac, superior mesenteric, and/or inferior mesenteric—established the diagnosis. Simultaneous surgical correction of associated vascular or gastrointestinal disease was performed in 14 of the patients. Concomitant lesions treated included abdominal aortic aneurysm in five patients, renal artery hypertension in three, and aortoiliac occlusive disease in three. Among these 25 patients, 38 arteries were revascularized. Two patients died, both deaths resulted from mesenteric infarction following unsuccessful revascularization procedures. In follow-up examination from five months to eight years, nine of the remaining 18 patients showed excellent results. Successful operative treatment of abdominal angina depends upon accurate preoperative diagnosis based on evaluation of the symptoms and correlation with anatomical disease.

From the Division of Surgery of the Texas Heart Institute, Houston, Texas

In 1918, a syndrome of chronic intestinal ischemia manifested by postprandial cramping abdominal pain was described.[1] Later, Conner[3] suggested that the syndrome was analogous to the angina of coronary artery disease, i.e., both were caused by decreased blood flow. Dunphy[6] reviewed the histories and the confirmed postmortem findings in 12 patients who died from mesenteric vascular occlusion. Of the 12 patients, seven experienced chronic recurrent abdominal pain that preceded the fatal attack by weeks, months, or years. Mikkelsen[10] suggested a possible surgical approach to obstructive lesions of the mesenteric arteries after analysis of two patients, both of whom died because of mesenteric vascular occlusion preceded by the classical signs of abdominal angina. Finally in 1958, Shaw and Maynard[16] were the first to successfully treat a patient with an obstructive lesion of the superior mesenteric artery. Other early reports of successful surgical treatment by Fry and Kraft[7] and Morris and associates[13] discussed operative techniques and suggested a possibly higher incidence of disease than

Presented at the Eighty-First Annual Meeting of the Western Surgical Association, Nov. 14-17, 1973, Houston, Texas.

Accepted for publication Feb. 22, 1974.

Reprint requests: Dr. D. A. Cooley, P.O. Box 20345, Houston, Texas 77025.

observed at the time of their report. Improved diagnostic techniques prompted Dunbar and associates[5] to describe the celiac axis compression syndrome or median arcuate ligament syndrome.[8, 17, 19] Since that time, other reports have appeared; yet, the significance of this syndrome remains controversial.[18] Despite renewed interest encouraged by improved diagnostic and vascular surgical techniques, other reports of the operative correction of intestinal angina have been infrequent.[4, 12, 14, 15] This report is an analysis of nine years' experience in the operative treatment of patients with intestinal angina.

CLINICAL MATERIAL

From January, 1964, through July, 1973, 25 patients underwent revascularization of the celiac (CA), superior mesenteric (SMA), and/or inferior mesenteric artery (IMA) primarily because of abdominal pain. The series included 17 women and eight men ranging in age from 19 to 72 years (Fig. 1). Most patients were in the seventh decade, although over half were less than 55 years of age. The predominant symptom in 23 of the 25 patients was abdominal pain (Table I). Each of the remaining two patients presented primarily with either coarctation of the abdominal aorta or nausea and vomiting. The abdominal pain was usually cramping in nature and occurred postprandially in 14 patients. It occurred from 15 minutes to two hours after ingestion of meals with an average of approximately one hour postprandially. The pain was located in the epigastrium in four patients, located in the lower abdomen in three patients, and was generalized in ten patients. Additional nausea and vomiting were present in ten patients. Severe diarrhea occurred in four patients. Only one patient had the malabsorption syndrome. Nine patients experienced a loss of weight within a range of ten to 40 pounds with an average of 21 pounds. The most frequent cause of the weight loss was not a problem of intestinal motility but failure to eat because of anticipated pain induced by meal ingestion. On physical examination, most patients had abdominal bruits; abdominal tenderness or other physical findings were infrequent.

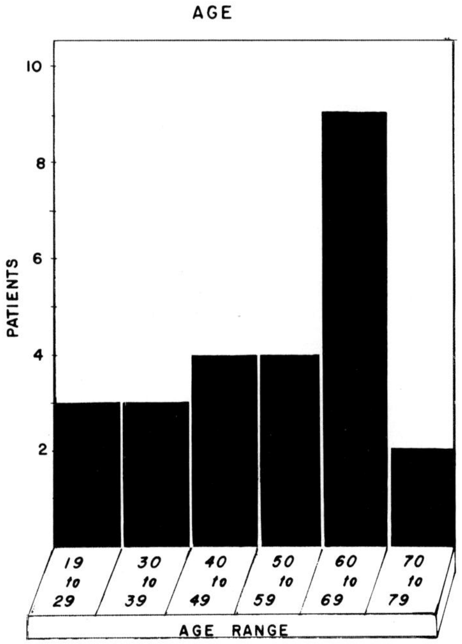

Fig. 1. Gastrointestinal arterial revascularization. Age distribution of 25 patients who had surgical treatment of abdominal angina. More than half were under the age of 55 years; most were from 60 to 69 years of age. Female:male ratio 17:8.

Table I. *Symptoms in 25 patients**

Symptom	*No. of patients*	
Postprandial pain	14	23
Abdominal pain	10	
Epigastric pain	4	
Lower abdominal pain	3	
Nausea and vomiting	3	8
Diarrhea	4	
Malabsorption	1	
Weight loss (10 to 40 lb.) (average, 21 lb.)	9	

*Duration: 0.5 to 60 mo. ($\overline{20}$ mo.)

Localized arteriosclerotic plaques at the origin of the SMA, CA, or IMA were the most frequent cause of obstruction of the mesenteric arteries (Table II). These patients frequently had associated arteriosclerotic occlusive disease of other arteries. Arteritis accounted for mesenteric occlusive disease in four patients. Two patients had ob-

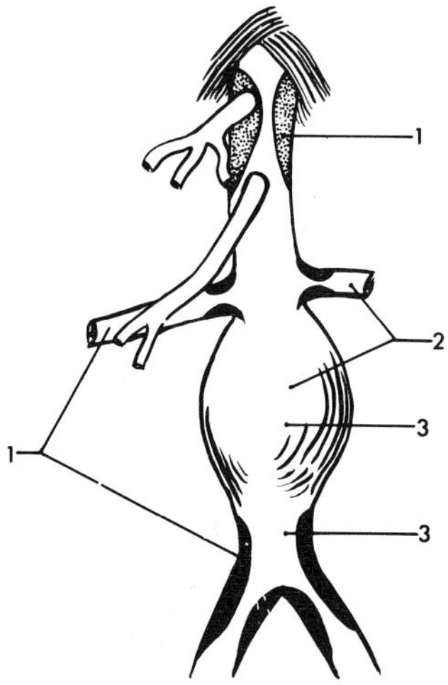

Fig. 2. Drawing showing associated arterial lesions which occurred in ten of 25 patients corrected concomitantly with mesenteric revascularization. Coarctation of the abdominal aorta, renal artery stenosis, abdominal aortic aneurysm and aortoiliac occlusive disease are shown.

struction of the CA by the median arcuate ligament which exerted external compression, probably resulting in significant intrinsic stenosis of the CA. Both patients were over the age of 60 and had experienced chronic gastrointestinal symptoms over several years. Fibrointimal hyperplasia was present in two patients, both of whom were young women. The remaining patient had coarctation of the abdominal aorta with obstruction of the CA and SMA.

Associated arterial and gastrointestinal diseases were present in 20 of the 25 patients and 14 underwent concomitant surgical treatment (Table III). Simultaneous resection of abdominal aortic aneurysm was performed in five patients (Fig. 2). Of these, two also had renal artery bypass. One patient had renal artery bypass and treatment of aortoiliac occlusive disease. Three patients had aortofemoral artery bypass grafts for aortoiliac occlusive disease. Another patient had correction of abdominal aortic coarctation in conjunction with mesenteric revascularization. Other localized arteriosclerotic disease processes were corrected either before the gastrointestinal revascularization or in the period following surgery.

Table II. *Etiology*

	No. of patients	*Average age (yr.)*	*Male: female ratio*
Arteriosclerosis	16	59	6/10
Arteritis	4	32	1/3
Arcuate ligament compression	2	66	0/2
Fibrointimal hyperplasia	2	28	0/2
Coarctation of abdominal aorta	1	23	1/0
Total	25		8/17

Table III. *Associated diseases*

Associated diseases	*No. of patients*	
Vascular		
Abdominal aortic aneurysm	5	(5)*
Aortoiliac occlusive disease	4	(2)
Renal hypertension	4	(3)
Carotid occlusive disease	4	(0)
Femoral popliteal occlusive disease	2	(0)
Reoperation—false aneurysm	1	(1)
Total	20	(11)
Gastrointestinal		
Cholelithiasis	2	(2)
Hiatal hernia	1	(1)
Total	3	(3)

*Numbers in parentheses indicate the number of patients who underwent simultaneous operative correction.

OPERATIVE TECHNIQUE

Satisfactory anatomical diagnosis was obtained in the 25 patients, correlating the clinical syndrome with the lateral translumbar aortogram or selective mesenteric arteriograms. In most patients, encroachment on the lumen of at least 75 percent or more in two of the three major mesenteric arteries (CA, SMA, IMA) was considered pathologically significant. Complete intra-abdominal aortic aneurysm and mesenteric vascular occlusive disease or renal artery hypertension were simultaneously corrected. Surgical correction of a single visceral artery was done in 14 patients and multiple arteries were revascularized in 11 patients (Fig. 3).

The technique of bypass graft was utilized in 26 of the 38 arteries revascularized (Fig.

4). The obvious simplicity of this technique made it more favorable than a direct attack on the diseased artery. Most lesions of the CA, SMA, and IMA were at the bifurcation of the artery and aorta. The distal artery was usually free of significant disease and also easier to expose surgically. This made an end-to-side anastomosis utilizing a bypass graft of Dacron or saphenous vein simple to perform. In addition, occlusion of the proximal abdominal aorta above the renal arteries is avoided. For use of a bypass graft, the aorta is clamped only below the renal arteries where the proximal end of the bypass graft is placed.

The conduit most frequently used was a 7 or 8 mm. tube graft of knitted Dacron. The graft was accurately beveled at the abdominal aortic anastomosis in order to avoid kinking. The distal end of the bypass graft was, on occasion, placed in one of the main branches of the CA rather than the CA itself which can be difficult to expose (Fig. 5). The hepatic artery was revascularized in four patients, the splenic artery was revascularized in three patients, and the CA itself was directly bypassed in seven patients. The SMA was bypassed in 12 patients.

A patch graft with or without endarterectomy was utilized in eight patients (Fig. 4). Three patients had direct patch of the celiac artery, four patients had a direct patch of the SMA, and one patient had a large Dacron patch of an abdominal aortic coarctation with simultaneous patching of the obstructing lesions of the SMA and CA.

The last technique employed was direct implantation of the artery. In one patient who had a stenotic CA probably caused by compression by the median arcuate ligament, the CA was reimplanted into the aorta at a lower level after excision of the stenotic area. Another patient underwent reimplantation of the splenic artery into the distal abdominal aorta after ligation of the distal splenic artery. This procedure allowed for retrograde revascularization of the celiac axis (Fig. 5). The IMA was directly reimplanted at the time of resection of the abdominal aortic aneurysm and revascularization of the

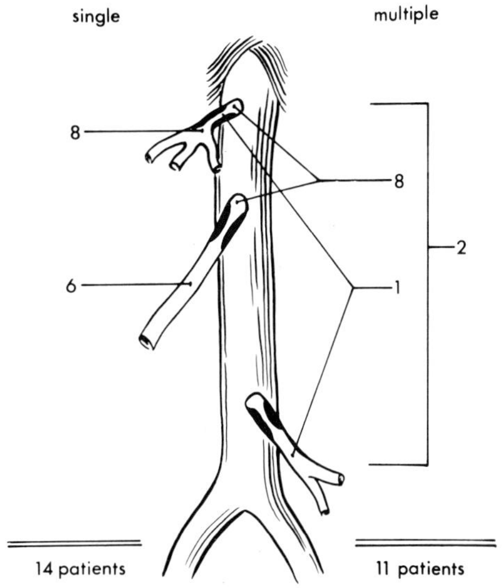

Fig. 3. Arteries involved in gastrointestinal arterial revascularization. Drawing indicating single and multiple arteries bypassed. Fourteen patients had single bypass grafts to either the superior mesenteric or celiac artery. Multiple grafts were done in the remaining 11 patients. Eight had bypass grafts to the superior mesenteric and celiac artery and one to the inferior mesenteric and celiac artery. Two patients had surgical treatment of all three major arteries.

CA and SMA in both patients. The disadvantages of direct reimplantation are obvious; however, it can be reserved for repair in some instances.

RESULTS

Among the 25 patients who underwent mesenteric revascularization procedures, two patients died following unsuccessful arterial bypass procedures (Table IV). One patient, a 30-year-old woman, presented with severe abdominal angina. She had experienced epigastric pain for the last two years with severe cramps occurring one to $1\frac{1}{2}$ hours after meals. A translumbar aortogram demonstrated generalized narrowing of the SMA and CA. Surgical exploration of the abdomen showed severe arteritis with narrowing of all the distal arteries. A long patch graft of the SMA was performed, with endarterectomy and dilation; however, backflow was very poor. The patient died after a protracted course because of mesenteric artery thrombosis. In retrospect, she was a

Table IV. *Operative deaths*

Patient	*Sex*	*Age*	*Etiology*	*Symptom*	*Procedure*	*Cause of death*
1	F	30	Severe arteritis	Epigastric pain, 2 yr. duration	SMA endarterectomy and long patch graft	Mesenteric infarction, poor distal artery
2	F	47	Generalized arteriosclerosis	Postprandial pain, 3 yr. duration	Bypass grafts to SMA and splenic artery (2 attempts)	Mesenteric infarction, poor distal artery

Table V. *Over-all results in 25 patients**

Over-all results	*No.*
Deaths	
Operative	2/25
Late (4 mo. to 4 yr.)	5/23
Abdominal pain	
Complete relief	9/18
Partial	4/18
Same	2/18
Worse	2/18
Malabsorption	1/18

*5 mo. to 8 yr. follow-up examination.

Table VI. *Postoperative complications in 23 survivors*

Complications	*No.*
Mild diarrhea	3
Postoperative hemorrhage and subphrenic abscess	1
Pancreatitis	1
Infarction gastric epiploica of cecum	1

poor candidate for mesenteric revascularization because of the small distal arteries.

The other patient was a 47-year-old woman who underwent Dacron bypass grafts from the aorta to the splenic artery and to the SMA because of severe stenosis of the CA, SMA, and occlusion of the IMA. On the first day after operation, she developed abdominal tenderness and shock. Exploration of the abdomen revealed occlusion of both grafts, and an autogenous saphenous vein graft was used to replace the Dacron grafts. Despite embolectomy, no backflow was present, and the patient died 24 hours later with mesenteric infarction. These two patients demonstrate the hazards of a technical failure because of improper selection of patients for operation. In retrospect, both patients were poor candidates for mesenteric revascularization.

Of the remaining 23 patients, five died four to 48 months after, one because of a bleeding gastric ulcer at four months; one died of pneumonia at four years; one died of hepatitis at four months; and sudden death occurred in another two at five months and 20 months (Table V).

On long-term follow-up examination of the 18 survivors, ranging from five months to eight years after surgery, nine patients were found to have an excellent result with relief of symptoms. Eight retained some degree of abdominal pain. Partial relief was afforded in four patients. Abdominal pain remained the same in two patients and had become worse in the remaining two patients. Postoperative aortograms demonstrated patency of the bypass grafts in the two patients who experienced increased pain after operation. One patient continued with severe malabsorption. He had a single high-grade occlusive lesion of the CA which was successfully bypassed. Apparently, his symptoms were not related primarily to the stenotic lesion.

Postoperative complications occurred in six patients (Table VI). A subphrenic abscess occurred in one patient after a second exploratory operation for postoperative hemorrhage. The patient was discharged in good condition but died four months later as the result of a bleeding gastric ulcer. Mild pancreatitis, presumably from manipulation of the pancreas in mobilizing the SMA and CA, occurred in the postoperative period in one patient. Peritonitis occurred in another patient after surgery and was secondary to a nonrelated infarcted gastric epiploica of the cecum which was resected without difficulty.

DISCUSSION

The clinical diagnosis of intestinal angina was apparent. The patient classically com-

OPERATIONS

	BYPASS	PATCH	DIRECT
Celiac	7	3	1
Hepatic	4		
Splenic	3		1
Superior mesenteric	12	4	
Inferior Mesenteric	--	-	2
Aorta	--	1	
TOTAL	26	8	4

Fig. 4. The three types of operation are shown. Bypass grafts were done in 26 of the 38 arteries. Direct implantation of the artery at a different location was done in four patients. A patch graft with localized endarterectomy was done in eight patients. Total was 38 arteries in 25 patients.

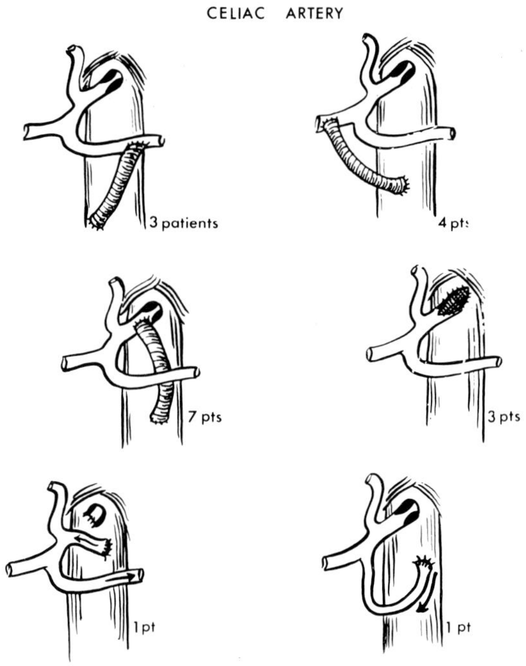

Fig. 5. Drawing showing different approaches used in surgical management of 19 patients with lesions of the celiac artery.

plained of cramping abdominal pain, occurring one hour postprandially. Loss of weight was moderate caused by anticipated fear of eating. The pain was relieved by narcotic agents and, in some instances, nitroglycerine. Early in the course of the disease, constipation occurred usually followed by diarrhea and finally by malabsorption if there was significant arterial insufficiency. Duration of pain was usually from months to years, although in two of our patients the pain was present for only two weeks before surgery. In these two patients, the pain was unrelenting and similar to the pattern of preinfarction angina in patients with coronary artery disease. Physical findings were generally minimal, except for an abdominal bruit which was found in all but four of our patients. In the patients with arteriosclerosis, repairable arteriosclerotic lesions were usually present.

The diagnosis of intestinal angina was based upon the correlation of clinical symptoms with arteriographic findings. Lateral translumbar aortogram demonstrated significant stenotic lesions in the visceral arteries. Selective arteriography allowed a more accurate demonstration of the distal runoff.

The significance of stenotic lesions without symptoms is questionable. Matz and Kahn[9] have described occlusion of the CA, SMA, and IMA in a patient without symptoms. Congenital absence of the celiac axis trunk has been described in a patient who developed symptoms in adult life.[11] Reports of pre-existing mesenteric artery disease in patients with subsequent mesenteric thrombosis vary greatly, although the incidence is thought to be approximately 50 percent.[6, 8, 10, 17, 19] Stenosis usually is localized to the proximal 2 cm. of the superior mesenteric artery.[2] The collateral patterns of the visceral arteries are adequate so occlusion of a single artery of the CA, SMA, or IMA should not result in symptoms or mesenteric infarction in most patients. However, lesions of two of the three major arteries (CA, SMA, IMA) have been considered significant.[12, 14] In the presence of arteriosclerosis, especially of the distal aorta with bilateral occlusion of the internal iliac arteries and IMA, the collateral patterns of the upper visceral arteries may be disturbed. Conversely, we have observed severe stenosis of one major artery, usually the CA, accompanied by gastrointestinal symptoms which were relieved by surgical treatment of the single arterial lesions. Thus, the clinical syndrome must be considered when reviewing the arteriographic findings. Prophylactic surgical treatment of stenotic lesions of the CA, SMA, or IMA, when encountered during other intraabdominal vascular procedures, usually is not indicated. When the IMA is detached from the aorta during placement of an abdominal aortic graft, reimplantation may be indicated if the IMA was not occluded originally and is of large caliber.

The most frequent and adaptable operation consisted of bypass grafts from the infrarenal abdominal aorta to the normal mesenteric artery beyond the area of stenosis. Long-term follow-up data failed to indicate that a knitted 8 mm. tube graft of Dacron has any greater tendency for thrombosis than a saphenous vein graft. Bypass grafts to the hepatic or splenic arteries for treatment of stenosis of the CA are especially useful. After returning the intestine and mesentery to the abdominal cavity, proper attention must be paid to angulation and tension.

Despite the large number of patients who undergo vascular surgical procedures, revascularization of the mesenteric arteries remains a somewhat infrequent operation. The rich collateral blood supply of the abdominal viscera accounts for this low incidence of symptomatic disease. On the other hand, constant awareness of the syndrome, as it is classically described and through modern arteriographic techniques, will lead to diagnosis in the small group of patients who are desperately ill.

In this series of 25 patients, death was directly related to the presence of distal runoff demonstrated on preoperative arteriograms. Selection of patients is important, and without evidence of good distal collateral vessels, revascularization proceduers should not be attempted. The late deaths (five patients) reflect the typical pattern of patients who are treated surgically for localized arteriosclerotic disease. Complete relief of abdominal symptoms by successful operative repair was dramatic in the nine patients. On the other hand, only partial relief in the four patients who had successful bypass procedures may be attributed to an improper relationship between the symptom complex and the arteriographic findings.

REFERENCES

1. Baccelli, F.: Cited by Goodman, E. H.: Angina abdominis, Am. J. Med. Sci., n.s. **155:** 524, 1918.
2. Carucci, J. J.: Mesenteric vascular occlusion, Am. J. Surg. **80:** 47, 1953.
3. Conner, L. A.: Discussion of role of arterial thrombosis in visceral diseases of middle life, based upon analogies drawn from coronary thrombosis, Am. J. Med. Sci. **185:** 13, 1933.
4. Dardik, H., Seidenberg, B., Parker, J. G., and Hurwitt, E. S.: Intestinal angina malabsorption treated with elective revascularization, J. A. M. A. **194:** 1206, 1965.
5. Dunbar, J. D., Molnar, W., Beman, F., and Marable, S. A.: Compression of the celiac trunk and abdominal angina: Preliminary report of 15 caes, Am. J. Roentgenol. **95:** 731, 1965.
6. Dunphy, J. E.: Abdominal pain of vascular origin, Am. J. Med. Sci. **192:** 109, 1936.
7. Fry, W. J., and Kraft, R. O.: Visceral angina, Surg. Gynecol. Obstet. **117:** 417, 1963.
8. Harjola, P. T., and Lahtiharju, A.: Celiac axis syndrome: Abdominal angina caused by external compression of the celiac artery. Am. J. Surg. **115:** 864, 1968.
9. Matz, E. M., and Kahn, P. C.: Occlusion of the celiac, superior mesenteric and inferior mesenteric arteries: Angiographic demonstration in an asymptomatic patient, Vasc. Dis. **5:** 130, 1968.
10. Mikkelsen, W. P.: Intestinal angina: Its surgical significance, Am. J. Surg. **94:** 262, 1957.
11. Morettin, L. B., Baldwin-Price, H. K., and Scheiber, M. H.: Congenital absence of the celiac axis trunk, Am. J. Roentgenol. **95:** 727, 1965.
12. Morris, G. C., Jr., and De Bakey, M. E.: Abdominal angina: Diagnosis and treatment, J. A. M. A. **176:** 89, 1961.
13. Morris, G. C., Jr., Crawford, E. S., Cooley, D. A., and De Bakey, M. E.: Revascularization of the celiac and superior mesenteric arteries, Arch. Surg. **84:** 113, 1962.
14. Morris, G. C., Jr., De Bakey, M. E., and Bernhard, V.: Abdominal angina, Surg. Clin. North Am. **46:** 919, 1966.

15. Rob, C.: Symposium on obliteration of visceral arteries: The indications for operation in occlusive disease of the visceral arteries, J. Cardiovasc. Surg. **3:** 223, 1962.
16. Shaw, R. S., and Maynard, E. P., III: Acute and chronic thrombosis of mesenteric arteries associated with malabsorption: Report of two cases successfully treated by thromboendarterectomy, New Engl. J. Med. **258:** 274, 1958.
17. Stoney, R. J., and Edwin, J. W.: Recognition and surgical management of visceral ischemic syndromes, Ann. Surg. **164:** 714, 1966.
18. Szilagyi, D. E., Rian, R. L., Elliott, J. P., and Smith, R. F.: The celiac artery compression syndrome: Does it exist? SURGERY **72:** 849, 1972.
19. Wylie, E. J., and Stoney, R. J.: Management of visceral arterial occlusion, *in* Management of arterial occlusive disease, Chicago, Ill., 1971, Year Book Medical Publishers, p. 291.

Congenital incomplete prepyloric diaphragm in infants and children

Dimitris C. Keramidas, M.D.,* *Athens, Greece*

One case of incomplete prepyloric diaphragm, with a submucosal abscess occurring proximal to the congenital abnormality, in a male child of 2½ years is described. Such an occurrence has not been recorded previously. Partial obstruction in the pylorus was compensated for by increased gastric tone. Nonprojectile bile-free vomiting was the main symptom. X-ray studies revealing distention of the stomach and prolonged retention of contrast material were suggestive of this abnormality. The diagnosis was confirmed at laparotomy and operative treatment was achieved by excision of the diaphragm and pyloroplasty. Review of the English literature showed that another 21 cases of incomplete pyloric or prepyloric diaphragms in neonates, infants, and children have been reported, with a predominance of 3:1 in the prepyloric area and a variety in onset, duration, and severity of obstructive symptoms.

From the Department of Surgery, Aglaias Kyriakou Children's Hospital, Athens, Greece

ATRESIA OF the pylorus has been classified into pyloric and prepyloric, each of which may be membranous or segmental.[11] The membranous form of atresia is the more common and consists of a mucosal diaphragm completely dividing the stomach from the duodenum.[4] Occasionally, the membranous diaphragm may retain an aperture, or it may perforate from the pressure of the gastric content resulting in a communication between the stomach and duodenum.[12] A congenital incomplete or perforated diaphragm is very rare. In the English literature, there are 21 reports of this abnormality occurring in neonates, infants and children. The reported cases are reviewed and one more case of an incomplete prepyloric diaphragm in a male child of 2½ years is added.

Accepted for publication Feb. 22, 1974.

Reprint address: Department of Surgery, Aglaias Kyriakou Children's Hospital, Athens 608, Greece.

*Present address: 1129 N. State St., Pediatric Pavilion (8E2), LAC/USC Medical Center, Los Angeles, Calif. 90033.

CASE REPORT

C. S., a 2½-year-old boy, was referred to the surgical department for persistent nonbilious vomiting following oral feeding for three days prior to referral. The patient was the first-born of a healthy mother who had an uncomplicated pregnancy and delivery. There was a history of episodes of nonprojectile bile-free vomiting, aggravated by eating solid foods during the last 12 months. The child was living mostly on milk and he appeared anemic and undernourished. On examination, there was distention of the upper abdomen extending to the lower intercostal spaces. Abdominal sounds were intensive in the epigastrium. The temperature was 37.6° C., and the respiratory rate was also higher than normal. Plain x-ray films of the abdomen showed excessive distention of the stomach and gas beyond the pylorus. The upper gastrointestinal series revealed a marked degree of pyloric obstruction, and barium was retained in the stomach after 24 hours (Fig. 1). Blood tests showed a hemoglobin of 8 Gm. per 100 c.c. and a white cell count of 16,000 with 81 percent polymorphonuclear leukocytes. The patient was prepared for surgery with correction of fluid and electrolyte deficits, transfusion of blood, administration of antibiotic agents and vitamins, and nasogastric suction.

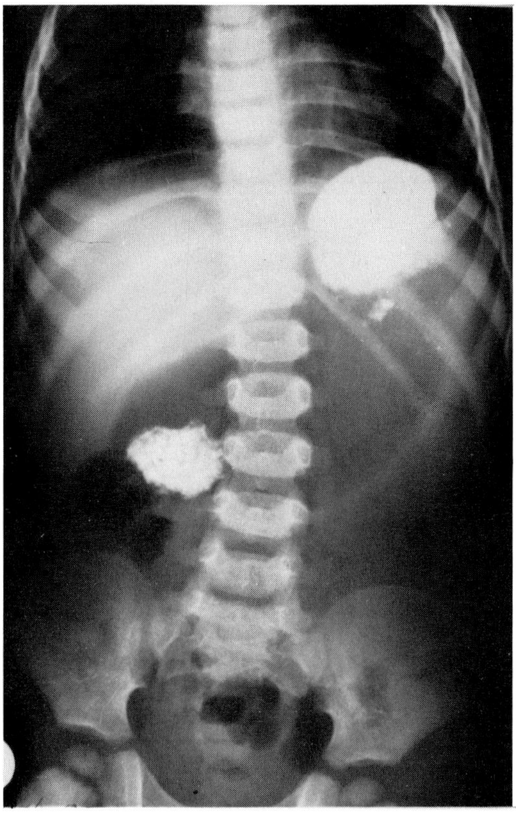

Fig. 1. Congenital incomplete prepyloric diaphragm. Preoperative barium study revealing gastric distention and prolonged retention of contrast medium in the stomach.

At operation 48 hours later, the stomach was found to be enlarged and its wall was hypertrophied. The pylorus was of normal appearance. A longitudinal gastrotomy was made up to the pylorus, and a thin prepyloric diaphragm with a small central aperture was found; a 3 mm. probe could not be passed through the aperture. An extension of the incision resulted in the evacuation of pus from within the antral wall proximal to the diaphragm. Eight cubic centimeters of pus was collected into a syringe from the submucosa, which was then irrigated with normal saline and antibiotic agents. Subsequently, the interior of the stomach was examined, and no other lesions could be found. The duodenum was proved to be patent by passing a soft rubber Foley catheter. The diaphragm was excised, and a Heineke-Mikulicz pyloroplasty was performed. The histology of the diaphragm was that of normal gastric mucosa in two layers with loose fibrous tissue between them. The postoperative recovery was uneventful. The nasogastric tube was removed on the third postoperative day, and oral feedings were gradually introduced and well tolerated. One week later, a barium study revealed patency into the duodenum (Fig. 2), and the child was discharged on the fifteenth postoperative day with a significant weight gain.

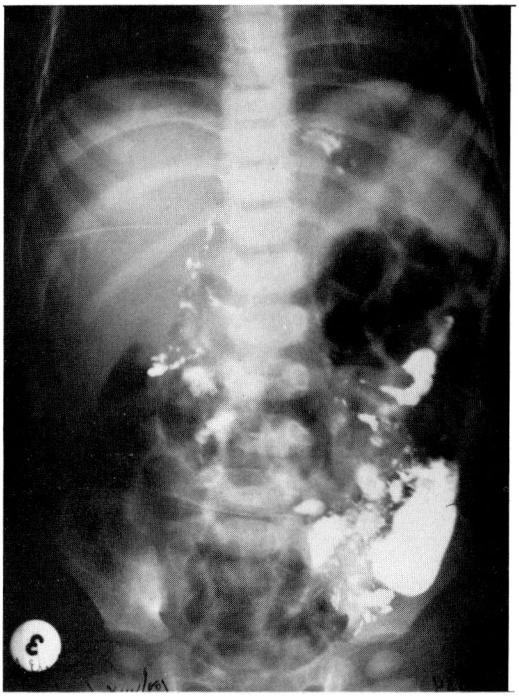

Fig. 2. Barium study showing patency into the duodenum after excision of the diaphragm and pyloroplasty.

DISCUSSION

There is uncertainty as to the embryology of the congentital incomplete or perforated pyloric and prepyloric diaphragm. It probably results from redundant endodermal lining and formation of epithelial fold which may or may not retain an aperture.[12] A thin membranous diaphragm may perforate from the pressure of the gastric content.[12] A fetal vascular accident may be causative along with the failure to recanalize.[16]

In our patient, the incomplete diaphragm was located proximal to the pylorus. In another 16 cases in a total of 21, the diaphragm was also classified as either prepyloric or antral (Table I). It is located more than three times more frequently in the prepyloric area than in the pyloric area.

Table I. *Collected reports of incomplete pyloric and prepyloric diaphragms in infants and children*

Author	*Year*	*Age at operation*	*Sex*	*Hydramnios*	*Site and size of incomplete diaphragm*	*Duration of symptoms*	*Surgical treatment*	*Result*
Bonner[3]	1912	1 mo.	—	—	Prepyloric	—	Gastrojejunostomy	D
Berman and Ballenger[2]	1942	2 yr.	M	No	Prepyloric; 1 mm. aperture	3 wk.	Incised; pyloroplasty	L
Despirito and Guthorn[8]	1957	3 wk.	M	No	Prepyloric; 5 mm. aperture	Life	Pyloroplasty	L
Wurtenberger[21]	1961	5 wk.	—	—	Pyloric	—	Excised	L
Benson[1]	1962	11 yr.	M	—	Prepyloric	9½ yr.	Excised	L
Dineen and Redo[9]	1963	33 days	M	No	Pyloric	3 wk.	Excised; Heineke-Mikulicz pyloroplasty	L
Liechti et al.[15]	1963	4 yr.	F	No	Prepyloric, 2-3 mm. aperture	Life	Incised; pyloroplasty	L
Slim et al.[19]	1964	2 wk.	F	No	Pyloric	Life	Heineke-Mikulicz pyloroplasty	L
Gerber[11]	1965	2½ yr.	M	No	Prepyloric; 3 mm. aperture	4 wk.	Incised; Heineke-Mikulicz pyloroplasty	L
DeBoer[7]	1965	11 yr.	F	—	Pyloric	Life	Excised?; pyloroplasty	L
Packard[17]	1965	5 yr.	F	—	Pyloric diaphragm?	2 mo.	Gastroenterostomy at 2 mo.; breakdown anastomosis/pyloroplasty at 5 yr.	L
Farman et al.[10]	1968	7 yr.	M	—	Antral	3 mo.	Antrectomy; Billroth 1 anastomosis	L
Parrish et al.[18]	1968	6 yr.	F	—	Antral; 2 mm. aperture	4 days	Excised; pyloroplasty	L
Cremin[6]	1969	3 days	F	—	Prepyloric; 2 mm. aperture	Life	Pylorectomy; end-to-end anastomosis	—
Cremin[6]	1969	4 days	M	Yes	Pyloric	Life	Pylorectomy; end-to-end anastomosis	—
Cremin[6]	1969	Neonate	—	—	Pyloric; pinhole meatus	Life	Resected	—
Willcoxon and Farha[20]	1970	10 wk.	M	Yes?	Prepyloric	4 wk.	Excised; Heineke-Mikulicz pyloroplasty	L
Campbell et al.[5]	1973	4 mo.	—	—	Antral	3 mo.	Excised; Heineke-Mikulicz pyloroplasty	L
Campbell et al.[5]	1973	4 mo.	—	—	Antral	3 mo.	Excised; Heineke-Mikulicz pyloroplasty	L
Campbell et al.[5]	1973	3 mo.	—	—	Antral	2 mo.	Excised; Heineke-Mikulicz pyloroplasty	L
Campbell et al.[5]	1973	4 yr.	F	—	Antral	6 mo.	Excised; Heineke-Mikulicz pyloroplasty	L

The histology of the diaphragm is that of normal gastric mucosa. Loose connective tissue or tunica muscularis mucosae can be found in the septum between the mucosal layers. As with the present case, the aperture does not dilate, although it is free from fibrous tissue; however, in one case, the gastric surface of the diaphragm was covered with squamous epithelium,[15] and in three other instances, the mucosal web was associated with muscular hypertrophy.[3, 10, 20]

Hydramnios was not reported with the present patient, nor was it with most of the cases in the literature. It was reported with only two cases.[6, 20] It seems that hydramnios may rarely be associated with the perforated pyloric or prepyloric diaphragm.

Nonbilious vomiting is the main symptom,

and in three instances, it led to diagnosis and/or surgery in the neonatal period.[6] The onset, duration, and severity of obstructive symptoms varied (Table I). Perforation and neonatal peritonitis in one instance were associated with a diaphragmlike obstruction of the prepyloric mucosa.[8] Usually, obstruction can be compensated for by increased gastric tone; in one half of the patients, symptoms did not start until adult life.[13] This phenomenon probably results from hypertrophy of the stomach with loss of its tone and from impaired mastication with increasing age, resulting in more compact boluses of food and gastric stasis. Chronic gastric stasis probably leads to excessive antral stimulation and ulcer formation proximal to the diaphragm.[18] A healed gastric ulcer was found proximal to a prepyloric diaphragm in a seven-year-old child.[10]

In the present case, the episodes of nonprojectile bile-free vomiting, aggravated after solid feedings, and the resultant malnutrition were typical of an abnormality in the pylorus with incomplete patency into the duodenum. Also, typical of the same abnormality were the preoperative barium studies revealing gastric distention and prolonged retention of contrast medium in the stomach. The patient's temperature and the laboratory findings before surgery were obviously related to the submucosal abscess found at operation. The occurrence of an abscess has not been recorded previously.

Standard radiologic techniques have been used for diagnosing high-grade outlet obstruction of the pylorus. Diaphragms causing low-grade obstruction need specific radiologic techniques.[5]

Excision of the diaphragm and pyloroplasty gave excellent results in the present patient. Incision or excision of the diaphragm and/or pyloroplasty were successfully performed in 17 other cases.[1, 2, 5, 6, 9, 11, 15, 17-21] Antrectomy and Billroth I anastomosis were performed in a seven-year-old boy with a healed ulcer proximal to the diaphragm,[10] and pylorectomy with end-to-end anastomosis was performed in two neonates.[6] This type of operation in neonates is probably better reserved for the treatment of the segmental type of pyloric atresia.[14] Excision or incision of the diaphragm and pyloroplasty is a lesser procedure for promoting gastric emptying, and it should be the operation of choice in complete or incomplete membranes of the pyloric area.

REFERENCES

1. Benson, C. D.: Congenital prepyloric atresia, *in* Benson, C. D., Mustard, W. T., Ravitch, M. M., Snyder, W. H., and Welch, K. J., editors: Pediatric surgery, Chicago, 1962, Year Book Medical Publishers, p. 660.
2. Berman, J. K., and Ballenger, F.: Prepyloric membranous obstruction, Q. Bull. Ind. Univ. Med. Center **4:** 14, 1942.
3. Bonner, A.: A unique case of intragastric congenital malformation simulating the clinical manifestations of pylorospasm, N. Y. Postgrad. Med. **27:** 118, 1912.
4. Bronsther, B., Nadeau, M. R., and Abrams, M. W.: Congenital pyloric atresia: A report of three cases and a review of the literature, SURGERY **69:** 130, 1971.
5. Campbell, D. P., Vanhoutte, J. J., and Smith, E. I.: Partially obstructing antral web: A distinct clinical entity, J. Pediatr. Surg. **8:** 723, 1973.
6. Cremin, B. J.: Congenital pyloric antral membranes in infancy, Radiology **92:** 509, 1969.
7. DeBoer, A.: *In* Discussion of Gerber, B. C.: Prepyloric diaphragm: An unusual abnormality, Arch. Surg. **90:** 472, 1965.
8. Despirito, A. J., and Guthorn, P. J.: Recovery from meconium peritonitis associated with diaphragm-like obstruction of the prepyloric mucosa, J. Pediatr. **50:** 599, 1957.
9. Dineen, J. P., and Redo, S. F.: Pyloric obstruction due to mucosal diaphragm, SURGERY **53:** 674, 1963.
10. Farman, J., Cywes, S., and Werbelaff, L.: Pyloric mucosal diaphragms, Clin. Radiol. **19:** 95, 1968.
11. Gerber, B. C.: Prepyloric diaphragm: An unusual abnormality. A case report, Arch. Surg. **90:** 472, 1965.
12. Gray, S. W., and Skandalakis, J. E.: Embryology for surgeons, Philadelphia, 1972, W. B. Saunders Company.
13. Hait, G., Esselstyn, C. B., and Rankin, G. B.: Prepyloric mucosal diaphragm (antral web): Report of a case and review of the literature, Arch. Surg. **105:** 486, 1972.
14. Keramidas, D. C., and Voyatzis, N.: Pyloric atresia: Report of a second occurrence in the same family, J. Pediatr. Surg. **7:** 445, 1972.
15. Liechti, R. E., Mikkelson, W. P., and Snyder, W. H., Jr.: Prepyloric stenosis caused by

squamous epithelial diaphragm—resultant infantilism, SURGERY **53:** 670, 1963.

16. Louw, J. H., and Barnard, C. N.: Congenital intestinal atresia: Observation on its origin, Lancet **2:** 1065, 1955.
17. Packard, G. B., Jr.: *In* Discussion of Gerber, B. C.: Prepyloric diaphragm: An unusual abnormality, Arch. Surg. **90:** 472, 1965.
18. Parrish, R. A., Canavage, C. B., Wells, J. A., and Moretz, W. H.: Congenital antral membrane, Surg. Gynecol. Obstet. **127:** 999, 1968.
19. Slim, M. S., Bitar, J. G., and Idriss, H.: Hypertrophy of the pyloric mucosa: A rare cause of congenital pyloric obstruction, Am. J. Dis. Child. **107:** 636, 1964.
20. Willcoxon, R. L., and Farha, G. J.: Prepyloric antral stenosis: Report of a case with muscular hypertrophy and mucosal web, J. Kan. Med. Soc. **71:** 353, 1970.
21. Wurtenberger, H.: Gastric atresia, Arch. Dis. Child. **36:** 161, 1961.

Diagnosis, pathology, and treatment of Buerger's disease

Shigehiko Shionoya, M.D., Ichiro Ban, M.D., Yukifumi Nakata, M.D., Junichi Matsubara, M.D., Kenzo Shinjo, M.D., Masafumi Hirai, M.D., Seiichi Kawai, M.D., Shoichi Suzuki, M.D., *and* Wen Hsiung Tsai, M.D., *Nagoya, Japan*

From our clinical and pathological studies on Buerger's disease, the following results were obtained: (1) In order to have a functional diagnosis of arterial occlusion in Buerger's disease, muscle blood flow of the leg should be measured in addition to angiography; (2) Buerger's disease is a separate clinicopathological entity, and the process of the thromboangiitis originates in small arteries in the extremities; and (3) direct arterial surgery is rarely feasible for patients with Buerger's disease, because of diffuse occlusion of the small vessels distal to the popliteal or brachial artery.

From the Department of Surgery, Nagoya University Branch Hospital, Nagoya, Japan

FOR MANY YEARS, Buerger's disease was recognized as a definite clinicopathological entity. However, recently published papers have raised the question whether Buerger's disease is an entity separate from atherosclerotic disease of the extremities and presented the conclusion that most cases represented atherosclerotic disease with secondary, more distal, arterial thrombosis or simple arterial thrombosis or embolism.[4, 13] Subsequently many investigators[2, 9] have defended its recognition as a clinical disorder.

These various reports of different viewpoints were the stimulus for us to examine our own experience in this disease.

A diagnostic category is of practical value to the clinician only if knowledge of the unique characteristics of the disorder provides a guide to prognosis and treatment. This information is divided into three categories: diagnostic, pathologic, and therapeutic.

Accepted for publication Feb. 22, 1974.

Reprint requests: Shigehiko Shionoya, M.D., Department of Surgery, Nagoya University Branch Hospital, 2-1 Higashimonzen-cho, Higashi-ku, Nagoya, Japan.

DIAGNOSIS

Of the series of 628 patients with peripheral vascular diseases, who had been treated in the department of Surgery at Nagoya University Branch Hospital from May, 1967, to June, 1972, 100 cases were Buerger's disease.

In our clinic, the number of cases of Buerger's disease was double that of arteriosclerosis obliterans. There is a distinct difference in the age at the onset of symptoms between Buerger's disease and arteriosclerosis obliterans. Of the 100 patients with Buerger's disease, 42 cases showed an involvement of the arteries of the upper limbs, and in 27 cases, superficial thrombophlebitis occurred.

The most common arteriographic finding of Buerger's disease was an occlusion of one or more large branches of the popliteal artery. Therefore, instep claudication is characteristic for patients with Buerger's disease,

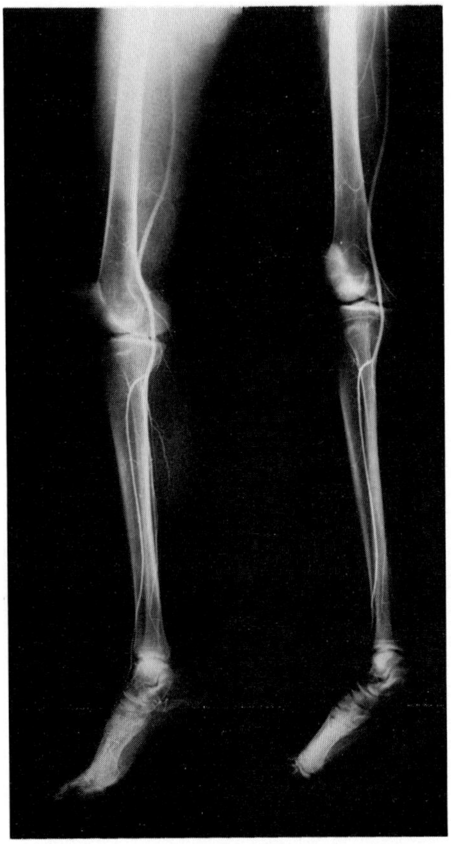

Fig. 1. The posterior tibial artery is occluded near its origin but the anterior tibial artery is patent in the two patients with Buerger's disease. However, the clearance curve of the anterior tibial muscle is abnormal on the right and normal on the left, as indicated below.

	MBFe	*MBFh*	*T-time*	*R-index*
Right	19.3	47.1	2.75	50.8
Left	30.6	27.4	2.0	12.8

but in the advanced stage, claudication of the calf occurs.

As arteriography gives only morphologic evaluation on the arterial occlusive process, it is desirable to have quantitative and functional evaluation on the arterial disorder.

In order to have a functional diagnosis of peripheral arterial diseases, muscle blood flow of the leg and distal blood pressure, namely, local perfusion pressure, should be measured in addition to angiography.[10]

A simple and reliable technique to determine muscle blood flow in ischemic limbs is Xe-133 clearance method.[8] The subjects are examined in the supine or prone position. Sterile isotonic solution of Xe-133 is injected into the leg muscle, and the disappearance rate of the tracer is measured. The subjects are instructed to exercise their feet.

The exercise of the feet is maximal dorsal flexion without arrested blood flow of the leg. We call this technique "non-ischemic work method."

From the clearance curves the following four parameters are calculated: (1) MBFe (maximal blood flow during exercise); (2) MBFh (maximal blood flow after exercise); (3) T-time (duration of postexercise hyperemic reaction measured in minutes): and (4) R-index (an index of the hyperemia that occurs one minute after the cessation of the exercise).

The clearance curve of the anterior tibial or gastrocnemius muscle is considered normal when the following criteria are fulfilled.[5] For the musculus tibialis anterior: (1) MBFe $\geqq$ 12.0 ml. per 100 Gm. per minute (34.0 $\pm$ 15.2); (2) T-time $<$ 2.6 minutes (1.5 $\pm$ 0.4); (3) R-index $<$ 22.0 percent (6.8 $\pm$ 5.6); and (4) when MBFe is under 24.0 ml. per 100 Gm. per minute, MBFe $\geqq$ MBFh, T-time $<$ 1.8 minutes, and R-index $<$ 10.0 percent. For the musculus gastrocnemius: (1) MBFe $\geqq$ 12.0 ml. per 100 Gm. per minute (23.9 $\pm$ 7.7); (2) T-time $<$ 3.1 minutes (1.5 $\pm$ 0.3; and (3) R-index $<$ 38.0 percent (9.5 $\pm$ 10.2).

As is indicated in Table I, there is a significant difference in blood flow of the anterior tibial muscle between Buerger's disease and arteriosclerosis obliterans.[6] This finding implies that ischemia of the leg muscle in Buerger's disease is more severe than that in arteriosclerosis obliterans.

Fig. 1 is an arteriogram taken in two patients with Buerger's disease. Although the anterior tibial arteries were patent, the one had normal clearance curve and the other had abnormal clearance curve of the anterior tibial muscle. In consideration of the fact that the process of Buerger's disease originates in small arteries in the extremities,

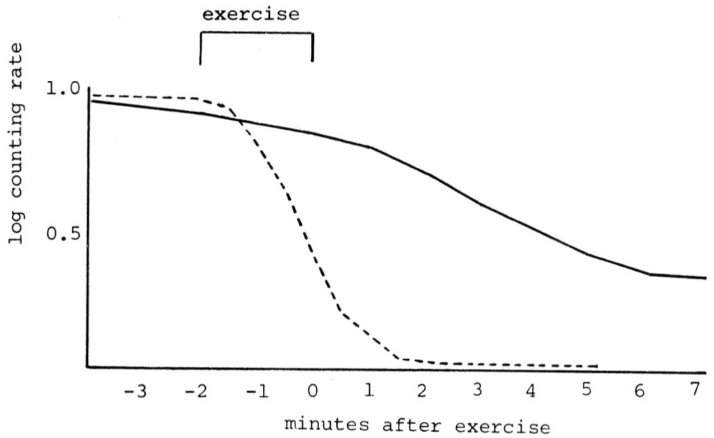

Fig. 2. Follow-up study of a 43-year-old patient with Buerger's disease, who underwent a ilio-popliteal bypass grafting. Successful reconstructive surgery converted pathological clearance curve of the anterior tibial muscle to normal. Solid line, preoperative clearance curve of musculus tibialis anterior; dashed line, postoperative clearance curve of musculus tibialis anterior.

	MBFe	*MBFh*	*T-time*	*R-index*
Preoperative	4.8	17.7	5.5	70.9
Postoperative	72.5	66.0	2.5	16.2

Table I. *Blood flow of the anterior tibial muscle*

	No. of legs	*MBFe*	*T-time*	*R-index*
Buerger's disease	19	8.8 ± 5.8	6.1 ± 3.5	71.0 ± 20.6
Arteriosclerosis obliterans	12	13.6 ± 7.1	4.1 ± 3.2	45.5 ± 33.5
		$P < 0.05$		$P < 0.02$

the muscle blood flow measurement seems to reveal a peripheral arterial insufficiency that could not be recognized by arteriography.

Successful reconstructive surgery converts pathologic clearance curve to normal, and follow-up study of the patients, with use of the muscle blood flow determination, is valuable in assessing the long-term results of surgery (Fig. 2).

After lumbar sympathectomy, there was no change in the clearance curve of the leg muscles.

The Xe-133 clearance method should be included in clinical evaluation of patients with peripheral arterial diseases, because it has shown to be a reliable, simple, and atraumatic procedure and because it clarifies the functional status of the occlusive process.

PATHOLOGY

Pathology of Buerger's disease is a nonspecific inflammation associated with thrombosis in the vessels of the extremities. Even skeptics will not deny distinctive characteristics of this disease, rather they dispute the specificity of the pathologic lesions. From the standpoint of pathology, the disease has certain outstanding characteristics which can be stated briefly as follows:

Macroscopic changes. Occluded vessels appear to be contracted and are definitely indurated. The artery and veins may be bound into a rather firm cord so that the vessels can be separated only with difficulty.

Microscopic changes. The lumen is occluded by a thrombus in which Langhans-typed giant cells are not rarely seen at the early phase. The internal elastic lamina is

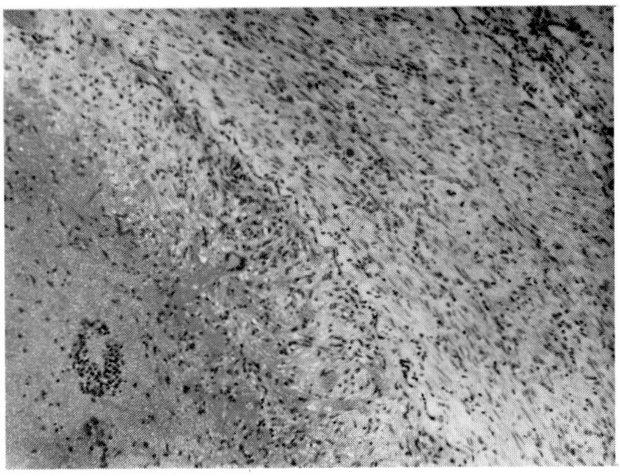

Fig. 3. Acute lesion of thromboangiitis obliterans of the brachial artery. Left lower corner is the lumen and right upper corner is the adventitia. The lesion shows panangiitis and there are a giant cell and collection of leukocytes in the margin of the organizing thrombus. (Hematoxylin and eosin. Original magnification ×125.)

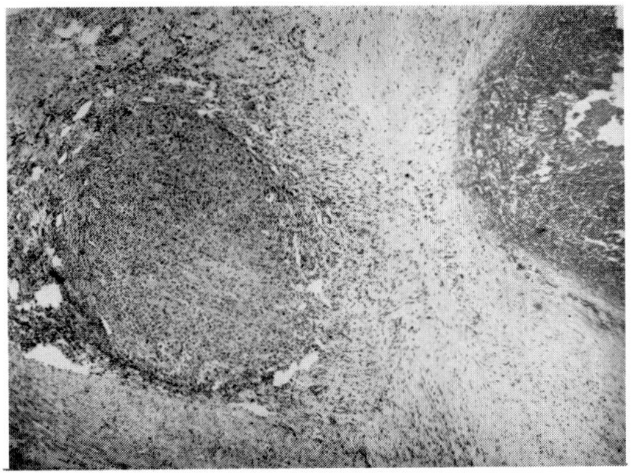

Fig. 4. On the right is the popliteal artery, and on the left is its branch artery. The former is occluded by fresh thrombus, and the latter is occluded by organizing thrombus. The branch artery shows moderately advanced lesions of thromboangiitis obliterans. (Hematoxylin and eosin. Original magnification ×50.)

relatively preserved, and marked proliferation of the intimal cells is noticed. The media contains fibroblasts and dilated capillaries, but the muscle fibers are usually well preserved.

In the adventitia, extensive fibroblastic proliferation and foci of lymphocytes appear around the vasa vasorum. Advanced lesions are characterized by minor canalization of the thrombus and an increased amount of fibrous tissue, but the general architecture of the vessel is preserved in old lesions.

Our knowledge concerning the early lesions of the arteries is limited by the fact that tissue is not usually available until the lesions have been present for some time. However, the early lesions can be sometimes observed in the superficial arteries.

A 34-year-old man, who, seven years ago, underwent an amputation of the left thigh as the result of occlusion of the left femoral artery, experienced a painful swelling along the right brachial artery, and pulsation of the right radial artery later disappeared. About one month after the onset of the symptoms, biopsy of the right brachial artery revealed recent thrombus with evidence of beginning of organization and inflammatory cell infiltration in all the arterial layers. In the thrombus, collection of leukocytes, so-called microabscess, and a giant cell were recognized (Fig. 3). It was very interesting that the skin over the radial artery of this patient reddened and blackened. This finding seems to imply marked periarterial inflammation.

In contrast to arteriosclerosis obliterans or simple arterial thrombosis, the thrombus in Buerger's disease is characterized by an early organization with intensive cellular infiltration. This phenomenon might be dependent upon activity of mesenchymal cells in the vessel wall, and it indicates a greater degree of inflammation of the vessel in the pathogenesis of Buerger's disease.

In Buerger's disease, little is known about where and how the process starts. A 34-year-old man sustained numbness, pain, and coldness of the left leg and cyanosis of the left toes three weeks previously. An arteriogram revealed a segmental occlusion of the left popliteal artery. The occluded segment was removed and autogenous vein was grafted. On serial histological sections of the specimen, the left popliteal artery was occluded by fresh thrombus, and its branch arteries were completely occluded by well-organized, more cellular thrombus accompanied by extensive cellular infiltration in the arterial walls (Fig. 4). These histologic findings sug-

Table II. *Follow-up results of eight thromboendarterectomies*

Site of procedure	No. of cases	No. of patent cases after operation 1st yr.	2nd yr.	3rd yr.
A. iliaca externa	3	1	1	1
A. femoralis–A. poplitea	1			
A. poplitea	3	2	1	1
A. radialis	1			

Table III. *Follow-up results of 17 bypass graftings*

Site of procedure	No. of cases	No. of patent cases after operation 1st yr.	2nd yr.	3rd yr.	4th yr.
A. iliaca externa–A. femoralis*	1	1	1	1	1
A. iliaca externa–A. poplitea	1	1	1		
A. iliaca externa–A. tibialis posterior	1				
A. femoralis–A. femoralis	1	1	1	1	
A. femoralis–A. poplitea	6	3	2	1	
A. femoralis–A. tibialis posterior	3	1			
A. femoralis–A. tibialis anterior	1				
A. femoralis–A. dorsalis pedis	1				
A. femoralis–A. femoralis (crossover)	1				
A. poplitea–A. peronea	1	1			

*All cases but one prosthetic grafting were autogenous vein bypass grafts.

gest that the process originated in the branch arteries of the popliteal artery and it then ascended. As a rule, when the thrombotic obliterative process reaches the medium-sized arteries, such as the anterior tibial, posterior tibial, radial or ulnar artery, ischemic symptoms in the extremities manifest themselves.

Thromboangiitis obliterans is primarily a disease of the blood vessels of the extremities. Typical lesions outside of the extremities are very rare and doubtful. Coronary and cerebral atherosclerosis or mesenteric arterial thrombosis have been reported in association with Buerger's disease.[1] Controversy continues as to the possible coexistence of Buerger's disease and arteriosclerosis. One aspect of many theories of atherogenesis is related to the hypothesis that there may be a defect in removal from the artery of plasma constituents or an increase in insudation from the blood stream, namely, a disturbance of perfusion in the arterial wall.[3]

Our autopsied case with Buerger's disease showed atheromatous changes of the coronary artery and abdominal aorta and slight cellular thickening of the intima in the visceral arteries.[11] It is evident that the aorta or visceral arteries of the patients with Buerger's disease are also susceptible to arteriosclerotic process.

TREATMENT

Although a procedure which arrests the progress of Buerger's disease can not be available, the response to tobacco abstentation is specific, and the treatment of Buerger's disease has, as its cornerstone, avoidance of tobacco.

As a procedure which produces vasodilatation, sympathectomy for Buerger's disease has been widely employed for relief of vasospasm, although it is agreed that no significant alteration occurs in muscle circulation after operation.[7] We prefer to perform lumbar sympathectomy during the time of reconstructive operation of the leg arteries with the expectation that there may be an increase in arterial flow through the revascularized segment as the result of a reduction in peripheral resistance.

Follow-up results of 57 lumbar sympathectomies were as follows: improved in 71.4 percent, same in 12.5 percent, and worse in 16.1 percent.

At the present time, direct arterial surgery is rarely feasible for patients with Buerger's disease, because of diffuse occlusion of the small vessels distal to the popliteal or brachial artery.

In our series of 100 patients with Buerger's disease, eight thromboendarterectomies and 17 bypass graftings were performed. As indicated in Tables II and III, as a whole, only five cases were patent at the end of three years.

About the postoperative administration of anticoagulant, there are widely divergent opinions.[12] We prefer to employ a combination consisting of heparin, low molecular dextran, and urokinase for one to two weeks postoperatively, in order to avoid early thrombotic occlusion of revascularized segments. However, it should be not forgotten that postoperative anticoagulant or fibrinolytic therapy will not salvage a poorly constructed vascular surgery.

REFERENCES

1. Asang, E., and Mittelmeier, H.: Die systematisierte Endangiitis obliterans (Zugleich ein Beirag zur Pathogenese der Arteriosklerose), Arch. Kreisl. **26:** 143, 1957.
2. Barker, N. W.: The case for retention of the diagnostic category "thromboangiitis obliterans," Circulation **25:** 1, 1962.
3. Doerr, W.: Perfusionstheorie der Arteriosklerose, Stuttgart, 1963, Thieme.
4. Gore, I., and Burrows, S.: A reconsideration of the pathogenesis of Buerger's disease, Am. J. Clin. Pathol. **29:** 319, 1958.
5. Hirai, M., and Shionoya, S.: Buerger's disease and insufficiency of muscle nutritive vessels, Med. Biol. **87:** 35, 1973.
6. Hirai, M., Shionoya, S., Ban, I., Nakata, Y., Matsubara, J., and Suzuki, S.: The diagnostic significance of Xe-133 clearance method in obliterative arterial diseases, J. Jap. Coll. Angiol. **12:** 365, 1972.
7. Hoffmann, D. C., and Jepson, R. P.: Muscle blood flow and sympathectomy, Surg. Gynecol. Obstet. **127:** 12, 1968.
8. Lassen, N. A., Lindbjerg, J., and Munck, O.: Measurement of blood-flow through skeletal muscle by intramuscular injection of Xe-133, Lancet **1:** 686, 1964.
9. McKusick, V. A., Harris, W. S., Ottensen, O. E., Goodman, R. M., Shelley, W. M., and Bloodwell, R. D.: Buerger's disease: A distinct clinical and pathologic entity, J. A. M. A. **181:** 5, 1962.
10. Nielsen, P. E., Bell, G., Augustenborg, G., Paaske-Hansen, O., and Lassen, N. A.: Reduction in distal blood pressure by sympathetic nerve block in patients with occlusive arterial disease, Cardiovasc. Res. **7:** 577, 1973.
11. Shionoya, S., Nakata, Y., Kamiya, K., Murakami, M., Yasui, S., Mizutani, T., and Miyajima, T.: An autopsy case of Buerger's disease. With special reference to clinical observations and systemic vascular lesions, Jap. Circ. J. **34:** 932, 1970.
12. Slätis, P.: Reconstructive surgery in obliterative atherosclerosis of the lower extremities: Experience of anticoagulant therapy, Acta Chir. Scand. **130:** 199, 1965.
13. Wessler, S., Ming, S.-C., Gruewich, V., and Freiman, D. G.: A critical evaluation of Thromboangiitis obliterans: The case against Buerger's disease, N. Engl. J. Med. **262:** 1149, 1960.

Effect of atropine on basal and food-stimulated serum gastrin levels in man

Horst D. Becker, M.D., David D. Reeder, M.D., *and* **James C. Thompson, M.D.,**
Galveston, Texas

Truncal vagotomy is known to increase basal and food-stimulated serum gastrin levels. We have studied the effect of atropine given intravenously on fasting serum gastrin levels and on the gastrin response of food. Eight normal subjects without evidence of gastrointestinal disease were studied. Atropine administration resulted in a significant diminution in basal serum gastrin concentrations. Since this is the opposite effect of the one noted after vagotomy, it appears to be independent of the anticholinergic action of atropine. Atropine caused an augmented serum gastrin response to food, which may result from a decrease in the acid-inhibition capacity of the released antral gastrin or from antral distention.

From the Department of Surgery, The University of Texas Medical Branch, Galveston, Texas

THE RELATIVE importance of nervous and local factors in the physiologic control of the release of gastrin is not known. In previous studies, we found that electrical stimulation of the antral branches of the vagus nerve caused a brisk release of gastrin from the antrum.[2] Furthermore, we found that in patients with duodenal ulcer disease, truncal vagotomy caused a significant increase in basal serum gastrin levels.[1]

Atropine has been found uniformly to be an effective inhibitor of basal[3, 10] or gastrin-stimulated[3, 8, 10, 11] gastric secretion. Although a number of toxic side effects occur at high dosage, the main action of atropine is anticholinergic.[5] Its effect on gastrin release from the antrum, however, is not totally understood.

In the present studies, we determined the effect of intravenous atropine sulfate on basal or food-stimulated serum levels of gastrin in man. Serum gastrin concentrations were measured directly by radioimmunoassay.

MATERIALS AND METHODS

The studies were performed in eight healthy volunteers, age 26 to 31 years, without known gastrointestinal disease.

Studies on the effect of atropine on basal serum gastrin levels were performed after the subjects had fasted overnight. Two basal blood samples were taken for serum gastrin determination by radioimmunoassay. Atropine sulfate* was then injected intravenously (0.5 mg.) at 15 minute intervals for one hour. Further blood samples were obtained at intervals throughout the study.

This study was supported by a grant from the National Institutes of Health (AM 15241) and General Clinical Research Centers Branch, RR 00073 and by a grant from the John A. Hartford Foundation, Inc.

Accepted for publication March 1, 1974.

Reprint requests: James C. Thompson, M.D., Department of Surgery, The University of Texas Medical Branch, Galveston, Texas 77550.

*Eli Lilly & Co., Indianapolis, Ind.

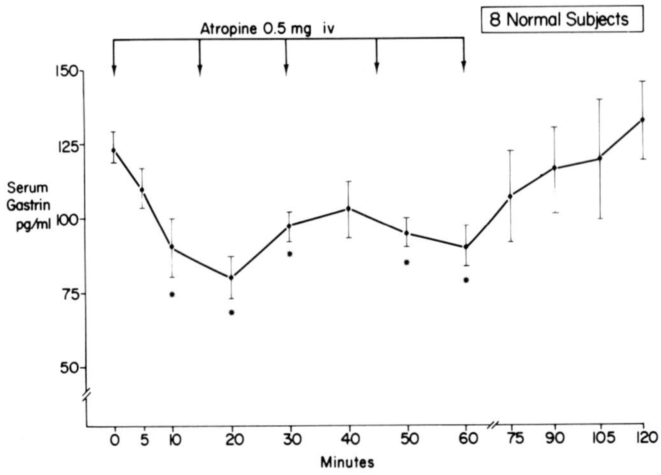

Fig. 1. Effect of intravenous atropine on fasting serum concentrations of gastrin. The level at zero time is the mean value of two basal samples. Asterisks identify values significantly lower than basal ($p < 0.05$).

The studies on the effect of atropine on food-stimulated serum gastrin levels were performed on separate days, and the sequence of control and test studies was alternated randomly. On the control day, each subject was given a 500 ml. liquid meal containing 52 Gm. of protein, 7 Gm. of fat, and 150 Gm. of carbohydrate. Blood samples for gastrin measurement were obtained in the basal state and at intervals for 150 minutes after the meal. On the day of the test study, this protocol was repeated, and additionally, 0.5 mg. of atropine sulfate* was injected intravenously at 10, 30, and 60 minutes after ingestion of the meal.

Gastrin concentrations in the serum were measured by radioimmunoassay. The technique used in our laboratory has been described previously.[9] Antibodies against gastrin were prepared in rabbits with synthetic human gastrin (residues 2 to 17) conjugated to bovine albumin used as immunogen. Synthetic human gastrin I was radioiodinated by means of the technique of Greenwood and associates.[6] The radioimmunoassay employs the double-antibody system described by Odell and co-workers.[14]

The results of these measurements are expressed as the serum concentration of gastrin at any given time or as the integrated gastrin response over the 150 minute test period.[16] Integrated gastrin is expressed as nanogram-minutes per milliliter (ng.-min./ml.). Comparison of serum gastrin concentrations and rates of gastric secretion in the various groups were made by the Student t test analysis. Differences with p values of less than 0.05 were considered to be significant.

*Eli Lilly & Co., Indianapolis, Ind.

RESULTS

In the study on the effect of atropine on basal gastrin, the mean basal serum gastrin level in these eight healthy volunteers was 121 ± 8 pg. (picograms) per milliliter (Fig. 1). Intravenous injection of atropine sulfate caused a significant decrease in serum gastrin concentration to a low of 80 ± 8 pg. per milliliter at 20 minutes after injection ($p < 0.02$). One hour after the last injection of atropine, serum gastrin concentration had returned to basal levels (132 ± 18 pg. per milliliter).

In the study of the effect of atropine on food-stimulated serum gastrin levels, the mean basal serum gastrin concentration was 117 ± 6 pg. per milliliter in the control study and 105 ± 5 pg. per milliliter in the test study (Fig. 2). The early serum gastrin response to food (i.e., during the first ten minutes) in the test studies was not signifi-

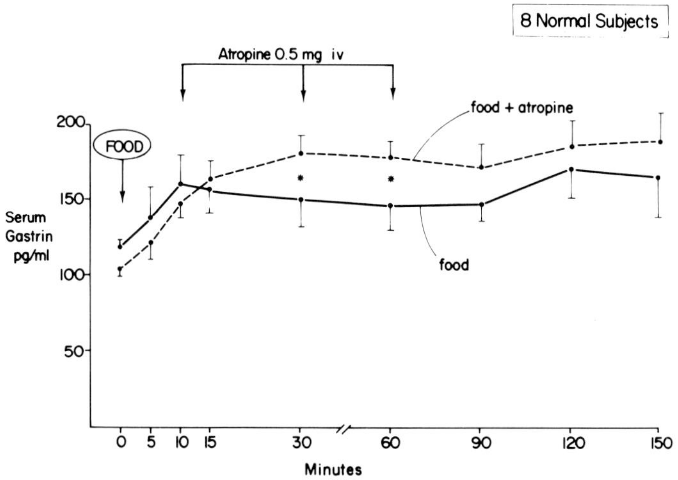

Fig. 2. Effect of intravenous atropine on the serum gastrin response to food. The level at zero time is the mean value of two basal samples. Asterisks identify times at which gastrin values were significantly augmented by atropine (as compared with control study, food alone).

cantly different from control studies; the test studies showed a 41 percent rise, and the control studies showed a 38 percent rise. After atropine administration, gastrin levels were consistently higher than those of the control study, e.g., at 30 minutes, gastrin was 181 ± 24 pg. per milliliter in the test study and 149 ± 21 pg. per milliliter in the control study, ($p < 0.05$). The 150 minute integrated serum gastrin response to the standard meal (Table I) was significantly higher when atropine was given (11.64 ± 1.97 ng.-min. per milliliter) than on the control day (5.97 ± 1.21 ng.-min. per milliliter).

Table I. *Effect of intravenous atropine on food-stimulated serum, gastrin levels in eight normal subjects (Integrated gastrin response measured for 150 minutes after food)*

	Basal serum gastrin (pg./ml.)	*Serum gastrin 60 min. after food intake (pg./ml.)*	*Integrated gastrin response to food (ng.-min./ml.)*
Food	117 ± 6	146 ± 16	5.97 ± 1.21
Food + atropine	105 ± 5	179 ± 14 $p < 0.05$	11.64 ± 1.97 $p < 0.05$

DISCUSSION

The results of the present study indicate that atropine significantly depresses basal levels of serum gastrin in normal man. The mechanism of this depression may involve a diminution in the tonic release or an increase in the catabolism of gastrin. Our studies do not allow us to choose between these two possibilities. Since it is well known that atropine reduces basal acid secretion in man, it might be expected that the lack of acid inhibition of the antrum would result in an increase in basal serum gastrin. Our results seem to indicate that this potential is overcome by the inhibitory effect of atropine. Since vagotomy, in man, causes an increase in basal gastrin levels,[1, 15] this action of atropine appears to be independent of its anticholinergic effects.

In previous studies somewhat different results have been reported. Korman and associates[12] reported that a single intramuscular injection of 0.6 mg. of atropine caused no significant change of basal serum gastrin levels. Walsh and colleagues[17] found no significant change of basal gastrin concentration in five healthy men and three patients with duodenal ulcer disease after intramuscular injection of 1 mg. of atropine. Nilsson and associates[13] found a small decrease of basal serum gastrin concentration in dogs after the intravenous injection of 1.25 mg. of atropine. A possible explanation for these controversial results are the different dosages used and the different kind of application; it is possible that with the lower dosages and intramuscular injection, locally ineffective concentrations of atropine were obtained at the antrum.

Atropine significantly increases the gastrin response to food. When atropine was given together with the test meal, the gastrin output was nearly doubled. These results confirm studies previously reported.[4, 12, 13, 17] Since it is known that atropine strongly inhibits the secretory response to endogenous gastrin by blocking the cholinergic synergism, a possible factor in this increased postprandial gastrin output may be the lack of acid inhibition. In addition, increased gastrin may be released as a result of antral distention and stasis after atropine. The possibility cannot be excluded, however, that gastrin release in response to food is partially mediated through an extracholinergic mechanism[7] and is, therefore, not affected by atropine.

REFERENCES

1. Becker, H. D., Reeder, D. D., and Thompson, J. C.: Effect of truncal vagotomy with pyloroplasty or with antrectomy on food-stimulated gastrin values in patients with duodenal ulcer, SURGERY **74:** 580, 1973.
2. Becker, H. D., Reeder, D. D., and Thompson, J. C.: Direct measurement of vagal release of gastrin, SURGERY **75:** 101, 1974.
3. Code, C. F., Hightower, N. C., and Hallenbeck, G. A.: Comparison of the effects of methantheline bormide (banthine) and atropine on the secretory responses of vagally innervated and vagally denervated gastric pouches, Gastroenterology **19:** 254, 1951.
4. Csendes, A., Walsh, J. A., and Grossman, M. I.: Effects of atropine and of antral acidification on gastrin release and acid secretion in response to insulin and feeding in dogs, Gastroenterology **63:** 257, 1972.
5. Ege, E. T.: Atropine, scopolamine and related compounds, Anesthesiology **23:** 365, 1962.
6. Greenwood, F. C., Hunter, W. M., and Glover, J. S.: The preparation of ^{131}I-labelled human growth hormone of high specific radioactivity, Biochem. J. **89:** 114, 1963.
7. Grossman, M. I.: How radioimmunoassay has added to our knowledge about gastrin, Metabolism, **22:** 1033, 1973.
8. Hirschowitz, B. T., and Sachs, G.: Atropine inhibition of insulin-histamine, and pentagastrin-stimulated gastric electrolyte and pepsin secretion in the dog, Gastroenterology **56:** 693, 1969.
9. Jackson, B. M., Reeder, D. D., and Thompson, J. C.: Dynamic characteristics of gastrin release, Am. J. Surg. **123:** 137, 1972.
10. Klein, E.: Gastric secretion. IV. The effect of atropine on the secretion of transplanted gastric pouches, Arch. Surg. **26:** 246, 1933.
11. Konturek, S. J., Olesby, J., and Wysocki, A.: Effect of atropine on gastric acid response to graded doses of pentagastrin and histamine in duodenal ulcer patients before and after vagotomy, Am. J. Dig. Dis. **13:** 792, 1968.
12. Korman, M. G., Soveny, C., and Hansky, J.: Serum gastrin in duodenal ulcer. Part I. Basal levels and effect of food and atropine, Gut **12:** 899, 1971.
13. Nilsson, G., Simon, J., Yalow, R. S., and Berson, S. A.: Plasma gastrin and gastric acid responses to sham feeding and feeding in dogs, Gastroenterology **63:** 51, 1972.
14. Odell, W. D., Rayford, P. L., and Ross, G. T.: Simplified, partially automated method for radioimmunoassay of human thyroid stimulating, growth, luteinizing and follicle stimulating hormones, J. Lab. Clin. Med. **70:** 973, 1967.
15. Stern, O. H., and Walsh, J. H.: Gastrin release in postoperative ulcer patients: Evidence for release of duodenal gastrin, Gastroenterology **64:** 363, 1973.
16. Thompson, J. C., Reeder, D. D., Bunchman, H. H., Becker, H. D., and Brandt, E. N.: Effect of secretin on circulating gastrin, Ann. Surg. **176:** 384, 1972.
17. Walsh, J. H., Yalow, R. S., and Berson, S. A.: The effect of atropine on plasma gastrin response to feeding, Gastroenterology **60:** 16, 1971.

Ureterosigmoid conduit urinary diversion

S. Martin Lindenauer, M.D., Joseph C. Cerny, M.D., *and* **George W. Morley, M.D.,**
Ann Arbor, Mich.

Supravesical urinary diversion by ureterosigmoid conduit was performed in 45 patients. In 41 patients, the procedure was done in conjunction with a total pelvic exenteration. The operative mortality rate was 2.2 percent. Renal complications occurred in 14 of the 45 patients. The ureterosigmoid conduit is the preferred method of urinary diversion in total pelvic exenteration since it shortens the operative procedure and eliminates a small bowel anastomosis. Because of the nature of the sigmoid mesentery, the conduit can be shorter in length and is more mobile. The larger sigmoid diameter significantly decreases cutaneous stoma problems. Conversion of an unsatisfactory ureterosigmoidostomy to an isolated sigmoid conduit is a very easy and highly satisfactory method of correcting the sepsis and electrolyte abnormalities frequently seen with ureterosigmoidostomy.

From the Department of Surgery, Section of General Surgery and Urology, and the Department of Obstetrics and Gynecology, University of Michigan Medical Center and Veterans Administration Hospital, Ann Arbor, Mich.

THE PERFECT means of supravesical urinary diversion has yet to be devised. The most successful method is the ureteroileal conduit described by Bricker[2] in 1950. The ureteroileal conduit has proved to be a reliable means of urinary diversion for a variety of urologic problems. Its use in total pelvic exenteration has made this operation clinically feasible.

The features which characterize the ideal form of supravesical urinary diversion are: (1) free drainage of the upper urinary tract; (2) minimal chance for stenosis at the ureterointestinal or intestinal-cutaneous junction; (3) low pressure efflux of urine from the conduit; (4) no ascending infection; (5) no electrolyte abnormalities; and (6) urinary continence. In general, the ureteroileal conduit has fulfilled these objectives reasonably well. However, it can be a lengthy and tedious procedure, particularly at the conclusion of a total pelvic exenteration. It seemed worthwhile, therefore, to consider alternate methods of urinary diversion in total pelvic exenteration, as well as for other urologic problems. A modification of the Bricker conduit utilizing an isolated segment of sigmoid colon has been described.[12-14] In our experience, the ureterosigmoid conduit provides all of the advantages of the ileal conduit and, in addition, does not require a small bowel anastomosis to restore intestinal continuity.

This report summarizes our experience with 45 patients in whom a ureterosigmoid conduit was constructed.

Accepted for publication March 11, 1974.

Reprint requests: S. M. Lindenauer, M.D., 2215 Fuller Rd., Ann Arbor, Mich. 48105.

CLINICAL MATERIAL

A total of 45 patients with ureterosigmoid conduit were studied. The patient's ages ranged from 12 years to 67 years; there were

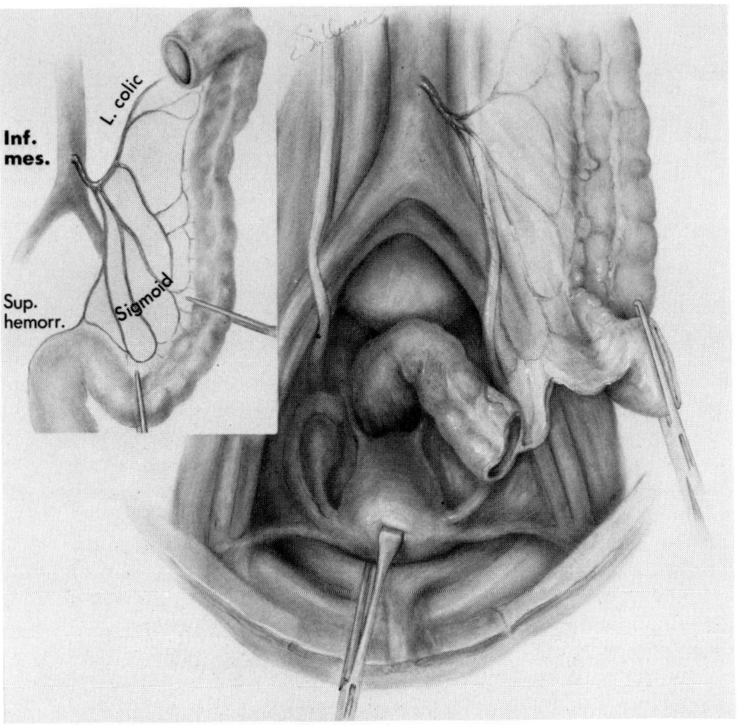

Fig. 1. Pelvic viscera in situ prior to exenteration. Branches of the inferior mesenteric artery *(Insert)*.

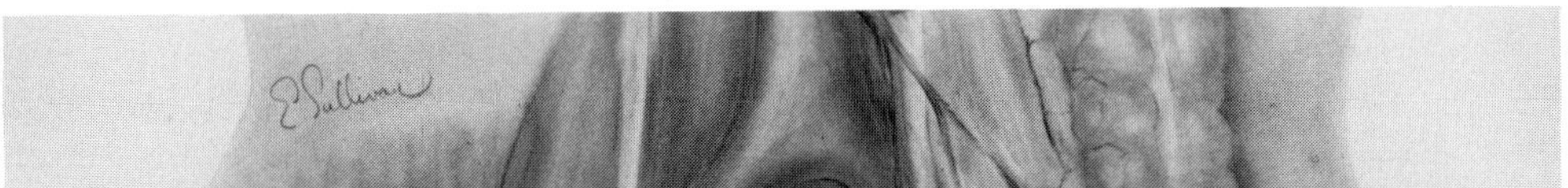

Fig. 2. Pelvis after exenteration illustrating distal ureters and 12 cm. segment of sigmoid colon selected for conduit.

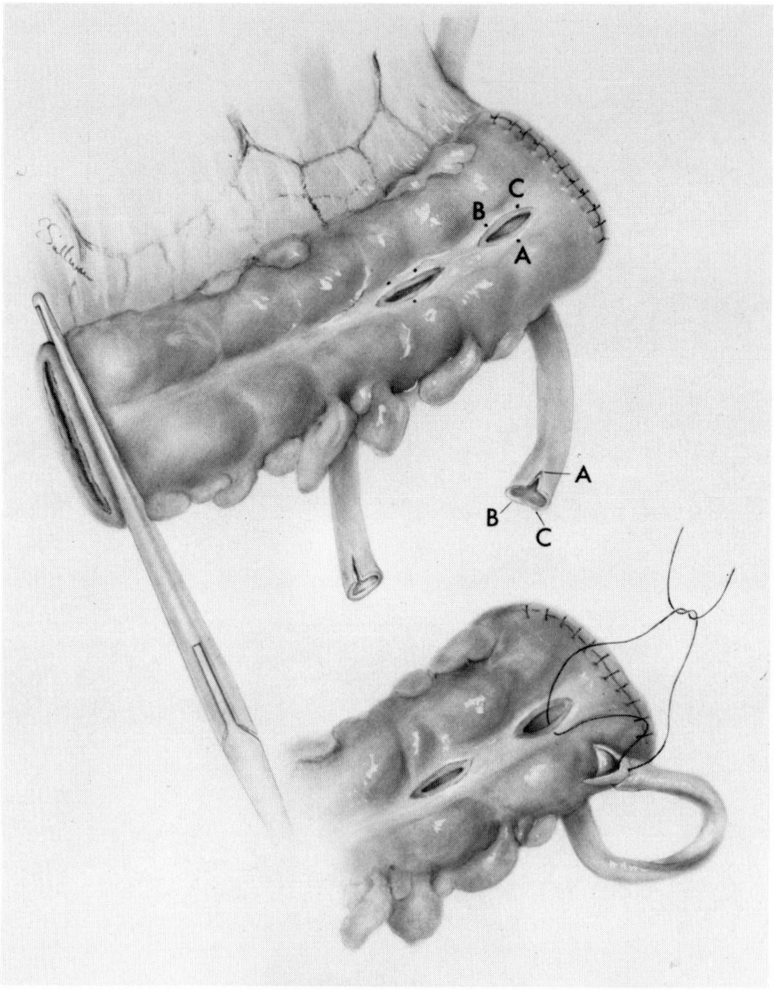

Fig. 3. Isolated sigmoid segment with proximal end closed. Note separate enterotomies for triangular one layer ureteral anastomoses. A = apex; B, C = base of triangular anastomosis.

42 females and three males. Forty-one patients underwent total pelvic exenteration. Forty of the 41 patients had previously undergone extensive radiation therapy to the pelvis with recurrence or persistence of their primary neoplasm. The primary lesion in the 41 patients was as follows: squamous cell carcinoma of the cervix, 33; adenocarcinoma of rectum, three; squamous cell carcinoma of the vagina, three; adenocarcinoma of the endometrium, two. Three other patients underwent conversion of a ureterosigmoidostomy to an isolated ureterosigmoid conduit because of persistent pyelonephritis, electrolyte abnormalities, and dilatation of the upper urinary tracts. A 12-year-old boy with progressive deterioration of the upper urinary tracts caused by congenital bladder neck and urethral obstruction also underwent ureterosigmoid conduit diversion.

OPERATIVE TECHNIQUE

A low transverse abdominal incision with the patient placed in the modified lithotomy or "ski position" is ideally suited for pelvic exenteration. Following removal of the pelvic viscera and iliac node dissection, the inferior vena cava is prophylactically plicated with staples to prevent major pulmonary embolism. The remainder of the sigmoid and left colon are mobilized to provide adequate length for the conduit. Occasionally, it is necessary to free the splenic flexure of the

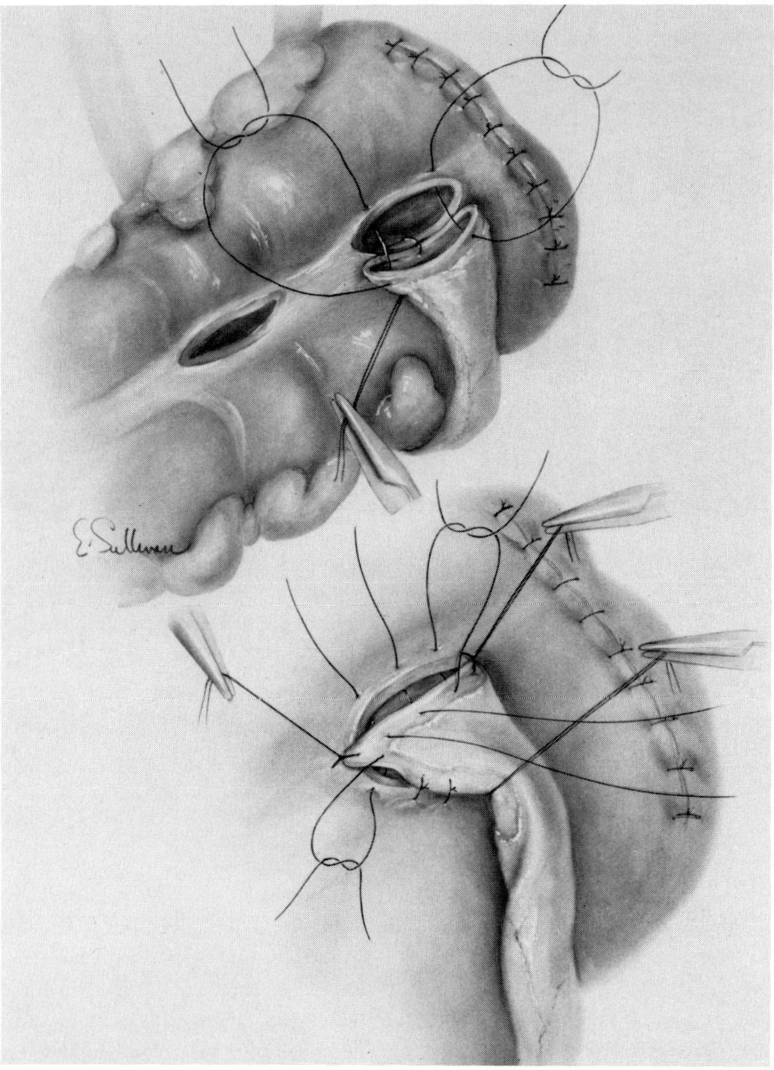

Fig. 4. Details of one-layer triangular ureterosigmoid anastomosis.

colon. This can be adequately performed through the lower abdominal transverse incision. A segment of proximal sigmoid colon or distal descending colon 12 to 15 cm. in length is chosen depending on the thickness of the abdominal wall. By means of transillumination, it is easy to ascertain the presence of two sigmoid artery branches to assure an adequate vascular supply to the conduit (Figs. 1 and 2). The colon is divided, and the proximal end which will become the left descending colostomy is laid aside. The proximal end of the sigmoid conduit is closed with continuous chromic catgut reinforced with interrupted silk. When the mesosigmoid is adequately divided, there is sufficient mobility to place the conduit in the right lower quadrant without tension and avoid possible impairment of its blood supply. The ureters are divided at the pelvic brim to avoid inclusion of previously radiated distal ureter. The ureters are dissected carefully to avoid undue trauma and to preserve the periureteral fascia. Their length is tailored to permit an anastomosis which is neither under tension nor redundant. The ureters are spatulated, and a 1 cm. incision is made in the conduit adjacent to the closed end, for separate anastomosis of the left and right ureters. A small "button" of sigmoid mucosa is exised to facilitate the anastomosis. A single-layer triangle anastomosis with interrupted No. 4-0 chromic catgut is performed with the use of full-thickness ureter and bowel wall with mucosal approximation and inversion of the edges (Figs. 3 and 4). Care must be exercised to include the ureteral fascia to avoid the sutures pulling out and subsequent leaks, etc. A grooved director and silver probe are sometimes useful to assure that the opposite side of the ureter or bowel are not inadvertently included in the sutures. Approximately 8 to 12 sutures are used if the ureters are not dilated. When both anastomosis are completed, they should be carefully inspected for defects. Areas of questionable viability cannot be tolerated and must be revised since most anastomotic problems are due to faulty blood supply. Anastomotic splints are unnecessary and potentially dangerous.

Proper placement of the conduit is essential. While it may be freely placed in either the right or left lower quadrants, the right lower quadrant is preferred. Ideally, the intraperitoneal portion of the conduit need not be more than 10 to 12 cm. in length. A 3 cm. diameter segment of skin fascia and peritoneum is excised, and the distal end of the conduit is drawn through the defect. The anterior fascia is sutured to the conduit to prevent retraction or herniation and the full-thickness conduit wall is anastomosed to the skin without eversion. The placement of the conduit stoma is carefully outlined preoperatively to provide a smooth, flat surrounding area of skin to allow reliable adherence of a urinary collecting device.

RESULTS

The 45 patients with ureterosigmoid conduit have been followed for an average of 1.7 years (three months to seven years). Thirty-three patients are living and well. Ten patients died of recurrent neoplasm; one patient died as the result of a second primary neoplasm; there was one operative death (2.2 percent) in a patient who died on the twenty-second postoperative day because of necrosis of the conduit, peritonitis, and renal failure.

Postoperative renal function was normal in 41 patients. Two patients had elevated serum creatinines (1.2 and 1.3) following revision of ureterosigmoid conduit strictures. Two patients with impaired renal function preoperatively had improved, but functioning was not normal postoperatively (creatinine, 1.4 and 1.6). Renal function in patients dying as the result of their neoplasm was normal prior to their death. Among the 45 patients, 44 had normal serum electrolytes postoperatively with no hyperchloremic acidosis. Three patients who had conversion of a ureterosigmoidostomy to an isolated ureterosigmoid conduit had hyperchloremic acidosis preoperatively. In two, the electrolyte pattern reverted to normal while one experienced a continuing but improved hyperchloremia.

All patients have been followed with postoperative excretory urograms at 3, 6, and 12 month intervals and then yearly thereafter. There were 86 renal units that could be evaluated (one postoperative death; two patients with solitary kidneys). Seventy-two

Table I. *Upper urinary tract (86 renal units)*

Preoperative	*Postoperative*	*No.*	*Percent*
Normal	Normal	65	76
Hydronephrosis	Normal or improved	9	10
Normal	Hydronephrosis	7	8
Hydronephrosis	Hydronephrosis	5	6

Table II. *Non-renal complications*

Complication	*No.*
Small bowel obstruction	9
Wound infection	4
Small bowel fistula	3
Pulmonary embolus	2
Thrombophlebitis	2
Hemolytic reaction	1
Pneumonitis	1
Postoperative hemorrhage	1
Pelvic abscess	1
Acute cholecystitis	1

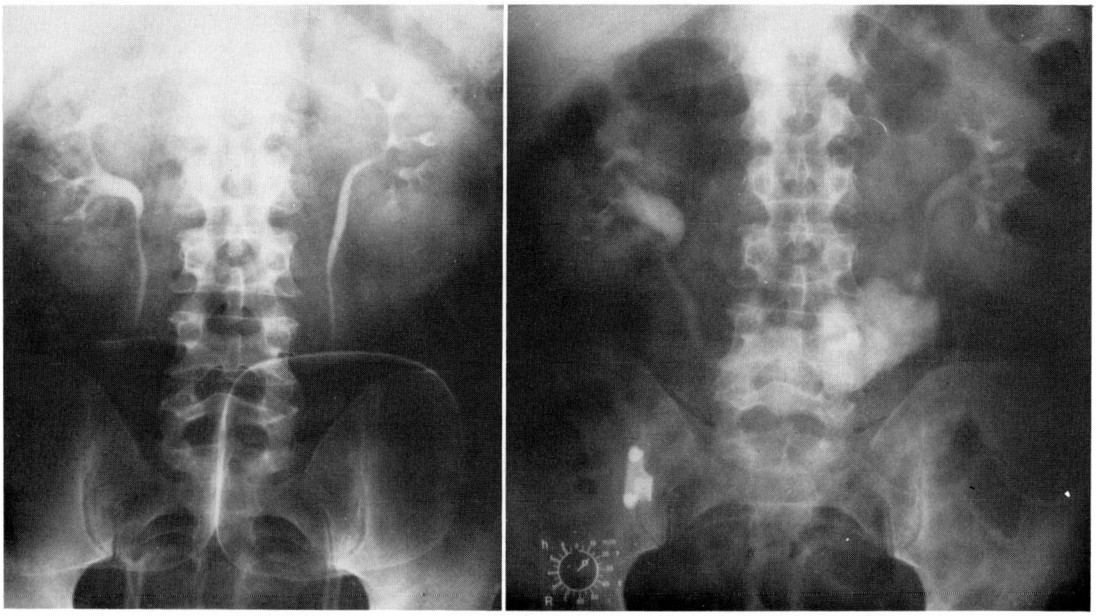

Fig. 5. Normal preoperative intravenous urogram *(left)* and essentially unchanged postoperative study *(right)*. Note short length of opacified sigmoid conduit.

Table III. *Renal complications*

Renal complications	*No.*	*Percent*
Pyelonephritis	9	20
Renal stones	3	6.6
Transient ureterosigmoid edema	2	4.4
High output renal failure	1	
Ureterosigmoid obstruction	2	2.3
Necrosis of conduit	1	
Stomal stenosis	0	

renal units were normal preoperatively and 90 percent of them (65 renal units) were normal postoperatively (Table I) (Figs. 5 and 6). Significant early and late complications occurred in 28 of the 45 patients. The non-renal complications are outlined in Table II. Two patients required reoperation for small bowel obstruction while seven were treated non-operatively. Two patients were reoperated upon to close a small bowel perineal fistula, and one patient was operated upon for control of postoperative bleeding. The remaining complications were managed non-operatively.

The renal complications are outlined in Table III. The incidence of pyelonephritis is similar to that reported by other authors.[4, 14, 18] The three patients with renal stones have remained asymptomatic. The two instances of obstruction at the ureterosigmoid junction occurred in one kidney in two patients. They both required surgical correction with subsequent improvement in the status of the upper urinary tracts. The one instance of necrosis of the conduit was due to a technical error early in our experience and resulted in the solitary operative death in the series. No patient experienced stenosis of the cutaneous stoma which is in marked contrast to the experience with ureteroileal conduits. There were no urinary leaks or fistulas in any patient.

In 44 patients studied, emptying of the conduit has been satisfactory. In most cases, excretory urograms were used to estimate conduit emptying time. In ten patients, contrast was placed directly in the conduit, and observed fluoroscopically. The length of time for emptying ranged from ten to 37 minutes. Fluoroscopically observed peristaltic activity, which ranged from poor to active, did not always correlate with the length of time required for the conduit to empty. In general, the degree of peristaltic activity observed

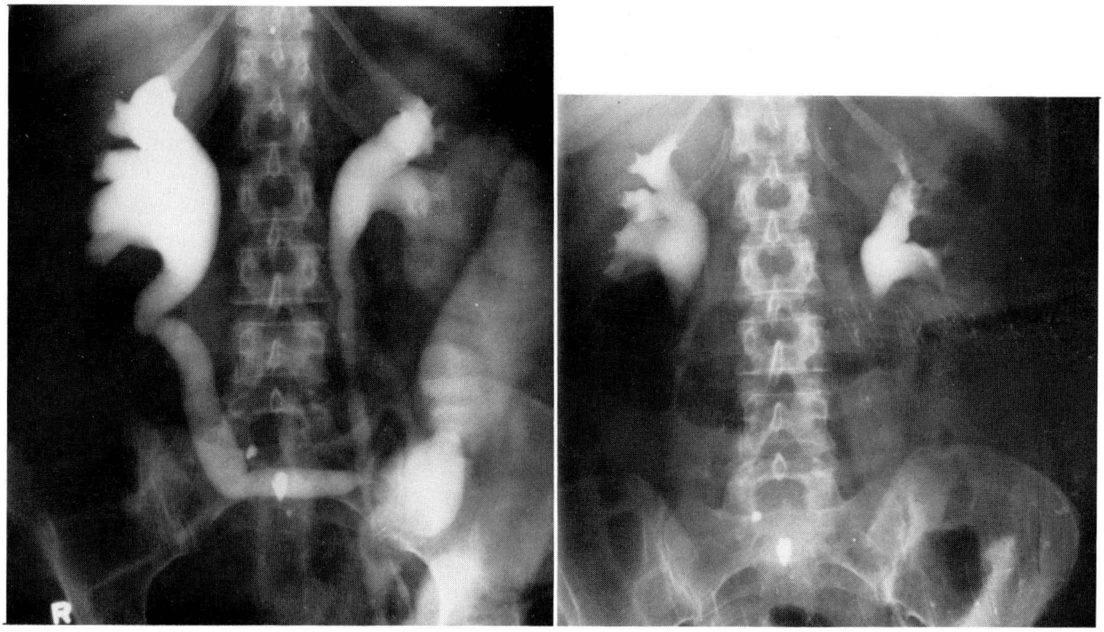

Fig. 6. Intravenous urogram in patient with ureterosigmoidostomy *(left)* converted to isolated ureterosigmoid conduit *(right)*. Note improvement in upper urinary tract.

was less than has been noted with uretero-ileal conduits. In all patients studied by contrast injection of the conduit, there was prompt reflux of contrast up both ureters except in the two instances of stricture at the ureterosigmoid junction. In the two patients with ureterosigmoid junction edema, the absence of reflux cleared within 48 hours.

Residual urine was studied in ten patients and ranged from 5 to 40 c.c.

Urine cultures from the conduit were generally positive and showed organisms present in quantities up to 100,000 colonies per cubic centimeter in asymptomatic patients while those with clinical pyelonephritis had positive cultures usually well in excess of 100,000 colonies per cubic centimeter.

DISCUSSION

The experience with ureterosigmoid conduit in this country is quite limited. Schmitz and associates[16] report the use of four sigmoid conduits in 40 patients requiring urinary diversion. Mattingly[9] describes his use of the sigmoid conduit, but does not record the number of cases. Rutledge and Burns[15] report the use of the sigmoid conduit in 16 patients out of a total of 97 requiring urinary diversion at the time of pelvic exenteration, and Mikuta and Murphy[10] discuss the use of the sigmoid conduit in four of 18 patients requiring urinary diversion. Recently, Kaplan and associates[8] described the use of the sigmoid conduit in eight patients requiring total pelvic exenteration and were pleased with the advantages of this type of urinary diversion. Symmonds and Gibbs[18] report a favorable experience with 26 sigmoid conduits and feel it is the preferred method of urinary diversion following total pelvic exenteration.

The ureterosigmoid conduit has received greater attention in Great Britain. Mogg[12-14] described the use of the sigmoid conduit in over 75 cases since 1952. Forty of his patients have been followed for over ten years. He has used the ureterosigmoid conduit in children with neurogenic bladders and in adults with vesical fistulas. He prefers the colon because it is thicker and feels it provides a safer anastomosis with less intraperitoneal manipulation and a smoother postoperative course. He has observed that the colon tends to distend and elongate less than the ileum and the long-term results are superior to those obtained with ureteroileal diversion. In his series, mortality with ureterosigmoid diversion has been nil and long-term complications are inferquent. Cook and associates[4] report the use of the sigmoid conduit in 17 children and note a much lower incidence of cutaneous stenosis.

The ureterosigmoid conduit, particularly when used with total pelvic exenteration, presents certain obvious advantages. The sigmoid mesentery allows considerable mobility, so that the conduit may be placed in either the right or left lower quadrants. The ureteral anastomosis to the sigmoid colon is technically quite satisfactory. The increased diameter of the colon allows a larger cutaneous stoma which is less prone to stricture. The sigmoid blood supply is somewhat less reliable than that of the ileum. This is not a problem if care is taken to include at least two arcades of sigmoidal arteries. The use of the sigmoid conduit in pelvic exenteration shortens the operative procedure by at least twenty to thirty minutes since a small bowel anastomosis and additional intraperitoneal manipulation are avoided. Furthermore, there is no potential for anastomotic complications in the ileum, and patients potentially may be alimented earlier since normal bowel function is likely to return more rapidly.

The significant number of postoperative complications reflect the magnitude of the operative procedure undertaken in heavily radiated patients with recurrent neoplasms. The renal complications, while significant, appear to be similar to those encountered by others with ureteroileal conduit diversions.[5, 7, 11] Cook and associates[4] noted a 20 percent early complication rate in both ileal and sigmoid conduits in children.

Symmonds and Gibbs[18] compared sigmoid conduit and ileal conduit urinary diversion in a group of 58 patients undergoing pelvic exenteration for recurrent pelvic neoplasms. The complications noted were entirely similar and were felt to be unrelated to the type of intestinal segment used for urinary diversion. In a comparison of ileal and colonic conduit urinary diversion in dogs, Spence and associates[17] found no major differences in terms of intravenous urograms, urine culture, renal tissue culture, ureteral reflux, residual urine, renal function, and serum electrolytes.

The results of sigmoid conduit urinary diversion noted in this study are similar. Postoperative renal function has been normal in all 41 patients who had a technically satisfactory result and who had normal renal function preoperatively. Only one patient had hyperchloremic acidosis postoperatively, and this was less than the hyperchloremia he had preoperatively. This is not surprising since Janknegt[6] noted that sodium chloride, potassium, and urea were absorbed less rapidly from the isolated sigmoid segment than from an isolated ileal segment in dogs.

The 20 percent incidence of pyelonephritis in this series compares to the 35 percent noted by Mogg and Syme[14] and the 15 percent noted by Symmonds and Gibbs[18] in patients with colonic conduits. The incidence of renal stones (6.6 percent) compares favorably to the five percent reported by Mogg and Syme[14] and the eight percent reported by Symmonds and Gibbs[18] in patients with colonic conduits. These results are similar to the incidence of pyelonephritis and renal stones in ileal conduits noted by Ellis and Hodges[5] and Minton and co-workers.[11]

Bricker,[2] in attempting to fashion a bladder substitute initially sought to devise an intra-abdominal urinary reservoir to allow the patient to be continent. However, he abandoned this concept in favor of an ileal conduit which he felt would peristalse satisfactorily, provide rapid emptying, avoid stasis of urine with subsequent bacterial overgrowth, and retrograde urinary infection. This concept has withstood the test of time rather well, and today the ureteroileal conduit is the preferred method of supravesical urinary diversion. The use of an isolated segment of colon theoretically could be less satisfactory because of diminished peristalsis and hence inadequate emptying with stasis and infection. However, when carefully examined, the peristaltic activity of isolated ileal conduits is less than expected.

Campbell and colleagues[3] studied 35 patients with ureteroileal conduits by means of cinefluoroscopy. The most frequent conduit activity was a churning, segmental, nonpropulsive, to and fro movement noted in 68 percent. Only 40 percent of the time was peristaltic or propulsive movements noted while in 23 percent only slight undulation was demonstrated with almost no peristaltic activity. A consistent finding in all cases in which any degree of peristalsis was observed was a complete lack of coordination between contraction of the ureters and the conduit.

Minton and associates[11] found that a spiking contractile pattern associated with vigorous peristaltic waves was most common but present in only 22 of 39 ureteroileal conduits studied (56 percent) Pressures ranged from 10 to 100 mm. Hg. Six conduits demonstrated frequent, rhythmic, weak, writhing, contractions with pressures of 3 to 15 mm. Hg, and 11 showed irregular, barely detectable contractions that were dysrhythmic with a pressure of only 1 to 10 mm. Hg. The latter two types were in general less satisfactory and associated with a higher incidence of urinary tract infection. They concluded, however, that the contractile pattern was not related to the length, configuration, or age of the conduit, nor to a history of previous irradiation, and they felt that loop contractility was unpredictable and due to inherent characteristics of the ileum which were extremely variable. Boyarsky and associates[1] studied ileal conduits and noted the same movements as in normal intact ileum: slow, rhythmic, churning, pendular movements; annular segmentation rings; and slow peristaltic movements with no rushes or antiperistaltic waves. The contractile patterns varied from hyperactive to almost no peristalsis except for slow writhing. They concluded that all of these forms of peristalsis were compatible with satisfactory conduit function.

Kafetsioulis and Swinney[7] found peristaltic contractions causing rapid propulsion of urine in ileal conduits in only 36 percent of 25 patients studied. The remainder had either ineffectual churning motions or minimal contractions with slow emptying. Also, there was no relationship between urinary infection and conduit-emptying time.

The emptying of the sigmoid conduits in this series was adequate. This is reflected in the minimal residual urines (5 to 40 c.c.) in patients tested and the low incidence of pyelonephritis. The peristaltic activity varied from poor to active but in general was less than in ileal conduits.

Kaplan and associates[8] noted residual urines of 7 to 36 c.c. and emptying times of 25 to 35 minutes in eight patients with ureterosigmoid conduits. The contraction pattern most often observed was regular contractions occurring every 1 to 1½ minutes and lasting 20 to 30 seconds with a force of 20 to 60 mm. of Hg.

Mogg and Syme[14] noted residual urines in sigmoid conduits of 10 to 40 c.c. and minimal urinary stasis in the absence of stomal obstruction. They noted peristaltic waves occurring every seven to ten minutes that were increased in frequency with greater urine flow. While peristaltic activity was felt to be less than in ileal conduits, it did not appear to adversely affect conduit function. Mogg and Syme[14] also state that some of their original sigmoid conduits were inserted in an anti-peristaltic fashion with no ill effects.

Thus, it would appear that propulsive peristaltic activity is present in ileal conduits only 36 to 56 percent of the time,[3, 7, 11] and the absence of peristalsis is not necessarily related to impaired function. The satisfactory utilization of the sigmoid colon as a ureterointestinal conduit despite its decreased peristaltic activity is consistent with these observations.

REFERENCES

1. Boyarsky, S., Kaplan, N., Martinez, J., and Elkin, M.: Cinefluorography of the urinary tract after ureter-ileostomy, J. Urol. **88:** 325, 1962.

2. Bricker, E. M.: Symposium on clinical surgery: Bladder substitution after pelvic evisceration, Surg. Clin. North Am. **30:** 1511, October 1950.
3. Campbell, J. E., Oliver, J. A., and McKay, D. E.: Dynamics of ileal conduits, Radiology **85:** 338, 1965.
4. Cook, R. C. M., Lister, J., and Zachary, R. B.: Operative management of the neurogenic bladder in children: Diversion through intestinal conduits, SURGERY **63:** 825, 1968.
5. Ellis, L. R., and Hodges, C. V.: Further clinical experience with intestinal segments for urinary diversion, J. Urol. **105:** 354, 1971.
6. Janknegt, R. A.: Absorption of urine products in jejunum, ileum, and sigmoid loops: A comparative study, Urol. Int. **22:** 435, 1967.
7. Kafetsioulis, A., and Swinney, J.: A study of the function of ileal conduits, Br. J. Urol. **42:** 33, 1970.
8. Kaplan, A. L., Hulme, G. W., Laskowski, T., and Calhoun, C. A.: The sigmoid conduit as a means of urinary diversion, South. Med. J. **60:** 688, 1967.
9. Mattingly, R. F.: Total pelvic evisceration, Clin. Obstet. Gynecol. **8:** 705, 1965.
10. Mikuta, J. J., and Murphy, J. J.: The team approach to pelvic exenteration for cervical cancer, Am. J. Obstet. Gynecol. **80:** 795, 1960.
11. Minton, J. P., Kiser, W. S., and Ketcham, A. S.: A study of the functional dynamics of ileal conduit urinary diversion with relationship to urinary infection, Surg. Gynecol. Obstet. **119:** 541, 1964.
12. Mogg, R. A.: Urinary diversion using the colonic conduit, Br. J. Urol. **39:** 687, 1967.
13. Mogg, R. A.: The treatment of urinary incontinence using the colonic conduit, J. Urol. **97:** 684, 1967.
14. Mogg, R. A., and Syme, R. R. A.: The results of urinary diversion using the colonic conduit, Br. J. Urol. **41:** 434, 1969.
15. Rutledge, F. M., and Burns, B. C.: Pelvic exenteration, Am. J. Obstet. Gynecol. **91:** 692, 1965.
16. Schmitz, R. L., et al.: Details of pelvic exenteration evolved during an experience with 75 cases, Am. J. Obstet. Gynecol. **8:** 43, 1960.
17. Spence, B., Esho, J., and Case, A.: Comparison of ileal and colonic conduit urinary diversions in dogs, J. Urol. **108:** 712, 1972.
18. Symmonds, R. E., and Gibbs, C. P.: Urinary diversion by way of sigmoid conduit, Surg. Gynecol. Obstet. **131:** 687, 1970.

Trends in the current management of primary hyperparathyroidism

Roderick C. Haff, Lieutenant Colonel, USAF, MC, *and* **Raymond G. Armstrong, Colonel, USAF, MC,** *Lackland Air Force Base, Texas*

Data were reviewed on 59 cases of primary hyperparathyroidism treated surgically at the Wilford Hall USAF Medical Center. As our series has progressed, several trends have appeared. The diagnosis of primary hyperparathyroidism is being made with increasing frequency and at an earlier stage in the disease, thus permitting earlier treatment. Chief cell hyperplasia has been recognized as the etiologic agent in this disease in 32 percent of the cases in our series, most of these appearing in the past 5½ years. We recently have adopted a policy of subtotal parathyroid resection in all cases, whether apparently due to hyperplasia or adenoma, with good success in avoiding recurrent hypercalcemia or permanent hypoparathyroidism.

From the Department of Surgery, Wilford Hall USAF Medical Center, Lackland Air Force Base, Texas

In recent years, surgeons have been called upon to manage increasing numbers of patients with primary hyperparathyroidism. Reports from a number of centers have shown a five- to tenfold increase in operations for this condition in the past five years.[6] This increase has been generated in large part by the introduction of routine screening techniques for serum calcium concentration.[9] Beyond this, however, is a generally increased awareness of the more subtle manifestations of hyperparathyroidism.

Associated with the increased frequency of diagnosis of primary hyperparathyroidism has been a change in the presenting symptoms of patients with this disease. Where earlier reports showed a predominance of complaints relating to bony resorption and renal calculi, more recent studies have shown a preponderance of neuromuscular and gastrointestinal symptoms, such as weakness, lethargy, mental deterioration, or abdominal pain of vague origin. Many of these complaints have been uncovered only by retrospective investigation after discovery of unsuspected hypercalcemia.

A third, and equally striking trend, has been the increased diagnosis of chief cell hyperplasia as the underlying pathologic entity in primary hyperparathyroidism. This condition was unknown prior to Cope's classic description in 1958.[5] Black[2] subsequently showed that the subtle differences between chief cell hyperplasia and parathyroid adenoma frequently defy detection by any technique short of electron miscroscopy. Because of this, many centers, including our own, have instituted a policy of subtotal parathyroid resection entailing removal of three to 3½ glands in all cases, regardless of gross and light microscopic appearance, in order to decrease the incidence of recurrent hypercalcemia.[8]

The current study was undertaken to ex-

Accepted for publication March 12, 1974.

Reprint requests to: Lt. Col. Roderick C. Haff, USAF, MC, General Surgery Service, Wilford Hall USAF Medical Center, Lackland AFB Texas 78236.

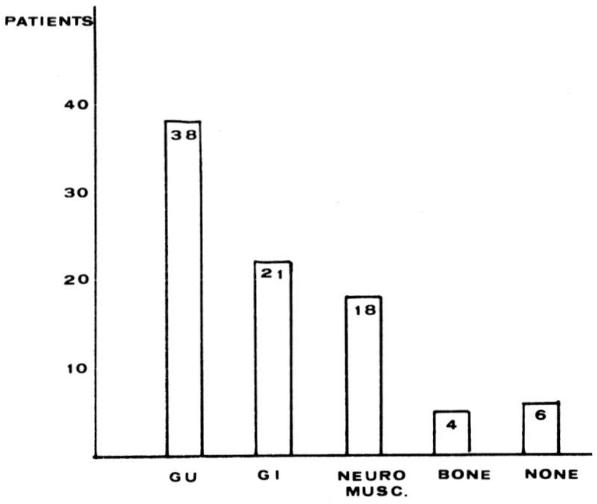

Fig. 1. Frequency of symptoms for the whole group. GU, urologic and GI, gastrointestinal.

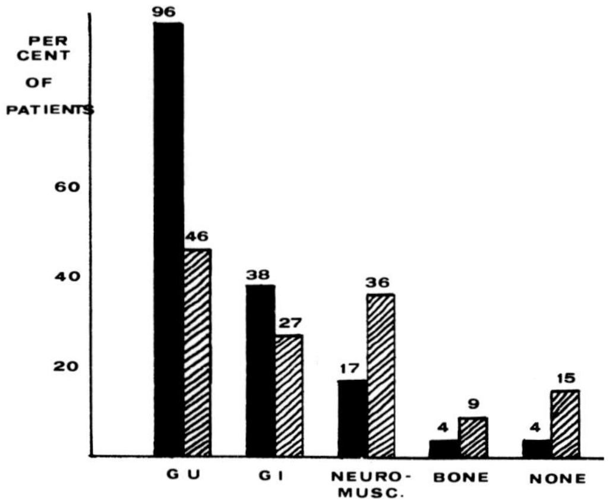

Fig. 2. Comparison of symptom frequency for the 1955 to 1967 group and the 1968 to 1973 group. Solid column, 1955 to 1967 group; striped column, 1968 to 1973 group.

Table I. *Pathologic diagnosis*

	Total group	*1958-1967*	*1968-1973*
Adenoma	38	18	20
Multiple adenoma	1	1	0
Chief cell hyperplasia	19	4	15
No pathologic diagnosis	1	1	0
Total	59	24	35

amine our own experience with primary hyperparathyroidism and to determine if these trends are manifested in that experience.

CLINICAL MATERIAL

The initial 24 cases of primary hyperparathyroidism operated upon at Wilford Hall USAF Medical Center were reported in 1968 by Evans and associates.[7] In the ensuing 5½ years, another 35 patients with this disease have been surgically treated in this institution. This study represents a compilation of data from both groups, obtained by reviewing the previously reported material and the clinical records of the last 35 patients. The 59 patients were managed over a 15 year period.

RESULTS

Fifty-nine patients underwent a total of 60 operations for primary hyperparathyroidism; thirty-two were male and 27 were female. Nineteen of our patients were 50 years of age or older at the time of surgery.

Fig. 1 shows the incidence of symptoms for the entire series. Patients presenting with urologic (GU) symptoms had either nephrolithiasis, nephrocalcinosis, or both. Those with gastrointestinal (GI) symptoms gave histories of either peptic ulcer, pancreatitis, constipation, or abdominal pain of undetermined origin. The neuromuscular problems included progressive lethargy, lassitude, depression, or muscular weakness. Bone signs or symptoms included either pain or subperiosteal resorption noted on x-ray films.

Fig. 2 compares the symptoms of the 35 patients operated upon more recently, with the group of 24 patients reported earlier.[7] As can be seen, the predominance of urologic symptoms, particularly nephrolithiasis, seen earlier, has decreased markedly in the more recent group, while neuromuscular symptoms have more than doubled in frequency. Further, the number of asymptomatic patients has now assumed greater significance. One of these latter patients was found to have hypercalcemia after hypocalcemic tetany was noted in her newborn daughter. Three others had significant family histories and were evaluated for this reason. A routine screening evaluation for serum

Table II. *Diagnosis, age, and symptoms*

Total group		Age (yr.)		Symptoms	
		50 or less	Over 50	No bone or GU	Bone or GU
Chief cell hyperplasia	15	10	5	8	7
Adenoma	20	11	9	9	11
Total	35	21	14	17	18

Table III. *Results of substotal and less than subtotal resections*

	Normal	Recurrent hypercalcemia	Hypocalcemia	Total
Chief cell hyperplasia				
Subtotal	8	1	2*	11
Less than 3 glands	3	2*	0	5
Adenoma				
Subtotal	10	0	0	10
Less than 3 glands	10	0	0	10

*One patient who had 2½ glands removed at an initial procedure, became permanently hypocalcemic after second operation in which a further gland was removed.

calcium concentration is not performed in our institution.

We use the operative technique of subtotal resection advocated by Ballinger and Haff.[1] All four glands are sought. If an apparent case of four-gland hyperplasia is encountered, a remnant of one gland near the size of a normal parathyroid is left in situ. If one large and three normal-sized glands are encountered, one normal-appearing gland is left untouched. If less than four glands are found, a remnant is left on the side where two have been discovered, and the opposite thyroid lobe and scalene fat pad are excised. Thus, subtotal resection implies removal of at least three parathyroid glands.

Table I lists the histologic diagnoses for the glands resected in this series. In comparing the earlier group with the more recent group, a marked increase in the incidence of chief cell hyperplasia was found in the latter.

In an attempt to determine whether or not chief cell hyperplasia and parathyroid adenoma represent points on the same continuum, with hyperplasia merely representing an earlier phase of the disease, data from the last 35 cases, relative to age and symptoms, were correlated in patients with these two diagnoses (Table II). An apparent increase in the number of older patients and of those with more advanced symptoms, such as nephrolithiasis and bone disease, is present in the patient group with adenoma. These differences are not statistically significant.

Data are not sufficient in the earlier group of patients to allow correlation of the influence of the number of glands excised with ultimate results. One patient with four normal biopsies had persistent hypercalcemia.

Table III relates the histologic diagnosis, operations performed (subtotal, as defined above, or less than subtotal) and recurrences in the more recent 35 patients in this series. All of the patients in this group have been followed at least six months after surgery, except for six who underwent operation within the past six months. Twenty patients have had subtotal parathyroid resections with one recurrence and one case of permanent postoperative hypocalcemia. Fifteen patients had less than three glands excised, and two had either persistent or recurrent hypercalcemia. One of these patients developed permanent hypocalcemia following a second procedure,

Table IV. *Trends in etiologic diagnosis*

Year	*Series*	*Adenoma (%)*		*Hyperplasia (%)*	*No. of cases*
		Single	*Multiple*		
1947	Norris[10]	94	6	0	322
1961	Black[2]	92	2.5	5	385
1958	Cope et al.[5]	76	5	11	206
1966	Cope[4]	77	1	15	343
1968	Schwarz and Hume[11]	65	6	19	52
1970	Black and Haff[3] Haff and Ballinger[8]	50	1	34	113
1973	Present series	65	2	32	59

during which one hyperplastic gland was excised. One patient, who underwent a subtotal parathyroid resection for obvious hyperplasia, has persistent hypoparathyroidism one year following his operation.

DISCUSSION

Our series mirrors well the current trends in the surgical management of primary hyperparathyroidism. The trend away from the diagnosis of this disease in its late stages is seen in the low numbers of patients with bone changes in our over-all series and, more particularly, in the striking decrease in the proportion of patients with urinary tract complaints in our more recent patients. This, coupled with the marked rise in the incidence of neuromuscular complaints seen in the latter group, is similar to the experience previously reported by one of us (R. H.)[8] The appearance of early, subtle symptoms of hypercalcemia in this series is due chiefly to an increased recognition of the clinical manifestations of hyperparathyroidism in its earlier stages, as we do not employ a routine serum calcium screening test.

It is of interest to speculate on the possibility that chief cell hyperplasia represents an early pathologic phase of a continuum culminating in parathyroid adenoma. The larger proportion of patients in our series with histologically demonstrable hyperplasia with early symptoms and under the age of 50, as opposed to those patients with adenomata, is suggestive in this regard. However, the differences represented are not statistically significant. Further, this theory does not address itself to the problem of recurrence, which seems to be the exclusive property of chief cell hyperplasia. We believe that the increasing incidence of chief cell hyperplasia seen in this series, as well as others, represents, rather, increasing recognition of a distinct and previously unknown entity.

Table IV compares our experience with several previous studies in which the increasing incidence of chief cell hyperplasia in primary hyperparathyroidism is shown. It is readily apparent that our series manifests the same marked increase in the recognition of chief cell hyperplasia seen by others in recent years. Based on this increase, we have come to accept Ballinger's policy of routine, subtotal parathyroid resection in all cases, regardless of gross or microscopic appearance.[1] The success of the subtotal resection is apparent in our series, with only one recurrence developing in eleven cases of verified chief cell hyperplasia so treated. We feel that this procedure will obviate persistent or recurrent disease in all cases save for those rare patients who have more than four glands and in whom the additional gland is diseased. We feel that our one recurrence in the subtotally resected group represents such a patient. The odds of such a case occurring are rare enough to demand individualized treatment.

The subtotal parathroid resection, when employed as a single operation, allows a much greater opportunity of avoiding postoperative hypoparathyroidism than does a repeat exploration. Only one of our 20 patients undergoing subtotal parathyroid resection developed persistent hypocalcemia. The only patient undergoing a second exploratory cervical operation for persistent hypercalcemia developed this complication. The anatomical distortion encountered at reoperation makes the meticulous dissection required to preserve the blood supply to the remaining parathyroid tissue difficult, if not impossible.

In conclusion, the approach to the management of our 59 patients with primary hyperparathyroidism matches the trends reported from other institutions. The number of surgically treated cases is markedly increasing. The disease is being diagnosed much earlier than was previously the case and the recognition of chief cell hyperplasia as a causative agent in primary hyperparathyroidism is increasing rapidly. With this recognition, the differentiation of adenoma from hyperplasia at the operating table has become tenuous. As a result, a policy of routine subtotal parathyroid resection in all cases, regardless of gross appearance, is being successfully and safely employed in an increasing number of cases.

REFERENCES

1. Ballinger, W. F., and Haff, R. C.: Hyperparathyroidism: Increased frequency of diagnosis, South. Med. J. **63:** 571, 1970.
2. Black, B. M.: Difficulties in the treatment of hyperparathyroidism, Surg. Clin. North Am. **43:** 1115, 1963.
3. Black, W. C., and Haff, R. C.: The surgical pathology of parathyroid chief cell hyperplasia, Am. J. Clin. Pathol. **53:** 565, 1970.
4. Cope, O.: The story of hyperparathyroidism at the Massachusetts General Hospital, N. Engl. J. Med. **274:** 1174, 1966.
5. Cope, O., Keynes, W. M., Roth, S. I., and Castleman, B.: Primary chief cell hyperplasia of parathyroid glands: New entity in surgery of hyperparathyroidism, Ann. Surg. **148:** 375, 1958.
6. Esselstyn, C. B., Jr., and Cribs, G., Jr.: Hyperparathyroidism—epidemic or endemic? Diagnosis and treatment, Cleve. Clin. Qt. **37:** 87, 1970.
7. Evans, W. E., Armstrong, R. G., and Dawson, R. G.: Hyperparathyroidism: Review of twenty-four cases, Am. J. Surg. **116:** 456, 1968.
8. Haff, R. C., and Ballinger, W. F.: Causes of recurrent hypercalcemia after parathyroidectomy for primary hyperparathyroidism, Ann. Surg. **173:** 984, 1971.
9. Haff, R. C., Black, W. C., and Ballinger, W. F.: Primary hyperparathyroidism: Changing clinical, surgical and pathologic aspects, Ann. Surg. **171:** 85, 1970.
10. Norris, E. H.: Collective review: Parathyroid adenoma—Study of 322 cases, Int. Abst. Surg. **84:** 1, 1947.
11. Schwarz, S. I., and Hume, D. M.: Thyroid and parathyroid, *in* Principles of surgery, ed. 1, New York, 1969, Blakiston Division, McGraw-Hill Book Co., pp. 1206-1369.

Increased gastrin release following penetrating central nervous system injury

John C. Bowen, M.D., *Houston, Texas,* **William H. Fleming, M.D.,** *Atlanta, Ga., and* **James C. Thompson, M.D.,** *Galveston, Texas*

Serum gastrin levels were determined by radioimmunoassay in 39 severely injured patients in Vietnam following either central nervous system (CNS) injury (16 patients) or non-CNS injury (23 patients). Serum gastrin was significantly higher ($p < 0.01$) after CNS injury than after non-CNS injury. Five patients with either penetrating cerebral or spinal cord injury had mean serum gastrin levels greater than 150 pg. per milliliter. There were no increased serum gastrin levels in the non-CNS injury group.

From the Division of Surgery, Walter Reed Army Institute of Research, Washington, D. C., and the Department of Surgery, University of Texas Medical Branch, Galveston, Texas

ACUTE gastroduodenal ulceration is a major problem in the postoperative management of the seriously injured patient. Despite numerous experimental and clinical investigations, the fundamental pathophysiology of this condition remains controversial. In an attempt to elucidate changes in gastric physiology that follow various types of trauma, we investigated serum gastrin levels after central nervous system (CNS) and non-CNS injury. The results of this study demonstrate a difference in the release of gastrin after certain types of CNS injury as compared to non-CNS injury and suggest that gastrin may play a role in the pathogenesis of CNS-related stress ulcer.

METHODS

The 2,720 patients who underwent major operations at the Twenty-fourth Evacuation Hospital in Long Binh, Vietnam, between Dec. 15, 1969, and June 30, 1970, were screened, after initial operation, by a member of the United States Army Medical Research Team to select those patients thought to be at high risk to develop stress ulcer. Patients were selected according to previously described criteria,[1] and, in addition, four patients with only closed-head injury were included in this study.

Serum gastrin concentrations were determined in 39 severely injured United States servicemen, ages 18 to 30 years. Sixteen patients had CNS injuries and 23 had non-CNS injuries. All CNS injury patients underwent either craniotomy or laminectomy for decompression and debridement and routinely received dexamethasone (usually 2 mg. every six hours) intravenously during the acute postoperative period. Patients with upper gastrointestinal injuries and patients who were not followed until convalescence or death were excluded from the study.

Initial serum gastrin values were obtained in 33 patients 12 to 48 hours after injury and determinations were repeated daily if

Accepted for publication March 12, 1974.

Reprint requests: Dr. Bowen, Program in Surgery, The University of Texas Medical School at Houston, Texas Medical Center, Houston, Texas 77025.

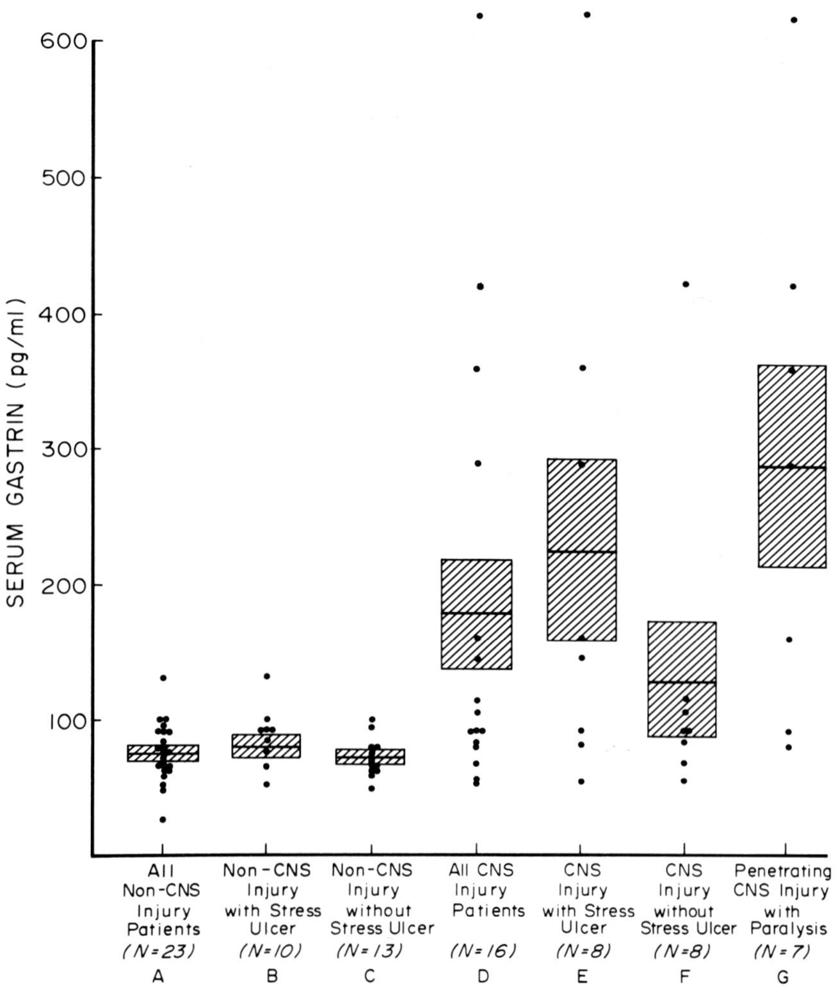

Fig. 1. Serum gastrin levels after CNS and non-CNS injury. The mean ± the standard error of the mean, represented by a horizontal line and hatched area, were calculated from mean serum gastrin values for each patient within the group. Statistical comparison of groups: A vs. D = $p < 0.01$; B vs. E = $p < 0.05$; E vs. F = N.S.; B vs. C = N.S.

gastric or duodenal bleeding occurred. The presence of any one of the following criteria were used to make the diagnosis of stress ulcer: (1) obvious hemorrhage via the nasogastric (NG) tube; (2) guaiac 4 plus NG aspirate on at least two occasions and, (3) gastric ulceration by gastroscopy.

Six patients (three with CNS injuries and three with non-CNS injuries) had only a single serum gastrin determination performed on blood drawn at the onset of stress ulcer bleeding. Fasting serum samples were drawn under uniform conditions, rapidly frozen, and later transported frozen to the United States, where all samples were measured simultaneously for gastrin by radioimmunoassay.

Radioimmunoassay of gastrin. Antibodies against gastrin were obtained in rabbits with the use of synthetic human gastrin (residues 2 to 17), conjugated to bovine serum albumin. The radioimmunoassay utilizes the double-antibody system described by Odell et al.[11] In the assay, gastrin I is radioiodinated by means of the technique of Greenwood and Hunter.[5] Additional details of the gastrin radioimmunoassay are described elsewhere.[7] Serum gastrin values are

Table I. *CNS injury patients with mean serum gastrin levels greater than 150 pg. per milliliter*

Patient	*Mean serum gastrin (pg./ml.)*	*No. of specimens*	*Stress ulcer*	*Injury and deficit*	*Associated injuries*
C. B.	362	3	Yes	Penetrating, cerebral right hemiparesis, decerebrate	Retroperitoneal hematoma and extremity wounds
L. D.	621	2	Yes	Penetrating, spinal, T-6 paraplegia	None
I. G.	162	3	Yes	Penetrating, cerebral and spinal, C-4 quadraplegia, decerebrate	None
H. G.	290	1	Yes	Penetrating, spinal, L-4 paraplegia	Intra-abdominal wound
H. P.	424	7	No	Penetrating, spinal, T-10 paraplegia	None

Table II. *Comparison of CNS- and non-CNS–related stress ulcers*

	CNS	*Non-CNS*
Location	Usually duodenal	Usually gastric
Gastric acidity	Increased	Normal or decreased
Mucosal barrier	Normal	Altered
Serum gastrin	May be increased	Normal

expressed as the mean concentrations (± 1 S.E.).

Student's t test for paired samples was used to determine the significance of differences between means of CNS and non-CNS injury groups. Differences with p values of less than 0.05 were considered significant.

RESULTS

The results are summarized in Fig. 1. The serum gastrin concentration was significantly higher after CNS injury than after non-CNS injury. Five patients with either penetrating cerebral or spinal cord injury had mean serum gastrin levels greater than 150 pg. per milliliter (Table I). In the non-CNS injury group, there were no increased serum gastrin levels. Although the data suggest that there may be a difference in serum gastrin levels between those with and without stress ulcer in the CNS injury group, the findings were not statistically significant. A single patient in the CNS injury group with consistently high serum gastrin levels (mean, 424 pg. per milliliter) did not develop evidence of upper gastrointestinal bleeding.

DISCUSSION

Because of the poorly understood pathophysiology of stress ulceration, acute upper gastrointestinal ulcerations occurring after all types of trauma have often been grouped together. However, several findings now suggest that the CNS-related stress ulcer is a distinct pathophysiological entity from the non-CNS related stress ulcer (Table II). Recent studies have demonstrated gastric acid hypersecretion after CNS injury in contrast to relatively low acid secretion after non-CNS injury.[10, 14, 15, 19] Stremple and coworkers[15] studied patients in Vietnam similar to ours and found that patients with only intra-abdominal injuries had very low initial outputs of gastric acid and, later, had lower mean acid outputs than patients with CNS injuries. Gordon and associates[4] studied alterations in gastric mucosal permeability and gastric acid secretion in patients with general surgical illness, patients with neurosurgical illness, and healthy male subjects. They found that patients with neurosurgical disease had normal gastric mucosal permeability and increased gastric acid secretion in contrast to the sickest group of general surgical patients who showed increased gastric mucosal permeability and normal gastric acid secretion. In addition, our study gives objective evidence of a physiological reaction, i.e., increased gastrin release, after CNS injury, that did not occur after non-CNS injury. Increased serum gastrin concentrations after CNS-related injuries may explain, at least in part, the increase in gastric acid secretion following CNS injury that has been found by other investigators.

Gastric hypersecretion and gastrin release after CNS injury is presumably mediated via the vagus nerves. The vagi directly influence gastric acid secretion by stimulation of the oxyntic glands and, indirectly, by the release of gastrin from the antral mucosa.[3] Release of gastrin by the vagus was first suggested by Uvnâs[17] in 1942 and, later, confirmed by Pe Thein and Schofield.[13] In recent experimental studies in dogs, Lanciault and co-workers[9] reported increases in immunoreactive gastrin, gastric acid secretion and gastric blood flow after electrical stimulation of the vagus nerve, and Orahood and colleagues[12] demonstrated a synergistic relationship between vagally released gastrin and cholinergic innervation of the oxyntic glands, suggesting that stimulation of gastric acid secretion by the vagus may be dependent, in part, on the concomitant release of gastrin by the vagus. Hansky and associates[6] found a serum gastrin response to insulin hypoglycemia in humans that was abolished by vagotomy. Our study demonstrates increased serum gastrin release in five of the 16 patients with CNS injury suggesting that the vagal release of gastrin has clinical significance in humans after some forms of CNS injury.

Since Cushing's[2] original suggestion of a relationship between CNS lesions and gastroduodenal ulceration in 1932, attention has been focused on the hypothalamus as the central neural control of gastric acid secretion. In this study, all serum gastrin levels greater than 150 pg. per milliliter occurred in patients with paralysis caused by penetrating CNS injuries; whereas, no elevations greater than 150 pg. per milliliter occurred after closed-head injuries without paralysis. Consistent with our findings, Watts and Clark[19] demonstrated higher gastric acid secretion in decerebrate comatose patients than in non-decerebrate comatose patients. Two of our five patients with elevated serum gastrin concentrations were decerebrate and all were at least partially paralyzed by penetrating cerebral or spinal cord injuries. However, it is interesting to note that three of the six CNS injury patients with elevated serum gastrin levels had only spinal cord injuries.

An important question raised by this study is whether or not the administration of dexamethasone may be responsible for the increased gastrin levels observed in five of the CNS injury patients. In a study by Watson and colleagues,[18] acute injections of hydrocortisone in anesthetized dogs caused no change in the level of serum gastrin in the antral venous blood; however, administration of hydrocortisone for five days caused an increase in Heidenhain pouch acid output, an increase in the basal levels of serum gastrin, and an increase in the gastrin response to a meal. At present, there is no information available on the effect of dexamethasone on serum gastrin levels in humans. In our study, all 16 CNS injury patients received dexamethasone and only five patients with severe penetrating injuries had hypergastrinemia. This suggests, but does not prove, that the type of injury, rather than the administration of steroids, caused an increase in the release of gastrin.

Gastrin release after CNS injury provides additional evidence that the pathogenesis of stress ulcers differs in patients with CNS injury as compared with non-CNS injured patients. In clinical studies of stress ulcer, it is important to clearly separate patients with these clinical entities. Although we cannot define the role of gastrin in CNS-related stress ulcers from this study, it suggests that gastrin may be involved in the genesis of CNS-related stress ulcers by potentiating direct vagal stimulation of the oxyntic glands to produce gastric acid hypersecretion. Further experimental and clinical studies will be necessary to determine the mechanism of gastrin release after CNS injury and the importance of hypergastrinemia in the pathophysiology of CNS-related stress ulcer.

REFERENCES

1. Bowen, J. C., and Fleming, W. H.: A prospective study of stress ulceration in Vietnam, South. Med. J. **67:** 156, 1974.
2. Cushing, H.: Peptic ulcers and interbrain, Surg. Gynecol. Obstet. **55:** 1, 1932.
3. Emas, S.: Vagal influences on gastric acid secretion, Scand. J. Gastroenterol. **8:** 1, 1973.
4. Gordon, M. J., Skillman, J. J., Zervas, N. T., and Silen, W.: Divergent nature of gastric mucosal permeability and gastric acid secretion in sick patients with general surgical and neurosurgical disease, Ann. Surg. **178:** 185, 1973.
5. Greenwood, F. C., and Hunter, W. M.: The preparation of ^{131}I-labeled human growth hormone of high specific radioactivity, Biochem. J. **89:** 114, 1963.
6. Hansky, J., Soveny, C., and Korman, M. D.: Role of the vagus in insulin-mediated gastrin release, Gastroenterology **63:** 387, 1972.
7. Jackson, B. M., Reeder, D. D., and Thompson, J. C.: Dynamic characteristics of gastrin release, Am. J. Surg. **123:** 137, 1972.
8. Korman, M. D., Soveny, C., and Hansky, J.: Radioimmunoassay of gastrin: The response of serum gastrin to insulin hypoglycemia, Scand. J. Gastroenterol. **6:** 71, 1971.
9. Lanciault, G., Adair, L. S., and Brooks, F. P.: Alterations in serum gastrin output in response to vagal stimulation in the isolated perfused stomach of the dog, Fed. Proc. **32:** 410, 1973.
10. McClelland, R. N., Shires, G. T., and Prager, M.: Gastric secretion and splanchnic blood flow studies in man following severe trauma and hemorrhagic shock, Am. J. Surg. **121:** 134, 1971.
11. Odell, W. D., Rayford, P. L., and Ross, G. T.: Simplified, partially automated method for radioimmunoassay of human thyroid-stimulation, growth luteinizing and follicle stimulating hormones, J. Lab. Clin. Med. **70:** 973, 1967.
12. Orahood, R. C., Beesley, W. H., Dutta, P., et al.: Gastrin release in vagally stimulated gastric acid secretion in dogs, Am. J. Surg. **125:** 39, 1973.
13. Pe Thein, M., and Schofield, B.: Release of gastrin from the pyloric antrum following vagal stimulation by sham feeding in dogs, J. Physiol. **148:** 291, 1959.
14. Robbins, R., Idjadi, F., and Stahl, H. W.: Studies of gastric secretion in stress patients, Ann. Surg. **175:** 555, 1972.
15. Stremple, J. F., Molot, M. D., McNamara, J. J., et al.: Posttraumatic gastric bleeding: Prospective gastric secretion composition, Arch. Surg. **105:** 177, 1972.
16. Stremple, J. F., Mori, H., Lev, R., et al.: The stress ulcer syndrome, Curr. Probl. Surg., April, 1973.
17. Uvnâs, B.: The part played by the pyloric region in the cephalic phase of gastric secretion, Acta Physiol. Scand. **4:** 1, 1942.
18. Watson, L. C., Reeder, D. D., and Thompson, J. C.: Effect of hydrocortisone on gastric secretion and serum gastrin in dogs, Surg. Forum **24:** 354, 1973.
19. Watts, C., and Clark, K.: Gastric acidity in the comatose patient, J. Neurosurg. **30:** 107, 1969.

Correction of coagulation in the hemophilic dog by transplantation of lymphatic tissue

Carl G. Groth, M.D., William E. Hathaway, M.D., Åke Gustafsson, M.D., W. Peter Geis, M.D., Charles W. Putnam, M.D., Christer Björkén, K. A. Porter, M.D., *London, England, and* **Thomas E. Starzl, M.D., Ph.D.,** *Denver, Colo.*

Available data concerning the non-hepatic source of plasma factor VIII are conflicting. In the present study, dogs with factor VIII deficiency hemophilia were transplanted with spleen or vascularized lymph node grafts obtained from normal donor dogs. Postoperative immunosuppression was done with azathioprine and heterologous antilymphocyte globulin. Four spleen transplants were successful and the recipients had positive technetium sulfide spleen scans along with adequate plasma factor VIII levels for three to eight weeks. Cessation of graft isotope uptake was accompanied by prompt disappearance of plasma factor in all four dogs. Histologically, the grafts were rejected at this time. In one dog, a second spleen graft immediately restored therapeutic factor VIII levels. Four lymph node transplants were successful and plasma factor VIII was detected for one, one, two, and ten weeks. Three dogs rejected their lymph node grafts with disappearance of factor VIII, while one had a viable transplant removed with loss of factor VIII within two days. The data suggest that factor VIII is produced in the lymphatic tissue of the dog.

From the Denver Veterans Administration Hospital, the Departments of Surgery and Pediatrics, Universary of Colorado School of Medicine, Denver, Colo., and the Department of Pathology, St. Mary's Hospital and Medical School, London, England

DATA PROVIDED by recent experiments with organ transplantation[10, 11, 19] has indicated a multiorgan site of synthesis of plasma antihemophilic factor (factor VIII). Thus, a major role of hepatic tissue in the process was established by the finding that transplantation of a normal liver into a hemophilic dog raised plasma factor VIII to an essentially normal level. But in the same studies, evidence of production of the antihemophilic factor in other organs was adduced by the observation that replacement of the liver in a normal dog with a hemophilic organ led to only a temporary decrease in plasma factor VIII. Available data concerning the nonhepatic source of the factor are conflicting. One group of investigators reported correction of hemophilia following splenic transplantation in dogs,[14, 17] but this finding could not be reproduced by others.[10-12, 19] In other canine experiments, transplantation of the kidney and the bone marrow were found not to cause detectable changes in the antihemophilic factor.[10, 19]

In the present study, canine hemophilic recipients of splenic or vascularized lymph node grafts were both found to maintain significant levels of plasma factor VIII. This result, in conjunction with the previous findings, indicates that canine antihemophilic

The work was supported by research grants from the Denver Veterans Administration; by grants AI-AM-08898 and AM-07772 from the National Institutes of Health; and by grants RR-00051 and RR-00069 from the General Clinical Research Centers Program of the Division of Research Resources, National Institutes of Health.

Accepted for publication March 12, 1974.

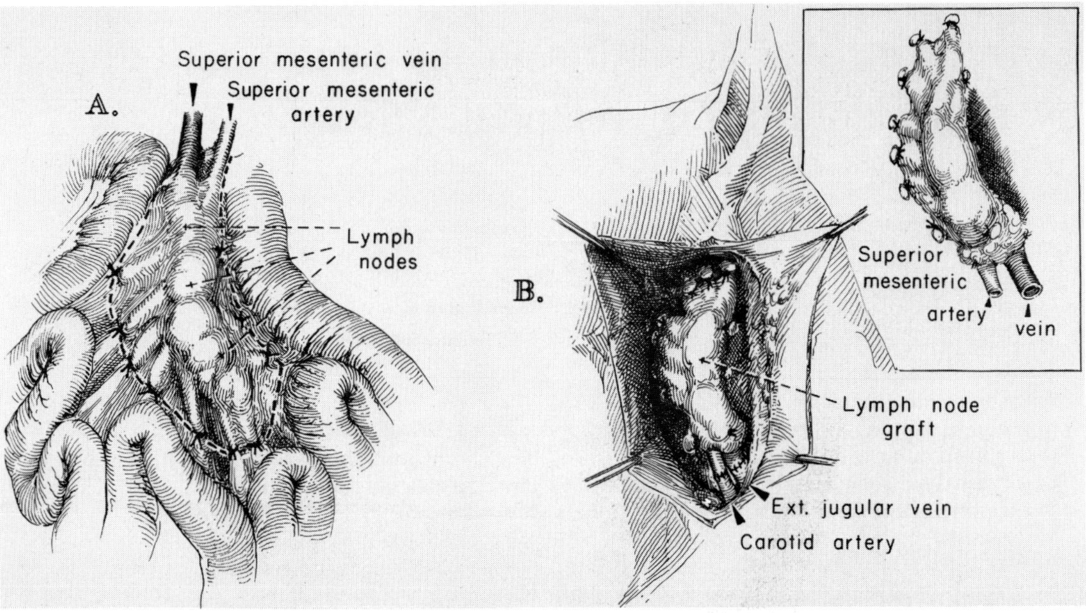

Fig. 1. Technique of vascularized lymph node transplantation. *A,* The root of the mesentery is dissected free from the small bowel in the donor, preserving the mesenteric vessels. *B,* The graft has been revascularized in the neck of the recipient. Vascular anastomoses are to the carotid artery and external jugular vein. The graft is placed in a subcutaneous pocket.

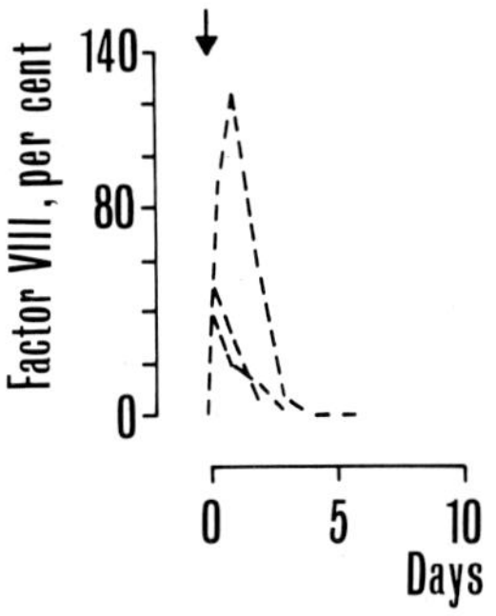

Fig. 2. Effect of plasma infusion on plasma factor VIII in three hemophilic dogs. In all instances, factor VIII returned to near zero in three days. One of the dogs received the immunosuppressive regimen used in the graft recipients but the effect of plasma infusion was not thereby prolonged.

factor is produced in tissues common to the liver, spleen, and lymph node.

METHODS

Eleven Labrador dogs with factor VIII deficiency hemophilia (four females and seven males, age 15 to 20 months, weighing 12 to 22 kilograms) were used.* All but two had had bleeding complications which ranged from simple surface hematomas to hemarthroses that had resulted in crippling arthritis. With blood drawing, the venipuncture site required prolonged compression. During observation in our laboratory for three to six months, plasma factor VIII was less than one percent when assayed on numerous occasions. Healthy, normal Labrador dogs served as graft donors; the animals were heparinized just prior to graft removal. The anesthetic agent was sodium pentobarbital supplemented with phencyclidine hydrochloride.

Whole organ splenic transplantation was achieved with vascular anastomoses to the

*The dogs were from the hemophilic colony developed by Dr. H. G. Downie of the Ontario Veterinary College, University of Guelph, Guelph, Ontario, by breeding which began in 1956. These dogs are not related to factor VIII–deficient dogs elsewhere in the United States or Canada. Pedigrees provided by Dr. F. Lotz of the Guelph Biomedical Science Department indicate a pattern of sex-linked inheritance identical to that seen in human classical hemophilia. The male dogs were hemizygous; the females were homozygous.

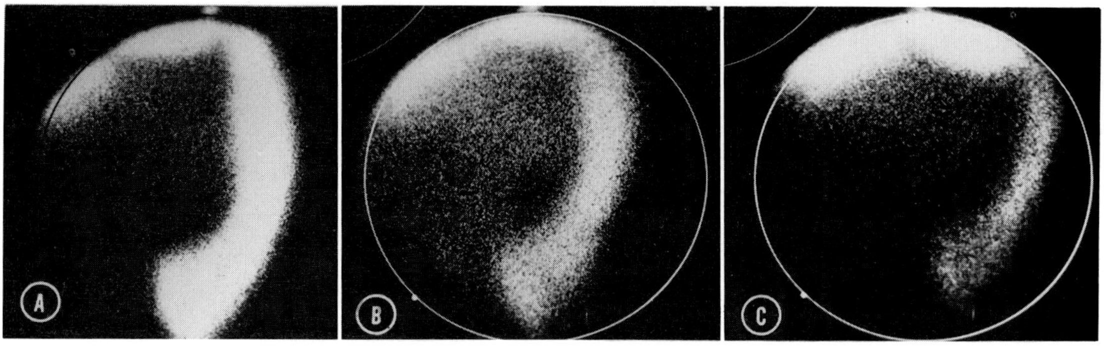

Fig. 3. Postoperative technetium disulfide scan in a splenic recipient (Dog No. 2). *A,* Eight days after transplantation. The graft which is visualized in the left lower abdomen shows an excellent uptake. The lower edge of the liver is also seen. The animal's own spleen was removed. *B* and *C,* Seventeen and 19 days after transplantation the uptake is decreasing rapidly. On day 21 the graft could no longer be visualized radiographically.

recipient iliac vessels as described previously.[9] Ischemia time for the grafts was 25 to 30 minutes. The recipient spleen was removed. Postoperatively, splenic graft function was assessed twice weekly by 99^{M}-technetium sulfide radioisotope scans.

Lymph node grafts were prepared from the root of the mesentery of the small bowel, preserving the superior mesenteric artery and vein (Fig. 1). In such a preparation, there are regularly two clusters of nodes, each having a size of approximately 1 by 1 by 5 cm. Revascularization in the recipient was done with end-to-end anastomosis of the mesenteric vessels to the carotid artery and external jugular vein. The graft was placed in a subcutaneous pocket in the neck (Fig. 1). Ischemia time was 21 to 33 minutes.

Prior to operation, each recipient dog was transfused with 25 ml. per kilogram of fresh, normal dog plasma. To prevent or reduce allergy-like transfusion reactions, intravenous hydrocortisone, 250 mg. was given simultaneously. Postoperative immunosuppression was achieved with a two-drug regimen. Azathioprine, 1 to 8 mg. per kilogram per day, was given orally; the daily dose was adjusted according to the peripheral white blood cell count. Horse antilymphocyte globulin (ALG) (leukoagglutinin titer 1:4000, cytotoxic titer 1:256), 10 mg. per kilogram per dose, was given subcutaneously daily for the first two postoperative weeks. The ALG was produced as described for the human material at our institution,[5] except that canine thymic lymphocytes were used for the immunization.

Factor VIII in citrated plasma samples was measured by the thromboplastin generation time assay of Pool and Robinson[15]; the normal reference plasma (100 percent activity) was pooled normal dog plasma. Unlike one-stage assays for factor VIII (partial thromboplastin time assays), this method is relatively insensitive to activated coagulation factors or traces of tissue thromboplastin or thrombin.[13] Assays for fibrinogen and factors II, V, and VII + X were done as previously described[6] with the use of pooled normal dog plasma as the normal standard. The whole blood clotting time, prothrombin time, thrombin time, euglobulin lysis time, platelet count, hematocrit, and total white cell count were performed by standard methods.

Biopsy and autopsy specimens from the grafts were stained with hematoxylin and eosin, methyl green pyronin, silver for reticulin, Weigert's for elastic, and periodic acid–Schiff reagent, and then they were examined by light microscopy.

RESULTS

Effect of plasma infusion and immunosuppression only. Infusion of fresh canine

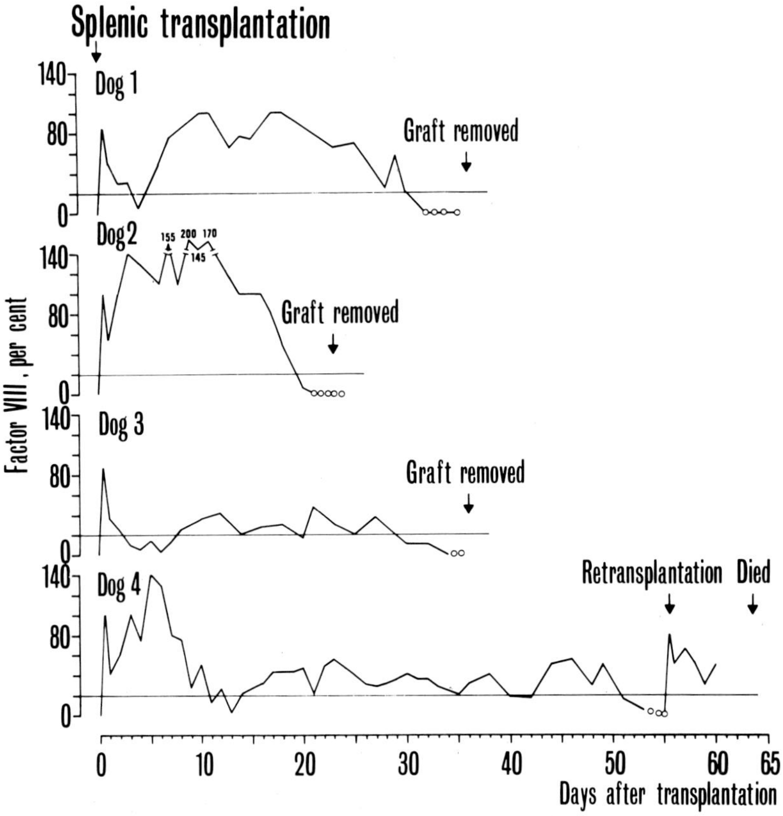

Fig. 4. Plasma factor VIII in four hemophilic dogs that received whole organ splenic grafts. The solid line denotes that there was isotope uptake on the splenic scan. The dotted line indicates that isotope uptake was no longer recorded. Horizontal lines mark the 20 percent level.

plasma, 25 ml. per kilogram, to three hemophilic dogs not undergoing concomitant transplantation caused a prompt rise in factor VIII. Maximum values recorded after transfusion were 40, 50, and 125 percent in the three dogs, respectively. Three days later the factor had returned to near zero in all instances (Fig. 2). One of the dogs was given the immunosuppressive regimen used in the graft recipients, starting at the day of transfusion. There was no apparent effect on the plasma factor VIII. The two other dogs were used as graft recipients six to eight weeks later.

Splenic transplantation. There were four hemophilic recipients of splenic transplants; one of the dogs received two consecutive grafts. Radioisotope scanning showed uptake in the grafts from the day of transplantation to day 28, 19, 32, and 50 after operation, respectively. During the last several days before disappearance of uptake, there was a gradual decline in the density of the radiological picture (Fig. 3). The dog (No. 4) in which the graft picture disappeared after 50 days, underwent retransplantation six days later. The second graft showed excellent isotope uptake, but the dog died nine days postoperatively with pneumonia.

On the day of transplantation, plasma factor VIII in the four *donor* dogs was 100, 40, 100, and 105 percent, respectively. In the recipients, preoperative antihemophilic factor was less than one percent in all instances. Postoperatively, an initial peak, caused by plasma infusion, was followed by a few days of wide fluctuations (Fig. 4). Following this, the plasma factor VIII was essentially normal during three to four weeks in two dogs (Nos. 1 and 2). In the other

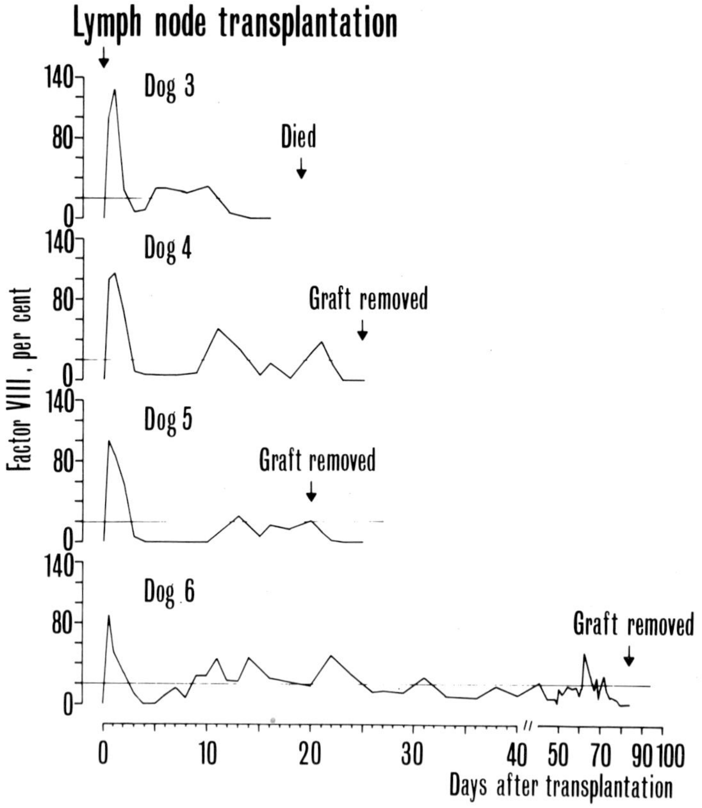

Fig. 5. Plasma factor VIII in four hemophilic dogs that recovered after receipt of a vascularized lymph node graft. Horizontal lines mark the 20 percent level.

two (Nos. 3 and 4) the level stabilized around 20 to 40 percent for four and eight weeks, respectively. There were no clinical clotting problems during or after surgery except that one dog (No. 4) had a brief period of wound bleeding 12 days after transplantation at a time when the factor was near zero. At the cessation of graft isotope uptake the plasma antihemophilic factor disappeared in all four dogs (Fig. 4). In the retransplanted dog, the provision of a second graft was again followed by a significant plasma level of factor VIII (Fig. 4).

On assay one week after transplantation, the previously prolonged clotting time was shortened to near normal. Several other clotting parameters studied were unaffected. The hematocrit and white blood cell count (WBC) had dropped moderately (Table I).

The four original splenic grafts were removed three to seven days after the cessation of their isotope uptake. Histologically, they showed end-stage rejection. There was necrosis of most of the lymphocytes in the white pulp; only a few large lymphoid cells with pyroninophilic cytoplasm survived immediately adjacent to the penicillary arterioles. The red pulp was necrotic and hemorrhagic, and there was fibrinoid necrosis of the walls of most of the arteries and arterioles.

At recipient death, nine days after retransplantation, the second graft of one dog (No. 4) showed a normal white pulp with abundant germinal centers, and a red pulp that was congested and filled with mononuclear cells possessing pyroninophilic cytoplasm. The arteries and arterioles were normal.

Lymph node transplantation. Six hemophilic dogs received vascularized lymph node grafts. In one dog, a severely congested graft was removed four days after transplantation; there was thrombosis at the venous anastomosis. Another recipient that had

Table I. *Hematological findings before and one week after splenic or lymph node transplantation (mean ± S.E. in the groups)**

	Splenic transplantation		Lymph node transplantation		
	Before	After	Before	After	Normal range
Whole blood clotting time (min.)	38 ± 10	13 ± 8	77 ± 25	24 ± 4	5–10
Prothrombin time (sec.)	7.5 ± 0.3	8.1 ± 0.3	7.8 ± 0.2	8.2 ± 0.3	6–7
Thrombin time (sec.)	9.1 ± 0.1	9.2 ± 0.3	9.0 ± 0.4	9.6 ± 0.5	7–9
Fibrinogen (mg./100 ml.)	571 ± 50	524 ± 23	604 ± 31	554 ± 46	400–600
Factor II (%)	95 ± 18	93 ± 5	93 ± 11	87 ± 7	70–100
Factor V (%)	125 ± 15	97 ± 3	115 ± 5	118 ± 2	70–100
Factor VII (%)	120 ± 19	111 ± 11	88 ± 15	85 ± 13	70–150
Platelets (1000/mm.^{3})	248 ± 75	198 ± 10	218 ± 44	194 ± 80	200–400
Euglobulin lysis time (min.)	122 ± 15	58 ± 13	123 ± 17	104 ± 33	90–300
Hematocrit (%)	41 ± 2	29 ± 3	42 ± 3	33 ± 2	—
White blood cell count (100/mm.^{3})	21.8 ± 3.0	14.0 ± 3.7	22.4 ± 3.1	14.1 ± 3.4	—

*Factor VIII depicted in Figs. 4 and 5.

operations on the first and second postoperative day because of bleeding from the graft site did not recover from anesthesia after the latter procedure. The other four dogs had an uneventful early postoperative course. Only these latter dogs will be discussed further.

On the day of transplantation, plasma factor VIII in the *donor* dogs used in the four technically successful experiments was 62, 100, 110, and 102 percent, respectively. Prior to transplantation, the antihemophilic factor was less than one percent in all recipient dogs. After operation, an initial peak caused by the plasma infusion was followed by a decline to levels around five percent except in one dog (No. 5) in which the level dropped to zero for several days (Fig. 5). At this time, there was a transient bleeding diathesis in this dog. Subsequently, factor VIII levels rose in every animal and then fluctuated between 10 and 40 percent. In one dog (No. 5), the graft was surgically removed 21 days after transplantation; in the next few days, the factor declined to less than one percent. In the other three dogs, the factor level was maintained between 10 and 40 percent for one, two, and ten weeks, respectively (Fig. 5).

There was a significant shortening in the previously prolonged clotting time on assay one week after transplantation. The findings in other clotting parameters and in hematocrit and WBC were similar to those found in the spleen transplant group (Table I).

Graft tissue was obtained on two different occasions when the recipient had circulating factor VIII; it was obtained in one dog (No. 6) by an open biopsy performed ten days after transplantation and in another (No. 5) when the whole graft was deliberately removed on the twenty-first postoperative day. Histologically, rejection was not apparent in the 10 day graft, which showed a normal cortex with many germinal centers and a normal paracortical zone and medulla. In the 21 day graft, rejection was occurring. The cortex contained fewer lymphocytes than normal and only occasional germinal centers, and there were a few focal areas of hemorrhagic necrosis. The paracortical zone was expanded and filled with a mass of lymphoid cells, many of them large and with pyroninophilic cytoplasm. Mitoses were frequent in this zone. The medulla contained many plasma cells.

Three lymph node transplants were examined three to seven days after plasma antihemophilic factor had returned to less than one percent. In one instance, the tissue became available at animal death 19 days after transplantation; in the two others the grafts were surgically removed. All showed marked rejection. In the two surgical specimens, the cortex was depleted of all lymphocytes, there were a few groups of large lymphoid cells with pyroninophilic cytoplasm in the paracortical zone, and the medulla contained some plasma cells. In the autopsy specimen, rejection was less advanced and small areas remained in which there were some cortical lymphoid cells, a prominent paracortical zone of pyroninophilic lymphoid cells, and abundant plasma cells in the medulla. In the two surgical specimens, the reticular cells survived and were the main cells in the cortex.

DISCUSSION

In 1967, Webster and colleagues[18] first reported on transplantation of the spleen in the hemophilic dog. Their animals were bred at the University of North Carolina, Chapel Hill, N. C. In this pioneer study, two recipient animals were found to have improved hemostasis and clotting tests for 52 and 72 hours after transplantation. More recently, the same investigators reported no sustained beneficial effect when studying similarly transplanted animals for weeks and months after operation.[19] They concluded that the role of the spleen is limited to the release of stored factor VIII as opposed to synthesis. Similar results were obtained by McKee and associates[12] and Marchioro and associates[10, 11]; both groups worked with dogs from the hemophilic beagle colony at Oklahoma State University, Stillwater, Okla. In McKee's series,[12] two spleen transplant recipients survived for seven and eight months, respectively; they displayed no postoperative rise in plasma factor VIII despite continuous and excellent isotope uptake by their grafts. Marchioro's group[11] reported on one dog in which the splenic graft remained viable as confirmed by biopsy for 93 days but with plasma antihemophilic factor levels never exceeding six percent.

In contrast to the findings of these investigators, Norman and associates[14] and Sise and co-workers[17] recorded significant levels of factor VIII in hemophilic canine recipients of splenic transplants which were also from the Oklahoma colony. This favorable finding was recorded in each of seven dogs and for a maximum length of 47 days after operation. Unfortunately, the use of normal human plasma as a reference in the factor VIII assay precluded a truly quantitative assessment of the degree of correction achieved in these experiments.

In the present study, therapeutic levels (exceeding 20 percent) of antihemophilic factor developed for at least three weeks in all recipients of splenic grafts, with the longest period being eight weeks. A close correlation between graft function and plasma factor VIII was indicated by the concomitant disappearance of radioisotope uptake in the graft and of the antihemophilic factor.

The reason for the discrepant findings with splenic transplantation in the hemophilic dog reported by different groups is obscure. The dogs used in the present study were from a different colony than those of the other investigators, but the sex-linked recessive pattern of our Guelph animals was the same. In our series, immunosuppression consisted of azathioprine in combination with antilymphocyte globulin while all earlier investigators used azathioprine and prednisone, but it seems unlikely that this difference affected the hematologic results.

The finding in the present study that the provision of a vascularized lymph node graft, as well as a splenic graft, was accompanied by a sustained increase in plasma factor VIII is evidence that lymphoreticuloendothelial tissue produces the factor. The initial lack of plasma antihemophilic factor in the lymph node recipients could be a reflection of a smaller storage capacity in this graft.

In 1971 Bouhasin and collaborators[2] reported a rise in plasma factor VIII in a hemophilic child that developed lymphoblastic leukemia and postulated a role of the lymphocyte in antihemophilic globulin production. Recent investigations[1, 8] indicate that factor VIII antigen can be localized to endothelial cells of blood vessels in many organs including lymph nodes and spleen. The lymphocyte could not be shown to have factor VIII antigens to any significant degree in these studies. In light of these new findings and the past publications, a unifying position might be that the degree of hematologic correction is proportional to the amount of tissue and/or blood vessels in grafts whether the grafts are primarily lymphatic (spleen, nodes) or not (liver). If this were true, it would not be surprising that the liver, spleen, and lymph node grafts were corrective in that order of effectiveness. Also, the finding of supernormal levels of factor VIII concomitant with very low levels of all other coagulation factors in a splenectomized liver transplant recipient with a failing graft indicates a site of synthesis of antihemophilic factor outside the liver and spleen.[3]

Of particular importance to our studies is the observations of Rickles and associates[16] that the prolonged clotting time of factor VIII–deficient plasma can be corrected by a lymphocyte procoagulant material characterized as tissue factor and not factor VIII. These authors used a partial thromboplastin time (PTT) test to demonstrate their findings. Our factor VIII assays were all done by a thromboplastin generation time test (two-stage). Studies in our laboratory, which are being prepared for publication, indicate that the two-stage factor VIII assay is not altered by the presence of thrombin or tissue factor and, therefore, probably measures factor VIII clotting activity specifically. In contrast, the PTT type VIII assay is extremely sensitive to small amounts of tissue thromboplastin. These technical considerations must be noted in determination of factor VIII activity after tissue transplantation.

The results of the present study keep open the question of feasibility of tissue transplantation in patients with severe hemophilia. Previous attempts at splenic transplantation for various disease entities in man have all resulted in graft rejection within months,[4, 7, 9] and the single attempt at transplantation for hemophilia was followed by graft rupture in seven days.[7] Nonetheless, the improvements in management introduced into the field of transplantation over the last few years may warrant a trial in carefully selected cases.

REFERENCES

1. Bloom, A. L., Giddings, J. C., and Wilks, C. J.: Factor VIII on the vascular intima: Possible importance in hemostasis and thrombosis, Nat. New Biol. **241:** 217, 1973.
2. Bouhasin, J. D., Monteleone, P., and Altay, C.: Role of the lymphocyte in antihemophilic globulin production: A rise in antihemophilic globulin levels in a hemophilic subject with acute leukemia, J. Lab. Clin. Med. **78:** 122, 1971.
3. Groth, C. G., Pechet, L., and Starzl, T. E.: Coagulation during and after orthotopic transplantation of the human liver, Arch. Surg. **98:** 31, 1968.
4. Groth, C. G., Hagenfeldt, L., Dreborg, S., Löfström, B., Öckerman, P. A., Samuelsson, K., Svennerholm, L., Werner, B., and Westberg, G.: Splenic transplantation in a case of Gaucher's disease, Lancet **1:** 1260, 1971.
5. Groth, C. G., Kashiwagi, N., Moore, G. E., Husberg, B., Björkén, C., Putnam, C. W., and Starzl, T. E.: Production of a standardized antilymphocyte globulin, *in* Seiler, F. R. and Schwick, H. G., editors: Behring Institute Mitteilungen (Behring Institute Workshop, Bad Soden [Ts], April 23-25, 1972), Marburg, 1972, Behringwerke AG, No. 51, pp. 86-89.
6. Hathaway, W. E., Belhasen, L. P., and Hathaway, H. S.: Evidence for a new plasma thromboplastin factor. I. Case report, coagulation studies, and physiochemical properties, Blood **26:** 521, 1965.
7. Hathaway, W. E., Mull, M. M., Githens, J. G., Groth, C. G., Marchioro, T. L., and Starzl, T. E.: Attempted spleen transplant in classical hemophilia, Transplantation **7:** 73, 1969.
8. Hoyer, L. W., de los Santos, R. P., and Hoyer, J. R.: Antihemophilic factor antigen: Localization in endothelial cells by immunofluorescent microscopy, J. Clin. Invest. **52:** 2737, 1973.
9. Marchioro, T. L., Rowlands, D. T., Jr., Rifkind, D., Waddell, W. R., Starzl, T. E., and Fudenberg, H.: Splenic homotransplantation, Ann. N. Y. Acad. Sci. **120:** 626, 1964.
10. Marchioro, T. L., Hougie, C., Ragde, H., Epstein, R. B., and Thomas, E. D.: Hemophilia: Role of organ homografts, Science **163:** 188, 1969.
11. Marchioro, T. L., Hougie, C., Ragde, H., Epstein, B., and Thomas, E. D.: Organ homo-

grafts for hemophilia, Transplant. Proc. **1:** 316, 1969.

12. McKee, P. A., Coussons, R. T., Buckner, R. G., Williams, G. R., and Hampton, J. W.: Effects of the spleen on canine factor VIII levels, J. Lab. Clin. Med. **75:** 391, 1970.
13. Niemetz, J., and Nossel, H. L.: Activated coagulation factors: in vivo and in vitro studies, Br. J. Haematol. **16:** 37, 1969.
14. Norman, J. C., Covelli, V. H., and Sise, H. S.: Transplantation of the spleen: Experimental cure of hemophilia, SURGERY **64:** 1, 1968.
15. Pool, J. G., and Robinson, J.: Assay of plasma antihaemophilic globulin (AHG), Br. J. Haematol. **5:** 17, 1959.
16. Rickles, F. R., Hardin, J. A., Pittick, F. A., Hoyer, L. W., and Conrad, M. D.: Tissue factor activity in lymphocyte cultures from normal individuals and patients with hemophilia, Am. J. Clin. Invest. **52:** 1427, 1973.
17. Sise, H. J., Joison, J., Pegg, C. A. S., and Norman, J. C.: Potential of the transplanted spleen in canine hemophilia, *in* Brinkhous, K. M., editor: Hemophilia and new hemorrhagic states, Chapel Hill, N. C., 1970. University of North Carolina Press, p. 106.
18. Webster, W. P., Penick, G. D., Peacock, E. E., and Brinkhous, K. M.: Allotransplantation of spleen in hemophilia, N. C. Med. J. **28:** 505, 1967.
19. Webster, W. P., Zukoski, C. F., Hutchin, P., Reddick, R. L., Mandel, S. R., and Penick, G. D.: Plasma factor VIII synthesis and control as revealed by canine organ transplantation, Am. J. Physiol. **220:** 1147, 1971.

Microangiography of the renal vasculature following total renal artery occlusion

Richard F. Brodman, M.D., Raymond L. Hackett, M.D., Birdwell Finlayson, M.D., Ph.D., *and* **William W. Pfaff, M.D.,** *Gainesville, Fla.*

Microangiography of the rabbit kidney following occlusion of the renal artery for 90 minutes demonstrates fluctuating focal malperfusion and hyperemia in the cortical microcirculation during reflow. The portion of microvasculature predominantly involved appears to be the efferent arteriole and postglomerular circulation. Persistent patchy malperfusion after establishment of reflow may contribute to the development of focal tubular necrosis.

From the Departments of Pathology and Surgery, University of Florida College of Medicine, Gainesville, Fla.

CESSATION or reduction of renal function is encountered in a variety of disease states. Assigned causes are many but frequently decreased or interrupted renal blood flow is a contributing factor. The result is a reversible injury, and this clinical and histological entity has been termed "acute tubular necrosis."

Experimentally, ischemic acute tubular necrosis has been produced by controlled hypotension,[2] splanchnic nerve stimulation,[27] tourniquet shock,[27] vasoactive agents,[15] and occlusion of the whole renal pedicle[4, 8, 13] or renal artery.[3, 14, 22] Occlusion of the rabbit renal artery for 90 minutes consistently produces a focal acute tubular necrosis, whereas shorter occlusion times are injurious only erratically. Occlusion in excess of two hours usually results in diffuse cortical necrosis.

When circulation is reestablished following arterial occlusion for 90 minutes, the kidney is initially mottled, but shortly it turns diffusely pink and the organ becomes tense. Subsequently, the kidney loses its turgor and the surface is irregularly cyanotic. These changes may reflect postocclusive ischemia, and this concept has been suggested in the literature.[3, 14, 18]

The purpose of the following study was to examine the microvasculature following renal artery occlusion.[5] The microangiographic changes suggest postocclusive focal malperfusion involving the postglomerular microvasculature.

METHODS

Forty-five New Zealand albino rabbits, male and female, weighing 2 to 5 kilograms were anesthetized with intravenous pentobarbital. The left kidney was exposed through a midline abdominal incision, freed from its peritoneal attachments, and the left renal artery, vein, and ureter were isolated. Ligatures were placed around the proximal aorta, the superior mesenteric artery, and the right renal pedicle. The left renal artery was then occluded with a serrafine clamp

This study was supported by a grant from the John A. Hartford Foundation, Inc.

Presented in part at the Surgical Forum, San Francisco, October, 1969.

Accepted for publication March 12, 1974.

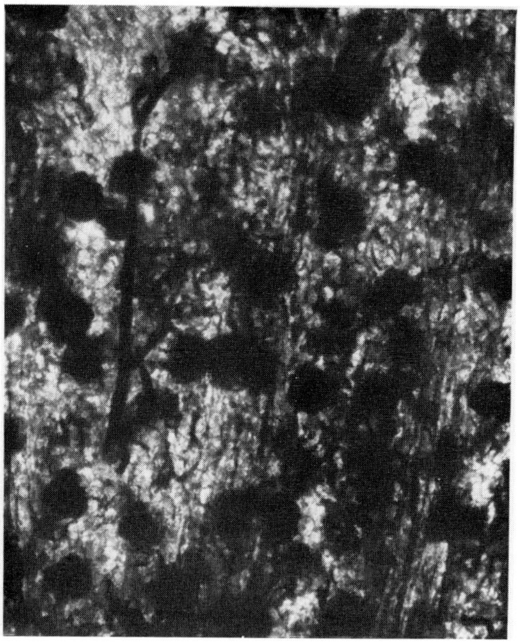

Fig. 1. Microvasculature of five-minute control rabbit demonstrating perfusion of interlobular artery, afferent arterioles and glomeruli. Post-glomerular circulation is represented by a background plexus of delicate vessels.

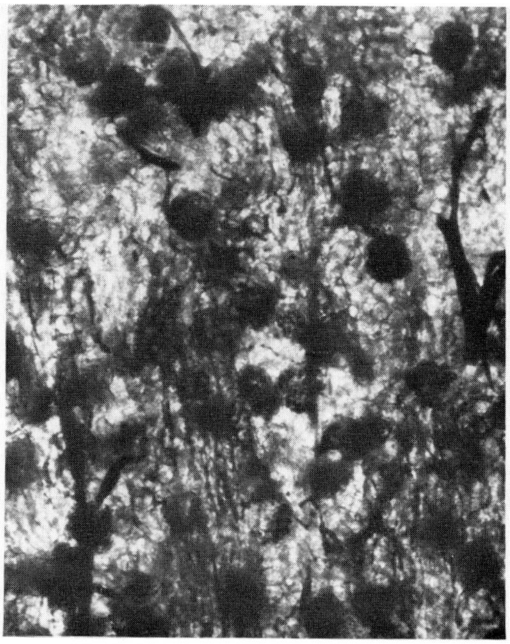

Fig. 2. Microvasculature of 15-minute control shows perfusion pattern comparable to five-minute control.

for 90 minutes. After release of the clamp, static renal angiography was performed at time intervals of 5, 15, and 30 minutes and 1, 2, 24, and 48 hours. Each group consisted of six animals.

Angiography was performed by cannulating the distal aorta with a large-bore polyethylene tube. The superior mesenteric and right renal arteries were occluded. Immediately after ligation of the proximal aorta, the left kidney was perfused for 20 minutes with a 22 percent aqueous suspension of Micropaque,* a barium sulphate suspension with particle size ranging from 0.015 to 10 μ. The interval from proximal aortic occlusion to initiation of contrast perfusion was approximately ten seconds. In varying series, static perfusion pressure was adjusted to 100 to 200, 150 to 180, and 150-200 mm. Hg. Sham operations including hilar dissections were performed using time intervals identical to the experimental groups; angiography perfusion pressure was 150 to 180 mm. Hg.

Following perfusion, the left renal pedicle was ligated and the kidney was fixed in buffered formalin for a minimum of two days. Cryostat sections were prepared at 800, 500 and 200 μ, stationed on photographic film,* and roentgenograms were prepared with a low kilovoltage apparatus.† The resulting transparencies were assessed by projection, microscopy, and print enlargements. Other sections were cleared with glycerine and examined by light microscopy. Representative samples were also imbedded in paraffin, sectioned and stained with hematoxylin and eosin.

The relative volume of perfused renal tissue was estimated from enlargements of microphotographs of the sections of four series, two control and two experimental. A lattice was placed over the print and the number of perfused areas coinciding to

*Micropaque powder, Damancy & Co. Ltd., Ware-Herts, England; distributed by the Picker X-Ray Corporation, 1275 Mamaroneck Ave., White Plains, N. Y.

*Kodak High Resolution Estar.

†General Electric Ca-7 Coolidge tube x-ray 20 kv., 20/Ma. for five minutes, plate being placed six inches from reflecting surface.

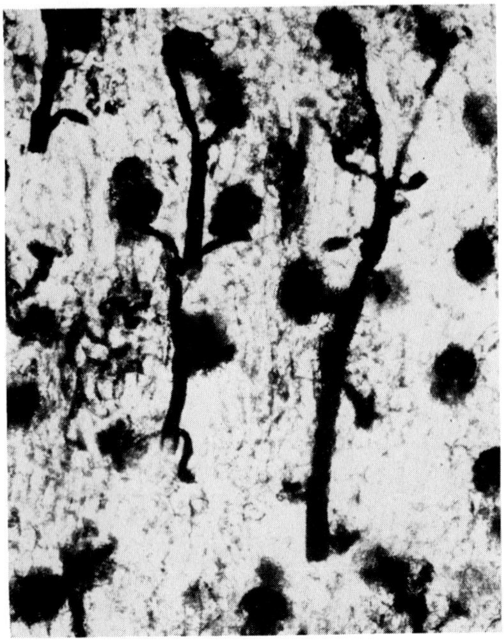

Fig. 3. Microvasculature of rabbit kidney cortex 5 minutes after resumption of circulation. Interlobular arteries, afferent arterioles and glomeruli are well perfused. Marked decrease in postglomerular perfusion is illustrated by lack of filling of cortical capillary network.

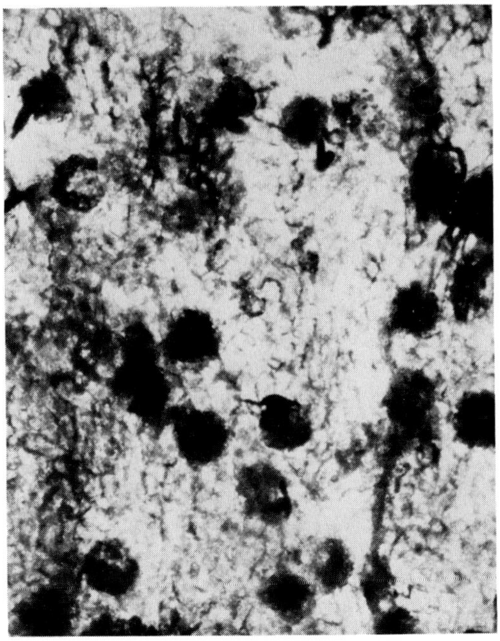

Fig. 4. Microvasculature of cortex, 15 minutes after resumption of circulation, demonstrating patchy filling of the cortical capillary network.

lattice sites was counted. If the lattice is coarse with respect to the feature being estimated and the feature is randomly distributed, this technique gives an unbiased estimate of the volume of the feature.[9]

RESULTS

When assessed by microscopy and projection, perfusion of a kidney from a sham-operated rabbit results in even filling of the arcuate and interlobular arteries and the afferent arterioles and glomeruli. The postglomerular circulation is a diffuse and evenly filled capillary plexus (Figs. 1 and 2). In each of the experimental series, irregular contrast distribution is seen five minutes (Fig. 3) and fifteen minutes (Fig. 4) after resumption of arterial circulation to an occluded kidney. While the interlobular arteries fill readily, the number of contrast-filled glomeruli is reduced focally, with accompanying minimal perfusion of the peritubular plexus. Further, glomerular filling could not be equated with perfusion of the adjacent cortical capillary network, suggesting obstruction at or beyond the efferent arteriole. After 30 minutes of arterial flow, perfusion of the entire cortex is strikingly improved, and progress of the Micropaque appears to be unimpeded. Perfusion of the cortical capillary network in the experimental kidney (Fig. 5) appears greater than the control (Fig. 6) and suggests reactive hyperemia. Perfusion of the 30 minute and one-hour control kidneys is even but demonstrates more irregularity than control animals subjected to lesser periods of anesthesia and visceral exposure. At one and two days, perfusion patterns of ischemic and control kidneys are indistinguishable.

The relative volumes of the perfused tree were estimated by overlaying photographic prints of whole kidney slice radiographs with a lattice. Ischemia caused reduction in perfusion in the early reflow periods (Table I). Statistical significance was noted only with kidneys allowed 15 minutes of blood reflow.

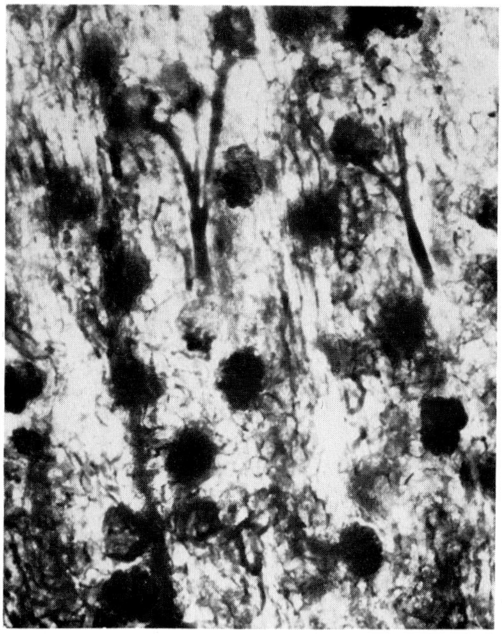

Fig. 5. Microvasculature of cortex after 30 minutes of reflow shows even filling of cortical capillary network; focal malperfusion is absent.

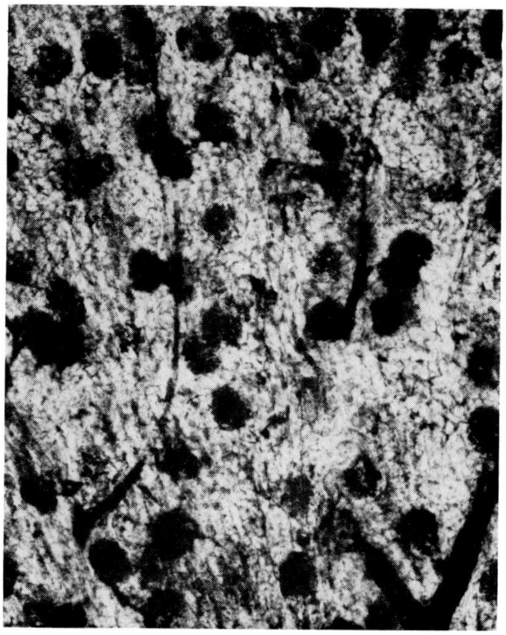

Fig. 6. Microvasculature of 30-minute control shows even perfusion of cortical capillary network.

Caution in interpretation relative to the microscopic descriptions is warranted, as the lattice technique gauges presence or absence of perfusion and neglects quantitative estimation in a given square.

Stained sections of fixed specimens of kidneys obtained 48 hours following occlusion showed characteristic focal acute tubular necrosis.

DISCUSSION

It is conceivable that the scattered necrosis that follows 90 minutes of ischemia is a simple, stochastic process, the manifestation of a randomized variable response in a biologic system. However, the described angiographic findings are of malperfusion with focal distribution and suggest correlative events, in that the pattern of tubular death in acute tubular necrosis is identical with the pattern of the angiographic defects.

While much of the kidney is insensible to 90 minutes of anoxia, the entire organ becomes necrotic with an additional 30 minutes of absolute ischemia. Accordingly it seems plausible that the malperfusion we have demonstrated may be equivalent to the additional 30 minutes of absolute ischemia necessary to produce cell death.

The exact limiting site of microvascular malperfusion is not discernible with these techniques, for either distal or proximal obstruction in a circulatory bed is equally effective in arresting contrast filling of the proximal vessels. However, the early postocclusive changes were reduced filling of the capillary network with minor changes in the glomeruli. A similar pattern was observed by Diethelm,[12] although the involved postglomerular vasculature in his experiments was limited to the juxtamedullary area. Obstruction of the efferent arteriole has also been postulated on the basis of India ink preparations in acute renal failure secondary to injection of glycerine into the rat.[24] Since some degree of flow is usually present in the malperfused regions, efferent arteriolar obstruction is either incomplete, or collateral flow from adjacent tubulovascular units occurs.

Table I. *Relative value of kidney occupied by perfusing blood vessels*

	Control		Experimental		
Duration of reflow	No. of samples*	Mean	No. of samples*	Mean	Statistical significance of difference†
5 minutes	8	0.59 ± 0.18‡	8	0.49 ± 0.19	NS§
15 minutes	8	0.50 ± 0.15	9	0.28 ± 0.10	P 0.05‖
30 minutes	8	0.42 ± 0.23	8	0.42 ± 0.19	NS
60 minutes	4	0.45 ± 0.05	8	0.53 ± 0.09	NS
120 minutes	5	0.39 ± 0.12	8	0.35 ± 0.12	NS
1 hour	8	0.32 ± 0.12	8	0.29 ± 0.09	NS
2 hours	8	0.37 ± 0.16	8	0.35 ± 0.15	NS

*Each sample contained from 283 to 610 points.

†Statistical significance evaluated by student's t-test.

‡Error is expressed as standard deviation.

§N.S. indicates the difference between control and experimental means is not statistically significant.

‖P is the probability that the difference between control and experimental means is a random result.

The shunting of blood away from the cortex, a mechanism described[27] after hemorrhage, was absent in our preparations. The medulla rarely perfused uniformly in any animal, and the technical differences between control and experimental groups were not observed. These findings are in contrast to those of Diethelm,[12] who described reflow failure as occurring predominantly in the medulla.

The cause of decreased flow remains conjectural. Intravascular sludging has been suggested as a mechanism in renal ischemia[18] and in necrosis in organs other than the kidney. Others have argued that intravascular thrombi interfere with the reestablishment of flow after an ischemic insult.[1, 6] Thrombi have not been observed in other models,[23] nor have we identified thrombi in histological sections from ischemic kidneys. In the comprehensive studies of Sheehan and Davis, clots were absent except for "wisps of thrombi" following 24 hours of total renal ischemia.[20]

Structural vascular damage has been described following renal ischemia and could contribute to areas of no reflow. Medial necrosis of arcuate and interlobular arteries was seen following occlusion of the rabbit renal pedicle from one to three hours, but occlusion for 90 minutes produced only occasional necrotic lesions.[21] Terry and associates[26] described vascular changes in rats after 75 minutes of ischemia induced by renal artery occlusion. Frequent medial necrosis in the renal, arcuate, and interlobular arteries, and the afferent arterioles was described at four hours after release of the occluding noose. The distribution of vessels with medial destruction does not appear similar to the distribution of malperfused areas described in this article.

Increased interstitial extravascular pressure has been implicated as a factor producing secondary hemodynamic changes in renal allotransplants.[10] The proposed site of action of increased pressure is upon the efferent arteriole resulting in vascular constriction. Little direct evidence exists for a similar mechanism in the reflow changes occurring after renal ischemia. Direct intrarenal pressures have been measured following renal arterial occlusion and found to be elevated, but determinations in the reported experiments were made several days after reflow and the results cannot be extrapolated to the early events we have described.[11, 17] The role of altered interstitial pressure in early postischemic events remains speculative.

Release of a vasoactive substance has been postulated on the basis of a measurable pressor response following prolonged ischemia[25] and by the finding that postocclusive ischemia is reversed by administration of exogenous agents such as acetylcholine[7] and phenoxybenzamine.[19] Vasoconstriction, increase in resistance, and loss of ability to autoregulate blood flow following renal ischemia[16] suggests response to a vasopressor. Liberation of a pressor material would not explain the focal nature of ischemic necrosis unless a randomly distributed differential response of the microvasculature is postulated.

The authors are grateful to John Rayl, M.D., and William C. Thomas, Jr., M.D., for their assistance in developing the radiographic procedures.

REFERENCES

1. Ames, A., III, Wright, R. L., Kowada, M., Thurston, J. M., and Majno, G.: Cerebral ischemia. II. The no-reflow phenomenon, Am. J. Pathol. **52:** 437, 1968.
2. Block, M. A., Wakim, K. G., Mann, F. C., and Bennett, W. A.: Renal lesions and function following prolonged experimental hypotension, Surgery **32:** 551, 1952.
3. Borcroft, J.: The respiratory function of the blood, 1914, Cambridge, University Press, p. 115. Cited by Stoll, J. E., and Carlson, A. J.: Am. J. Physiol. **67:** 153, 1923.
4. Brake, C. M., Reins, D., and Wittmers, L. E.: Intrarenal hemodynamic changes following acute partial renal artery occlusion, J. Trauma **7:** 48, 1967.
5. Brodman, R. F., Hackett, R. L., and Pfaff, W. W.: Microangiography of the renal vasculature following ischemia (abstr.), Surg. Forum **20:** 46, 1969.
6. Chiang, J., Kowada, M., Ames, A., III, Wright, R. L., and Majno, G.: Cerebral ischemia. III. Vascular changes, Am. J. Pathol. **52:** 455, 1968.
7. Coelho, J. B., Ruiz-Guinazu, A., and Lanari, A.: Effect of acetylcholine on the increased renal resistance consecutive to renal ischemia, Acta Physiol. Lat. Am. **17:** 207, 1967.
8. Cuppage, F. E., Neagoy, D. R., and Tate, A.: Repair of the nephron following temporary occlusion of the renal pedicle, Lab. Invest. **77:** 660, 1967.
9. DeHoff, R. T., and Rhines, F. N.: Quantitative microscopy, New York, 1968, McGraw-Hill Book Co., chap. 3.
10. Dempster, W. J.: Hypertension and acute rejection processes in allotransplanted kidneys, Br. J. Exp. Pathol. **51:** 149, 1970.
11. DeWardener, H. E.: Intrarenal pressure in experimental tubular necrosis, Lancet **1:** 580, 1955.
12. Diethelm, A. G.: Effect of ischemia upon the renal microcirculation, Am. Surg. **35:** 833, 1969.
13. Eisendroth, D. N., and Strauss, D. C.: The effect on the kidney of temporary compression of its vessels, J. A. M. A. **55:** 2286, 1910.
14. Friedman, S. M., Johnson, R. L., and Friedman, C. L.: The pattern of recovery of renal function following renal artery occlusion in the dog, Circ. Res. **2:** 231, 1954.
15. Hatcher, C. R., Jr., Gagnon, J. A., Clarke, R. W., and Geever, D. R.: Acute reversible and irreversible renal insufficiency in the dog, J. Surg. Res. **2:** 36, 1967.
16. Hinshaw, L. B., Archer, L. L., Parry, W. L., and Shires, T. K.: Renal hemodynamics and function in response to renal artery occlusion in canine and primate kidneys, Invest. Urol. **7:** 422, 1970.
17. Miles, B. E., and DeWardener, H. E.: Intrarenal pressure, J. Physiol. **123:** 131, 1954.
18. Neely, W. A., and Turner, M. D.: The effect of arterial, venous and arteriovenous occlusion on renal blood flow, Surg. Gynecol. Obstet. **108:** 669, 1959.
19. Sakai, K., Yasuda, K., and Hashimoto, K.: Role of catecholamine and adenosine in the ischemic response following release of a renal artery occlusion, Jap. J. Physiol. **18:** 673, 1968.
20. Sheehan, H. L., and Davis, J. C.: Complete permanent renal ischemia, J. Pathol. **76:** 569, 1958.
21. Sheehan, H. L., and Davis, J. C.: Renal ischemia with good reflow, J. Pathol. **78:** 351, 1959.
22. Stoll, J. E., and Carlson, A. J.: The anuria following temporary anemia of the kidneys, Am. J. Physiol. **67:** 153, 1923.
23. Strock, P. E., and Majno, G.: Microvascular changes in acutely ischemic rat muscle, Surg. Gynecol. Obstet. **129:** 1213, 1969.
24. Suzuki, T., and Mostofi, F. K.: Electron microscopic studies of acute tubular necrosis: Vascular changes in the rat kidney after subcutaneous injection of glycerine, Lab. Inv. **23:** 29, 1970.
25. Taquini, A. C.: The production of a pressor substance by the totally ischemic kidney, Am. Heart J. **19:** 513, 1940.
26. Terry, B. E., Jones, D. B., and Mueller, C. B.: Experimental ischemic renal arterial necrosis with resolution, Am. J. Pathol. **58:** 69, 1970.
27. Trueta, J., Barclay, A. E., Daniel, P. M., Franklin, K. J., and Pritchard, M. M. L.: Studies of the renal circulation, Oxford, 1947, Blackwell Scientific Publications, Ltd.

Non-simultaneous bilateral breast carcinoma

Sukawat Watanatittan, M.D., *and* **M. D. Ram, M.D., M.S.(Surg.), F.R.C.S., F.A.C.S.,**
Cleveland, Ohio

The incidence of non-simultaneous bilateral breast carcinoma among 688 patients with breast cancer was 3.5 percent. The carcinoma in the second breast was similar to the primary in the first breast, in its location, histologic type, degree of axillary node involvement, and prognosis. The interval between the development of the cancers in the two breasts ranged from less than one year to 22 years with a mean of 6.1 years. The prognosis of the patient was not affected by the length of interval between the development of the two carcinomas but was dependent on the stage of the tumor. Carcinoma developed more frequently in the second breast in those patients who had a good prognosis after the treatment of the first breast tumor than in those who had a poor prognosis after the first tumor. Patients who had mastectomy for carcinoma should be carefully screened for a tumor in the second breast at follow-up examination. Physical examination alone is inadequate, and mammography or xerography should be employed. At present, there is not enough justification for routine prophylactic contralateral mastectomy. The risk to the opposite breast should be assessed by random biopsy.

From the Department of Surgery, Huron Road Hospital, Cleveland, Ohio

THE MOST FREQUENT precancerous lesion of the breast is a cancer of the opposite breast.[18]

The risk of developing a second primary carcinoma in the remaining breast of a woman who has undergone unilateral mastectomy is well recognized. In the past, the tumors in the remaining breast were considered metastatic, but it is now realized that some of these are truly primary tumors and should be treated as such.

Carcinomatous changes in breast tissue occur at more than one site and multicentricity of breast carcinoma has been demonstrated by whole organ section.[5, 16] With the use of such techniques, multiple independent carcinomas of different stages and histologic patterns were found in 54 percent of 157 breasts removed for carcinoma.[16] Some of these lesions were microscopic foci which were not detectable by palpation or by naked eye examination. Similar foci may exist or appear in the apparently normal opposite breast.

The incidence of bilateral breast carcinoma has been reported to be one to 16 percent in the literature,[3, 13, 17] and the variation in figures is probably due to differences in criteria used in distinguishing metastases from a new primary, age group of patients, methods of data retrieval, duration of follow-up study, and related factors.

Cutler[3] suggested criteria based on (1) differences of histologic patterns, (2) the

Accepted for publication March 13, 1974.

Reprint requests: M. D. Ram, M.D., Director Department of Surgery, Huron Road Hospital, Cleveland, Ohio 44112.

presence of local hyperplasia or in situ carcinoma adjacent to the second breast carcinoma, (3) absence of local recurrence or distant metastases from the first breast carcinoma, and (4) time interval between the appearance of the two carcinomas. Robbins and Berg[17] based their distinction on (1) location of tumor, (2) behavior of tumor, and (3) histologic pattern of the tumor. Primary carcinoma is usually found in the breast parenchyma while metastatic lesions are usually found in the fat surrounding the breast. They also emphasized the presence of in situ carcinomatous changes accompanying the lesion as the most important evidence in favor of diagnosing an independent primary carcinoma. Despite all these criteria, it may still be difficult to distinguish metastases from a new primary tumor. It has also been reported that evidence of lymphatic spread from the first primary was seen in areas adjoining non-invasive carcinoma in the second breast and that the two may co-exist.[5]

This report presents our experiences with bilateral primary breast carcinomas.

MATERIAL AND METHODS

The records of all the patients who had mastectomy for breast carcinoma at Huron Road Hospital during the years 1953 to 1971 were reviewed. Of the total 688 patients, 24 were found to have a new primary carcinoma in the second breast. The criteria on which we based the diagnosis of a primary were (1) the patients did not have clinical or radiological evidence of local recurrence or distant metastases from the first primary tumor at the time of mastectomy for second breast carcinoma, (2) the time interval between the two independent primary carcinomas was greater than six months, and (3) histologically, the tumor in the second breast was in the parenchyma of the gland and appeared to be a primary tumor.

During the same period, there were five patients who had mastectomy of the remaining breast for carcinoma, within six months of the first mastectomy and these were grouped as simultaneous bilateral breast carcinoma. Four of these patients died within three years of the second mastectomy, and the fifth is alive at present, one year after surgery.

Table I. *Age at the time of diagnosis of first breast carcinoma*

Age (yr.)	*All patients with breast cancer*	*Patients with non-simultaneous bilateral breast cancer*
< 30	3	0
30–39	67	1
40–49	170	9
50–59	150	7
60–69	146	6
70–79	111	1
80 over	41	0
Total	688	24
Mean age	58 yr.	54 yr.

The clinical features of the 24 patients in the category of non-simultaneous bilateral breast carcinoma were studied with particular reference to age, time interval between the two primary tumors, location of tumor, degree of nodal involvement, histologic type, treatment, and survival.

FINDINGS

Incidence. Twenty-four patients fulfilled the criteria for non-simultaneous bilateral breast carcinoma, giving an incidence of 3.5 per cent in the total group. During the same period, the incidence of simultaneous bilateral carcinoma was 0.7 percent.

Age. The age distribution of the whole group and of the 24 patients with non-simultaneous bilateral breast carcinomas is shown in Table I. The mean age at time of diagnosis of the first tumor among the 24 patients was 54 years, while it was 58 years in the whole group of 688 patients. It has been reported that those patients who go on to develop a separate primary in the second breast, develop their first primary at a younger age than in the over-all group of women who develop breast cancer.[4, 6, 17]

Time interval between the first and second carcinomas. The mean interval between the diagnosis of the two tumors was 6.1 years. Two patients developed the second

Table II. *Location of carcinoma*

Location	*First breast (%)*	*Second breast (%)*
Upper outer quadrant	45.5	41.7
Upper inner quadrant	22.7	20.8
Lower inner quadrant	4.5	4.2
Lower outer quadrant	13.6	4.2
Central	13.6	29.1

Table III. *Involvement of axillary nodes*

	First breast cancer (No. of patients)	*Second breast cancer (No. of patients)*
Positive axillary nodes	14	11
Negative axillary nodes	9	8
Unknown*	1	5

*These patients underwent simple mastectomy, and hence the lymph node status is not known.

primary within one year of the first, seven between one and three years, six between three and five years, five between five and ten years, and four patients developed the second tumor ten years or more after the first. The longest interval was 22 years.

Location of lesion. The most frequent location of the tumors in both breasts was the upper outer quadrant (Table II). The distribution of the second tumors was in general similar to those of unilateral breast carcinoma. About one third of the tumors in the second breast were located in a mirror-image quadrant of their mates in the first breast.

Axillary node status and clinical stage. Axillary node involvement as shown by histologic study is noted in Table III. Involvement of axillary nodes was noted in 61 percent at time of the first carcinoma and in 58 percent at time of the second carcinoma.

At time of diagnosis of the first breast cancer, eighteen patients were in Stage I and five were in Stage II. The stage of tumor in one patient was unknown since she underwent simple mastectomy. When diagnosed of a tumor in the second breast, fifteen patients were in Stage I and four were in Stage II. Five patients were in Stage III.

It is noteworthy that the carcinomas in the second breast were not diagnosed at an earlier stage than those in the first breast. This, despite the fact that these patients were being followed up, emphasizes the inadequacy of clinical examination in making an early diagnosis. Similar findings were noted in other studies.[13, 17]

Histologic types. The histologic types of the tumors in the two breasts is shown in Table IV. Infiltrating ductal carcinoma was the most frequent type in both groups.

Treatment. The treatment of carcinoma of the breast at this hospital in the first half of the period under study was almost always a conventional radical mastectomy; in recent years, modified radical mastectomy is performed more frequently. Postoperative radiotherapy is given to all patients with histologic evidence of axillary node involvement. Simple mastectomy is generally performed for Stage III or IV tumors.

For the first breast carcinoma, radical mastectomy was done in 21 patients, and modified radical mastectomy in two. Simple mastectomy was done for one patient for reasons other than the stage of the tumor. When the women developed a tumor in the second breast, thirteen underwent conventional radical mastectomy, six underwent a modified radical mastectomy, and five patients with Stage III tumors were treated by simple mastectomy.

Over-all survival. The over-all survival data after each mastectomy are shown in Table V. If survival is calculated from the first mastectomy, 90.9 percent survived five years, 70 percent survived ten years, and 37.5 percent survived 15 years. These results are well above the over-all survival rates for patients with unilateral breast carcinoma in general and is in agreement with others' experiences.[7-9, 13, 17] The figure simply reflects the fact that the longer a woman survives after mastectomy for unilateral breast cancer, the more likely she is to develop a second carcinoma in the remaining breast.

Survival after mastectomy for second breast cancer was 47.4 percent at five years and 27.7 percent at ten years. If the five patients with Stage III tumors in the second breast were excluded, the survival rate was 60 percent at five years, and 36 percent at ten years for all Stage I and II tumors. These are comparable to those of unilateral breast carcinoma in general. Of the five patients with Stage III carcinoma, three died within one year, one died three years after the second mastectomy, and one was lost to follow-up study.

Although the development of carcinoma in the second breast may appear to worsen the prognosis of the patient, the results in the group were comparable to that of the group with unilateral breast carcinoma.

Survival related to interval between tumors. To determine the effect of the time interval between the diagnosis of the two tumors, on survival, the patients were divided into two groups: (1) those that developed the second breast tumor within three years after the first and (2) those that developed the second tumor more than three years after the first. At five and ten years, no differences in survival rates were found in the two groups, and the interval had no effect on the outcome.

While the later appearance of a new primary in the remaining breast may appear not to affect the prognosis, the group with simultaneous bilateral breast carcinoma had a poor outcome. Four of the five died within three years, and the fifth one is alive at one year after her second mastectomy.

COMMENTS

The incidence of carcinoma in the second breast among patients who had mastectomy for unilateral carcinoma has been estimated to be from one to 10 percent.[17] The woman who had unilateral carcinoma has a risk of developing cancer of the remaining breast, which is three to seven times that of the risk of the general female population.[6, 11, 17] This is not surprising since the same factors that induce carcinogenesis in one breast continue to be operative on the other breast.

Table IV. *Histologic types*

Type	*First breast cancer (No.)*	*Second breast cancer (No.)*
Infiltrating ductal	15	20
Medullary	3	2
Non-infiltrating ductal	2	1
Colloid	1	0
Infiltrating lobular	1	0
Tubular	0	1
Undetermined	2	0

Table V. *Survival*

No. of yr.	*Survival after first mastectomy*		*Survival after second mastectomy*	
	No. of patients	*Percent survival*	*No. of patients*	*Percent survival*
5	20/22	90.9	9/19	47.4
10	14/20	70.0	5/18	27.7
15	6/16	37.5	1/14	7.1

Among all such patients at risk, different groups of workers have tried to identify a "high-risk" population that are more prone to bilateral breast cancer in an effort to offer early diagnosis and treatment. Many factors which may affect the high risk group have been identified.

Age at time of diagnosis of first breast cancer. Robbins and Berg[17] estimated that if carcinoma developed in the first breast under the age of 50 years, the risk of developing contralateral breast carcinoma in this group is ten times of that of the general female population of the same age group, while Haagensen[6] estimates the risk to be seventeen times. In contrast, the risk falls to less than two[17] to six times[6] the corresponding age-related female population, if the women were over 50 years of age at time of diagnosis of first breast cancer. The younger women, particularly if they have a good prognosis after the first breast cancer, are more likely to live longer and develop carcinoma in the remaining breast while the older women may die either of the tumor or of other diseases.

Stage of the carcinoma in the first breast. Those patients with an earlier stage of the tumor in the first breast carry a better prognosis and are more susceptible to the risk of developing a second tumor.[6, 11, 13, 17]

Histologic type of tumor. Robbins and Berg[17] found a high risk of contralateral primary tumors among those whose first primary was a comedocarcinoma, medullary carcinoma, or a colloid carcinoma. A high incidence of bilaterality, ranging from ten to 56 percent, has been documented among patients with in situ lobular carcinoma.[14, 19] About nine to ten percent of these patients with in situ lobular carcinoma have been known to have developed invasive carcinoma at a later date. However, in our material, none of these histologic types were frequent.

Multicentricity. If the lesion in the first breast was multicentric, there is a higher risk of developing another carcinoma in the second breast.[6]

Family history. Patients with a family history of carcinoma of the breast carry a higher risk of bilateral tumors.[1, 2, 11, 12] We did not find a strong family history in the patients reviewed.

The importance of these risk factors should be kept in mind in the management of all women who had mastectomy for cancer. Our results show that if the carcinoma in the second breast is diagnosed at an early stage, the prognosis is no worse than that of patients with unilateral carcinoma. The problem is in making the diagnosis early enough, and in this respect clinical examination alone is inadequate. Five of the patients in our group had Stage III carcinoma in the second breast at time of diagnosis. The frequency of axillary nodal involvement was equal in both the first and second breast tumors. Similar experiences have been reported by others.[12, 17]

Mammography, xeroradiography, and thermography have been useful in suspecting and diagnosing subclinical breast cancer. These methods would have a greater application in women who had breast cancer and frequent periodic assessment should be recommended. In the future, hormonal tests based on steroid patterns or immunologic tests may be helpful.

The management of the remaining breast is a matter of controversy. Prophylactic contralateral mastectomy was first suggested by Bloodgood[2] in 1921 and was later supported by Pack.[15] Delayed selective prophylactic mastectomy in the "high-risk" group was advocated by Hubbard[10] and Leis.[13] In the "high-risk" group Hubbard[10] found unsuspected carcinoma in two of 16 asymptomatic breasts. Leis[12] found unsuspected carcinoma in 16 of 91 asymptomatic breasts. The incidence of such unsuspected lesions in the second breast needs further investigation.

In a different approach, Urban[19] claimed to have found a high incidence of carcinoma in the opposite breast by random biopsy, and he found a six to ten percent incidence of simultaneous bilateral carcinoma. If these figures are confirmed, the management of the contralateral breast could be based on more solid grounds. However, it is questionable whether the foci of malignancy noted microscopically in the biopsy material would develop into overt clinically significant carcinomas. Further data is needed.

The woman's view on whether bilateral mastectomy is acceptable or not, has not received due consideration. At present we do not feel justified in advocating prophylactic contralateral mastectomy for all women presenting with unilateral carcinoma of the breast. The procedure may have a place for women in the "high-risk" group. Meanwhile one should try and improve our methods for early diagnosis.

REFERENCES

1. Anderson, D. E.: Some characteristics of familial breast cancer, Cancer **28:** 1500, 1971.
2. Bloodgood, J. C.: Discussion of Trout, H. H.: The remaining breast after radical removal of the opposite side for carcinoma, J. South. Surg. Assoc. **34:** 223, 1921.
3. Cutler, M.: Tumors of the breast, Philadelphia, 1962, J. B. Lippincott Co., pp. 211-217.
4. Finney, G. G., Jr., Finney, G. G., Montague, A. C. W., Stonesifer, G. L., and Brown, C. C.: Bilateral breast cancer: Clinical and pathological review, Ann. Surg. **175:** 635, 1972.
5. Gallagher, H. S., and Martin, J. E.: Early

phases in the development of breast cancer, Cancer **24:** 1170, 1969.
6. Haagensen, C. D.: Disease of the breast, ed. 2, Philadelphia, 1971, W. B. Saunders Company, p. 449.
7. Haagensen, C. D., Lane, N., and Lattes, R.: Neoplastic proliferation of the epithelium of the mammary lobules, Surg. Clin. N. Am. **52:** 497, 1972.
8. Harrington, S. W.: Survival rates of radical mastectomy for unilateral and bilateral carcinoma of breast, SURGERY **19:** 154, 1946.
9. Harrington, S. W.: Fifteen year to 40 year survival rates following radical mastectomy for cancer of breast, Ann. Surg. **137:** 843, 1953.
10. Hubbard, T. B., Jr.: Non-simultaneous bilateral carcinoma of breast, SURGERY **34:** 706, 1953.
11. Kilgore, A. R.: Incidence of cancer in second breast; after radical removal of one breast for cancer, J. A. M. A. **77:** 454, 1921.
12. Leis, H. P., Jr.: Selective elective prophylactic contralateral mastectomy, Cancer **28:** 956, 1971.
13. Leis, H. P., Jr., Mersheimer, W. L., Black, M. M., and Chabon, A. D.: The second breast, N. Y. State J. Med. **65:** 2460, 1965.
14. Newman, W.: In situ lobular carcinoma of breast: Report of 26 women with 32 cancers, Ann. Surg. **157:** 591, 1963.
15. Pack, G. T.: Argument for bilateral mastectomy, SURGERY **29:** 929, 1951.
16. Qualheim, R. E., and Gall, E. A.: Breast carcinoma with multiple sites of origin, Cancer **10:** 460, 1957.
17. Robbins, G. F., and Berg, J. W.: Bilateral primary breast cancers: A prospective clinicopathological study, Cancer **17:** 1501, 1964.
18. Stewart, F. W.: Tumors of the breast, Atlas of tumor of pathology, Sec. 9, Fasc. 34, Washington, D. C., 1950, Armed Forces Institute of Pathology, p. 9.
19. Urban, J. A.: Bilateral breast cancer, Cancer **24:** 1310, 1969.

Obturator intestinal obstruction following renal allotransplantation: Relief with hyperosmolar enemas

Michael Berger, M.D., John S. Schuessler, M.D., Hugo F. Carvajal, M.D., William B. Lorentz, Jr., M.D., Luther B. Travis, M.D., *and* **Kenneth R. T. Tyson, M.D.,** *Galveston, Texas*

Three pediatric renal allograft recipients developed obturatory intestinal obstruction in the immediate posttransplant period. Administration of large doses of aluminum hydroxide, peritoneal dialysis, and intestinal ileus secondary to the transplant procedure were all temporally related to the onset of fecal impaction in these patients. Aggressive administration of the routine type of enemas and stool softeners was uniformly unsuccessful in relieving the impactions. Because of the high risk in operative intervention in this group of patients, hyperosmolar radiographic contrast material (sodium diatrizoate) was given by rectal enema in an attempt to alleviate the obstruction by producing an osmotic diarrhea. Such a technique has been utilized successfully in infants with meconium ileus. Its successful application in these patients prevented hazardous operative intervention.

From the Departments of Surgery and Pediatrics, The University of Texas Medical Branch at Galveston, Galveston, Texas

INTESTINAL OBSTRUCTION secondary to fecal impaction has been observed in three pediatric renal allograft recipients. The osmotic gradient created by the rectal administration of hypertonic radiographic material has been utilized previously to promote the passage of tenacious stool in patients with meconium ileus.[3, 6] By producing a similar osmotic diarrhea, we were able to relieve the obstruction in these patients by conservative means and thus avoid laparotomy.

REVIEW OF CASES

Patient 1. J. G., a four-year-old boy, presented with nephrotic syndrome in March, 1973, approximately five months after a two-year-old sister died of renal failure secondary to congenital nephrotic syndrome. The patient's clinical condition deteriorated rapidly and peritoneal dialysis was necessary by June, 1973.

Renal transplantation was performed on Aug. 16, 1973, when a suitable cadaveric kidney became available. The postoperative period was complicated by a transient episode of disseminated intravascular coagulation and infarction of the transplanted ureter requiring reimplantation on Aug. 19, 1973. Following reimplantation, the patient continued to experience acute tubular necrosis and required intermittent peritoneal dialysis. In addition, he required high-dose aluminum hydroxide suspension for control of hyperphosphatemia. On Aug. 23, he developed abdominal distention that progressed in spite of aggressive therapy with stool softeners, bisacodyl suppositories, glycerin suppositories, and various types of enemas. Five days later, fecal material could be palpated in the right lower quadrant and abdominal x-ray films showed an obturator obstruction extending into the small bowel (Fig. 1). Air-fluid levels were present and there was little colonic air. A sodium diatrizoate* enema was ad-

Supported in part by Grant No. DHEW 5PO1 CA14109-04.

Accepted for publication March 13, 1974.

*Hypaque, Winthrop Laboratories, New York, N. Y.

ministered under fluoroscopy but the contrast material did not pass the splenic flexure. A second enema resulted in the passage of much stool and decompression of the abdomen. There was no change in the patient's vital signs; hematocrit and electrolytes remained stable. Intravenous fluids were increased prophylactically in both instances. He had no further bowel symptoms as the acute tubular necrosis resolved.

Patient 2. D. R., a 12-year-old girl, was in apparent good health until May, 1973, when she presented with a two-week history of fatigue, facial edema, shortness of breath, and subsequent seizure activity. She was found to have a high blood urea nitrogen (BUN) level (153 mg. percent) and was referred to the University of Texas Medical Branch Hospitals, where dialysis was instituted. Evaluation revealed the patient to have end-stage renal disease, the etiology of which was undeterminable. After discharge, the patient received conservative medical therapy until that time that she was readmitted in August for elective transplantation from a living related donor source. During the two weeks prior to renal transplantation, she received aluminum hydroxide suspension (300 mg. four times daily) as part of her renal failure regimen. Renal transplantation was performed on Aug. 22, 1973. Three days later aluminum hydroxide suspension (30 c.c. four times daily) was instituted because of persistent hyperphosphatemia (11.1 mg. percent). Renal vein thrombosis necessitated removal of the renal allograft on the seventh posttransplant day, and peritoneal dialysis was reinstituted. On Sept. 4, she complained of severe abdominal pain and was noted to be passing much flatus. Roentgenograms of the abdomen revealed little colonic air; there was small bowel dilatation and a large collection of fecal material in the right colon. Iron bile salts, Fleet brand enemas, bisacodyl suppositories, and mineral oil retention enemas were unsuccessful in relieving the fecal impaction. Hypaque enema was at first unsuccessful in alleviating the obstruction, because the dye would not pass the site of impaction during fluoroscopy. A second enema was, however, successful in relieving the fecal impaction. There was no change in hematocrit or serum electrolytes following administration of the enemas.

Patient 3. J. C., a 15-year-old boy, first presented at the University of Texas Medical Branch at the age of 8 years with clinical and biopsy features of a rapidly progressive glomerulonephritis. Following intensive therapy, his renal function stabilized at about 50 percent of normal (as measured by serial clearances of inulin) until May, 1973, when in association with severe dehydration secondary to gastroenteritis, renal function fell, necessitating peritoneal dialysis. Renal function failed to recover and preparation for renal allotransplantation from a living related donor was undertaken. In the three-week period prior to transplantation, the patient received aluminum hydroxide in a dosage of 600 mg. three times daily and underwent daily peritoneal dialysis. Renal transplantation was performed on Aug. 29, 1973. The postoperative course was complicated by a transient ileus, although good renal function was prompt. On the ninth posttransplant day, the patient complained of severe abdominal pain. Bowel sounds were decreased, and the rectal ampulla was free of stool. Roentgenograms of the abdomen revealed a large collection of fecal material in the right colon consistent with an obturator obstruction (Fig. 2). Bisacodyl suppositories, Fleet brand enemas, iron bile salts tablets, and use of a rectal tube were ineffective in relieving the obstruction. An initial 500 c.c. Hypaque enema per rectum was also unsuccessful in relieving the obstruction. A second enema resulted in the passage of large amounts of stool and abdominal decompression. In neither instance did a change in vital signs occur following administration of the enema.

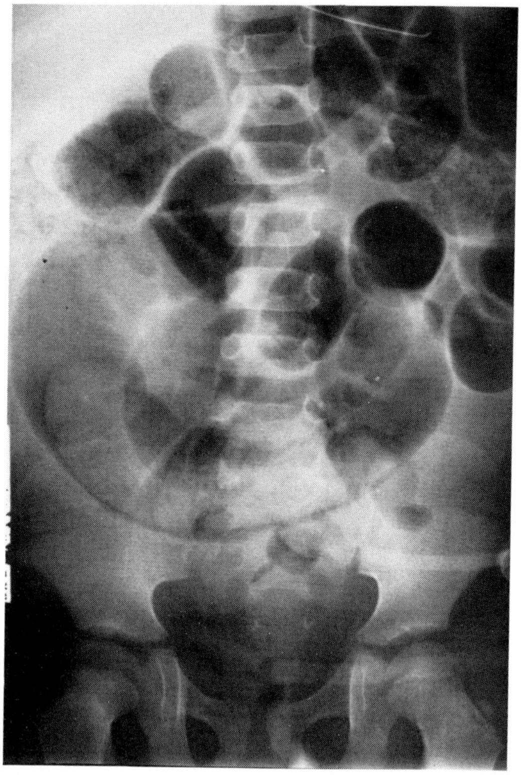

Fig. 1. Obturator intestinal obstruction is confirmed in Patient J. G. by the presence of air-fluid levels, dilated loops of small bowel, and the absence of colonic air.

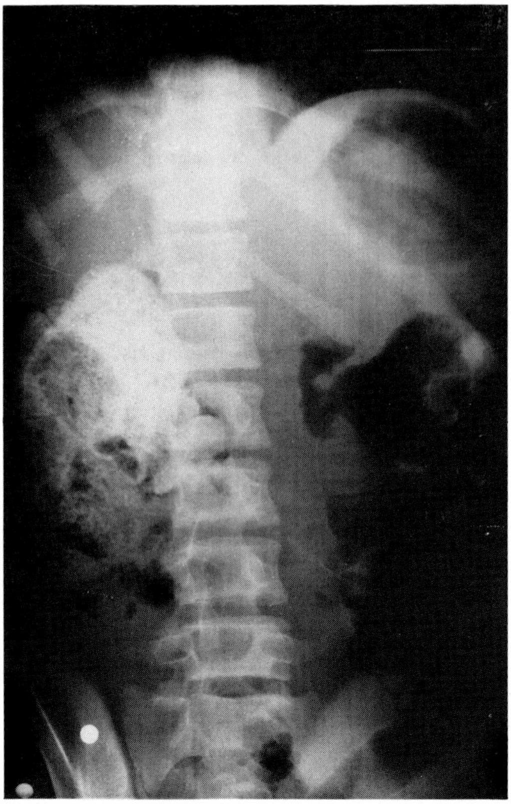

Fig. 2. Roentgenogram of the abdomen in patient J. C. at the time he developed severe abdominal pain. A large fecal impaction is present in the right colon.

DISCUSSION

Townsend and associates[5] recently reported the occurrence of obturator intestinal obstruction in three adult patients with renal failure. They attributed this complication to the administration of large doses of aluminum hydroxide suspension, changes in the patient's state of hydration with repeated dialysis, and intestinal inactivity. Similarly, peritoneal dialysis, aluminum hydroxide administration, and intestinal ileus secondary to the transplant procedure were all temporally related to the onset of fecal impaction in our renal allograft recipients. Since this complication is not commonly observed during the management of chronic renal failure in patients receiving aluminum hydroxide and intermittent dialysis, it may be that the ileus secondary to extraperitoneal dissection was the precipitating factor. In none of these children did their previous history or physical examination suggest bowel abnormalities.

Recently, Baliah and co-workers[1] described the occurrence of intestinal obstruction secondary to the administration of aluminum hydroxide in a child who had previously undergone renal transplantation. A significant decrease in renal function was noted following operation to relieve the obstruction.

While the patients of Townsend and coworkers[5] and Baliah and colleagues[1] required laparotomy for relief of obstruction, high-dose immunosuppression in the immediate posttransplant period added to the hazard of operative intervention in our patients. Since meglumine diatrizoate* has been employed to relieve intestinal obstruction in infants with meconium ileus,[3, 6] we used Hypaque in an attempt to induce a similar osmotic effect. Because of the potential problems related to extracellular volume depletion when such hyperosmolar compounds are employed,[2, 4] the contrast material was diluted with isotonic saline, reducing the osmolarity from 3,000 mOsm. per kilogram of water to approximately 1,300 mOsm. per kilogram of water. In this manner, the threat of dehydration produced by osmotic diarrhea was lessened. Prophylactic increase in fluids, frequent monitoring of vital signs, and serial hematocrits served as further safeguards against unrecognized dehydration. In two of our patients, the contrast material was injected under fluoroscopy, as has been recommended for infants.[3, 6] The size of one of our patients enabled us to administer the contrast material by gravity drainage without fluoroscopic control.

In all instances, the enema was administered through an appropriately sized Foley catheter with the balloon inflated and the patient's buttocks taped together. After retention of the fluid for fifteen minutes, the Foley catheter was withdrawn and the enema evacuated. The results of the initial enema were uniformly unsatisfactory, probably because the contrast material could not pass

*Gastrograffin, E. R. Squibb & Sons, Princeton, N. J.

the fecal mass causing the obstruction. The second enema always resulted in the passage of large amounts of stool. At no time were changes in vital signs or symptoms of extracellular volume depletion noted. In two patients, the rate of intravenous fluid administration was increased for a brief period during administration of the enema and following its evacuation to protect against undetected fluid loss secondary to osmotic diarrhea. In our oldest patient, an increased volume of oral fluids was given. Although the size of our patients gave us some range with regard to the aggressiveness of fluid replacement, one must be aware of the potential for acute dehydration and shock when this method is employed in infants without adequate fluid replacement.

REFERENCES

1. Baliah, T., Kim, K. H., Anthone, S., Anthone, R., Montes, M., and Andres, G. A.: Recurrence of Henock-Schönlein purpura (HSP) glomeruonephritis in transplanted kidney, Presented at the Sixth Annual Meeting of the American Society of Nephrology, Nov. 19-20, 1973, Washington, D. C.
2. Harris, P. D., Neuhauser, E. B. D., and Gerth, R.: The osmotic effect of water soluble contrast media on circulating plasma volume, Am. J. Roentgenol. **91:** 694, 1973.
3. Noblett, H.: Treatment of Uncomplicated meconium ileus by Gastrograffin enema: A preliminary report, J. Pediatr. Surg. **4:** 190, 1969.
4. Roe, M. I., Furst, A. J., Altman, D. H., and Poole, C. A.: The neonatal response to Gastrograffin enema, Pediatrics **48:** 29, 1971.
5. Townsend, C. M., Remmers, A. R., Sarles, H. R., and Fish, J. C.: Intestinal obstruction from medication Bexoar in patients with renal failure, N. Engl. J. Med. **288:** 1058, 1973.
6. Wagget, M. B., Johnson, D. G., Borns, P., and Bishop, H. C.: The non-operative treatment of meconium ileus by Gastrograffin enema, J. Pediatr. **77:** 407, 1970.

Factors altering pulmonary capillary perfusion

Michael L. Schwartz, M.D., William R. C. Murphy, M.D., Demetre M. Nicoloff, M.D., *and* **Edward W. Humphrey, M.D., Ph.D.,** *Minneapolis, Minn.*

The fraction of pulmonary capillaries perfused (FPCP) was determined in dogs by the ratio of pulmonary extravascular water (PEVW) measured by simultaneous indicator dilution curves of I^{125} radioiodinated serum albumin (RISA) and I^{131} iodoantipyrene to total weighed lung water. Cardiac output (CO) was varied by opening or closing chronic bilateral A-V fistulas. Lobar atelectasis was produced by obstructing the bronchus with an intrabronchial balloon. In control animals, the FPCP was 0.6 to 0.7 with a cardiac index (CI) of 3 to 4 L. per miunte per square meter. During hemorrhage, with a CI of 0.6 L. per minute per square meter, the FPCP was 0.54. During high blood flow (fistula open and CI, 5.2 L. per minute per square meter) the FPCP approached 1.0. Left lower lobar atelectasis (LLLA) had no effect on the FPCP, although the shunt fraction increased from 16 to 32 percent. These data indicate that pulmonary capillary recruitment is a linear function of CO between a cardiac index of 2 and 5 L. per minute. Over a short period, atelectasis does not change FPCP.

From the Department of Surgery, Minneapolis Veterans Administration Hospital and the University of Minnesota Hospital.

THE DOUBLE-INDICATOR dilution technique for the measurement of pulmonary extravascular water (PEVW) has been used by several investigators as evidence for a change in the water content of the lung in various pathological conditions. Prior work from this laboratory[10, 11, 13] has shown that radioiodinated serum albumin (RISA) used as the reference indicator and iodoantipyrene used as the diffusible indicator would indeed accurately measure a change in PEVW in an in vitro model up to a 100 percent increase in volume. However, the interpretation of data showing an increase in volume of PEVW in vivo with the use of this method has been unclear. Because indicator dilution methods can measure the volume of *perfused* capillary beds only, it is possible (and indeed likely) that an increase in the volume of PEVW calculated by this method represents principally an increase in the fraction of pulmonary capillaries that are perfused (FPCP). In the present work, this fraction is represented by the ratio of PEVW, calculated from RISA and iodoantipyrene indicator dilution curves, to the total lung water measured by the difference between the wet and dry weights of the lung after the death of the animal. We are interested in determining what effect an increase or decrease in pulmonary blood flow would have on this ratio and, additionally, to determine if the ratio changed with lobar atelectasis.

Accepted for publication March 13, 1974.

METHODS

All groups were anesthetized with pentobarbital and allowed to breath spontaneous-

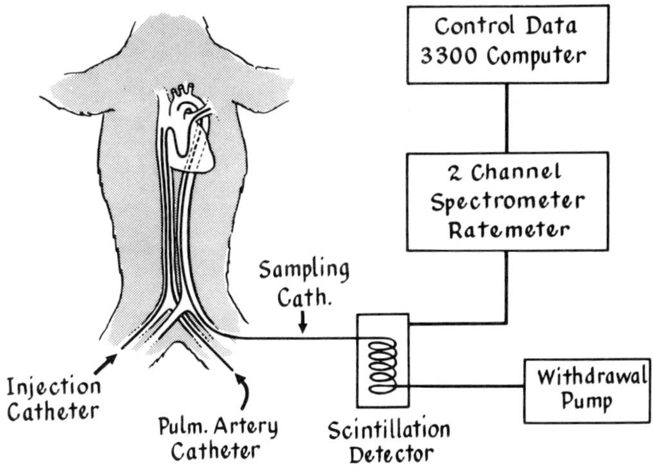

Fig. 1. Schematic representation of experimental apparatus.

ly. Sampling and injection catheters were placed in the ascending aorta and in the right atrium. A Swan-Ganz catheter was positioned in the pulmonary artery for withdrawal of mixed venous blood and to measure pulmonary artery and pulmonary wedge pressures. Four groups of dogs were studied.

Group 1. Atelectasis of the left lower lobe was produced in six dogs by inflating a balloon, under bronchoscopic control, in the left lower lobe bronchus. The completeness of atelectasis was always verified at autopsy. Prior to inflating the balloon and 30 minutes afterward, the pulmonary shunt fraction, $\dot{Q}s/\dot{Q}t$, the PEVW, the central blood volume (CBV), and cardiac output (CO) were measured.

Group 2. A group of 12 dogs underwent creation of bilateral femoral arteriovenous (AV) fistulas three weeks prior to the study. During the experiment, the CO was changed acutely by opening and closing these fistulas. After each of these maneuvers, 15 minutes was allowed for the CO to become stable, and then the PEVW, the CO, and the CBV were measured.

Group 3. In a group of six dogs, the CO was decreased by acutely bleeding the animals through a femoral artery catheter to a mean systemic pressure of 50 mm. Hg. The PEVW, CO, and CBV were determined 15 minutes after this pressure was obtained.

Group 4. This group of seven dogs had indicator dilution measurements both while breathing room air and while breathing 100 percent oxygen.

Shunt flow was determined by allowing the dogs to breath 100 percent oxygen for ten minutes, then withdrawing blood anaerobically from the aortic and pulmonary artery catheters. The pH, Pco_2, and Po_2 were measured on a Instrumentation Laboratory Blood Gas Analyzer. Hemoglobin was determined by the cyanomethemoglobin method. Oxygen saturation was determined from a Severinghaus dog slide rule, and the oxygen content was calculated from the sum of combined and dissolved oxygen. $\dot{Q}s/\dot{Q}t$ was calculated by the standard shunt equation.

Pulmonary extravascular water was measured by injecting a mixture of I^{125} RISA and I^{131} iodoantipyrene into the right atrium (Fig. 1). An effluent blood sample was continuously withdrawn from the aortic catheter through a flow-through cuvette in a well-type scintillation detector. The output of this detector went to a dual-channel spectrometer–ratemeter connected on line to a Control Data 3300 Digital Computer. The computation programs made use of the usual assumption of exponential decay of each indicator. The PEVW was calculated from the relationship PEVW $= \dot{Q}\ (\overline{T}_d - \overline{T}_r)$, where $\dot{Q}$ is the cardiac output, $\overline{T}_d$ is the mean transit time of the diffusible indicator, and $\overline{T}_r$ is the mean transit time of the reference indicator. Because the distribution coefficient of iodoantipyrene in blood is 1.0, no cor-

Table I. *Atelectasis**

Parameters†	*Control*	*Atelectasis*
Pa_{O_2} (torr)	488.0 ± 11.0	170.0 ± 43.0‡
Pa_{CO_2} (torr)	34.0 ± 0.9	33.8 ± 3.1
pH	8.34 ± 0.01	7.33 ± 0.03
$\dot{Q}s/\dot{Q}t$	0.16 ± 0.03	0.32 ± 0.06‡
PA (mm. Hg)	12.2 ± 2.2	12.7 ± 1.5
Wedge (mm. Hg)	3.0 ± 1.2	2.6 ± 0.6
BP (mm. Hg.)	122.0 ± 5.0	114.0 ± 9.0
CO (L./min.)	1.73 ± 0.18	1.70 ± 0.19
CBV (c.c.)	236.0 ± 20.0	220.0 ± 12.0
PEVW (c.c.)	69.6 ± 8.0	69.8 ± 9.2
FPCP	0.81 ± 0.09	0.81 ± 0.11

*Values are mean and standard error of the mean for the control period and one-half hour after atelectasis.

†$\dot{Q}s/\dot{Q}t$, shunt fraction; PA, mean pulmonary artery pressure; Wedge, pulmonary artery wedge pressure; BP, systemic arterial pressure; CO, cardiac output; CBV, central blood volume; PEVW, pulmonary extravascular water; FPCP, fraction of pulmonary capillaries perfused.

‡Significant at 0.05 level.

Table II. *A-V fistulas**

Parameters†	*Fistula open*	*Fistula closed*
$\dot{Q}s/\dot{Q}t$	0.20 ± 0.01	0.13 ± 0.02‡
PA (mm. Hg)	18.8 ± 0.8	14.6 ± 1.4‡
Wedge (mm. Hg)	7.0 ± 0.06	7.1 ± 0.08
BP (mm. Hg)	153.0 ± 10.0	155.0 ± 6.0
CI (L./min./M.^{2})	5.2 ± 0.6	3.1 ± 0.6‡
CBV (c.c.)	728.0 ± 76.0	533.0 ± 75.0‡
PEVW (c.c./Kg.)	6.3 ± 0.8	3.7 ± 0.4‡
FPCP	1.05 ± 0.10	0.62 ± 0.07‡

*Mean and standard error of the mean with fistula open and closed.

†$\dot{Q}s/\dot{Q}t$, shunt fraction; PA, mean pulmonary artery pressure; Wedge, pulmonary artery wedge; BP, systemic arterial pressure; CI, cardiac index; CBV, central blood volume; PEVW, pulmonary extravascular water; FPCP, fraction of pulmonary capillaries perfused.

‡Significant at 0.05 level.

Table III. *Hypovolemia**

Parameters†	*Control*	*Hypotension*
Pa_{O_2} (torr)	82.0 ± 5.0	86.8 ± 6.9
Pa_{CO_2} (torr)	26.4 ± 1.6	22.7 ± 2.4
pH	7.47 ± 0.03	7.27 ± 0.05‡
PA (mm. Hg)	9.8 ± 1.2	5.2 ± 0.8‡
BP (mm. Hg)	133.0 ± 12.0	54.0 ± 2.0‡
CI (L./min./M.^{2})	3.4 ± 0.2	0.6 ± 0.1‡
CBV (c.c.)	203.0 ± 16.0	122.0 ± 16.0‡
PEVW (c.c./Kg.)	3.2 ± 0.6	2.8 ± 0.4
FPCP	0.59 ± 0.11	0.54 ± 0.08

*Values are mean and standard error of the mean for control period and two hours of hypotension.

†Pa_{O_2} and Pa_{CO_2}, partial pressure of O_2 and CO_2 in arterial blood (Note animals in this group were on room air); PA, mean pulmonary artery pressure; BP, mean blood pressure; PEVW, pulmonary extravascular water; FPCP, fraction of pulmonary capillaries perfused.

‡Significant at the 0.05 level.

rection for hematocrit was necessary. At the conclusion of each experiment, the dogs were exsanguinated, the lungs were excised, blotted, weighed, dried for 48 hours, and then reweighed. This difference was considered total lung water (TLW). Because the corrections for retained blood was smaller than the variation in PEVW, no such correction was used. The fraction of pulmonary capillaries perfused was assumed to equal the ratio PEVW: TLW.

RESULTS

Left lower lobe atelectasis in a group of six dogs caused a mean fall of P_aO_2 from 488 to 170 torr (Table I). This corresponded to an increase in the shunt fraction from 0.16 to 0.32. Over the ensuing 30 minutes, pulmonary artery wedge pressures were unchanged, and within this period of time, there was no significant change in the calculated PEVW or in the FPCP.

The CO was changed acutely in Group 2 of 12 dogs by opening and closing chronic A-V fistula and in a Group 3 of seven dogs by hemorrhage (Tables II and III). Closure of the A-V fistula caused a mean fall in the cardiac index (CI) from 5.2 to 3.1 L. per minute per square meter. Pulmonary artery pressure decreased significantly, the PEVW decreased acutely from 6.3 to 3.7 c.c. per kilogram, and the FPCP decreased from a mean of 1.05 to 0.62. Valid data could not be obtained from several dogs with A-V fistula open because the rapid recirculation interfered with the calculation of the downslope of the indicator dilution curves. Table II, however, represents data from eight dogs which we believe to be valid.

Hemorrhage caused a fall in the CI from a mean of 3.4 to 0.6 L. per minute per square meter. Both pulmonary artery and pulmonary artery wedge pressures fell slightly during this time. The PEVW decreased from 3.2 to 2.8 c.c. per kilogram while the FPCP decreased from 0.59 to 0.54.

The relationship between the FPCP and the CI is given in Fig. 2. A linear regression performed on all the data has a correlation coefficient of 0.5. When the data from 2 to 5 L. per minute per square meter are analyzed alone, the correlation coefficient is 0.81. Below a CI of 2 L. per minute, the FPCP does not appear to decrease below a value of 0.5. Above 5 L. per minute, the FPCP stayed near 1.0.

Six dogs of Group 4 were placed on 100 percent oxygen to determine if this would affect the measurement of PEVW. After ten minutes, the CO changed from 1.76 to 1.44 L. per minute and the mean PEVW decreased from 45.3 to 43.4 ml. Neither of these changes are significant.

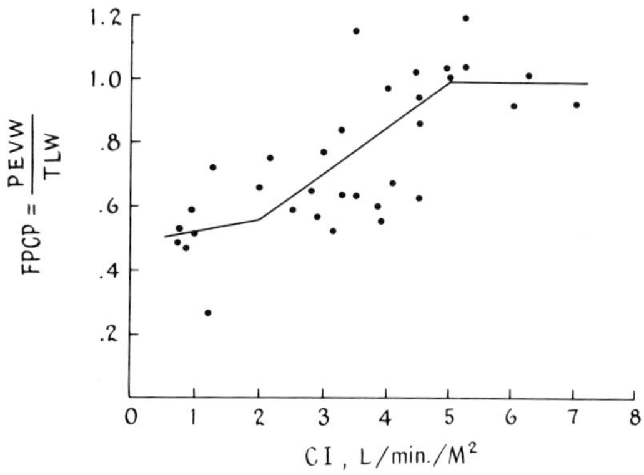

Fig. 2. Fraction of pulmonary capillaries perfused (FPCP) vs. cardiac index (CI). (See text for discussion.)

DISCUSSION

The control values of PEVW in this study are comparable to those of Chinard and Enns,[1] Goresky and associates,[5] Gump and colleagues,[6] English and co-workers,[2] and others who use tritiated water as a diffusible indicator and tagged red cells, albumin, or cardio-green as a nondiffusible indicator.

Atelectasis did not cause an immediate (30 minute) change in pulmonary capillary perfusion when determined by the indicator dilution curves. Since the left lower lobe receives 16 percent of the pulmonary blood flow,[14] atelectasis is expected to increase the shunt fraction by a similar percentage. In this study, the shunt fraction increased by 19 percent when atelectasis was induced. The amount of shunting generally decreases with time, but from the work of Fishman[3] and a recent study by Wahrenbrock and associates,[14] this decrease takes several hours to develop.

Changes in the calculated PEVW can represent either an actual change in lung water or a change in the size of perfused capillary beds. Previous investigations into the relationship of PEVW to pulmonary blood flow have revealed contradictory results. Goresky and associates[5] found PEVW increased with exercise in awake dogs. Marshall and colleagues[12] and Korsgren and associates[8] have confirmed these findings in humans. Levine and associates[9] found no change in the PEVW of dogs infused with dextran to increase CO. Kirk[7] reported that changing the blood flow by hemorrhage, hypoxia, or isoproterenol resulted in no change in PEVW. However, previously reported studies from this laboratory[13] on dogs have shown that isoproterenol seems to have a direct action on the pulmonary vasculature to prevent the usual increase in PEVW that occurs with prolonged anesthesia or with hemorrhagic hypotension and reinfusion.

Fishman[4] found the inflection in the flow-pressure curve of the pulmonary circulation to occur at an increase of 250 percent of control resting blood flow. The two inflections in the flow-FPCP curve from the present study occurred at cardiac indices of 2 and 5 L. per minute. This is a 250 percent increase in blood flow between the two plateaus of capillary perfusion; however, the resting blood flow in these animals averaged 3 L. per minute. The difference between the pressure-flow data and the PEVW data may represent additional vasodilatation of the precapillary pulmonary vessels after all capillaries are open.

The present data seem to give validity to the use of the ratio: calculated PEVW: weighed TLW as an estimate of lung capillary perfusions in those instances in which no increase in weighed lung water is found. The ability to make this estimate may prove to be a valuable tool in the study of pulmonary function.

REFERENCES

1. Chinard, F.P., and Enns, T.: Transcapillary pulmonary exchange of water in the dog, Am. J. Physiol. **178:** 197, 1954.
2. English, T. A. H., Digerness, S. B., Kirklin,

J. W., and Karp, R. B.: Pulmonary capillary blood volume and lung water in pulmonary edema, Surg. Gynecol. Obstet. **132:** 93, 1972.
3. Fishman, A. P.: Repiratory gases in the regulation of the pulmonary circulation, Physiol. Rev. **41:** 214, 1961.
4. Fishman, A. P.: Dynamics of the pulmonary circulation, *in* The handbook of physiology, Vol. 2, Hamilton, W. F., section editor: Sect. 2: Circulation, The Williams & Wilkins Co., Baltimore, Md., 1963, p. 1667.
5. Goresky, C. A., Cronin, R. F. P., and Wangel, B. E.: Indicator dilution measurement of extravascular water in the lungs, J. Clin. Invest. **48:** 487, 1969.
6. Gump, F. E., Mashima, Y., and Kinnex, J. M.: Water balance and extravascular lung water in surgical patients, Am. J. Surg. **119:** 515, 1970.
7. Kirk, B. W.: The effect of alterations in pulmonary blood flow in lung-exchangeable water in the dog, J. Appl. Physiol. **27:** 607, 1969.
8. Korsgren, M., Luepker, R., Lander, R., and Varnavskas, E.: Pulmonary intra- and extravascular fluid volume changes with exercise, Cardiovasc. Res. **3:** 1, 1969.
9. Levine, O. R., Mellins, R. B., and Senior, R. M.: Extravascular lung water and distribution of pulmonary blood flow in the dog, J. Appl. Physiol. **28:** 166, 1970.
10. Lindsay, W. G., and Humphrey, E. W.: The sodium space in pressure-induced pulmonary edema, Curr. Top. Surg. Res. **2:** 351, 1970.
11. Lindsay, W. G., and Humphrey, E. W.: Measurement of pulmonary extravascular water, Surgery **71:** 650, 1972.
12. Marshall, B. E., Teichner, R. L., Kallos, T., Sugerman, H. J., Wyche, M. W., and Tantum, K. R.: Effects of posture and exercise on the pulmonary extravascular water volume in man, J. Appl. Physiol. **31:** 375, 1971.
13. Murphy, W. A., Nicoloff, D. M., and Humphrey, E. W.: Factors influencing the measurement of pulmonary extravascular water, J. Surg. Res. **14:** 331, 1973.
14. Wahrenbrock, E. A., Carrico, C. J., Amundsen, D. A., Trummer, M. J., and Severinghaus, J. W.: Increased atelectatic pulmonary shunt during hemorrhagic shock in dogs, J. Appl. Physiol. **29:** 615, 1970.

The effect of endogenous secretin and cholecystokinin on pentagastrin-stimulated innervated and denervated gastric mucosa

John A. Dorighi, M.D., Donald L. Kaminski, M.D., *and* **Vallee L. Willman, M.D.,**
St. Louis, Mo.

The inhibition of pentagastrin-stimulated hydrogen ion output by endogenous secretin and cholecystokinin (CCK) was evaluated in dogs with chronic gastric fistulas (innervated mucosa) and Heidenhain pouches (denervated mucosa). Endogenous secretin release was stimulated by intraduodenal HCl, and endogenous CCK release was stimulated by intraduodenal elemental amino acids. The effectiveness of these methods to stimulate duodenal hormone release was confirmed in dogs with chronic pancreatic fistulas. We found that endogenous CCK produced no inhibition of pentagastrin-stimulated hydrogen ion output from innervated or denervated mucosa. The intraduodenal amino acids produce a pancreatic response similar to, but greater than 2 U. per kilogram per hour of exogenous CCK, but they do not inhibit an acid secretory response. Endogenous secretin is an effective enterogastrone significantly inhibiting a pentagastrin-stimulated hydrogen ion response from innervated and denervated mucosa. The percent inhibition in innervated mucosa was significantly greater at all doses of intraduodenal hydrogen ion than that produced in denervated gastric mucosa. The results indicate that vagal section decreases the effectiveness of the duodenal enterogastrone.

From the Department of Surgery, St. Louis University School of Medicine, St. Louis, Mo.

RECENT STUDIES have demonstrated the ability of exogenous secretin to act as an enterogastrone and inhibit gastric acid secretion.[4, 6, 12, 22] The influence of vagal innervation of the parietal cell mass on these enterogastrone mechanisms is not well understood.

Code and Watkinson[3] evaluated the effect of intraduodenal acid on gastric acid output stimulated by alcohol and a test meal and concluded that significant inhibition of gastric secretion by acid in the duodenum only occurs when the vagal nerve supply to the gastric mucosa is intact. This result is in contrast to that obtained by Brooks and associates,[2] who found that secretin inhibition of food-stimulated gastric acid secretion was significantly increased in denervated pouches compared to innervated pouches.

Exogenous cholecystokinin (CCK) has been shown to be an effective enterogastrone, producing a significant inhibition of pentagastrin-stimulated hydrogen ion output from a denervated Heidenhain pouch.[4, 13, 24] Konturek and colleagues[17] have found that endogenous CCK, released by duodenal perfusion with elemental amino acids, was effective as an enterogastrone only when acting on innervated gastric mucosa. Others[23] have also found that endogenous CCK is not effective as an enterogastrone when acting on denervated gastric mucosa.

Accepted for publication March 13, 1974.

Address all correspondence to: Donald L. Kaminski, M.D., Department of Surgery, St. Louis University Hospital, 1325 S. Grand Blvd., St. Louis, Mo. 63104.

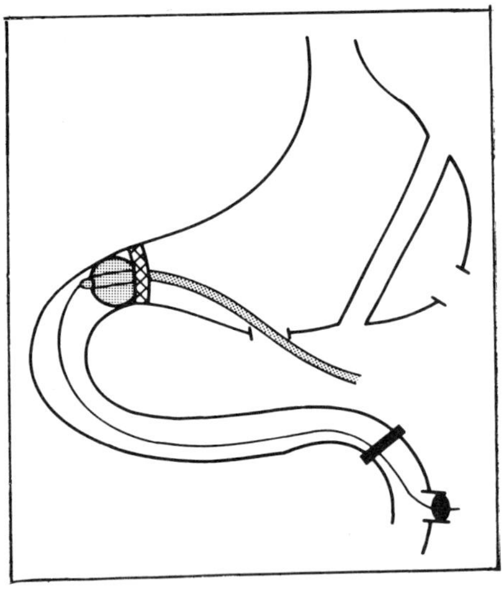

Fig. 1. Schematic drawing of the preparation used to stimulate endogenous duodenal hormone release.

This study was designed to compare the enterogastrone properties of endogenous secretin and CCK on innervated and denervated gastric mucosa.

METHOD

Part 1. Preliminary evaluation of the methods utilized to release secretin and CCK was performed.

Pancreatic fistulas were created in four female dogs with the use of a modification of the apparatus described by Herrera and co-workers.[10] Two weeks following the operative procedures, the experiments were begun. Prior to each experiment, the animals were fasted for 18 hours. During each experiment, a continuous intravenous infusion of 0.15 M NaCl solution (60 ml. per hour) was delivered by a peristaltic pump.* In addition, the duodenum was continuously perfused through the pancreatic cannula. The perfusate was 0.15 M NaCl solution at a rate of 150 ml. per hour until three consecutive 15 minute basal collections from the pancreatic fistula of less than 2.5 ml. per 15 minute collection were obtained.

Following the three control periods, the pancreatic fistulas were stimulated for nine 15 minute periods. The stimulus was either intraduodenal, 160 mM HCl at 150 ml. per hour (24 mEq. per hour); intraduodenal, 127 mM L-phenylalanine* at 150 ml. per hour (19 μM per hour); or intraduodenal, 0.15 M NaCl solution plus intravenous commercial CCK† in a dose of 2 U. per kilogram per hour. The phenylalanine perfusate was prepared just prior to infusion, made isosmolar (300 mOsm. per kilogram) with mannitol and adjusted to pH 7.0 with dilute NaOH. Two experiments for each variable were performed in random order on each of four dogs.

*Auto-Analyzer, Technicon Corp., Tarrytown, N. Y.

Pancreatic secretions were collected and measured every 15 minutes. Pancreatic protein concentration was determined and equated with pancreatic enzyme secretion. The protein concentration was determined by measuring fluorescence at 280 nm. using an Auto-Analyzer (Technicon). The standard was bovine serum albumin, and concentration is expressed as milligrams per milliliter of pancreatic juice. Hydrogen ion concentration in gastric juice was determined by titrating 0.2 ml. samples with 0.2N NaOH to pH 7.0 on an automatic titrator and pH meter.† Pancreatic bicarbonate concentration was estimated by adding 0.5 ml. of pancreatic juice to 1 ml. of 0.1 N HCl, heating and back-titrating the residual HCl with 0.2N NaOH.

Part 2. Four dogs were prepared each with a Gregory cannula[7] in a Heidenhain pouch and a Thomas[25] cannula in the main stomach. In addition, a second small cannula was placed in the jejunum just distal to the ligament of Trietz. A plastic cuff was anchored around the pylorus to facilitate securing a No. 18 Fr. Foley catheter in place. For the experiments, the Foley catheter was drawn from the gastric fistula into the duodenum by a string left in the bowel between the gastric and jejunal fistulas (Fig. 1). During the experiments, the balloon of the Foley catheter was inflated and pulled tightly against the plastic cuff. Duodenal perfusion was performed through the Foley

*Sigma Chemical Co., St. Louis, Mo.
†Radiometer, Copenhagen, Denmark.

catheter. A marker (methylene blue) in the perfusate demonstrated that no perfusate refluxed back into the stomach.

The experiments were begun three weeks after surgery and performed on alternate days. After an 18 hour fast, the fistulas were opened and duodenal perfusion was instituted. Throughout each experiment, the animals received a continuous intravenous infusion delivered by a peristaltic pump* of 0.15 M NaCl solution at a rate of 60 ml. per hour for two 15 minute periods followed by 0.15 M NaCl solution with pentagastrin,† 4 μg per kilogram per hour for three hours.

The duodenum was perfused with 0.15 M NaCl solution for eight 15 minute periods at a rate of 150 ml. per hour, after which time the test substances were infused into the duodenum for six 15 minute periods. Control experiments were performed when 0.15 M NaCl solution was infused into the duodenum throughout the study. Two control and two experiments with each duodenal perfusate were performed in random order on each of four dogs. The acid solutions infused were 160, 120, and 60 mM HCl, delivering H^+ loads of 24, 18, and 12 mEq. per hour, respectively. The amino acid perfusate consisted of 127 mM L-phenylalanine given as described previously.

Gastric fistula and Heidenhain pouch secretions were collected continuously, divided into 15 minute samples and measured to the nearest 0.1 ml. Hydrogen ion content was determined as described previously.

Statistical analysis was performed by a Student's t test for non-paired values. As used in the text, "significant" indicates $p < 0.05$, unless otherwise indicated.

RESULTS

The effectiveness of the methods utilized in this study to produce endogenous secretin and CCK release are indicated in Figs. 2 and 3. Intraduodenal HCl (24 mEq. per hour) produced a mean pancreatic bicarbonate output during periods 10, 11, and 12 of 1,720 ± 128 μEq per 15 minutes (control, 37 ± 9 μEq per 15 minutes). Intraduodenal amino acid perfusion produced pancreatic volume and protein output and concentrations greater than 2 U. per kilogram per hour of exogenous CCK.

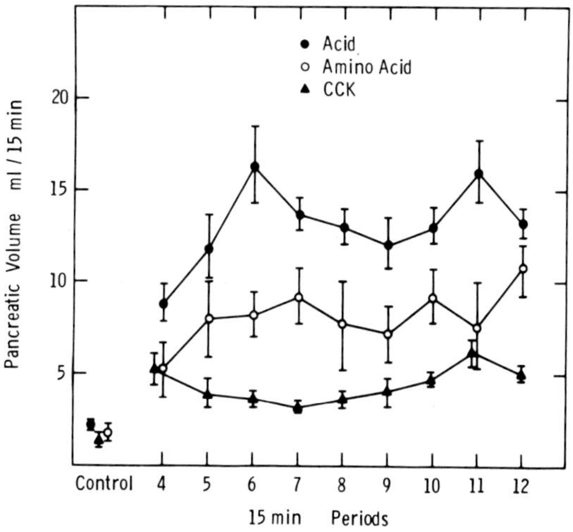

Fig. 2. Pancreatic volume response produced by the various stimuli indicated. Control points represent the mean of 24 values obtained from three 15 minute periods from two experiments on each of four dogs. Test points represent the mean of eight values obtained from two experiments on each of four dogs. Bars indicate one S.E.M.

The effect of intraduodenal hydrogen ion on pentagastrin-stimulated Heidenhain pouch acid output is illustrated in Fig. 4. When the mean of the values produced during periods 10, 11, and 12 were used as representing maximal inhibition, a significant decrease in acid output, as compared to corresponding control values, was produced by infusing 24 and 18 mEq. per hour, but not 12 mEq. per hour.

The effect of intraduodenal hydrogen ion on pentagastrin-stimulated gastric fistula output is illustrated in Fig. 5. By utilizing the mean values of periods 10, 11, and 12, significant inhibition of pentagastrin-stimulated gastric fistula acid output occurred with all three doses of intraduodenal hydrogen ion when compared to corresponding control values.

The percentage of inhibition of pentagastrin-stimulated acid secretion from the

*Auto-Analyzer, Technicon Corp., Tarrytown, N. Y.
†Ayerst Labs., New York, N. Y.

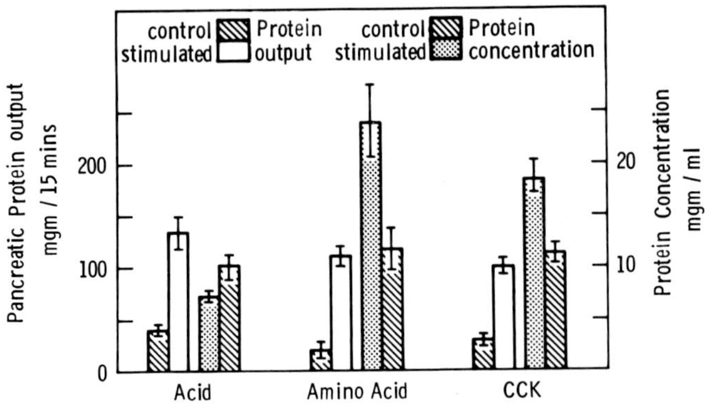

Fig. 3. Pancreatic protein output and concentration in response to the various stimuli indicated.

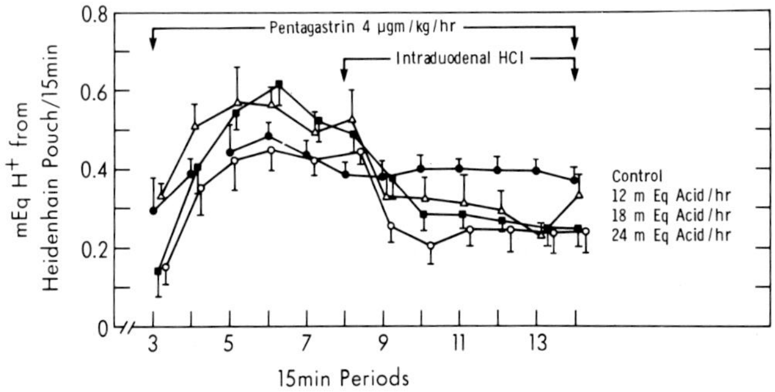

Fig. 4. The effect of infusion of various concentrations of acid into the duodenum on Heidenhain pouch secretion stimulated by 4.0 μg per kilogram per hour of pentagastrin. Control received pentagastrin and intraduodenal 0.15 M NaCl solution. In this figure and Figure 5, each point represents the mean and one S.E.M. of eight values obtained from two experiments on each of four dogs.

gastric fistulas and Heidenhain pouches was calculated by subtracting the mean of the values obtained during periods 10, 11, and 12 from the mean acid outputs of the corresponding control periods, dividing by the control values, and multiplying by 100 to give percent inhibition. In Fig. 6, the percent inhibition of hydrogen ion output from the gastric fistula is compared to the percent inhibition from the Heidenhain pouch. The percent inhibition of acid from both the gastric fistula and Heidenhain pouch appears to be dependent on the dose of H^+ delivered to the duodenum. At each dose of hydrogen ion administered, the percent inhibition of acid output from the innervated mucosa of the gastric fistula is significantly greater than the percent inhibition of acid output from the denervated mucosa of the Heidenhain pouch.

The effect of duodenal perfusion with L-phenylalanine on the inhibition of pentagastrin-stimulated gastric fistula and Heidenhain pouch acid output is presented in Fig. 7. There was no evidence of an inhibitory response produced by the release of endogenous CCK.

DISCUSSION

Others have previously presented evidence which indicates that the release of endogenous secretin from the duodenum is stimulated primarily by hydrogen ion in the duodenum and that hydrogen ion is the only strong releaser of secretin.[9] Preshaw and associates[20] demonstrated that only at high

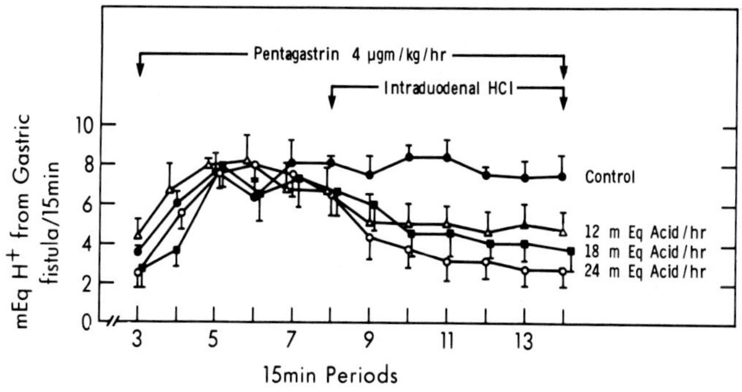

Fig. 5. The effect of infusion of various concentrations of acid into the duodenum on gastric fistula secretion stimulated by 4 μg per kilogram per hour.

rates of hydrogen ion infusion was there evidence that acid in the duodenum stimulated CCK release, and Meyer and Grossman[18] have postulated that the ratio of secretin to CCK released by acid in the duodenum is approximately 24:1.

Go and associates[5] demonstrated in man that neutral L-form amino acids are effective stimulants of CCK release, and Meyer and co-workers[19] have presented evidence in dogs that such amino acids release CCK, but not secretin. In view of the apparent capability of amino acids in the duodenum to release CCK selectively and intraduodenal hydrogen ion to release practically only secretin, it should be possible to define the relative capabilities of the two hormones to act as enterogastrones by stimulating their release selectively.

The data presented in this study suggests that endogenous CCK is not an effective enterogastrone; it inhibits neither innervated nor denervated pentagastrin-stimulated gastric mucosa. This result agrees with that of Spingola and Grossman[23] and Konturek and associates,[17] who found that release of endogenous CCK by intraduodenal amino acids did not inhibit the acid output from a pentagastrin-stimulated Heidenhain pouch. In a similar study, however, Konturek and colleagues[15] found that endogenous CCK did inhibit acid output from a pentagastrin-stimulated, innervated Pavlov pouch. The differences in the results obtained may be due to the use in Konturek's

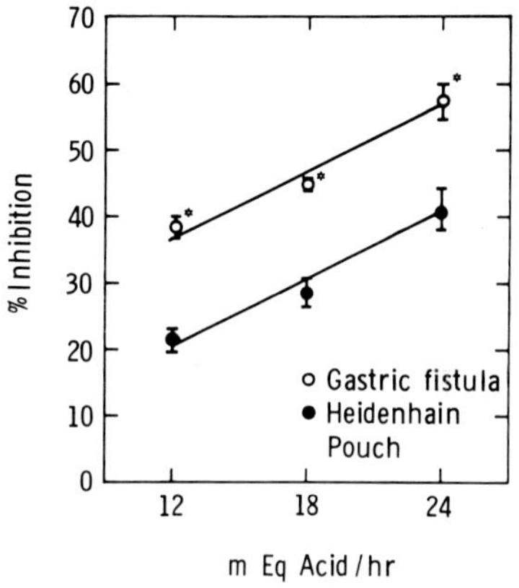

Fig. 6. Percent inhibition of pentagastrin-stimulated hydrogen ion output from the gastric fistulas and Heidenhain pouches produced by various concentrations of intraduodenal acid. Lines were drawn by the method of least squares. The equation for the line representing inhibition of gastric fistula output is $y = 18.33 + 1.56X$, $r = 0.98$. The equation of the line representing inhibition of Heidenhain pouch acid output is $y = 0.60 + 1.66X$, $r = 0.98$. Asterisk indicates that the percent inhibition obtained from gastric fistula is significantly greater than that obtained from the Heidenhain pouch.

study,[15] of an amino acid mixture (leucine and tryptophan) which possibly released more CCK. It may also be due to the larger parietal cell mass subjected to inhibition in our study where gastric fistulas, rather than Pavlov pouches were utilized. Also parietal cell stimulation in the study by Konturek was accomplished by 2 μg per kilogram per hour of pentagastrin, one half the pentagastrin dose employed in our study. It is

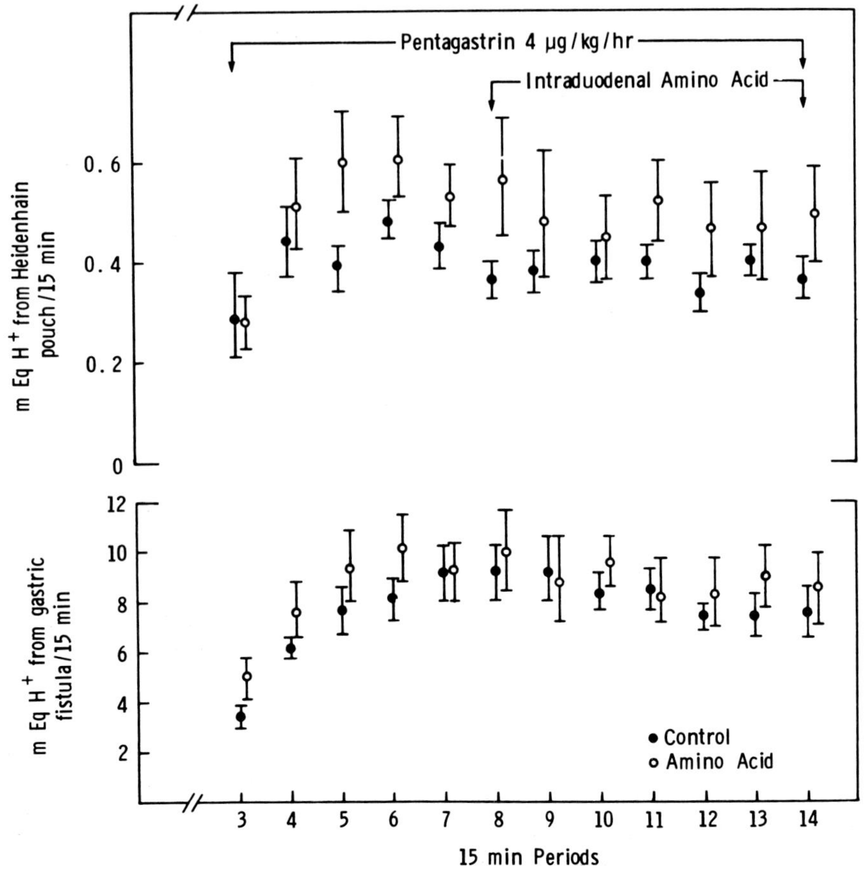

Fig. 7. Response of pentagastrin-stimulated gastric fistulas and Heidenhain pouches to the intraduodenal infusion of 127 mM L-phenylalanine. During the control experiment, 0.15 M NaCl solution was infused into the duodenum. Each point represents the mean and S.E.M. of eight values obtained from two experiments on each of four dogs.

possible that a larger endogenous CCK load, effecting inhibition on a smaller parietal cell mass, stimulated by a smaller pentagastrin dose, may produce significant inhibition of acid output in innervated gastric mucosa.

The effectiveness of exogenous CCK as an enterogastrone inhibiting acid output from denervated Heidenhain pouches has been well demonstrated.[4, 13, 14, 24] The reason for the lack of inhibition by endogenous CCK is unclear. The possibility that pentagastrin administration interferes with CCK release has been eliminated by studies presented by Konturek and associates.[16] Using stimulation of pancreatic protein or enzyme secretion as an index of CCK release, they demonstrated that endogenous CCK significantly augments the pancreatic protein response produced by pentagastrin. The data in Figs. 1 and 2 indicates that the mechanism utilized to release CCK in this study produces a pancreatic response greater than 2 U. per kilogram per hour of exogenous CCK, a dose which others[13] have found maximally inhibits pentagastrin-stimulated acid output.

Preliminary studies[21] with radioimmunoassay of CCK have demonstrated significant increases in serum CCK levels by perfusion of jejunal loops with L-phenylalanine while similar perfusion of duodenum failed to elicit the response, suggesting a possible reason for our failure to elicit an inhibitory response with intraduodenal amino acids. This data, however, does not agree with that of Konturek and associates,[16] who found by bioassay that the amount of releasable CCK in the small intestine decreases as the distance from the pylorus increases. The data presented suggests that in the denervated stomach and possibly in the innervated stomach of the dog, the hormonal receptor mechanism[8] which stimulates the parietal cell to secrete hydrogen ion is receptive to the pentagastrin molecule (stimulation) and to exogenous porcine CCK (inhibition), but not to endogenous canine CCK.

The inhibition of a pentagastrin-stimulated gastric acid secretory response by secretin is significantly greater when the mucosa is innervated in contrast to denervated gastric mucosa. While it is clear from this study that innervation of the gastric mucosa enhances inhibition, the study does not define the exact mechanism by which this enhancement occurs. It is possible that a regional vagal mechanism inhibiting acid output is stimulated by acid in the duodenum, although no evidence of such a mechanism has been presented. Similarly, local cholinergic factors may enhance the humoral response. Again, there is no evidence supporting such a hypothesis; however, we do know that secretin will not decrease direct cholinergic stimulation of the parietal cell.[26] Also, Grossman[9] has suggested that the responsiveness of the parietal cell to gastrin stimulation is reduced by vagotomy and that the diminished response is due to reduced affinity of the gastrin molecule for the receptor sites. It is possible that vagotomy similarly reduces the affinity of the receptor site for secretin, thus decreasing the acid inhibition and rendering secretin inhibition of pentagastrin-stimulated hydrogen ion output greater in innervated gastric mucosa than in denervated mucosa.

Pentagastrin was donated by John D. Stevens, M.D., Ayerst Laboratories, New York, N. Y.

REFERENCES

1. Anderson, S.: Inhibitory effects of hydrochloric acid in the duodenum on gastrin-stimulated gastric secretion in Heidenhain pouch dogs, Acta Physiol. Scand. **50:** 105, 1960.
2. Brooks, A. M., Stening, G. F., and Grossman, M. I.: Effect of gastric vagal denervation on inhibition of acid secretion by secretin, Am. J. Dig. Dis. **16:** 193, 1971.
3. Code, C. F., and Watkinson, G.: Importance of vagal innervation in the regulatory effect of acid in the duodenum on gastric secretion of acid, J. Physiol. (Lond.) **130:** 233, 1955.
4. Gillespie, I. E., and Grossman, M. I.: Inhibitory effect of secretin and cholecystokinin on Heidenhain pouch response to gastrin extract and histamine, Gut **5:** 342, 1964.
5. Go, V. L. W., Hofmann, A. F., and Summerskill, W. H. J.: Pancreozymin bioassay in man based on pancreatic enzyme secretion: potency of specific amino acids and other digestive products, J. Clin. Invest. **49:** 1558, 1970.
6. Greenlee, H. B., Longhi, E. H., Guerrero, J. D., et al.: Inhibitory effect of pancreatic secretin on gastric secretion, Am. J. Physiol. **190:** 396, 1957.
7. Gregory, R. A.: Gastric secretory responses after portal venous ligation, J. Physiol. (Lond.) **144:** 123, 1958.
8. Grossman, M. I.: Gastrin, cholecystokinin and secretin act on one receptor, Lancet **1:** 1088, 1970.
9. Grossman, M. I.: Hormone-hormone, and vagus hormone interactions on gastric acid secretion, Symposium on "Frontiers in Gastrointestinal Hormone Research" (Special Nobel Symposium series, Uppsala, Sweden), Stockholm, 1973, Almqvist and Wiksell, p. 203.
10. Herrera, F., Kemp, D. R., and Tsukamoto, M., et al.: A new cannula for the study of pancreatic function, J. Appl. Physiol. **25:** 207, 1970.
11. Johnson, L. R., and Grossman, M. I.: Secretin: The enterogastrone released by acid in the duodenum, Am. J. Physiol. **215:** 885, 1968.
12. Johnson, L. R., and Grossman, M. I.: Characteristics of inhibition of gastric secretion by secretin, Am. J. Physiol. **217:** 1401, 1969.
13. Johnson, L. R., and Grossman, M. I.: Analysis of inhibition of acid secretion by cholecystokinin in dogs, Am. J. Physiol. **218:** 550, 1970.
14. Kaminski, D. L., Rose, R. C., and Nahrwold, D. L.: Effect of pentagastrin on cholecystokinin and secretin choleresis in the dog, J. Surg. Res. In press.
15. Konturek, S. J., Tasler, J., and Obtulowicz, W.: Duodenal mechanisms for inhibition of gastric acid secretion in the dog, Am. J. Physiol. **220:** 918, 1971.
16. Konturek, S. J., Tasler, J., and Obtulowicz, W.: Localization of the cholecystokinin release in intestine of the dog, Am. J. Physiol. **222:** 16, 1972.

17. Konturek, S. J., Tasler, J., and Obtulowicz, W.: Role of gastric vagal innervation in the action of cholecystokinin on gastric secretion, *in* Demling, L., editor: Gastrointestinal hormones, New York, 1972, Intercontinental Medical Book Corporation, p. 69.
18. Meyer, J. H., and Grossman, M. I.: Release of secretin and cholecystokinin, *in* Demling, L., editor: Gastrointestinal hormones, New York, 1972, Intercontinental Medical Book Corporation, p. 43.
19. Meyer, J. H., Spingola, L. J., and Grossman, M. I.: Endogenous cholecystokinin potentiates exogenous secretin on pancreas of dog, Am. J. Physiol. **221:** 742, 1971.
20. Preshaw, R. M., Cooke, A. R., and Grossman, M. I.: Quantitative aspects of response of canine pancreas to duodenal acidification, Am. J. Physiol. **210:** 629, 1966.
21. Reeder, D. D., Becker, H. D., Smith, N. J., et al.: Radioimmunoassay of cholecystokinin, Surg. Forum **23:** 361, 1972.
22. Wormsley, K. G., and Grossman, M. I.: Inhibition of gastric acid secretion by secretin and by endogenous acid in the duodenum, Gastroenterology **47:** 72, 1964.
23. Spingola, L. J., and Grossman, M. I.: Failure of endogenous cholecystokinin to inhibit pentagastrin stimulated acid secretion, Gastroenterology **60:** 804, 1971.
24. Stening, G. F., Johnson, L. R., and Grossman, M. I.: Effect of cholecsytokinin and caerulein on gastrin- and histamine-evoked gastric secretion, Gastroenterology **57:** 44, 1969.
25. Thomas, J. E.: An improved cannula for gastric and intestinal fistulas, Proc. Soc. Exp. Biol. Med. **46:** 260, 1941.
26. Way, L. W.: The effect of secretin on acid secretion in response to cholinergic stimuli, Clin. Res. **18:** 175, 1970.

Hypermetabolism in sepsis: Correlation with fever and tachycardia

D. F. J. Halmagyi, M.D., D.Sc., J. Broell, M.S., F. E. Gump, M.D., *and*
J. M. Kinney, M.D., *New York, N. Y.*

Metabolic rate (M) is a fundamental parameter but the difficulty of its measurement led to attempts to predict it from body temperature and heart rate. The validity of such estimates of M has been examined in five afebrile (Group A) and 18 febrile surgical patients. Rectal temperature (T) and heart rate (R) were measured at two to four hourly intervals; O_2 uptake and CO_2 output were measured in our canopy system over 30 minutes, five times daily at set intervals. More than 25,000 individual observations extending over 1,314 patient days were stored on tape and mean daily values of M (Kcal./m.^{2}), R (per minute), and T (°C.) were calculated. In Group A, both M (785 ± 53) and R (79 ± 8) were normal. The regression equations for M and R on T were significant in all febrile patients, but in ten of these (Group B) M was normal (866 ± 63) and R was high (103 ± 8) at 37 °C.; hospital stay was 51 ± 9 days and all recovered. In eight febrile patients (Group C) both R (105 ± 17) and M (1,103 ± 144) were elevated at 37° C.; four died and four spent 105 ± 37 days in the hospital. At 39° C., both M and R were identical in Groups B and C. We conclude: (1) Tachycardia may occur in the absence of fever and hypermetabolism; (b) hypermetabolism at normothermia occurs in the more severely ill (these patients are likely to benefit less from antipyresis); (3) during fever, these groups cannot be separated; (d) separate factors need to be identified to account for the hypermetabolism and tachycardia in these conditions.

From the Department of Surgery, College of Physicians and Surgeons, Columbia University, New York, N. Y.

IT HAS BEEN reported that in sepsis, particularly when it involves the large serous cavities, resting caloric expenditure is high.[2, 5] The measurement of caloric expenditure in severely ill patients is technically difficult, and it was probably for this reason that the original observations were based on a limited number of patients and were never repeated by others.

Septic patients are usually febrile and metabolic rate is known to increase by 12 percent for each 1° C. increment in body temperature,[3] but Roe and Kinney[5] expressed the opinion that in their septic patients the degree of hypermetabolism was in excess of that expected from this relationship, suggesting that causes other than fever are operative in increasing the oxygen requirements in sepsis. The availability of improved technical facilities to measure metabolic rate prompted us to reinvestigate this phenomenon by studying the regression of metabolic rate on body temperature in a larger group of septic patients.

We found that persistent severe tachycardia is another constant clinical feature

Accepted for publication March 20, 1974.

Address all correspondence to D. F. J. Halmagyi, M.D., Dept. of Surgery, College of Physicians and Surgeons, Columbia University, 630 W 168th St., New York, N. Y. 10032.

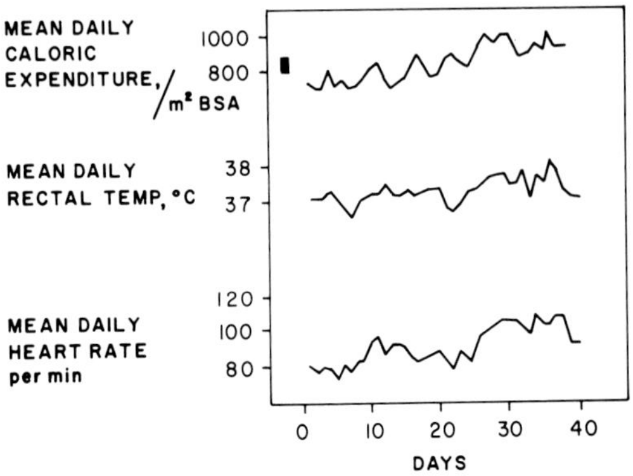

Fig. 1. Clinical course in a non-septic patient (Patient 2, Table I) who had granulomatous colitis and protein depletion. ■, Expected normal. (See text for explanation.)

Table I. *Non-septic patients*

Patient No.	*Diagnosis*	r_1*	r_2†
1	Duodenal ulcer	0.57	NS
2	Granulomatous colitis; depletion	0.44	0.43
3	Malabsorption; peripheral neuropathy	0.51	0.45
4	Obesity	0.64	NS
5	Rectovaginal fistula; depletion	NS‡	NS

*r_1 = correlation coefficient of heart rate and rectal temperature.

†r_2 = correlation coefficient of caloric expenditure and rectal temperature.

‡NS = not statistically significant.

Table II. *Septic patients*

Patient No.	*Diagnosis*	r_1*	r_2†
1	Burn	NS§	0.29
2	Sepsis after appendectomy	0.84	0.50
3	Skeletal + soft tissue trauma; shock	0.53	0.36
4	Small bowel fistulas	0.70	0.62
5	Hemorrhagic pancreatitis	0.88	0.85
6	Acute pancreatitis	0.54	0.52
7	Gunshot wounds of chest + abdomen	0.68	0.67
8	Perforated appendix; ileus	0.41	0.30
9	Sepsis after hysterectomy	0.40	0.57
10	Abdom. stab wound; pancreatic necrosis; shock	0.47	0.61
11†	Peritonitis; diabetes; respiratory failure	NS	NS
12‡	Renal failure	0.56	NS
13	Small bowel fistula; desmoid tumor	0.87	0.50
14	Sclerosing cholangitis; respiratory failure	0.79	0.27
15‡	Burn	NS	0.37
16‡	Sepsis	0.72	0.27
17	High intestinal obstruction; depletion	0.84	0.28
18	Subphrenic abscess	0.51	0.50

*r_1 = correlation coefficient of heart rate and rectal temperature.

†r_2 = correlation coefficient of caloric expenditure and rectal temperature.

‡ Died.

§NS = not statistically significant.

of sepsis. This tachycardia was unrelated to volume depletion or heart failure and was not accompanied by any specific electrocardiographic abnormalities. Here, again, the possible role of fever had to be assessed.

The technical difficulties in measuring caloric expenditure in severely ill patients led to attempts to predict metabolic rate from temperature and heart rate. However, for reasons outlined above, the validity of this shortcut needed to be established, and here we determined the interrelation of caloric expenditure, heart rate, and body temperature in sepsis.

METHODS AND MATERIAL

Five non-septic (Group A) and 18 septic patients admitted to the Surgical Metabolic Unit were studied. Their diagnoses are listed in Tables I and II.

Mean daily rectal temperature and heart rate were calculated from measurements taken at two to four hourly intervals during day and night. Oxygen consumption and CO_2 output were measured in our ventilated head-canopy system[6] over 20 to 30 minutes five times daily at 05.00 to 06.00, 09.00 to 10.00, 13.30 to 15.00, 18.00 to 19.00 and 22.00 to 23.00 hours. Mean daily values were calculated, converted into daily caloric expenditure by using the conventional tables and expressed per square meter of body surface area (BSA). Body weights were measured daily on precision bed scales. The values obtained for caloric expenditures were compared with normal values for the pa-

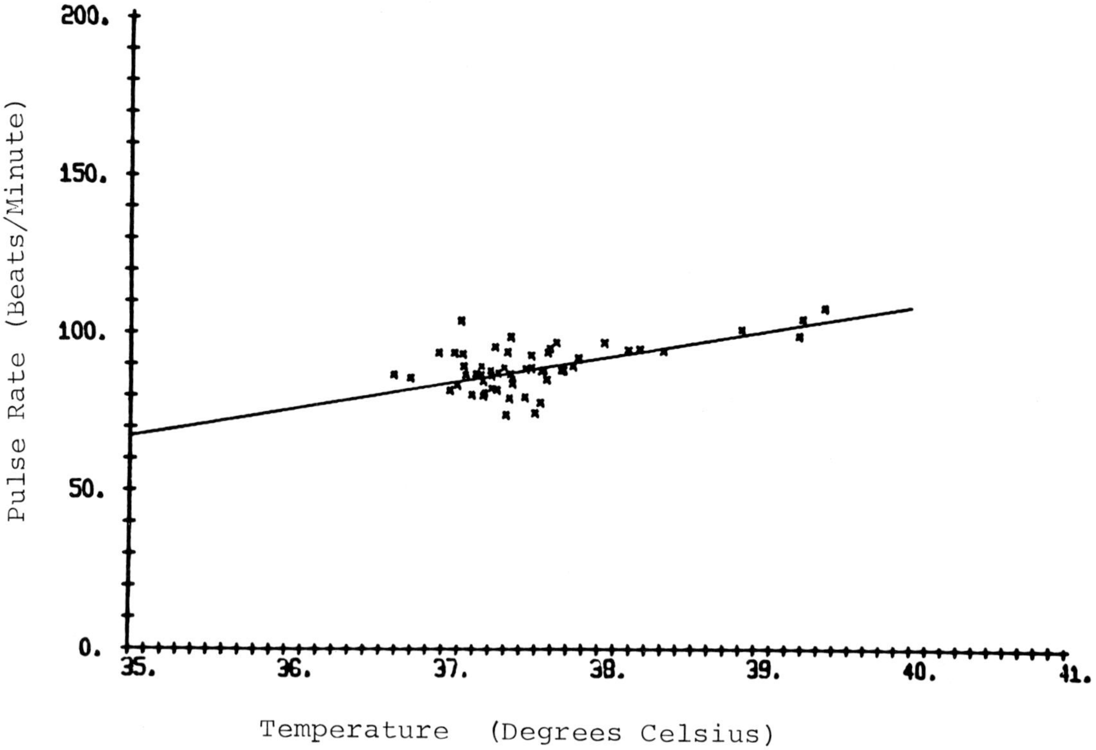

Fig. 2. Regression of mean daily heart rate on mean daily rectal temperature in a non-septic cally significant. Note that at 37° C. heart rate is normal. Equation of line is Y = 0.84264E 01X + −0.22772E 03. Correlation coefficient = 0.5131.

tients' age and sex.[1] All results were stored on tape and calculations were carried out with the use of an IBM 1130 computer.

The least squares fit was calculated to determine the regression of heart rate and caloric expenditure on rectal temperature: linear, semilogarithmic, and logarithmic relationships were considered but, invariably, the linear relationship was found equal to, or better, than the other two.

RESULTS

The course of a non-septic patient is shown in Fig. 1 (Patient 2, Table I). During the first week, when both nitrogen and caloric balances were negative, caloric expenditure was less than predicted; restoration of positive nitrogen and caloric balances coincided with an increase in caloric expenditure to normal. On the twenty-fifth day, the onset of a mild urinary tract infection was accompanied by a minor rise in temperature, heart rate, and caloric expenditure. Such short periods of fever caused by trivial infections widened the range of body temperature and revealed, in two patients, a positive correlation with metabolic rate as shown in Figs. 2 and 3, in which heart rate and metabolic rate were plotted against rectal temperature. Calculation of the individual regression equations indicated that heart rate at 37° C. was 79 ± 8 and caloric expenditure was also normal (785 ± 53 Kcal. per 24 hours per square meter of BSA).

In septic patients, both heart rate and metabolic rate increased with fever but, more importantly, calculation of the individual regression equations revealed that while heart rate was already elevated (104 ± 13) at 37° C. in all patients, caloric expenditure at 37° C. was normal in some and increased in others. On this basis, we divided our septic patients in two groups: those whose caloric expenditure was normal at 37° C. (Patients 1 through 10, Table II) comprised Group B, and those whose caloric expenditure was

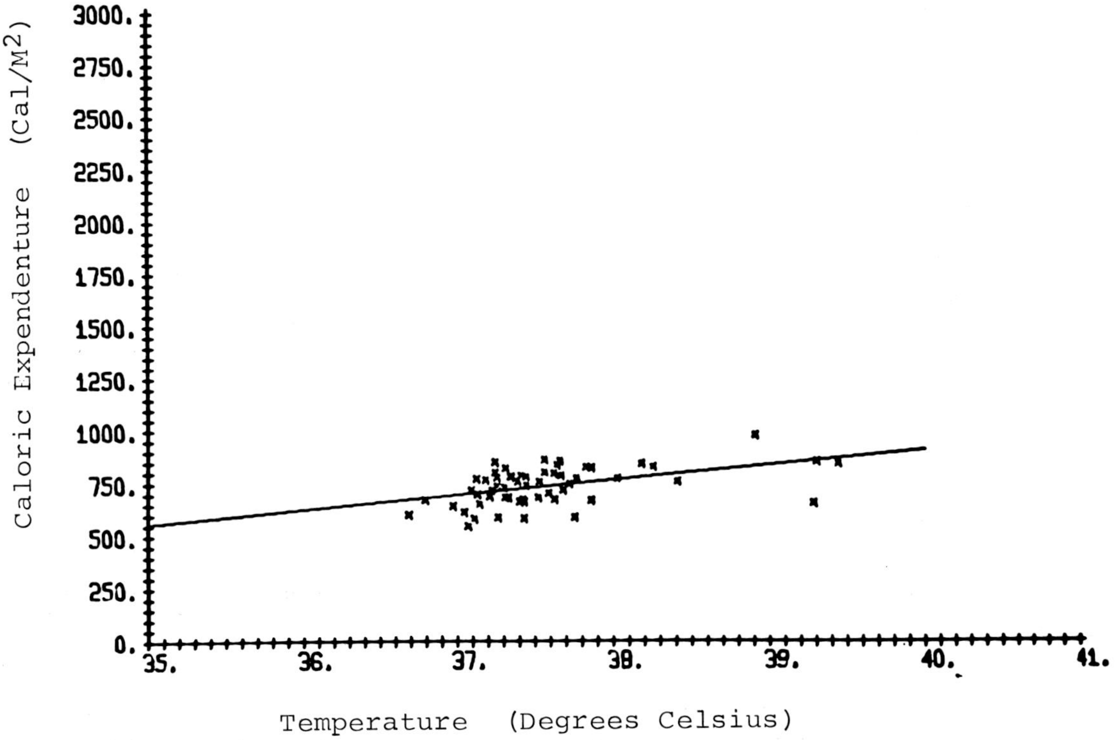

Fig. 3. Regression of mean daily caloric expenditure on mean daily rectal temperature in a non-septic patient who had malabsorption and peripheral neuropathy. Correlation coefficient is statistically significant. Note that at 37° C. caloric expenditure is normal. Equation of line is Y = 0.69899E 02X + –0.18872E 04. Correlation coefficient = 0.4539.

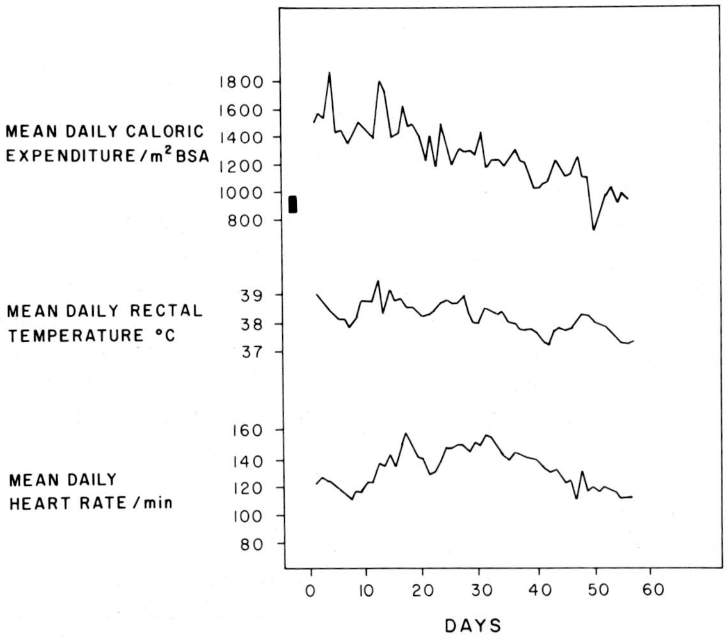

Fig. 4. Clinical course in a septic patient who had undergone a hysterectomy. Note that metabolic rate and body temperature, both high at admission, gradually decreased while the heart rate remained high. ■, Expected normal.

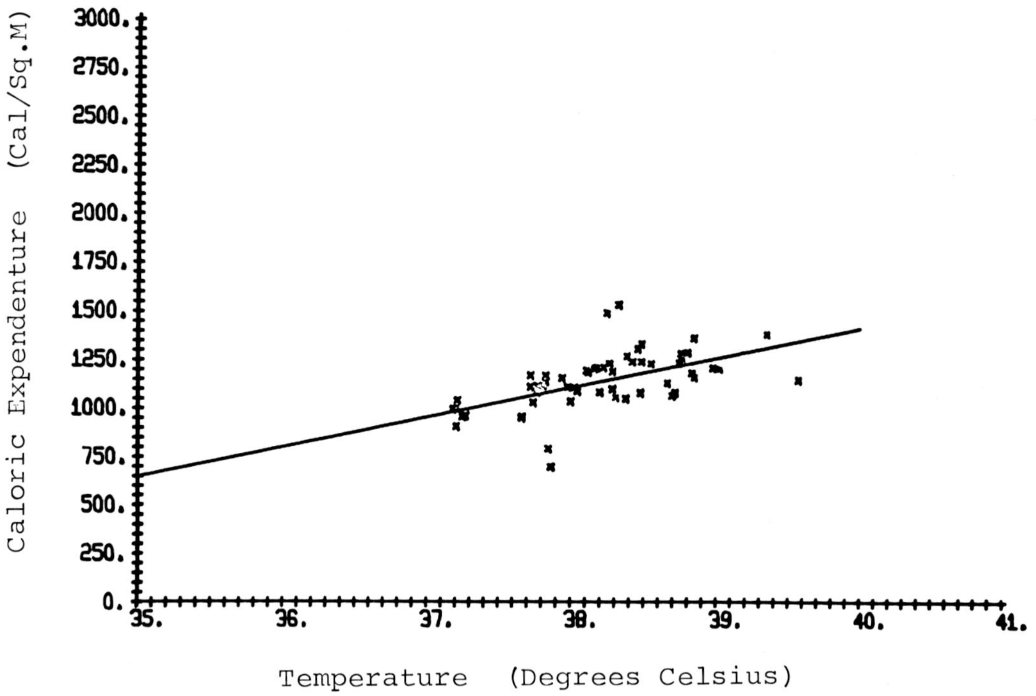

Fig. 5. Regression of mean daily heart rate on mean daily rectal temperature in the post-hysterectomy septic patient shown on Fig. 4. Correlation coefficient is statistically significant but of a smaller magnitude than that of the non-septic patient shown in Fig. 2. Note that at 37° C. heart rate is elevated. Equation of line is Y = 0.15361E 03X + −0.24728E 04. Correlation coefficient = 0.5667.

elevated at 37° C. (Patients 11 through 18, Table II) comprised Group C.

The course in a patient of Group B (Patient 9, Table II) is shown in Fig. 4. At admission, she was febrile and tachycardic, with a mean daily caloric expenditure of about twice the predicted normal. Over the next few weeks, both caloric expenditure and fever decreased gradually while heart rate increased during the first month and commenced to decrease after about 30 days. Caloric expenditure and heart rate plotted against rectal temperature are shown in Figs. 5 and 6. The correlation coefficients of both relationships were statistically significant, but the correlation coefficient for caloric expenditure was of higher magnitude. Calculation of the regression equations revealed that at normal body temperature (37° C.) caloric expenditure was normal while heart rate was increased.

The course in one patient of Group C (Patient 16, Table II) is shown in Fig. 7. At admission, she was febrile, tachycardic, and somewhat hypermetabolic. During most of the observation period (three months) fever and tachycardia remained virtually unchanged while caloric expenditure gradually increased and after 90 days she died. The correlation coefficient of mean daily caloric expenditure and rectal temperature was low (Fig. 8), because hypermetabolism was not dependent upon fever.

Clinical course in these two groups was markedly different. Patients in Group B spent an average of 51 ± 19 days in the hospital and they all recovered, while half of the patients in Group C died and the remaining four were hospitalized for 105 ± 37 days.

The above findings are summarized in Fig. 9.

DISCUSSION

Body temperature is determined by the balance between heat production (measured as oxygen consumption) and heat dissipation (usually not measured). In steady states and in a thermoneutral environment when the

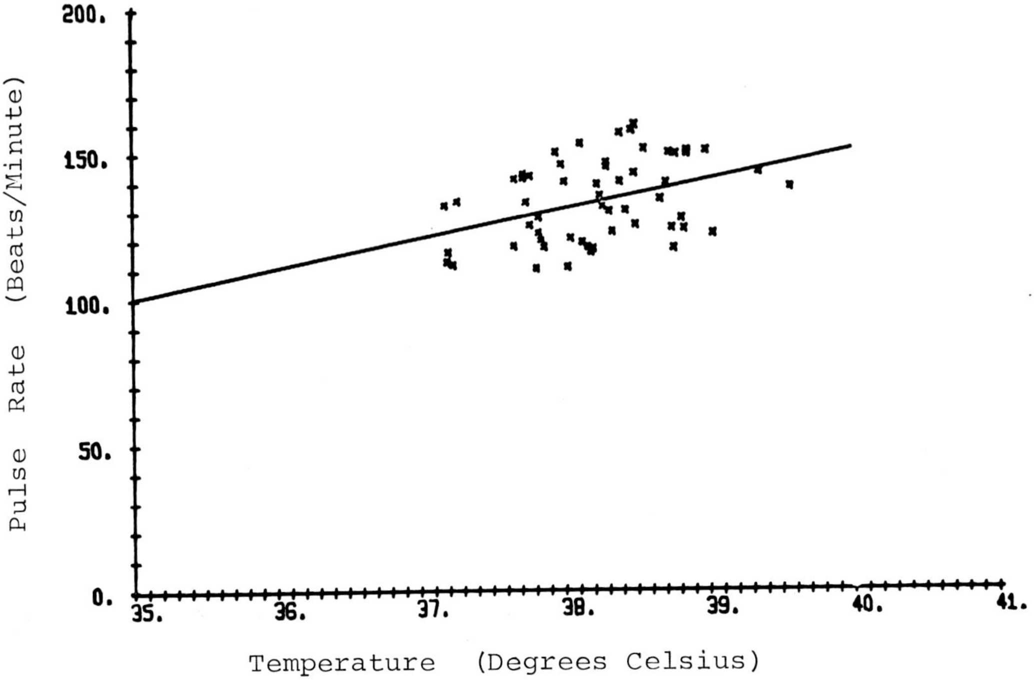

Fig. 6. Regression of mena daily caloric expenditure on mean rectal temperature in the posthysterectomy septic patient shown on Fig. 4. Correlation coefficient is statistically significant. Note that at 37° C. caloric expenditure is normal. Equation of line is Y = 0.10166E 02X + −0.25548E 03. Correlation coefficient = 0.3959.

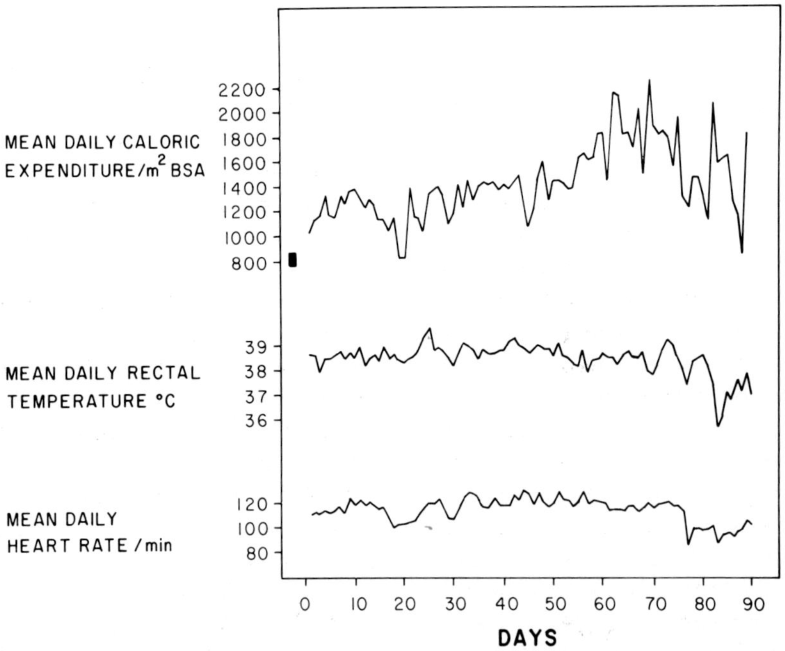

Fig. 7. Clinical course in a septic patient who died. Note that heart rate and body temperature remained largely unchanged during the entire course while mean daily caloric expenditure gradually increased and showed large fluctuations over the days preceding death. ■, Expected normal.

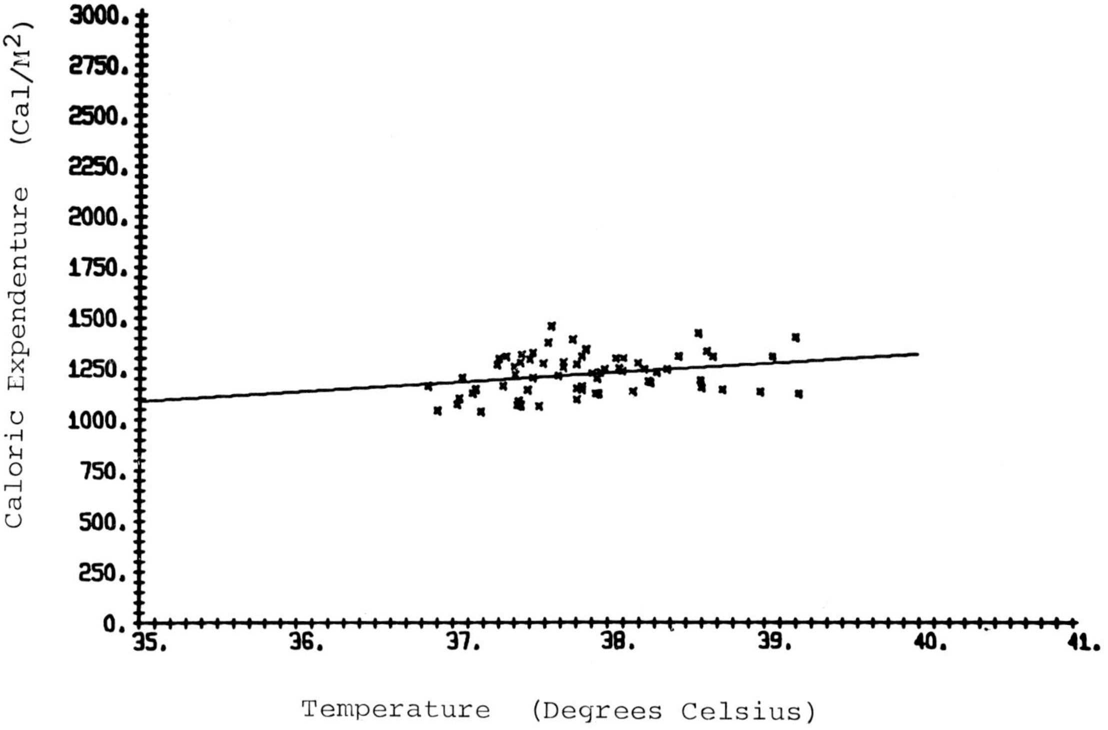

Fig. 8. Regression of mean daily caloric expenditure on mean daily rectal temperature in the septic patient shown on Fig. 7. Note flat slope of the regression line. Caloric expenditure was elevated at 37° C. Equation of line is Y = 0.46919E 02X + −0.55431E 03. Correlation coefficient = 0.2719.

body temperature is stable, heat loss is assumed to be constant and oxygen uptake is proportional to body temperature, but in unsteady states, this relationship may be distorted. In spiking fever, the rise in metabolic rate precedes the increase in body temperature, and during rapid defervescence, the fall in temperature lags behind the reduction in metabolic rate, both phenomena being related to heat storage in the body.[4] In sepsis, body temperature often shows rapid fluctuations and the time-lag between changes in body temperature and metabolic rate could affect calculations of the correlation between these two functions. It was for this reason that we used mean daily values for all parameters, hoping that this would cushion the effect of the time-lag.

Although heart rate increased with rising temperature, all septic patients were tachycardic even at normothermia, suggesting the need to consider causes other than fever. Infections, antibiotic drugs, and nutritional deficiencies, ever present in sepsis, may occasionally produce various forms of cardiomyopathies which cause tachycardia. However, these conditions ultimately result in cardiac enlargement and heart failure, and these we have never seen in our patients. Finally, tachycardia may be the consequence of increased sympathetic activity, and although we do not know of any evidence suggesting sustained sympathetic stimulation in longstanding sepsis, this possibility would merit more detailed exploration.

Metabolic rate was increased in all febrile patients, but only some were hypermetabolic at normothermia, and it is tempting to speculate that the 40 percent rise in resting energy expenditure at normal body temperature was causally related to the unfavorable clinical course. Our ventilated head-canopy system allows measurement of caloric expenditure when the inhaled gas is air and the

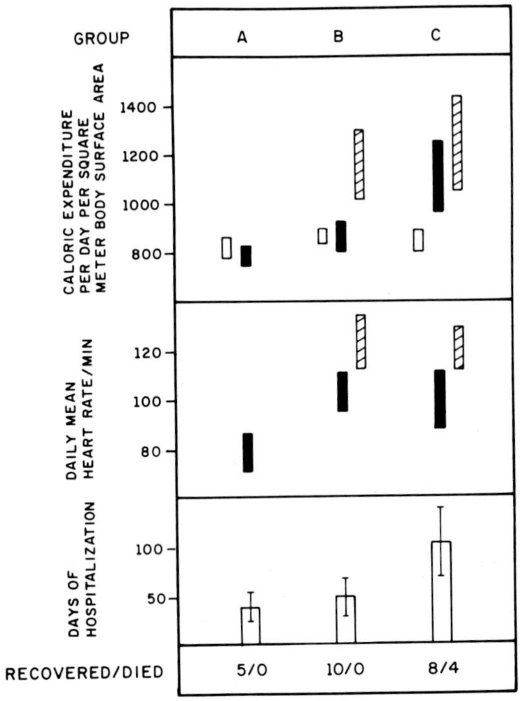

Fig. 9. Summary of the relationship of caloric expenditure and heart rate to body temperature in non-septic and septic patients. Note the more severe clinical course in patients with normothermic hypermetabolism. Group A, nonseptic; Groups B and C, septic. ▯, Expected values at 37° C.; ▮, observed values at 37° C.; ▨, observed values at 39° C.

patient is breathing spontaneously; yet in the more severe forms of sepsis, oxygen breathing and assisted ventilation are required. If hypermetabolism is, indeed, proportional to the clinical severity of sepsis, metabolic rate in septic patients with respiratory failure may be even higher. This study is presently in progress.

Du Bois[3] asserted that the 12 percent rise in metabolic rate per 1° C. increment in body temperature was applicable only to some types of fever, while in other types the increase was less. Our observations are consistent with this statement. During fever, metabolic rate was similar in all septic patients (Fig. 9), while in normothermia some were hypermetabolic (Group C) and others were not (Group B). Consequently, the slope of the regression line of metabolic rate on body temperature was flat in Group C (Fig. 8), suggesting that not the type of fever but the severity of the disease determines this response.

Similar to tachycardia, normothermic hypermetabolism may also be the result of increased sympathetic activity further emphasizing the necessity to explore this aspect of sepsis.

High resting metabolic expenditure in normothermia and its additional increase in fever should be given serious consideration when calculating daily caloric requirements in sepsis.

REFERENCES

1. Albritton, E. C.: Standard values in nutrition and metabolism, Philadelphia, 1954, W. B. Saunders Company, p. 241.
2. Cole, O., Nardi, G. L., Quijano, M., Rovit, R. L., Stanbury, J. B., and Wight, A.: Metabolic rate and thyroid function following acute thermal trauma in man, Ann. Surg. **137:** 165, 1953.
3. Du Bois, E. F.: Basal metabolism in health and disease, Philadelphia, 1927, Lea & Febiger, Publishers.
4. Liebermeister, C.: Handbuch der Pathologie und Therapie des Fiebers, Leipzig, 1875, Vogel.
5. Roe, F. C., and Kinney, J. M.: The caloric equivalent of fever. II. Influence of major trauma, Ann. Surg. **161:** 140, 1965.
6. Spencer, J. L., Zikria, A. A., Kinney, F. M., Broell, J. R., Michailoff, T. M., and Lee, A. B.: A system of continuous measurement of gas exchange and respiratory functions, J. Appl. Physiol. **33:** 523, 1972.

Extraperitoneal endarterectomy for unilateral iliofemoral occlusive disease

Toshio Inahara, M.D., *and* **Jose D. Pineda, M.D.,*** *Portland, Ore.*

For the treatment of unilateral iliofemoral occlusive disease, several procedures are commonly employed. Among these procedures, the more common are the femoral-to-femoral, axillary-to-femoral, and crossover external iliac–to-femoral grafts. In addition to these techniques, a more direct reconstruction by endarterectomy has been presented employing a similar extraperitoneal approach and using the eversion method. Over the past seven years, 15 patients and 17 limbs have been treated by this method with successful restoration of circulation in all cases for the immediate and long-term patency. There has been no acute or late vascular complications. Eversion method of endarterectomy seems well suited for the treatment of unilateral external iliac and common femoral disease and is recommended as the treatment of choice. Advantages and limitations are discussed.

From St. Vincent Hospital, Portland, Ore.

UNILATERAL occlusive disease of the common and external iliac and common femoral arteries in more recent years has been treated with the bypass procedures in which limb salvage is the primary aim. Emphasis has been placed on minimizing the operative procedure because, frequently, it is the poor-risk patient who presents with a severely ischemic limb. It is generally acknowledged that the expediency of the bypass procedure is less hazardous than that of a major limb amputation, and use of the procedure is justified because it preserves the ischemic limb.

In minimizing the operative procedure, several extraperitoneal procedures have been described. The more common are the femoral-to-femoral graft by Vetto,[7, 8] the iliofemoral crossover graft by McCaughan and Kahn,[4] and the axillofemoral graft by Blaisdell and Hall[1] and Louw.[3] Sauvage and Wood[6] have modified the axillofemoral-to-bilateral femoral anastomosis. The greatest expediency of these methods are that the procedures may be performed after the administration of local anesthesia.

More recently, Parsonnet and co-workers[5] have suggested that the femoral-to-femoral graft might be considered the procedure of choice in the elective patient. This concept is somewhat controversial,[5] as there is a relatively higher incidence of immediate and long-term failures, as well as the uncertainty of the longevity of the donor vessel.

Endarterectomy for unilateral iliofemoral occlusion has not been described except as performed electively in conjunction with aortoiliofemoral endarterectomy. As this procedure is a major intra-abdominal operation, endarterectomy has not been entertained as a procedure of expediency where it might be applied to the poor-risk patient or even to elective patients with unilateral external iliac occlusion.

Accepted for publication March 20, 1974.

*Present address: Barrio La Guadalupe, Tegucigalpa, Honduras, C. A.

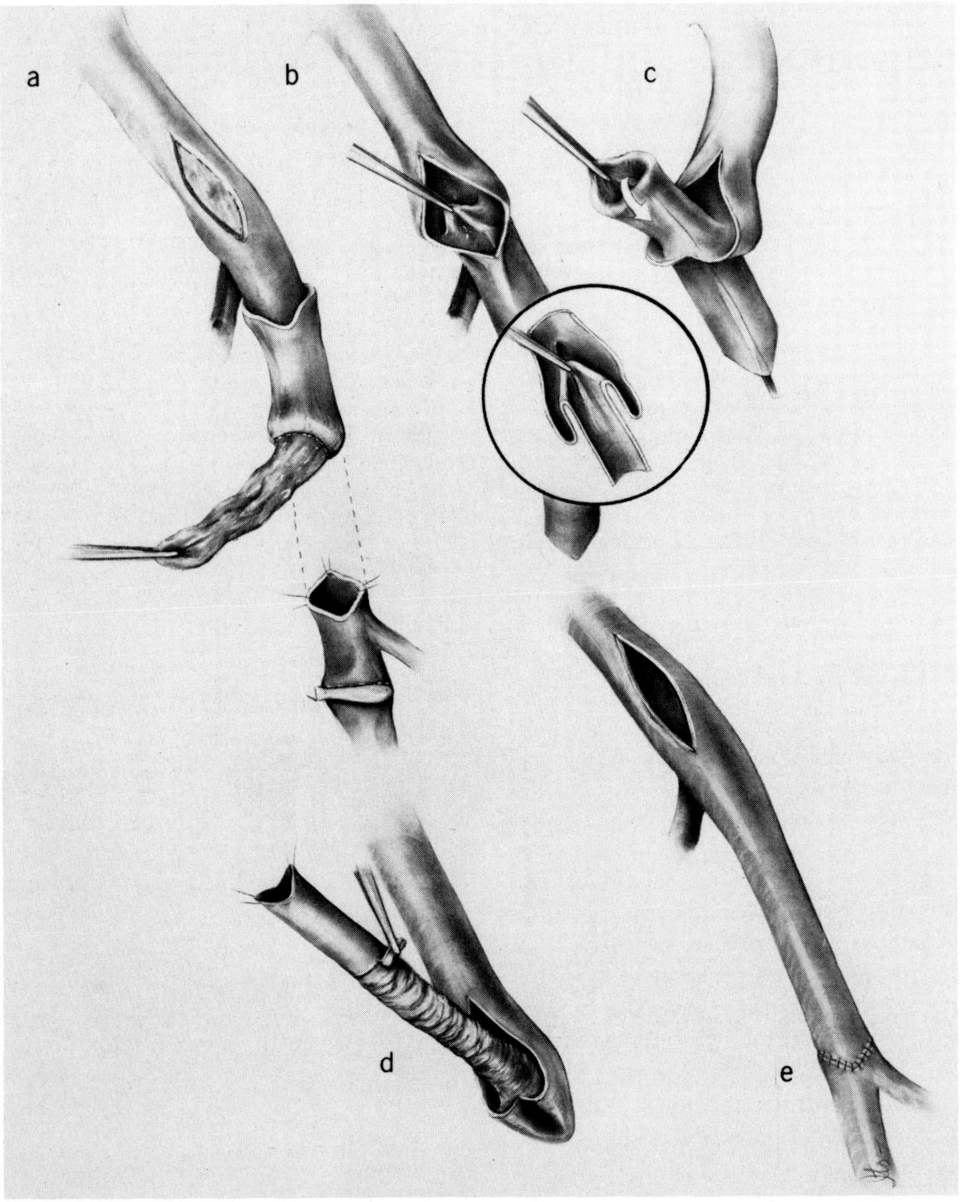

Fig. 1. Technique of eversion endarterectomy.

The purpose of this report is to describe the application of endarterectomy for occlusive disease of a unilateral iliac and common femoral artery with minimal operative trauma so that it can be readily applied to the poor-risk patient. Lower quadrant extraperitoneal exposure is ideally suited to approach the iliac vessels. Additionally, inguinal exposure is made for the common femoral artery. The method of endarterectomy is by the eversion technique described in an earlier report.[2]

Fig. 1 briefly depicts the technique. After complete mobilization of the external iliac and common femoral segment, the common femoral artery is transected obliquely just proximal to its bifurcation. Longitudinal arteriotomy is made in the distal common iliac artery. Endarterectomy is then performed from both ends. Eversion is first started at the distal end with removal of the atheromatous core. The proximal external iliac is next everted from the common iliac opening over the full length of the segment to complete the endarterectomy and debridement. The vessel is turned right side out and reconstructed by end-to-end anastomosis to the endarterectomized femoral bifurcation.

CLINICAL MATERIAL AND RESULTS

Extraperitoneal endarterectomy by eversion method was started in 1966, and the series totals 15 patients and 17 endarterectomies. There were 11 men and four women. Ages ranged from 47 to 80 years, with the average age of 65 years (Table I). Presenting symptoms and indications for operation were disabling claudication of less than one block in seven limbs, rest pain in eight, and ischemic necrosis in two.

Arteriography revealed occlusions of the external iliac in six limbs, occlusions of external iliac and common femoral in six, occlusions of common femoral in two, and severe stenosis of the external iliac in three. Associated distal femoral popliteal occlusions were present in 11 limbs.

Diabetes mellitus, coronary artery disease, hypertension, and cerebral vascular disease were present in 11 patients. Eight patients were considered to be poor operative risks.

Anesthesia of choice was either a spinal or continuous epidural anesthesia. Adequate exposure was obtained combining an oblique lower quadrant incision with extraperitoneal approach and an inguinal incision. Using the eversion method, endarterectomy of the common and external iliac and the common femoral was performed through two arteriotomies regardless of the severity of the disease. Endarterectomy was carried into the superficial femoral in one and the profunda femoral in eight limbs, of which four required vein patch grafts. Average operating time was slightly less than three hours. Blood replacement was 1,000 ml. in three patients in whom

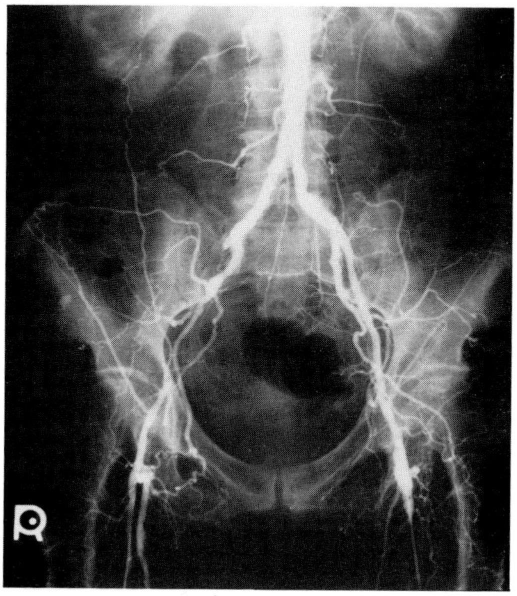

Fig. 2. Preoperative aortogram.

Table I. *Extraperitoneal ilieofemoral endarterectomy: 1966 to 1973*

No. of patients		*No. of limbs*	*Average age (yr.)*
Men	11	12	65
Women	4	5	

it was necessary to endarterectomize the common iliac artery to the aortic bifurcation. Concomitant femoral popliteal grafts were not placed in any patient.

Femoral pulses were restored in all limbs. There were no acute postoperative occlusions, hemorrhages, false aneurysms, or infections (Table II). The only morbidity was an occurrence of a transient pulmonary atelectasis in one patient. All patients were discharged with restored femoral pulses.

Fifteen patients have been followed from four months to 7½ years with the mean follow-up period of 26 months. There have been two late deaths from myocardial infarctions, both with patent recostructions. All surviving endarterectomies have remained patent. One patient has required a femoral popliteal bypass graft for progressive distal disease. No further operations have been

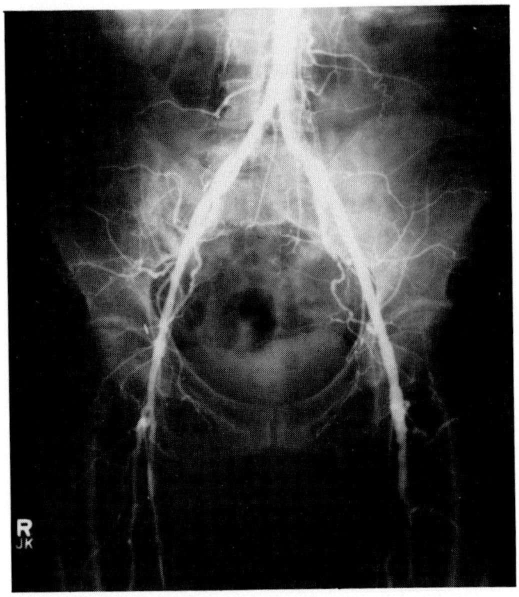

Fig. 3. Postoperative aortogram following bilateral extraperitoneal eversion endarterectomies.

Table II. *Extraperitoneal ilieofemoral endarterectomy (1966 to 1973): Results*

Results	*No.*
Early	
Thrombosis	0
Infection	0
False aneurysm	0
Amputations	0
Morbidity	1
Deaths	0
Late	
Thrombosis	0
Reoperations	0
Amputation	0
Femoropopliteal graft	1
Deaths	2

needed beyond the original endarterectomy in any patient, and there has been no amputation (Figs. 2 and 3).

DISCUSSION

The technique of endarterectomy for the external iliac and common femoral arteries evolved from endarterectomy of the aortoiliac and femoral arteries by altering the exposure to an extraperitoneal approach. Exposure of the iliac arteries is quite simple and adequate, and it is even more direct than by the transabdominal route, particularly to the segment beneath the inguinal ligament. This was first performed electively on the average-risk patient and later applied to the poor-risk patient. This method of revascularization has produced reliable and reproducible results for both the immediate and long-term patency; this operation has therefore become the procedure of choice for certain indications.

This method of reconstruction provides certain advantages. First, it is simple, direct, and minimally traumatic so that it is well suited to the poor-risk patient. Second, the reconstruction is not dependent upon a subcutaneously positioned graft subject to its usual problems. Third, the inflow source is not depenlent upon a small donor vessel, which often is concomitantly diseased, as seen in the contralateral external iliac artery. This allows the donor vessel to be treated later and independently on its own merits without interfering with the first repair. Fourth, it provides advantages inherent to endarterectomy with less susceptibility to infection, and the reconstruction is hemodynamically sound with linear flow without the end-to-side anastomosis.

However, there are certain limitations in this method. One of the more common indications for use of the bypass procedure is to bypass the site of graft infection. Endarterectomy is precluded under these conditions, as it is designed primarily for relief of obstruction in an uncontaminated site.

The presence of severe occlusive disease of the common iliac artery may compound the problem by prolonging the operation, and the exposure is a little more difficult. However, endarterectomy can be extended to the aortic bifurcation with the use of a balloon catheter in the terminal aorta for proximal control. With the eversion method, the distal half of the common iliac is routinely endarterectomized so that it may be extended proximally as indicated.

Another relative contraindication for invasion of the retroperitoneal space is the presence of metastatic malignancy in the pelvis and along the course of the iliac vessels. Here it would be prudent to resort to one of the bypass procedures.

This procedure is not well suited to the use of infiltration local anesthesia. However, by using spinal anesthesia under the careful management of a concerned anesthesiologist, it can be even more effective in minimizing anesthetic trauma and will expedite the operative procedure with a more cooperative patient.

REFERENCES

1. Blaidsdel, F. W., and Hall, A. D.: Axillary-femoral artery bypass for lower extremity ischemia, SURGERY **54:** 563, 1963.
2. Inahara, T.: Surgical treatment of aortoiliac atherosclerosis, Am. J. Surg. **58:** 960, 1965.
3. Louw, J. H.: Splenic to femoral and axillary to femoral bypass graft in diffuse atherosclerotic occlusive disease, Lancet **1:** 1401, 1963.
4. McCaughan, J. J., Jr., and Kahn, S. F.: Cross-over graft for unilateral occlusive disease of the iliofemoral arteries, Ann. Surg. **151:** 26, 1960.
5. Parsonnet, V., Alpert, J., and Brief, D. K.: Femorofemoral and axillofemoral grafts—compromise or preferred, SURGERY **67:** 26, 1970.
6. Sauvage, L. R., and Wood, S. J.: Unilateral axillary bilateral femoral bifurcation graft: A procedure for the poor-risk patient with aorto-iliac disease, SURGERY **60:** 573, 1966.
7. Vetto, M. R.: The treatment of unilateral iliac artery obstruction with a transabdominal subcutaneous, femorofemoral graft, SURGERY **52:** 342, 1962.
8. Vetto, M. R.: The femorofemoral shunt: An appraisal, Am. J. Surg. **112:** 162, 1966.

A broadening of vision: Observation on the practice of surgery in a university hospital in Great Britain

Nicholas L. Tilney, M.D., *Boston, Mass.*

A series of observations collected during a year spent in the practice of surgery at a university hospital in Great Britain are recorded. Various facets of this specialty as performed within the National Health Service are described, and general aspects of the philosophy of the surgeon and the surgical patient are discussed.

From the Department of Surgery, Harvard University Medical School, Peter Bent Brigham Hospital, Boston, Mass.

Every man takes the limits of his own field of vision for the limits of the world.
Schopenhauer (c. 1840)

SINCE MUCH OF THE impetus of medical knowledge and technology has emanated from the United States in recent decades, relatively few American doctors spend time abroad working clinically within other health systems. When the opportunity arose for me to spend a year in surgery at a British university hospital following my formal training, it offered the chance to gain direct experience into the workings of one facet of the National Health Service (NHS) and to explore at leisure mechanisms of health care based upon tenents quite different from those with which I was familiar. The timing seemed fortuitous, as I would experience the last of a program set up 25 years previously, which at the present time is undergoing reorganization and change on a major scale in an effort to increase efficiency and to broaden and deepen the liason between the local medical authority, the general practitioner, and the hospital consultant.

The following is a series of observations on surgery, the surgeon, and the surgical patient gathered during a years' work at a major teaching hospital in Scotland. Scotland has been well served by the NHS and may differ relatively from England in the surgical thrust and interpretation of the system. This may be due to the somewhat Calvinistic approach to the profession of medicine and the notable de-emphasis of private practice. Little effort is made in this paper to provide generalities regarding surgery as a whole throughout Great Britain, and there is no intention of drawing parallels between surgery in this small, relatively homogenous, and socially oriented country, to that of a large, diffuse, and consumer-oriented country such as the United States. However, various approaches to surgery and to health care in general may be of interest.

Accepted for publication March 20, 1974.

THE INSTITUTION AND ITS ORGANIZATION

The Western Infirmary in Glasgow is a large flamboyantly Victorian complex, embellished in the Scottish architectural tradition with corner turrets and steep roofs. It is associated educationally and geographi-

Vol. 75, No. 5, pp. 776-782

cally with the University of Glasgow, a venerable institution of the fifteenth century. The hospital serves the western side of Glasgow, an industrial city of about a million people, and receives patients from the entire west coast of Scotland, the Hebrides, and all other coastal islands. Medicine and surgery are represented with their ancillary specialties, while obstetrics, pediatrics, and plastic surgery are practiced at nearby institutions. The hospital has 220 general surgical beds, subdivided into four non-university units and a Department of Surgery. In keeping with the Scottish emphasis on education and traditions in medicine, its surgical past is proud and includes Lister, MacEwan, and Illingworth among its leaders. Physically, the buildings are large and airy, clean, and well kept. Accommodations and facilities are plain, and some equipment is rather dated, although modern units such as Intensive and Cardiac Care are amply supplied. Pleasant touches of a more gentle era are present; the garden, a large conservatory with palm trees and flowers, and a comfortable doctors' dining room and lounge.

The organization of the Western Infirmary and other affiliated hospitals is under the control of a Board of Management of medical professionals and laity. A medically qualified administrator organizes the hospital on a day-to-day basis. Although the NHS body responsible ultimately for all hospitals in this area of the country has been the Western Regional Hospital Board, the current restructuring of the Health Services in Britain is changing this administrative machinery. The eventual effects of such changes are not as yet clear.

As in most British hospitals, the institution is organized into a Unit system. These are self-contained divisions which run autonomously, each with their own consultants, house staff, and nursing and operating theatre staff. Over-all decisions and surgical policy are made through a committee of consultant representatives from each of the five Units. The Professor, as head of the Department of Surgery, has but an equal voice in this group. His responsibilities are varied; he has a clinical commitment combined with organizing clinical and laboratory investigative programs within his Department and he has duties in the College of Surgeons with work on national committees. He has no private practice. The present professor, Sir Andrew Watt Kay, is of considerable national and international stature. He is presently the president of the Royal College of Physicians and Surgeons in Glasgow, and he has held primary positions in the organization of the biomedical sciences in Britain, in the Medical Research Council, and as Chief Scientist to the Scottish Home and Health Department. His Unit is somewhat larger than the others with a proportionately larger staff of those remaining in academic surgery with positions on the University faculty. The several areas of special emphasis within the Department serve to attract research fellows or visitors with similar interests and expertise.

Each non-university Unit supports two to three consultants, one of whom is the titular head. Every surgeon has one to two operating sessions a week and runs a weekly clinic in which he and the house staff see 20 to 30 patients who are both new and for follow-up examination. One consultant is on call and makes rounds on weekends. Although the Senior Registrar or Registrar generally performs emergency surgery on Receiving Nights, which each Unit accepts in turn, a consultant is available and will provide help if asked. In addition to his NHS commitments, he may attend private patients in smaller private hospitals or nursing homes. Upon acceptance of his Health Service appointment, he may arrange his contract regarding time spent in private practice. His salary is adjusted accordingly. Private practice is remarkably downplayed in Scotland, a situation contrasting to that of London with its strong traditions of Harley Street. Although a patient is free to consult a surgeon on a private basis, most elect to stay within the NHS. Although this choice may be largely financial, the majority of patients actively desire national care. Monetary benefit for the surgical consultant is not particularly great in private practice, and many Scottish surgeons consciously play a small private role.

The Units include two open wards and an operating theatre suite. Each large, multi-windowed ward holds 25 patients divided by sex. Several three- to four-bed rooms are also available. Armchairs placed in the center around electric fires act as a focus where ambulatory patients gather to read or converse. A long table is set three times a day, and meals are served by two maids attached to each ward. Patients in bed are helped individually, while many of their ordinary wants, tea, newspapers, companionship, are attended to by the others. Privacy for examinations, nursing, and treatment is gained by curtains. Two bathrooms service each ward. Hot water is plentiful and baths are routine.

The two head nurses, the Ward Sisters, are the dominant figures on the Unit. Fully within the Nightingale tradition, each combines surgical knowledge and expertise with administrative command, tact in handling the patients and their families with sympathetic rapport with the staff. In addition to nursing training and several years of practical experience on the wards, each Sister has been trained in midwifery. This extensive practical experience is obvious in their competent attention toward the patients. Their primary responsibility is patient welfare: easing their lot, organizing convalescence, and arranging transport. One sister controls all admissions to the Unit and maintains a flexible and personal approach to a dynamic biological system. Even more than the doctors, the Sisters do much to determine the personality of each Unit. Many patients respond to this by visiting the Sister and the ward, even years later. Two staff nurses and several student nurses comprise the remainder of personnel on each ward. Nursing care is their major responsibility, and one runs the recovery room each morning. All ancillary procedures are performed by Sister and her staff, and they include dressing changes, suture removal, abscess drainage, and tube placement. For a doctor to interfere with daily wound care is anathema. Such nurses seem to represent the essential professional calmly and competently assuming duties for which they have been trained.

An operating suite lies immediately adjacent to each Unit. The theatre is a high-ceilinged airy room which is considerably larger than the more cramped operating rooms of more contemporary design. Anesthesia is induced rapidly in an induction room by an anesthetist who has worked extensively with the particular consultant, and the intubated patient is immediately transferred to the operating table. Routine monitoring devices are few. Upon removal of one patient from the theatre, the next, already anesthetized, is brought in. Little washing or cleaning of the room is done between cases. By the time the surgeon rescrubs and regowns, the following patient is ready for skin preparation and draping. In this way, the flow of surgery is continuous and the volume of operations considerable. Despite beginning the first operation at 9:00 A.M. and breaking for coffee, three to five major cases can be completed comfortably by lunchtime. An afternoon session might then begin for another consultant and his team. Several variations in surgical technique decrease operative time. Midline incisions are employed frequently in the strikingly thin patient population. The cautery is used extensively for hemostasis of the abdominal wall and subcutaneous tissues. Finger dissection along anatomical tissue planes is a primary method of dissection. The suture lines of all enteric anastomoses, excluding esophageal repairs and some colon resections are continuous, as are all abdominal wall closures. One Assistant is present, and self-retaining retractors are used to advantage. Because of the extensive number of cases performed by one consultant each year, each surgical routine is standard and invariable. The smooth, rapid, but unhurried completion of even extensive dissections is noteworthy.

Like the Ward Sister, the Theatre Sister has been a member of the Unit for a long period. Her ultimate familarity with operative techniques and idiosyncracies of each consultant and her technical expertise and knowledge of each procedure increases the rate and efficiency of the caseload. The theatre orderly catalyzes the rapid and efficient operative turnover by fetching and preparing the patients, assisting the anesthesist, and acting as general factotum. Both he and the Theatre Sister see the patients pre- and postoperatively, and they contribute to the personal and individual atmosphere of each Unit.

PATIENT ATTITUDE AND CARE

The patients seemed unanimous in their enthusiasm for the NHS and its ancillary social benefits. In an economic system where money is scarce and salaries low, lack of financial pressure on the sick and on their families is important. Little abuse of the system at the hospital level is evident, and the relatively spartan conditions on the wards are accepted good naturedly. A camaraderie of a shared situation is engendered by the surroundings which serves to assuage individual discomfort and ease acceptance of illness. Professional decisions and aims or methods of diagnosis are rarely questioned, and appreciation of attention and care by the staff is often mentioned. Although the turnover rate is high, pressure for beds is not serious. Many diagnostic procedures are performed on an outpatient basis, while most surgical patients remain in hospital until removal of sutures. Many are discharged a few days later following operation than I was accustomed to; since most families work, it seemed convenient to allow them to remain for a somewhat longer period. While the majority are discharged directly home it is not uncommon for the elderly or those recovering from major procedures to enter recuperative centers for varying periods. Such homes maintain good standards and help to free acute hospital beds. Home Care or the Visiting Nurses are used frequently for older patients or others with particular disabilities. Social workers are intensely practical and effectively catalyze placement and disposition of difficult patients. Psychological evaluations have little place. Fleets of ambulance-buses ferry patients to and from clinic visits or outpatient treatments. A light plane is available to remove the sick from the offshore islands and to return them home at the end of hospitalization.

Extensive waiting periods for much elective surgery is uncommon in the Western Infirmary and many hospitals in Scotland. This situation may contrast to that in various areas in England, where long delays are reputedly more frequent. For routine procedures, such as thyroidectomy, cholecystectomy, and ulcer operations, the time varies between two and six weeks. If the urgency of a problem such as a suspicious breast mass is warranted, the patient will be admitted within a few days. Emergency situations are dealt with immediately. A waiting period for cosmetic surgery, such as excision of nevi or removal of varicose veins, may be as long as three years in some hospitals. As a result, the use of injections for varicosities is common practice. As the public seems relatively undemanding and less oriented toward rapid treatment, such delays are accepted quietly. Although it was never apparent to me, an obvious potential hazard of this system may be conscious prolongation of scheduling particular procedures as the result of either lack of interest on the part of a salaried surgeon or as means to force patients to accept private treatment.

Practically every person in Britain is assigned to a general practitioner under the NHS. Since one of his roles is to act in a screening capacity, the majority of patients seen in hospital clinics and in the Casualty Department have been referred with a covering letter. One of the criticisms of the system as it now stands has been lack of information between the general practitioner and the hospital, although in my experience, stress was laid on continuous and open communication between hospital doctors and the primary physician who is given detailed reports of any hospitalization and notified of significant variations in the patient's course. A summary of each clinic visit is transmitted to him and a duplicate entered in the permanent record. Thus, continuity of care is achieved and numbers of patients in outpatient and emergency departments lessened. One of the aims of the reorganization of the NHS is to allow the general practitioner hospital beds and increased facilities in his regional hospital, as another major complaint has been his lack of admitting privileges. His pay has improved during the past few years, as has his free time with the formation of group practices and emergency clinics.

SURGICAL DISEASE AND DEATH

Variations in the spectrum of surgical disease is of interest when comparing Glasgow and Boston. Despite generous use of alcohol and tobacco among both populations, ulcer disorders present quite differently. The incidence of perforated duodenal ulcers, although reputedly diminishing, seems extraordinarily high among the Glaswegians, whereas surgical intervention for bleeding ulcers is relatively uncommon. Esophagitis is frequent. Cirrhosis and esophageal varices are a noticeable rarity as are acute and chronic pancreatitis. Crohn's disease seems almost endemic. Diverticulitis and diverticulosis present infrequently, while carcinoma of the colon is relatively common. Carcinoma of the pancreas and of the breast are all too prevalent.

The postoperative management of the majority of patients is relatively uncomplicated. Although the incidence of minor pulmonary complications is about 25 percent because most patients are heavy smokers with chronic bronchitis, the strenuous efforts of physiotherapists are of significant aid. Mechanical ventilatory devices, except in the Intensive Care Unit, are not generally used. Much attention is paid to getting the patient active after surgery, and formal morning exercises are performed in some wards. Nasogastric tubes, when used, are kept in place for only short periods and liquids are started soon postoperatively. Hyperalimentation is used only as necessary. Postoperative thrombophlebitis is noted infrequently, and pulmonary embolism is rarely diagnosed clinically. The overall incidence is probably considerably higher, however, as noted in various postmortem studies.

The approach to serious disease, especially in old age or in those with cancer, is of interest. Until relatively recently, the majority of people in Britain died at home, although increasing numbers now enter hospital or other medical facilities for terminal care. A "good death" with the family at the bedside, while certainly not as stylized as in Victorian time, remains an integral facet of life. Many families still gather in hospital, and professional concern seems more atuned to sustaining the patient in comfort and dignity than continuing the struggle against the inevitable. A realistic approach to the particular disease process is combined with discriminate treatment. Relief of pain and of dismay is aided by use of "Brompton's mixture" or "Mist Euphoria," a cocktail including heroin, morphine, and glycerin, which the terminal patient is given to sip as needed. Surgical or chemotherapeutic heroics are few especially in the face of advanced cancer. A philosophy of kindly sympathy and comfort is maintained by the professional staff as the inevitable end of life becomes apparent.

MEDICAL EDUCATION AND SURGICAL TRAINING

The majority of British medical students undertake a six-year course financed by skimpy government grants. The students seem remarkably well educated, having covered extensively various general courses while in school. Thirty to forty percent of the students are women. Few notes of dissatisfaction or social protest are apparent, and the majority are polite, interested, and sympathetic toward the study of medicine and toward the patients they see. They approve of the aims of a NHS and are openly skeptical of any fee-for-service system. Anatomy and physiology are of primary importance in the preclinical years, and physical diagnosis stressed later on, as much of the tradition of British clinical teaching entails discussions in small groups around the bedside. About 80 percent of the medical graduates enter general practice, while only a few opt for the various specialties. This lack of specialization may be on a financial basis, an unwillingness to enter a long training period, or the relative dearth of consultant openings.

Although the years of training are long in surgery, the pace is controlled and time is available for other interests. Upon completion of medical school, each student spends a year as Resident divided between medicine and surgery. His total responsibility is patient care, and he rarely enters the operating room. He has been issued a temporary license to practice within the confines of a hospital, and he becomes fully licensed at the end of the year. During this initial period, he may decide to spend an extra year training for general practice or may apply for specialty training. As Senior House Officer, he spends much time in the operating room, usually with a single consultant. He sees surgical problems in the Casualty Department on Receiving Nights and performs emergency surgery with the Senior Registrar. After two to three years at this level, during which time he has taken the primary part of the Surgical Fellowship, he applies for position of Registrar. The Registrar completes the Fellowship and gains increasing clinical and operative responsibility and experience. During the three- to four-year period, he must decide whether to enter a Department of Surgery as an academic or remain in a non-university capacity. Having rotated through various subspecialties, he applies for Senior Registrar. At this level he may work in various Units to fill gaps in his training as noted by him or by the Senior Registrar Committee. Finally he applies for consultant posts as they become available and usually will be accepted within three years about age 40. The surgeon generally spends his professional career in the particular institution in which he obtains consultant rank.

With the attraction of surgery and the limited numbers of consultant positions throughout the country, there is a significant glut of Registrars waiting for advancement, although in other specialties such as radiology, psychiatry, and anesthesia, consultant positions are more freely available and are obtained years earlier. A manpower committee has recently been formed to study this problem and to assimilate numbers of surgical Registrars with available surgical consultant posts. Those Registrars unassured of a future position may emigrate at this juncture, or enter subspecialties or general practice. This overcrowding of young professionals is increased by many foreign graduates who come to Britain to try to gain the Surgical Fellowship. The likelihood of eventual consultant status in surgery for these individuals is remote. Staying about three years, they staff many county hospitals which are fully dependent upon them. A poor grasp of the language combined with medical education of different emphasis, cause distinct problems both for these doctors and for the patients.

All beyond the stage of Resident take a months' holiday each year, and cross-coverage within each unit is assured. Pay at lower levels is lean, but increases in graded increments to consultant status. While consultant earnings are toward the top of the Civil Service pay scale in Britain, surgeons in general are unquestionably underpaid in relationship to their training and experience. Their salaries are similar to that of a general practitioner, although this difficulty may in part be resolved by the present changes in the NHS. Many older consultants may gain substantial increases in salary by a system of merit awards. These awards are based on reputation and may vary widely in amount depending upon recognition of the contributions, authority, and expertise of the individual surgeon.

OBSERVATIONS ON THE SYSTEM

For the doctor working within a system that is organized, financed and answerable to the government, the absence of recognizable bureaucratic overlay is remarkable. Such silent underwriting may stem from respect for the medical profession in combination with long traditions of a competent and effective Civil Service. While one reads of continuous interchange between the British Medical Association and government, especially during the present period of reorganization and restructuring of the Health Services, it all seems distant from those practically involved with patient care. There is little day-to-day harrassment by committees, forms and signatures. The ease of performing one's role with judicious use of ancillary services is most noticeable, and ordinary problems of organization, scheduling, and care run smoothly. The absence of financial overtones compounding the effects of illness is of importance to the doctor who is not pressed by cost or rapid disposition of the sick. The daily pace is unhurried and uncluttered with trivial tasks, yet large amounts of work can be accomplished. The number of hours spent on patient care each week by the surgeon are not excessive, but are used conscientiously and competently. Although most consultants use only modest opportunity for private practice, little professional abuse of the system is evident.

Two medical organizations serve to catalyze and translate administrative theory into practical reality. The British Medical Association is organized both at a local and national level. Representative of the great majority of doctors in the country, it speaks to governmental administrators essentially for the entire profession. Through such dialogue, the practitioner has an important voice in the organization of medical care. Although initiated in the sixteenth century, the General Medical Council was formalized by the Medical Act of 1956. It is a system of "peer review" which aims at uniform standards of medical care. Run by doctors under the law, it involves itself in registration, undergraduate and postgraduate education, and occasional censure. Hospital review and accreditation, per se, are only now evolving.

The threat of litigation is almost unknown. The law suit is an uncommon feature of British life in general, while trust on the part of the public toward the medical profession diminishes further any threat. Medical law suits are screened by a Medical Defense Union, a defense and insurance organization funded and managed by doctors with legal advisors. The majority of cases of malpractice are defended by the Union and either cancelled or settled out of Court. As a result, only a few well-deserved suits are tried in Court each year. This seems to control spread of litigation and increases the efficiency of the courts. The contingency fee system is unknown, and membership of the Defense Union costs around $60 each year for each doctor.

Several aspects of surgery in the Health Service are of considerable practical appeal as viewed from a university hospital. Although the system is obviously uneconomic, and its increasing expense in a period of serious inflation worries its organizers and planners, it seems obvious that the majority of the public and the doctors support it enthusiastically. Over-all care is of good quality, and the various social programs are of benefit to all. A philosophy is often expressed that a civilized country must be responsible for the welfare of its citizens. As the British have committed themselves to such a program during the past 25 years, they accept the inevitable inconveniences and rigors with good faith and seem pleased and heartened with the results.

Clinical review

Measurement of hepatic blood flow in man

E. L. Bradley, III, M.D., *Atlanta, Ga.*

The various techniques currently employed to measure hepatic blood flow are examined from logical, mathematical, and procedural standpoints. Limitations of these existing methods are discussed. Criteria for an idealized technique are proposed and the importance of volumetric evaluation of nutritive perfusion in the establishment of hepatic physiopathology is stressed.

From the Department of Surgery, Emory University School of Medicine, Atlanta, Ga.

THE MEASUREMENT of hepatic blood flow has been a highly desirable if somewhat elusive goal in the establishment of hepatic physiopathology. Today, thirty years following the original methodologic description, it is uncertain whether any technique can produce reliable flow data under all circumstances. Yet many investigators continue to interpret the results strictly from such techniques, perhaps in some cases without full realization of underlying limitations.

The importance of quantitative hemodynamic data regarding hepatic perfusion under varying pathologic circumstances is clear, having wideranging diagnostic and therapeutic implications. Nowhere are these implications more evident at present than in the area of portal hypertension, where the degree of preoperative hepatic perfusion may determine the response to portasystemic shunting.[25] The apparent confusion with regard to the choice of a particular operative procedure in these patients is directly attributable to the inability to test this hemodynamic premise objectively.

Accepted for publication March 20, 1974.

It will be the purpose of this paper to examine the logical foundations of the various methods of estimating blood flow and, where appropriate, to designate limitations of such methods.

In general, all methods claiming to measure hepatic perfusion may be grouped into one of three broad categories: (1) techniques relying on the hepatic clearance of a substance from the circulation; (2) techniques depending upon indicator-dilution methodology; and (3) a group of miscellaneous techniques applying a form of physical measurement (Table I).

CLEARANCE TECHNIQUES

The initial attempt at a clinically useful method of measuring hepatic blood flow was reported by Bradley and colleagues[1] in 1945. Their method was based upon the indirect Fick principle, involving the selective removal of BSP dye by the hepatocytes from blood perfusing the liver. Dye was injected into a peripheral vein and sampled via hepatic vein catheterization. Application of the Fick principle involves knowledge of the concentration of bromsulphalein (BSP) in blood

Table I. *Methods for the determination of volumetric total hepatic blood flow*

Methods
Clearance techniques
Hepatocyte excretory clearance
Bromsulphalein
Indocyanine green
^{131}I-rose bengal
Hepatocyte metabolic clearance
Ethanol
Galactose
Reticuloendothelial particle clearance
^{33}P-chromic colloid
^{198}Au
^{59}Fe-saccharate
^{99m}Tc-sulfur colloid
^{131}I-heat denatured serum albumin
Miscellaneous
^{133}Xe
Indicator-dilution techniques
^{131}I-serum albumin
^{51}Cr-red blood cells
Miscellaneous physical techniques
Electromagnetic flowmetry
Lipiodol velocity
Heat transfer

entering the liver, the concentration of BSP in blood leaving the liver, and the total amount of BSP removed per minute by the organ. With these values known, the blood flow through the liver may be calculated by dividing the total amount of BSP removed per minute by the amount of BSP removed from each milliliter of blood passing through the liver. Mathematically, this can be represented as:

$$\text{THPF*} = \frac{B}{C_I - C_o} \qquad (1)$$

where:

THPF = total hepatic plasma flow per minute.
B = total amount of BSP removed by liver per minute.
C_I = concentration of BSP per milliliter entering liver.
C_o = concentration of BSP per milliliter leaving liver.

Since the concentration of BSP entering the liver was not directly measured, this value was indirectly approached by varying the infusion rate to maintain a constant peripheral blood concentration of BSP. The rationale was that BSP infusion rate was then equal to the hepatic extraction rate (B). Concentration of BSP entering the liver (C_I) was then calculated as being equal to the peripheral concentration, and the concentration of BSP leaving the liver (C_o) was determined by the hepatic venous catheter.

Similar principles have been applied to the measurement of hepatic blood flow by other materials dependent upon hepatocyte extraction. Caesar and co-workers[2] used indocyanine green, which they believed to be more reliable, while Combes[5] was an early advocate of ^{131}I-rose bengal. Others have described clearance methods dependent upon hepatocyte uptake and metabolism using ethanol[26] and galactose.[21] No doubt other materials specifically removed from the circulation by the hepatocyte will be suggested as possible determinants of hepatic blood flow in the future.

The accuracy of all clearance techniques dependent upon hepatocyte extraction is based upon several assumptions; the material is removed from the blood *only* by the liver, single hepatic vein sampling is representative of the total venous efflux, extrahepatic shunting does not exist, and perhaps most important, the efficiency of hepatocyte clearance is not spontaneously variable or affected by the presence of hepatic disease. While the validity of solitary hepatic vein sampling as representative of total hepatic venous concentration has been established,[10, 18] unfortunately for the hepatocyte clearance method, many of the other assumptions have proved false. Some materials supposedly extracted solely by the liver are subject to varying amounts of extrahepatic removal.[2] The occurrence of spontaneous extrahepatic portasystemic shunts in cirrhosis is well known. Under these circumstances, marker concentration in the hepatic vein (C_o in equation 1) will be artificially low, resulting in an underestimation of hepatic flow if the marker is not lost in a concentration equal to that remaining in the portal vein. Finally, the major limitation to these techniques would

*Convertible to total blood flow with knowledge of hematocrit and appropriate corrections.

appear to be that hepatocyte extraction diminishes markedly and becomes quite variable in the presence of hepatic cellular disease.[3, 4] In this instance these techniques become less valuable for measuring hepatic flow, but they become increasingly valuable as hepatic function tests.

Realizing some of the problems inherent in clearance techniques dependent upon extraction by hepatocytes, in 1952, Dobson and Jones[6] formulated a method of determining total hepatic blood flow related to hepatic reticuloendothelial cell function. He observed that following the intravenous injection of a particulate material, chromic ^{32}P, clearance of the circulating concentration of the substance at any given time could be described by an exponential function. This can be expressed as:

$$C_t = C_o e^{-kt} \qquad (2)$$

where:

C_t = particulate concentration at time t.
C_o = original particulate concentration.
k = disappearance constant.

Liver blood flow was then related to the disappearance constant:

$$\text{THBF} = \frac{V}{E}(k) \qquad (3)$$

where:

THBF = total hepatic blood flow.
V = blood volume.
E = efficiency of hepatic particulate removal.

Hepatic efficiency was defined as:

$$E\% = \frac{C_a - C_{hv}}{C_a} \times 100 \qquad (4)$$

where:

C_a = arterial particulate concentration.
C_{hv} = hepatic vein particulate concentration.

Since the original description of this method, many other colloidal and particulate materials have been used to measure hepatic blood flow in this fashion: ^{198}Au,[23] ^{59}Fe-saccharate,[7] ^{99m}Tc-sulfur colloid,[12] and ^{131}I-heat denatured serum albumin.[18] In addition to this method, others[20, 22] have related the hepatic accumulation rate of colloidal material as measured by external counting to total hepatic blood flow.

Because approximately 90 percent of the reticuloendothelial cells are found lining the liver sinusoids under normal conditions, particulate clearance methods would seem quite applicable to volumetric determination of blood flow. However, the accuracy of this form of clearance methodology is dependent upon several assumptions: All of the marker is removed on the first pass through the liver or the extraction efficiency can be accurately measured by hepatic vein catheter; extrahepatic portasystemic shunting does not occur; particulate material is cleared from the blood only by the liver; the disappearance constant is independent of the initial colloid concentration; and reticuloendothelial cell function is not affected by the presence of hepatic disease.

Since all particulate material is *not* cleared from the blood on the first pass through the liver, any clearance method which assumes complete removal and relies upon peripheral venous sampling without measuring extraction efficiency will be in error. As can be seen by an examination of equation 3, if E is assumed to be unity (complete extraction), then blood flow is simply the product of the disappearance constant and the blood volume. However, if E is not in fact 100 percent, then total hepatic blood flow will be underestimated by the exact percentage by which the extraction efficiency differs from unity. Therefore, whether internally or externally monitored, any method not using a hepatic vein catheter to actually measure particulate extraction is subject to potentially large errors.

Even when hepatic venous catheterization is employed to measure extraction efficiency, difficulties may arise if any material present in the portal vein does not traverse the hepatic veins. Extrahepatic portasystemic shunting is known to exist spontaneously in addition to shunts created surgically. It would appear that the use of this method under such conditions would result in an artificially high extraction efficiency, since the shunted particulate matter would not appear in the hepatic veins when in fact the particulate material was not extracted by the liver. This consideration demands that any material lost by extrahepatic shunts be lost in the same concentration to that concentration remaining in the portal vein. Continuing, since more particulate material will then be presented to the extrahepatic reticuloendothelial system (RES), it can no longer be assumed that the liver is the only site of RES extraction. It then follows that the disappearance constant (k) would be a composite rate of all RES extraction, and not primarily hepatic. In all likelihood, this would tend to lower the disappearance constant, adding to the possibility of spuriously low calculated values for hepatic blood flow by this method. Significant extrahepatic RES extraction is known to exist under conditions of cirrhosis; in fact, it is of such degree that the amount of extrahepatic uptake of particulate material has been advocated as an index of the degree of portal hypertension,[8] suggesting that extrahepatic particulate uptake is a function of the degree of portasystemic shunting. Therefore, this method would seem least reliable in evaluating hepatic blood flow whenever spontaneous or surgically induced portasystemic shunting exists.

Other potential difficulties with this method are less clearly defined. Dobson has shown that the extraction efficiency of the hepatic RES can be reduced if sufficient particulate material was presented to these cells; i.e., k is *not* independent of C_0 (equation 2). Sufficient experimentation to establish the function relating k to C_0 was not done, but it was felt that the hepatic RES would not be "overwhelmed" if the total dose of particulate material were kept below 1 mg.[6] Further work seems to be needed supporting the independence of the disappearance constant to low mass presentations of any specific particulate material. Second, and of primary clinical importance, is whether hepatic RES function is affected by the presence of hepatic disease. A disease-produced failure of particulate phagocytosis would amount to an "intrahepatic shunt" unrelated to actual blood flow. While the extraction efficiency (E) could still be measured, more particulate material would be available to the extrahepatic RES leading to a composite "k," as previously noted. What little information that is available bearing upon this problem seems to suggest that hepatic RES function continues in the face of significant hepatic cellular disease.[18] Further work is needed in this area. Finally, Dobson[6] suggested that the actual colloidal particle size was of critical importance to the efficiency of hepatic RES extraction and that larger particles were more efficiently extracted. This observation has been subsequently confirmed.[13] However, the function relating particle size to extraction efficiency has not been determined. This is of some importance as it has been shown that smaller particles are removed by the extrahepatic RES. Under such circumstances, the disappearance constant, not being exclusively hepatic in origin, would be invalid.

Shizgal and Goldstein[19] have described an ingenious clearance method, seemingly independent of hepatic cellular extraction, relating the disappearance of a known mass of ^{133}Xe placed into the small bowel lumen to total hepatic blood flow. However, in addition to being subject to the general criticisms of clearance techniques as noted above, xenon is known to have a high solubility constant in fat. In the presence of fatty deposition in the liver, one might expect that concentrations of xenon reaching the hepatic vein would be artificially low, resulting in spuriously low calculations of hepatic blood flow (see equation 3).

INDICATOR DILUTION TECHNIQUES

Reichman and co-workers[16] were the earliest investigators attempting to apply the Stewart-Hamilton principle to the volumetric determination of hepatic blood flow. The indicator, ^{131}I-serum albumin, was injected into the spleen and monitored in a hepatic vein. Other studies based upon indicator dilution principles but using different indicators, ^{51}Cr-red blood cells, have been subsequently reported.[10] This method is also an extension of the Fick principle and, in essence, requires knowing only the total amount of indicator injected and the ability to determine the concentrations of the indicator immediately after the indicator has passed through the organ. The mathematical expression is:

$$\text{THBF} = \frac{I}{\int_0^\infty C_t \cdot dt} \qquad (5)$$

where:

I = total amount of indicator injected.
C_t = concentration of indicator at any time t.

Results are based upon the integration of the concentrations of the specific indicator appearing at a hepatic vein catheter during the first circulation through the liver. Several assumptions underlie this method. Two of the most important are that the indicator remains in the vascular space and is neither metabolized nor excreted prior to the sampling site and that the hepatic circulation is in a "steady state."

The existence of spontaneous or surgically induced extrahepatic portasystemic shunting permits indicator to bypass the hepatic vein sampling site. In order to permit meaningful calculations under these circumstances, the amount of indicator lost through shunts must be similar in concentration to that remaining in the portal vein and subsequently sampled at the hepatic vein. Data supporting this assumption do not seem to be available.

Second, the accuracy of indicator-dilution methodology in general has been questioned. Marked discrepancies between actual flow values and those determined by indicator-dilution techniques have been noted in carefully controlled model systems.[11] In an elegant analysis, Visscher and Johnson[24] have shown that the Fick principle presupposes that blood flow is constant, i.e., steady state, and not pulsatile. Under these circumstances, in order to apply Fick techniques to calculations, it is necessary to postulate that either the flow or the marker concentrations are equal on each side of the organ at each instant of time.[24] Such a set of conditions seems highly unlikely.

Finally, the realization that this method permits only estimation of total volumetric blood flow is of paramount clinical importance. The fraction of hepatic perfusion actually nourishing cells is of greater importance than total hepatic flow rates. Few statements concerning nutritive or effective cellular perfusion can be made from data presenting total volumetric flow. It is conceivable that organ dysfunction may exist as a result of inadequte cellular perfusion while maintaining "normal" total flow rates. Since both venovenous and arteriovenous shunts are numerous in cirrhosis,[14] total flow values may not be meaningfully comparable between cirrhotic patients without the nutritive perfusion fraction being known.

MISCELLANEOUS PHYSICAL TECHNIQUES

With careful attention to technique, the results of hepatic blood flow derived from the placement of electromagnetic flowmeters seems clinically reliable.[17] However, the need for anesthesia represents an uncontrolled variable which may also adversely affect values when compared to those obtained under more physiologic conditions. Clearly, the necessity for operative exposure severely restricts repeatability and clinical usefulness.

Reichle and associates[15] have suggested a method for quantitation of portal blood flow which involves determining the cross-sectional area of the portal vein by biplane fluoroscopy and multiplying this value by the velocity of portal venous flow obtained by cineradiographic mapping of Lipiodol droplets introduced into the portal system via umbilical vein catheterization. While theoretically acceptable, perhaps the complexity of this method and the need for umbilical vein catheterization have limited widespread clinical use.[15]

Graf[9] has applied thermodynamic principles to the determination of total hepatic blood flow. An almost linear relationship has been shown to exist between thermal conductivity and vascular perfusion when thermocouples were placed in the liver. However, it was also shown that hepatic temperatures were not solely dependent upon blood flow.

It should be clear that none of these techniques are capable of measuring nutritive or effective hepatic perfusion.

REQUIREMENTS OF AN IDEAL TECHNIQUE

From the foregoing comments, it is clear that any technique purporting to measure hepatic blood flow should also be primarily capable of measuring nutritive perfusion. This provision requires that the method take into account not only intrahepatic shunting, but also spontaneous and surgically induced extrahepatic portasystemic collateral vessels. Such considerations would then result in a volumetric estimation of total hepatic blood flow, a volumetric measure of effective or nutritive perfusion, and an objective valuation of the shunt fraction.

The method should also be capable of use in the face of hepatocellular disease, capable of determination without anesthesia or operative procedures, safe and repeatable, simple in concept and procedure, available for widespread use without resort to complicated and expensive instrumentation, and finally, validated against the most objective means currently available.

Whether such a method will ever be found, the superiority of such an idealized technique over currently available methods forces us to recognize the limitations to the strict interpretation of data derived from our present procedures. Great advances in hepatic physiopathology await the development of such a technique.

REFERENCES

1. Bradley, S. E., Inglefinger, F. J., Bradley, G. P., et al.: Estimation of hepatic blood flow in man, J. Clin. Invest. **24:** 890, 1945.
2. Caesar, J., Shaldon, S., and Sherlock, S.: The use of indocyanine green in the measurement of hepatic blood flow as a test of hepatic function, Clin. Sci. **21:** 43, 1961.
3. Christie, J. H., and Chaudhuri, T. K.: Measurement of hepatic blood flow, Semin. Nucl. Med. **2:** 97, 1972.
4. Cohn, J. N., Khatri, I. M., Groszman, R. J., et al.: Hepatic blood flow in alcoholic liver disease measured by an indicator dilution technique, Am. J. Med. **53:** 704, 1972.
5. Combes, B.: Estimation of hepatic blood flow in man and dogs by ^{131}I-labeled rose bengal, J. Lab. Clin. Med. **56:** 537, 1960.
6. Dobson, E. L., and Jones, H. B.: The behavior of intravenously injected particulate matter: Its rate of disappearance from the blood stream as a measure of liver blood flow, Acta Med. Scand. **144:** Suppl. 273, 1952.
7. Fellinger, K., Gisinger, E., and Vetter, H.: Der Stoffwechsel Fe 59—Markierten Kolloidalen Eisen-Saccharates beim Menschen, *in* Fellinger, K., and Vetter, H., editors: Radioaktive Isotope in Klinik und Forschung, vol. II, München, 1956, Urban and Schwarzenberg, p. 13.
8. Gourgoutis, G. D., Das, G., and Lindsay, N.: Splenic uptake of ^{99m}Technetium sulfur colloid as an index of portal hypertension, Am. J. Gastroenterol. **57:** 435, 1972.
9. Graf, W.: Patterns of human temperature, Acta Physiol. Scand. **46:** Suppl. 160, 1959.
10. Huet, P. M., Lavoie, P., and Viallet, A.: Simultaneous estimation of portal and hepatic blood flows by an indicator dilution technique, J. Lab. Clin. Med. **82:** 836, 1973.
11. Jacobs, R. R., Schmitz, A., Heydon, W. C., et al.: A comparison of the accuracies in the electro-magnetic flowmeter and in the cardiogreen dilution blood flow measurement techniques in a model, Surg. Forum **19:** 113, 1968.
12. Mundschenk, H., Hromec, A., and Fisher, J.: Phagocytic activity of the liver as a measure of hepatic circulation. A comparative study using ^{198}Au and ^{99m}Tc-sulfur colloid, J. Nucl. Med. **12:** 711, 1971.
13. Playoust, M. R., McRae, J., and Boden, R. W.: Inefficient hepatic extraction of colloidal gold: Resulting inaccuracies in determination of hepatic blood flow, J. Lab. Clin. Med. **54:** 728, 1959.
14. Popper, H., Elias, H., and Petty, D. E.: Vascular pattern of the cirrhotic liver, Am. J. Clin. Pathol. **22:** 717, 1952.
15. Reichle, F. A., Sovak, M., Soulen, R. L., et al.: Portal blood flow determination in the unanesthetized human by umbilicoportal cannulation, J. Surg. Res. **12:** 146, 1972.
16. Reichman, S., Davis, W. D., Storaasli, J. P., et al.: Measurement of hepatic blood flow by indicator dilution techniques, J. Clin. Invest. **37:** 1848, 1958.
17. Schenk, W. G., McDonald, J. C., McDonald, K., et al.: Direct measurement of hepatic blood flow in surgical patients, with related

observations on hepatic flow dynamics in experimental animals, Ann. Surg. **156:** 463, 1962.

18. Shaldon, S., Chiundussi, L., Guevara, L., et al.: The estimation of hepatic blood flow and intrahepatic shunted blood flow by colloidal heat-denatured human serum albumin labeled with ^{131}I, J. Clin. Invest. **40:** 1346, 1961.
19. Shizgal, H. M., and Goldstein, M. S.: Measurement of portal and total hepatic blood flow by the intestinal xenon technique, SURGERY **72:** 83, 1972.
20. Torrance, H. B., and Gowenlock, A. H.: Radioactive colloidal clearance techniques to measure liver blood flow in man, Clin. Sci. **22:** 413, 1962.
21. Tygstrup, N., and Winkler, K.: Galactose blood clearance as a measure of hepatic blood flow, Clin. Sci. **17:** 1, 1958.
22. Ueda, H., Unuma, T., Iio, M., et al.: Measurement of hepatic arterial and portal blood flow and circulation time via hepatic artery and portal vein with radioisotope, Jap. Heart J. **3:** 154, 1962.
23. Vetter, H., Falkner, R., and Neumayr, A.: The disappearance rate of colloidal radiogold from the circulation and its application to the estimation of liver blood flow in normal and cirrhotic subjects, J. Clin. Invest. **33:** 1594, 1954.
24. Visscher, M. B., and Johnson, J. A.: The Fick principle: analysis of potential errors and its conventional applications, J. Appl. Physiol. **5:** 635, 1953.
25. Warren, W. D., Restrepo, J. E., Respess, J. C., et al.: The importance of hemodynamic studies in management of portal hypertension, Ann. Surg. **158:** 387, 1963.
26. Winkler, K., Larsen, J. A., Munkner, T., et al.: Determination of the hepatic blood flow in man by simultaneous use of five test substances measured in two parts of the liver, Scand. J. Clin. Lab. Invest. **17:** 423, 1965.

Brief clinical reports

Lipoma, a cause of paralysis of deep radial (posterior interosseous) nerve: Report of a case and review of the literature

Kwang-Tzen Wu, M.D., Francis R. Jordan, M.D., *and* **Charles Eckert, M.D.,** *Albany, N. Y.*

Ten cases, including one case we observed, of posterior interosseous nerve paralysis caused by compression of a lipoma in the proximal portion of the forearm were reviewed. The lesion occurred in seven men and three women ranging in age from 40 to 77 years. The onset of paralysis was usually insidious, and in seven cases it preceded awareness of the presence of the mass. Duration of nerve paralysis ranged from a few months to twelve years before the diagnosis was made and treatment was instituted. There was no set pattern of which fingers were involved first. The nerve paralysis was progressive and weakness of the wrist eventually developed in four cases. In five of the six patients who had roentgenographic study, it was possible to establish the diagnosis preoperatively. In all six patients who had paralysis for less than five years, recovery was noted after the treatment. On the other hand, in two patients who had paralysis for eight and twelve years no significant recovery was noted. Early excision of lipoma is recommended and complete recovery of the extensor mechanism of the finger and hand is expected when this is done.

From the Surgical Service, Veterans Administration Hospital, and the Department of Surgery, Albany Medical College, Union University, Albany, N. Y.

PARALYSIS OF the posterior interosseous nerve (a motor branch of the radial nerve) may be caused by space-occupying lesions, such as lipoma[7] or ganglion,[2] trauma, bicepital bursitis,[5] or compression of fibrous superior edge of supinator muscle (Arcade of Frohse).[12]

Richmond[10] in 1953 reported a case of parosteal lipoma of the neck of the radius causing radial nerve palsy. Since then, sporadic reports of lipoma causing radial nerve palsy have appeared.[3, 7, 8] A review of the literature published in the English language yields eleven cases. As the total number of such cases that have been reported is limited, it is our purpose to report one such case and to review the literature on this subject.

Accepted for publication Feb. 22, 1974.

CASE REPORT

A 77-year-old white male veteran, a retired painter, was admitted to the hospital in July, 1972, because of pain in the neck, wrist drop on the right, and swelling of the right forearm. Twelve years prior to admission, he noted a sudden onset of tightness and inability to extend the fingers of his right hand. The diagnosis was "nerve palsy" owing to cerebrovascular accident. A few months later he noticed painless swelling at the proximal portion of the right forearm which gradually increased in size with concomitant gradual increase in the difficulty of extending his fingers. His right wrist started to drop five years prior to his admission and gradually became worse. Apparently there was no loss in his grasping power and he continued to work as a painter until two years prior to admission. Four years prior to admission, he underwent a resection of the left colon for carcinoma. Since late 1971 the patient suffered from neck pain radiating to both arms attributed to cervical spondylosis.

Pertinent physical findings include a large painless ill-defined swelling approximately 10 by 5 cm. at the radial aspect of proximal right forearm. There was a deep radial nerve paralysis on the right manifested by wrist drop and involuntary flexion of the fingers. He could not extend his fingers voluntarily, but they could be extended passively although with great resistance. No sensory loss was present. The results of routine laboratory examinations were all within normal limits. X-ray film of cervical spine revealed degenerative changes of the fourth to seventh cervical vertebrae, and that of the right forearm showed a large radiolucent area at the proximal forearm suggestive of lipoma (Fig. 1). In October, 1972, the swelling was explored through an incision made on the anterolateral aspect of the proximal forearm. The brachioradialis muscle was retracted laterally, and the mass was noted to be a lipoma located deeper to the brachioradialis and supinator muscles, lateral to the flexor muscles, and attached to the periosteum of the proximal radius. The posterior interosseous nerve was stretched by the lipoma, and there were fibrous bands along the superior edge of the supinator crossing and compressing the nerve. On palpation, the proximal portion of the nerve was cordlike in consistency. After releasing the fibrous band, the compression on the nerve was found to be localized and sharply demarcated, and the consistency of the proximal portion of the nerve became as soft as that of the distal portion. The lipoma measured 6 by 4 cm. in size, and it was excised without difficulty. One day after the operation, a photograph of the right wrist and hand was taken in maximal flexion and extension (Fig. 2). A nerve conduction study done six days after the operation showed evidence of conduction block in the right radial nerve distal to the elbow with normal conduction proximally. Since the operation, the patient could "relax" his fingers and grasp objects with less difficulty.

Follow-up examination performed fourteen months after the excision of lipoma revealed minimal recovery of the extensor mechanism of his right fingers and hand (Fig. 3). Electromyogram study showed no action potential in the extensor muscles innervated by deep radial nerve.

Comment. The present patient probably is the oldest and also had the longest duration of posterior interosseous nerve paralysis before diagnosis was made and treatment was instituted. It is unlikely that either cervical spondylosis or cancer of the colon were related to the radial nerve palsy. Delay in diagnosis and the institution of proper treatment in this patient has been associated with very slow recovery. A localized linear compression of the posterior interosseous nerve by the superior edge of the supinator against the lipoma and cordlike consistency of the proximal portion of the nerve before the release of the fibrous bands do not appear to have been previously reported.

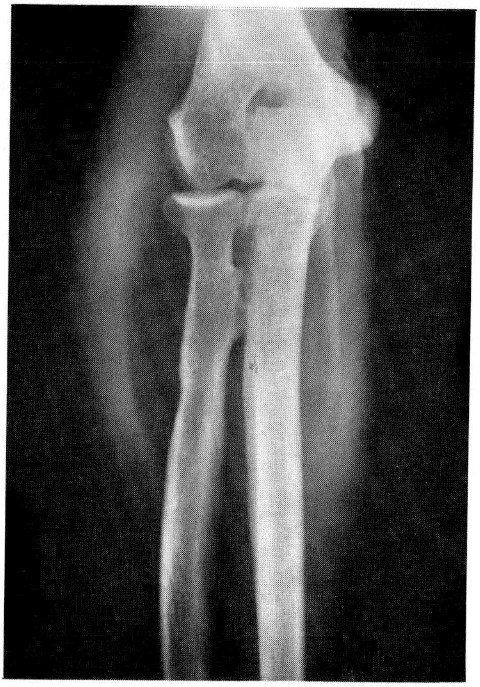

Fig. 1. X-ray film of the proximal portion of the right forearm showing a distinct area of radiolucency.

LITERATURE REVIEW

Smith[11] in 1868 was the first to report a lipoma located at the radial neck, and the term "parosteal lipoma" was introduced by Power[9] in 1888. The radial nerve paralysis caused by parosteal lipoma was not described until 1953 by Richmond.[10] He reported a painter unable to extend his left index fingers and thumb with progressive paralysis for twelve weeks. The patient had complete recovery of muscular function of the involved extensors 16 months after the excision of lipoma.

Campbell and Wulf[3] in 1954 reported a case of radial nerve palsy caused by lipoma in a 40-year-old white female church worker.

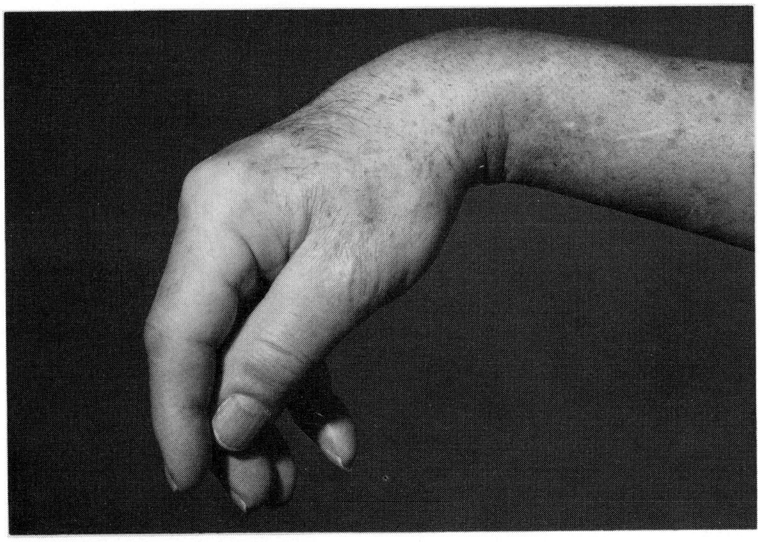

Fig. 2. Photograph taken one day after the excision of the lipoma. The wrist was in maximal extension when this photograph was taken. It illustrates apparent wrist drop caused by deep radial nerve paralysis.

Table I. *Posterior interosseous nerve paralysis caused by lipoma*

Case No.	*Year reported*	*Author*	*Age (yr.)*	*Sex*	*Profession*	*Duration of motor paralysis*
1	1953	Richmond[10]	62	M	Painter	3 mo.
2	1954	Campbell and Wulf[3]	40	F	Church worker	3 mo.
3	1955	Hustead et al.[6]	63	F	Housewife	1½ yr.
4	1955	Hustead et al.[6]	56	M	Laborer	1½ yr.
5	1962	White and Hanna[13]	65	F	Clerk	5 yr.
6	1964	Moon and Marmor[7]	73	M	Not stated	8 yr.
7	1966	Capener[4]	58	M	Company director	2 mo.
8	1971	Phalen et al.[8]	56	M	Not stated	5 yr.
9	1971	Phalen et al.[8]	62	M	Not stated	1 yr.
10	1974	Wu et al. (present case)	77	M	Painter	12 yr.

No long-term follow-up was included in this report.

Hustead and associates[6] in 1955 reviewed 16 cases of non-traumatic progressive paralysis of the posterior interosseous nerve reported in the literature and added two cases of their own. In both of their cases, the paralysis was caused by lipomas. Surgical exploration was carried out in seven of these 18 cases. Benign neoplasms were found in four; three of these were lipomas and one was an atypical lipoma. Diseased bursae were found in two cases, and an anomalous course of the deep radial nerve was found in one case. In the remaining eleven cases, the etiologic factors remained obscure.

Lipomas are usually asymptomatic but occasionally they may become troublesome. White and Hanna[13] in 1962 reported 24 patients with troublesome lipoma located in

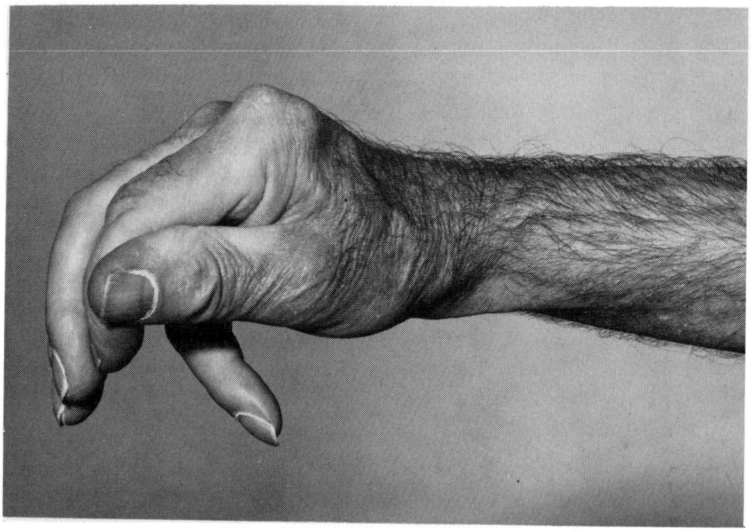

Fig. 3. Photograph taken 14 months after the excision of the lipoma. The wrist was in maximal extension when this photograph was taken. It illustrates minimal recovery of the paralysis of the posterior interosseous nerve.

Paralysis pre- :edes or suc- eeds awareness of mass	*Pattern of involvement*	*Size*	*Roentgenogram*	*Recovery*
Precedes	Left thumb and index finger	Not stated	Diagnostic	Complete, 16 mo.
Same time	Left thumb and index finger	Not stated	Not done	Not stated
Precedes	Left thumb, then all fingers and wrist weakness	4 cm.	Diagnostic	Complete, 9 mo.
Precedes	Right midfinger, then all fingers and wrist drop	20 Gm.	Not done	Not stated
Succeeds	Right little and ring fingers	4 × 2 × 2 cm.	Not done	Complete, 4½ mo.
Precedes	Left thumb, then all fingers and wrist weakness	4 cm.	Diagnostic	No recovery, 1 yr.
Same time	Left thumb and fingers, then all fingers	7 cm.	Not done	Complete, 5 yr.
Precedes	Left index finger then all fingers	6.5 × 4 × 2 cm.	Not diagnostic	Complete, 1½ yr.
Precedes	Right middle, ring, and little fingers	3 × 2.5 × 1 cm.	Diagnostic	Almost complete, 2 yr.
Precedes	All fingers, then wrist drop, right side	6 × 4 cm.	Diagnostic	Minimal, 1 yr., 2 mo.

the upper extremity. Among the 24 cases, 21 patients complained of discomfort ranging from tickling, itching, heaviness, and local tingling to aching and pain. Eleven patients presented functional disturbances, four of whom had some alteration in nerve function caused by pressure of the neoplasms on one of the peripheral nerves. In three of these, the lipoma was found to be in contact with the ulnar nerve, and in the remaining one, it was in contact with the radial nerve. The patient with posterior interosseous nerve palsy was unable to extend her right ring and little fingers following a minimal trauma. In this case, the presence of the mass at her upper forearm was noted for five years before the appearance of nerve palsy. Four and one-half months after the removal of the lipoma, the patient had complete return to digital extension.

Barber and associates[1] in 1962 reviewed 32 benign extraneural soft tissue tumors of the extremities causing compression of nerves. Included were four cases of lipoma located at the proximal forearm causing compression of the radial nerve. Two of these cases were included in the above-mentioned report by Hustead and associates.[6] No details of the other two cases were given.

Parosteal lipoma is not always associated with paralysis of the posterior interosseous nerve. In 1964, Moon and Marmor[7] reviewed the literature and found 18 cases of parosteal lipoma of the proximal part of the radius and added two of their own cases, making a total of 20. In nine of these 20 cases, there was involvement of the posterior interosseous nerve causing some degree of paralysis; in one case, the superficial radial nerve was compressed; while in the remaining ten cases there was no nerve involvement at all.

Capener[4] in 1966 added one case of posterior interosseous nerve paralysis caused by lipoma, and he described in detail his method of approaching the posterior interosseous nerve.

Lipomas located in the upper extremity seem to cause more symptoms of nerve compression than that of the lower extremity. Phalen and associates[8] in 1971 reviewed their experience with lipomas of the upper extremity and reported six cases with nerve involvement. Of these six cases with nerve involvement, three had a lipoma located in the proximal portion of the forearm. The remaining one had lipoma located in the upper arm. The other three of the six cases had only sensory disturbance. They consider that lipoma located in the upper extremity is more apt to cause sensory rather than motor disturbance.

Excluding the three cases published in non-English literature which appeared in the review by Moon and Marmor[7] and the two cases observed by Barber and associates,[1] and by adding the present one case, the authors have tabulated ten cases of posterior interosseous nerve palsy caused by lipoma located in the proximal forearm (Table I). This disease occurs in middle-aged to older individuals with variable duration of nerve compression. The presence of parosteal lipoma in the proximal forearm does not necessarily cause the symptoms of posterior interosseous nerve paralysis, but it is interesting to note that the functional loss often precedes awareness of the mass. Among ten cases, only one case had a tumor mass noticeable in the proximal portion of the forearm before the onset of motor paralysis. The onset of the symptom usually is insidious, but occasionally it may be relatively sudden as in one of the cases reported by Hustead and associates.[6] It may occasionally be associated with trauma.[4, 7] The nature of the patient's occupation does not appear to bear a definite relationship to the development of a deep radial nerve palsy. There is no set pattern of which finger(s) will be involved first. In all the cases, once weakness of the extensors of the fingers has started, if untreated, the symptom appears to progress, and the involvement will advance from one or two fingers to all fingers, with the eventual possibility of developing wrist drop. In four of the ten cases, there was some weakness in extension at the wrist joint. The diagnosis can usually be made with radiographic examination. In one of the six patients who had roentgenographic study was the result nondiagnostic. As the nerve paralysis often precedes the awareness of the presence of lipoma, it is important to suspect such a lesion.

The surgical approach is by either an anterior incision, dissecting the space between brachioradialis and brachialis, or by an incision over the groove between the extensor carpi radialis brevis and the extensor digitorum communis. After the lipoma is removed, the prognosis appears to be excellent. The duration of the follow-up varied from a few months to five years and recovery usually followed early excision. If removal is delayed, however, functional loss may be permanent.

We would like to thank Miss Lucia Battistello for typing the manuscript and Mr. Kenneth C. Perry and Mr. Robert Szembrot for photographing the figures.

REFERENCES

1. Barber, K. W., Jr., Bianco, A. J., Jr., Soule, E. H., and MacCarty, C. S.: Benign extraneural soft-tissue tumors of the extremities causing compression of nerves, J. Bone Joint Surg. **44A:** 98, 1962.
2. Bowen, T. L., and Stone, K. H.: Posterior interosseous nerve paralysis caused by a ganglion at the elbow, J. Bone Joint Surg. **48B:** 774, 1966.
3. Campbell, C. S., and Wulf, R. F.: Lipoma producing a lesion of the deep branch of the radial nerve, J. Neurosurg. **11:** 310, 1954.
4. Capener, N.: The vulnerability of the posterior interosseous nerve of the forearm, J. Bone Joint Surg. **48B:** 770, 1966.
5. Esposito, G. M.: Peripheral entrapment neuropathies of upper extremity, N. Y. State J. Med. **72:** 717, 1972.
6. Hustead, A. P., Mulder, D. W., and MacCarty, C. S.: Nontraumatic, progressive paralysis of the deep radial (posterior interosseous) nerve, Arch. Neurol. Psychiat. **79:** 269, 1958.
7. Moon, N., and Marmor, L.: Parosteal lipoma of the proximal part of the radius, J. Bone Joint Surg. **46A:** 608, 1964.
8. Phalen, G. S., Kendrick, J. I., and Rodreiguez, J. M.: Lipomas of the upper extremity, Am. J. Surg. **121:** 298, 1971.
9. Power, D'A.: A parosteal lipoma or congenital fatty tumour, connected with the periosteum of the femur, Trans. Pathol. Soc. London **39:** 270, 1888.
10. Richmond, D. A.: Lipoma causing a posterior interosseous nerve lesion, J. Bone Joint Surg. **46A:** 83, 1953.
11. Smith, T.: Fatty tumor growing from the neck of the radius, Trans. Pathol. Soc. London **19:** 344, 1868.
12. Spinner, M.: The arcade of Frohse and its relationship to posterior interosseous nerve paralysis, J. Bone Joint Surg. **50B:** 809, 1968.
13. White, W. L., and Hanna, D. C.: Troublesome lipomata of the upper extremity, J. Bone Joint Surg. **44A:** 1353, 1962.

Interscapulothoracic amputation for the complications of breast cancer: A new approach

Peter I. Pressman, M.D., F.A.C.S., *New York, N. Y.*

Following radical mastectomy and radiation therapy for breast cancer, necrosis in the subclavicular area can produce an ulcerative wound overlying the brachial plexus and axillary blood vessels. This is usually associated with lymphedema, intractable pain, infection, and hemorrhage. Interscapulothoracic amputation can accomplish significant palliation and cure in selected patients. The strategic location of the wound requires a different surgical approach to forequarter amputation, and the operative technique is described.

From the Department of Surgery, Beth Israel Medical Center and Mt. Sinai School of Medicine, New York, N. Y.

SUCCESS in the treatment of cancer of the breast generally depends on the results of surgical excision, with or without radiation therapy. Extension beyond the pectoral area generally presages salvage failure. Radical limb amputation has a limited but accepted place in the palliation of advanced and recurrent breast cancer. In certain cases, radiation necrosis, with or without demonstrable local tumor recurrences produces an ulcerative wound overlying the brachial plexus and axillary blood vessels. Interscapulothoracic amputation is the only satisfactory method of completely extirpating the local pathology and providing adequate skin coverage. In the absence of disseminated disease, not only can palliation and rehabilitation be accomplished, but the possibility of cure also exists. The role of radical surgery in treating recurrent breast cancer was discussed by Holleb and Lucas.[3] Two recent cases, prompted us to review the subject and to develop a technique for managing the particular problem of necrosis in the axillary area which differs from the standard forequarter amputation for tumors distal to the shoulder.

Accepted for publication March 20, 1974.

Reprint requests: Dr. Peter I. Pressman, 50 East 79th St., New York, N. Y. 10021.

CASE STUDIES

Case 1. M. C., a 55-year-old nurse had a right radical mastectomy in 1967. The lymph nodes were free of tumor, and x-ray therapy was given because of the medial location of the tumor. A subclavicular ulceration developed in 1968. Multiple biopsies of the progressively enlarging wound were negative for recurrent tumor, and plastic surgical attempts at skin grafting and closure were unsuccessful, including construction of a thoracoabdominal tube pedicle. In January, 1970, the arm had become lymphedematous and was virtually useless, and narcotics were required for pain. The ulcerated area extended to the axillary vessels and the brachial plexus, and carcinoma was demonstrated in the wound which was heavily infected with Pseudomonas (Fig. 1). There was no evidence of distant metastases and internal mammary nodal biopsies were negative. In March, 1970, right interscapulothoracic amputation was done. No tumor was found in the specimen. The wound healed per primum. The patient has been successfully rehabilitated and is currently free of disease. (Fig. 2).

Case 2. C. S. is a 67-year-old woman who had a right radical mastectomy and x-ray therapy in 1966. In 1969, a chest wall recurrence appeared at the operative site, and additional radiation therapy was given. This was followed by edema of the arm and numerous episodes of cellulitis. In January, 1971, a small ulceration over the anterior axilla appeared, progressing rapidly to become a large necrotic wound. It was debrided in February, 1971, and tumor cells were present. By September, 1971, the right upper extremity was paralyzed and massively lymphedematous. The anterolateral chest wall was denuded of skin and the subclavicular area was an adherent, foul-smelling ulceration infected with Pseudomonas (Fig. 3). There was recurrent bleeding requiring transfusions, and narcotics were required for control of pain. A right interscapulothoracic amputation was done in September, 1971. There was no residual tumor found in the specimen. Delayed healing at the midportion of the wound required skin grafting. The patient was returned to an ambulatory status (Fig. 4), and in September, 1973, underwent a left modified radical mastectomy for a second primary breast cancer.

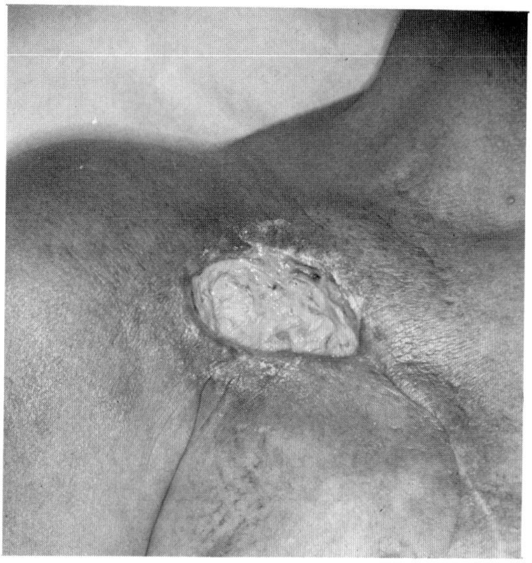

Fig. 1. Subclavicular ulceration in Case 1 (M. C.). At the base of this infected wound is the necrotic brachial plexus and the axillary artery. The arm is paretic and lymphedematous.

OPERATIVE TECHNIQUE

Preoperative preparation should include roentgenographic studies to rule out distant metastases and, most importantly, spreading beyond the planned operative field. Apical lung views are recommended to differentiate between radiation fibrosis and the presence of contiguous tumor. Eradication of infection is not possible because the necrotic tissue often includes the brachial plexus and overlies the axillary blood vessels, limiting debridement. Antibiotics to which the organisms are sensitive should be started systemically 24 hours prior to planned surgery. Pseudomonas has been the dominant organism in our cases and we have used gentamicin (Garamycin) singly and in combination with carbenicillin (Geopen).

The technique of interscapulothoracic amputation for tumors of the upper extremity has been described by Pack and associates,[5] Beattie and Economou,[1] and El-Domeiri and Miller.[2] Specific modifications are necessary where the skin has been heavily irradiated and when there are tissue defects high in the axilla, as may occur in the necrosis of radiation therapy following radical mastectomy and radiation therapy. The problems of exposing and controlling the subclavian blood vessels and of providing healthy skin coverage will be discussed.

The patient should be positioned on the operating room table midway between a full lateral and supine position and draped to expose the entire thorax and with the arm free to rotate the scapula. The incision is basically an ellipse which encompasses the shoulder girdle, with the apex at the medial aspect of the clavicle and lowest point in the mid axillary line (Fig. 5). It is designed to preserve the skin overlying the shoulder and the scapula, creating a long and broadly based posterior flap. In these cases (Fig. 3), the anterolateral thorax may already be denuded of skin and the ribs bared in areas by progressive infection and loss of tissue. The flap, although composed of tissue from a lymphedematous extremity can be rotated medially following interscapulothoracic amputation and utilized to provide primary skin coverage of the anterior chest wall. The incision is outlined with methylene blue and planned to encompass the pathology. The skin of the upper arm is included, and any redundancy can be excised at the end of the operative procedure. The incision is

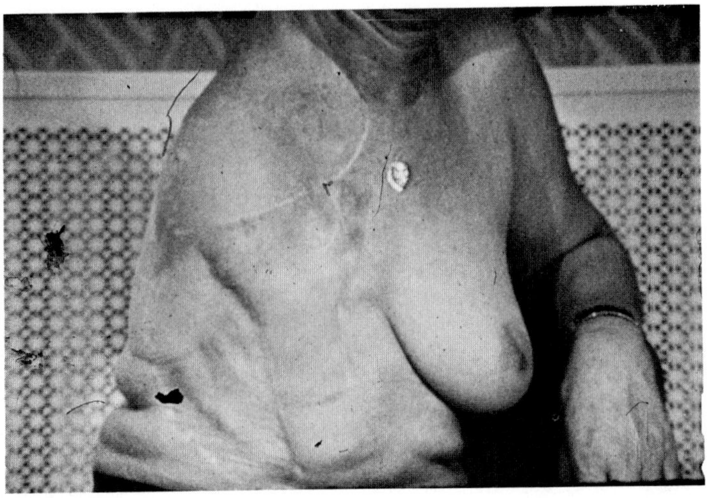

Fig. 2. Appearance of the patient M. C., 2½ years following interscapulothoracic amputation and five years following right radical mastectomy.

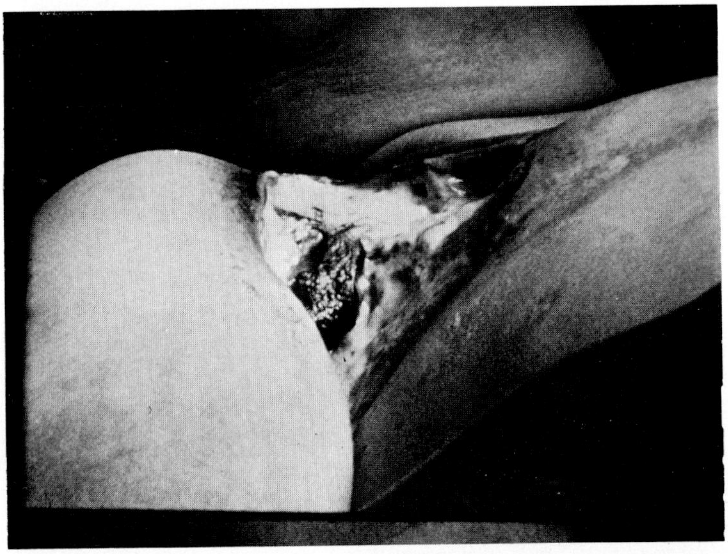

Fig. 3. Subclavicular ulceration in Case 2 (C. S.) which progressed to involve the anterolateral chest wall, axilla, and arm. It is heavily infected with Pseudomonas; the shoulder is fixed and the arm is paralyzed.

started at the apex, and paralleling the superior aspect of the clavicle, it is directed laterally over the shoulder. The omohyoid and sternocleidomastoid muscles are divided cephalad to the clavicle. The clavicle is removed in its entirety because of its proximity to the pathology and to gain access to the tough, costocoracoid membrane and the underlying subclavian vessels. Since the subclavian vessels emerge from beneath the medial aspect of the clavicle, subperiosteal excision is safer. A Gigli saw can facilitate this maneuver by first dividing the clavicle at its midpoint and then carefully excising the two segments of bone. The supraclavicular and scalene lymph nodes are excised en bloc with the specimen, and the thyrocervical trunk is divided. On the left side, the thoracic

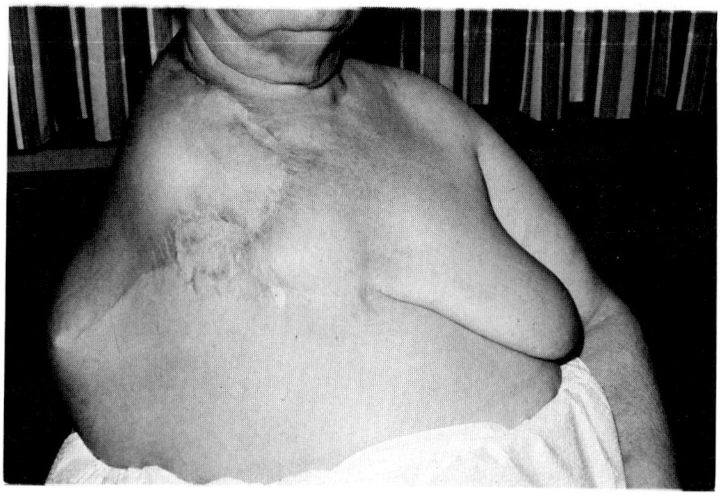

Fig. 4. Appearance of the patient C. S., one year following interscapulothoracic amputation and six years following right radical mastectomy.

duct should be sought and ligated. Isolation and division of the subclavian artery and vein is desirable at this stage in the operation, but because of radiation, the tissues are usually stony hard and fused and normal tissue planes are obscured. We have found that the subclavian vein which is superficial following removal of the clavicle can now be ligated and divided, leaving the artery to be dealt with later in the operation. This differs from previously described techniques for forequarter amputation which emphasize the necessity for dividing the axillary artery and brachial plexus as the initial part of the operative procedure.

The lateral aspect of the incision is completed, coursing over the scapula and downward along the lateral axillary border. A full-thickness flap is developed from the lymphedematous tissues of the upper arm and the shoulder. It is reflected posteriorly toward the midline, exposing all of the muscular attachments of the scapula in the midline (Fig. 6). These are the trapezius, levator scapulae, and rhomboid major and minor muscles, and they are transected close to the vertebral border of the scapula. The cutting cautery is used to divide all the muscles, conserving blood and operating time. By next dividing the serratus anterior and

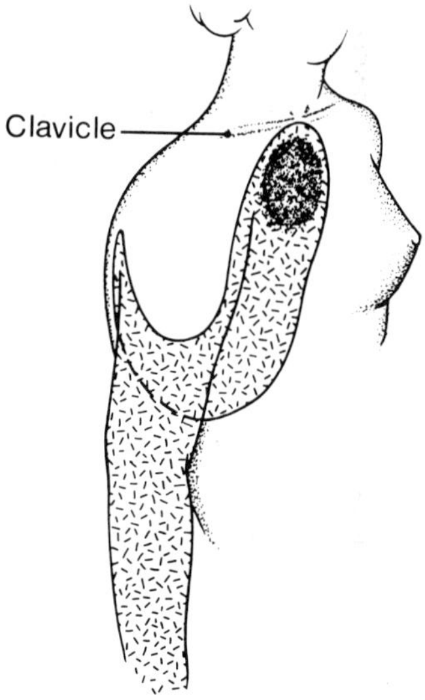

Fig. 5. Drawing demonstrating operative technique. (See text for explanation.)

lattisimus dorsi muscles inferiorly, the scapula is completely mobilized. Because these patients have had radical mastectomies, the pectoralis major and minor muscles are absent and the specimen is now attached to the trunk by the skin and subcutaneous scar tissue of the anterior chest, the brachial plexus, and the subclavian artery. The shoulder can now be reflected anteriorly like opening a book (Fig. 7), affording clear

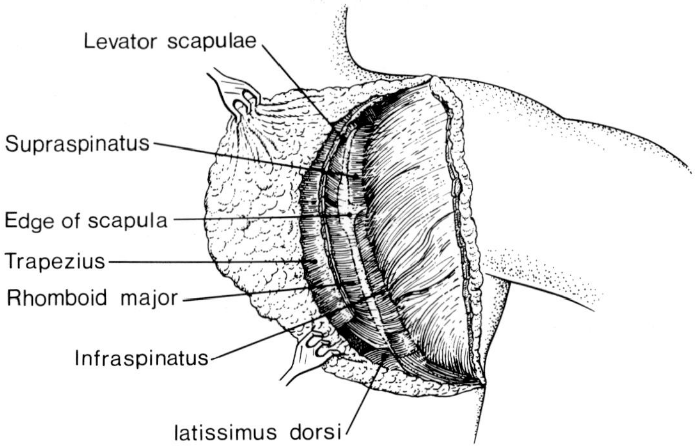

Fig. 6. Drawing demonstrating operative technique. (See text for explanation.)

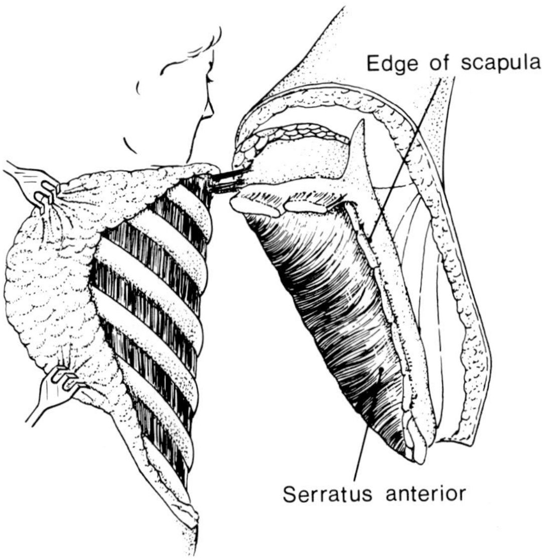

Fig. 7. Drawing demonstrating operative technique. (See text for explanation.)

visualization of the subclavian artery, which can now be safely ligated and divided, and the brachial plexus, which is then divided. We have not found it necessary to enter the chest posteriorly to obtain intrathoracic control of the major vessels, as described by Nadler and Phelan.[4] The theoretic objection of losing blood into the extremity by ligating the artery last has not been realized. In all probability, considerable venous return is accomplished by collateral vessels which remain intact during most of the operative procedure. Finally, the anterior skin incision is completed, elevating the specimen with sharp dissection so that all the dense scar tissue overlying the ribs is removed en bloc with the specimen, accomplishing exarticulation. The skin flap is then rotated medially and approximated to the anterosuperior margins of the wound. Utilizing the tissues of the arm as described, there is ample skin to cover the defect. Hemovacs are used to drain the wound and a dressing of gauze fluffs and Elastoplast is applied. The antibiotics given intraoperatively are continued for one week. Blood transfusions are administered as needed by estimation of blood loss and monitoring of the blood pressure and central venous pressure.

DISCUSSION

Interscapulothoracic amputation has a definite, although limited, role in the palliation of the complications of breast cancer. The operation can be safely performed even with necrosis involving the axillary blood vessels and the brachial plexus. By eliminating sepsis, pain, and a source of hemorrhage, a bedridden and malodorous patient can be resuscitated and returned to an ambulatory condition.

Two patients who have undergone interscapulothoracic amputation for the complications secondary to the treatment of breast cancer have been presented. The management of these cases and the operative technique employed have been described. Where radiation necrosis has been the dominant pathology and in the absence of disseminated disease, interscapulothoracic amputation can accomplish worthwhile palliation and provide the real hope of "cure."

REFERENCES

1. Beattie, E. J., Jr., and Economou, S. G.: An Atlas of advanced surgical techniques, Philadelphia, 1968, W. B. Saunders Company.
2. El-Domeiri, A. A., and Miller, T. B.: The role of interscapulothoracic amputation in the treatment of malignant tumors, Surg. Gynecol. Obstet. **129:** 1203, 1969.
3. Holleb, A. I., and Lucas, J. C.: Palliative interscapulothoracic amputation in the management of the breast cancer patient, Cancer **12:** 643, 1959.
4. Nadler, S. H., and Phelan, J. T.: A technique of interscapulothoracic amputation, Surg. Gynecol. Obstet. **122:** 359, 1966.
5. Pack, G. T., Ehrlich, H. E., and Gentil, F.: Radical amputation of extremities in treatment of cancer, Surg. Gynecol. Obstet. **84:** 1105, 1947.

Letters to the editors

Scientists and medical writing

To the Editors:

Lois DeBakey provided a convenient review, in her paper (SURGERY 75:38, 1974) about ghostwriting, of all the conventional objections to the practice of concealing editorial aid in preparing papers for submission, or resubmission, to scholarly journals like SURGERY.

Her passion for purity, however, seems to have led her to ignore some of the facts of life in medical reporting, as well as a possible means of abolishing the practice she deplores, without sacrificing editorial aid to those who sorely need it.

The facts I refer to are these: (1) Many physicians and biomedical scientists are outstandingly able in the care of sick people and in research but awkward bunglers in English composition, either because they have been passed along in our schools at all levels despite their lack of proficiency or because English is not their native tongue. (2) There is no logical reason to suppose that a competent physician or scientist is ipso facto a competent expository writer. (3) The ghostwriter does not falsify, nor does the illiterate physician or scientist, the statements or the diction of the "aided" paper—the editorial aide suggests to the original author certain improvements in the logic, organization, and rhetoric of the report, which will aid significantly in communication with readers; and the signing of the physician's or scientist's name means that he or she agrees with the report's form and content and thereby makes it his own.

The possible means of abolishing, or greatly reducing, ghostwriting is to give credit by name to all who have materially aided in the work, including the reporting of it. This could and should be done in all papers whose authors have received substantial aid. The acknowledgement could appear in the "Acknowledgements" section of the printed paper; it could appear in a footnote; or, when indicated, joint authorship or semiauthorship could be recognized in the byline. The following might be appropriate:

John Doe, M.D., and Richard Roe, Ph.D.,

with the assistance of Nathaniel Poe, Ph.D., and William Coe, M.Sc.

Either Nat Poe or Bill Coe might be a chemist or an editorial worker; both would have rendered important aid in the work, and neither would be a ghost.

Naming one's major collaborators, it seems to me, could not injure the authenticity of the work. I agree with DeBakey that collaboration should be acknowledged. Sometimes, as DeBakey must know, it *is* acknowledged.

Perhaps the editors of SURGERY could help —not to lay to rest, but to revive—the many ghosts of whom DeBakey complains, by requiring that all major collaborators be named by the principal authors. As a ghostwriter of some decades of wraithing and writhing, I would be happy to see my work correctly attributed, and I would hope that this requirement would spread.

William F. Hewitt, Ph.D.
Box 5
Smyrna, N. Y. 13464

Reply: Honesty in authorship

To the Editors:

Dr. Hewitt, by his easy interchange of the terms "ghostwriting" and "editorial aid," blurs a clear and important distinction that I made in my article, which was published in the January, 1974, issue of SURGERY.[1] Writing and editing are two separate activities: one consists in composing; the other, in preparing a completed manuscript for publication. I disapproved of writing that is done by one person in the name of another; I did not condemn minor editing.

Vol. 75, No. 5, pp. 802-804

If, as Dr. Hewitt indicates, some physicians and scientists, however competent in their fields of specialization, are "awkward bunglers in English composition," why should they present themselves to readers as skillful literary craftsmen? Is there not something ignoble about such an imposture? And how far is it from ghostwriting to ghost data? It is difficult to justify fraudulence of any kind in a field, such as biomedical science, which prizes intellectual honesty and the pursuit of truth. The person who presents the writings of another as his own is, by definition, a plagiarist, and plagiarism is frowned upon in scholarly circles. The clandestine nature of ghostwriting suggests that the participants themselves do not view it with pride.

A few other bold souls have taken a firm stand against auctorial forgery, among them D. Price Jones,[3] who wrote: "As for regular ghosting of scientific papers: may heaven preserve us from such an imposition. . . . We may grant him [the scientist] the help of a dictionary, typewriter, computer and even a secretary, but never a stooge communicator! Save us from stale tobacco smoke dressed up as mountain freshness!" An editorial in *The New England Journal of Medicine* takes a similar position: ". . . for an investigator simply to turn his material over to a professional 'ghost,' as politicians are forced to do with their speeches, seems not quite cricket. . . . To have a paper on the use of a proprietary drug prepared for the investigator by the editorial staff of the pharmaceutical house that manufactures it suggests the possibility of a conflict of interest and is certainly questionable."[2]

How far removed is ghostwriting in the biomedical sciences from the peddling of student papers on campuses? So pernicious did that practice become a couple of years ago that several states passed legislation to ban it. Firms such as "Quality Bull" and "Write-on" sprang up all over the country, contracting to write student papers of any length and on any subject. One "ghost" explained the ease and speed with which he could crank out the pieces by pointing out that structure and organization are far more important than content; once you master the style that pleases professors, he explained, "you zing."

The logic that consumers and producers of ghosting activities use in dismissing ethical questions is that only a faulty system of values nurtures or tolerates such duplicity. There is some truth in that charge, but reform of that system is hardly to be achieved by sanctioning the deception that it spawns.

Dr. Hewitt contends that "There is no logical reason to suppose that a competent physician or scientist is ipso facto a competent expository writer." I maintain that there is no logical reason to suppose that he cannot *become* one. If a ghostwriter, who generally has less scientific knowledge, education, and experience than a medical scientist, can learn to write readable prose, so can the scientist. The basic principles of good scientific exposition are simply not that difficult to master. The tacit assumption is not, however, sound that one who hires out as a "writer" necessarily has superior literary skills. Unfortunately (or fortunately, depending on your vantage point), no licensing or certifying boards exist for ghostwriters or manuscript editors. Anyone who can find customers can ply the trade, and, as in other vocations, skills vary from one practitioner to the next.

A writer who can earn a livelihood composing under his own name is not likely to forego the gratification that authorship provides. The question naturally arises, then, whether one who employs a ghostwriter might not be settling for second-rate talent. It is doubtful that many ghostwriters compose immortal prose. The uninformed ghostwriter who mechanically transcribes or paraphrases what the scientist relates to him lacks the knowledge and the insights that an authority can draw on to resolve problems regarding appropriate sequence of ideas, extent of explanation needed by a scientific audience, and other questions of structure and content that arise during composition. Although the ideal reading material consists in brilliant thoughts couched in flawless language, I would prefer the honest, awkward phraseology of a creative thinker any day to the vulgarized, slick style of the uncomprehending ghost.

Because of differences in objectives, motivation, point of view, responsibility, and literary standards and style, the ghostwriter is rarely a satisfactory literary stand-in for the medical scientist whose thoughts deserve publication in a *scholarly* journal. The primary objective of the medical scientist is the accurate presentation of information; that of the ghostwriter, readability. At best, the medical scientist is motivated by the desire to share his knowledge with his colleagues and at worst to gain professional prestige; the ghostwriter writes for money. Scholarly writing is a profession; ghostwriting, a trade. The medical scientist offers authoritative, first-hand information; the ghostwriter delivers second-hand or more remote opinions. The medical scientist is held responsible—intellectually, morally, and legally—for what he writes; the disembodied writer escapes all responsibility (and relinquishes credit). Writing published in a learned journal is expected to be enlightened and erudite; the writing of the invisible author is usually uninspired and journalistic.

Those who employ ghostwriters deny themselves the intellectual gratification that competent writing provides. But even more important than that, they forfeit the intellectual dividends accruing from the conversion of mental concepts to verbal symbols. As one who sees thought and language as mutually reinforcing and enriching, I cannot endorse a practice that clearly separates the two. Anyone who has labored for verbal exactitude knows how such precision clarifies thought.

I am not advocating the annihilation of literary mercantilism; I ask only that the by-line be reserved for the name of the *actual* writer. Lay reporting of medical science has unquestioned educational value, but it belongs in popular, not learned, publications. Those who wish to publish in scholarly journals should do their own composing. My plea, then, is for *honesty* in authorship. Is honesty too much to ask of those who deal with human life and health?

Lois DeBakey, Ph.D.
Professor of Scientific Communications
Baylor College of Medicine
Houston, Texas 77025

REFERENCES

1. DeBakey, L.: Rewriting and the by-line, SURGERY **75:** 38, 1974.
2. Editorial: Controversies in medical communication, N. Engl. J. Med. **271:** 1067, 1964.
3. Jones, D. P.: Science writing (Letter to the Editor), New Scientist **57:** 625, 1973.

Volume 75 *Number* 6

SURGERY

JUNE, 1974

Society of University Surgeons

Functional characteristics of surgically induced jejunal neomucosa

H. Bradley Binnington, M.D., Hatton Sumner, M.D., Peggy Lesker, B.A., David A. Alpers, M.D., *and* **Jessie L. Ternberg, M.D.,** *St. Louis, Mo.*

Growth of new jejunal mucosa was induced in four dogs by patching a jejunal defect with intact colon. Three of the dogs had nearly complete coverage of the colon by neomucosa 36 weeks postoperatively; the fourth had 50 to 60 per cent coverage. Histologically, the neomucosa had some normal villi; others were short and blunt. Several brush border enzymes were assayed: levels of aminopeptidase, maltase, and lactase activities were normal; alkaline phosphatase, sucrase, and trehalase activities were significantly less active than in normal adjacent mucosa. Amino acids were concentrated intracellularly to the same degree by neomucosa and normal mucosa. The neomucosa was sufficiently similar to normal jejunal mucosa to warrant further studies to determine its usefulness in ameliorating severe forms of the short gut syndrome.

From the Departments of Surgery, Pathology, and Medicine, Washington University School of Medicine, St. Louis, Mo.

New small intestinal mucosa can be grown on the serosa of small bowel[3] and colon.[2] If this new tissue is capable of digesting and absorbing food, a way might become available to improve the condition of patients having a severe form of the short gut syndrome. This new mucosa was therefore tested to define some of its in vitro functional characteristics.

Morphologic integrity was examined with the use of routine histology and histochemistry. Brush border enzyme activities[5, 10] and the ability to concentrate amino acids intracellularly were determined as parameters of gastrointestinal mucosal function.

Supported in part by Veterans Administration Training and Research Grant No. TR 192.

Presented at the Thirty-fifth Annual Meeting of the Society of University Surgeons, St. Louis, Mo., Feb. 14-16, 1974.

Reprint address: Jessie L. Ternberg, M.D., 4960 Audubon, St. Louis, Mo. 63110.

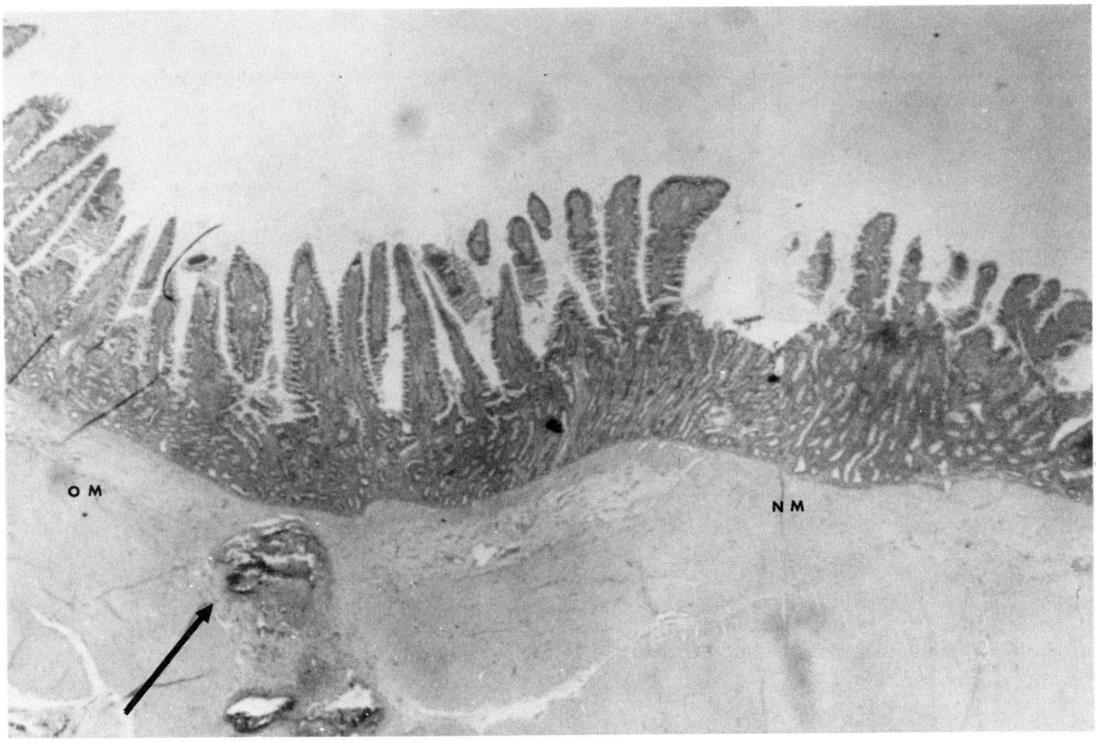

Fig. 1. Low-power view showing both original mucosa (*OM*) and new mucosa (*NM*). Anastomotic site indicated by arrow.

METHODS

Four adult mongrel dogs weighing between 20 and 25 kilograms had the proximal jejunum incised along its anti-mesenteric border for a distance of 12 to 15 cm. The resultant defect was patched as previously described[2] by suturing it to the descending colon, leaving an elliptical area (1.5 to 2.0 cm. wide) of colonic serosa exposed to the jejunal lumen. The dogs were fed dog chow for 36 weeks and then examined. The jejunum was opened along the mesenteric border parallel to the patch. Scrapings of neomucosa and adjacent normal mucosa were quick frozen in liquid nitrogen for later determination of enzyme activities (sucrase, maltase, trehalase, and lactase[4]; aminopeptidase[1]; alkaline phosphatase[6]; non-collagen protein[8]). Two assays were performed on each homogenate, and the average value was reported. Pieces of neomucosa and normal mucosa were sharply dissected from underlying tissue, cut into 5 by 5 mm. slices, placed in freshly oxygenated Krebs-Ringers-bicarbonate buffer, and then appropriately incubated to determine the ability to concentrate leucine, lysine, glycine, and 3-0 methyl glucose intracellularly.[7, 12] Results are reported as the ratio (partition coefficient) of intracellular to extracellular concentration of the particular labeled amino acid. Paired t test analysis was used to evaluate enzyme activity and partition coefficient data.

Thin cross-sections of the patched area, with colon cut away, were placed on foil-wrapped ice cubes; a short time later, cryostat sections were cut, placed on glass slides, and stained for alkaline phosphatase activity.[11] Finally, cross-sections of the patched area were fixed in neutral buffered formalin and routinely processed for light microscopy. The stains employed were hematoxylin and eosin, mucicarmine, alcian blue at pH 2.6, and Kossa's method for calcium.[9]

RESULTS

On gross examination, dogs 1 and 4 had new mucosa covering the entire exposed co-

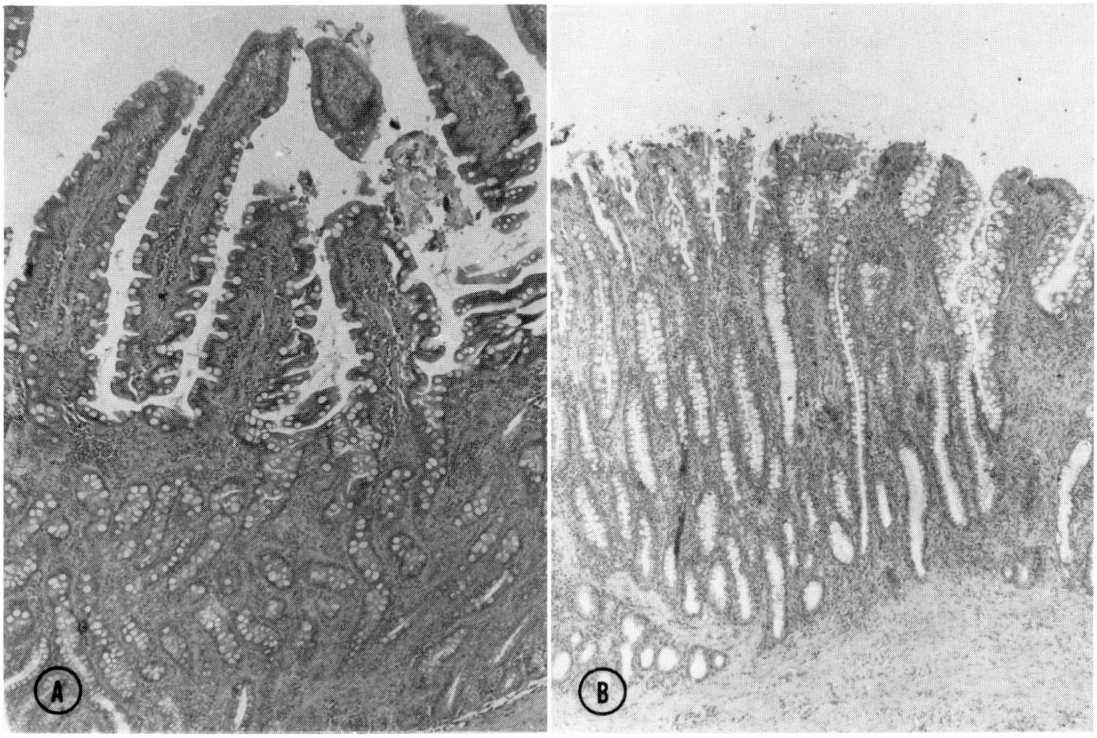

Fig. 2. Variations in surface appearance of the new mucosa: *A*, well-developed villi; *B*, markedly shortened villi. (Hematoxylin and eosin. Original magnification ×40.)

lonic serosa except for focal 0.1 to 0.9 cm. strips. The colonic serosa of dog 2 was wholly covered with mucosa except for one 0.1 to 1.0 cm. strip. Dog 3 had non-mucosal covered areas measuring from 0.5 to 1.5 cm. and in no area was the entire width of colon bridged. The areas of incomplete coverage were not necessarily located where the jejunal gap was widest.

The new surface, when viewed under the dissecting microscope, had a somewhat variable pattern. In general, the neomucosa immediately adjacent to original mucosa had a villous surface pattern. These villi were sligthly shorter than normal. Some centrally located neomucosal areas had a cerebroform appearance.

Microscopic examination confirmed the presence of new jejunal epithelium (Fig. 1). Between it and the colon musculature was a layer of collagen containing many blood vessels. In dogs 1 and 4 only small areas without complete epithelial coverage were seen; in dog 2, none was seen. The new epithelium of dog 3 extended only 2 to 4 mm. from the old mucosal margins, with no areas of total coverage. Where epithelialization was incomplete, an acute inflammatory infiltrate was present. The goblet cell–to–columnar cell ratio was the same in the new villi as in the normal villi; columnar cells appeared to have a normal height and morphology; and a well-developed brush border was present on the new villi (Fig. 2, *A*). Most of the new mucosa present in dogs 1, 2, and 4 had well-formed villi that were slightly shorter than those of adjacent normal mucosa. Some central areas had villi that were quite short and broad based (Fig. 2, *B*). This corresponded to the cerebroform areas seen under the dissecting microscope. Total mucosal thickness was 80 to 100 percent of normal. In dog 3, the neomucosa present had short, broad villi. Alkaline phosphatase activity was normally distributed, with no differences between old and new mucosa (Fig. 3).

A few of the hematoxylin and eosin–

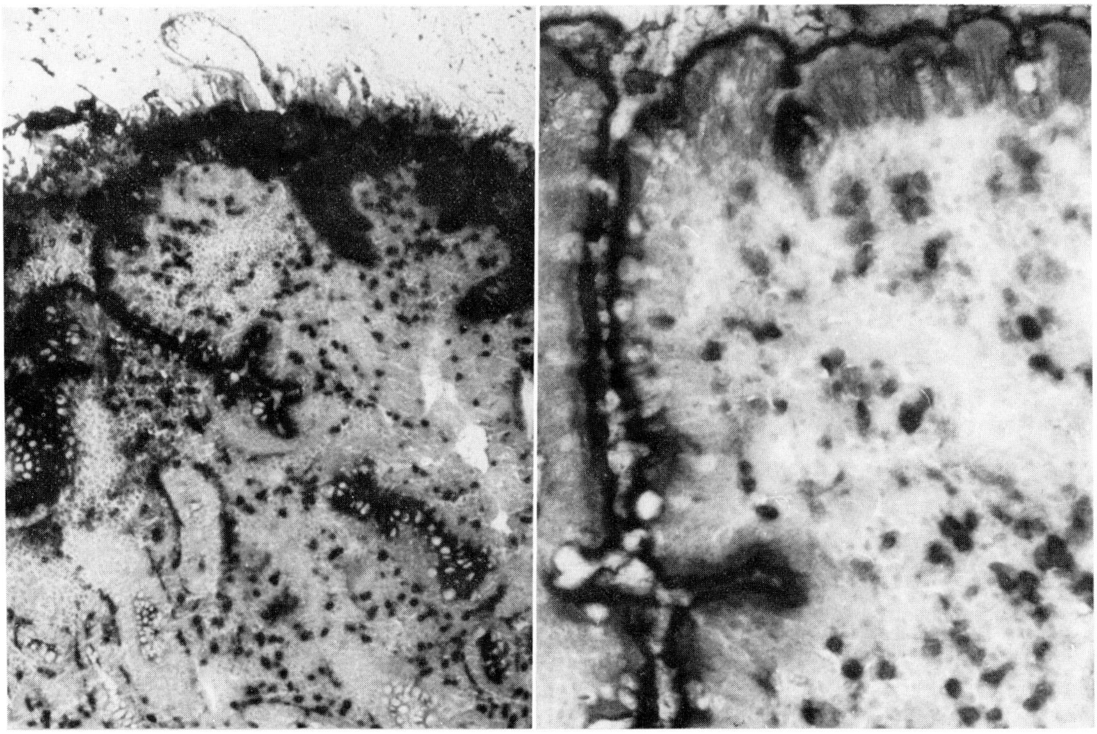

Fig. 3. Alkaline phosphatase staining of the new mucosa. (Right, ×40; left, ×250.)

Table IA. *Brush border enzyme activities*

	Alkaline phosphatase (mM indicator released/Gm. non-collagen protein/hr.)		*Aminopeptidase (% hydrolysis/hr.)*	
	Control	*Neomucosa*	*Control*	*Neomucosa*
Dog 1	10.51	5.99	108	285
Dog 2	10.99	5.09	291	243
Dog 3	5.33	2.39	271	202
Dog 4	11.43	4.93	270	140
Mean difference	4.96		17.5	
SEM	0.792		67.1	
p	< 0.025		N.S.	

stained sections from dogs 2 and 4 had deposits which, upon specific staining, were determined to be calcium. In dog 2, they were located beneath an intact neoepithelium; in dog 3, they were located beneath the inflammatory surface. These deposits were, for the most part, located in small vessels and were infrequently seen.

The results of direct enzyme activity assays are recorded in Tables IA and IB. Aminopeptidase, maltase, and lactase activities were the same in neomucosa and normal jejunum. Alkaline phosphatase, sucrase, and trehalase showed less activity in the neomucosal samples than in the normal. Partition coefficients for leucine, lysine, glycine, and 3-0 methyl glucose (Table II) were the same for neomucosa as for control jejunal mucosa.

DISCUSSION

The new jejunal mucosa that can be grown on colon serosa in dogs looks healthy. The villi have a well-formed brush border,

Table IB. *Glycosidase activities (Gm. indicator released/mg. non-collagen protein/hr.)*

	Sucrase		*Maltase*		*Trehalase*		*Lactase*	
	Control	*Neo-mucosa*	*Control*	*Neo-mucosa*	*Control*	*Neo-mucosa*	*Control*	*Neo-mucosa*
Dog 1	4.22	2.43	11.95	12.69	1.02	0.752	0.791	1.11
Dog 2	6.52	2.80	9.57	9.80	1.37	0.406	2.43	0.649
Dog 3	6.99	1.39	12.28	7.35	1.06	0.345	1.18	0.732
Dog 4	5.16	1.97	13.32	12.14	1.68	0.933	0.735	1.11
Mean difference	3.58		1.28		0.676		0.384	
SEM	0.788		1.28		0.146		0.501	
P	< 0.05		NS		< 0.01		NS	

Table II. *Partition coefficients (intracellular concentration/extracellular concentration)*

	Leucine		*Lysine*		*Glycine*		*3-0 Methyl glucose*	
	Control	*Neo-mucosa*	*Control*	*Neo-mucosa*	*Control*	*Neo-mucosa*	*Control*	*Neo-mucosa*
Dog 1	1.16	12.38	5.56	6.03	2.76	3.96	2.28	2.43
Dog 2	9.16	12.47	3.44	15.70	3.34	5.70	2.05	4.98
Dog 3	19.81	12.94	28.48	11.65	7.60	5.30	7.79	2.71
Dog 4	8.78	7.23	14.76	5.69	3.92	3.67	2.66	2.30
Mean difference	– 1.53		3.29		– 0.095		0.590	
SEM	3.84		6.28		0.901		1.66	
p	N.S.		N.S.		N.S.		N.S.	

staining normally for alkaline phosphatase; and there is no increase in the number of goblet cells. Functionally, in vitro concentration of amino acids and glucose is normal, and aminopeptidase, maltase, and lactase activities are the same as those of adjacent normal mucosa.

There are, however, differences. The average height of the new villi is less than normal, and some are abnormally shaped. Activity levels of alkaline phosphatase, sucrase, and trehalase are depressed, most probably because of the shorter average villus length. There is no particular pattern in these enzyme deficiencies.

Functionally, the neomucosa should be capable of some degree of digestion and absorption of carbohydrates and peptides. We did not examine fat absorption as it is passive and therefore depends on surface area rather than active cell processes.

An additional finding was that neo-epithelialization is not always complete in dogs when colon serosal areas of 2 by 12 cm. are exposed to the jejunal lumen. This finding is contrary to the report of Cywes,[3] who found complete epithelialization by using smaller areas and small bowel patches.[3] The distance to be bridged does not seem to be the major factor, since lack of complete epithelialization occurred both in narrow and wide areas of serosal exposure.

The finding of calcification in a few vessels of the bed of the new mucosa is not readily explainable. It is not related to the degree of mucosal generation. It occurs early postoperatively and is not progressive, since it has the same frequency at three weeks as at 36 weeks.

The new jejunal mucosa grown on the colon serosa of dogs has, therefore, histologic and functional characteristics which are similar to those of normal jejunal mucosa. Deficiencies are present. To ascertain whether such mucosa will be of help in treating severe forms of the short gut syndrome, direct in vivo application must be made and seems warrented.

Special thanks to Ms. Nancy Grimme for extensive technical assistance.

REFERENCES

1. Barber, V. T., Stern, K., Askonas, B.A., and Cullen, A. M.: Peptidases in human serum, Proc. Soc. Exp. Biol. Med. **67:** 421, 1948.
2. Binnington, H. B., Siegel, B. A., Kissane, J. M., and Ternberg, J. L.: A technique to increase jejunal mucosa surface area, J. Pediatr. Surg. **8:** 765, 1973.
3. Cywes, S.: The surgical management of massive small bowel resection, J. Pediatr. Surg. **3:** 740, 1968.
4. Dahlqvist, A.: Assay of intestinal disaccharidases, Anal. Biochim. **22:** 99, 1968.
5. Eichholz, A.: Structural and functional organization of brush border of intestinal epithelial cells. III. Enzymic activities and chemical composition of various fractions of tris-disrupted brush borders, Biochem. Biophys. Acta **135:** 475, 1967.
6. Fernley, H., and Walker, P. G.: Kinetic behavior of calf-intestinal alkaline phosphatase with 4-methylumbilliferyl phosphate, Biochem. J. **97:** 95, 1965.
7. Kinzie, J. L., Ferrendelli, J. A., and Alpers, D. H.: Adenosine cyclic 3′:5′-monophosphate –mediated transport of neutral and dibasic aminoacids in jejunal mucosa, J. Biol. Chem. **248:** 7018, 1973.
8. Lowry, O. H., Rosebrough, N. J., Farr, A. L., and Randall, R. J.: Protein measurement with the Folin phenol reagent, J. Biol. Chem. **193:** 265, 1951.
9. Luna, L. G.: Manual of histologic staining methods of the Armed Forces Institute of Pathology, New York, 1968, McGraw-Hill Book Company.
10. Maroux, S., Louvard, D., and Baratti, J.: The amino peptidase from hog intestinal brush border, Biochim. Biophys. Acta **321:** 282, 1973.
11. Pearse, A. G. E.: Histochemistry, Boston, 1960, Little, Brown & Co., p. 868.
12. Rosenberg, L. E., Blair, A., and Segal, S.: Transport of amino acids by slices of rat kidney, Biochim. Biophys. Acta **54:** 479, 1961.

DISCUSSION

Dr. Charles F. Zukoski (Tucson, Arizona). Do you think that the short brush border that you saw was in the middle, or were these lateral areas where the mucosa was growing in? Did you look at any of them before 36 weeks to see what progress you were making and, perhaps with fiberoptics or another method, to see how rapidly it reepithelialized?

Dr. M. David Tilson (New Haven, Conn.). The decrease in alkaline phosphatase to a shortened villus, but the disaccharidases, sucrase and maltase, of course, are also brush border enzymes. If that's the correct explanation for the alkaline phosphatase, one would expect the sucrase and maltase also to be low.

Dr. H. B. Binnington (closing). By three weeks the neomucosa has grown and the brush border that we saw by light microscopy appeared normal on all the villi that we examined. The villi that were shortened were primarily those in the central areas. In those areas where there were short villi, villi close to the normal jejunum looked normal.

There were two disaccharidases which were decreased and two which were normal. The most logical explanation seemed to be that it had to do with the shortened villi in the central areas of the neomucosa.

Depletion of brain norepinephrine in acute hepatic coma

John M. Dodsworth, M.B., F.R.C.S.E.,* J. Howard James, B.S., Michael C. Cummings, B.S., *and* **Josef E. Fischer, M.D.,** *Boston, Mass.*

When acute hepatic coma is produced in rats by a two-stage ligation of hepatic blood supply, octopamine, a false neurotransmitter, is accumulated more rapidly in the brain than in the periphery. Norepinephrine depletion occurs more rapidly in the brain as well, suggesting a local phenomenon. In turnover studies of intracisternally injected norepinephrine, disappearance occurs at a normal rate. The results suggest that in acute hepatic coma, brain norepinephrine synthesis is decreased.

From the Department of Surgery, Massachusetts General Hospital and Harvard Medical School, Boston, Mass.

PREVIOUS WORK from this laboratory has documented the accumulation of false neurochemical transmitters, such as octopamine, in the brains of animals in acute hepatic coma. Fischer and Baldessarini[12] have suggested that in the presence of detrioration in hepatic function and shunting of blood around the liver, two situations are usually present in hepatic encephalopathy[11]; amines or their precursors, normally catabolized by the liver and arising in the gut, enter into the portal circulation, bypass the failing liver, and accumulate in the central and peripheral nervous systems replacing the normal adrenergic transmitters, norepinephrine, and dopamine. Evidence for the hypothesis has been forthcoming from several sources. Fischer and Baldessarini[12] and Fischer and James[13] demonstrated a rapid rise in brain octopamine in rats made essentially anhepatic by a two-stage ligation of hepatic blood supply. Increased amounts of urinary octopamine were recovered in patients with hepatic encephalopathy.[12, 13] The excretion of octopamine appeared to correlate with the state of the patient, increased urinary octopamine being present in patients with profound hepatic coma. Subsequently, increased serum and urinary octopamine in patients with hepatic encephalopathy was reported by Lam and co-workers[28] working independently.

Implicit in the hypothesis is the depletion of putative transmitters, dopamine and norepinephrine, in the central nervous system and norepinephrine in the peripheral sympathetic adrenergic system, by the accumulation of false neurochemical transmitters. As yet, there has been little evidence for this, either in man or in experimental animals. Mashford, Mahon, and Chalmers[30] using a tyramine infusion test (tyramine being an indirectly acting amine that produces its effects by release of endogenous norepinephrine) found evidence for diminished endogenous stores of norepinephrine in hypotensive oliguric patients with terminal hepatic failure.

Supported in part by United States Public Health Service Grant No. AM-15347.

Presented at the Thirty-fifth Annual Meeting of the Society of University Surgeons, St. Louis, Mo., Feb. 14-16, 1974.

Reprint address: Josef E. Fischer, M.D., 16 Charles River Square, Boston, Mass. 02114.

*Present address: John M. Dodsworth, M.D., 6 Sherbourne Walk, Farnham Common, Slough—SL 23TZ, Bucks, England.

As they suggested, possible causes of diminished norepinephrine may be either secondary to displacement of norepinephrine, or what seemed more likely, decreased synthesis on the basis of the toxic state.

In the following experiments, the time course of accumulation of the neurotransmitters and false neurotransmitters were measured in brains of animals in acute hepatic coma and compared with a variety of controls, including hepatic artery ligation, acute portacaval shunts, and sham operation.

MATERIALS AND METHODS

Female Sprague Dawley rats (175 to 200 grams) fed on water and Purina Chow ad libitum were used throughout. End-to-side portacaval anastomoses were performed under ether-air anesthesia either by use of a silk suture technique or the use of a stainless steel button. The procedure takes 15 to 20 minutes. The animals recover rapidly from the anesthetic in approximately 10 minutes and behave normally. Survival following this procedure is normally over three months, although the animals lose weight. Overt signs of deterioration appear at approximately six to eight weeks. To produce acute hepatic coma, the portacaval anastomosis is followed at 48 hours by repeat laparotomy and ligation of the hepatic artery. At the same time, a No. 23 gauge butterfly needle is inserted into a suitable tail vein to allow repeated glucose infusions. These animals recover more slowly from the anesthetic and appear normal for a period of four to six hours. At six to eight hours following ligation, the animals become comatose and unresponsive to all but severe stimuli, remaining immobile in the corner of the cage. Urine is extremely dark, containing bile, and smells offensive. In the final one to three hours of life, the rats lie on their side breathing stertorously, passing further quantities of heavily bile-stained urine. During the entire period following ligation, rats were kept warm with incandescent lamps and every 2 hours, 2.5 ml. of 7.5 percent dextrose and saline was administered by tail vein. Control animals were divided in four groups: (1) normal weight matched female rats. (2) Sham-operated rats in which two laparotomies of similar proportions and duration to those experienced by the coma rats were performed at intervals of 48 hours; but these rats recover more rapidly from the anesthetic on both occasions. The surgical trauma involved is similar in the two groups. (3) Portacaval shunt alone with repeat laparotomy 48 hours later. (4) Hepatic artery ligation alone. These animals recover rapidly from the anesthetic and appear normal, and generally have a life-span equivalent to normal animals. At 48 hours, repeat laparotomy is performed.

All rats were killed at stated time intervals following the second procedure, six or nine hours following hepatic artery ligation in the hepatic coma rats, or when they appeared moribund. Since numerous experiments were performed in this series, and the moribund condition is reached at various times from 9 to 12 hours following the hepatic artery ligation, some of the animals in the moribund group were killed at time periods of approximately nine hours. After death, hearts and brains were rapidly weighed and frozen on Dry Ice prior to assay procedure. In certain instances, blood was also collected for octopamine assay or biochemical testing by guillotining the animals and exsanguination over a chilled beaker with 1,000 U. of heparin added.

Turnover studies. In order to assess the release and displacement of norepinephrine from both central and peripheral binding sites, labeled norepinephrine was injected. It was assumed that the injection of labeled tritiated norepinephrine either intracisternally or via tail vein when taken up into the peripheral and central nervous system would give some indication of the rate of displacement of endogenous norepinephrine, an assumption which may not be completely correct.[26] Accordingly, animals in acute hepatic coma and various control animals were reanesthetized with light ether anesthesia, three hours following hepatic artery ligation and 2 μCi of 1-^{3}H norepinephrine (S.A. 7 Ci per millimole) in a volume of 20 μl was injected intracisternally. Simultaneously, 10 μCi of 1-^{3}H norepinephrine was injected intravenously. The peripherally administered nor-

Table I. *Octopamine levels in rats in acute hepatic coma**

	Brain (ng./Gm.)	Serum (ng./ml.)	Heart (ng./Gm.)
Normal	3.83 ± 0.41	2.35 ± 0.54	172.8 ± 10.9
Hepatic artery ligation	2.78 ± 1.47	2.74 ± 0.45	124.7 ± 13.5
Acute shunt	6.44 ± 1.39†	3.17 ± 0.39	162.3 ± 18.5
Sham operation	3.47 ± 0.78	2.90 ± 0.69	180.5 ± 14.2
Hepatic coma			
6 hour	10.4 ± 0.4‡	2.94 ± 0.41	298 ± 19.1‡
9 hour	11.3 ± 0.65‡	5.85 ± 0.39†	334.7 ± 42.1‡
Moribund	13.4 ± 0.82‡	11.73 ± 1.02‡	379.1 ± 28.2‡

*Octopamine levels in serum, brain, and heart in rats in acute hepatic coma and in various controls produced as described in the text. Results are given as mean ± S.E.M. for 8 to 30 animals.

†$p < 0.05$ as compared with various controls.

‡$p < 0.01$.

epinephrine does not cross the blood-brain barrier in significant amounts. After a predetermined period of time, 30 or 90 minutes or 4.5 hours, animals were killed and specific activities of tritiated norepinephrine in both brain and heart were measured.

In other experiments, in order to ascertain nonspecific effects on the turnover of tritiated norepinephrine in the brain, a mixture of DL-^{3}H norepinephrine (S.A. 6.9 Ci per millimole), 5 μCi in 20 μl, was injected intracisternally and 10 μCi intravenously in a volume of 1 c.c. Animals were killed at 10 or 30 minutes and three hours and specific activities of norepinephrine determined. Only the results in brain turnovers will be discussed.

Assay of octopamine. Octopamine was assayed by the method of Molinoff and coworkers[32, 33] with minor modifications. Thus, portions of the tissues were homogenized in Tris buffer, pH 8.6, containing pargyline, a potent inhibitor of monoamine oxidase. The homogenates were heated to 95° C. for five minutes, and centrifuged at 10,000 × g. Next, 0.5 ml. portions of the supernatant were incubated with [^{14}C-methyl] S-adenosylmethionine (SAMe, 1 Ci. per mole, New England Nuclear Corporation) and a preparation of beef adrenal phenylethanolamine N-methyltransferase (PNMT) partially purified by the method of Axelrod[3] and concentrated by pressure dialysis. A duplicate sample with added authentic octopamine (Cal-Biochem Company) was included with each sample to permit estimates of recovery of each amine. After 30 minutes of incubation, the reaction was stopped with borate buffer, pH 10, and the radioactive N-methylated products were extracted into a 66 percent mixture (volumes) of isoamylol in toluene. Samples assayed for octopamine were first evaporated to dryness, then taken up in ethanol and toluene solution and counted by scintillation spectrometry. Radioactive toluene was then added as an internal standard to correct for quenching.

The products were further identified by incubating additional portions of homogenates of both brain and heart with the PNMT preparation and more intensely labeled [^{3}H-methyl] SAMe (10 Ci. per millimole, New England Nuclear Corporation). After extraction into the 66 percent isoamylol:toluene mixture, the labeled products were chromatographed with authentic N-methyl-phenylethanolamine or N-methyl-octopamine as well as N-methyl derivatives of several other β-hydroxylated amines on thin-layer silica gel plates in *i*-propanol:ammonia:water (8:1:1, volumes) or *n*-butanol saturated with 1 *N* HCl. The radioactive products were found to migrate in a single peak of radioactivity at Rf positions identical to those of the authentic reference compounds.

Assay of norepinephrine. The method used is that of Haggendähl[27] with minor modifications. Acidwashed glassware rinsed with triple-distilled water is used throughout.

"Dr. Roth"-type columns are filled to 2 cm. with washed alumina. Samples are homogenized in 12 ml. of 0.4 N $HClO_4$ and centri-

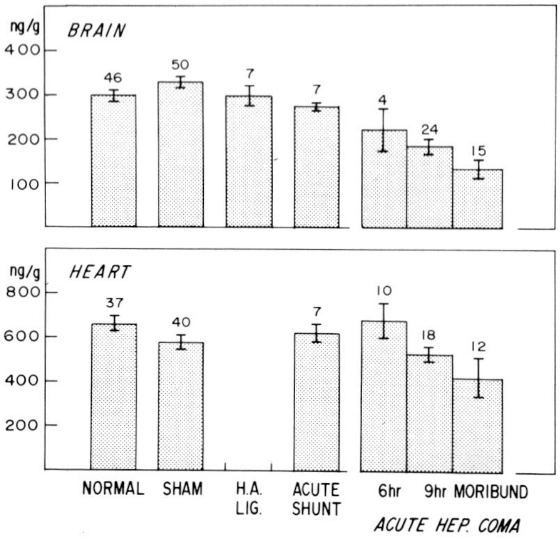

Fig. 1. Norepinephrine content of brain and heart in rats at various stages of hepatic coma and sham-operated control animals. Numbers of animals are given in histograms. Differences are significant for brain at six and nine hours and moribund groups and for nine hours and moribund for heart.

fuged at 15,000 r.p.m. for 30 minutes. Eight milliliters of supernatant, 2 ml. of 5 percent EDTA and 0.2 ml. of Tris (pH 8.4) are mixed and then poured over the columns. The columns are washed four times with 10 ml. of distilled water and blown dry. Norepinephrine is then eluted with 5 ml. of 0.2 N acetic acid and the column blown dry with N_2. An aliquot is counted for labeled norepinephrine. NaH_2PO_4 (0.5 N) and 0.75 percent $ZnCl_2$ are added and the pH is adjusted to 6.5. A standard curve is prepared. K_3FeCn_6 is used to initiate the reaction and three minutes later a mixture of sodium bisulfite and British Anti-Lewisite (BAL) in NaOH is added to stop the reaction. Twenty-five minutes later, fluorescence is read at 450/515 mμ on a spectrophotofluorometer.

RESULTS

Octopamine levels in acute hepatic coma. Octopamine determinations in brain, heart, and serum are presented in Table I. Although brain octopamine levels did not differ significantly between sham-operated animals and normal unoperated animals, some decrease in brain octopamine was seen following hepatic artery ligation. Forty-eight hours after acute shunt, however, brain octopamine increased, suggesting that the diversion of portal blood past the liver alone brings about conditions sufficient to increase brain octopamine.

Following hepatic artery ligation in an already shunted animal, brain octopamine is increased further in the "coma animals" and rises progressively thereafter to approximately 300 to 400 percent above those levels seen in hepatic artery ligation. In contrast, octopamine in the heart of rats with end-to-side shunts alone does not differ significantly from normal animals, animals with sham operations, or hepatic artery ligation. Heart octopamine, however, increases markedly at six hours into acute hepatic coma and rises gradually until the animals are moribund. The rise in cardiac octopamine preceded that of the serum which is only increased in an advanced state of acute hepatic decompensation (Table I).

Norepinephrine. Brain norepinephrine does not differ significantly in normal, sham-operated animals, animals with hepatic artery ligation alone, or acute portacaval shunt alone. When animals become symptomatic at six hours, brain norepinephrine begins to decrease, reaching a final depletion of approximately 50 percent when the animal is moribund. Operation itself does not appear to influence or decrease brain norepinephrine, since all of the animals that were operated on in the control groups had two procedures over a similar time course. Similarly, heart norepinephrine, taken in these experiments as representing the peripheral sympathetic nervous system, is decreased to a significant extent when the animals become moribund, although some decrease is seen at six and nine hours following the hepatic artery ligation in the "coma animals" (Fig. 1).

Turnover studies. In the animals injected with ^{3}H-d,l-norepinephrine, no difference was seen in initial uptake or turnover, whether expressed in terms of turnover or specific activity (Fig. 2). In the animals injected with 1-^{3}H norepinephrine, uptake was greater in the brains of animals in coma (Fig. 3). Dis-

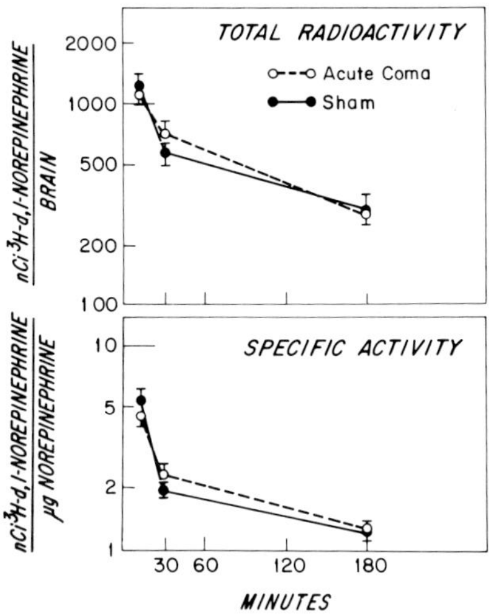

Fig. 2. Disappearance of ^{3}H-d,1-norepinephrine from rat brain in acute hepatic coma. 5 μCi ^{3}H-d,1-norepinephrine was injected in 20 μl intracisternally under light ether anesthesia at three and seven hours and animals were killed at 10, 30, and 180 minutes. Disappearance is similar in coma and sham-operated animals whether expressed as labeled norepinephrine alone, or specific activity. Results are mean ± S.E.M. for groups of five to six animals.

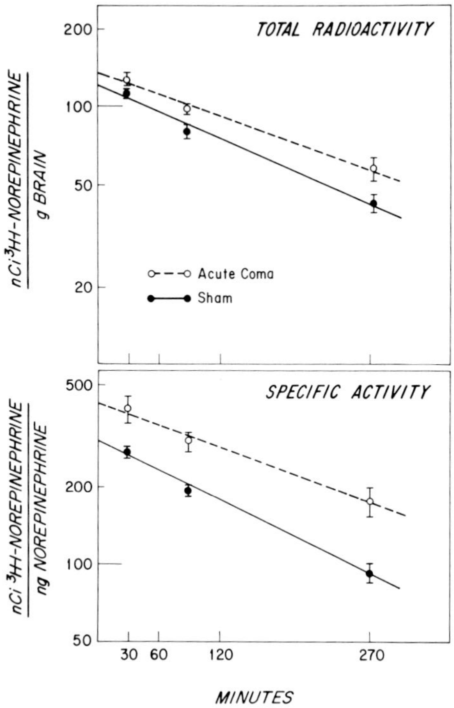

Fig. 3. Disappearance of 2 μCi of intracisternally injected ^{3}H-1-norepinephrnie from brains of rats in acute hepatic coma and sham-operated control animals. Uptake is greater in brains of "coma" animals possibly because of decreased content, but slopes of disappearance are parallel, whether expressed as labeled norepinephrine or specific activity.

appearance slopes were parallel in all experiments (Figs. 2 and 3), whether expressed as labeled norepinephrine or in terms of specific activity. These results strongly suggest that there is no difference in the rate of release of norepinephrine from the brains of animals in acute hepatic coma. Thus, it appears that norepinephrine is being depleted at a normal rate.

DISCUSSION

Any hypothesis concerning the pathophysiology of the symptoms of hepatic failure must take into account several well-known clinical axioms: (1) Deterioration of hepatic function is usually present in hepatic coma.[41] (2) Shunting of blood around the liver is generally present.[41] (3) The substance(s) involved in the production of symptomatology of hepatic encephalopathy in hepatic failure appeared to arise in the gut. Bacteria have some role in causation in that decreasing bacterial flora ameliorates the symptoms of hepatic encephalopathy. (4) Those substances involved in the causation of hepatic coma appeared to be of nitrogenous origin. Hepatic coma may be provoked by increased dietary protein or gastrointestinal bleeding. (5) While ammonia is generally regarded as not being the etiologic agent in the pathogenesis of hepatic coma, serum ammonia levels generally reflect the cerebral state of the patient with hepatic encephalopathy, although the correlation is by no means exact.[17]

Several years ago, an hypothesis was proposed which suggested that in the presence of hepatic failure and/or shunting of portal blood around the liver, amines or their precursors arising in the gut and normally catabolized by the liver, flood the peripheral and central nervous system and accumulate in adrenergic neurons, displacing the putative transmitters, norepinephrine, and dopamine.

On the basis of evidence previously derived in the peripheral sympathetic nervous system,[14, 25] and more recently in the central nervous system,[4, 25, 26] it has been established that such potential false neurochemical transmitter amines have a phenolic ring with at least one ring hydroxyl group and a carbon side chain which may include a β-hydroxyl group. Other side-chain and ring-appended groups might be present. The toxicity of methionine in patients with cirrhosis, for example, suggests a possible involvement of methylated or methoxy groups on the side chain or phenolic ring as well.

Such amines or their precursors have their origin in the gut; amines are produced by bacterial amino acid decarboxylases[18] from gut protein. Subsequent findings in animals[7, 11, 12, 13, 15] as well as in man[12, 13, 28] have confirmed the increased accumulation or excretion of such amines in the blood and urine of patients as well as in the brain and peripheral sympathetic nervous system in animals in acute hepatic coma. In these experiments, rats with acute hepatic coma produced by a two-stage ligation of hepatic blood supply are seen to accumulate octopamine more rapidly in their brain than can be explained by the accumulation in the periphery or in the plasma. This finding is not entirely unexpected, since the blood-brain barrier is generally thought to be relatively impermeable to amines, at least in normal animals. (The possibility that the blood-brain barrier may be defective in acute hepatic coma has not been examined in these experiments.) It has generally been assumed that the accumulation of false neurochemical transmitters such as octopamine may produce symptoms of hepatic encephalopathy by interference with the release of the true transmitter, norepinephrine, and dopamine. To date, we have only evoked a presynaptic mechanism in which octopamine is released instead of norepinephrine, although a postsynaptic competitive mechanism or a direct effect of octopamine on the postsynaptic receptor is entirely possible. According to this hypothesis, one would expect that the brain concentrations of dopamine and norepinephrine would be diminished in acute hepatic coma, a finding partially confirmed by these experiments.

The decrease in brain norepinephrine may take place by two mechanisms. (1) The accumulation of false neurochemical transmitters may displace norepinephrine from its binding sites causing a more rapid release. (2) The accumulation of false neurochemical transmitters is a result of increased synthesis of false neurochemical transmitters brought about by alterations in synthetic pathways of catecholamines and phenylethylamines.

These experiments suggest that the first mechanism, displacement of norepinephrine by accumulation of false neurochemical transmitters, is not the principal mechanism by which depletion of norepinephrine occurs, since increased displacement of norepinephrine on the basis of specific activity was not found in the brains of animals in acute hepatic coma at three to seven hours. These results, however, are not conclusive for the following reasons: (1) The decrease in whole-brain norepinephrine and the unchanged turnover of norepinephrine determined on a whole-brain basis may not be completely valid for specific pools of norepinephrine or regional concentrations of norepinephrine. The concentration of norepinephrine in the brain stem, for example, may be more important in determining the consciousness of the animal than, for example, more nonspecific norepinephrine stores in the cortex. (2) Since octopamine is known to be a more rapidly turning over amine[33] than norepinephrine, the octopamine may accumulate preferentially in a small but metabolically active neurotransmitter pool. The increased octopamine displaces a greater amount of functionally important and more easily released norepinephrine than one would expect in the mere stoichiometry of the observed results.

However, these experiments do suggest that the synthesis of norepinephrine, within the limits of the experimental design, is decreased in acute hepatic coma. Since Mashford, Mahon, and Chalmers[30] found evidence of peripheral norepinephrine depletion in pa-

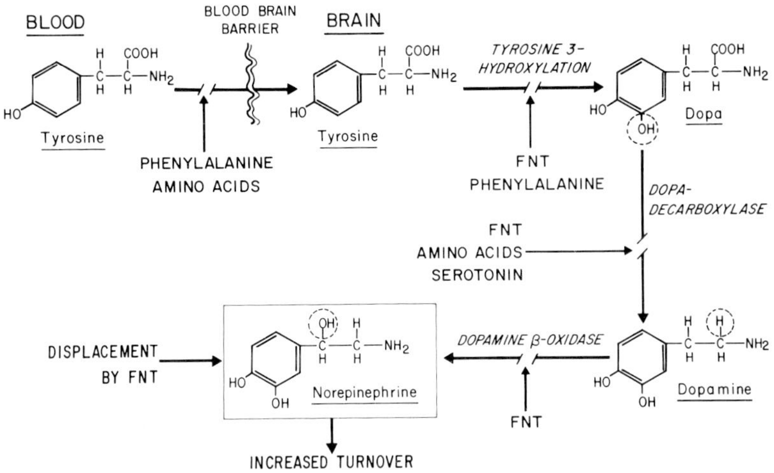

Fig. 4. Hypothetical scheme of catecholamine synthesis showing various points at which synthesis may be blocked by excesses of amino acids, amines, or false neurochemical transmitters (FNT).

tients with chronic liver disease, it is possible that in man a similar mechanism of decreased synthesis of norepinephrine occurs as well.

It is interesting to speculate on the possible mechanism of a decreased synthesis. The synthetic pathways of catecholamines and phenylethylamines are rather similar. Whereas, tyrosine is thought to be the amino acid precursor of catecholamine synthesis,[39] phenylalanine may be preferentially synthesized to phenylethylamine by decarboxylation. At each given point along the pathway (Fig. 4) it is possible that tyrosine instead of being hydroxylated to dopa, may be shunted aside, decarboxylated to tyramine, then to octopamine or a variety of other phenylethylamines. Being similar in structure, phenylalanine and tyrosine compete at points in the synthesis of catecholamines, beginning at the blood-brain barrier. Phenylalanine and tyrosine, among other neutral amino acids, including tryptophan and the branched-chain amino acids, valine, leucine and isoleucine, are competitive across the blood-brain barrier for entry into the brain.[20] It is possible that phenylalanine, known to be present in a large excess in animals and man with hepatic encephalopathy[2, 16, 21, 31, 37] prevents the adequate entry of tyrosine into the brain.[16] Once within the brain, the excess phenylalanine competes with tyrosine hydroxylase, since phenylalanine and tyrosine have a similar Km for this enzyme.[23, 24] Under such circumstances, one might expect that an excess of phenylalanine within the brain would cause tyrosine hydroxylase to preferentially hydroxylate phenylalanine, thus causing an accumulation of brain tyrosine. Up to a point, this would appear to favor the increased synthesis of catecholamines. However, if tyrosine hydroxylase, present in limited concentrations is occupied, as it were, synthesizing tyrosine from phenylalanine, the accumulation of tyrosine will then shift the synthetic pathway from tyrosine-3-hydroxylation to dopa and then to chatecholamines to decarboxylation of tyrosine to tyramine and subsequent synthesis of octopamine and other β-hydroxylated amines. Preliminary experiments suggest that this in fact may be the case.[11] Although some have claimed that phenylalanine is the true precursor of catecholamines within the brain,[23, 24] recent experiments utilizing mass spectrometry suggest that phenylalanine is hydroxylated to tyrosine, and once hydroxylated, the tyrosine joins the general typrosine pool available for a variety of metabolic fates, and not necessarily only the synthesis of catecholamines.[39] Furthermore, in patients with phenylketonuria, evidence of diminished catecholamine synthesis on high phenylalanine diets, when blood levels of phenylalanine are increased, has been presented.[6] It appears that patients with impaired hepatic function have the same defect in phenylalanine hydroxylase as the patients with phenylketonuria, causing an increase in plasma phenylalanine.[16, 31, 37] Thus, as phenylalanine accumulates in plasma and brain, decreased norepinephrine synthesis may result. Further along the synthetic pathways, other inhibitors, competitive and noncompetitive, may also contribute to decreased synthesis (Fig. 4).

Finally, some therapeutic implications if this conjecture is correct. First, the quality of protein, i.e., amino acid composition of protein may be more important than the total amount of protein in a patient with hepatic encephalopathy. This is especially feasible in the area of total parenteral nutrition where the advent of synthetic amino acid mixtures makes it possible to tailor solutions to individual disease states. Preliminary results obtained in our laboratory with a new amino acid mixture specifically designed for patients with hepatic insufficiency, appears to be better tolerated by animals with chronic hepatic insufficiency on the basis of an end-to-side portacaval shunt than the standard amino acid mixtures available, suggesting that if one decreases the amounts of aromatic amino acids including phenylalanine, amino acid profile in the brain may be considerably more appropriate to normal neurotransmitter synthesis than the amino acid profile present in the brains of animals and man in hepatic encephalopathy.

Finally, these results may help explain the recently reported efficacy of L-dopa in both acute[13, 15, 35, 36, 38] and chronic hepatic encephalopathy.[29] A variety of mechanisms for the efficacy of L-dopa has been suggested, including the release of serotonin[5, 19, 34] and the prevention of further serotonin synthesis,[5, 19] the release of accumulated false neurochemical transmitters,[12-15, 22] the decrease in SAMe available for S-adenyl methionine,[35] the decreased absorption of phenylalanine as dopa competes across the intestinal barrier with both phenylalanine and tyrosine,[40] and finally, the replenishment of normal putative transmitters, norepinephrine, and dopamine.[13, 15]

One finding which has remained unexplained to date, is that while the administration of L-dopa to normal animals elevates brain dopamine, but not norepinephrine,[8] the administration of L-dopa to animals in acute hepatic coma brings about an increase in not only dopamine, but in brain norepinephrine.[15] The results reported herein may help explain this discrepancy. If synthesis of catecholamines is blocked at a variety of levels along the catecholamine synthetic pathway, including tyrosine hydroxylase which is normally responsible for the synthesis of dopa, the administration of L-dopa which crosses the blood-brain barrier in large amounts thereby circumvents the synthetic block and by increasing the amount of substrate available for both dopa decarboxylase and subsequently, dopamine β-oxidase, may help obviate the metabolic consequences of this blocked sympathetic pathway.

As usual, experiments in the area of hepatic coma generate more questions than they manage to answer. It should be possible, however, by the application of gas chromatographic techniques as well as tracer techniques of both synthesis and turnover to obtain specific information on the lateral ventricular cerebrospinal fluid thought to be representative of brain metabolism in order to confirm or deny some of the speculative points raised in these experiments.

REFERENCES

1. Abel, R. M., Beck, C. H., Jr., Abbott, W. M., Ryan, J. A., Barnett, G. O., and Fischer, J. E.: Improved survival from acute renal failure following treatment with intravenous essential L-amino acids and glucose, N. Engl. J. Med. **288:** 695, 1973.
2. Aguirre, A., Yoshimura, N., Westman, T., and Fischer, J. E.: Plasma amino acids in two experimental forms of liver damage, J. Surg. Res. In press, 1974.
3. Axelrod, J.: Purification and properties of phenylethanol-amine N-methyl transferase, J. Biol. Chem. **237:** 1657, 1962.
4. Baldessarini, R. J.: Release of aromatic amines from brain tissues of the rat in vitro, J. Neurochem. **18:** 2509, 1971.
5. Baldessarini, R. J., and Fischer, J. E.:

Serotonin metabolism in rat brain after surgical diversion of the portal venous circulation, Nature New Biol. **254:** 25, 1973.

6. Curtius, H.-Ch., Baerlocher, K., and Vollinins, J. S.: Pathogenesis of phenylketonuria: Inhibition of dopa and catecholamine synthesis in patients with phenylketonuria, Clin. Chem. Acta **42:** 235, 1972.
7. Dodsworth, J. M., Cummings, M. G., James, J. H., and Fischer, J. E.: The effects of intestinal sterilization on brain amines, Gastroenterology **64:** 881, 1973.
8. Everett, G. M., and Borcherding, J. W.: L-Dopa: Effect on concentrations of dopamine, norepinephrine and serotonin in brains of mice, Science **168:** 849, 1970.
9. Fischer, J. E.: Hepatic coma in cirrhosis, portal hypertension and following portacaval shunt—Its etiologies and the current status of its treatment. (*In* Orloff, M., editor: Symposium on progress in liver disease), Arch. Surg. **108:** 325, 1974.
10. Fischer, J. E.: Acute hepatic failure, *in* Becker, F. F., editor: The liver—The molecular biology of its disease, Marcel Dekker, New York. In press, 1974.
11. Fischer, J. E.: False neurotransmitters and hepatic coma, New York, 1974, Raven Press.
12. Fischer, J. E., and Baldessarini, R.: False neurotransmitters and hepatic failure, Lancet **2:** 75, 1971.
13. Fischer, J. E., and James, J. H.: Treatment of hepatic coma and hepatorenal syndrome: Mechanism of action of L-dopa and aramine, Am. J. Surg. **123:** 222, 1972.
14. Fischer, J. E., Horst, W. D., and Kopin, I. J.: β-Hydroxylated sympathomimetic amines as false neurotransmitters, Br. J. Pharmacol. **24:** 477, 1965.
15. Fischer, J. E., James, J. H., and Baldessarini, R. J.: Changes in brain amines following portal flow diversion and acute hepatic coma: Effects of L-dopa and intestinal sterilization, Surg. Forum **23:** 348, 1972.
16. Fischer, J. E., Yoshimura, N., James, J. H., Cummings, M. G., Abel, R. M., and Deindoerfer, F.: Plasma amino acids in patients with hepatic encephalopathy: Effects of amino acid infusions, Am. J. Surg. **127:** 40, 1974.
17. Gabuzda, G. J., and Davidson, C. S.: Hepatic coma, *in* Schiff, L., editor: Diseases of the liver, ed. 3, Philadelphia, 1969, J. B. Lippincott Company, p. 387 ff.
18. Gale, F. F.: The bacterial amino acid decarboxylases, Adv. Enzymology **6:** 1, 1946.
19. Goldstein, M., and Frenkel, R.: Inhibition of serotonin synthesis by dopa and other catechols, Nature New Biol. **233:** 179, 1971.
20. Guroff, G., and Udenfriend, S.: Studies on aromatic acid uptake by rat brain in vivo, J. Biol. Chem. **237:** 803, 1962.
21. Iber, F. L., Rosen, H., Levenson, S. M., and Chalmers, T. C.: The plasma amino acids in patients with liver failure, J. Clin. Lab. Med. **50:** 417, 1957.
22. James, J. H., and Fischer, J. E.: Release of octopamine and α-methyl octopamine by L-dopa, Gastroenterology **66:** 887, 1974.
23. Karobath, M.: Catecholamines and the hydroxylation of tyrosine in synaptosomes isolated from rat brain, Proc. Nat. Acad. Sci. **68:** 2370, 1971.
24. Karobath, M., and Baldessarini, R. J.: Formation of catechol compounds from phenylalanine and tyrosine with isolated nerve endings, Nature New Biol. **236:** 206, 1972.
25. Kopin, I. J.: False adrenergic transmitters, Ann. Rev. Pharmacol. **8:** 377, 1968.
26. Kopin, I. J.: Aminergic neurons and substitute transmitters in the brain, *in* Kopin, I. J., editor: Neurotransmitters, Proceedings ARNMD, Baltimore, 1972, The Williams & Wilkins Company, p. 207.
27. Haggendähl, J.: An improved method for fluorometric determination of small amounts of adrenaline in plasma and tissues, Acta Physiol. Scand. **59:** 242, 1963.
28. Lam, K. C., Tall, A. R., Goldstein, G. B., and Mistilis, S. P.: Role of a false neurotransmitter, octopamine, in the pathogenesis of hepatic and renal encephalopathy, Scand. J. Gastroenterol. **8:** 465, 1973.
29. Lunzer, M., James, I. M., Weinman, J., and Sherlock, S.: Treatment of chronic hepatic encephalopathy with levodopa, Gut **14:** 816, 1973.
30. Mashford, M. L., Mahon, W. A., and Chalmers, T. C.: Studies of the cardiovascular system in the hypotension of liver failure, N. Engl. J. Med. **267:** 1071, 1962.
31. McMenamy, R. H., Vang, J. H., and Drapanas, T.: Amino acids and α-keto acid concentrations in plasma and blood of the liverless dog, Am. J. Physiol. **209:** 1046, 1956.
32. Molinoff, P. B., and Axelrod, J.: Octopamine: Normal occurrence in sympathetic nerves of rats, Science **165:** 428, 1969.
33. Molinoff, P. B., Landsberg, L., and Axelrod, J.: An enzymatic assay for octopamine and other β-hydroxylated phenylethylamines, J. Pharmacol. Exp. Therap. **170:** 253, 1969.
34. Ng, K. Y., Chase, T. N., Colburn, R. W., and Kopin, I. J.: L-Dopa induced release of cerebral monoamines, Science **170:** 76, 1970.
35. Parkes, J. D., Sharpstone, P., and Williams, R.: Levodopa in hepatic coma, Lancet **II:** 1341, 1970.
36. Posado, J. G., Penicha, J. H., and Tirado-

Arroyava, S.: Effect of 3-4 dihydroxyphenylalanine (L-dopa) in hepatic coma, Arch. Invest. Med. **3:** 1, 1972.

37. Richmond, J., and Girdwood, R. H.: Observations on amino acid absorption, Clin. Sci. **22:** 301, 1962.
38. Sarrazin, A., Emerit, J., Olivier, L., Rebelo, R., and Bousquet, O.: Présentation d'une malade guérié d'un coma hépatique par un traitement à la L-dopa, Rev. Neurol. **125:** 391, 1971.
39. Sedvall, G., Mayevsky, A., Fri, C. G., Sjoquist, B., and Samuel, D.: The use of stable oxygen isotopes for labelling of homovanillic acid in rat brain *in vivo, in* Advances in biochemistry and psychopharmacology, New York, 1973, Raven Press, vol. 7, p. 57.
40. Van Woert, H. M.: Phenylalanine and tyrosine metabolism in Parkinson's disease treated with levodopa, Clin. Pharmacol. Therap. **12:** 368, 1971.
41. Webster, L. T., Jr.: Hepatic coma: A biochemical disorder of the brain, Gastroenterology **49:** 698, 1965.

DISCUSSION

Dr. Leon Forrest (Baltimore, Md.). Central nervous system epinephrine or catecholamine is subject to explicit pharmacologic regulation; levels of norepinephrine can be manipulated by the use of the decarboxylase inhibitors, MK-45 or RO 4-4602. If the problem with hepatic coma is norepinephrine depletion per se, then the administration of L-dopa should tend to reverse that state. If, on the other hand, the problem with hepatic coma is the formation of a false transmitter, then you might be able to pick that apart with L-dopa and a central nervous system decarboxylase inhibitor.

Dr. Jeremiah George Turcotte (Ann Arbor, Mich.). Six or seven years ago at the Toronto meeting we presented this model in the evaluation of exchange transfusion. The model was originally described by Dr. Rapaport, who is a professor at Toronto.

Since then, I think it has become a fairly common model. There is quite a variation in response, however. What I want to emphasize is an extension of that model: if you ligate the gastroduodenal artery, and not only temporarily occlude the hepatic artery, you can get a much more precise model in terms of animal survival and biochemical change.

There are a few survivors, and you can, several weeks or months later, take down the end-to-side portacaval shunt and reconstruct the portal vein and reverse your biochemical changes.

Dr. William V. McDermott, Jr. (Boston, Mass.). Although this hasn't really established the final metabolic pathway that accounts for all the symptoms, it sheds a lot more biochemical light on a very complicated disorder. Would Dr. Fischer please comment on the rather haphazard work done on monoamine oxidase about a decade ago?

Dr. Josef E. Fischer (closing). Dr. Drapanas raised a very interesting point in his paper in the American Journal of Physiology in 1956, when he pointed out that the branched chain amino acids—no matter how many are given in acute hepatic insufficiency—it is difficult to raise the peripheral levels of branched chain acids. These appear to be going into the muscle and being chewed up for calories.

It would be very nice if L-dopa had only one mechanism of action. There are at least five ways that L-dopa may actually ameliorate the symptoms of hepatic coma. One cannot predict which patients L-dopa will arose from hepatic coma; about 50 to 60 per cent show a response. When you give L-dopa to an animal with acute hepatic coma, you get increased brain norepinephrine, but if you give L-dopa to a normal animal, you don't get increased brain norepinephrine. It may be that with the pathway blocked up the line, with dopa you are just bypassing the entire block, and you are increasing brain norepinephrine because all the other enzymes are intact. L-dopa releases about 90 to 95 per cent of the accumulated false transmitters in both heart and brain. L-dopa also releases serotonin and prevents its further synthesis, prevents the accumulation of phenylalanine by the gut, and transport across the gut, if given orally, and decreases SAMe levels in the brain, perhaps decreasing toxic methylamines.

Sheila Sherlock's paper about monoamine oxidase inhibitors and the dissociation of ammonia did not do any better actually, some of them became worse—which gave me the whole idea of false transmitters.

This is a very severe model, and it may or may not have anything to do with chronic human hepatic encephalopathy. I would be much happier if we had a chronic model or if we could have access to the brain in a larger animal.

Effect of small bowel bypass on gastric secretory function: Postintestinal exclusion hypersecretion, a phenomenon in search of a syndrome

Henry Buchwald, M.D., Ph.D., John J. Coyle, M.D., *and* **Richard L. Varco, M.D., Ph.D.,** *Minneapolis, Minn.*

Patients undergoing partial ileal bypass for hyperlipidemia and jejunoileal bypass for massive obesity were studied pre- and postoperatively: Group A consisted of fourteen jejunoileal bypass patients, restudied at one year; Group B consisted of seven partial ileal bypass patients, restudied at three months; and Group C was composed of seven partial ileal bypass patients, restudied at one year. There were significant differences in only the Group B posthistalog volume (−46.14 ± S.E. 15.28 ml. per 30 minutes, $p < 0.05$) and in Group A postHistalog peak acid output (+4.07 ± S.E. 1.32 mEq. per 30 minute peak, $p < 0.01$). Two of three Group A preoperative hypersecretors showed a better than 2 S.E. increase (other patient unchanged), and four normal secretors became hypersecretors (with an increase greater than +2 S.E.). Only one of 14 partial ileal bypass patients became a hypersecretor. None of the patients with hypersecretion manifested clinical evidence of acid-peptic disease. We conclude: (1) There is a significant decrease in Histalog-stimulated gastric juice volume three months following partial ileal bypass, this effect is not present at one year. (2) There is a significant increase in free acid in Histalog-stimulated gastric juice one year after jejunoileal bypass. (3) There is a difference in postoperative stimulation of gastric secretion between partial ileal bypass and jejunoileal bypass patients. (4) Gastric hypersecretion rarely occurs following partial ileal bypass. (5) Gastric hypersecretion frequently occurs following jejunoileal bypass, with an incidence rate as high as 43 percent.

From the Department of Surgery, University of Minnesota Medical School, Minneapolis, Minn.

In the German literature of 1914, Stassoff[17] first described gastric hypersecretion following massive small bowel resection in the dog. This interesting physiological phenomenon was to search for a clinical syndrome until 1965, when Frederick and associates[5] described a patient they had seen in 1963 and in whom they had documented marked hypersecretion following massive intestinal resection. Previously, Shelton and Blaine[16] published a suggestive case report of a patient with a perforated marginal ulcer after a massive bowel resection. Additional case reports were subsequently provided by Osborne and co-workers.[8, 9] However, the true incidence rate of gastric hypersecretion following small bowel loss in the human remained and still remains unknown.

How much intestine must be excluded and what particular segment of the intestinal tract is associated with hypersecretion have been the subjects of several investigations. In dogs, Reul and Ellison[11] found an increase in Heidenhain pouch secretion after a 75

Supported in part by a State of Minnesota Legislative Grant.

Presented at the Thirty-fifth Annual Meeting of the Society of University Surgeons, St. Louis, Mo., Feb. 14-16, 1974.

percent distal small bowel resection. Frederick and associates[5] showed fairly conclusively that the increase in gastric secretion is proportional to the length of the removed small intestine. Quintana and co-workers[10] showed an increase in gastric secretion from a Heidenhain pouch after excision of the duodenum. Sabsai[14] and, independently, Westerheide and associates[20] were able to produce in dogs a greater increase in gastric secretion after excision of the proximal half of the small intestine than that which followed excision of the distal half. The exact opposite result was recorded by Osborne and associates[8] in Heidenhain pouch dogs. Santillana and co-workers,[15] in the dog, very convincingly demonstrated that there was no difference in the gastric secretory effect following bypass or excision of an identical bowel segment, that exclusion of the proximal third of the small bowel caused marked gastric hypersecretion, that the gastric secretory response to exclusion of the middle third of the small intestine was variable, and that there was no significant change in gastric secretion after distal third small bowel exclusion. We[2] confirmed these findings with respect to the distal bowel when we published, in 1971, a study which demonstrated that there was no hypersecretion following a one-third or better distal small intestinal bypass (performed in management of a hyperlipidemia) ; indeed, there appeared to be evidence for an actual decrease in volume and a decrease in gastric acid secretion following this procedure.

This study seeks to explore further the effect of partial ileal bypass (approximately distal one-third) on gastric secretion and to compare the effects of partial ileal bypass and jejunoileal bypass (over 90 percent) on gastric secretory function.

METHODS

Three groups of small bowel bypass patients, with ostensibly normal intestinal tracts, underwent gastric analyses pre- and postoperatively.

Group A. This group consisted of 14 patients who were managed by jejunoileal bypass for their marked morbid exogenous obesity; they were studied preoperatively and one year postoperatively.

Group B. Consisting of seven hyperlipidemic, non-obese patients who received a partial ileal bypass operation, this group underwent preoperative gastric analysis and repeat gastric analysis at three months.

Group C. The composition of this group was identical to Group B, but these patients had follow-up gastric analysis at one year.

Our standard jejunoileal bypass operation consists of anastomosis of the proximal 40 cm. of jejunum beyond the ligament of Treitz, end to end, to the terminal 4 cm. of ileum. The intervening bypassed bowel is closed proximally and anastomosed for drainage distally, end to side, to the cecum. Thus, better than 90 percent of the normal bowel length is bypassed by this procedure. Our standard partial ileal bypass operation consists of bypass of the distal 200 cm. of the small intestine with bowel continuity restored by end-to-side anastomosis of the proximal bowel to the cecum. This procedure is, therefore, approximately a distal one-third small intestinal bypass.

Gastric secretory studies at the preoperative and postoperative evaluation consisted of analysis of gastric juice collected during a one-hour basal period followed by 2½ hours of collections after Histalog* stimulation. The postHistalog samples were collected at 15 minute intervals. Histalog was administered subcutaneously at a dose of 2 mg. per kilogram, with a maximum dose of 200 mg. The volume and free acid content of each gastric juice sample were determined. Free acid was determined by titration of a 2 ml. aliquot of a gastric aspirate sample against 0.1N NaOH after addition of two drops of Topfer's agent had been added as the indicator (pH 3.5). The gastric volume was expressed in milliliters per time interval and the acid output was expressed as milliequivalents of free acid per time interval.

The parameters of evaluation consisted of the basal one-hour volume and free acid

*A β-aminoethyl heterocyclic nitrogen analogue of histamine, Eli Lilly and Co., Indianapolis, Ind.

Table I. *Preoperative and postoperative acid and volume output for all subjects*

	Preoperative values				Postoperative values			
	Basal		Histalog		Basal		Histalog	
	ml./hr.	mEq. FA/hr.	ml./30 min.	mEq. FA/30 min.	ml./hr.	mEq. FA/hr.	ml./30 min.	mEq. FA/30 min.
Group A								
1	96	5.47	125	12.66	89	2.67	119	9.82
2	97	3.59	235	28.78	84	6.05	213	27.11
3	52	0.00	132	16.00	97	3.49	162	22.00
4	56	3.75	105	10.54	55	2.04	184	18.29
5	46	0.00	98	11.36	58	0.00	107	13.23
6	85	1.53	122	13.67	29	0.26	125	14.50
7	82	2.46	151	13.57	80	4.40	213	27.11
8	92	0.92	229	13.88	117	0.59	130	11.34
9	78	3.90	144	16.49	84	3.53	204	23.45
10	50	1.75	155	20.35	87	5.66	292	28.29
11	80	0.40	100	11.02	26	0.44	124	12.15
12	45	0.00	101	3.02	72	0.00	120	8.35
13	15	0.83	62	5.31	82	2.46	157	15.13
14	62	1.86	133	17.84	70	2.87	155	20.65
Group B								
1	20	1.75	160	15.43	77	0.00	182	5.44
2	150	1.06	216	5.92	72	0.00	160	14.00
3	89	8.32	139	34.24	73	4.40	185	19.70
4	81	3.13	178	10.18	40	2.80	188	11.90
5	50	3.00	208	24.27	176	0.28	270	20.54
6	50	0.15	115	5.08	37	0.92	123	4.12
7	77	0.00	134	8.32	27	1.08	170	11.45
Group C								
1	50	0.00	175	13.85	27	2.08	95	20.26
2	53	0.00	63	16.89	46	0.00	134	14.32
3	114	3.56	274	18.61	110	2.04	167	20.72
4	34	1.46	74	17.06	40	1.08	84	18.98
5	120	4.00	204	27.21	55	0.74	172	34.25
6	22	1.45	45	14.89	27	1.22	38	15.01
7	31	3.54	153	11.29	36	0.35	117	12.60

content and also the volume and free acid content for the peak 30 minute secretory response to Histalog. Selection of these parameters was based on the work of Laudano and Roncoroni.[7] The mean and standard error of peak secretory response to Histalog in our laboratory is 15.3 ± 0.7 mEq. per 30 minutes. When two standard errors above the mean were used as the criteria for judging an individual to be a gastric hypersecretor, a 30 minute Histalog response greater than 16.7 mEq. is defined as representing chemical hypersecretion.

RESULTS

In Table I, the acid and volume output for all subjects is shown. In Table II the mean group difference ± S.E. for the pre- and postoperative test pairs are given for the basal and Histalog response for both acid output and gastric aspirate volume. Calculation of the confidence interval for these data focuses attention on the Group A postHistalog acid output and the Group B postHistalog volume output. With the use of matched pair Student's t test analysis, significant differences occurred in Group A Histalog acid output ($p < 0.01$) and in Group B Histalog volume output ($p < 0.05$). The other paired analyses were not significant at the $p < 0.05$ level. Thus, jejunoileal bypass apears to elicit a mean increase in Histalog-stimulated free acid output, whereas, this response is not found as part of the mean gastric aspirate response to partial ileal bypass. A decrease in peak Histalog-stimulated gastric volume three

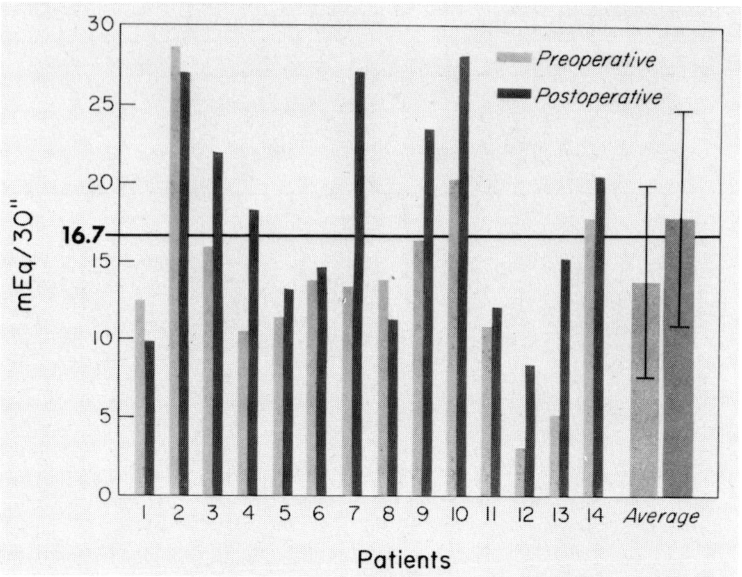

Fig. 1. Bar graphs of the 30 minute peak Histalog acid response of jejunoileal bypass patients (Group A) both preoperatively and postoperatively and the mean group response ± S.E.

Table II. *Matched pair analysis of the mean difference ± S.E. (postoperative to preoperative) with Student's t test*

Group	No.	Acid output		Volume output	
		Basal (mEq./hr.)	Histalog (mEq./30 min.)	Basal (ml./hr.)	Histalog (ml./30 min.)
A	14	+ 0.45 ± 0.57	+ 4.07 ± 1.32*	− 1.14 ± 9.3	+ 30.21 ± 15.32
B	7	− 1.13 ± 0.68	− 2.33 ± 2.95	− 11.86 ± 9.66	− 46.14 ± 15.28†
C	7	+ 0.5 ± 1.2	+ 2.33 ± 1.28	+ 17.86 ± 26.09	+ 18.29 ± 14.39

*$p < 0.01$.
†$p < 0.05$.

months following partial ileal bypass is no longer apparent one year after this procedure.

Fig. 1 gives bar graph plots for the acid output response to Histalog for each individual jejunoileal bypass patient (Group A), preoperatively and postoperatively. The same material is plotted for each partial ileal bypass patient (Groups B and C) in Fig. 2. When the value of a peak response greater than 16.7 mEq. per 30 minutes was used to judge an individual a hypersecretor at the time of that particular analysis, the following results can be derived.

Of the patients who underwent jejunoileal bypass, three patients can be classified as hypersecretors preoperatively and seven were hypersecretors postoperatively. Of the three preoperative hypersecretors, two increased the degree of their response to Histalog significantly (20.35 to 28.29, a +7.94 change and 17.84 to 20.65, a +2.81 change), with an increase greater than two standard errors (the S.E. for these data is 1.32 [see Table II]); the Histalog response of the third preoperative hypersecretor remained essentially unchanged (28.78 to 27.11, a −1.67 change). Four patients in Group A became hypersecretors with the following response changes: 16.00 to 22.00, a +6.00 change; 10.54 to 18.29, a +7.75; 13.57 to 27.11, a +13.54 change; and 16.49 to 23.45, a +6.96

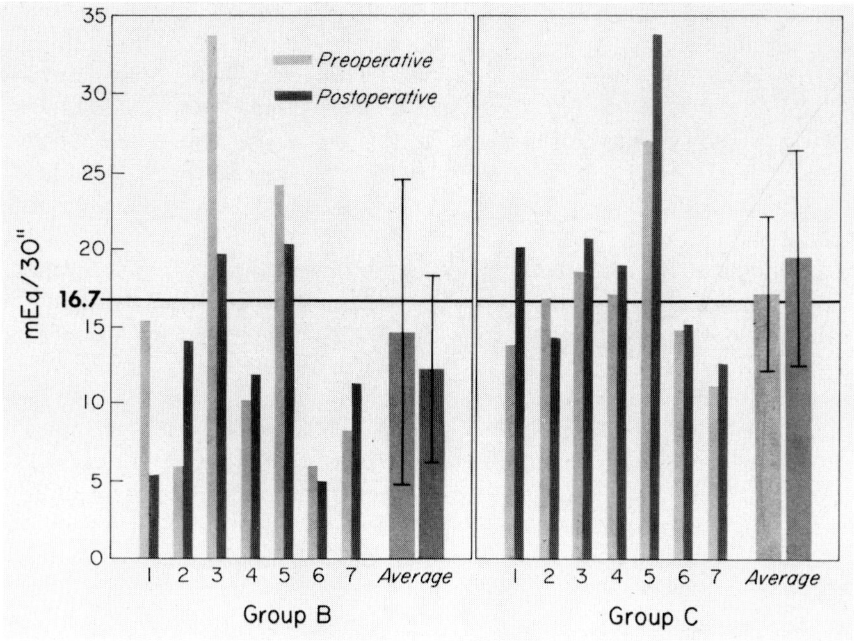

Fig. 2. Bar graphs of the 30 minute peak Histalog acid response of partial ileal bypass patients (Groups B and C) both preoperatively and postoperatively and the mean group responses ± S.E.

change; all these increases to Histalog stimulation are greater than two standard errors above the mean. Thus, a significant increase in Histalog-stimulated acid output with a postoperative value greater than 16.7 mEq. per 30 minutes was found in six of the seven postoperative hypersecretors, or 43 percent of the total group of 14 individuals.

Of the patients who underwent partial ileal bypass (Groups B and C), six patients can be classified as hypersecretors (i.e., peak Histalog response greater than 16.7 mEq. per 30 minutes) preoperatively and six postoperatively. Only one (a Group C patient) with a preoperative normal response to Histalog became a hypersecretor (13.85 to 20.26, a +6.41 change), with an increase greater than two standard errors (the S.E. for these data are 2.95 for Group B and 1.28 for Group C [see Table II]). Of the six preoperative hypersecretors in combined Groups B and C, only one (an individual in Group C) increased the level of his response greater than two standard errors (27.21 to 34.25, a +7.04 change); three patients had insignificant changes in their Histalog response (24.27 to 20.54, a −3.73 change for one patient in Group B and 18.61 to 20.72, a +2.11 change, and 17.06 to 18.98, a +1.92 change for two patients in Group C); and two individuals had a significant fall in their peak Histalog response postoperatively (34.24 to 19.70, a −14.54 change for one in Group B and 16.89 to 14.32, a −2.57 change for one in Group C), with one falling below the 16.7 mEq. per 30 minutes level of response. This individual patient breakdown corroborates the matched-pair analysis in showing no significant hypersecretory response as a result of partial ileal bypass.

Statistical analysis of the difference of the pre- and postoperative means in Groups A, B, and C, contrary to the finding for matched-pair analysis in Group A, shows no significant difference for Histalog-stimulated acid secretion at the $p < 0.05$ level.

None of the patients in Groups A, B, and C with hypersecretion preoperatively or postoperatively manifested clinical evidence of acid-peptic disease. Neither was the expected postoperative diarrhea of these hypersecretors noticeably more severe than the diarrhea experienced by the bypass patients who were not hypersecretors.

DISCUSSION

This study with respect to the partial ileal bypass patients, differs in methodology from our previous human study[2]; we previously analyzed a different parameter of secretion, namely, overnight gastric aspirates. We failed to confirm the data based on the overnight analyses showing that partial ileal bypass is associated with a statistically significant decrease in gastric juice volume and acid content. On the other hand, both studies agree, and are in agreement with the animal experiments of Santillana and co-workers,[15] in demonstrating that distal one-third small intestinal bypass does not cause gastric hypersecretion.

This study does show that jejunoileal bypass, or a bypass of greater than 90 percent of small bowel, in humans is frequently associated with gastric hypersecretion. Yet, this effect is variable and unpredictable and occurs in less than 50 percent of patients with this massive bypass procedure. To date, the clinical implications of gastric hypersecretion, in those jejunoileal bypass patients with the hypersecretion syndrome, have not become manifest; it is premature to draw any definitive conclusions regarding the eventual effect of the hypersecretion on the state of health of these individuals. Indeed, repeat studies over a prolonged period of time will be necessary to ascertain if the postjejunoileal bypass hypersecretion persists or is transitory and if other jejunoileal bypass patients develop the hypersecretion syndrome at a later date.

The phenomenon of gastric hypersecretion following massive loss of the small intestine was first described in the animal laboratory[17] and only after 40 years was the syndrome documented clinically.[5] To this time (60 years after its discovery), we still do not know why it occurs. It is time to return to the laboratory, where many animal models have produced gastric hypersecretion as a result of small bowel loss, and to initiate additional clinical studies in order to find a definitive answer. Let us briefly review what we do know with respect to causation.

The evidence that the gastric hypersecretion is largely postprandial,[8] coupled with the fact that most animal models measure gastric secretion in denervated pouches, leads one to believe that a hormone is responsible for the gastric hypersecretion. Gastric secretogogues, as well as inhibitors, have been postulated to explain this mechanism.

Gastric secretogogues have been found in the small intestine. Chandler and associates[3] have isolated a peptide of low-molecular weight from pig intestinal mucosa which is a potent gastric secretory stimulant when injected into dogs. Complete diversion of thoracic duct lymph has been shown by Yakimets and Bondar[22] to eliminate postenterectomy hypersecretion in dogs. Becker and colleagues[1] found release of gastrin from proximal duodenum and proximal jejunum of dogs, when these isolated intestinal segments were perfused with acetylcholine. It is difficult, however, to implicate a gastric secretogogue elaborated primarily by the small intestine following small bowel loss, unless one can adequately explain the mechanism for this release effect. It is easier for us to postulate that a secretogogue, normally released into the portal circulation by the postprandial stomach, duodenum, or upper jejunum and normally degraded in the upper small intestine, continues to exert its influence in the absence of the upper small bowel or secondarily to atrophy of the upper small intestine. This theory is essentially the same as that of Temperley and associates,[18] who in 1971 demonstrated that gastrin is inactivated in the small bowel, probably as the result of the action of a specific enzyme. Again, the hypothesis is in keeping with the results reported in a recent paper of Wickbom and co-workers[21] which demonstrated an elevation of gastrin levels in the two-hour postprandial sera of dogs. The data showing no hypersecretion secondary to loss of distal small bowel and the variability of the hypersecretory response in the jejunoileal bypass patients are compatible with the inadequate gastrin degradation concept.

There is also strong evidence for loss of a small intestinal inhibitor of gastric secretion by excision or atrophy of the proximal small intestine. Ruderman and co-workers[12, 13] have shown that a thermolabile substance contained in the jejunal, but not in the ileal, homogenate of rats when injected intraperitoneally will inhibit the acid hypersecretion caused by a jejunectomy and return acid output to near preresection levels. These studies can explain the lack of gastric hypersecretion following a distal small bowel bypass; however, the variability of the response of patients to a standard jejunoileal bypass poses a problem in fitting this mechanism to the human situation. What are the known gastric secretory inhibitors? Serotonin[15] was proposed as the involved inhibitor but the work of Fischer and associates[4] fairly convincingly excludes both serotonin and histaminase as the inhibitory agent involved. Enterogastrone[6] (if there is such a unique substance) has been implicated as the inhibitor, as has secretin. It has been shown that the intestinal secretin concentration diminishes with increasing distance from the pylorus.[19]

In summary, no animal-derived data verify a specific theory or a definitive secretogogue or inhibitor mechanism; human hypersecretion investigation is in the earliest stage of development. Furthermore, though transfer of animal experimental conclusions to the human situation can be warranted, methodology has not been comparable. Animal studies, to this time, primarily rely on measuring postprandial gastric secretion in a standardized Heidenhain pouch. The human investigations have, on the other hand, employed basal or artificially stimulated gastric aspirate analysis. Thus, we not only lack a clear definition of the extent of the postintestinal exclusion hypersecretion syndrome, but we also have no clear answer to the question of causation.

REFERENCES

1. Becker, H. D., Reeder, D. D., Evans, J. C., and Thompson, J. C.: Gastrin release from duodenum and jejunum in dogs, Surg. Forum **23:** 3, 1972.
2. Buchwald, H., and Varco, R. L.: Human gastric secretory studies following distal small bowel bypass, Curr. Top. Surg. Res. **3:** 409, 1971.
3. Chandler, J. G., Rosen, H., Kester, R. C., and Orloff, M. J.: Isolation of the hormone responsible for intestinal phase of gastric secretion from pig intestinal mucosa, Surg. Forum **23:** 382, 1972.
4. Fischer, J. E., Snyder, S. H., James, J. H., and Baldessarini, R.: Histamine and serotonin metabolism following massive small bowel resection, Ann. Surg. **175:** 260, 1972.
5. Frederick, P. L., Sizer, J. S., and Osborne, M. P.: Relation of massive bowel resection to gastric secretion, N. Engl. J. Med. **272:** 509, 1965.
6. Kosaka, T., and Lim, R. K. S.: Demonstration of humoral agent in fat inhibition of gastric secretion, Proc. Soc. Exp. Biol. Med. **27:** 890, 1930.
7. Laudano, O. M., and Roncoroni, E. C.: Determination of the dose of histalog that provokes maximal gastric secretory response, Gastroenterology **49:** 372, 1965.
8. Osborne, M. P., Frederick, P. L., Sizer, J. S., Blair, D., Cole, P., and Thum, W.: Mechanism of gastric hypersecretion following massive intestinal resection: Clinical and experimental observations, Ann. Surg. **164:** 622, 1966.
9. Osborne, M. P., Sizer, J., Frederick, P. L., and Zamcheck, N.: Massive bowel resection and gastric hypersecretion: Its mechanism and a plan for clinical study and management, Am. J. Surg. **114:** 393, 1967.
10. Quintana, R., Kohatzu, S., Woodward, E. R., and Dragstedt, L.: Mechanisms of duodenal inhibition of gastric secretion, Arch. Surg. **89:** 585, 1964.
11. Reul, G. F., and Ellison, E. E.: Effect of seventy-five percent distal resection on gastric secretion, Am. J. Surg. **111:** 772, 1966.
12. Ruderman, R. L., and Kamel, I.: The effect of intestinal resection on gastric acidity in the rat, Surg. Forum **21:** 312, 1970.
13. Ruderman, R. L., and Nagy, E. J.: Intestinal control of gastric acid secretion in rats, Surg. Forum **23:** 331, 1972.
14. Sabsai, B. I.: The effect of extensive resections of the proximal and distal portions of the small intestine on canine gastric secretion, Biull. Ekap. Biol. Med. (Moscow) **55:** 287, 1963.
15. Santillana, M., Wise, L., Schuck, M., and Ballinger, W. F., II: Changes in gastric acid secretion following resection or exclusion of different segments of the small intestine, Surgery **65:** 777, 1969.
16. Shelton, E. L., Jr., and Blaine, M. H.: Mas-

sive small bowel resection in post-gastrectomy patients, Texas J. Med. **50:** 96, 1954.

17. Stassoff, B.: Experimentelle Untersuchungen über die Kompensatorischen Vorgange bei Darmresektionen, Beitr. Klin. Chir. **89:** 527, 1914.
18. Temperley, J. M., Stagg, B. H., and Wyllie, J. H.: Disappearance of gastrin and pentagastrin in the portal circulation, Gut **12:** 372, 1971.
19. Weaver, M. M.: Distribution of pancreatic secretin in the gastrointestinal tract, Am. J. Physiol. **82:** 106, 1947.
20. Westerheide, R. L., Elliott, D. W., and Hardacre, J. M.: The potential of the upper small bowel in regulating acid secretion, SURGERY **58:** 73, 1965.
21. Wickbom, G., McGuigan, J. E., and Landor, J. H.: Role of gastrin in short-bowel gastric hypersecretion, Surg. Forum **24:** 353, 1973.
22. Yakimets, W. W., and Bondar, G. S.: Hormonal stimulatory mechanism producing gastric hypersecretion following massive small-intestinal resection, Can. J. Surg. **12:** 241, 1969.

Transient kwashiorkor: A cause of fatty liver following small bowel bypass

John J. White, M.D., C.M., Richard T. Moxley, III, M.D.,* Thomas Pozefsky, M.D., *and* **Dean H. Lockwood, M.D.,** ** *Baltimore, Md.*

Changes in protein nutrition have been compared with alterations in hepatic morphology and function in 18 patients undergoing small bowel bypass for morbid obesity. Moderate to marked hepatic fat accumulation occurred during the periods of intense weight loss, with return to preoperative levels after weight stability was attained. These changes were accompanied by significant depressions in the fasting serum values of most of the essential and nonessential amino acids and with elevation in glycine and serine. Reduced absorption of lysine and leucine and less absorption of glycine were observed during oral amino acid tolerance tests. Improvements in protein absorption were observed in patients who had achieved weight stability and reduction in fatty metamorphosis of the liver toward normal levels. These studies demonstrate that a state of protein malnutrition develops during the period of intense weight loss following jejunoileal bypass and that protein nutrition returns toward normal level coincident with attainment of weight stability. Significant fatty infiltration of the liver develops during intense weight loss, as well. The morphologic similarity between these changes and those noted in the livers of patients with kwashiorkor and in those of laboratory animals made protein deficient suggests that their etiology may also be similar. The improvement in both fatty metamorphosis of the liver and protein absorption with the attainment of weight stability is presumably due to functional adaptation by the bowel. The occasional occurrence of liver fibrosis and failure following small bowel bypass for obesity may be due to an additional hepatic insult superimposed upon persistent marked hepatic steatosis secondary to persistent protein malnutrition and insufficient intestinal adaptation.

From the Departments of Surgery and Medicine, The Johns Hopkins University School of Medicine, Baltimore, Md.

JEJUNOILEAL BYPASS is being utilized increasingly in the therapy of morbid obesity. Widespread acceptance of this treatment has been limited chiefly by uncertainty regarding ultimate development of serious metabolic and anatomic sequelae. One organ of major concern is the liver. Following small bowel bypass, significant fatty changes in the liver occur, which usually revert to preoperative levels with weight stabilization. Such changes have not been noted with prolonged starvation. The etiology of these fatty changes has been unclear; whether they might be associated with development of the hepatic fibrosis that is occasionally seen following intestinal bypass is of serious concern.

Supported in part by Pediatric Clinical Research Unit Grant No. 5-MO1-RR-00052, by General Clinical Research Unit Grant No. RR-00035, by United States Public Health Service Grant AM 14754, and by a Grant from Weight Watchers Foundation, Inc.

Presented at the Thirty-fifth Annual Meeting of The Society of University Surgeons, St. Louis, Mo., Feb. 14-16, 1974.

*Supported by Special Traineeship Award (FN 02 IF11NS2617) from the National Institute of Neurological Diseases and Stroke.

**Recipient of United States Public Health Service Career Development Award (AM 42579).

Fatty metamorphosis of the liver also accompanies kwashiorkor, a severe protein malnutrition state. In view of the similarity in hepatic morphology, changes in protein and carbohydrate nutrition and in hepatic morphology and function were studied in 18 patients following small bowel bypass for morbid obesity.

CLINICAL MATERIAL

Only patients with true morbid obesity (weight at least twice normal, failure of medical management, and significant physiologic or socioeconomic impairment) have been treated with jejunoileal bypass and studied in our series. All patients were screened medically and psychologically, and the advantages and disadvantages of operative therapy were fully explained.

Only the first patient in our series had the proximal jejunum 14 inches from the ligament of Treitz anastomosed end to side to the terminal ileum, 4 inches from the ileocecal valve. Subsequently, end-to-end anastomosis of the proximal jejunum to the terminal ileum has been carried out. One early patient had 12 inches of proximal jejunum anastomosed to 12 inches of terminal ileum; the remainder had a standardized 14 to 15 inches of proximal jejunum anastomosed to 4 to 5 inches of terminal ileum. A right transverse incision has been favored. Halothane anesthesia was used in ten patients, five in each study group; subsequent to one death from apparent halothane hepatitis, a combination of other anesthetic agents has been used. Postoperatively, all patients received oral multivitamins, parenteral folate, and vitamin B_{12}; diet was as desired. Potassium and magnesium supplements were added as necessary. Diphenoxylate (Lomotil) and deodorized tincture of opium were used to control diarrhea.

Protein nutrition and hepatic morphology were studied in 18 patients. Patients were compared at two postoperative periods: during intense weight loss, the "weight-losing" group, and after weight eventually had reached plateau for at least three months, the "weight-stable" group.

Thirteen patients, five males and eight females, with an average age of 31 years (range, 23 to 41 years) comprise the weight-losing group. All were studied preoperatively and then restudied four months post-jejunoileal bypass. Their initial weights had been 357 ± 19 pounds (range, 290 to 520 pounds), or 240 percent of the ideal weight. Their weights at the 4-month period examination averaged 292 ± 16 pounds, or 192 percent of ideal weight, for an average weight loss of 65 pounds, or 18 percent of their preoperative weight.

Five patients, four males and one female, with an average age of 29 years (range, 22 to 35 years) comprise the weight-stable group. Their initial weights had been 387 ± 50 pounds (range, 275 to 522 pounds), or 223 percent of the ideal weight. All were studied 12 to 36 months postoperatively, at which time their weights had reached a constant plateau averaging 252 ± 24 pounds, or 144 percent of ideal weight. Their average weight loss was 135 pounds, or 35 percent of their initial weight.

METHODS

Hepatic morphology and function. Wedge biopsies of the liver were obtained at the time of jejunoileal bypass in all patients. Subsequently, needle biopsies were obtained. The extent of hepatic fat was estimated from hematoxylin and eosin–stained sections as "slight" when up to 30 percent of the hepatocytes were vacuolated with fat; a "moderately" fatty liver had 30 to 60 percent hepatocyte vacuolization; a "markedly" fatty liver had more than 60 percent vacuolization. Hepatic fibrosis was determined in all biopsies by Masson staining techniques. Alkaline phosphatase, serum glutamic oxaloacetic transaminase (SGOT), total bilirubin, serum albumin, and prothrombin time were measured by standard clinical laboratory methods. Bromsulfphthalein retention tests were not performed because of the large quantity of dye required for the massive size of the patients.

Carbohydrate nutrition and intestinal absorption. Hepatic glycogen was estimated by

Table I. *Hepatic fat content*

	No.	Slight (< 30%)	Moderate (30%–60%)	Marked (> 60%)
Preoperative	18	12	6	0
Weight-losing group	12*	1	4	7
Weight-stable group	5	2	3	0

*One patient refused follow-up liver biopsy.

periodic acid–Schiff (PAS) staining of biopsies from five patients in each group. Fasting blood glucose levels were measured by routine clinical laboratory methods, as were serum cholesterol values. Fecal fat was assayed on serial 24 hour stool collections, and D-xylose absorption tests were performed in routine fashion.

Protein nutrition. Plasma amino acid profiles were obtained both preoperatively and four months postoperatively in the 13 patients in the weight-losing group, and they were obtained postoperatively after plateau had been reached in the weight-stable group. Postabsorptive (overnight fasted) concentrations of individual amino acids were determined from venous plasma after three days of a standardized diet. Protein-free supernatants were prepared with sulfosalicylic acid,[2] and amino acids were measured by an automated chromatographic technique.[26] Values were obtained for seven essential amino acids and for 12 nonessential amino acids.

An oral tolerance test for selected amino acids was carried out in five patients from the weight-losing group, both pre- and postoperatively, as well as in the five patients composing the weight-stable group. After an overnight fast, 75 mM. each of leucine (a neutral amino acid), glycine, and lysine (a basic amino acid), dissolved in 400 ml. of 0.1N HCl and neutralized to pH 7.4, were given orally. Venous blood samples were collected at 0, 30, 60, 120, 180, and 300 minutes, and the plasma was separated for amino acid analysis.

RESULTS

Weight loss was satisfactory. The weight-stable group lost an average of 35 percent of their preoperative weights (range, 21 to 55 percent), and leveled off at an average of 45 percent above ideal weight (range, 26 to 66 percent). The weight-losing group had lost an average of 18 percent (range, eight to 27 percent) of their preoperative weights by four months, approximately half of their anticipated total weight loss, based on the experience of the weight-stable group. One female patient in the weight-losing group required intestinal reanastomosis because of relentless weight loss without stabilization (326 pounds preoperatively to 156 pounds 14 months postoperatively, a 52 percent reduction), refractory hypokalemia and hypomagnesemia, progressive deterioration of protein nutrition, and progressive hepatic steatosis with severe fibrosis.

Weight loss was accompanied by intestinal malabsorption. Fecal fat excretion (normal < 6.0 Gm. per day) averaged 2.7 Gm. per day (range, 0.6 to 5.1 Gm. per day) preoperatively in each group. There was a tenfold increase to an average excretion of 27.3 Gm. per day (range, 3.4 to 66.1 Gm. per day) in the weight-losing group. Significant steatorrhea persisted in the weight-stable group: fecal fat excretion averaged 20.3 Gm. per day (range, 12.4 to 29.6 Gm. per day). Serum cholesterol values inversely paralleled the extent of steatorrhea. From a preoperative average of 189 mg. per cent (range, 140 to 250 mg. percent), serum cholesterol diminished to 130 mg. percent (range, 70 to 198 mg. percent) in the weight-losing group, and leveled off at 140 mg. percent (range, 65 to 175 mg. percent) in the weight-stable group. D-xylose excretion averaged 6.8 Gm. per five hours (range, 2.9 to 9.2 Gm. per five hours) preoperatively and was significantly depressed in the weight-losing group to an average value of 2.4 Gm. per five hours (range, 1.6 to 3.7 Gm. per five hours). In the weight-stable group, nearly

Table II. *Amino acid profiles in weight-losing and weight-stable groups**

Amino acid†	*Preoperative*	*Weight-losing group*	*Weight-stable group*
Essential			
Valine	271 ± 11	168 ± 10 (↓ 39%)‡	187 ± 15 (↓ 31%)
Lysine	226 ± 11	140 ± 8 (↓ 38%)	172 ± 17 (↓ 24%)
Leucine	150 ± 7	99 ± 6 (↓ 34%)	123 ± 6 (↓ 18%)
Isoleucine	77 ± 3	58 ± 4 (↓ 25%)	65 ± 4 (↓ 16%)
Phenylalanine	68 ± 2	52 ± 2 (↓ 22%)	63 ± 11
Threonine	143 ± 6	124 ± 9 (↓ 13%)	123 ± 15 (↓ 14%)
Methionine	24 ± 1	23 ± 1	25 ± 2
Nonessential			
Glycine	183 ± 14	232 ± 15 (↑ 27%)	249 ± 26 (↑ 36%)
Serine	99 ± 4	137 ± 12 (↑ 38%)	109 ± 9
A-aminobutyrate	26 ± 2	19 ± 2 (↓ 37%)	16 ± 2 (↓38%)
Tyrosine	78 ± 4	55 ± 4 (↓ 29%)	58 ± 5 (↓ 26%)
Ornithine	75 ± 6	55 ± 7 (↓ 27%)	51 ± 4 (↓ 32%)
1/2 Cystine	123 ± 4	97 ± 6 (↓ 37%)	102 ± 10
Taurine	55 ± 4	48 ± 4	43 ± 6
Arginine	79 ± 5	54 ± 4 (↓ 32%)	84 ± 4
Citrulline	27 ± 1	20 ± 1 (↓ 35%)	30 ± 2
Alanine	402 ± 19	324 ± 21 (↓ 19%)	369 ± 25
Proline	200 ± 14	198 ± 22	199 ± 30
Histidine	82 ± 4	83 ± 7	88 ± 1

*Modified from Moxley, R. T., et al.: N. Engl. J. Med. 290: 921, 1974.

†Amino acid concentrations presented as mean ± SEM in μmoles per liter.

‡Percentage change from preoperative values is given when significant. Changes from preoperative mean were tested for significance ($p < 0.05 - 0.001$) by paired t test for weight-losing group and unpaired t test for weight-stable group.

normal levels were observed; they averaged 4.2 Gm. per five hours (range, 2.97 to 6.18 Gm. per five hours).

Hepatic morphology and function. Preoperatively, slight fat accumulation was present in 12 patients, and moderate accumulation was present in six. Increased hepatic fat was present in the weight-losing group; eleven of the 12 patients studied changed categories toward increased fat accumulation (Table I). In none of the weight-stable patients was there marked fat accumulation; only two of the five showed an increase over their preoperative levels.

Among the several tests of functional status of the liver, the SGOT values appeared to be the most meaningful. From the average preoperative level of 11.7 mIU. per milliliter (range, 8 to 23 mIU. per milliliter), the average SGOT value of the weight-losing group was elevated to 29.7 mIU. per milliliter (range, 16 to 39 mIU. per milliliter), and that of the weight-stable group rose from 14.6 to 42.6 mIU. per milliliter (range, 15 to 110 mIU. per milliliter) at four months postoperatively. After weight plateau had been reached, the SGOT values of the weight-stable group averaged 15 mIU. per milliliter (range, 9 to 18 mIU. per milliliter). In 17 of the patients, the alkaline phosphatase rose from an average normal preoperative value of 20.7 mIU. per milliliter (range, 9 to 32 mIU. per milliliter) to a high normal value of 29 mIU. per milliliter (range, 12 to 39 mIU. per milliliter) in both groups at four months; it had decreased slightly to 26.8 mIU. per milliliter in the weight-stable group. The liver studies of one patient in the weight-stable group had grossly abnormal results preoperatively: the SGOT was 37 mIU. per milliliter, and the alkaline phosphatase was 104 mIU. per milliliter; bilirubin and albumin were normal. He has demonstrated some hepatic fibrosis postoperatively. Total bilirubin values were within the normal range throughout in both groups; some patients had low serum albumin levels.

Carbohydrate nutrition. Fasting blood glucose levels were normal and unchanged throughout in all patients in both the weight-losing and weight-stable groups. Hepatic glycogen, based on estimations of PAS-stained

Table III. *Oral amino acid tolerance tests. Pre- and postjejunoileostomy for obesity**

	Time (min.)				
	30	60	120	180	300
Lysine					
Preoperative	454 ± 80	853 ± 117	855 ± 129	509 ± 102	224 ± 28
Weight losing	152 ± 32†	321 ± 39†	328 ± 53†	227 ± 41†	160 ± 31
Weight stable	266 ± 59	470 ± 58†	525 ± 124	207 ± 46†	115 ± 22†
Leucine					
Preoperative	480 ± 74	718 ± 136	510 ± 90	301 ± 102	130 ± 52
Weight losing	213 ± 35†	344 ± 37†	322 ± 55†	278 ± 47	155 ± 33
Weight stable	343 ± 77	502 ± 35	391 ± 110	190 ± 53	89 ± 32
Glycine					
Preoperative	112 ± 25	194 ± 30	128 ± 30	77 ± 42	27 ± 16
Weight losing	58 ± 10	106 ± 10†	105 ± 20	79 ± 18	58 ± 15†
Weight stable	96 ± 34	217 ± 19	167 ± 25	83 ± 19	41 ± 10

*All values reflect change from base line and are expressed in μmoles per liter as mean ± SEM.
†Significant by t test compared to preoperative values.

sections of the liver biopsies remained normal throughout in both groups. Ketosis was absent.

Protein nutrition. Amino acid profiles in the weight-losing group showed significant depressions in six of seven essential amino acids with only methionine unchanged (Table II). Among the 12 nonessential amino acids assayed, significant reductions occurred in six; proline, taurine, and histidine were unchanged; and serine and glycine levels were significantly elevated. In the weight-stable group, five of seven essential amino acids remained depressed, though to a much lesser extent than in the weight-losing group (except for threonine). Only three of the nonessential amino acids continued to be significantly depressed, and glycine remained significantly elevated.

Peak increments in plasma of the three selected amino acids during the oral tolerance test in the weight-losing group was less than half the observed preoperative values (leucine $P < 0.005$; glycine $P < 0.005$; lysine $P < 0.05$) (Table III). The slope of decline from peak values was also considerably flatter (Fig. 1). In the weight-stable group, the glycine tolerance curve paralleled the preoperative curve; leucine and lysine peaks had improved considerably. For all three, the slope of the curve of decline from peak value was nearly normal.

DISCUSSION

Morbidly obese patients generally show mild to moderate hepatic steatosis preoperatively. Following intestinal bypass, the degree of steatosis increases during the intense weight-losing period and returns to preoperative levels on attainment of weight stability. Such a pattern, observed commonly before, was seen in our patients.[3, 4, 9, 10, 20, 24]

Hepatomegaly and hepatic dysfunction are also well recognized in kwashiorkor, in which protein malnutrition is extreme.[6, 16] In this condition, most serum enzyme assays are normal, except for SGOT, serum glutamic pyruvic transaminase (SGPT), and isocitric dehydrogenase (ICD).[8] A similar pattern was noted for those enzymes tested in our patients. In kwashiorkor, striking hepatocellular fatty changes occur, which may be reversible with improvement in protein nutrition.[13, 15] These histologic changes in the liver appear to be similar to those reported following jejunoileal bypass for obesity.

In contrast, treatment of obesity by caloric restriction or by starvation produces progressive diminution of hepatic steatosis.[7, 19] Similarly, fatty liver and hepatomegaly are not characteristic of marasmus, in which protein and caloric deficiency is extreme,[16] nor does liver enzyme derangement occur.[19]

Assay of free amino acids in the plasma of patients with kwashiorkor has shown a

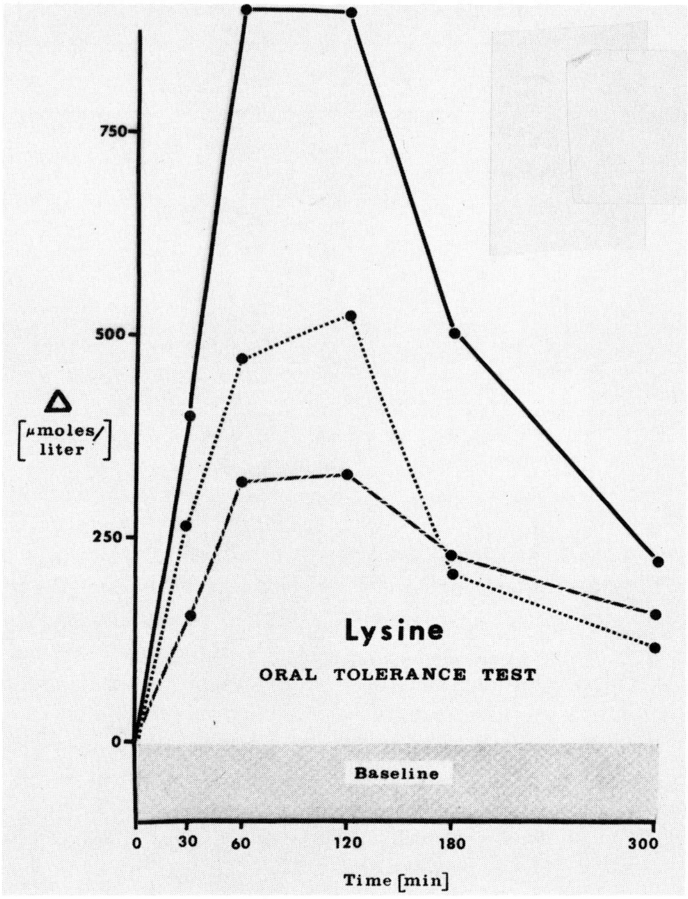

Fig. 1. Oral amino acid tolerance test. Absorption curves up to five hours following ingestion of lysine preoperatively (solid line), during intensive weight loss (hatched line), and following weight stabilization (dotted line). Values are presented as elevations above basal levels.

constant pattern with depression of certain essential amino acids, in particular, valine, leucine, isoleucine, and methionine, and usually with elevation of the nonessential amino acids serine and glycine.[17, 22] The plasma amino acid profiles of our patients, especially during the intense weight-losing period, resemble the pattern of kwashiorkor. A return toward a normal profile is apparent in our weight-stable patients. Concomitantly, a return toward the preoperative degree of hepatic steatosis also occurred.

Oral tolerance tests for two of the essential amino acids which are usually deficient in kwashiorkor, lysine and leucine, showed significant impairment during the period of intense weight loss in our bypass patients. The leucine absorption curve was insignificantly impaired in the weight-stable group. Lysine absorption, however, has remained moderately impaired in the weight-stable group. Oral tolerance tests for glycine showed moderate impairment at four months and were normal in the weight-stable group. The significance of these findings is uncertain. Follow-up studies are continuing.

Experimentally, fatty livers have been produced in normal laboratory animals fed diets deficient in specific amino acids, particularly lysine, isoleucine and threonine.[1, 12, 25, 29] The fat level of the diet appears to have no effect upon accumulation of hepatic lipids; the liver lipid content is higher, however, when sucrose rather than glucose is used as a carbohydrate source.[1] Since fat absorptive and serum lipid levels are significantly de-

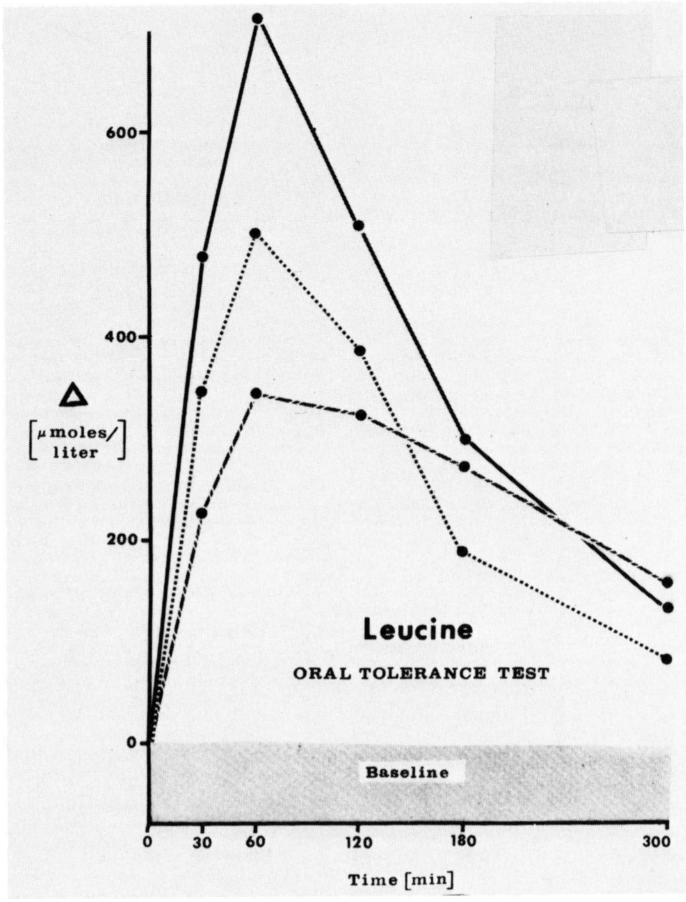

Fig. 2. Oral amino acid tolerance test. Absorption curves up to five hours following ingestion of leucine preoperatively (solid line), during intensive weight loss (hatched line), and following weight stabilization (dotted line). Values are presented as elevations above basal levels.

creased[11] following small bowel bypass for obesity, it is likely that hepatic steatosis probably results from increased intrahepatic synthesis of triglycerides with storage. C^{14}-labeled dietary carbohydrate has been shown to lead to labeling of liver lipids in experimental threonine deficiency.[29] This increased hepatic fat synthesis in experimental kwashiorkor is in the form of triglycerides[12, 29]; similarly, triglycerides form the main component of the increased hepatic lipid in man following small bowel bypass.[9]

As in kwashiorkor, carbohydrate nutrition following small bowel bypass appears to be relatively well maintained. Although glucose tolerance curves have been reported to be flattened for a prolonged period following operation,[28] improvement in carbohydrate nutrition has been noted with improved K values,[18] with normalization of prediabetic glucose tolerance curves,[23] and with correction of hyperinsulinism.[18]

Weight stability following jejunoileostomy is achieved presumably in part by intestinal adaptation. This phenomenon has been noted following massive intestinal resection and has been credited to increased numbers of cells,[5] rather than to increased cellular function.[30] A similar villous hypertrophy has been seen in the functioning intestine following small bowel bypass for obesity.[21]

Relentlessly progressive amino acid deficiencies associated with steady deterioration in liver function and morphology prompted intestinal reanastomosis in one of our patients. A similar pattern has been noted in

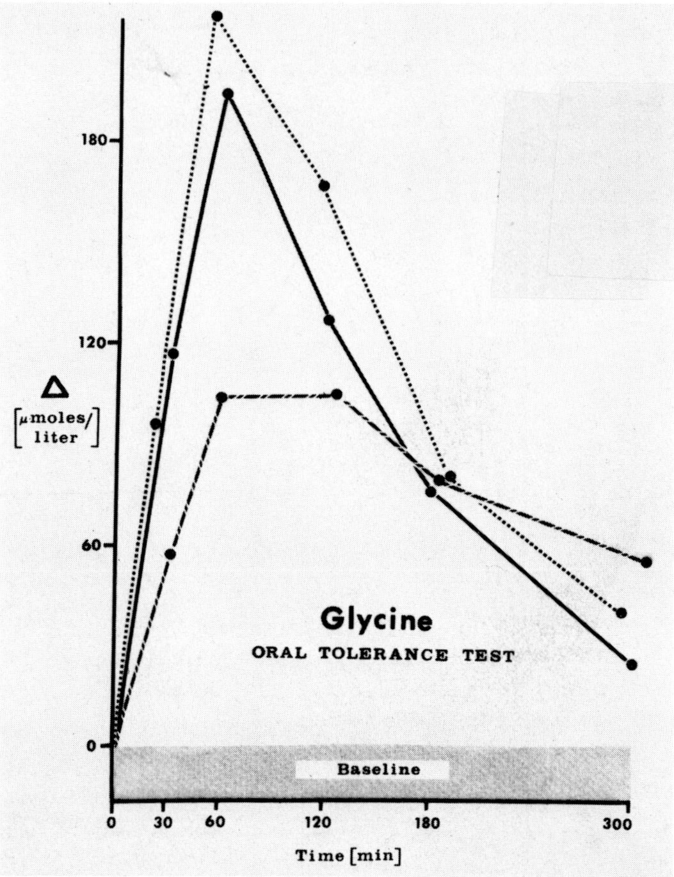

Fig. 3. Oral amino acid tolerance test. Absorption curves up to five hours following ingestion of glycine preoperatively (solid line), during intensive weight loss (hatched line), and following weight stabilization (dotted line). Values are presented as elevations above basal levels.

one patient by Warren.[27] Presumably, intestinal adaptation following small bowel bypass was insufficient in these patients so that a state of severe residual protein malnutrition occurred. It should be pointed out, however, that improvement in protein nutrition and, by inference, adequate intestinal adaptation has been observed in the vast majority of the patients we have studied and in those reported in the literature.

Hepatic fibrosis is not common in patients with kwashiorkor and has been reported only infrequently following small bowel bypass for obesity. Experimentally, hepatic fibrosis has been more easily produced in nutritionally deprived animals with fatty livers than in otherwise normal animals. Whether a state of continuing severe hepatic steatosis and protein malnutrition permits fibrosis to supervene under the influence of hepatotoxic substances, such as certain bile salts, is under investigation. Whatever the reason for the hepatic fibrosis which may supervene in a small percentage of bowel bypass patients, a careful watch must be maintained for those at risk. Such patients are characterized by severe rapid weight loss, significant electrolyte disturbances, and progressive deterioration of liver function demonstrated by test results. Continued marked hepatic steatosis without reversion to preoperative morphology and with addition of significant fibrosis on serial liver biopsies should encourage plasma amino acid assay. Evidence of continued protein malnutrition without improvement in the face of continued hepatic damage and progressive fibrosis should prompt reanastomosis.

Finally, if protein malnutrition underlies the fatty liver changes following small bowel bypass, then amino acid supplementation should help avoid or improve them. McClelland and associates have shown in laboratory and limited clinical studies[14] that this may apply. Such supplementation is under investigation.

REFERENCES

1. Aoyama, Y., Nakanishi, M., and Ashida, K.: Effect of methionine on liver lipid metabolism of rats fed a protein-free diet, J. Nutr. **103:** 54, 1973.
2. Block, W. D., Markovs, M. E., and Steele, B. F.: Comparison between free amino acid levels in plasma deproteinated with picric acid and with sulfosalicylic acid, Proc. Soc. Exp. Biol. Med. **122:** 1089, 1966.
3. Brown, R. G., O'Leary, J. P., and Woodward, E. R.: Hepatic effects of jejunoileal bypass for morbid obesity, Am. J. Surg. **127:** 53, 1974.
4. Buchwald, H., Lober, P. H., and Varco, R. L.: Liver biopsy findings in seventy-seven consecutive patients undergoing jejunoileal bypass for morbid obesity, Am. J. Surg. **127:** 48, 1974.
5. Bury, K. D.: Carbohydrate digestion and absorption after massive resection of the small intestine, Surg. Gynecol. Obstet. **135:** 177, 1972.
6. Chanda, N. K.: Pathological study of the liver in kwashiorkor, Br. Med. J. **1:** 1263, 1958.
7. Drenick, E. J., Simmons, F., and Murphy, J. F.: Effect on hepatic morphology of treatment of obesity by fasting, reducing diets and small bowel bypass, N. Engl. J. Med. **282:** 829, 1970.
8. Edozien, J. C.: Enzymes in serum in kwashiorkor, Pediatrics **27:** 325, 1961.
9. Holzback, R. T., Wieland, R. G., Lieber, C. S., DeCarli, L. M., Koepke, K. R., and Green, S. G.: Hepatic lipid in morbid obesity, N. Engl. J. Med. **290:** 296, 1974.
10. Juhl, E., Christoffersen, P., Baden, H., and Quaade, F.: Liver morphology and biochemistry in eight obese patients treated with jejunoileal anastomosis, N. Engl. J. Med. **285:** 543, 1971.
11. Lewis, L. A., Turnbull, R. B., and Page, I. H.: Effects of jejunocolic shunt on obesity, serum lipoprotenis, lipids, and electrolytes, Arch. Intern. Med. **117:** 4, 1966.
12. Lyman, R. L., Cook, C. R., and Williams, M. A.: Liver lipid accumulation in isoleucine-deficient rats, J. Nutr. **82:** 432, 1964.
13. MacDonald, I., Hansen, J. D. L., and Bronte-Stewart, B.: Liver, depot, and serum lipids during early recovery from kwashiorkor, Clin. Sci. **24:** 55, 1963.
14. McClelland, R. N., DeShazo, C. V., Heimbach, D. M., Eigenbrodt, E. H., and Dowdy, A. B. C.: Prevention of hepatic injury after jejuno-ileal bypass by supplemental jejunostomy feedings, Surg. Forum **21:** 368, 1970.
15. McLaren, D. S., Faris, R., and Zekian, B.: The liver during recovery from protein-calorie malnutrition, Am. J. Clin. Nutr. **20:** 271, 1968.
16. McLean, A. E. M.: Hepatic failure in malnutrition, Lancet **2:** 1292, 1962.

16a. Morley, R. T., et al.: N. Engl. J. Med. **290:** 921, 1974.

17. Padilla, H., Sanchez, A., Powell, R. N., Umezana, C., Swendseid, M. E., Prado, P. M., and Sigala, R.: Plasma amino acids in children from Guadalajara with kwashiorkor, Am. J. Clin. Nutr. **24:** 353, 1971.
18. Rehfeld, J. F., Juhl, E., and Quaade, F.: Effect of jejunoileostomy on glucose and insulin metabolism in ten obese patients, Metabolism **19:** 529, 1970.
19. Rozental, P., Biava, C., Spencer, H., and Zimmerman, H. J.: Liver morphology and function tests in obesity and during total starvation, Am. J. Dig. Dis. **12:** 198, 1967.
20. Salmon, P. A.: The results of small intestine bypass for operations for the treatment of obesity, Surg. Gynecol. Obstet. **132:** 965, 1971.
21. Sanders, G. B.: In Discussion of Scott, H. W., Jr., et al.: New considerations in use of jejunoileal bypass in patients with morbid obesity, Ann. Surg. **177:** 733, 1973.
22. Saunders, S. J.: Plasma-free amino acid pattern in protein-calorie malnutrition, Lancet **2:** 795, 1967.
23. Scott, H. W., Jr., Dean, R., Shull, H. J., Abram, H. S., Webb, W., Younger, R. K., and Brill, A. B.: New considerations in use of jejunoileal bypass in patients with morbid obesity, Ann. Surg. **177:** 723, 1973.
24. Shibata, H. R., Mackenzie, J. R., and Huang, S.: Morphologic changes of the liver following small intestinal bypass for obesity, Arch. Surg. **103:** 229, 1971.
25. Singal, S. A., Hazan, S. J., Sydenstricker, V. P., and Littlejohn, J. M.: The production of fatty livers in rats on threonine- and lysine-deficient diets, J. Biol. Chem. **200:** 867, 1973.

26. Spackman, D. H., Stein, W. H., and Moore, S.: Automatic recording apparatus for use in the chromatography of amino acids, Anal. Chem. **30:** 1190, 1958.
27. Warren, W. D.: In Discussion of Scott, H. W., Jr., et al.: New considerations in use of jejunoileal bypass in patients with morbid obesity, Ann. Surg. **177:** 734, 1973.
28. Weismann, R. E.: Surgical palliation of massive and severe obesity, Am. J. Surg. **125:** 437, 1972.
29. Wilfred, G., and Sekhara Varma, T. N.: The mechanism of hepatic infiltration in acute threonine deficiency, Biochem. Biophys. Acta **187:** 442, 1969.
30. Wilmore, D. W., and Holtzapple, G.: Structure and function of intestinal epithelial cells from compensated small bowel following massive intestinal resection, J. Surg. Oncol. **4:** 454, 1972.

DISCUSSION

Dr. Marshall J. Orloff (San Diego, Calif.). I am not sure that small bowel bypass is going to result in permanent benefit to morbidly obese patients. However, one thing is certain: It presents one of the most elegant models for the study of gastrointestinal physiology in man that we have come upon in recent years, and it certainly is the human counterpart of the traditional experimental model that has been studied so much in the dog for evaluating gastric hypersecretion.

We have studied a small number of patients who have had the bypass; we have measured basal acid and Histalog-stimulated acid, much as this other group has. We have found no increases in basal or in Histalog-stimulated acid secretion, and I think that Dr. Buchwald would agree that even though they found a statistically significant increase in Histalog-stimulated secretion, it really was not a very impressive increase, and a sizable number of their patients had no increase at all.

But I think that both of us have gone about this in the wrong way. What we should be studying is the intestinal phase of gastric secretion. We are talking about the possibility of one or more jejunal or jejunal and ileal hormones which influence gastric secretion; yet we study the patients in the fasting state or after Histalog stimulation.

Therefore I would like to urge the Minnesota group, which now has accumulated a large experience with these operations, both for hypercholesterolemia and for obesity, to take advantage of the opportunity to study the patients in the intestinal phase, either by studying their response to a meal, for which the technique is now well established and which we had not been able to use for years, or by evaluating gastric secretion stimulated by installing food into the jejunum by means of a long tube of some sort. I think that we might find some very striking increases in gastric secretion.

Prof. Richard Welbourne (London, England). Kwashiorkor is very rare in the adult, and I had the opportunity of studying several patients in detail some years ago. Our patients, like Dr. White's, had deficiency of essential amino acids. They had quite a number of other things which I would like to ask Dr. White about. Ours had very low total protein and albumin levels in the blood. You did not give us your data on these. Could you tell us, Dr. White?

Second, ours had a constant pattern of clinical features, and I wonder if these patients did too. They had, of course, loss of weight, and your patients lost weight, because that is what you were intending to do. They also had weakness, a protein deficiency anemia, edema, mental changes which were characteristic, changes in the hair, including partial baldness and loss of pigment in the remaining hair. They also had diarrhea, stomatitis, and a dry skin.

You told us the results of many studies of hepatic function. Our patients also had increased retention of BSP. They had a deficiency of the enzyme urokinase, which is rather characteristic of kwashiorkor in infants, and they all had evidence of impaired synthesis of protein by the liver.

Now, our patients had all had a gastrectomy, and either a stagnant loop with intestinal overgrowth in it or pancreatic insufficiency was found. It seems to me possible that after these operations the remaining small bowel, or the defunctioning small bowel, might become colonized with bacteria.

You mentioned the possibility that the liver might go on to fibrosis. If you are worried that it is doing harm, if it is producing any of these rather distressing clinical features, it might be worthwhile infusing the patients with albumin intravenously. We did this, and we found that it caused complete cure of this syndrome temporarily, until we put it right permanently either by operation or by replacement of pancreatic enzymes.

I think it would be very nice indeed to look at GIP, the gastric inhibitory peptide, and VIP, the vasoactive intestinal polypeptide in Dr. Buchwald's patients. We can measure both of them, and both are capable of inhibiting gastric secretion.

Dr. James C. Thompson (Galveston, Texas). The first question is whether or not these patients hypersecrete. It seems to me that 16.7 mEq. per hour is a very particular way of defining hypersecretion, and it may have to do with the control series that was utilized in establishing that level in the laboratory. Across the country, I think a level of something like 35 mEq. would be required to designate hypersecretion, which would be more than twice that.

If, indeed, there is a hypersecretion, there is very likely a mechanism that may be involved, and that is: In some recent studies in our laboratory that Dr. Becker reported in *Gastroenterology,* the small bowel is found to be an important catabolic site for gastrin. It does not catabolize basal levels of gastrin, but it does catabolize stimulated levels of gastrin by about 40 percent.

Dr. McGuigan's group reported recently that resection of 90 percent of the dog's small bowel caused a hypergastrinemia, and Rosiello has a paper that will come out in *Gastroenterology* next month that reports high levels of gastrin in patients following massive small bowel resection. It may well be that the small bowel is a major site of gastrin catabolism and that loss of it by resection or diminished circulation following defunctionalization may result in a diminished level of gastrin, and I would like to know if Dr. Buchwald has gastrin levels on these patients pre- and postoperatively.

I do not mean that this problem is simple. We have resected 90 percent of the dog's small intestine and can show hypergastrinemia in only about a third of our animals.

Dr. John R. Benfield (Torrance, Calif.). Have your patients had the same decrease in appetite and changes in the types of foods for which they crave as ours? If your patients have had these changes, I wonder whether such changes in appetite might in part account for the hepatic failure or the hepatic sequelae which you and others are observing.

Prof. Lars Semb (Oslo, Norway). It might be that there is a low serum potassium in some of Dr. Buchwald's patients, explaining why some were not becoming hypersecretors.

I would like to ask if there are any dose-response curves in these patients, to see if their sensitivity to any of the commonly used stimulants is changed.

Dr. Henry Buchwald (closing). I agree that jejunoileal bypass may not cause clinically significant hypersecretion. I think that was one of the very points of our paper. It has, unfortunately, been assumed by many people, that hypersecretion will occur in a large number of individuals, if not all individuals, after massive small intestinal loss. This unwarranted conclusion is based on patients who come in with hypersecretion in the postoperative state, having catastrophically lost their intestinal tract.

Our patients were studied pre- and postoperatively. We did not see a hypersecretion syndrome that is predictable, that is clinically significant, and that may even be chemically significant.

We are performing additional studies at this time on gastrin release mechanisms and on the serum gastrin level in our patients.

One of the purposes of showing the slides of secretogogues versus inhibitor substance is that, at this time, to us, there is no theory that can explain it all. All are inferential. By definition, three quarters of the work that was presented has to be discredited in the future; and we will see who ends up on the side of the angels.

The main purpose of our presentation was not to take any side whatsoever, but just to show that in a unique human model this hypersecretion occurred. If we take that 16.7 level when you have a massive bypass situation, and it does not occur in a limited distal one-third bypass. And I think either the secretogogue or the inhibtor theory could fit.

Our experience at this time with jejunoileal bypass for obesity extends to approximately 300 patients, and we have not been impressed that these individuals changes their dietary habits postoperatively. On the contrary, I think many of them eat more. They have a cetrain sense of liberty and freedom, and we have measured their calorie counts in the hospital, and this can go as high as 8,000 to 9,000 calories per day.

The electrolytes in these patients were not abnormal at any time of their determinations pre- or postoperatively.

Dr. John J. White (closing). We have looked at the proteins and the albumins, but these have not been significantly altered in our series. We did not do BSP tests because of the large quantities of dye that are required in these large people. We did not study the urokinase deficiencies.

I have no feeling for whether the bypass loop is colonized. I agree with Dr. Buchwald that in 95 percent of the patients who have the bypass and in 90 percent of patients who have kwashiorkor, the fatty liver itself does no harm. Fibrosis is not unknown. We had only one patient who showed signs of persistent kwashiorkor. I think the reason why it usually does no harm is that kwashiorkor is a transient phenomenon that improves as bowel adaptation takes place. Our one patient was a lady who relentlessly lost and progressively lost weight. Her liver biopsies did show some fibrosis. At this point, she is one of the few of our patients who have shown fibrosis, and her amino acid profiles kept going downhill till they had reached the profile of the patient with severe kwashiorkor. We did an intestinal reanastomosis on her, and she has done well.

I think that I would suggest that in those patients in whom serial biopsies are showing progression or maintenance of the marked hepatic metamorphosis, amino acid curves or tolerance profiles be obtained; if you have a persistent picture of kwashiorkor, this might be another indicator of the group that may require anastomosis.

We have, noticed that there is a decrease in the appetite of most of our patients. This decrease seems to take place immediately following the operation, and I do not know whether it is due to loss of a large segment of functioning gut, whether it is psychologic, or whether it is for other reasons. We do know, too, that in many of our patients there is a tremendous loss of sexual appetite. As you are aware, most of these very obese people have voracious appetites sexually as well. This appetite is also lost and constitutes one of our main psychosocial problems postoperatively with the group of patients we have treated.

Serum calcium, serum gastrin, and gastric acid secretion before and after parathyroidectomy for hyperparathyroidism

John F. Stremple, M.D., F.A.C.S., *and* **Charles G. Watson, M.D., F.A.C.S.,** *Pittsburgh, Pa.*

One patient with hyperparathyroidism had a mean systemic serum gastrin before parathyroidectomy of 2,035 pg. per milliliter, a parathyroid adenoma tissue gastrin content of 16,216 pg. per milligram (16,216,000 pg. gastrin per 1 Gm. adenoma); and a postoperative mean systemic serum gastrin level of 350 pg. per milliliter. The high tissue gastrin content in the parathyroid adenoma removed from this patient with hyperparathyroidism, as determined by radioimmunoassay and immunofluorescence, and the decrease in serial serum gastrin measurements after its removal demonstrated that this parathyroid adenoma was also the source of gastrin; it was a parathyroid gastrinoma. Fourteen other patients with hyperparathyroidism but without duodenal ulcer had a decrease in mean serum calcium which was accompanied by a decrease in mean serum gastrin after parathyroidectomy. Gastric acid secretion was low and not significantly different both before and after parathyroidectomy. Three other patients with hyperparathyroidism and duodenal ulcer had gastric secretory findings markedly different than those without ulcer. Their gastric secretory findings were similar to those associated with peptic ulcer without hyperparathyroidism.

From the Department of Surgery, University of Pittsburgh, Pittsburgh, Pa.

HYPERPARATHYROIDISM (HPT) has been associated with increased gastric acid,[6, 9] pepsin,[5] and serum gastrin.[9] After parathyroidectomy, gastric acid,[6, 9, 24] pepsin,[5] serum gastrin,[9] and calcium[2] (Ca^{++}) all decrease, but peptic ulcer may or may not be ameliorated.[1, 3, 21, 22, 26, 30, 38] A causal relation between these changes in serum calcium, serum gastrin, and gastric acid,[9, 39] and the increased incidence of peptic ulcer (eight to 87 percent)[1] in association with HPT has been suggested.[9, 38] Dent and co-workers[9] have found that serum gastrin falls after parathyroidectomy and suggested an extragastric source of gastrin in HPT. Friesen[10] and others[18-20, 22, 23, 30-32, 41] have reviewed the variety of unusual clinical manifestations of multiple endocrine adenomatosis (MEA) and pointed out the genetic, embryologic,[40] and cytochemical[27] similarities which may result in the production of the same hormone by many different tumors. So far, parathyroid tumors have been found to secrete parathyroid hormone (PTH) and possibly ACTH.[29] The purposes of this study are to determine if a parathyroid adenoma like the nonbeta-islet cell tumor of the pancreas might also produce gastrin and, in addition, to determine the relation of serum Ca^{++}, serum gastrin, and gastric acid secretion to the presence or absence of associated ulcer in patients with HPT.

Presented at the Thirty-fifth Annual Meeting of the Society of University Surgeons, St. Louis, Mo., Feb. 14-16, 1974.

Reprint requests: J. F. Stremple, M.D., Veterans Administration Hospital, University Drive, Pittsburgh, Pa. 15240.

PATIENTS AND METHODS

A total of 19 patients with primary HPT were studied before and after parathyroidec-

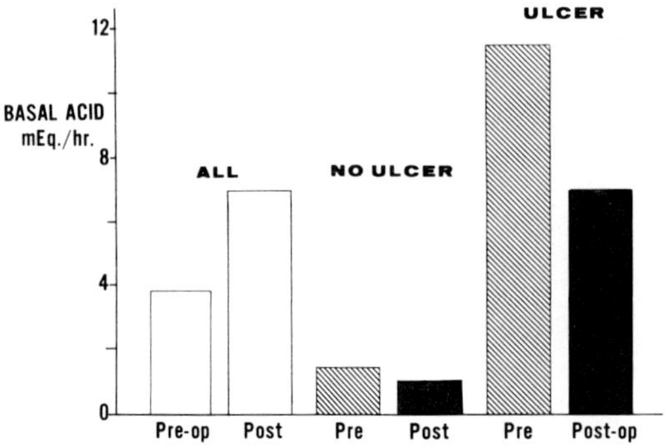

Fig. 1. Mean basal gastric acid secretion in patients (n = 17) with HPT. Note the low acid levels both before and after parathyroidectomy in patients without ulcer as compared to those with duodenal ulcer.

tomy. There were ten women (average age, 51 years) and nine men (average age, 44 years). Fourteen patients had HPT without gastric (GU) or duodenal ulcers (DU). Three of these 14 patients had primary parathyroid hyperplasia rather than adenoma. Three patients had HPT as the result of adenoma with DU. In addition, there were two individuals who are considered separately because they had elevated basal serum gastrins. One of these with elevated serum gastrin had HPT and both GU and DU. Another patient had markedly elevated serum gastrin levels in the Zollinger-Ellison (ZE) range with HPT but no basal acid or ulcer.

Each patient had both basal (BAO) and maximum histamine-stimulated (MAO) gastric acid secretion rate determined at least once both before and after parathyroidectomy. Nasogastric tubes were positioned in the stomach with the use of fluoroscopy. Basal gastric juice secretion was collected for two hours. Each patient was then given Benadryl (50 mg., given intramuscularly) and then histamine acid phosphate (0.04 mg. per kilogram of body weight) subcutaneously. Gastric juice specimens were collected separately for eight consecutive 15 minute periods. Determinations of gastric acid output per hour were made from the volume and titration with 0.1 NaOH to pH 7 with a pH meter. Samples of peripheral venous blood were taken for serum gastrin determinations during the basal period and at the peak acid output after histamine stimulation. Serum samples were frozen so that all serum gastrin determinations could be done simultaneously. Each gastrin determination was done in triplicate and repeated twice by two different technicians. Each patient had at least four determinations of serum gastrin, PTH, and Ca^{++} before parathyroidectomy and again after parathyroidectomy over a period up to one year. The methods used for the radioimmunoassay of serum gastrin[33] and PTH[8, 28] have been published elsewhere. Parathyroid tumor was obtained in the operating room in seven of the 19 patients. A portion of the parathyroid tumor was immediately frozen. Several sections were saved for formalin fixation and examination by light microscopy. The remainder of the frozen parathyroid tumor was used for determination of tissue gastrin content by the radioimmunoassay and immunofluorescent methods of Greider and McGuigan.[15] PTH is a polypeptide which contains 84 amino acid residues; the first 45 are those necessary for biologic and immunologic activity.[14] PTH should not cross-react with gastrin in our radioimmunoassay system because the amino acid sequences of these two hormones are known and entirely different.[4]

RESULTS

The normal serum PTH is less than 4.0 ng. per milliliter. In patients with HPT without DU, the preoperative mean serum PTH was elevated at 6.2 ± S.E. 2.8 ng. per milliliter and postoperatively decreased to 3.8 ± 1.0 ng. per milliliter. In patients with HPT accompanied by DU, the preoperative mean serum PTH was elevated at 6.7 ± 2.5 ng. per milliliter and postoperatively decreased to 2.5 ± 0.8 ng. per milliliter, as did the patients without ulcer.

In those patients with HPT but without DU, the preoperative mean serum Ca^{++} was increased at 12.2 ± 0.07 mg. per 100 ml. and postoperatively decreased to 9.1 ± 0.5 mg. per 100 ml. In patients with both HPT and DU, the preoperative mean serum Ca^{++} was

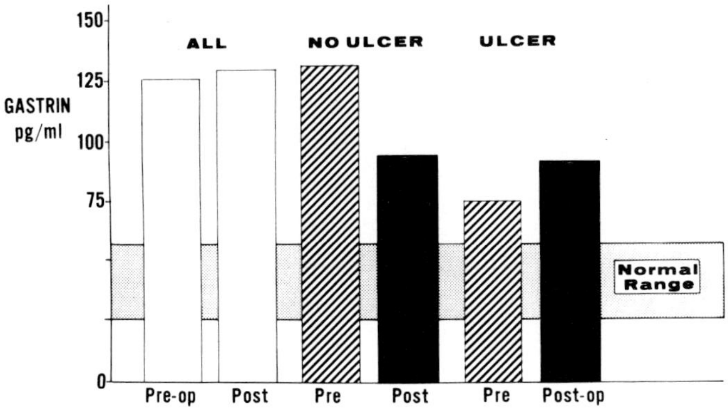

Fig. 2. Mean basal serum gastrin in patients (n = 17) with HPT. Note the decrease in mean serum gastrin after parathyroidectomy in patients without ulcer as compared to the slight increase in those with ulcer.

increased at 11.8 ± 1.0 mg. per 100 ml. and decreased postoperatively to 9.2 ± 0.7 mg. per 100 ml., exactly as did the patients without ulcer.

The normal BAO in our laboratory is 2.1 ± 1.5 mEq. per hour and 4.6 ± 2.1 mEq. per hour in patients with proved DU without HPT. In patients with HPT but no DU, the preoperative mean BAO was 1.4 ± 0.8 mEq. per hour, and postoperatively the mean BAO did not change, remaining at 1.0 ± 0.6 mEq. per hour. In three patients with both HPT and DU, the preoperative mean BAO was markedly elevated at 11.5 ± 3.2 mEq. per hour, and the postoperative mean BAO fell moderately to 6.6 ± 0.9 mEq. per hour (Fig. 1). MAO was elevated only in those with both HPT and DU before operation and not significantly different after parathyroidectomy.

The normal mean basal serum gastrin in our laboratory is 36 ± 18 pg. per milliliter. In 37 patients with proved DU, but without HPT the mean basal serum gastrin is 47 ± 31 pg. per milliliter in our laboratory. Levels above 1,000 pg. per milliliter are found in Zollinger-Ellison (ZE) syndrome and pernicious anemia. In those patients with HPT, but without DU, the preoperative mean basal serum gastrin was 132 ± 20 pg. per milliliter. Postoperatively, the mean basal serum gastrin decreased moderately to 94 ± 10 pg. per milliliter. In three patients with both HPT and DU, the preoperative mean basal serum gastrin was 75 ± 18 pg. per milliliter. Postoperatively, the mean basal serum gastrin increased to 93 ± 15 pg. per milliliter, in contrast to HPT patients without DU, in which the postoperative level fell (Fig. 2). Histamine-stimulated mean serum gastrin levels were not significantly different from basal levels in either group and did not change after parathyroidectomy.

The three patients with HPT due to parathyroid hyperplasia without DU had a preoperative mean basal serum gastrin of 50 pg. per milliliter and a postoperative mean basal serum gastrin of 65 pg. per milliliter, essentially no change. In contrast, the 11 patients with HPT due to parathyroid adenoma without DU had a preoperative mean basal serum gastrin of 140 pg. per milliliter and postoperatively decreased to a mean basal serum gastrin of 105 pg. per milliliter. These results indicate that serum gastrin decreases postoperatively in those patients with HPT and parathyroid adenoma but not in those with HPT and parathyroid hyperplasia.

There were two patient with elevated serum gastrins considered separately. One of these, patient G. L., a 45-year-old woman with HPT and both GU and DU had a mean serum gastrin of 400 pg. per milliliter, a BAO of 14.7 mEq. per hour, and a mean serum Ca^{++} of 11.9 mg. per 100 ml. before operation. After parathyroidectomy, this patient had a mean serum gastrin of 572 pg. per milliliter, a BAO of 15.8 mEq. per hour, and a mean serum Ca^{++} of 10.0 mg. per 100 ml. This patient continued to have severe

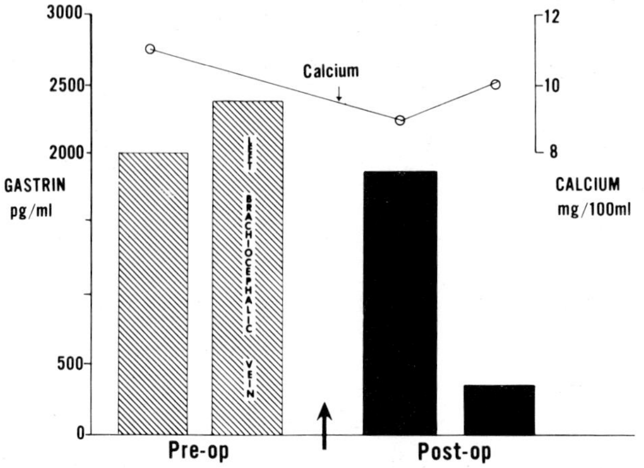

Fig. 3. Changes in serum gastrin levels in patient O. C. before and after parathyroidectomy. This patient had a gastrinoma of the parathyroid gland.

Table I. *Serum vs. tissue gastrin in hyperparathyroidism**

	Hyperparathyroidism			
Gastrin	*ZE syndrome range*	*Duodenal ulcer*	*No ulcer*	*No hyperthyroidism—with ZE syndrome*
Patients	1	2	4	1
Preop. serum (pg./ml.)	2,035	75	132	2,400
Tissue				
Parathyroid (pg./mg.)	16,216	4	5	
Per 1 Gm. adenoma	16,216,000	4,000	5,000	
Pancreas (pg./mg.)				136-
ZE tumor (pg./mg.)				133,000

*Mean serum and tissue content, as determined by radioimmunoassay, in patients with normal levels of basal serum gastrin and HPT compared to patient O. C. with HPT and a patient without HPT but with the ZE syndrome.

ulcer symptoms and required a vagotomy and antrectomy ten months after parathyroidectomy. In this patient with HPT in whom the serum gastrin levels and gastric acid secretion did not fall after parthyroidectomy, the ulcer apparently was not causally related to the HPT.

The second patient considered separately, O. C., a 54-year-old woman, had HPT and a markedly elevated mean basal serum gastrin (Fig. 3). Before parathyroidectomy, mean serum Ca^{++} was 11.0 mg. per 100 ml. and mean basal systemic serum gastrin was 2,035 pg. per milliliter. The patient had basal achlorhydria but was not stimulated by histamine because of severe asthma. Upper gastrointestinal and gastroscopic examinations showed no evidence of ulcer. The patient had a family history of ulcer diathesis but had no history of HPT. The patient did not have the hematologic stigmata of pernicious anemia. One week before removal of a left parathyroid adenoma, a blood sample from the left brachiocephalic vein was obtained with a serum gastrin level of 2,375 pg. per milliliter while in a peripheral vein the level was significantly lower at 2,035 pg. per milliliter. On Nov. 22, 1972, the left parathyroid adenoma was removed. The left parathyroid adenoma had a tissue gastrin content of 16,216 pg. per milligram or 16,216,000 pg. per 1 Gm. of adenoma. Three

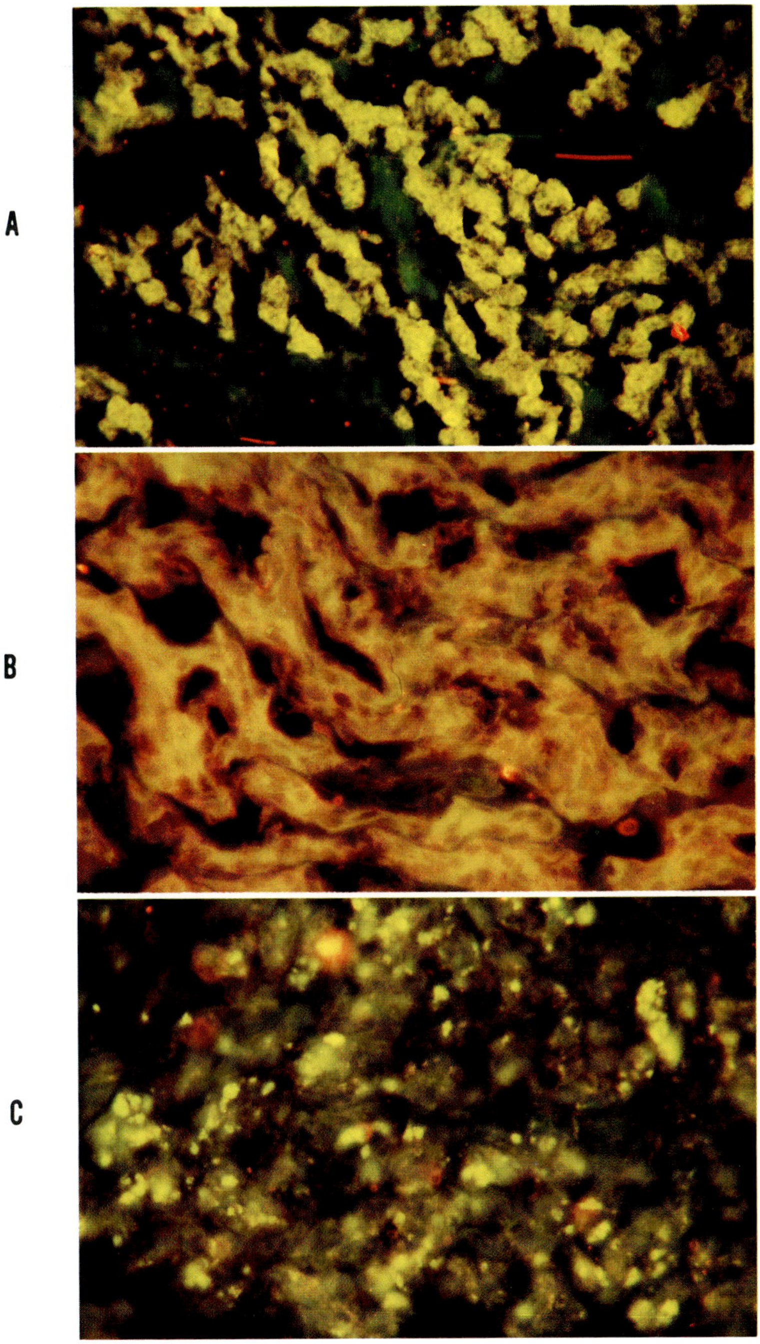

Fig. 4. Fluorescent micrographs of unfixed, cryostat-cut sections stained with fluorescinated antibodies to gastrin. *A,* Parathyroid gastrinoma removed from patient O. C. with HPT and markedly elevated serum gastrin. The cytoplasm of cells corresponding to chief cells by hematoxylin and eosin stain were brightly fluorescent specifically due to the presence of gastrin. (×53.) *B,* Parathyroid adenoma removed from a different patient with HPT and relatively normal serum gastrin. The cytoplasm of the cells showed only reddish-yellow nonspecific background autofluorescence. (×132.) *C,* Gastrinoma of the pancreas removed from a different patient with the Zollinger-Ellison syndrome without HPT. The cytoplasm of the tumor cells were brightly fluorescent specifically due to the presence of gastrin. (×53.)

months after removal of the parathyroid adenoma, mean basal serum gastrin had fallen slightly to 1,757 pg. per milliliter and mean serum Ca^{++} was normal at 8.7 mg. per 100 ml. Twelve months following removal of the parathyroid adenoma, the patient continued to have basal achlorhydria, but mean basal serum gastrin had fallen significantly in three separate determinations to 350 pg. per milliliter. Serum Ca^{++} remained normal at 10.0 mg. per 100 ml.

Table I shows the mean of determinations of serum gastrin and parathyroid tissue gastrin content in patient O. C. with HPT and markedly elevated serum gastrin. Her findings are compared to those of six other patients with HPT and normal serum gastrin levels, two with and four without DU. Table I also included the serum gastrin and tissue gastrin content found in a patient with a ZE syndrome without HPT.

Parathyroid tissue gastrin content determined by radioimmunoassay correlated with the intensity of gastrin immunofluorescence of the same parathyroid tumors (Fig. 4). Light microscopy showed no cytologic differences.

DISCUSSION

The variety of reported changes in gastric acid secretion and serum gastrin levels before and after parathyroidectomy for HPT has suggested a complex relationship.[9] This relationship becomes somewhat less complex if patients with HPT are separated into those with and without ulcer instead of being grouped together. Those with parathyroid adenoma should be also separated from those with hyperplasia. Patients with HPT and with elevated serum gastrin levels must also be studied separately.

Our data confirm the previously reported[9] increase in serum gastrin in patients with HPT without ulcer and the decrease in serum gastrin after parathyroidectomy. Our data do not confirm an increased BAO in patients with HPT without ulcer before parathyroidectomy or a significant decrease in BAO after parathyroidectomy associated with the fall in serum Ca^{++}. Similar to the findings of Ward and colleagues,[38] our three patients with both HPT and DU had gastric secretory findings markedly different from those without DU both before and after parathyroidectomy. Gastric secretory findings were similar to those associated with duodenal ulcer without HPT.[33, 36] In our patients with both HPT and DU, the calcium fell postoperatively, but serum gastrin and gastric acid levels remained elevated. It seems unlikely that HPT is causally related to the peptic ulcer through hypercalcemia. Duodenal ulcer may be a coincidental event in conjunction with HPT.

Decreases in gastric acid and serum gastrin have also been reported after parathyroidectomy in patients with both HPT and the ZE syndrome.[36, 37] Patient G. L. with HPT and both GU and DU had elevated gastric acid secretion and serum gastrin levels not definitely diagnostic for the presence of a ZE tumor. After parathyroidectomy and also vagotomy and antrectomy, both gastric acid secretion and serum gastrin remained elevated, and the patient has continued to have ulcer symptoms. This patient may yet prove to have an occult gastrinoma of the pancreas. This patient may also fit into the MEA–peptic ulcer complex described by Ballard and associates,[1] in whom 87 percent had HPT and peptic ulcer. In patients with this syndrome, the clinical picture is similar to those with the ZE syndrome. The ulcers are multiple and in atypical locations, and they are complicated even in the absence of a gastrinoma of the pancreas.

Decreases in gastric acid and serum gastrin have also been reported in patients after parathyroidectomy for HPT with either achlorhydria or acid hypersecretion and hypergastrinemia in the ZE range but without gastrinoma of the pancreas (pseudo-ZE).[9] Patient O. C. first presented with a markedly elevated serum gastrin in the ZE range, basal achlorhydria, and HPT before removal of a parathyroid adenoma, but postoperatively her serum gastrin has fallen significantly. The parathyroid adenoma was found to have a very high tissue gastrin content. Because the patient had no gastric acid, it is unlikely that there was concomitantly present a ZE tumor which secreted gastrin. It is also unlikely that elevated serum gastrin levels before parathyroidectomy were entirely due to failure of acid inhibition of antral gastrin release.[7, 12] Serum gastrin levels decreased to very low levels, considering that the patient remained achlorhydric. The time lag for a marked decrease in serum gastrin may be accounted for by an initial release of feedback inhibition of the antrum after removal of the parathyroid gastrinoma.[10] Antral gastrin (G)-cell hyperplasia and increased antral gastrin release may accompany peptic ulcer or hyperparathyroidism.[10a, 12a, 27a] The later decrease to near normal serum gastrin may be speculated as reverse corollary to the reported visible regression of gastrinoma of the pancreas and the slow decline in elevated serum gastrin levels to near normal after total gastrectomy or parathyroidectomy.[25, 36]

It seems clear that patients with HPT may occasionally present with elevated serum gastrin levels similar to those found with the ZE syndrome. This may suggest to the clinician a need for total gastrectomy. Others[9, 37] have suggested that a parathyroidectomy should be done first, and patients with elevated serum gastrin after parathyroidectomy should be followed closely for the possibility of harboring a gastrinoma of the pancreas. In view of our additional evidence that a parathyroid adenoma associated with HPT may also produce gastrin, this seems to be good advice.

A gastric secretagogue has not been found in the parathyroid gland by gastrin bioassay techniques previously used.[17, 34, 43] The more sensitive gastrin radioimmunoassay technique has been used by several investigators to quantitate the gastrin content of normal[15] and tumor tissue[35] from the pancreas. Our results with pancreatic tissues have been similar (Table I). These techniques have now been applied to parathyroid tissue. We have found a patient with HPT whose parathyroid tumor, the vein draining it, and the systemic blood have contained excessive amounts of gastrin. The amount of gastrin found in the parathyroid adenoma and serum was elevated to levels comparable to those in gastrinoma of the pancreas (ZE syndrome). After removal of the parathyroid adenoma, serum gastrin returned to normal. Gastrin was found only in the cytoplasm of the chief cells and not in the oxyphil cells of this parathyroid adenoma by immunofluorescence. Gastrin can now be added to the list of hormones secreted by a parathyroid adenoma.

ADDENDUM

On March 6, 7, and 8, 1974, now 17 months after removal of the parathyroid gastrinoma, patient O. C. had additional studies. Mean serum Ca^{++} has remained normal at 9.2 mg. per 100 ml. for these three consecutive days. Mean basal serum gastrin has decreased from 350 to 125 pg. per milliliter for three separate determinations. Fifteen minutes after beef broth stimulation, mean serum gastrin was 295 pg. per milliliter for three separate determinations. Basal and Histalog-stimulated gastric acid determinations were performed. Again, bile reflux but no measurable gastric acid was found. Gastroscopy showed grossly normal appearing gastric mucosa. Five separate gastric mucosal biopsies from the fundus and three from the antrum showed chronic gastritis. Numerous parietal cells were found in the fundus. Antral gastrin (G)-cell hyperplasia was demonstrated by both toluidine blue staining and gastrin immunofluorescence. Results of serum vitamin B_{12} level and Schilling test were normal. The chronic gastritis was probably due to bile reflux.

REFERENCES

1. Ballard, H., Frame, B., and Harstock, R: Familial multiple endocrine adenoma—peptic ulcer complex, Medicine **43:** 481, 1964.
2. Berreras, R.: Calcium and gastric secretion, Gastroenterology **64:** 1168, 1973.
3. Black, B.: Primary hyperparathyroidism and peptic ulcer, Surg. Clin. North Am. **51:** 955, 1971.
4. Brewer, H., and Ronan, R.: Bovine parathyroid hormone: Amino acid sequence, Proc. Natl. Acad. Sci. **67:** 1862, 1970.
5. Christiansen, J.: Gastric secretion of pepsin in patients with primary hyperparathyroidism before and after removal of parathyroid adenomas, Scand. J. Gastroenterol. **8:** 337, 1973.
6. Christiansen, J., and Aagaard, P.: Parathyroid adenoma and gastric acid secretion, Scand. J. Gastroenterol. **7:** 445, 1972.
7. Creutzfeldt, W., Arnold, R., and Creutzfeldt, C.: Gastrin and G-cells in the antral mucosa

of patients with pernicious anemia, acromegaly and hyperparathyroidism and in Zollinger-Ellison tumor of pancreas, Eur. J. Clin. Invest. **1:** 461, 1971.
8. Desbuquouis, B., and Aurbach, G.: Use of polyethylene glycol for radioimmunoassay, J. Clin. Endocrinol. Metab. **33:** 732, 1971.
9. Dent, R., James, J., Wang, C., Deftos, L., Talamo, R., and Fischer, J.: Hyperparathyroidism: Gastric acid secretion and gastrin, Ann. Surg. **176:** 360, 1972.
10. Friesen, S.: Zollinger-Ellison syndrome, *in* Ravitch, M., editor: Current problems in surgery, Chicago, 1972, Year Book Medical Publishers, Inc., p. 29.
10a. Friesen, S.: Personal communication.
11. Friesen, S., Bolinger, R., Pearse, A., and McGuigan, J.: Serum gastrin levels in malignant Zollinger-Ellison syndrome after total gastrectomy and hypophysectomy, Ann. Surg. **172:** 504, 1970.
12. Ganguli, P., Cullen, D., and Irvine, W.: Radioimmunoassay of plasma gastrin in pernicious anemia, achlorhydria without pernicious anemia, hypochlorhydria and in controls, Lancet **1:** 155, 1971.
12a. Ganguli, P., Polak, J., Pearse, A., Elder, J., and Hogarty, M.: Antral-gastrin-cell hyperplasia in peptic ulcer disease, Lancet **1:** 583, 1974.
13. Gleeson, M., Bloom, S., Polak, J., Henry, C., and Dowling, R.: Endocrine tumour in kidney affecting small bowel structure, motility, and absorptive function, Gut **12:** 773, 1971.
14. Goldman, L., Gordan, G., and Roof, B.: The parathyroids: Progress, problems and practice, *in* Ravitch, M., editor: Current problems in surgery, Chicago, 1972, Year Book Medical Publishers, Inc., p. 10.
15. Greider, M., and McGuigan, J.: Cellular localization of gastrin in the human pancreas, Diabetes **20:** 389, 1971.
16. Grossman, M.: Gatrointestinal hormones: Some thoughts about clinical applications, Scand. J. Gastroenterol. **7:** 97, 1972.
17. Hallenbeck, G. A.: Gastrin-like activity of tumors: A review, *in* Grossman, M., editor: Gastrin, Berkeley and Los Angeles, 1966, University of California Press, pp. 285-308.
18. Huizenga, K., Goodrick, W., and Summerskill, W.: Peptic ulcer with islet cell tumor, Am. J. Med. **37:** 564, 1964.
19. Isenberg, J., Walsh, T., and Grossman, M.: Zollinger-Ellison syndrome, Gastroenterology **65:** 140, 1973.
20. Kaplan, E., Sizemore, G., Peskin, G., and Jaffe, B.: Humoral similarities of carcinoid tumors and medullary carcinomas of the thyroid, SURGERY **74:** 21, 1973.
21. Kerr, G., and Smith, R.: Hypercalcemia and gastric hypersecretion in the familial endocrine-adenoma syndrome, Lancet **1:** 1074, 1967.
22. Moldawer, M., Nardi, G., and Raker, J.: Concommitance of multiple adenomas of the parathyroids and pancreatic islets with tumor of the pituitary: A syndrome with familial incidence, Am. J. Med. Sci. **228:** 190, 1954.
23. O'Neal, L., Kipnis, D., Luse, S., Lacy, P., and Jarett, L.: Secretion of various endocrine substances by ACTH-secreting tumors—gastrin, melanotropin, norepinephrine, serotonin, parathormone, vasopressin, glucagon, Cancer **21:** 1219, 1968.
24. Passaro, E., and Gordon, H.: Gastric secretory tests, Am. J. Surg. **114:** 333, 1967.
25. Passaro, E., Basso, N., and Walsh, J.: Calcium challenge in the Zollinger-Ellison syndrome, SURGERY **72:** 60, 1972.
26. Patterson, M., Wolma, F., Drake, A., and Ong, H.: Gastric secretion and chronic hyperparathyroidism, Arch. Surg. **99:** 9, 1969.
27. Pearse, A.: The cytochemistry and ultrastructure of polypeptide hormone–producing cells of the APUD series and the embryologic, physiologic, and pathologic implications of the concept, J. Histochem. Cytochem. **17:** 303, 1969.
27a. Pearse, A., Coulling, I., Weavers, B., and Friesen, S.: The endocrine polypeptide cells of the human stomach, duodenum, and jejunum, Gut **11:** 649, 1970.
28. Potts, J., Sherwood, L., O'Riordan, J., and Aurbach, G.: Radioimmunoassay of polypeptide hormones, Adv. Intern. Med. **23:** 183, 1967.
29. Robinson, W.: Need for further study as the role of the parathyroids in Cushing's syndrome (abstr.), J. Clin. Endocrinol. Metab. **14:** 811, 1954.
30. Sanzenbacher, L., Mekhjian, H., King, D., and Zollinger, R.: Studies on the potential role of secretin in the islet cell tumor diarrheagenic syndrome, Ann. Surg. **176:** 394, 1972.
31. Sizemore, G., Go, U., Kaplan, E., Sanzenbacher, L., Holtermuller, K., and Arnaud, C.: Relationships of calcitonin and gastrin in the Zollinger-Ellison syndrome and medullary carcinoma of the thyroid, N. Engl. J. Med. **288:** 641, 1973.
32. Steiner, A., Goodman, A., and Powers, S.: Study of a kindred with pheochromocytomas, medullary thyroid carcinoma, hyperparathyroidism, and Cushing's disease: Multiple endocrine neoplasia, type 2, Medicine **47:** 371, 1968.
33. Stremple, J., and Meade, R.: Radioimmunoassay of hormones associated with the pancreas, *in* Carey, L. C., editor: The pancreas,

St. Louis, 1973, The C. V. Mosby Company, chap. 6, p. 130.
34. Summerskill, W. H., Code, C. F., Hallenbeck, G. A., and Priestley, J. T.: Intractable peptic ulcer in hereditary endocrine-ulcer disease: Gastrin content of endocrine tissues, Proc. Mayo Clin. **36:** 611, 1961.
35. Thompson, J., Reeder, D., and Bunchman, H.: Clinical role of serum gastrin measurements in the Zollinger-Ellison syndrome, Am. J. Surg. **124:** 250, 1972.
36. Trudeau, W., and McGuigan, J.: Effects of calcium on serum gastrin in the Zollinger-Ellison syndrome, N. Engl. J. Med. **281:** 862, 1969.
37. Turbey, W., and Passaro, E.: Hyperparathyroidism in the Zollinger-Ellison syndrome, Arch. Surg. **105:** 62, 1972.
38. Ward, J., Adesola, A., and Welbourn, R.: The parathyroids, calcium and gastric secretion in man and the dog, Gut **5:** 173, 1964.
39. Wang, C.: Surgery of the parathyroid glands, Adv. Surg. **5:** 109, 1971.
40. Weichert, R.: Neural ectodermal origin of peptide-secreting endocrine glands, Am. J. Med. **49:** 232, 1970.
41. Wermer, P.: Genetic aspects of adenomatosis of endocrine glands, Am. J. Med. **16:** 363, 1954.
42. Wilder, W., Frame, B., and Haubrich, W.: Peptic ulcer in hyperparathyroidism, Ann. Intern. Med. **55:** 885, 1961.
43. Zollinger, R. M., Elliott, D. W., Endahl, G. L., Grant, G. M., Goswitz, J. T., and Taft, D. A.: Origin of the ulcerogenic hormones in endocrine induced ulcer, Ann. Surg. **156:** 575, 1962.

DISCUSSION

Dr. Josef E. Fischer (Boston, Mass.). I personally think that these divisions that have been pointed out are far too rigid and far too arbitrary in a disease that is as complicated as hyperparathyroidism. We have been able to identify at least five different categories of patients with hyperparathyroidism: (1) some of whom have normal basal acids; (2) some of whom have high basal acids; (3) some of whom have what we call calcium-independent Zollinger-Ellison tumors; (4) some of whom have what we call calcium-dependent Zollinger-Ellison tumor categories; and (5) this very interesting group of patients with the very high levels of serum gastrin. These patients in this category are high-volume achlorhydrics and produce anywhere between 80 and 100 c.c. an hour of a very thick, viscid gastric secretion, and they are histamine-fast achlorhydrics.

In our series, three out of the four patients who have this high-volume achlorhydria are patients with hyperplasia; these patients did not have an adenoma as the source of their gastrin, although, in truth, the parathyroid glands were not examined for gastrin.

I also think that it is arbitrary to separate patients with ulcers from patients without ulcers, since in hyperparathyroidism some of the most symptomatic patients are patients who do not have ulcers at all. I can recall three patients without ulcers who couldn't eat because of severe gastritis. One patient's basal acid secretion dropped from 70 mEq. per hour in the preoperative weeks to 5 mEq. per hour in the postoperative weeks. This patient, rightly, should probably be included in the ulcer-type patient.

Prof. Richard Welbourn (London, England). There is one thing that worries me a little bit. Are those levels of 1,757, 2,035, and 2,375 really different? I would have thought that if this adenoma were really producing the gastrin, then the concentration of gastrin in the vein which was near the tumor should have been very much higher than that; it should have had double or more the concentration in the peripheral vein.

And again, if the parathyroid adenoma were producing the gastrin, surely the level should have fallen precipitously immediately after it had been removed. As I understood from that slide, the fall was not found until about a year afterwards.

The following is data from one patient: She had multiple endocrine adenopathy. She had hyperinsulinism, acromegaly, and hyperparathyroidism. When we studied her acid secretion, both basal and peak in response to pentagastrin, before we did anything to her, the levels were normal, 2.1 and 18.3. I then took out two insulinomas, which cured her hyperinsulinism. Shortly after this she had a massive hemorrhage from a duodenal ulcer which had not been there before; I did a vagotomy and pyloroplasty.

Basal acid went up to 11, and peak acid was more or less unchanged. The high basal level may have been the result of stasis after vagotomy.

Three weeks later she bled again, and this time I did an antrectomy. This procedure brought the basal level down, but still it was higher than it had been initially; and the peak acid came down a bit, but it was still a good deal higher than you would expect in a patient who has had a vagotomy and antrectomy. The insulin test was negative, suggesting that the vagotomy had been complete. After she had had her parathyroids out, the basal output fell to zero, and the peak output came down much further than it had been before.

The initial gastrin level was 200, which is rather above the upper limit of normal in our laboratory, but not really in the ZE range. I did not know these results, because they had not come back from the lab until after I had done the first three operations. But after we had done the antrectomy, plasma gastrin went up to double what it had been before, after we had removed, of course, what is the normal source of gastrin in the body.

And after the parathyroidectomy, when the acid secretion had come right down, her plasma gastrin went up still further. Now, where on earth was this gastrin coming from? There was no sign of it in the insulinoma on immunofluorescence. The details in the pancreas, again, looked entirely normal. The G-cells in the antrum looked entirely normal. We biopsied her jejunum and found a few G-cells present there. We think those are normal, but we do not really have enough data in man to know whether they were normal or high.

She had four large parathyroids with chief cell hyperplasia which were loaded with parathormone in the chief cells. But the gastrin was present, as shown on immunofluorescence in the oxyphil cells.

Now, I still find it hard to believe that these parathyroids were the source of the gastrin any more than I think they were in Dr. Stremple's case, and I think there is another source of gastrin in both our patients—perhaps a gastrinoma in the pancreas which we have so far missed—and the parathyroid is acting as a sponge and mopping it all up.

Dr. James C. Thompson (Galveston, Texas). I think it is improper to speak about serum gastrin being in the ZE range, giving these cases the significance of the Zollinger-Ellison syndrome, because this patient does not secrete acid, and as long as the patient is not secreting acid, you cannot even speak of the Zollinger-Ellison syndrome. Patients with pernicious anemia are the other group that have high levels of serum gastrin.

Now, we need to know: Did this patient have parietal cells? If the patient does have any parietal cells, why is she secreting this very high level of gastrin? If the patient does not have parietal cells, why does she not have pernicious anemia.

This is not like any other previously reported gastrinoma. The gastric biopsy for parietal cells needs to be done; and also, I think, we need to find out if infusion of this serum into a dog causes that dog to secrete, or causes an isolated sheet of frog gastric mucosa to secrete. And the question is: Is this biologically active gastrin?

I think we are now learning that there are at least eight, and perhaps ten, molecular forms of gastrin, two of which are probably biologically inert; the so-called big, big gastrin. That form which has a molecular weight of about that of albumin does seem to react quantitatively with the gastrin antibody but perhaps does not have any biologic significance. And it is probably the major contributor to basal levels of gastrin. That is the reason people carry anywhere from 25 to 70 pg. of basal gastrin and yet may secrete no acid at all. The reason for this is that the basal level of gastrin is probably mainly made up of a biologically inert form and that may well be what we have detected here.

Is the patient truly achlorhydric? We know that she was not tested with histamine, but a pentagrastrin infusion would easily have established that. If the patient is achlorhydric, that means that she has no parietal cells. And if there are no parietal cells, why does this patient not have pernicious anemia, since intrinsic factor is secreted by parietal cells?

Dr. David Scharp (St. Louis, Mo.). In reviewing some of the pathology in our cases here, we have seen that parathyroids which look normal grossly often have microscopic abnormalities. And I was concerned, in the data of those cases that had the adenomata, that the serum gastrin postoperatively did not fall to normal. What I am asking is: Could this, in fact, be coming from some of the small glands that may be abnormal that were left behind?

Dr. John F. Stremple (closing). Dr. Fischer stated that my division of hyperparathyroid patients into those with and without ulcer was too rigid and arbitrary. He stated that there were several different categories of patients with hyperparathyroidism, some of whom have high basal acids. Dr. Fischer's group reported basal acid output data without separating their five patients with peptic ulcer. He also combined those with parathyroid adenoma with those having primary parathyroid hyperplasia. When we studied our data, we found that the standard error for both basal acid and serum gastrin before and after parathyroidectomy was quite high when all patients were taken together. This suggested to us that we should separate those with proved duodenal ulcer from those without ulcer. Although we had only three patients with proved duodenal ulcers, it is quite evident from our data that the changes in basal acid and serum gastrin were markedly different in those patients with ulcer and similar to those associated with peptic ulcer without hyperparathyroidism. Therefore, I believe this separation may be necessary, but more patients need to be studied.

Prof. Welbourn asked if the difference between the gastrin levels of 2,375 pg. per milliliter from the brachiocephalic vein and 2,035 pg. per milliliter from the peripheral vein was significant. The sample taken from the left brachiocephalic vein was closer to the left parathyroid gastrinoma, but it was not from the primary vein draining this tumor. Nevertheless, there was a difference of 340 pg. per milliliter which is quite significant since the sample from the brachiocephalic vein could be almost considered systemic. I would suspect that if the catheter had been placed directly into the primary vein draining the adenoma, the difference in gastrin levels would have been greater. Second, Prof. Welbourn noted that the level of serum gastrin three months following removal of the parathyroid adenoma had not fallen precipitously. I believe that antral-gastrin (G)-cell hyperplasia which has been found both with hyperparathyroidism and peptic ulcer was present. The serum gastrin level of 1,757 pg. per milliliter three months after removal of the parathyroid gastrinoma could be due to antral (G)-cell gastrin. Finally, Prof. Welbourn showed that in his case, gastrin was found by immunofluorescence in the oxyphil cells of the parathyroid tumor removed. He commented that it was his opinion the tumor was acting as a sponge. It may be that the parathyroid tumor in his case was acting as a sponge, but because of the high tissue gastrin content in the parathyroid adenoma from our patient determined both by radioimmunoassay and immunofluorescence and the marked decrease in serial serum gastrin levels after its removal, I believe that in our case the parathyroid adenoma was the source of gastrin. The gastrin immunofluorescence in our case was in the cytoplasm of the chief cells and not in the oxyphil cells as it was in the case shown by Prof. Welbourn. I question the evidence for his hypothesis that either the chief cells or the oxyphil cells act as a sponge rather than as the source of gastrin secretion. It may be that, in the human, either the chief cell or the oxyphil cell could be responsible for hypergastrinemia.

Dr. Thompson mentioned that we have not proved that our patient was truly achlorhydric since we were not able to stimulate this patient with histamine or determine if parietal cells were present. We plan to bring this patient back for further studies to answer this question. Dr. Thompson also questioned the biologic activity of the gastrin secreted by the parathyroid adenoma. This also must be determined. I realize that this is not like any previously reported gastrinoma, but should not be surprising considering the many common characteristics shared by the parathyroid and the pancreas as has been related by Pearse.

Dr. Sharp asked if the serum gastrin found after parathyroidectomy could not come from small glands left behind. We will continue to follow this patient's parathyroid function for this possibility.

Influence of vasopressin and topical bile salts on the gastric mucosal barrier of the subhuman primate

W. P. Ritchie, Jr., M.D., Ph.D., *Washington, D. C., and Charlottesville, Va.*

Based on studies in the rabbit and dog, mucosal ischemia, regurgitation of bile, and an incompetent gastric mucosal barrier (GMB) have all been implicated in the pathogenesis of posttraumatic stress ulcer. The present study was designed to determine the effect of mucosal ischemia alone and in combination with topically applied bile salts on the GMB properties of an animal phylogenetically closer to man, the rhesus monkey (Macaca mulatta). Animals (n=4) were prepared with internally drained, vagally denervated fundic pouches (HP). Each HP was cannulated and exposed first to acid test solution (ATS) alone (ATS = 80 mM. HCl, 80 mM. NaCl, 2 Gm. PEG per liter) and then to ATS containing 10 mM. sodium taurocholate (TC). Electrical potential difference (PD) was continuously monitored, and the net fluxes of H_2O, H^+, and Na^+ were assessed at 15 minute intervals with ATS and ATS + TC during (1) the continuous intra-arterial infusion of 0.9 percent NaCl into the celiac axis (CA) and (2) infusion of the CA with vasopressin, 0.05 U. per kilogram-minute. With ATS alone, mucosal ischemia markedly reduced net Na^+ and H_2O flux and significantly impaired the ability of the mucosa to maintain electrical gradients, findings more consistent with inhibition of active transport processes and contraction of the extracellular space than with alterations in mucosal permeability. With ATS + TC, mucosal ischemia did not further alter the PD vs. ATS alone and did not increase net H^+ flux vs. the non-ischemic mucosa. In the subhuman primate, ischemia per se does not markedly affect mucosal permeability and does not significantly enhance damage to the GMB induced by topical bile salts.

From the Division of Surgery, Walter Reed Army Institute of Research, Walter Reed Army Medical Center, Washington, D. C., and the Department of Surgery, University of Virginia School of Medicine, Charlottesville, Va.

THE NORMAL mammalian stomach maintains a low intraluminal pH despite the presence of a large hydrogen ion concentration gradient between lumen and blood. A variety of topically applied agents, including bile salts, can damage this gastric mucosal barrier (GMB) to hydrogen ion diffusion, resulting in (1) increased net luminal loss of hydrogen ion, (2) increased net luminal gain of sodium, and (3) an associated fall in electrical potential difference (PD; lumen negative vs. blood).[5] Evidence suggests that these changes are a direct consequence of a physical increase in gastric mucosal permeability.[1]

Studies in the dog and rabbit have implicated gastric mucosal ischemia, regurgitation of upper intestinal content, and an incompetent GMB in the pathogenesis of acute posttraumatic hemorrhagic gastritis.[7, 15, 16] By using an animal phylogenetically much closer to man, the rhesus monkey, the present study was designed to determine (1) if gastric

Supported in part by Contract No. DAMD 17-74-C-4014.
Presented at the Thirty-fifth Annual Meeting of the Society of University Surgeons, St. Louis, Mo., Feb. 14-16.

mucosal ischemia itself increases mucosal permeability, and (2) whether or not the permeability changes regularly induced by topical application of bile salts are enhanced by mucosal ischemia. It is assumed that mucosal blood flow was reduced significantly by the continuous infusion of vasopressin,* 0.05 U. per kilogram-minute, into the celiac axis. This assumption is reasonable because Dorricott and associates[6] have demonstrated a fall in gastric mucosal blood flow to 16 percent of control levels during splenic artery perfusion with a smaller dose (0.01 U. per kilogram-minute with the use of conscious dogs. In addition, also using a smaller dose, Swan and Reynolds,[18] have shown a sustained reduction in superior mesenteric artery flow in the Anubis baboon, a closely related species.

METHODS†

Four healthy rhesus monkeys *(Macaca mulatta),* weighing 3.4 to 5.2 kilograms, were used. First, a vagally denervated fundic pouch pedicled on the short gastric vessels was fashioned in each. The pouch was drained internally by a six-inch Roux-en-Y limb of jejunum, as previously described,[13] because conventionally drained pouches frequently develop patchy areas of gastric atrophy which might interfere with the experimental parameters.[12] Three weeks later, following a 48 hour fast (water was allowed ad libitum), the animals were anesthetized with chlorolose-urethane (50 mg. per kilogram given intravenously) and subjected to laparotomy. The pouch was cannulated with a multiperforate, plastic cannula through a small distal enterotomy and was secured with an umbilical ligature to produce a watertight seal. A three-way stopcock and a verticle plastic sidearm were placed on the cannula, and the enterotomy was closed. The descending branch of the left gastric artery was identified, through which a polyethylene tube (PE 60) was advanced to the celiac axis. This was connected to a constant infusion pump* and infused with 0.11 ml. per minute of 0.9 percent NaCl. Systemic arterial blood pressure and pulse rate were monitored via a femoral artery cannula connected to a calibrated transducer† and a balanced recorder.‡ In order to monitor the PD, a femoral vein was cannulated with polyethylene tubing (PE 160) containing saturated KCl in 4 percent agar. Agar-KCl tubing was also passed into the lumen of the pouch via the sidearm on the intraluminal cannula. These bridges were immersed in beakers of saturated KCl containing balanced calomel electrodes which were connected to a recording potentiometer.§ Basal secretion of HCl was assessed by instilling 10 ml. of 0.9 percent NaCl into the pouch. Fifteen minutes later, the pouch was evacuated and the volume of the aspirate was determined. An aliquot was titrated, and total acid output per 15 minutes was calculated. This maneuver was repeated twice. Background secretion of HCl (±SEM) was 7 ± 2 μEq. per 15 minutes determined in this way. Fifteen milliliters of an acid test solution (ATS = 80 mM. HCl and 80 mM. NaCl) were then instilled into the pouch. This volume produced an intraluminal pressure of 8 ± 3 cm. H_2O as measured in the sidearm. Thereafter, the PD was monitored at three-minute intervals.

Once the PD had stabilized, net hydrogen ion, sodium, and water fluxes in non-ischemic mucosa in contact with acid alone (ATS) were determined. This was accomplished by instilling 15 ml. of ATS containing 2 Gm. per liter of polyethylene glycol (PEG) as a non-absorbable marker into the pouch. An aliquot was withdrawn, its volume was determined, and the flux study period was begun. Fifteen minutes later, the pouch was evacuated and washed with ATS containing

*Pitressin, Parke-Davis & Co., Detroit, Mich.

†"In conducting the research described in this report, the investigators adhered to the 'Guide for Laboratory Animal Facilities and Care,' as promulgated by the Committee on the Guide for Laboratory Animal Facilities and Care of the Institute of Laboratory Animal Resources, National Academy of Sciences–National Research Council."

*Harvard Apparatus Company, Cambridge, Mass.

†Statham, Hato Rey, Puerto Rico.

‡Sanborn, Waltham, Mass.

§Model 601, Keithley Instruments, Cleveland, Ohio.

no indicator. The flux study and subsequent wash were then repeated. Net ion and water fluxes in non-ischemic mucosa in contact with topical bile salts (ATS + TC) were then assessed. Fifteen milliliters of ATS containing PEG and 10 mM. sodium taurocholate* were instilled into the pouch and a 15 minute flux study performed. The pouch was washed with indicator-free ATS solution and the PD was allowed to return to base-line levels. A second flux with ATS containing sodium taurocholate was then performed. Following recovery of the PD to base-line levels, mucosal ischemia was induced by perfusing the celiac axis with 0.9 percent NaCl containing vasopressin delivered at a rate of 0.05 U. per kilogram-minute. Once the PD had restabilized, the entire sequence of fluxes was repeated.

At the conclusion of the study, the pouch was rapidly excised, and the animal was put to death by injecting saturated KCl intravenously. The pouch mucosa was dissected from the muscular layers by sharp dissection. The mucosa was flattened on drawing paper, its circumference was carefully traced, and the area was determined with the use of planimetry.

The equations used to calculate the net fluxes of ions and water have been described previously.[11] The concentration of hydrogen ion was measured by titration to pH 8 with phenolphthalein as an indicator; the concentration of sodium was determined by using a flame photometer bracketed by appropriate standards†; and the concentration of PEG was assessed with the use of the turbidometric technique of Hyden.[8] All fluxes were corrected to a standard mucosal area of 50 cm.[2] A positive value for net flux indicates gain of material by the lumen, while a negative value indicates net luminal loss.

The results were subjected to statistical analysis by using Student's t test for paired observations.[17] The level of statistical significance used was the 95 per cent confidence limits.

*Mann Chemical Company, New York, N. Y.
†Instrumentation Laboratory, Watertown, Mass.

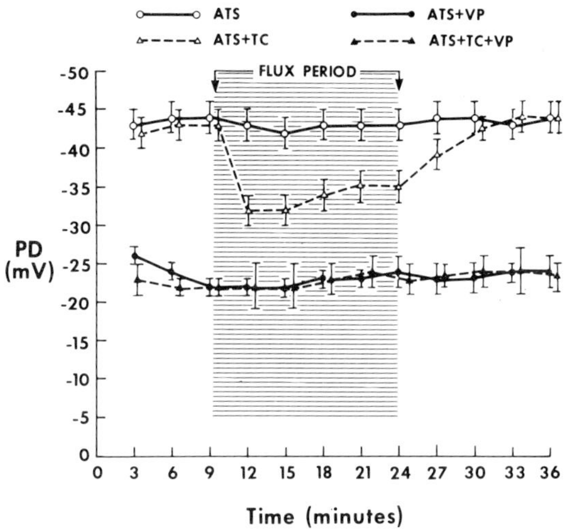

Fig. 1. Effect on potential difference (PD; lumen negative vs. blood) of various intraluminal solutions in non-ischemic and ischemic mucosa. The shaded area indicates the time during which concomitant flux studies were performed. ATS, acid test solution; TC, sodium taurocholate (10 mM.); VP, vasopressin infusion.

RESULTS

Effect of ischemia and bile salts on PD. As Fig. 1 indicates, the PD of non-ischemic mucosa in contact with ATS alone varied between –42 and –45 mv. During the topical application of 10 mM. sodium taurocholate (ATS + TC), the potential fell within three minutes, stabilizing at between –32 and –35 mv. Following evacuation of the taurocholate solution from the pouch, the potential returned to base-line levels within six minutes. In contrast, during vasopressin perfusion, when the mucosa was in contact with ATS alone (ATS + VP), the PD fell at a rate of approximately 2 mv. per minute, ultimately stabilizing at between –22 and –25 mv. The subsequent topical application of 10 mM. sodium taurocholate (ATS + TC + VP) resulted in no further decrease in the PD, and no tendency toward recovery was noted following evacuation of the bile salt solution from the pouch.

Effect of ischemia on net ion and water fluxes in the presence of ATS alone. As indicated in Fig. 2, in the presence of ATS alone, the non-ischemic mucosa demonstrated a net gain of water and sodium and a net

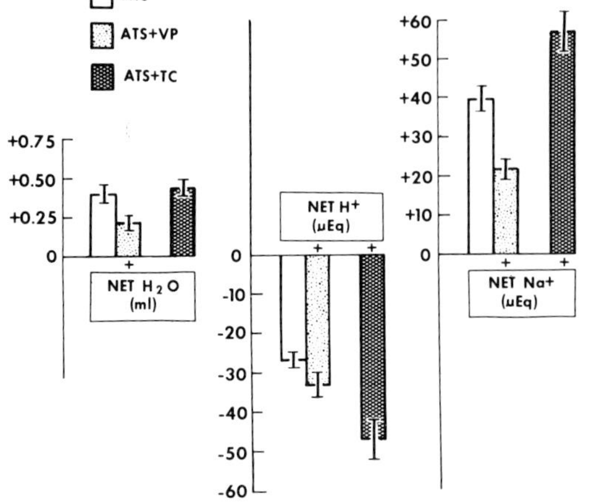

Fig. 2. Effect of vasopressin (VP) infusion on net flux (±SEM) per 15 minutes per 50 cm.^{2} mucosal area when acid test solution alone (ATS) was used.

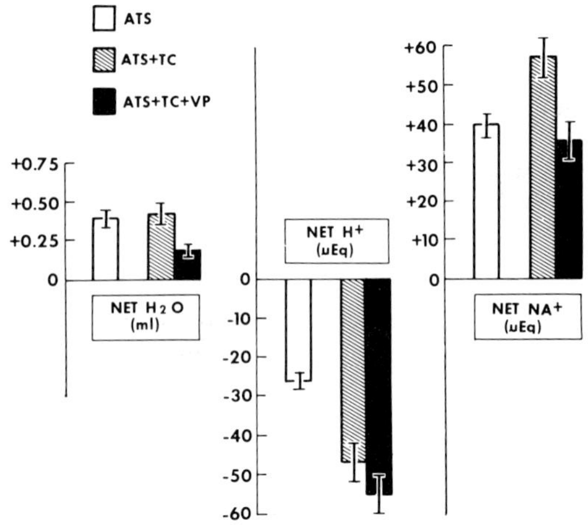

Fig. 3. Effect of vasopressin (VP) infusion on net flux (±SEM) per 15 minutes per 50 cm.^{2} mucosal area when acid test solution +10 mM. Na taurocholate (TC) was used.

loss of hydrogen ion. When the mucosa was made ischemic (ATS + VP), a marked reduction in net water and sodium flux occurred ($p < 0.01$ and $p = 0.01$, respectively), and a small, but significant, increase in net hydrogen ion flux ($p = 0.05$) was observed. As Fig. 2 also indicates, these changes were unlike those observed when mucosal permeability was increased by sodium taurocholate in the absence of ischemia (ATS + TC), i.e., no change in net water flux and a significant increase of considerable magnitude in both net sodium gain and net hydrogen ion loss (< 0.01 in each instance).

Effect of ischemia on net ion and water fluxes in the presence of bile salts. The effects of 10 mM. sodium taurocholate applied to non-ischemic (ATS + TC) and ischemic (ATS + TC + VP) mucosa are illustrated in Fig. 3, and are compared to the effects of ATS alone in normally perfused tissue. As indicated, in non-ischemic mucosa, the topical application of the bile salt solution resulted in no change in net water flux and a significant increase in both net sodium and net hydrogen ion flux when compared to ATS alone. In ischemic mucosa (ATS + TC + VP), on the other hand, significantly reduced net water and sodium flux were noted ($p < 0.01$ and $p = 0.01$, respectively) accompanied by an insignificant increase in net hydrogen ion flux ($p = 0.2$).

No significant alterations in mean systemic arterial pressure or pulse rate were noted during the infusion of vasopressin into the celiac axis. There was no evidence of intraluminal bleeding at any time during the experiment.

DISCUSSION

It is widely believed that acute posttraumatic hemorrhagic gastritis is a consequence of increased gastric mucosal permeability. The "back diffusion" hypothesis postulates that, as a consequence of gastric mucosal ischemia, the GMB is damaged, permitting excessive enterosorption of H^+ and pepsin with resulting autodigestion of the gastric mucosa.[16] Experimentally, this thesis is based on observations in rabbits that a brief period of hypoperfusion, induced by hemorrhage, results in excessive "back diffusion" of hydrogen ion associated with the development of linear fundic ulcers and intraluminal bleeding in the intact stomach.[15] These data have not proved reproducible in other species. Using chambered segments of canine fundic mucosa, Moody and Aldrete[9] could demonstrate no evidence of an impaired

Table I

*Period**	*H+ flux ratio (±SEM)*		*Na+ flux ratio (±SEM)*	
(ATS) (ISCHEMIA) / (ATS)	1.39 ± 0.16	N.S.†	0.57 ± 0.05	N.S.
(ATS) (TC) (ISCHEMIA) / (ATS) (TC)	1.37 ± 0.28		0.73 ± 0.18	
(ATS) (TC) / (ATS)	1.85 ± 0.22	N.S.	1.49 ± 0.16	N.S.
(ATS) (TC) (ISCHEMIA) / (ATS) (ISCHEMIA)	1.72 ± 0.14		1.56 ± 0.09	

*ATS = acid test solution; TC = 10 mM. sodium taurocholate.
†N.S. = Differences not statistically significant.

GMB in dogs subjected to hemorrhagic shock, despite the development of punctate erosions and a marked reduction in amniopyrine clearance, an index of gastric mucosal blood flow. Similarly, Ritchie and Fischer[11] could find no evidence of increased mucosal permeability in the denervated fundic pouch of the dog during a 3.5 hour period of hemorrhagic shock, even though the ability of the mucosa to maintain an electrical gradient was markedly impaired. Recently, Dorricott and co-workers[6] have shown that the infusion of vasopressin, 0.01 U. per kilogram per minute, directly into the arterial supply of canine denervated fundic pouches markedly reduced aminopyrine clearance but did not significantly alter the net fluxes of hydrogen ion and sodium.

The present study used a different species and a dose of vasopressin five times greater than that employed by Dorricott and colleagues.[6] Although significant changes in net water and ion fluxes were observed in ischemic mucosa exposed to ATS alone (markedly reduced net water and sodium flux and a small but significant increase in net hydrogen ion flux), these alterations are not a reflection of increased mucosal permeability as exemplified by the circumstance observed when non-ischemic mucosa is in contact with 10 mM. sodium taurocholate solution (no change in net water flux and a marked increase in both sodium and hydrogen ion flux). Although the kinetics of water and sodium movement into the gastric lumen are unclear, it is probable that both are ultimately derived from extracellular sources.[4] Shires and associates,[14] using the hind limb of the primate, have demonstrated that hemorrhagic shock causes a marked reduction in extracellular water and sodium content. If a similar situation pertains in gastric mucosa subjected to pharmacologically induced ischemia, it is possible that the reduced net sodium and water flux observed are a consequence of contracted extracellular sodium and water spaces. The small increment in hydrogen ion flux noted during ischemia could be the result either of inhibition of background secretion or of changes in the electrochemical potential of the ion produced as a consequence of the altered electrical gradient.

Since the factors responsible for the maintenance of PD under normal circumstances are not completely understood, no precise explanation is available for the changes observed in ischemic mucosa exposed to ATS alone (ATS + VP) and in non-ischemic mucosa exposed to topical bile salts (ATS + TC). In each instance, a fall in PD was noted. The magnitude of the change (21 ± 2 mv. with ATS + VP, 10 ± 3 mv. with ATS + TC) were different, however, suggesting that the mechanisms responsible may also be dissimilar. Of interest in this regard is the observation of Chou and associates[3] that dogs subjected to hemorrhagic shock or endotoxemia demonstrated a fall in PD associated with a rise in electrical resistance of the tissue, suggesting altered active transport mechanisms. Birkett and Silen,[1] on the other hand, using in vivo rabbit mucosa, have demonstrated that the topical application of 10 mM. sodium taurocholate also caused a fall in PD, but, in this instance, an associated decrease in tissue resistance was apparent.

When compared to the alterations observed in non-ischemic mucosa exposed to bile salts, a marked reduction in both net water and sodium flux was noted when 10 mM. sodium taurocholate was applied during vasopressin administration. No significant differences in net hydrogen ion flux were apparent. In addition, no additive change in PD was observed under these circumstances relative to ischemic mucosa exposed to ATS alone. These data suggest that mucosal ischemia does not enhance damage to the GMB induced by the topical application of this concentration of sodium taurocholate. Examination of hydrogen ion and sodium flux ratios (Table I) obtained by comparing the appropriate flux periods supports this conclusion. No significant differences were noted between the hydrogen ion flux ratios ATS + VP:ATS and ATS + TC + VP:ATS + TC, which indicated that the increment in hydrogen ion flux caused by ischemia was similar in bile salt–treated and bile salt–free mucosa. The hydrogen ion flux ratios ATS + TC:ATS and ATS + TC + VP:ATS + VP also were not different, showing that the enhanced hydrogen ion movement noted in the presence of sodium taurocholate was of the same magnitude in both the ischemic and non-ischemic states. Similarly, no differences were observed between the appropriate sodium flux ratios, indicating that the reduction in net sodium flux noted during ischemia was similar irrespective of the presence of topical bile salts and that the increment in sodium flux caused by bile salt application was similar in ischemic and non-ischemic mucosa.

These data suggest that, under the conditions of the present experiment, in the subhuman primate, mucosal ischemia per se (1) does not significantly affect gastric mucosal permeability and (2) does not significantly enhance permeability changes induced by the topical application of 10 mM. sodium taurocholate. Since this study was not designed to evaluate the ulcerogenic potential of concomitant bile salt application and mucosal ischemia, this conclusion does not imply that "back diffusion" of hydrogen ion plays no role in the development of acute posttraumatic hemorrhagic gastritis. Hamza and DenBesten[7] have shown that topically applied bile salts enhance ulcer formation in the intact stomach of the dog subjected to hemorrhagic shock, even though increased net loss of luminal hydrogen ion was not observed during the shock period. In addition, this induced ulcerogenesis could be prevented by the concomitant administration of cholestyramine, an exchange resin which binds bile salts, renders them unabsorbable, and prevents "back diffusion" of hydrogen ion of any magnitude.[19] A synergistic relationship may exist, therefore, between impaired gastric mucosal blood flow, ulcerogenesis, and "back diffusion" of intraluminal acid, even though the magnitude of the hydrogen ion loss is "normal" under these circumstances.

The technical assistance of Sp 4 Henry Sullivan, Jr., is gratefully acknowledged.

REFERENCES

1. Birkett, D., and Silen, W.: Alteration of physical pathways through gastric mucosa by bile and ASA, Gastroenterology **64:** 701, 1973.
2. Birkett, D., and Silen, W.: Effect of severe anoxia and sodium taurocholate on H+ loss from luminal surface of in vitro gastric mucosa, Surg. Forum **24:** 421, 1973.
3. Chou, A. C., Miller, J., Jacobson, E. D., and Shanbour, L. L.: Effects of endotoxin on gastric mucosal active transport processes. Gastroenterology **64:** 710, 1973.
4. Davenport, H. W.: Physiological structure of the gastric mucosa, *in* Handbook of Physiology, Alimentary Canal II, American Physiological Society, Washington, D. C., 1967.
5. Davenport, H. W., Warner, H. A., and Code, C. F.: Functional significance of the gastric mucosal barrier to sodium, Gastroenterology **47:** 142, 1964.
6. Dorricott, N. J., Eisenberg, H., and Silen, W.: Effect of intra-arterial vasopressin on

canine gastric mucosa permeability, Gastroenterology **65:** 625, 1973.

7. Hamza, K. N., and DenBesten, L.: Bile salts producing stress ulcers during experimental shock, Clin. Res. **19:** 393, 1971.
8. Hyden, S.: A turbidometric method for the determination of higher polyethylene glycols in biologic materials, Ann. R. Agric. Coll. Sweden **22:** 139, 1955.
9. Moody, F. G., and Aldrete, J. S.: Hydrogen permeability of canine gastric secretory epithelium during formation of acute superficial erosions, SURGERY **70:** 154, 1971.
10. Ritchie, W. P., Jr., and Fischer, R. P.: Studies on the pathogeneous of "stress ulcer": Electrical potential difference and ionic fluxes across canine gastric mucosa during hemorrhagic shock, J. Surg. Res. **3:** 173, 1972.
11. Ritchie, W. P., Jr., and Fischer, R. P.: Effect of metabolic inhibitors in the gastric mucosal barrier, SURGERY **73:** 614, 1973.
12. Ritchie, W. P., Jr., Delaney, J. P., Barzilai, A., Molina, E., Wangensteen, O. H.: Histological differences between Heidenhain pouches and their parent stomachs. SURGERY **60:** 1224-1228, 1966.
13. Ritchie, W. P., Jr., Butler, B. A., and Delaney, J. P.: Studies on the pathogenesis of benign gastric ulcer: Increased "back diffusion" of hydrogen ion in experimental atrophic gastritis, Ann. Surg. **175:** 594, 1972.
14. Shires, G. T., Cunningham, J. N., Baker, C. R. F., Reeder, S. F., Illner, H., Wagner, I. Y., and Maher, J.: Alterations in cellular membrane function during hemorrhagic shock in primate, Ann. Surg. **176:** 288, 1972.
15. Skillman, J. J., Gould, S. A., Chung, R. S. K., and Silen, W.: The gastric mucosal barrier: Clinical and experimental studies in critically ill and normal man and in the rabbit, Ann. Surg. **172:** 564, 1970.
16. Skillman, J. J., and Silen, W.: Stress ulcers, Lancet **2:** 1303, 1972.
17. Snedecor, G. W., and Cochran, W. G: Statistical methods, ed. 6, Ames, Iowa, 1967, Iowa University Press.
18. Swan, K. G., and Reynolds, D.: Personal communication.
19. Zike, W. L., Safaie-Shirazi, S., Paluska, G., and DenBesten, L.: The role of cholestyramine in the prevention of stress ulcers, Gastroenterology **64:** 826, 1973.

DISCUSSION

Dr. John Joakim Skillman (Boston, Mass.). This data is really supported by observations that have been published by Davenport, and also by a recent publication of Dorricott and Silen, who used vasopressin in an experimental preparation in which the vasopressin was infused directly into the pouch blood supply and who found that they could not detect back diffusion in these experiments in which vasopressin was the source of the ischemia. It seems quite clear that at least this form of mucosal ischemia is not associated with increased back diffusion.

Now, although the dose of vasopressin which was used in Dr. Ritchie's experiments was, I think, five times greater than that which was used by Dorricott and Silen, I have some question about whether the vasopression—or how much of the vasopressin—was really getting to the pouch, since, in fact, as Dr. Ritchie pointed out, the exact mucosal blood flow was not measured in these experiments.

I would like to ask Dr. Ritchie about the controlled experiments that he showed with acid test solution, in which there was a decrease in the potential difference. I noticed the control values were significantly lower than those animals where the acid test solution was used alone, without the vasopressin. I wonder if you would comment whether in some experiments vasopressin was infused after using the acid test solution. Did the vasopressin itself produce a decrease in the potential difference?

I think that I would agree with the conclusion that mucosal ischemia by itself—while it does not produce a very dramatic or, perhaps, even a very small change in mucosal permeability—may in fact have a considerable potential for the production of acute ulceration, since in those cells which are ischemic, the effect of even a small amount of acid, especially when associated with another injurious agent such as bile salts, may be additive, and in combination produce acute ulceration.

Dr. L. DenBesten (Iowa City, Iowa). The title of the paper, as you see, is the effect of vasopressin and topical bile salts on mucosal barrier. And the hypotheses to be tested are (1) does the mucosal ischemia change permeability and (2) are permeability changes produced by bile salts enhanced by ischemia?

Now, from this Dr. Ritchie seems to go on to design some experiments which will obtain or produce data primarily concerning flux of volume and ions, and then go from there on, flux of volume and ions to conclusions concerning the permeability of the mucosa.

It is assumed, I think, that there are certain definite assumptions in this sort of inferential conclusion. It is assumed, for instance, that the pH on the mucosal and the serosal sides remains the same during ischemia as during the time of application of topical bile salts. Now, rather than this, let us assume that ischemia causes total permeability of the gastric mucosa with ions diffusing freely from mucosa to serosa. And then assume that the ischemia induced by vasopressin is effective, so that these ions are no longer removed. A gradient, then, would no longer exist between mucosa and serosa; and if one attempted to measure flux, or motion of ions out of the mucosa, no flux would be detected in these instances.

The point I am trying to make is that I think Dr. Ritchie's data concerning flux of ions as measured is totally correct and accurate. I question, however, whether these data say anything, really, about the integrity or lack of integrity of the mucosal barrier under these circumstances.

I have two smaller questions. The paper continuously refers to "water flux," and somewhat from the purist's point of view, I do not think we really know that it is water. I wonder if "volume flux" would not be a more accurate term here.

And then, finally, Dr. Ritchie does not report his data on potassium flux. Normally, potassium and sodium flux should be parallel, unless there has been injury to mucosal cells; and data as to whether these do parallel each other might be some index as to whether there has been cellular damage induced by the experiment.

President Drapanas. Have you studied any of your vasoactive mucosal amines following pitressin infusion? As you know, this has been implicated as one of the possible mechanisms of producing back diffusion.

Dr. W. P. Ritchie, Jr. (closing). Answering your question first, Dr. Drapanas, I have not studied it. Dr. Wise and Dr. Ballinger have presented evidence a couple of years ago that this, indeed, may play a role. I think that those experiments deserve repetition because of the way the results were expressed—they were not quite comparable to how other persons have approached the problem—and because I believe the whole stomach preparation is used, as opposed to the pouch.

Dr. Skillman indicates quite correctly—and we freely admit—that we did not measure flow. We wish we had. We did not have the capacity at the time. I believe that mucosal blood flow was reduced, for the reasons enumerated, for the fact that we did observe changes which were sustained in the case of the potential difference.

Furthermore, in some studies that we are carrying out now, in which we have finally the capacity to do aminopyrine clearances, this dose of vasopressin, delivered in precisely the same way into a dog, unfortunately, does result in sustained reduction of aminopyrine clearance over a period of 2½ hours.

The blood pressure change was not noted in our experiment. Others, including Dorricott, did note a slight increase in mean systemic arterial pressure associated with bradycardia. I really do not know why we did not.

Do I feel that the potential difference is related to the vasopressin? I think, quite clearly, that is true. There is experimental evidence from many years ago to indicate that if you clamp the blood supply of a denervated fundic pouch in a dog, the potential falls. It returns when you unclamp it. Potential difference is a rather interesting parameter of gastric function, which perhaps needs more emphasis. Before it is applied clinically, however, I think we need to know precisely what it reflects.

I think it reflects at least two things: physical increase in mucosal permeability, and alterations in mucosal flow, with whatever attendant reactions that induces.

Both Dr. DenBesten and Dr. Skillman really questioned whether or not combined ischemia and bile salt application might not have a potential for ulceration. I very strongly believe that it does, but, of course, that was not the purpose that we set out to attain. The purpose was to see whether or not, using these parameters of gastric function, there was increased mucosal permeability or whether damage by bile salts to these parameters was enhanced by ischemia, and our conclusions are as outlined.

I do believe, however, it would be a great mistake to take away the feeling from this study that the combination of ischemia and bile salts is not potentially very injurious.

Dr. DenBesten raises, really, an excellent point. While we talk rather glibly about changes in mucosal permeability, we very rarely measure it directly, although that has been done. We measure the consequences of it. I would submit, however, that if combined ischemia and acid do change the permeability, which you cannot measure because of the altered gradient, the change must be very small, because, assuming that the gradients are precisely the same when we add bile salts, we find very typical changes associated with increased permeability: namely, the increased hydrogen ion flux and the sodium flux ratio data that I gave you. I think his point may be a real consideration when we talk about the combination of bile salts and ischemia; but again I tend to doubt it, because there is no additive change in the potential difference.

I would also suggest to Dr. DenBesten that each man is entitled to his own assumptions, and what you indicate is as assumptive as what I indicate.

I will concede that "volume flux" is an excellent term, and I will attempt to rectify that in the future. The potassium fluxes do not parallel the sodium fluxes, and I do believe that your interpretation that this respresents cellular damage is correct.

Physiologic factors in the selection of patients for superficial temporal artery–to–middle cerebral artery anastomosis

George Austin, M.D., David Laffin, *and* William Hayward, *Loma Linda, Calif.*

Occlusion of the internal or common carotid artery in the neck, stenosis of the internal carotid artery at the syphon, or distally, and occlusion or stenosis of the middle cerebral artery are not amenable to endarterectomy. The possibility of a bypass procedure, using a superficial temporal artery (STA) to middle cerebral artery (MCA) anastomosis, in such cases, poses the problem of optimal physiologic selection of patients. CBF, using the intravenous bolus injection technique (^{133}xenon), was measured in this type of patient. If the patients are not hemiplegic or aphasic, have one or more TIA's per week, and have at least a 25 percent reduction in gray matter blood flow, in the frontal area, on the side of the lesion, they may be considered as suitable candidates. Of 35 such patients who have undergone microsurgical anastomoses of the STA-MCA for cerebral ischemia, the CBF was studied before and after surgery in 22 patients. Control cerebral blood flow in gray matter (CBFG) = 75 ± 9 ml. per 100 Gm. The mean CBFG, on the side of pathology, was 53 ± 13 preoperatively, and 64 ± 15 postoperatively ($p = 0.02$). All patients showing this degree of improvement by CBF measurement have improved significantly, in terms of psychometric testing and decrease in TIA's. No patient has developed a stroke postoperatively.

From the Section of Neurological Surgery, Loma Linda University School of Medicine, Loma Linda, Calif.

A LARGE PROPORTION of extracranial occlusive disease is inaccessible to the vascular surgeon. This includes internal carotid artery occlusion, or high stenosis involving the distal internal carotid artery or the syphon. Intracranial attempts at endartrectomy of the middle cerebral arter have rarely been successful. In 1967, Donaghy and Yasargil[4] proposed a new form of bypass operation to provide an additional collateral circulation for the above groups of patients. This consisted of an end-to-side anastomosis of the superficial temporal artery to the middle cerebral artery performed under the operating microscope.

Most patients with extracranial or intracranial occlusive disease have numerous preliminary warnings before a major stroke occurs; these warnings consist of transient ischemic attacks (TIA's), which last seconds or minutes. It has been reported that between 20 and 25 percent of patients with TIA's develop a major stroke within 44 months.[14] Also, in a small group of patients with TIA's who were diagnosed angiographically as having internal carotid occlusion, 45 percent had a major stroke within three years of the onset of TIA's.[15] These statistics support the serious regard one should have for the symptoms of TIA's. Other than TIA's and an occlusion or stenotic lesion demonstrable by angiography, there has been no satisfactory physiologic means of selecting patients for a superficial temporal artery–to–middle cerebral artery (STA-MC) bypass anastomosis. The purpose of this presentation is to

Presented at the Thirty-fifth Annual Meeting of the Society of University Surgeons, St. Louis, Mo., Feb. 14-16, 1974.

Table I. *Average values for gray and white matter in a series of ten controls*

	Gray	*White*
Normal (intravenous method)	75 ± 9	25 ± 2
Reproducibility (intravenous method)	± 14%	± 14%
Relative tissue weights (intravenous method)	48%	52%
Pathologic (intravenous method)	55 ± 13	22 ± 2
Pathologic (internal carotid method)	58 ± 15	19 ± 4
Normal (internal carotid method)[8]	79.7 ± 11	21 ± 2.6

consider the use of the gray matter cerebral blood flow (CBFG) as a physiologic factor in selecting patients for surgery.

TRANSIENT ISCHEMIC ATTACKS (TIA's)

These have varied in different patients in our series but for a given patient, the same TIA's seem to recur. They are due to a decrease in blood flow below a critical level, and it is assumed that the regional tissue Po_2 decreases to the point that oxygen utilization is impaired. This decreases the saturation of cytochrome oxidase with decrease in oxidative phosphorylation. The resulting diminished ATP production causes failure of the ion pump mechanisms with a resulting fall in membrane resting potential.[9] The latter is manifested by altered neuronal firing patterns and clinically by the symptomatology of TIA's. It is well known that cerebral tissue Po_2 decreases with a decrease in blood flow as shown in Fig. 1. However, it is also likely that most patients with TIA's have some additional small vessel disease or regions of borderline tissue profusion. These regions would already have maximum tissue capillary perfusion and hence could not tolerate the occlusive effects of microemboli or transient drops in blood pressure due to decreased cardiac output or postural hypotension.

Focal symptoms of decrease in cerebral blood flow (CBF) are first manifest when the CBF falls to 75 percent of normal,[8] while the initial symptoms of impaired consciousness have been reported when the CBF falls to approximately 60 percent of normal.[5, 11] The fact that relatively few symptoms of TIA's are of localizing value is due partially to the frequent asymmetry of the branches of the Circle of Willis and its inability to provide adequate collateral flow. In other cases, an intracerebral steal mechanism may account for symptoms of TIA's in a distal region.

Since cerebral blood flow is such a critical factor in the development of TIA's, it seems important to attempt to use it as one physiologic factor in the selection of patients for surgery.

MEASUREMENT OF CEREBRAL BLOOD FLOW (CBF)

Method. This was done by the intravenous bolus injection method with the use of ^{133}xenon.[1, 2] The gamma emission was measured for 35 minutes over both sides of the head by using two scintillation detectors per side, over the frontal and parietal regions. In addition, the gamma activity in the patient's end-expired air (EEA) was monitored with a face mask leading to a scintillation detector and gas-counting chamber, approximately three feet from the patient's face.

From the gas-counting chamber the air was evacuated through a hood to the outside atmosphere. A brief injection of 10 mCi of ^{133}xenon was made into any convenient arm vein. A record of the gamma activity in the EEA and from the head probes was permanently stored on magnetic tape for future analysis. Also, an inkwriter recording was made following the injection of isotope for immediate monitoring.

Since ^{133}xenon is 10 to 15 times more soluble in air than in blood, the envelope of the EEA curve is approximately proportional to the arterial concentration.[10, 12] The two main problems of this method are extracerebral contamination and recirculation of isotope for roughly four minutes. In addition to the usual assumptions made for the internal carotid injection technique,

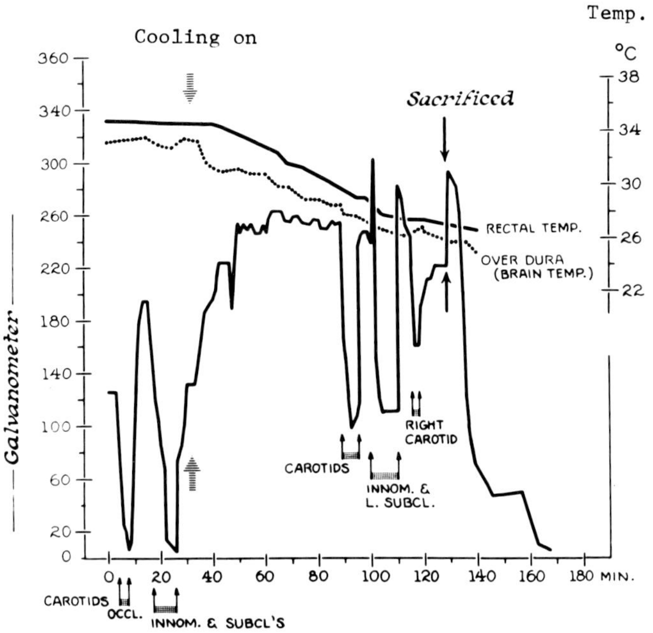

Fig. 1. Decrease in frontal cerebral Po_2 (ordinate) when carotid arteries are occluded in the monkey. Po_2 measured by 25 μ tip platinum-iridium electrode in Rt. frontal cortex. Time in minutes on abscissa. (Unpublished observations by Austin and Sayen.)

Table II. *Site of lesion with pre- and postoperative CBFG (ml./100 Gm./min.)*

Pathology	*No. of patients**	*Preoperative CBFG*	*Postoperative CBFG*	*P*
Unilateral internal carotid occlusion	12	59	63	< 0.07
High internal carotid stenosis	3	47	70	—
Middle cerebral stenosis	4	44	63	—
Bilateral internal carotid occlusion	1	38	74	—
Unilateral common carotid occlusion	2	67	63	—

*The number of patients having had pre- and postoperative measurements with each pathologic grouping.

namely that (1) there is complete mixing of isotope in the blood; (2) free diffusion of isotope occurs between blood and brain, and (3) the brain is composed predominantly of two main compartments; a fast compartment (gray matter flow), and a slow compartment (white matter flow), an additional three assumptions are made: (1) The CBF remains approximately constant over the 35 minute recording period. (2) The extracerebral component is assumed to be a single, slow compartment. (3) The white matter component is assumed to approach 0 after 16 minutes, and the gray matter component approaches 0 after eight minutes.

The Fick equation with a time-varying arterial function is assumed to hold for each compartment. In its voltage-simulated form, it is solved separately for each compartment by a special purpose analogue computer modified after that described by Crawley.[3] The solution for each compartment is displayed separately on a cathode ray oscilloscope and projected down through a lens onto an inkwriter record of the head curve.

The average values for gray and white matter in a series of ten controls, between the age of 18 and 57 years, compared closely with those published by the internal

Table III. *Pre- and postoperative CBFG in 21 patients*

*Area**	*Pre-operative CBFG*	*Post-operative CBFG*	*P*
Frontal (operated)	53 ± 13	64 ± 15	< 0.02
Parietal (operated)	53 ± 15	65 ± 14	< 0.015
Frontal (nonoperated)	60 ± 14	68 ± 16	< 0.07

*Describes frontal or parietal head probes on the operated or non-operated side.

carotid injection method of Ingvar and Lassen[7] (Table I).

Similarly, the reproducibility of ±14 percent determined by repeating the flow studies one week later in the same group of controls, compares closely with the internal carotid method.[13] Comparison of CBF done by the intravenous method and by the internal carotid method, in the same patient, showed a close correlation between the two methods, and especially for the gray matter flow (Table I). The intravenous bolus technique was used as a screening test in all patients considered as possible candidates for STA-MC anastomoses.

Preoperative CBF results.

Unilateral internal carotid artery (ICA) occlusion. This comprised a total group of 22 patients, 12 of whom had pre- and postoperative measurement of CBFG and also symptoms of TIA's. A small number of patients had gray matter flows that were considered to be within normal limits. In these cases, it was apparent that maximum collateral flow had developed through the ophthalmic artery, the pial anastomosis, and possibly a small amount through the middle meningeal and occipital arteries. In most patients showing a decrease in ipsilateral flow, there was likewise a decrease in flow on the side opposite the occlusion, although of lesser degree. In some patients, there was a significant difference in the two probes on the side of the occlusion. This was probably due to a regional area of ischemia on the basis of atherosclerosis or microemboli in which there was inadequate collateral flow. In most cases, the gray matter CBF reduction was greater than that in the white matter. The values of CBF for this group were CBFG = 60 ml. per 100 Gm. per minute, and CBFW = 22 ml. per 100 Gm. per minute. This was a 21 percent reduction in CBFG and a 12 percent reduction in CBFW.

High internal carotid artery stenosis. In three of four cases, CBF was measured. These stenotic lesions occurred below and at the carotid syphon. In two cases, they involved the distal internal carotid artery (between the takeoff of the posterior communicating artery and the bifurcation of the anterior and middle cerebral arteries). The stenotic lesions considered in this group always occluded greater than half the diameter of the vessel so that we were considering flow in vessels which had approximately 25 percent, or less, of the normal cross-sectional area at the stenotic site. The cause of the stenotic lesion was probably atherosclerotic with one caused by arteritis and at least one caused by trauma (Table II).

Middle cerebral artery stenosis. There are five cases in this group of patients, and in all the etiology remains unknown. In four patients, CBF was measured pre- and postoperatively. In none of these cases was there a history of valvular heart disease. In virtually all of these cases, the TIA's were more localizing than in patients with internal carotid pathology. They consisted primarily of brief episodes of numbness or weakness of the opposite hand. When the stenotic lesion involved the dominant hemisphere, there was invariably slurring of speech. Cerebral blood flow reduction was reduced significantly, more so in the gray matter than in the white. The average gray matter flow was 45 ml. per 100 Gm. per minute, and the average white matter flow was 22 ml. per 100 Gm. per minute (Table II). This was a 41 percent reduction in CBFG, and a 12 percent reduction in CBFW. Collateral flow was present to a limited degree through the pial anastomosis from anterior and posterior cerebral artery.

Unilateral common carotid occlusion. There were only two cases in this group, and

Table IV. *Site of pathology and surgical results in 35 patients undergoing STA-MC anastomoses*

	Excellent	*Good*	*Fair*	*Poor*	*No. of deaths*
Unilateral internal carotid occlusion	11	5	1	1	3
Middle cerebral stenosis	3	2			
High internal carotid stenosis	3	1			
Bilateral internal carotid occlusion	3				
Common carotid occlusion	1	1			

only one showed significant reduction in cerebral blood flow, with the greater reduction being in the gray matter. One case was the result of a previous common carotid ligation for intracranial aneurysm. The cause of occlusion in the other case remains unknown. Both had very small but palpable superficial temporal arteries that presumably were filled through a contralateral facial anastomosis.

Bilateral internal carotid artery occlusion. Only one of three patients in this group had a pre- and postoperative CBF with CBFG = 38 ml. per 100 Gm. per minute, and CBFW = 24 ml. per 100 Gm. per minute. These three men all were extremely hard working and highly tense individuals. The presumable etiology was atherosclerosis. In one patient who had only a preoperative CBF, the flow was normal. The collateral flow which permitted these people to function was due to a large vertebral artery input with good forward collateral flow through the post communicating arteries. The TIA's in these patients were associated with postural hypotension and involved brief episodes of dizziness, faintness, confusion, recent-memory loss and slurred speech.

Patients with TIA's and normal CBF. There were seven patients in this group; five of the seven had unilateral internal carotid occlusion, and there was one case each of common carotid occlusion and bilateral internal carotid occlusion. All except one case of unilateral internal carotid occlusion and one case of bilateral internal carotid occlusion had multiple and severe TIA's. The gray matter blood flow was within normal limits in every case. White matter flow was also normal, except in one patient, in whom flow was reduced by 24 percent. The TIA's were usually associated with postural hypotension or cardiac abnormalities.

CLINICAL RESULTS OF SURGERY

Results at this time must be classified to some extent as preliminary since no follow-up study lasted longer than 1½ years. No patient has had a stroke since discharge from the hospital. Results were classified as "excellent" if the patient had zero to three TIA's postoperatively; "good" if the patient had three to ten TIA's postoperatively; "fair" if the patient had fewer TIA's than preoperatively; and "poor" if the patient was unimproved. In none of the patients was the neurological status worsened. In five patients with some fixed neurologic deficit, there was improvement. This was more marked in motor and sensory speech deficit. In two patients with monoplegias of the hand, there was no improvement in function.

"Excellent" or "good" results. These were obtained in 29 patients, or 83 percent (Table III).

"Fair" or "poor" results. "Fair" or "poor" results occurred in three patients, and in two instances, they resulted from faulty selection. The one poor result occurred in a patient with severe and poorly controlled diabetes whose blood sugar rose to 738 mg., 24 hours after surgery. In the case of a "fair" result, the patient had diffuse and severe atherosclerosis and had previously undergone coronary bypass surgery. His intracranial anastomosis was later shown to have occluded several weeks following surgery.

Surgical death, i.e., patient died in the hospital within 30 days of surgery, occurred in three patients. In two of these, faulty selec-

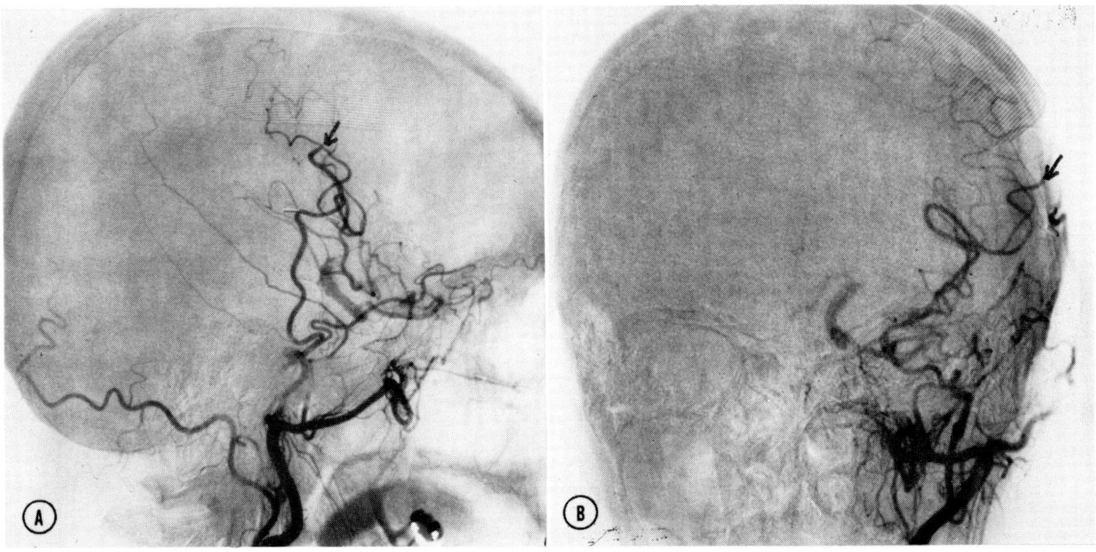

Fig. 2. *A,* Lateral postoperative angiogram shows filling of middle cerebral and internal carotid by STA-MC anastomosis. (Case No. 22-70-58: bilateral internal carotid occlusion.) Arrow at site of anastomosis. *B,* Anteroposterior postoperative angiogram shows filling of middle cerebral and internal carotid by STA-MC anastomosis. (Case No. 22-70-58.) Arrow at site of anastomosis.

tion was attributed as a major factor. One patient had a coronary occlusion 24 hours postoperatively. He gave a history of two previous myocardial infarctions and was having four to five anginal attacks per day requiring nitroglycerin. A second patient of 69 years had two previous strokes, with some recovery, and he had a third stroke during the operative closure and died several days later. The third death occurred in a patient with cirrhosis and a massive spleen (620 Gm.) who succumbed to a Serratia septicemia.

In the group of seven patients with TIA's but normal preoperative CBFG, six patients had "excellent" results postoperatively.

POSTOPERATIVE CBF STUDIES

In the 12 cases of internal carotid occlusion, there was a modest but significant improvement in CBFG and CBFW, with $p < 0.07$. In the other groups, there was a much larger degree of improvement but since the groups were too small for statistical analysis, we have compared the values of all patients ($N = 22$), preoperative CBFG with postoperative CBFG. This was done for both the operated side and the nonoperated side (Tables III and IV). Unfortunately, it is impossible to get postoperative angiograms on all patients because of the discomfort and the patient's awareness of the hazards involved. We have used palpation and the Doppler flow meter in some cases, and angiograms in cases where we suspected possible occlusion. At present, we only know of four cases of occlusion. Typical postoperative angiograms are seen in Fig. 2.

From the Tables the following observations are pertinent: (1) CBFG was more significantly reduced than CBFW. (2) CBFG was not only significantly reduced from 22 to 50 percent on the side of the lesion, but to a lesser extent on the opposite side. (3) With the use of t tests, there was postoperative increase in CBFG on the side of the lesion of approximately 23 percent in both the frontal and parietal flows with $p < 0.02$. (4) There was a smaller but significant increase postoperatively on the side opposite the lesion of approximately 14 percent with $p < 0.07$.

DISCUSSION

In general the clinical improvement was parallel to the increase in CBFG. However, in the six patients who had a normal CBFG, before surgery, but with severe and frequent TIA's, the postoperative improvement was excellent. This was probably due to the fact that they had no reserve capacity preoperatively with maximum vasodilatation of the capillary bed and hence there was no tolerance to decreased CBF on any etiologic bases. Postoperatively, their CBFG remained normal or was increased, giving them some physiologic reserve in cases where there were regions of lost autoregulation of CBF.

The decrease in CBFG on the side opposite the lesion is explained as partly due to cross-over of CBF to the pathologic side through the anterior communicating artery and forward flow to the pathologic side from the post communicating artery. Hence, this is a form of intracerebral steal. This is supported by the observation that postoperatively CBFG was also improved but to a lesser extent in the non-operated side. This may explain why TIA's of brief episodes of slurred speech were present in such a high proportion of cases.

Although the mean increase in CBFG on the operated side of 11 ml. per 100 Gm. per minute does not seem large, its significance lies in the fact that it brings the CBFG to the point that the patient can better tolerate drops in perfusion pressure without the discouraging symptoms of TIA's and probably with less chance of a stroke. In three patients, maximum flow in the STA was measured in the operating room before the anastomosis, giving an average of 38 c.c. per minute. When equal weights of gray and white matter are assumed, this would amount to an increase of roughly 19 ml. per 100 Gm. per minute in CBFG in the middle cerebral distribution. This checks reasonably well with the measured increase in perfusion CBFG.

CONCLUSIONS

1. A preliminary study of 35 patients (total number is now 41) undergoing superficial temporal to middle cerebral artery (STA-MC) anastomoses has been made and the incidence of various TIA's was noted to be largely non-localizing in value.

2. A study of the cerebral blood flow pre- and postoperatively done in 22 patients showed the gray matter flow (CBFG) to be much more significantly reduced than white matter (CBFW).

3. There was also a significant decrease in CBFG on the side opposite the lesion.

4. Postoperatively, as demonstrated with the use of t test, there was an improvement in CBFG on the side of the lesion of 23 percent ($p < 0.02$), and on the opposite side of 14 percent ($p < 0.07$).

5. Approximately 83 percent of the patients had a good or excellent result in terms of improvement, in frequency of TIA's, and no patient had a stroke in the postoperative follow-up period of less than 1½ years.

6. We suggest that in addition to a history of TIA's and an angiographically visualized lesion that is inaccessible to the vascular surgeon, a reduction of greater than 20 to 25 percent in CBFG, on the side of the lesion, may be one good physiologically positive indication for STA-MC anastomosis.

7. However, in certain patients with the above criteria but with a normal CBFG, we suggest that surgery may also be indicated to increase the reserve capabilities of CBF and improve autoregulation, if severe TIA's are present.

REFERENCES

1. Austin, G., Horn, N., Rouhe, S., and Hayward, W.: Description and early results of an intravenous radioisotope technique for measuring cerebral blood flow in man, *in* Proceedings of International Symposium on Cerebral Blood Flow, Rome-Seina, October, 1971.
2. Austin, G., Laffin, D., Rouhe, S., and Hayward, W.: Intravenous isotope injection method of cerebral blood flow measurement: Accuracy and reproducibility, *in* Proceedings of The International Symposium on Cerebral Circulation and Metabolism, Philadelphia, Pa., June 6-9, 1973. In press.
3. Crawley, J. C. W.: An analogue computer

for calculating blood perfusion rates, Biomed. Eng. **3:** 256, 1968.
4. Donaghy, P., and Yasargil, G.: Extrain-tracranial blood flow diversion (abst.), American Association of Neurological Surgeons, Chicago, Ill., April, 1968.
5. Finnerty, F. A., Witkin, L., and Fazekas, J. F.: Cerebral hemodynamics during cerebral ischemia produced by acute hypotension, J. Clin. Invest. **33:** 1227, 1954.
6. Hoedt-Rasmussen, K., Sveinsdottir, E., and Lassen, N. A.: Regional cerebral blood flow in man determined by intra-arterial injection of radioactive inert gas, Circ. Res. **18:** 237, 1966.
7. Ingvar, D. H., Cronquist, S., Ekberg, R., Risberg, J., and Hoedt-Rasmussen, K.: Normal values of regional cerebral blood flow in man, including flow and weight estimates of grey and white matter, presented at the International Symposium of Regional Cerebral Blood Flow, Lund, Sweden, 1965, Acta Neurol. Scand. Suppl. **14:** 72, 1965.
8. Jennett, W. B., and Harper, M. A.: Measurement of regional cerebral blood flow during carotid ligation, Lancet **11:** 1162, 1966.
9. Kerkut, G., and York, B.: The electrogenic sodium pump, Bristol, U. K., 1971, Scientclinica, p. 51.
10. Mallett, B. L., and Veall, N.: The measurement of regional cerebral clearance rates in man using ^{133}xenon inhalation and extracranial recording, Science **29:** 179, 1965.
11. McHenry, L. C., Fazekas, J. F., and Sullivan, J. F.: Cerebral hemodynamics of syncope, Am. J. Med. Sci. **241:** 173, 1961.
12. Obrist, W. D., Thompson, H. D., King, C. H., and Wang, H. S.: Determination of regional cerebral blood flow by inhalation of ^{133}xenon, Circ. Res. **20:** 124, 1967.
13. Prencipe, M.: Reproducibility of cerebral blood flow determinations: Cerebral blood flow and intracranial pressure, Proc. Fifth International Symposium, Rome-Seina, 1971. European Neurology. Part I, Vol. 6: 234-235. 1971/1972.
14. Siekert, R. G., editor: Cerebrovascular Survey Report for Joint Council Subcommittee on Cerebrovascular Disease–National Institute Neurological Diseases and Stroke and National Heart and Lung Insitute, revised, Rochester, Minn., July, 1970, Whiting Printers & Stationers.
15. Ziegler, D. K., and Hassanein, R. S.: Prognosis in patients with TIA's Stroke. **4:** 666, 1973.

DISCUSSION

Chairman Zuidema. As you have developed the technique, to what extent have your indications for operation changed and how extensive do you feel that this can be? How extensively do you feel this can be employed in the future management of patients with TIA? I mean, is this going to be a large segment of the population, or is this going to be very limited?

Dr. George M. Austin (closing). About 35,000 patients each year, we believe, are possible, or potential, candidates for the surgery, in terms of preventing major strokes.

The present predictions are that if a patient has transient ischemic attacks, he has about a 24 percent chance of having a major stroke in four years. If a patient has a transient ischemic attack and undergoes four-vessel angiography, and this shows an internal carotid occlusion, he has a 45 percent chance of having a major stroke in three years.

The follow-up period in our group has been short, about 1½ years. No patient has had a stroke postoperatively. Of course, we are going to have to wait another few years before we can prove anything. The improvement we recorded was a decrease in frequency of TIA's, and, without going into it, if they had zero to three transient ischemic attacks postoperatively, we considered them an excellent result; three to ten in the total postoperative period, are a good result, and so forth.

Altered action of parathyroid hormone by chlorpropamide

Patricia J. Numann, M.D., *and* **Arnold M. Moses, M.D.,** *Syracuse, N. Y.*

Chlorpropamide (CP), in addition to augmenting insulin release, produces an antidiuresis by increasing both the release and the peripheral action of antidiuretic hormone (ADH). The antidiuretic activity of CP is sufficient to treat most patients with central diabetes insipidus and to produce dilutional hyponatremia in some patients with diabetes mellitus. Since the biochemical action of parathyroid hormone (PTH) on the renal tubule is similar to that of ADH, except the former acts at the cortical tubular level and the latter at the medullary level, we investigated whether CP might produce an augmentation of the renal action of PTH. In experiments on parathyroidectomized rats, the expected phosphaturia which resulted from the administration of either commercial Lilly PTH or synthetic Beckman PTH was increased by the administration of CP ($p < 0.005$). Since the action of PTH, like ADH, is mediated by cyclic AMP (CAMP), CAMP was measured in the urine. CP inhibited the PTH-induced CAMP response ($p < 0.005$). These data suggest that CP may be of use in treating patients with para thyroid disease and perhaps might have to be avoided in patients with disorders of calcium deficiency. Chlorpropamide may alter cyclic AMP production in many areas of the body and thus may have widespread effects in many cellular functions that are mediated by cyclic AMP.

From the Syracuse Veterans Administration Hospital and the Departments of Surgery and Medicine, State University of New York, Upstate Medical Center, Syracuse, N. Y.

CHLORPROPAMIDE, which is used in the treatment of adult onset diabetes mellitus because of its ability to release insulin, has a well-known antidiuretic action. Some patients with diabetes mellitus (DM) treated with chlorpropamide develop a deleterious water retention state. The antidiuretic effect of chlorpropamide is used therapeutically in some patients with diabetes insipidus (DI). Chlorpropamide produces its antidiuretic effect by increasing the release of antidiuretic hormone (ADH)[2, 9, 13] and by augmenting the peripheral action of ADH.[1, 11, 13] Chlorpropamide apparently augments the peripheral action of ADH by increasing the renal medullary adenyl cyclase production in response to ADH.[7, 8] Since the effect of parathyroid hormone (PTH) on the renal tubule is also mediated by way of adenosine 3′,5′ monophosphate (cyclic AMP),[3] we carried out experiments to see if chlorpropamide also affected the action of PTH.

Supported by Veterans Administration Research Funds, Grants No. 5855-01 and 6152-02.

Presented at the Thirty-fifth Annual Meeting of the Society of University Surgeons, St. Louis, Mo., Feb. 14-16, 1974.

MATERIALS AND METHODS

Adult Charles River rats were surgically parathyroidectomized. Serum calcium levels of less than 7 mg. percent were considered indicative of total parathyroidectomy. To detect possible recovery of parathyroid function, serum calcium concentrations were measured weekly during the study period. The rats were housed in metabolic cages during the four-hour study period with no access to additional food or water to avoid

Table I. *Effect of chlorpropamide, parathyroid hormone, and combined treatment in parathyroidectomized rats*

	No treatment	*Chlorpropamide*	*Parathyroid hormone*	*Chlorpropamide and parathyroid hormone*
Serum calcium (mg. %)	6.03 ± 0.17	6.09 ± 0.36	7.98 ± 0.29*	6.98 ± 0.24†
Serum phosphorus (mg. %)	13.58 ± 0.34	13.05 ± 0.55	7.95 ± 0.34*	10.36 ± 0.51‡
Urine volume (ml./4 hr.)	3.52 ± 0.31	7.04 ± 0.48*	2.42 ± 0.18*	5.83 ± 0.76‡
Urinary sodium (mEq./4 hr.)	0.370 ± 0.60	0.590 ± 0.85§	0.254 ± 0.33§	0.718 ± 0.48‡
Urinary potassium (mEq./4 hr.)	0.424 ± 0.047	0.396 ± 0.035	0.467 ± 0.037	0.522 ± 0.032
Urinary phophorus (mg./mg. creatinine)	2.27 ± 0.26	4.78 ± 0.38*	3.13 ± 0.27§	7.00 ± 0.95†
Phosphorus clearance (ml./4 hr.)	27.2 ± 5.16	48.24 ± 5.72	96.24 ± 13.08*	160.2 ± 20.4†
Urinary cyclic AMP (nanomoles/4 hr.)	14.1 ± 1.59	13.54 ± 3.60	28.66 ± 2.88‖	15.70 ± 1.87†

*$p < 0.001$ when compared to Column 1.
†$p < 0.005$ when compared to Column 3.
‡$p < 0.001$ when compared to Column 3.
§$p < 0.05$ when compared to Column 1.
‖$p < 0.005$ when compared to Column 1.

error in urinary phosphate determinations.

The chlorpropamide powder was diluted in NaOH and then titrated to a pH of 7.4. The parathyroid hormone was dissolved in sterile saline. In order to assure the effects were due to PTH and not a contaminant in the Lilly parathyroid injection. Beckman synthetic PTH was used in one group and Lilly parathyroid injection was used in another group. The paired data were analyzed and found to be the same, so the data were pooled. Lilly parathyroid injection was used for the remainder of the study to decrease expense.

The parathyroidectomized rats were divided into four groups for each week of the study. One group received no treatment. One group received chlorpropamide, 20 mg. per 100 Gm. of rat per day intraperitoneally, for five days. The third group received Lilly parathyroid injection, 40 U. per day subcutaneously, on the third, fourth, and fifth days. The fourth group received chlorpropamide, 20 mg. per 100 Gm. of rat per day intraperitoneally, daily and on the third, fourth, and fifth days received Lilly parathyroid injection, 40 U. per day. Each week the groups received a different therapy until each rat had received all four types of therapy so each rat could be used as its own control.

Four-hour urine collections were begun as soon as the PTH had been injected. The four-hour total volume of urine was measured for phosphorous, creatinine, sodium, potassium, and cyclic AMP. At the end of the fifth day of each study week, blood was drawn from the retro-orbital plexus for serum phosphorous, calcium, and creatinine determinations.

Sodium and potassium concentrations were determined by flame photometry. Serum and urinary creatinine concentrations were performed with the Jaffee reaction. Phosphorous determinations were performed colorimetrically with the use of the phosphomolybdic acid reaction. Calcium determinations were carried out colorimetrically by using the cresolphthalein complexone reaction. Urinary cylcic AMP determinations were performed with a modification of the competitive protein-binding assay of Gilman.[6]

The data were analyzed with the use of the t test for paired data. Comparisons were made between chlorpropamide and no treatment, between PTH and no treatment, and between PTH plus chlorpropamide and PTH alone.

RESULTS

Untreated parathyroidectomized rats showed the findings of low serum calcium, high serum phosphorous, and low urinary cyclic AMP concentration (Table I), that are expected after parathyroidectomy.

Chlorpropamide treatment did not change the serum calcium or serum phosphorous concentration, urinary cyclic AMP, or urinary potassium excretion (Table I). Chlorpropamide did increase urinary sodium excretion, urinary volume, and urinary phosphorous excretion (Table I).

Parathyroid hormone treatment produced the expected increase in serum calcium concentration and urinary phosphorous and cyclic AMP excretion, and it did produce the expected decrease in serum phosphorous (Table I).

When the rats were pretreated with chlorpropamide prior to PTH injection, the effect of PTH was significantly altered. The elevation of serum calcium produced by PTH was significantly reduced, and the decrease in serum phosphorous was significantly less (Table I). Urinary volume and sodium were significantly greater with the combination of PTH and chlorpropamide than with chlorpropamide alone. Chlorpropamide did not obliterate the phosphaturic effect of PTH (Table I). Chlorpropamide did significantly decrease the rise in cyclic AMP which had been produced by PTH (Fig. 1 and Table I).

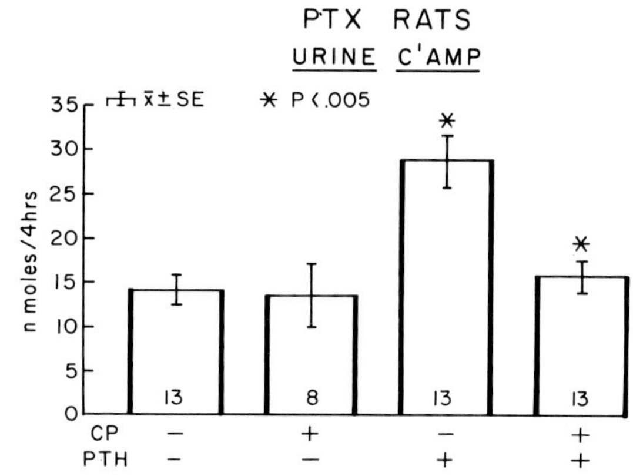

Fig. 1. The effect of chlorpropamide treatment on the PTH-induced cyclic AMP excretion in the parathyroidectomized rat. CP, chlorpropamide powder (20 mg. per 100 Gm. per rat); PTH, parathyroid injection (40 U. per rat). PTH significantly increases cyclic AMP excretion. This effect is significantly less when the rats are pretreated with CP.

DISCUSSION

Antidiuretic hormone (ADH) and parathyroid hormone (PTH) have certain similarities in their mechanism of action in the kidney. Although the ADH receptor site is in the distal renal tubule and the PTH receptor site is in the proximal renal tubule, both hormones activate adenyl cyclase which converts ATP to cyclic AMP within the cell. The cyclic AMP is then responsible for subsequent chemical changes which result in the physiologic action of the hormones. The major action of ADH in the renal tubule is to enhance the reabsorption of water while the major action of PTH is to decrease the tubular reabsorption of phosphate, thereby increasing the urinary phosphate excretion. The serum changes induced by ADH are due to the concentrating effect on the renal tubule, whereas PTH also has a major action on bone, mobilizing calcium, in addition to its action on the renal tubule.

Chlorpropamide has no intrinsic antidiuretic action. It does, however, result in an ADH-like effect in most patients with diabetes insipidus and in some patients with diabetes mellitus.This action is a result of increasing the release of ADH from the pituitary[2, 9, 13] as well as augmenting the peripheral action of ADH[1, 11, 13] as demonstrated in the DI rat[11] and the toad bladder.[10] Chlorpropamide produces an antidiuresis in normal adult volunteers who are water loaded and undergoing maximal diuresis.[13] This peripheral augmentation may be due to an increase in the ADH-induced activation of adenyl cyclase.[7, 10] In contrast to its augmentation effect of urinary adenyl cyclase in response to ADH, chlorpropamide appears to interfere with the cyclic AMP excretion in response to PTH. Since the physiologic effects of PTH on both bone and kidney are at least in part due to cyclic AMP, an inhibition of PTH effect would be expected to occur in conjunction with chlorpropamide treatment. Chlorpropamide does interfere with the rise in serum calcium and the fall in serum phosphorous, indicating a physiologic response in bone to the inhibition of PTH-induced change in cyclic AMP.

Although chlorpropamide alone produces significant phosphaturia when the altered creatinine clearance is taken into consideration, the phosphaturic response to PTH administration in the rats pretreated with chlorpropamide was not inhibited despite the decrease in urinary cyclic AMP. The mechanism by which chlorpropamide produces phosphaturia and fails to inhibit the phosphaturic response to PTH could be explained in many ways since the mechanisms of phosphate excretion by the kidney are very complex. The inorganic phosphate load, which is produced by ingestion and metabolism of phosphorous bound to numerous compounds, may change the degree of phosphaturia. Phosphorous excretion, which is an intimate part of acid-base regulation in the kidney, can be altered by changes in the carbonic anhydrase system. Although PTH is the hormone that most drastically alters phosphate excretion, cortisone, glucagon, thyroid hormone, thyrocalcitonin, and vitamin D also produce increases in phosphate excretion.[14] Chase and associates[5] have noted in normal subjects the phosphaturic response to parathyroid hormone was more variable than the change in cyclic AMP. The data presented here, which show augmentation of the phosphaturic effect of PTH and yet inhibition of cyclic AMP production in response to PTH, raise the possibility that the phosphaturic effect of parathyroid hormone is not simply a direct effect of cyclic AMP. Chlorpropamide may affect the metabolism of cyclic AMP in the kidney to allow a prolonged effect of cyclic AMP without an increase in production; however, unpublished data suggest that the changes in the kidney cyclic AMP parallel the change in the urine which would preclude altered metabolism of cyclic AMP as the cause of the augmented phosphaturia. The minimal elevation in cyclic AMP excretion seen which occurs in response to combined PTH and chlorpropamide therapy may be sufficient to produce a maximal increased phosphaturic effect. This divergent effect of PTH on phosphaturia and cyclic AMP production suggests that measuring the phosphaturic effect as the only indication of PTH effect, as has been done in many physiologic studies of PTH, may not have given valid data and raises many interesting questions related to the phosphaturic effect of PTH.

Chlorpropamide also appears to be a proximal tubular diuretic as indicated by the natriuretic, diuretic, and phosphaturic effect produced in these hypoparathyroid rats. Miller and Moses[12] have also shown an increase in sodium and water excretion in normal Brattleboro rats and heterozygous Brattleboro rats with congenital diabetes insipidus treated with chlorpropamide.

In parathyroidectomized rats, chlorpropamide significantly inhibits the effect of parathyroid hormone on urinary cyclic AMP excretion and interfers with the PTH-induced changes in serum calcium and phosphorous concentration but not in urinary phosphorous excretion. Although the clinical applications have not been determined, chlorpropamide may well be of use in the treatment of patients with parathyroid disease and perhaps should be avoided in patients with disorders of calcium deficiency. A very important consideration is that chlorpropamide may alter cyclic AMP production in many areas of the body and thus have widespread effects on many cellular functions that are mediated by cyclic AMP.

The authors wish to thank Pfizer Corporation for their generous supply of chlorpropamide powder. We also wish to acknowledge the expert technical assistance of Miss Janice Hager.

REFERENCES

1. Berndt, W. O., Miller, M., Keltyle, W. M., and Valtin, H.: Potentiation of the antidiuretic effect of vasopressin by chlorpropamide, Endocrinology **86:** 1028, 1970.
2. Bode, H. H., Harley, B. M., and Crawford, J. D.: Restoration of normal drinking behavior by chlorpropamide in patients with hypodipsia and diabetes inspidus, Am. J. Med. **51:** 304, 1971.
3. Chase, L. R., and Aurbach, G. D.: Para-

thyroid function and the renal excretion of 3′,5′-adenylic acid, Proc. Natl. Acad. Sci. USA **58:** 518, 1967.

4. Chase, L. R., and Aurbach, G. D.: Cyclic AMP and mechanism of action of parathyroid hormone, *in* Talmadge, R. V., and Belanger, L. F., editors: Parathyroid hormone and thyrocalcitonin (calcitonin), Amsterdam, 1968, Exerpta Medica Foundation, pp. 247-257.
5. Chase, L. R., Melson, G. L., and Aurbach, G. D.: Pseudohypoparathyroidism: Defective excretion of 3,5-AMP in response in parathyroid hormone, J. Clin. Invest. **48:** 1832, 1969.
6. Gilman, A. G.: A protein binding assay for adenosine 3′,5′-cyclic monophosphate, Proc. Natl. Acad, Sci. **67:** 305, 1970.
7. Inglefinger, J. R., and Hays, R. M.: Evidence that chlorpropamide and vasopressin share a common site of action, J. Clin. Endocrinol. **29:** 738, 1969.
8. Lozada, E. S., Gauaux, J., Franklin, N., et al.: Studies of the mode of action of the sulfonureas and phenylacetamides in enhancing the effect of vasopressin, J. Clin. Endocrinol. **34:** 704, 1972.
9. Mahoney, J. H., and Goodman, A. D.: Hypernatremia due to hypodypsia and elevated threshold for vasopressin release, N. Engl. J. Med. **279:** 1191, 1968.
10. Mendoza, S. A.: Effect of chlorpropamide on the permeability of the urinary bladder of the toad and the response to vasopressin, adenosine 3′,5′-monophosphate and theophylline, Endocrinology **84:** 411, 1969.
11. Miller, M., and Moses, A. M.: Potentiation of vasopressin action by chlorpropamide in vivo, Endocinology **86:** 1023, 1970.
12. Moses, A. M., and Miller, M.: Personal communication.
13. Moses, A. M., Numann, P., and Miller, M.: Mechanism of chlorpropamide-induced antidiuresis in man: Evidence for release of ADH and enhancement of peripheral action, Metabolism **22:** 59, 1973.
14. Mudge, G. H., Berndt, W. O., and Valtin, H.: *in* Orloff, W., and Berliner, R. W., editors: Handbook of Physiology, Section 8: Renal Physiology, American Physiologic Society, Baltimore, Md., 1973, The Williams & Wilkins Company, pp. 605-619.

DISCUSSION

Dr. Edwin L. Kaplan (Chicago, Ill). Is it possible that you can interpret these data in a different way? Is it possible that chlorpropamide gives the phosphaturia, as noted in your parathyroidectomized rats, and then the synergistic effect may be two separate actions, rather than PTH effect. In other words, you have a decrease in urinary cyclic AMP. You have a decrease in the serum calcium. And what you have really shown is an increase in urinary phosphate. Is it possible that this is really not increased effect of PTH, but just the action of the drug iself?

Dr. Joshua Miller (St. Louis Park, Minn.). We have tertiary hyperparathyroidism occurring after our renal transplants, and sometimes we are faced with the problem of having to operate at a time when we do not want to. I was just wondering if anybody has considered using chlorpropamide to control hypercalcemia.

We also have done some diabetic transplants and run into a problem of diuresis, despite the fact that insulin is controlling diabetes. I just wonder whether we are seeing something akin to what you are describing that may be controlled by the use of this agent.

Dr. Patricia J. Numann (closing). We were concerned that the phosphaturic effect also might be an independent action of the drug, rather than an augmentation of the effect of parathyroid hormone. So we have done this study with other doses of the drug that do not appear to give a phosphaturic effect in and of themselves, and we still do produce an augmentation of the phosphaturia produced by PTH; yet in the low-dose studies do not seem to interfere with the cyclic AMP production.

We have been very interested in the number of people who have water metabolism problems related to the treatment of their diabetes and to the use of many other drugs that also interfere with the effect and the action of antidiuretic hormone, and, actually, some of the first people who aroused our interest in this subject were patients who were on Diabinese and who appeared to develop an inappropriate ADH syndrome in response to their treatment. We really could not figure out what was wrong with them until we stopped their Diabinese and put them on insulin coverage, and then they did diurese very nicely.

I wonder if the patients who have diabetes might not have been treated with chlorpropamide preoperatively, and you are seeing the diuresis in response to the cessation of the use of the drug. If you are having troube with diuresis and want to stop it, you can stop it with chlorpropamide, and we actually treat, now, the majority of our patients with diabetes insipidus with chlorpropamide, without any problem at all.

Gas tensions in healing tissues of traumatized patients

R. Bruce Heppenstall, M.D., Fred N. Littooy, M.D., Richard Fuchs, George F. Sheldon, M.D., *and* **Thomas K. Hunt, M.D.,** *San Francisco, Calif.*

Recent studies in animals show that abnormally low Po_2 and high Pco_2 in wounds, both of which are demonstrated consequences of trauma, delay repair and increase susceptibility to infection. For this reason, the Po_2 and Pco_2 of wounds in humans were measured in seven traumatized patients, six uninjured controls, and ten operative patients. All trauma patients had multiple system injuries requiring extensive resuscitation. Severe trauma induces a defect in oxygen transport to injured tissue. This defect is only partially responsive to changes in cardiac index, arterial Po_2, and intrinsic red cell function. The data give objective support to the observation that wounds in trauma patients are particularly slow to heal and are unusually susceptible to pyogenic and anaerobic infection.

From the Department of Surgery, University of California, San Francisco, and The Trauma Center, San Francisco General Hospital, San Francisco, Calif.

OXYGEN HAS a direct effect on the rate of repair in injured tissue. Previous studies have defined the role of oxygen in the rate of collagen synthesis, energy production, cellular proliferation, and ability to combat infection within a wound.[4, 5, 7-11, 13, 15-17] A diminished oxygen supply to an area of injured tissue decreases the rate of repair and increases the susceptibility to infection.[11, 16] The available oxygen supply in an area of reparative tissue is governed by the following factors: (1) an adequate ambient oxygen supply (FiO_2); (2) pulmonary exchange; (3) blood flow (CI); (4) adequate number of functional red blood cells; (5) presence or absence of peripheral shunting; (6) a functional capillary pattern within the wound. Oxygen delivery in injured and healing tissue is unique in that the degree of capillary regeneration is initially important, since it influences the distance in the wound across which oxygen must diffuse to reach the reparative cell. The long diffusion distances in the wound place an important emphasis on the arterial Po_2 and blood flow in maintaining an oxygen gradient within the reparative tissue. Oxygen delivered to the advancing wound edge is rapidly utilized, and consumption increases with additional oxygen supply.[9, 10]

This study was designed with the following goals in mind: to evaluate the effect of remote trauma on the oxygen and carbon dioxide tensions within minor wounds in humans and to investigate the application of the present method as a clinical tool.

MATERIALS AND METHODS

Three groups of patients were studied.

Group 1. The first group consisted of six normal subjects, including some of the authors and several healthy volunteers, who served as controls.

Supported by United States Public Health Service Grant No. GM-12829, United States Army Contract DADA 17-72-C-2030, and National Institutes of Health Grant No. GM-18470.

Presented at the Thirty-fifth Annual Meeting of the Society of University Surgeons, St. Louis, Mo., Feb. 14-16, 1974.

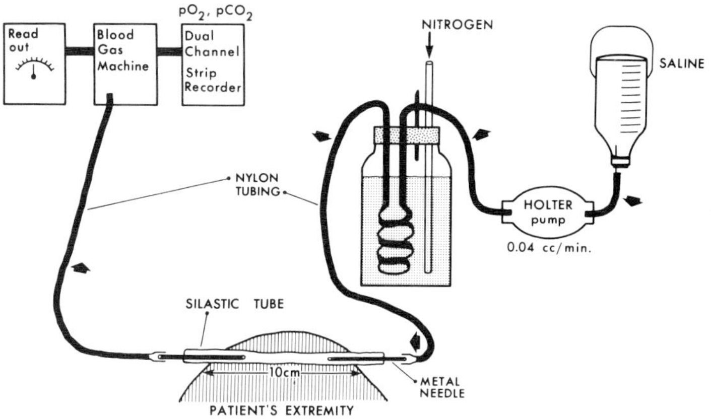

Fig. 1. Schematic diagram of the gas-monitoring apparatus.

Group 2. The second group was ten patients who were investigated prior to, during, and following various elective surgical procedures in an attempt to evaluate the effect of minor trauma on wound oxygen values.

Group 3. The third group was composed of seven patients who suffered severe trauma with multiple system injuries requiring extensive fluid and blood replacement.

A minor subcutaneous wound was produced in all subjects by the insertion of a silicone rubber tissue tonometer in an extremity, as described previously by Niinikoski and Hunt.[13, 14] In the control group, the tonometer was placed in the lateral aspect of the upper extremity between the shoulder and elbow. In the group with minor trauma (Group 2), the tonometer was placed in an extremity which did not interfere with the surgical procedure. In patients with multiple trauma (Group 3), it was placed in an uninvolved extremity.

The tissue tonometer was introduced subcutaneously through a No. 14 gauge spinal needle six inches long. Local anesthetic was injected at the entrance and exit sites of the needle, which was inserted so that 10 cm. of silicone rubber tubing (0.6 mm., internal diameter, 1.19 mm., outside diameter) threaded through it would remain within the subcutaneous tissue, following removal of the needle. A metal connector was inserted to a depth of 1 cm. into each end of a 12 cm. silicone rubber tube prior to implantation. Following implantation, the metal inserts extended from deep in the dermis to the exterior. This prevented atmospheric oxygen from influencing the tissue measurements. To further ensure against atmospheric or bacterial contamination, the entrance and exit sites were sealed with a tissue bond, Loctite. Physiological saline, or 5 percent dextrose and water, buffered to a pH of 4 to 5 was used to perfuse the tonometer (Fig. 1). The solution was buffered after in vitro testing in fluid baths of known gaseous concentration revealed that this particular pH resulted in optimal carbon dioxide tension equilibration without affecting the oxygen across the silicone rubber membrane. The perfusing solution was delivered to a deoxygenating bottle by a Holter pump at a flow rate of 0.4 ml. per minute. The bottle contained a long silicone rubber coil immersed in saline through which nitrogen was bubbled. The perfusing solution passed through the silicone rubber tubing and equilibrated with the surrounding saline solution, which was deoxygenated by the bubbling nitrogen gas mixture. The perfusate then flowed through nylon tubing, previously demonstrated by testing to be impermeable to oxygen and carbon dioxide. The nylon tubing was connected by the metal connectors to the silicone rubber tonometer in the patient. Once the perfusate traversed the tonometer, it was delivered by nylon tubing to calibrated oxygen and carbon dioxide electrodes* which, in turn, were connected to an oxygen and carbon dioxide

*BMS 3 MK 2 microsystem, Radiometer.

Table I. *Correlation table**

	P_{50}	Lactate	CI	Pv_{O_2}
% P_tO_2	−0.38†	−0.36†	0.56‡	0.33†
P_{50}		0.19 (N.S.)	−0.48‡	0.29 (N.S.)
Lactate			−0.48‡	−0.35†
CI				0.48‡

*Y = % P_tO_2; R_2 = 0.356; n = 41; F = 4.45.
†p < 0.05.
‡p < 0.01.

Table II. *P_{50}: Hemoglobin-oxygen affinity*

Day	N*	Mean ± S.E.M.†
1	13	24.24 ± 0.61
2	13	24.82 ± 0.49
3	11	24.24 ± 0.67
4	8	25.29 ± 0.63
5	5	25.68 ± 0.66

*N = number of determinations.
†S.E.M. = standard error of the mean.

monitor* and a dual-channel recorder.† Extensive testing of the apparatus through in vitro fluid baths of known gaseous concentrations revealed an equilibration of 95 percent with oxygen and 85 percent with carbon dioxide. Following insertion, daily values were obtained in each group of patients. In addition, the response of tissue and blood Po_2 to systemically administered oxygen was determined. In the severely traumatized patients, several parameters were measured, including cardiac index, arterial gas tensions, red blood cell 2-3 diphosphoglycerate (DPG), hemoglobin-oxygen affinity (P_{50}), and serum lactate. Cardiac index was determined by the dye dilution method. Arterial gases were determined in the above Radiometer system. Determinations of 2-3 DPG were done by a modification of Keitt's method.[11a] P_{50} oxyhemoglobin curve was spectrophotometrically‡ determined after whole blood had been equilibrated with gases containing low concentrations of oxygen which were balanced by CO_2 (5.25 percent) and nitrogen. P_{50} was calculated by the Hill equation. Serum lactate (micromoles per gram of hemoglobin) was measured by the Boehringer kit. The tonometer was placed in the majority of the patients 12 to 24 hours following their admission; therefore, Day 1 following implantation corresponds to Day 2 after traumatic injury.

*PHA 729, Radiometer.
†Leeds and Northrup Co., North Wales, Pa.
‡Co-Oximeter 182, Instrumentation Laboratory, Inc., Lexington, Mass.

RESULTS

As we have found previously, the gas tensions in this particular type of wound differ somewhat from those of the surgically incised wound.[13, 14] However, the gas tensions measured reflect the average extracellular oxygen tension at a tissue level at a site of relatively minor injury. No significant difference in the tissue oxygen levels was noted between the control subjects and the patients undergoing elective surgical procedures (herniorrhaphy, plastic procedures, vagotomy-pyloroplasty, splenectomy, jejunoileal bypass, and total hip replacement).

Correlations within the trauma patient group were performed on multiple regressions with percentage P_tO_2 as a dependent variable (Table I). A direct correlation was found when compared with cardiac index (CI) and central venous oxygen (P_vO_2). A significant inverse correlation was found with P_{50} and lactate. Cardiac index appeared to be a major determinant of tissue oxygen levels. However, an elevated cardiac index did not ensure an elevated or even normal P_tO_2. Although P_{50} and 2-3 DPG were correlated, the relationship of P_tO_2 to 2-3 DPG was not significant (R = −0.175).

The summary data of P_{50} in the first five days after injury are shown in Table II. The correlation coefficients indicate that when tissue Po_2 is low, P_{50} tends to rise. In time, however, the mean P_{50} tends to rise as the patients improve. Thus, the data by the fourth and fifth days are heavily influenced by patients who have survived long enough for the transfusion effects to be minimized.

In Fig. 2, the daily positive values for the severely traumatized patients are individually compared to the grouped controls. In Fig. 3, the two groups are compared. The tissue oxygen levels were significantly decreased in the patients with multiple trauma for at least four days following injury. The tissue oxygen data are more abnormal than they appear be-

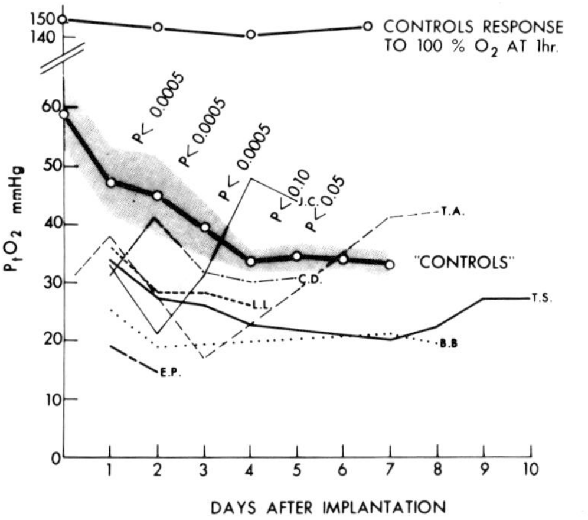

Fig. 2. Daily base-line values for the individual trauma patients compared to the grouped controls.

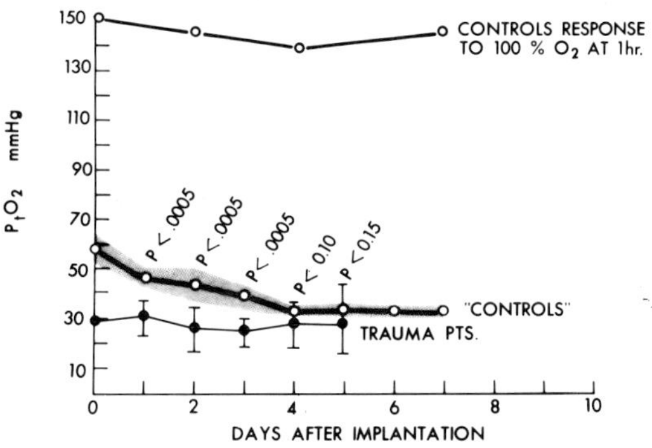

Fig. 3. Mean P_tO_2 values for control and trauma patients. Standard errors of the mean are shown by brackets for trauma patients and shading for controls. Differences at 1, 2, and 3 days were statistically significant above the 0.05 level by Student's t test.

cause the arterial Po_2 in these patients had to be maintained in a normal or elevated range, and most of the patients were breathing oxygen-enriched atmospheres when studied.

Many investigators have found increased cardiac index in response to multiple injury. Our experience is similar. Table III shows that cardiac index was significantly elevated by almost 50 percent by the third day and remained elevated. Despite this major response, wound-tissue Po_2 was depressed by a similar amount. Therefore, in the first day, Po_2 and CI diverged from their normal relationship. Thereafter, however, further elevations in CI brought elevations in P_tO_2. By the time mean tissue P_tO_2 became normal on the fifth day, the average cardiac index was still elevated by about 50 percent.

The response of tissue Po_2 by one hour after administration of pure oxygen to normal controls is recorded in Figs. 2 and 3. The response of tissue Po_2 to the breathing of pure oxygen was not systematically measured in patients undergoing elective surgery. The tissue response in the trauma patients was strikingly depressed. The data are difficult to analyze statistically because it was therapeutically necessary to maintain adequate and varying base-line oxygen breathing mixtures in trauma patients. Several patients failed to respond at all at the tissue level to changes of several hundred millimeters of mercury in arterial oxygen, and in only one case did the response to elevated arterial Po_2 rise above the normal values obtained for the control subjects who were breathing room air.

Table III. *Cardiac index*

Day	*N**	*Mean ± S.E.M.†*
1	13	3.37 ± 0.39
2	13	3.94 ± 0.37
3	11	5.01 ± 0.32
4	8	4.68 ± 0.18
5	5	4.86 ± 0.22

*N = number of determinations.
†S.E.M. = standard error of the mean.

Tissue carbon dioxide levels seemed responsive to arterial Pco_2. Wound tissue Pco_2 did not differ significantly between the trauma and control groups. The findings were consistent with those of Furuse and co-workers.[6]

DISCUSSION

The clinical application of measuring tissue oxygen by the present technique has been derived from previous experimental work.[13-15] The method has at least two useful clinical applications. First, by definition, it is a minor wound since it involves an invasive technique; therefore, it can be utilized as a method of measuring the average extracellular oxygen and carbon dioxide content in an area of injured tissue. Second, it may be applied to the "monitoring" of critically injured patients.

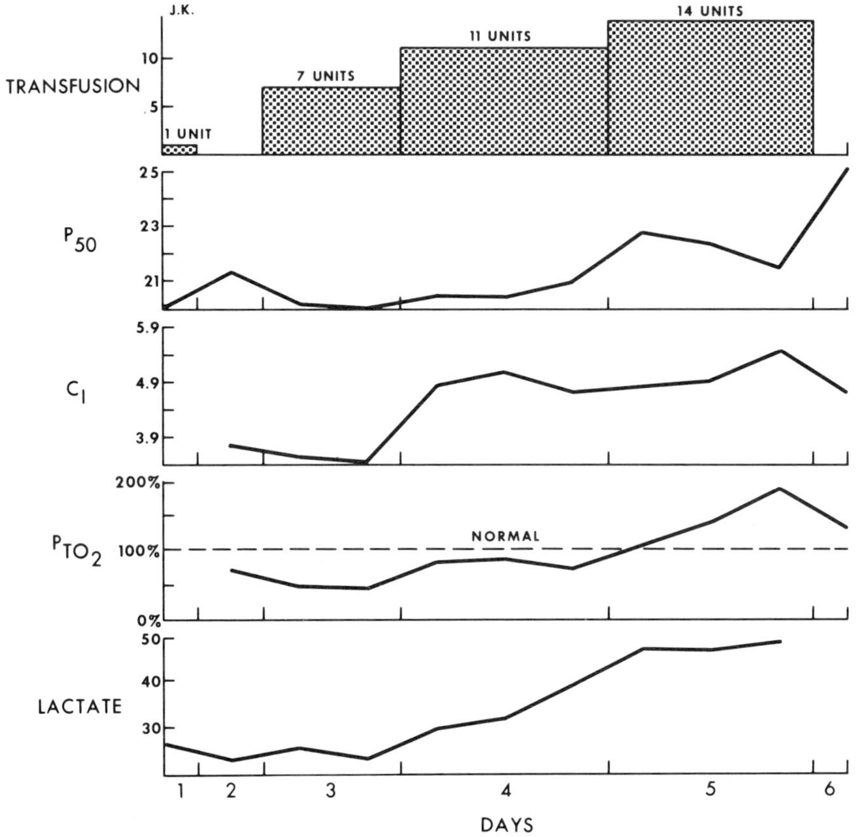

Fig. 4. Daily determinations of (1) transfused blood, (2) blood P_{50}, (3) cardiac index (CI), (4) tissue oxygen tension (P_tO_2), (5) serum lactate in patient J. K., who developed clostridial sepsis following massive soft tissue injury. On days 3, 4, and 5 several determinations were made.

The most striking finding of this study is the low wound tissue Po_2 found in severely injured patients. The tissue oxygen was depressed despite a major elevation of cardiac index above that expected for controls. There is, apparently, a major obstacle to the delivery of oxygen to the tested tissue. The nature of this obstacle cannot be proved by the results of this study. On the first day, one component of the low P_tO_2 would seem to be depressed hemoglobin function as shown by a depressed P_{50}. Thereafter, however, the negative correlation coefficient seems to imply that hemoglobin-oxygen affinity falls more as a compensating mechanism. This also implies that P_{50} changes are not a primary factor in the poor tissue oxygenation. Obviously, there are many possible reasons for depressed tissue oxygen delivery. We have not measured local capillary flow and have no means of estimating the degree of peripheral shunting. No information we have developed allows us to rule out peripheral flow problems as a cause of the poor tissue oxygen delivery.

We were, in most cases, unable to elevate the tissue oxygen levels that significantly increase F_iO_2. Although the arterial oxygen usually responded normally to systemically administered oxygen, the tissue response was slow and incomplete or nil. In other words, arterial Po_2 bore little relationship to wound Po_2. The patient illustrated below failed to elevate tissue oxygen significantly despite increasing arterial Po_2 by administering higher percentage of oxygen in the inspired air. Merely elevating arterial Po_2 increases tissue gases in normal patients, but increased arterial Po_2 is, by itself, not sufficient to increase tissue oxygen supply in severely injured patients. The poor tissue Po_2 response, despite increased arterial Po_2, clearly places the majority of the obstacle to oxygen delivery at the microcirculatory-cellular level. Our findings are consistent with existing theories about rheologic response to injury, as well as theories about capillary endothelial swelling due to shock. It is also possible that the arrival of some added oxygen in the wound is obscured by increased utilization of oxygen by the inflammatory cells and fibroblasts in the tissue. These cells can increase oxygen consumption when supplied with oxygen at an increased Po_2; but normally, this effect is overcome when arterial Po_2 increases to approximately 200 mm. Hg. Arterial Po_2 surpassed this level in most of the patients tested for Po_2 response in tissue.

A summary of one patient is found in Fig. 4. This patient was admitted with gas gangrene and ultimately died of it. The tissue Po_2 in the first few days was low despite an elevated cardiac index and normal or elevated arterial Po_2. When the cardiac index rose even further, tissue Po_2 remained below normal and finally rose above normal only after massive transfusion with fresh blood and elevation of blood P_{50}. Unfortunately, the patient was in septic shock in the last few days and the rising tissue oxygenation could have been due to any number of hemodynamic changes. In this patient, lactate rose as peripheral gangrene became worse. He also received a major load of lactate in the 25 units of blood given in the last two days. In the other patients, the correlation with lactate was in most cases in the other direction. Perhaps in this patient, the lactate load may have driven the P_{50} higher.

The depressed oxygen delivery at a tissue level as demonstrated in this study is of particular importance since most of these patients are subjected to a number of surgical procedures shortly after their initial injury and admission to the hospital. An additional surgical procedure might compound the insult. This may result in a delay in wound repair and an increased susceptibility to infection. Because most surgical procedures performed on these patients are essential to correct the threat to life or limb, we normally accept the increased risk. However, other unnecessary surgical procedures should probably be delayed until hemodynamic and metabolic factors are corrected.

This study was designed with a second major goal in mind: testing of the technique of measuring "tissue Po_2" for clinical use. The method has previously demonstrated its ability to measure changes in tissue oxygen with alteration of blood volume in animals.[12] It has also shown its ability to respond to arterial Po_2 changes in the normal person and patients following elective relatively minor surgery without blood replacement. When this study is compared with that of Furuse and colleagues,[6] it demonstrates the suitability of measuring *subcutaneous* Po_2 with this inexpensive technique as a representative monitor of tissue oxygenation. The present study clearly reveals that the control of tissue Po_2 is a complex process for which we may not yet know all the determinants. In this setting a measure of tissue Po_2 would seem valuable. Certainly, we are just beginning to appreciate the individual significance of some of the determinants in this study, since a correction of cardiac index and arterial Po_2 did not necessarily ensure a normal tissue Po_2. The method, performed well, was reliable and inexpensive, was tolerated by the patient, and produced no significant damage. It seems to qualify for further assessment as an adjunct to patient care. Its major advantage seems to be that it can be used with equipment readily available in any intensive care unit. The method is currently undergoing further simplification.

CONCLUSIONS

1. The means and standard deviations of Po_2 in a reproducible wound in normal subjects over a one-week period of time are presented.

2. The normal response of wound tissue Po_2 to 100 percent systemically administered oxygen in the wound is recorded.

3. Wound tissue gases in patients undergoing elective surgical procedures were similar to those in control, unoperated subjects.

4. Severe trauma is associated with a defect in oxygen delivery to injured tissue as evidenced by a depressed wound tissue oxygen in the trauma patients as compared to

the controls for at least four days after injury. This deficit exists despite major elevations of cardiac index.

5. Changes in tissue oxygen in trauma patients are correlated with changes in cardiac index, P_{50}, and serum lactate.

6. The data may explain the observation that traumatic wounds heal slowly and are unusually susceptible to infection.

7. The method may also be used as a clinical tool in the monitoring of critically ill patients.

REFERENCES

1. Benesch, R., and Benesch, R. E.: The effect of organic phosphates from the human erythrocyte on the oxygen equilibrium of human erythrocytes, Biochem. Biophys. Res. Commun. **26:** 162, 1967.
2. Brewer, C. J.: Clinical implications of variation in erythrocyte oxygen affinity, *in* Rorth, M., Astrup, P. L., editors: Oxygen affinity of hemoglobin and red cell acid base status, New York, 1972, Academic Press, pp. 629-646.
3. Chanutin, A., and Curnish, R. R.: Effect of organic and inorganic phosphates on the oxygen equilibrium of human erythrocytes, Arch. Biochem. Biophys. **121:** 96, 1967.
4. Conolly, W. B., Hunt, T. K., Sonne, M., and Dunphy, J. E.: Influence of distant trauma on local wound infection, Surg. Gynecol. Obstet. **128:** 713, 1969.
5. Ehrlich, H. P., Grislis, G., and Hunt, T. K.: Metabolic and circulatory contributions to oxygen gradients in wounds, SURGERY **72:** 578, 1972.
6. Furuse, A., Brawley, R. K., Struve, E., and Gott, V. L.: Skeletal muscle gas tension: Indicator of cardiac output and peripheral tissue perfusion, SURGERY **74:** 214, 1973.
7. Heughan, C., Niinikoski, J., and Hunt, T. K.: Effect of saline infusion on tissue oxygen transport, Surg. Gynecol. Obstet. **135:** 257, 1972.
8. Heughan, C., Zederfeldt, B. H., Grislis, G., and Hunt, T. K.: Effect of dextran solutions on oxygen transport in wound tissue, Acta Chir. Scand. **138:** 639, 1972.
9. Hunt, T. K., and Pai, M. P.: The effect of varying ambient oxygen tensions on wound metabolism and collagen synthesis, SURGERY **135:** 561, 1972.
10. Hunt, T. K., Zederfeldt, B., and Goldstick, T. K.: Oxygen and healing, Am. J. Surg. **118:** 521, 1969.
11. Hunt, T. K., Linsey, M., Sonne, M., and Jawetz, E.: Oxygen tension and wound infection, Surg. Forum **23:** 47, 1972.

11a. Keitt, A. S.: Reduced nicotinamide adenine dinucleotides linked analysis of 2,3-diphosphoglycemic acid, J. Lab. Clin. Med. **77:** 470, 1971.

12. Maxwell, T. M., Lim, R. C., Fuchs, R., and Hunt, T. K.: Continuous monitoring of tissue gas tension and pH in hemorrhagic shock, Am. J. Surg. **126:** 249, 1973.
13. Niinikoski, J., and Hunt, T. K.: Measurement of wound oxygen with implanted Silastic tube, SURGERY **71:** 22, 1972.
14. Niinikoski, J., Heughan, C., and Hunt, T. K.: Oxygen tensions in human wounds, J. Surg. Res. **12:** 77, 1972.
15. Niinikoski, J., Hunt, T. K., and Dunphy, J. E.: Oxygen supply in healing tissue, Am. J. Surg. **123:** 247, 1972.
16. Niinikoski, J., Grislis, G., and Hunt, T. K.: Respiratory gas tensions and collagen in infected wounds, Ann. Surg. **175:** 588, 1972.
17. Pai, M. P., and Hunt, T. K.: Effect of varying oxygen tensions on healing of open wounds, Surg. Gynecol. Obstet. **135:** 756, 1972.

DISCUSSION

Dr. Richard Morse Peters (San Diego, Calif.). Is there a possible alternative explanation, in that there is also a correlation in the tissue Po_2 with the venous Po_2? Is it possible that this represents increased tissue use of oxygen in a severely injured patient, rather than a failure of delivery of oxygen to the patient?

Dr. Clarence Dennis (Bethesda, Md.). Would it be helpful to determine what the pH is adjacent to this device in the tissues, in view of the fact that this might shift the oxygen dissociation curve? I ask because some very interesting work has been done by Dr. Harry Leveen at the Brooklyn Veterans Hospital, in which the bacteria which happen to involve the tissues may not be productive of obvious evidences of infection but can produce enough ammonia to shift this so that it makes a very real difference in the oxygen tension.

Dr. R. Bruce Heppenstall (Closing). We did measure the tissue Po_2 and found that it did not elevate. Therefore, we can have some evidence to assume that there is no increased oxygen utilization. Two patients were in septic shock, and the A/V difference was not substantial in those patients; we assume that this is not due to increased consumption. However, we do not have a direct measurement of consumption at a tissue level, and, obviously, this would be important.

As far as the pH adjacent to the tissue we are measuring, we did do muscle pH right adjacent to the tonometer with a different technique, and we found that it was slightly acidotic, so that there is some slight influence by the pH, obviously.

Pulmonary changes due to hemorrhagic shock resuscitation with isotonic and hypertonic saline

Robert L. Fulton, M.D., *Louisville, Ky.*, and **Ronald P. Fischer, M.D., Ph.D.**, *Albuquerque, N. M.*

Three groups of dogs were submitted to Wiggers' type of hemorrhagic shock modified by mechanically controlled respiration. In the control group only shed blood was returned; in a second group, shed blood plus 0.9 percent saline was given to maintain carotid artery flow at initial value. The third group received shed blood plus 1.8 percent saline according to the same criterion. There was a 100 mm. Hg increase in alveolar-arterial Po_2 gradient and a 20 percent decrease in pulmonary compliance during hypovolemia which reversed in all groups during immediate resuscitation. Lung function remained normal in the group receiving only shed blood but hemodynamic function deteriorated. Pulmonary function (alveolar-arterial Po_2 gradient, compliance, and shunting) worsened in the group receiving normal saline and hemodynamic function was maintained. Lung function and hemodynamic function were nearly normal in the group receiving hypertonic saline. Lung weights and lung water increased in all groups with the most severe increase in the group receiving normal saline. Little pulmonary dysfunction occurs as the result of hemorrhagic hypotension. Large volumes of normal saline required for resuscitation produce pulmonary changes, and hemodynamic stability is better acquired without pulmonary injury when hypertonic saline rather than isotonic saline is infused.

From the Department of Surgery, the University of Louisville School of Medicine and the Price Institute of Surgical Research, Health Sciences Center, Louisville, Ky., and the Department of Surgery, University of New Mexico School of Medicine and Albuquerque Veterans Administration Hospital, Albuquerque, N. M.

Rapid and substantial infusions of sodium solutions such as Ringer's lactate have been shown to enhance survival following prolonged and refractory hemorrhagic hypotension.[9, 30, 35] Pulmonary insufficiency may occur following major trauma and volume resuscitation in man.[17, 23, 36, 37] Some studies indicate that both the hypotensive episode[21, 22, 34] and the necessary resuscitation with blood and sodium solutions may alter pulmonary structure and function.[1, 16, 19, 33] Other investigations suggest that hemorrhage is associated with only moderate pulmonary dysfunction and that saline infusions have only minimal effects upon the lung.[7, 26]

Clinically, it has been noted that at least in the first several days following resuscitation from hemorrhagic hypotension, many patients have arterial desaturation[1, 23] and the water content and the weight of the lungs are increased significantly.[17, 18]

This study was undertaken to re-explore the pulmonary effects of hemorrhagic hypotension and the infusion of large volumes of saline solutions and to determine if hypertonic saline may be less damaging to pul-

Presented at the Thirty-fifth Annual Meeting of the Society of University Surgeons, St. Louis, Mo. Feb. 14-16, 1974.

Reprint requests: Dr. R. Fulton, Department of Surgery, University of Louisville School of Medicine, Louisville, Ky. 40201.

monary function than normal saline or Ringer's lactate solution.

METHODS

Preliminary study showed that dogs became apneic or bradypneic during severe hypotension or if only shed blood was returned, obviating the determination of various parameters. Some dogs died in the apneic state with little demonstrable pulmonary dysfunction. In a second group, the shed blood was supplemented with 65 ml. per kilogram of normal saline, with blood pressure returning to normal, but cardiac output approximating only 70 percent of normal.[13] Respiration was, therefore, controlled mechanically, and solutions were given at a rate to maintain normal cardiac output.

Thirty-two mongrel dogs weighing 15 to 30 kilograms were given 25 mg. per kilogram of pentobarbital intravenously and intubated. A Harvard respirator (Series 600) connected to a Collins spirometer was used for ventilation. The system, filled with 100 percent O_2, was airtight, allowing measurements of volume changes and oxygen consuption ($\dot{O}_2$). The respirator was initially set at 250 to 350 ml. tidal volumes (depending on size of dog) at a rate of 20 r.p.m. and not altered subsequently except for compliance determinations.

Airway pressure was measured with a small-bore catheter inserted into the cuffed endotracheal tube and attached to a Statham strain gauge (P 23db) and Beckman Dynograph. The dogs were given 20 mg. of succinylcholine, and compliance wa s determined from the endotracheal pressure resulting from step-wise 200 ml. increases in intrathoracic volume produced by clamping the exhaust line of the respirator. Compliance was calculated as the average of six to eight $\Delta V/\Delta P$ determinations. This average gives the compliance on the more nearly vertical limb of the $\Delta V/\Delta P$ curve. Several determinations made on the horizontal limb produced severe hypotension and erratic results.

Pulmonary artery (PAP), central venous (CVP), and systemic mean arterial pressure (MAP) measurements were made using Statham strain gauges and an Electronics for Medicine amplifier and galvanometer. The right femoral vessels were cannulated with large catheters attached through a Y-connector to a collection bottle. Left carotid artery flow rate was measured with a Statham flow meter. Blood gases (P_{O_2}, P_{CO_2} and pH) were measured with a Radiometer pH meter and gas analyzer (Model No. 127). Hemoglobin concentration was found using the cyanmethemoglobin method. Cardiac output was calculated from the Fick principle:

$$\text{Cardiac output} = \frac{\dot{O}_2}{\Delta AV_{O_2} \times 10}\ \text{L./min.}$$

where ΔAV_{O_2} is the arterial-venous O_2 content difference.

$$\text{Blood } O_2 \text{ content} = \{[\text{Hgb}] \times 1.34 \times \text{percent } O_2 \text{ Sat.}\} + 0.0031\ P_{O_2}$$

The pulmonary shunt fraction (Qs/Qt) was calculated:

$$Qs/Qt = \frac{C_E - C_a}{C_E - C_v}$$

where C_E, C_a, and C_v are the oxygen contents of end-capillary, arterial, and venous blood, respectively. End-capillary P_{O_2} was assumed to be the same as alveolar P_{O_2}. Using 100 percent O_2, the alveolar P_{O_2} is[8]:

$$(\text{Barometric pressure—47 mm. Hg}) — \text{arterial } P_{CO_2}$$

Barometric pressure (approximately 627 at the altitude of the laboratory) was determined daily. Alveolar-arterial gradient $(\Delta A - a)\ P_{O_2}$ is the difference between alveolar P_{O_2} and arterial P_{O_2}.

Vascular resistance (TPR) was determined in arbitrary units:

$$\text{TPR} = \frac{\text{MAP} - \text{CVP}}{\text{C.O.}}$$

After initial values were obtained, the dogs were given heparin (5,000 units) and bled rapidly into the collection bottle to a MAP of 50 to 60 mm. Hg, which was maintained for 90 minutes by the addition or removal of blood. The MAP was then lowered to 30 mm. Hg for 60 minutes after which all measurements were repeated. Shed blood was returned over a 30 minute period in 12 dogs (SBG). A second group of ten dogs (NSG) was given the shed blood and 10 mEq. of sodium per kilogram (65 ml. per kilogram) as normal saline (0.9 percent in the first 30 minutes. A third group of ten dogs (HSG) was given the shed blood and 10 mEq. of sodium per kilogram (32.5 ml. per kilogram) as 1.8 percent saline in the first 30 minutes. After infusion, all variables were remeasured. The first group received no further solutions. The carotid flow rate in the latter two groups was kept at 95 to 100 percent of initial value by additional saline infusion. All variables were measured at one and two hours following infusion of shed blood. The experiment was arbitrarily terminated two hours after infusion of the blood at which time both hemithoraces were opened with the dogs alive. The hilum of each lung was quickly clamped, and the lung excised and weighed. Small portions were excised, weighed, and dried to constant weight at 250° C. Then:

$$\text{Percent lung water} = \frac{\text{wet weight} - \text{dry weight}}{\text{wet weight}}$$

RESULTS

The expected survival rate for the dogs in the shed-blood group (SBG) is 20 to 50 percent and in the normal saline group (NSG) 70 to 80 percent.[9, 35] Monafo, Blanke, and Deitz[24] demonstrated that 1.8 percent saline is as effective as normal saline in enhancing survival of murine hemorrhagic shock.[24] No dog died, but one dog in the normal saline group had pulmonary edema with hypoxia at two hours. Two dogs in the hypertonic saline group (HSG) took inordinately large amounts of solution to maintain carotid flow because of necrotic intestines found at autopsy. Hemodynamic parameters of the SBG indicate that the dogs were dying as expected.[9, 35]

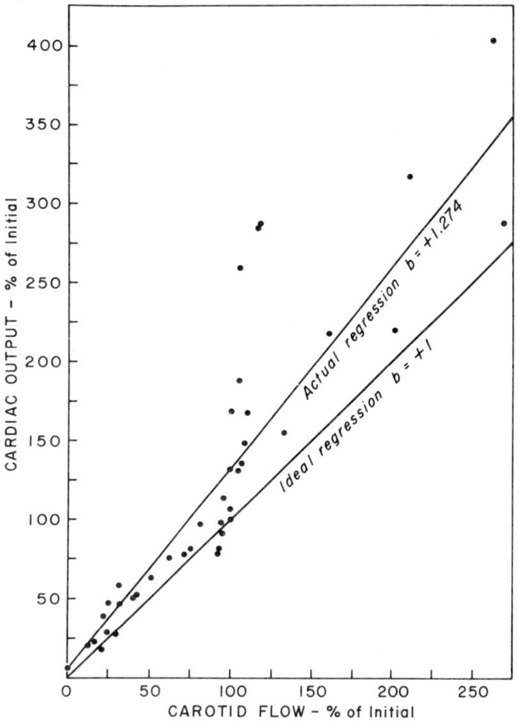

Fig. 1. Regression line of cardiac output and carotid flow. Values expressed as percent of initial flow rate.

Fig. 1 shows regression analysis of cardiac output on carotid flow. For carotid flows of 0 to 100 percent of initial value, changes in carotid flow rate reflected nearly ideal correlation to cardiac output. At the higher transient cardiac output, the correlation was not so close. Correlation of cardiac output to carotid flow was +0.856. The slope was ±1.274. Presumably, carotid flow was representative of cardiac output.

Hemodynamic parameters are depicted in Figs. 2 and 3. The immediate response to infusion of blood and saline was a return toward normal MAP (return to normal only in HSG) and an overshoot in cardiac output during rapid infusion (most marked in the NSG). Cardiac output declined in the SBG, returned to normal in the HSG, but remained elevated in the NSG. The nearly normal MAP in the SBG resulted from severe, increasing vasoconstriction, while TPR (total peripheral resistance) was normal in the HSG and subnormal in the NSG.

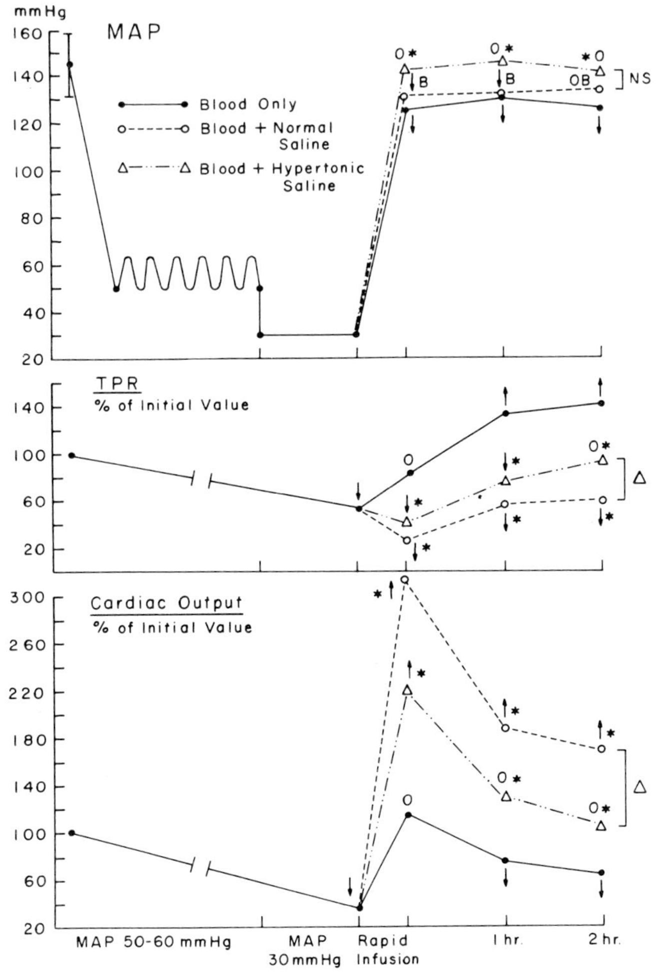

Fig. 2. Alterations of mean arterial pressure (MAP), total peripheral resistance (TPR), and cardiac output caused by hemorrhage and resuscitation. Statistics code: O, no difference from initial value ($p > 0.05$); ↑ or ↓, difference from initial value ($p < 0.05$); *, difference from SBG ($p < 0.05$); B, no difference from SBG ($p > 0.05$); NS, no difference between HSG and NSG at 2 hr. ($p > 0.05$); and Δ, difference between HSG and NSG at 2 hr. ($p < 0.05$).

Carotid flow paralleled changes in cardiac output: normal in NSG and HSG but 50 percent of control value in SBG at two hours. During rapid infusion PAP rose significantly in all groups, being highest in NSG. PAP returned to normal levels in SBG and HSG but remained elevated in the NSG. Central venous pressure rose significantly in all groups, remained above normal in SBG and NSG, but was normal at two hours in HSG. Hemoglobin concentration increased in SBG following infusion of blood but declined in HSG and NSG.

Arterial P_{CO_2} was low in all groups because of the relative mechanical hyperventilation (15 to 30 mm. Hg). No difference between groups ($p > 0.2$) occurred at any time. Arterial pH essentially reflected the lowered P_{CO_2}—slightly below normal except during the period of hypotension when it was severely depressed.

At two hours, the SBG had severe vasoconstriction, lowered cardiac output, carotid flow and MAP, and hemoconcentration. The NSG had normal MAP and carotid flow but elevated PAP, cardiac output, and CVP, and lowered resistance and hemodilution. The HSG had normal MAP, cardiac output, re-

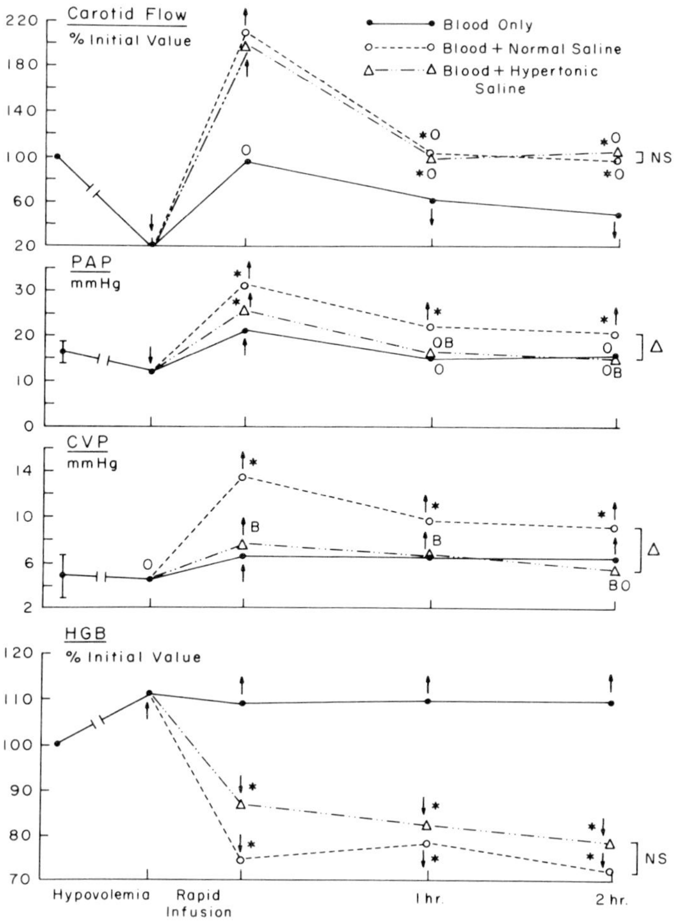

Fig. 3. Changes in carotid flow, pulmonary artery pressure (PAP), central venous pressure (CVP), and hemoglobin concentration (HGB) which occurred during the experiment.

sistance, PAP, CVP, and carotid flow, but hemodilution. Apparently, 1.8 percent saline restores hemodynamic parameters to normal levels without as wide deviations as occur with normal saline.

The data in Table I show that twice the volume of 0.9 percent saline as 1.8 percent saline was required for resuscitation. The amount of sodium required was the same in both groups showing again that it is most likely sodium rather than excess volume which restores normal function following hemorrhagic shock.[9, 13] The hemodynamic data indicate that the excessive water administered in the NSG increases the vasular volume, but that the increase is not necessarily beneficial.

Lung weight and percent water increased in all groups, especially in the NSG (Table II). The NSG lung weights varied so widely that the mean was not different from the other two groups. Percent water in the NSG was higher than normal as well as higher than in the other groups. The HSG had a higher lung water content than the SBG but less than the NSG.

Table I. *Comparison of water and sodium infused in the normal saline group and the hypertonic saline group*

Substance given	*Blood + normal saline*	*Blood + hypertonic saline*	*P*
H_2O ml./Kg.	152 ± 51	78 ± 31	< 0.001
Na^+ mEq./Kg.	23 ± 8	24 ± 9	> 0.8

Fig. 4 shows that during hemorrhagic hypotension ($\Delta A - a$), P_{O_2} increased and com-

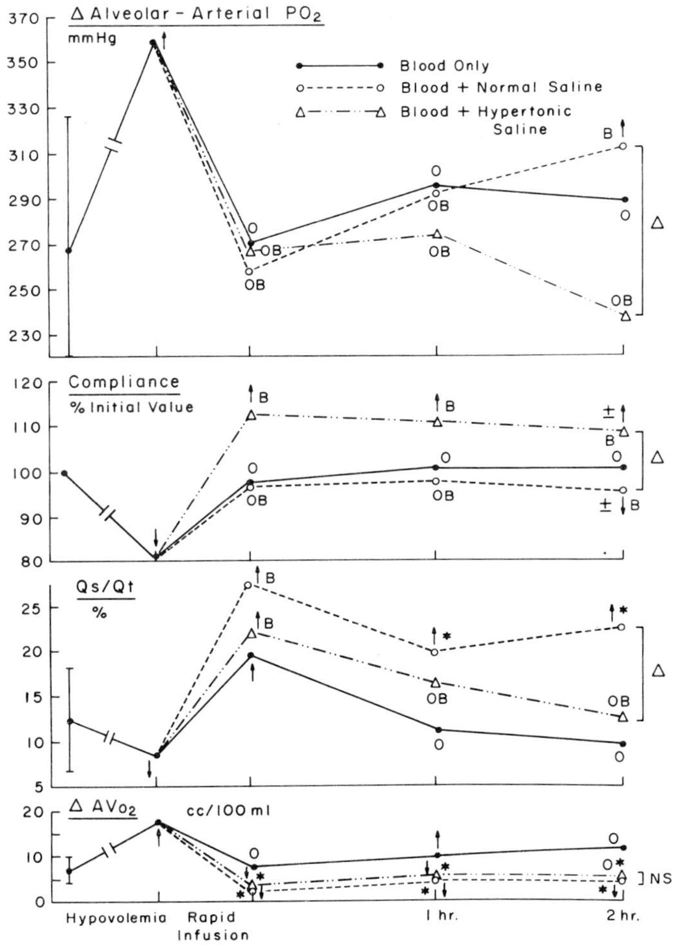

Fig. 4. Representation of alterations in alveolar-arterial P_{O_2} gradient, compliance, shunting (Qs/Qt), and arterial venous O_2 content difference which occurred with shock and resuscitation.

pliance and Qs/Qt decreased. The Qs/Qt decrease was attributable to the increase in the $\Delta A - V_{O_2}$. Following initial resuscitation in all groups, the $(\Delta A - a)$ P_{O_2} and compliance returned to normal. The $(\Delta A - a)$ P_{O_2} remained normal in the SBG and the HSG, but widened significantly in the NSG. The NSG had a much larger $(\Delta A - a)$ P_{O_2} than the HSG at two hours. Compliance was slightly below normal ($P < 0.10$) in the NSG and slightly above normal in the HSG ($P < 0.10$); these two groups were different ($P < 0.05$) at two hours. Qs/Qt alterations in the SBG were slight, reflecting changes in $\Delta A - V_{O_2}$. The HSG had a transient increase in Qs/Qt because of lowered $\Delta A - V_{O_2}$, but both variables returned to normal at two hours. Shunting persisted in the NSG, increasing from one to two hours and being significantly higher than normal as well as higher than in the other groups. There was no difference in $\Delta A - V_{O_2}$ between the NSG and the HSG.

The second rise in PAP seen only in the NSG is probably a result of perivascular edema,[12, 40] leading to increased resistance and a rise in PAP. Although hypoxemia does raise the PAP,[15] true hypoxemia did not occur in this group. Changes in $(\Delta A - a)$ P_{O_2} and compliance during the hypotensive period were reversed when shed blod was returned, remaining normal despite declining cardiovascular function. Except for a slight increase in lung weight and lung water, no

Table II. *Comparison of lung weights and percent water between groups and to normal dogs**

	Normal lung†	Shed blood only	Blood + normal saline	Blood + 1.8% saline
Lung weight (Gm./Kg.)	12.4 ± 1.3	14.1 ± 2.0 ↑	19.0 ± 10.1 ↑ B	14.5 ± 2.0 B ↑ NS
Lung H_2O (%)	79.0 ± 1.3	80.0 ± 1.2 ↑	85.5 ± 1.6 ↑ ‡	83.0 ± 1.3 ↑ Δ †

*Symbols used : ↑, experimental group vs. normal value $P < 0.05$; B, experimental group vs. shed blood only $P > 0.05$;
†Obtained from 29 other normal dogs specifically for this data.[11, 12]
‡Experimental group vs. shed blood only $P < 0.05$; NS, NSG vs. HSG $P > 0.05$; Δ, NSG vs. HSG $P < 0.05$.

gross pulmonary damage resulted from hemorrhagic shock and inadequate resuscitation.

Pulmonary function became increasingly worse in the NSG despite normal hemodynamic parameters. As there was no difference between the $A - V_{O_2}$ in the NSG and the HSG, the increased Qs/Qt in the NSG was probably caused by pulmonary changes. The large volumes of normal saline needed in addition to shed blood for resuscitation of hemorrhagic shock led to an increase in lung water (weight) which is detrimental to lung function.

For the period studied, hypertonic saline restored hemodynamic parameters to normal without grossly altering lung function. The lungs of the HSG were normal except for slightly increased percent water and lung weight. Increased water may be attributable to the hemodiluted blood trapped in the lung at the end of the experiment.

DISCUSSION

This study and others[20, 26] show that little permanent pulmonary dysfunction results from hemorrhagic hypotension. Moss and associates[28] microscopically demonstrated reversal of interstitial alterations with resuscitation. Lowery and Sugg[22] demonstrated that moderate pulmonary dysfunction due to hemorrhagic hypotension is worsened by infusion of shed blood. Despite findings of arterial desaturation in wounded men in Vietnam,[23] hemorrhage without resuscitation probably does not lead to overt pulmonary distress. Two reasons are likely. First, the lung has a large functional reserve, and such phenomena as platelet emboli,[2, 4] fatty emboli,[31] and vasoactive substances,[3] that may occur in wounding and are known to alter lung function either do not exist in pure hemorrhagic states or are of such minor extent that functional reserve is not overcome. Second, no animal lives long enough in pure hemorrhagic shock for such mechanisms to be operative. The Vietnam experience is different in that the injury and shock were usually the result of massive contusing trauma with much tissue damage,[36, 37] whereas the experimental animal undergoes no mechanical tissue destruction. Furthermore, even though pulmonary dysfunction occurs with hypotension, it apparently reverses with resuscitation.[20]

The question of the effect of hemorrhage upon the lung is clinically trivial, as no patient is treated for long without the intravenous infusion of blood and usually a sodium solution, be it Ringer's lactate, dextran in saline, plasma, or normal saline. Gump and co-workers[17] noted that in early deaths following such therapy, lung weight, lung water, and lung albumin were increased greatly. Jenkins and others[19] described respiratory insufficiency as the result of massive fluid infusion. Sugg and colleagues[39] demonstrated congestive atelectasis in shocked dogs following rapid infusion of blood. Collins, Braitberg, and Butcher[7] showed a transient increase in lung water and weight following shock and saline infusion. Gaisford, Pandey, and Jensen[16] found mild-to moderate functional and compositional pulmonary derangements as the result of Ringer's lactate infusions.

Certainly, following pulmonary injury[6, 14, 15] large saline loads have adverse effects on pulmonary function. Fulton and Peter[14] confirmed the findings of Rutherford and Valenta[32] that normal lung, as well as contused lung, becomes functionally impaired with moderate saline loads.

This experiment demonstrates that therapeutically appropriate loads of saline solutions do adversely alter lung function. Damage may occur because of the rise in PAP seen during rapid fluid infusion. Previously, we have shown that pulmonary edema will result if pulmonary hypertension is caused by increased precapillary forces with lowered resistance.[12] We have also correlated numerically the deterioration of lung function several hours after infusion of blood and/or saline with the rise in PAP during infusion.[11, 14] The increased pressure is not accommodated well in the lung. Motsay and colleagues[28] have shown that filtration is outward when pulmonary capillary pressure exceeds 7.6 mm. Hg. The outward pressure gradient results in increased extravascular water. If the capacity of the capillaries is exceeded under the increased pressure, congestive atelectasis or hemorrhage into the interstitium and alveoli may occur.[11, 12] Functionally, the increased interstitial water should result in decreased compliance and some deterent to oxygen diffusion as implied by this study. Moyer and Butcher[29] questioned the importance of plasma oncotic pressure in the regulation of capillary exchange of water and implied that a positive load of salt and water will distribute freely through the vascular and interstitial space regardless of the administration of colloids. It cannot be assumed from their work that the effect of the normal saline was attributable to simple hemodilution, nor conversely that the hypertonic solution was beneficial because of osmotic forces.

Moss and co-workers[25] and Fulton[10] have shown that collagen adsorbs sodium and water during hemorrhagic shock; more importantly, Moss and associates[25] showed that this occurs in the lung and that this phenomenon reverses during resuscitation with saline solutions.[26] Reversal of an interstitial accumulation of sodium and, presumably, water could explain the reversal of decreased oxygen diffusion and compliance seen in this and similar experiments.[20] Continued administration of salt solution may not allow reversal as other changes such as increased PAP and capillary distention take place.

Pulmonary dysfunction apparently is related more to the volume of water infused and the initial rise in PAP than to any other factor. Hemodynamic stability following hemorrhagic hypotension seems more dependent upon the sodium infused than upon the volume of solutions, which is in accord with our previous work[13] and that of Dillon and co-workers.[9] The amount of solution infused seems large, but it is not rare to see injured patients requiring over 20 mEq. of sodium per kilogram (11 liters of Ringer's lactate) in addition to transfusions exceeding their blood volume for resuscitation.[1] Albeit, the solutions are not usually given in two and one-half hours. Other investigators have used 16 to 23 mEq. of sodium per kilogram in experimental resuscitation.[9, 27]

CONCLUSION

The clinical duration of pulmonary effects of such shock therapy is unknown. It is unlikely that pulmonary dysfunction as seen in this experiment could be equated with posttraumatic pulmonary insufficiency. However, it may be enough to require intubation and respiratory support, with their inherent dangers of oxygen toxicity[38] and pulmonary sepsis,[5] thus setting the stage for the clinical syndrome commonly referred to as "shock lung." Hypertonic saline prevented the lung changes in this experiment, while achieving equivalent resuscitation, suggesting that this solution may be more efficacious than isotonic salt solutions in the resuscitation of shock.

The conclusions reached are: (1) little pulmonary damage occurs in hemorrhagic shock; (2) moderate alterations of pulmonary function and composition occur as the result of resuscitation with large volumes of normal saline; (3) hemodynamic stabilization occurs as well with hypertonic saline as with normal saline; and (4) pulmonary dysfunction is minimized with hypertonic saline.

REFERENCES

1. Abrams, J. S., Deane, R. S., and Davis, J. H.: Adverse effects of salt and water retention on pulmonary function in patients with multiple trauma, J. Trauma **13:** 788, 1973.

2. Bergentz, S. E., Ljungqvist, U., and Lewis, D. H.:The distribution of platelets, fibrin, and erythrocytes in various organs following thrombin infusion: an experimental study in dogs with and without antifibrinolytic therapy, SURGERY **71:** 190, 1972.
3. Berk, J. L., Hagen, J. F., Koo, R., Beyer, W., Dochat, G. R., Rupright, M., and Nomoto, S.: Pulmonary insufficiency caused by epinephrine, Ann. Surg. **178:** 423, 1973.
4. Blaisdell, F. W., and Schlobohm, R. M.: The respiratory distress syndrome: a review, SURGERY **74:** 251, 1973.
5. Bryant, L. R., Trinkle, J. K., Moblin-Uddin, K., Baker, J., and Griffen, W. O.: Bacterial colonization profile with tracheal intubation and mechanical ventilation, Arch. Surg. **104:** 647, 1972.
6. Burford, T. H., and Burbank, B.: Traumatic wet lung, J. Thorac. Surg. **14:** 415, 1945.
7. Collins, J. A., Braitberg, A., and Butcher, H. R.: Changes in lung and body weight and lung water content in rats treated for hemorrhage with various fluids, SURGERY **73:** 401, 1973.
8. Comroe, J. H., Forster, R. E., Dubois, A. B., Briscoe, W. A., and Carlsen, E.: The Lung, Chicago, 1962, Year Book Medical Publishers, Inc., p. 125.
9. Dillon, J., Lynch, L. J., Myers, R., Butcher, H. R., and Moyer, C. A.: A bioassay of treatment of hemorrhagic shock, Arch. Surg. **93:** 537, 1966.
10. Fulton, R. L.: The adsorption of sodium and water by collagen during hemorrhagic shock, Ann. Surg. **172:** 861, 1970.
11. Fulton, R. L., and Peter, E. T.: Compositional and histologic effects of fluid therapy following pulmonary contusion, J. Trauma. In press, 1974.
12. Fulton, R. L., and Peter, E. T.: The effects of pulmonary arterial hypertension in the isolated lung, J. Surg. Res., Dec. 1973.
13. Fulton, R. L., and Peter, E. T.: The metabolic and physiologic effects of sodium in the treatment of hemorrhagic shock, Am. Surg. **40:** 152, 1974.
14. Fulton, R. L., and Peter, E. T.: Physiologic effects of fluid therapy after pulmonary contusion, Am. J. Surg. **126:** 773, 1973.
15. Fulton, R. L., Peter, E. T., and Wilson, J. N.: The pathophysiology and treatment of pulmonary contusions, J. Trauma **10:** 719, 1970.
16. Gaisford, W. D., Pandey, N., and Jensen, C. G.: Pulmonary changes in treated hemorrhagic shock. II. Ringer's lactate solution versus colloid solution, Am. J. Surg. **124:** 738, 1972.
17. Gump, F. E., Mashima, T., Ferenczy, A., and Kinney, J. M.: Pre- and postmortem studies of lung fluids and electrolyes, J. Trauma **11:** 474, 1971.
18. Gump, F. E., Mashima, Y., Jorgensen, S., and Kinney, J. M.: Simultaneous use of three indicators to evaluate pulmonary capillary damage in man, SURGERY **70:** 262, 1971.
19. Jenkins, M. T., Jones, R. F., Wilson, B., and Moyer, C. A.: Congestive atelectasis: a complication of the intravenous infusion of fluids, Ann. Surg. **132:** 327, 1950.
20. Kallos, T., Wyche, M. Q., and Marshall, B. E.: Effects of hemorrhagic shock on pulmonary diffusion and capillary blood volume of the dog, J. Trauma **13:** 218, 1973.
21. Kim, S. I., and Shoemaker, W. C.: Role of acidosis in the development of increased pulmonary vascular resistance and shock lung in experimental hemorrhagic shock, SURGERY **73:** 723, 1973.
22. Lowrey, B. D., and Sugg, J. H.: Pulmonary dysfunction after shock and trauma, Adv. Exp. Med. Biol. **23:** 415, 1972.
23. Martin, A. M., Simmons, R. L., and Heisterkamp, C. A.: Respiratory insufficiency in combat casualties. I. Pathologic changes in the lungs of patients dying of wounds, Ann. Surg. **170:** 30, 1969.
24. Monafo, W. W., Blanke, T., and Deitz, F.: Effectiveness of hypertonic saline solutions in the treatment of murine hemorrhagic shock, Surg. Forum **20:** 42, 1969.
25. Moss, G. S., Das Gupta, T. K., Newson, B., and Nyhus, L. M.: Effect of hemorrhagic shock on pulmonary interstitial sodium distribution in the primate lung, Ann. Surg. **177:** 211, 1973.
26. Moss, G. S., Das Gupta, T. K., Newson, B., and Nyhus, L. M.: The effect of saline solution resuscitation on pulmonary sodium and water distribution, Surg. Gynecol. Obstet. **136:** 934, 1973.
27. Moss, G. S., Siegel, D. C., Cochin, A., and Fresquez, V.: Effects of saline and colloid solutions on pulmonary function in hemorrhagic shock, Surg. Gynecol. Obstet. **133:** 53, 1971.
28. Motsay, G. J., Alho, A. V., Schultz, L. S., Dietzman, R. H., and Lillehei, R. C.: Pulmonary capillary permeability in the posttraumatic pulmonary insufficiency syndrome: comparison of isogravimetric capillary pressures, Ann. Surg. **173:** 244, 1971.
29. Moyer, C. A., and Butcher, H. R.: Burns, Shock, and Plasma Volume Regulation, St. Louis, 1967, The C. V. Mosby Company, Chapter 1.
30. Penfield, W.: The treatment of severe and progressive hemorrhage by intravenous injections, Am. J. Physiol. **48:** 121, 1919.
31. Pomerantz, M., and Eiseman, B.: Experi-

mental shock lung model, J. Trauma **8:** 782, 1968.
32. Rutherford, R. B., and Valenta, J.: An experimental study of traumatic wet lung, J. Trauma **11:** 146, 1971.
33. Schloerb, P. R., Hunt, P. T., Plummer, J. A., and Cage, G. K.: Pulmonary edema after replacement of blood loss by electrolyte solutions, Surg. Gynecol. Obstet. **135:** 893, 1972.
34. Sealy, W. C., Ogino, S., Lesage, A. M., and Young, W. G.: Functional and structural changes in the lung in hemorrhagic shock, Surg. Gynecol. Obstet. **122:** 754, 1966.
35. Shires, T., Coln, D., Carrico, J., and Lightfoot, S.: Fluid therapy in hemorrhagic shock, Arch. Surg. **88:** 688, 1964.
36. Simmons, R. L., Heisterkamp, C. A., Collins, J. A., Bredenberg, C. E., Mills, D. E., and Martin, A. M.: Respiratory insufficiency in combat casualties. IV. Hypoxemia during convalescence, Ann. Surg. **170:** 53, 1969.
37. Simmons, R. L., Heisterkamp, C. A., Collins, J. A., Genslar, S., and Martin, A. M.: Respiratory insufficiency in combat casualties. III. Arterial hypoxemia after wounding, Ann. Surg. **170:** 45, 1969.
38. Soloway, H. B., Castillo, Y., and Martin, A. M.: Adult hyaline membrane disease: relationship to oxygen therapy, Ann. Surg. **168:** 937, 1968.
39. Sugg, W. L., Webb, W. R., Nakae, S., Theodorides, T., Gupta, D. N., and Cook, W. A.: Congestive atelectasis: an experimental study, Ann. Surg. **168:** 234, 1968.
40. West, J. B., Dollery, C. T., and Heard, B. E.: Increased pulmonary vascular resistance in the dependent zone of the isolated dog lung caused by perivascular edema, Circ. Res. **17:** 191, 1965.

DISCUSSION

Dr. Gerald S. Moss (Northbrook, Ill.). The thrust of the paper is twofold: (1) that normal saline normalizes circulation, but produces lung damage, whereas hypertonic saline normalizes circulation but does not produce lung damage. These results with regard to normal saline resuscitation are obviously part of a long controversy about the effect of saline on the lung, but most of the recent data seems to suggest that normal saline resuscitation does not injure the lungs. The work from Schloerb's lab in Kansas and Collins' lab here in St. Louis, and ours in Chicago suggests that the lungs are not injured during resuscitation.

I think the differences can be reconciled if one looks at the volume used for resuscitation. I would suggest that the animals were given excess amounts of saline in the normal saline group, and I base this on the data which show that the cardiac output at the end of the thirty-minute resuscitation period in the normal saline group was 300 percent of normal, and the pulmonary artery pressure was also considerably above normal.

In our studies in the baboon, we have learned that it is extraordinarily difficult to raise cardiac output to levels above normal following shock. In fact, this is one of the initial criticisms of normal saline, that it is difficult to maintain the circulation in the hyperdynamic state. So, to achieve triple the initial cardiac output and double the initial output at the end of the study to me would imply that fluids way in excess of what would be required for resuscitation were given, and I think the use of the carotid artery flow was probably the reason for this overshooting. There was an enormous scatter of values, and I suspect that what happened was that the normal saline animals fell into that group above the line.

If you look at the volume of fluid given, it was 150 c.c. per kilogram in about two hours, which is equivalent to about 10 L. in man in that length of time. This would also suggest that an excess amount of fluid was given.

Thus, I suggest that the compliance data and the shunting data, which showed deterioration in the normal saline group, reflect the extent of pulmonary edema. This was also reflected in the 85 percent lung water data, again indicating pulmonary edema, and again on the basis of overinfusion.

If adequate amounts of saline were given, enough to restore the circulation, but not to produce a hyperdynamic state, lung water values would have been normal.

With regard to hypertonic saline, the objective of reducing the total volume of fluid infused is obviously a valuable one, and one that all of us would wish for. The big question I think we should ask is: How does an animal handle that load of sodium? The problem is that the concentration of sodium in 1.8 percent saline is 380 mEq. per liter. Again, using the analogy of man, that would be 10 L. of that solution in a short period of time. Does this produce hypernatremia? And, if so, would that be dangerous in man?

Dr. William Monafo (St. Louis, Mo.). As Dr. Moss implied, the experiments are obviously complex, and one has to be very cautious about interpreting the data. However, the real thrust of the paper—that is, the sodium that was given obviously was the most important determinant of restoration of hemodynamic function—I think, still remains clear.

Now, obviously, the water loads which are given are going to distribute themselves everywhere, and to a certain extent in the lungs. What Dr. Fulton is beginning to look at is: What is the optimum? What is the optimal relationship between sodium and water that one should give in an effort to restore hemodynamic function, yet not produce corporeal water overloads with possible pulmonary functional disadvantages?

I would like to know what the morphology of those lungs was, and whether there were any sodium analyses in the tissue.

Dr. Herbert Benjamin Hechtman (Boston, Mass.). I would like to ask the authors whether they made any measurements of colloid osmotic pressure.

Second, I would like to ask whether, in their experience, the elevated pulmonary arterial pressure does not correlate with elevated pulmonary arterial wedge pressures, which has been our customary experience in patients and in animals.

Third, I wonder whether the mechanics of breathing could be correlated in any way with the measured increases in lung water. It appears that in both the saline and hypertonic saline animals there was an increase in lung weights. However, the mechanics of breathing did not appear to correlate with that.

Finally, the use of intrapulmonary shunt as a measure of respiratory insufficiency is hazardous when you abruptly reduce hemoglobin concentration in half, since the intrapulmonary shunt is very sensitive to the drop in hemoglobin.

Dr. Robert L. Fulton (closing). Dr. Collins did show an increase in water in the lung in his experiments. He questioned that this was of functional importance in rats, but those rats did have an increase in water.

Gump has shown that patients resuscitated with large volumes of fluid, as was done in this experiment, do have an increase in the amount of water in their lungs. The question is: Was there an excess of saline? That's hard to answer.

In a study performed two years ago, Dr. Monafo showed that perhaps the optimal amount of sodium to be given in an experiment such as this is about 17 mEq. per kilogram. However, in his studies the rats were shocked for one hour. The dogs in this study were shocked for two and one-half hours. So the amount of sodium may not be in excess.

In Dr. Moss' baboon studies the amount of sodium that was taken to effect resuscitation in his animals was exactly the same as the amount given in these dogs. Now, he did it over a much longer period of time, and that is probably important.

One of the purposes of this study was to show that the rapid infusion of saline, as we all do in a shock situation, is perhaps deleterious to the lung. I would quibble with Dr. Moss that 10 L. of Ringer's lactate is a lot of fluid to give somebody in hemorrhagic shock.

This is the lesion that is produced. Now, this was not the lung lesion from these dogs, it was from a dog that was given a rapid saline infusion. This is congestive atelectasis; it is not pulmonary edema.

I think Dr. Monafo answered Dr. Moss' question of how does an animal handle a saline load. The water is distributed fairly equally, perhaps, between the blood, the extracellular space, and some of it certainly goes intracellularly. The sodium probably follows. Dr. Shires has shown that the membrane potential decreases during hemorrhagic shock. If that happens, sodium has to move into the cell.

In Dr. Monafo's studies—and this applies mainly to burn shock—the patients had a mild hypernatremia following resuscitation with hypertonic saline. I did not measure the serum sodium in the dogs.

I think we answered one of Dr. Monafo's questions by showing the morphology of this lung. No, I did not perform sodium analysis of the tissue.

We did not measure the colloid osmotic pressure. In the interest of time I would rather not go into that, but refer you to the work that Dr. Moyer did on colloid pressure in the resuscitation of shock. Briefly, I do not think that it is of too much importance.

The pulmonary artery pressure is not equal to the wedge pressure. This shows in a very similar experiment what the effect of pulmonary artery pressure during resuscitation is on shunting. They were numerically equivalent. The regression curve is significantly good.

I am aware that the QS-QT wave is a function of the hemoglobin concentration, but you will recall that the hemoglobin concentrations were no different in the normal saline group and the hypertonic saline group.

Topical lipid protection of burned subjects and their wounds

Carl Jelenko, III, M.D., Mogan L. Wheeler, B.S., Ann P. Anderson, Dianne Callaway, B.S., *and* **Robert A. Scott, Jr.,** *Augusta, Ga.*

We evaluated the naturally occurring cutaneous water-holding lipid, ethyl linoleate (ethyl-[9,12]-cis, cis-octadecadienoate) for its water-holding, metabolic, healing, and toxic properties in groups of unburned and burned rabbits and its toxic potentials in this species and mice. The lipid appears to reduce evaporative water loss in "full-thickness" burned rabbits. Associated with this effect is a proportional and related lowering of metabolic heat production. The topical application of the lipid at any time after burn appears to be associated with a significant healing incidence in lesions that, histologically, at least, would be interpreted as full-thickness. The material is highly toxic if applied daily to mice or rabbits. Chronic exposure of EL to air may result in the formation of hydroperoxides and epoxides. Use of EL on a daily basis (±1.5 Gm. per kilogram) in mice or rabbits is associated with an extremely high mortality rate and/or exfoliative dermatitis. Potential uses of this agent in the therapy of human burn lesions are great, but at present the toxicity of the agent is such that the material cannot be thought of other than as an experimental preparation.

From the Department of Surgery, Medical College of Georgia, Augusta, Ga.

IN THIS communication, the authors extend and amplify observations resulting from a continuum of studies[9-16] in which attempts have been made to control postburn hypermetabolism by decreasing excessive postburn evaporative water loss through the burn eschar. Data will be presented that suggests that a topical agent, ethyl linoleate (ethyl-9,12-cis-cis octadecadienoate (EL), has been delineated which has this potential and, in addition, may enable "healing" of wounds that formerly would have been considered full-thickness burns.

Research supported in part by National Institutes of Health Grant GM-16973-04 and in part by the Defense Civil Preparedness Agency, Office of the Secretary of the Army, Contract No. DAHC-20-68-C-0163.

This article does not represent the official opinions of the United States Army, the Secretary of Department of Defense, or the Defense Civil Preparedness Agency. Opinions expressed are solely those of the authors, or of authorities cited in references.

In conducting the research reported herein, the investigators adhered to the "Principles of Laboratory Animal Care" as established by the National Society for Medical Research.

Presented at the Thirty-fifth Annual Meeting of the Society of University Surgeons, St. Louis, Mo. Feb. 14-16, 1974.

GENERAL INFORMATION

We studied the metabolic effects of topical EL on 41 subjects, the healing effects on 55 New Zealand albino male rabbits, and the toxic effects in 149 male albino mice and eight rabbits.

All rabbit burns were histologically confirmed, 20 percent body surface area (BSA),[12] full-thickness lesions created by 15 second (timed) application of 730° C. heat to the premeasured, clipped abdomen, flanks, and back.

All studies were conducted in unanesthetized subjects with the exception of the burning itself, which was accomplished while the subjects were under intraperitoneal Surital anesthesia. With the exception of biopsies for bacteriologic purposes or toxicity studies requiring injection of material, no attempt was made to maintain sterility.

Animals were divided at random into five groups for the metabolic and healing studies. Rabbits weighed 2.19 ± 0.09 kilograms. Groups comprised: (1) Untreated, burned control (control); (2) subjects treated within one hour of burning (immediate); (3) at 12 hours after burn (12 hours); (4) at 18 hours after burn (18 hours); and (5) at 24 hours after burn (24 hours).

Treatment comprised topical application of a Freon-driven aerosol (0.01 ml. per square centimeter of eschar) of commercial grade 75 percent pure EL (Nu-Check-Prep, Inc., Elysian, Minn.) protected from oxidation/hydrolysis by the addition of 5 p.p.m. of tertiary-butyl hydroquinone (TBHQ: Eastman Organic Chemical, Rochester, N. Y.). The single application of EL to the wound at the time indicated was the *only* treatment given. The animals were allowed food and water ad libitum and were not exogenously resuscitated. In the metabolic studies, food was removed 12 hours before each calorimetric evaluation.

METABOLIC STUDIES

Materials and methods. Composition of the subject group is given in Table I. Animals were studied in the unburned state; the burned state (first 24 hours after burn); and burned-treated state (days 2 to 21, inclusive). Study comprised partitional calorimetric evaluation of the subjects in a constant temperature (wall = 27.16 ± 0.03° C.) environment in a double-wall chamber, which has been described elsewhere, along with the specific techniques and mathematics of the method.[7, 8, 19, 20, 22] Each subject was studied for three hours in the environmental chamber. Selection of the period for mathematical evaluation has been described by several authorities.[7, 8, 19, 20, 22] After the initial "steady-state" evaluation of the subject in the unburned state and collection of calorimetric data in this condition, the subject was burned. Following recovery from anesthesia (usually within one hour after burn), the subject was again studied in the burned and burn-treated states. Partitional calorimetry was conducted at 24 hours after burn and at intervals of 3 days through the 21 day postburn period.

Table I

Groups	Total No.	No. of subjects: Metabolic study	No. of subjects: Healing study
Untreated	24	11	13
Treated	72		
Immediately after burn		5	5
At 12 hours		11	5
At 18 hours		7	25
At 24 hours		7	6

Parameters evaluated comprised: (1) ΔW, mean weight change (grams); (2) O_2, oxygen consumption (grams per hours); (3) CO_2, carbon dioxide production (grams per hours); (4) RR, respiratory rate (per minute); (5) AR, activity rate (per minute); (6) WR, respiratory water loss (grams); (7) T_r, rectal temperature (°C.); (8) W_{ev}, evaporative water loss (grams), a calculated value in which algebraic summation of all intake and output is made and subtracted from ΔW; (9) T_s, surface temperature (°C.) (with evaluation including continual electronic thermometric evaluation from multiple point; the technique is described in detail elsewhere[8, 9, 20, 22]).

Certain values were also derived mathematically: D, dry heat loss (kilocalories per square meter per hour); E_v, evaporative heat production (kilocalories per square meter per hour); ΔS, change in heat storage (kilocalories per square meter per hour); and M, metabolic heat production, evaluated in kilocalories per square meter per hour, watts per square meter, and watts per kilogram.

Evaluation of the parametric data within

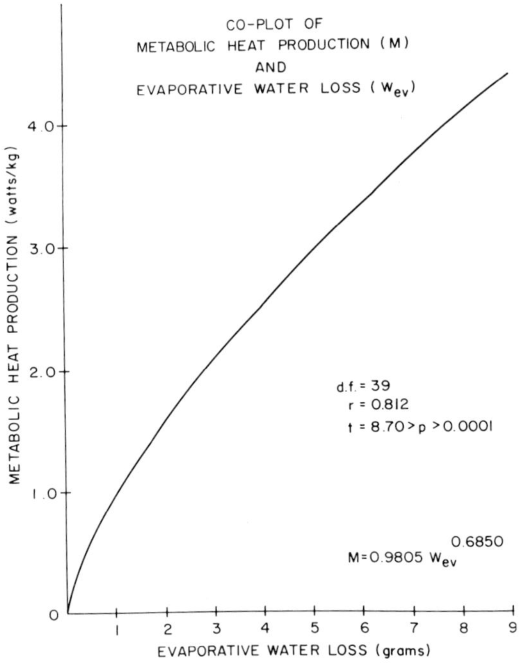

Fig. 1. The relationship between evaporative water loss (W_{ev}) and metabolic heat production (M).

and between groups was by standard statistical methods.

Results of metabolic studies. The results of these studies are summarized in Table II and Fig. 1.

For convenience in mathematical consideration and because of the homogeneity of the respective data, the evaluations at the several days could be grouped into unburned, burned, and burn-treated sets. The "burn" values comprise those observations made during the first 24 hours after burn. The "burn-treated" values comprise the mean (±1 S.E.M.) of all evaluations from day 2 to 21, inclusive, in subjects whose burns had been treated with EL.

We found that certain of the parameters measured increased in the "burned" state and returned to or toward normal in the "burn-treated" state, i.e., AR, W_{ev}, E_v, ΔS, and M. Another group of parameters decreased in the "burned" and returned to or toward normal in the "treated" state, i.e., O_2, CO_2, RR, T_s, T_r, and D.

It was observed that the subjects treated "immediately" exhibited significant changes in the "burned" state in O_2, RR, D, AR, and ΔS. Following treatment, these subjects had significant changes only in O_2, CO_2, and T_r. All other parameters had returned to (statistical) "normal."

In the subjects treated at 12 hours after burn, significant changes occurred in the burned, untreated state in all areas evaluated except CO_2, T_r, and E_v. All values returned to the normal range following treatment, with the exception of O_2 which stayed slightly, but significantly, below the preburn control value.

Among the subjects treated at 18 and 24 hours after burn, virtually all metabolic parameters were significantly altered in the untreated, burned state. In these subjects, significant and important changes occurred after treatment. Most particularly, evaporative water loss and evaporative heat production remained above normal, although both had markedly and significantly returned toward the control level. In these subjects, also, heat storage and metabolic heat production returned to a level within the preburn range. It is also significant that, although a return toward the control levels was observed in dry heat loss, the predominant component of metabolic heat production remained evaporative heat loss.

In Fig. 1 is a coplot of evaporative water loss and metabolic heat production. It will be observed that there is a highly statistically significant ($t = 8.70 > P > 0.001$) relationship between these two functions such that:

$$M = 0.9805 W_{ev} 0.6850 \qquad (1)$$

A highly significant relationship also existed (at the 99.9 percent confidence level) between evaporative water loss and evaporative heat loss and also between evaporative heat loss and metabolic heat production.

We evaluated the day-to-day weight change in the various treatment groups and also the change in weight loss during the calorimetric run. There was virtually no difference in early gross weight change between the unburned and treated animals. By day 14 the treated group had gained significantly more weight ($t = 3.19 > P > 0.001$) and this weight gain was maintained through day 21, at which time the group weighed approxi-

Table II. *Percent change of various metabolic parameters**

Parameter†	*No. Rx*	*Immediate*	*12 hr.*	*18 hr.*	*24 hr.*
From "unburned" to "burned" state: $\left(\frac{U\text{-}B}{U}\right) \times 100.$					
O_2	*10.7*	*20.9*	*18.6*	15.3	*18.5*
CO_2	*7.6*	*(21.1)*	*(18.0)*	22.5	*14.8*
RR	*14.4*	*16.7*	*12.3*	*16.2*	*(10.6)*
T_s	2.6	*(4.0)*	*5.4*	*5.9*	*(1.8)*
T_r	1.7	*(1.0)*	*(2.6)*	*4.3*	*1.3*
D	(15.5)	*23.8*	(47.6)	*33.2*	*(9.5)*
AR	33.6	15.6	12.7	56.0	*(22.7)*
W_{ev}	57.8	(18.3)	74.6	99.1	153.5
E_v	29.4	(16.5)	(45.0)	224.9	435.9
%D	*(3.3)*	*22.9*	*19.0*	*61.3*	*50.6*
ΔS	92.7	354.8	394.1	174.6	153.8
M	39.7	(28.0)	97.48	(17.1)	139.9
From "unburned" to "treated" state: $\left(\frac{U\text{-}T}{U}\right) \times 100.$					
O_2	—	9.8	*6.0*	21.5	*1.8*
CO_2	—	*28.6*	*(19.8)*	(12.8)	*(17.8)*
RR	—	*(10.1)*	*(5.3)*	*(2.7)*	*(9.2)*
T_s	—	*(1.2)*	(2.4)	*(0.2)*	(1.8)
T_r	—	*1.6*	(2.4)	(1.4)	1.5
D	—	*(9.8)*	(49.3)	(14.5)	21.5
AR	—	*(5.5)*	*(6.1)*	86.9	*27.3*
W_{ev}	—	(0.0)	(19.5)	133.6	62.5
E_v	—	*(17.4)*	*(0.7)*	63.7	58.3
%D	—	*(6.2)*	32.1	*38.2*	*(9.9)*
ΔS	—	*(21.7)*	(71.3)	(31.2)	(24.4)
M	—	*(13.1)*	*(8.0)*	62.1	54.5

*Percentages in italics are negative; those in brackets are not statistically significant.
†Definitions for parametric symbols are found in the "Metabolic studies" section (see text).

Table III. *Healing: Summary of statistical analysis**

	Statistics	*Chi-square distribution*
Controls	2/13 healed in excess of ±12.46% BSA (15.39% of subjects) 4/13 died	X^2 healing = 11.62 > P > 0.0001
Treated	29/42 healed in excess of ±12.46% BSA (69.04% of subjects) 0/42 died	X^2 death = 766.52 > P > 0.0001
Healing	Mean (±1S.E.M.) area: Control: 12 ± 5 Treated: 64 ± 5	t = 7.21 > P > 0.001

*No significant difference between (1) areas healed among treated subjects and (2) areas healed: controls vs. untreated areas in one-half treated wounds.

mately 50 grams more than the untreated subjects (significant at $t = 2.24 > P > 0.05$).

HEALING STUDIES

Materials and methods. Composition of the subject group is given in Table I. Twenty-five animals were treated; six each were treated on only the front, back, right, or left half of the wound, and all at 18 hours after burn. Study was composed of biopsies of the burn for histologic appearance and quantitative bacteriologic study at burn and every third day and serial observation of mortality and gross appearance.

Except for those animals that died or spontaneously separated their eschar, the animals were killed with pentobarbital and debrided at the twenty-first postburn day. At that time, an estimate was made, on a diagram representing the burned surface, of

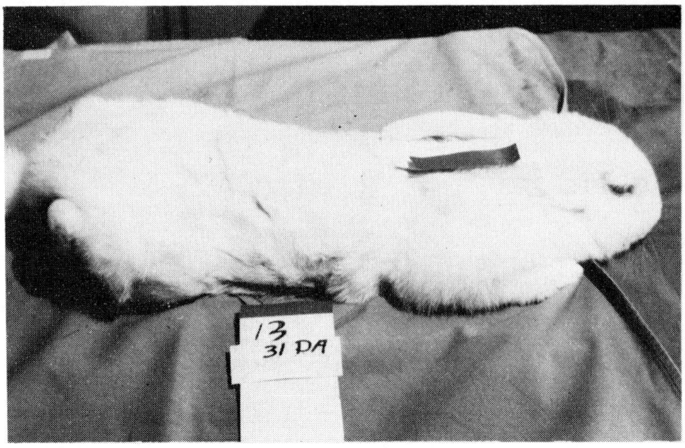

Fig. 2. Lesion at 31 days.

the percentage of the treated area healed. Simultaneously, cultures and photographs were obtained.

Results. Results of these studies are summarized in Table III and Fig. 2.

We observed marked contracture and some anterior and posterior epithelization (12.46 ± 4.86 percent at day 21) in the wounds of the 13 control rabbits. Four of the 13 control rabbits died (at ±day 3). Among the treated subjects, 29 of 42 (69 percent) healed 63.96 ± 5.20 percent of their wounds. No treated rabbit died. Evaluation of 441 biopsy wound cultures of the treated rabbits revealed only 41 cultures (9.3 percent) positive: 31 for staphylococci, and four each for *E. coli* and diphtheroids. Four contained other organisms.

TOXICITY STUDIES

Methods and material. For these studies we used 149 male albino Swiss-Webster mice (weight: 27.21 ± 0.94 Gm.) and eight rabbits. Drug and dosage are given in Table IV.

The group of mice whose treatment began on day 5 after excision was studied for 15 days or until death. Gross characteristics of the surfaces were observed, and at the termination of the experiment, appropriate observations were made at autopsy.

Results. Results of these studies are included in Table IV. The daily application of EL to 72 mice and eight rabbits resulted in the death of 62 mice and three rabbits. Approximately 1.52 ± 0.04 Gm. per kilogram of EL was applied daily to the surface of our subjects, with 1.2 ± 0.05 × 10^{-4} mg. per kilogram of TBHQ. Most deaths occurred on or about the fourth to sixth posttreatment day.

COMMENT

Considerable speculation and discussion have ensued since the first suggestion in 1963[6] that postburn hypermetabolism resulted from a demand for increased caloric work in order to provide the heat to evaporate the supranormal evaporative water lost through burn-damaged skin.[1-4, 9, 17, 21, 25]

A major portion of postburn hypermetabolism is related to evaporative heat loss, which is in turn related to evaporative water loss. The efficiency of EL at controlling evaporative water loss seems to be time-related and to have a critical period of optimum effectiveness. EL at any time up to 24 hours after burn exerts a pronounced effect on metabolic heat production.

The occurrence of significant healing in lesions that were heretofore considered "full-thickness" burns was, to say the least, unanticipated. The histological material suggested that the lesions involved all layers of the skin; and in our control subjects, the lesions extended at times even into the subdermal muscle.

Our first speculation was that the material acted as an antibacterial substance. However, the material is not an antibacterial: If the material was sprayed onto already-growing cultures of staphylococci, streptococci, *E. coli*,

Table IV. *Toxicity studies on ethyl linoleate*

Animal	Purity of lipid	Dosage	Animal conditions	No. of subjects	Deaths No.	Deaths %	Cutaneous reaction	Comment
Rabbits (N = 94)	75%	Single	1 dose to 30% burn	73	0	—	0	Lowered H_2O loss and metabolic heat production, significant healing
		Daily	(No Rx of 30% burn)	13	4	31	0	From sepsis
			Daily to unexcised surface	4	1	25	4	*
			Daily to 10% excision	4	2	50	4	†
Mice (N = 149)			Control	6	0	—	–	
			10% excised control	24	7	29	–	Sepsis
	75%	Daily	As 10% w/w in Unibase daily					
			to 10% excised	6	3	50	–	†
			to unexcised	6	0	—	5	*
			With propyl gallate 5ppm					
			to 10% excised	6	6	100	0	†
			to unexcised	6	6	100	0	†
			With TBHQ 5ppm					
			to 10% excised	24	24	100	0	†
			to unexcised	12	12	100	0	†
	100%		With TBHQ 5ppm					
			to 10% excised	6	6	100		†
			to unexcised	6	5	83	4	*†
			Castor oil					
			to 10% excised	6	6	100	0	†
			to unexcised	6	0	—	0	—
	75%	Single	To intact skin	15	0	—	0	—
	100%	Single	(25% body wt.) intraperitoneal	20	2	10	0	Hemorrhage from vessel laceration

*Marked inanition, dehydration, hypothermia, with hepatocellular and proximal renal tubular necrosis.
†Severe exfoliative dermatitis.

pseudomonas, serratia, klebsiella, or proteus, the organisms continued to grow. Likewise, if the plate was sprayed with the lipid before implanting the organisms, no inhibition of organism viability was noted.

It has been stated that "irreversible damage to all dermal epithelial elements constitutes a full-thickness burn."[1] It would seem that we cannot exclude the possibility that there are viable cells present in the surface even after so severe a thermal challenge as in our burn model. Indeed, earlier in this century we called many burns "full-thickness" (under the definition above) although they ultimately proved to be partial-thickness when treated with an appropriate topical antibacterial agent. It is not unreasonable to presume that the diagnosis of burn wound depth must be made post hoc in patients treated with these topical agents today. Burns that heal are, by definition, "partial thickness"; those that do not heal are, by definition, "full-thickness." The topical antibacterial agents exert their effect by minimizing bacterial growth in and beneath the burn wound, thereby eliminating competitive metabolizing organisms which utilize the nutrients present to their own advantage at a cost of converting a potentially partial-thickness wound into a full-thickness one. It is not unreasonable to suspect that, whatever its mode of action may be, ethyl linoleate exerts an analogous protective effect on still-living cells in the burn surface.

We must, therefore, suspect that the burn wound we induce with a 15 second contact application of 730° C. heat leaves behind some surface cells that are viable, however marginally. The wound is not, therefore, by definition full-thickness. This experience causes us to seriously wonder how much caloric input is required to induce a full-thickness lesion if optimal circumstances are provided for surface survival.

Curreri[5] performed a series of experiments in which rats were challenged with 75 percent pure EL applied daily to their excised wounds. Eighty percent of Curreri's EL-treated rats died within the ten-day study period; eighty-six percent of our daily-treated mice died.

It is important to note that all of the deaths observed in our laboratory occurred in animals treated without washing off old lipid. All of the untoward cutaneous reactions were also associated with daily topical use of the material.

On chronic exposure to air, many oils, including EL, produce variable quantities of hydroperoxides and epoxides. These are highly toxic agents in very small quantities.[18a] Ingestion of these materials is sometimes lethal, but transcutaneous absorption and toxicity is not defined. Although we used a collar designed to prevent our mice from licking their skins and kept the animals in separate cages, we cannot rule out the possibility of lipid ingestion. We suspect the material is toxic by the transcutaneous route because of the significant development of exfoliative dermatitis in many subjects with intact skins and the death of some. Clearly, we must find a way to prevent the formation of the hydroperoxides and epoxides of the lipid. It is probable that ingestion of only 0.4 mg. of the hydroperoxides and/or epoxides would be fatal to a 26 Gm. mouse. The quantity present in each topical dose used may be as much as twice this amount.

REFERENCES

1. Artz, C. P., and Moncrief, J. A.: The treatment of burns, Philadelphia, Pa., 1969, W. B. Saunders Co., pp. 27-28.
2. Bradham, G. B.: Direct measurement of total metabolism of a burned patient, Arch. Surg. **105:** 410, 1972.
3. Caldwell, F. T., Jr.: Personal communication.
4. Caldwell, F. T., Jr., Hammel, H. T., and Dolan, F.: A calorimeter for simultaneous determination of heat production and heat loss in the rat, J. Appl. Physiol. **21:** 1665, 1966.
5. Curreri, W. P.: Personal communication.
6. Fallon, R. H., and Moyer, C. A.: Rates of insensible perspiration through tape-stripped and epidermally denuded living human skin, Ann. Surg. **158:** 915, 1963.
7. Gonzalez, R. R., Kluger, M. J., and Hardy, J. D.: Partitional calorimetry of the New Zealand white rabbit at temperatures 5-35° C., J. Appl. Physiol. **31:** 728, 1971.
8. Huckaba, C. E.: Personal communication.
9. Jelenko, C., III: Studies in burns. I. Water-loss from the body surface, Ann. Surg. **165:** 83, 1967.
10. Jelenko, C., III, and Wheeler, M. L.: Effects of antoxidants on the long-term utility of ethyl linoleate as a water-holding lipid for topical use post burn, J. Surg. Res. **12:** 161, 1973.
11. Jelenko, C., III, Smulyan, W. I., and Wheeler, M. L.: Studies in burns. VI. The role of lipids in the transmissivity of membranes, Ann. Surg. **167:** 521, 1968.
12. Jelenko, C., III, Ginsburg, J. M., and Anderson, A. P.: Studies in burns. VIII. The role of cutaneous water-holding lipid in post-burn thermoregulation, Ann. Surg. **174:** 109, 1971.
13. Jelenko, C., III, Anderson, A. P., Scott, T. H., Jr., and Wheeler, M. L.: Organ weights and water composition of the New Zealand albino rabbit, Am. J. Vet. Med. **32:** 1637, 1971.
14. Jelenko, C., III, Wheeler, M. L., and Scott, T. H., Jr.: Studies in burns. X. Ethyl linoleate: The water-holding lipid of skin. A. The evidence, J. Trauma **12:** 968, 1972.
15. Jelenko, C., III, Wheeler, M. L., and Scott, T. H., Jr.: Studies in burns. XI. Ethyl linoleate: The water-holding lipid of skin. B. Effects on in-vivo burn eschar, J. Trauma **12:** 974, 1972.
16. Jelenko, C., III, Wheeler, M. L., Anderson, A. P., Callaway, D., and Scott, R. A.: Unpublished data.
17. Miksche, L. W., and Caldwell, F. T., Jr.: Energy balance in the immediate post-burn period, Ann. N. Y. Acad. Sci. **150:** 755, 1968.
18. Johnson, W. C.: Oral elemental diet, Arch. Surg. **108:** 32, 1974.

18a. Shue, G. M., Douglass, C. D., Firestone, D., et al.: Acute physiological effects of feeding rats non-urea-adducting fatty acids (urea-filtrate), J. Nutr. **94:** 171, 1968.

19. Stitt, J. T., and Hardy, J. D.: Thermal regulation in the squirrel monkey, J. Appl. Physiol. **221:** 48, 1971.
20. Stolwijk, J. A., and Hardy, J. D.: Partitional calorimetric studies of responses of man to thermal transients, J. Appl. Physiol. **19:** 967, 1963.
21. Stoner, H. B.: Mechanism of body tempera-

ture changes after burns and other injuries, Ann. N. Y. Acad. Sci. **150:** 722, 1968.

22. Stolwijk, J. A., and Hardy, J. D.: Temperature regulation in man—a theoretical study, Pflugers Arch. **291:** 129, 1966.
23. Winitz, M., Adams, R. F., Seedman, D. A., and Graff, J.: Regulation of intestinal flora patterns with chemical diets (abstr.), Fed. Proc. **25:** 343, 1966.
24. Winitz, M., Seedman, D. A., and Graff, J.: Studies in metabolic nutrition employing chemically defined diets, Am. J. Clin. Nutr. **23:** 525, 1970.
25. Zawacki, B. E., Spitzer, K. W., Mason, A. D., Jr., and Johns, L. A.: Does increased evaporative water-loss cause hypermetabolism in burned patients? Ann. Surg. **176:** 171, 1970.

DISCUSSION

Chairman Zuidema. As I understand it, you sprayed the wound surface one time only. Did you perform any studies to see how long the surface coating remained—in other words, what its decay rate might be?

Dr. Thomas Knight Hunt (San Francisco, Calif.). I think there is an explanation for your healing results. As we have said quite often, at the time an injury occurs is the time when the tissue—particularly skin—needs the most circulation and has the least. It is the time when the energy demand is the greatest, but the circulation has been destroyed. Therefore, the energy available to this area is extremely limited; what energy is subtracted in the form of heat is unavailable for repair, synthesis of collagen, epithelial tissues, and so forth. Your ethyl linoleate is an energy-saver, essentially, and you proved that very well. It merely leaves more energy available for the healing process; I suppose that is the reason why you got, apparently, less necrosis of the deeper tissue in your treated as opposed to the control, because the energy demand was so much less.

Dr. Basil A. Pruitt (Fort Sam Houston, Texas). Very few of the control rats healed spontaneously, and since a bit more than half of the treated rats did, suggesting there was a systematic difference in the severity of the inflicted wound, does Dr. Jelenko feel that that explains at least the metabolic changes?

In early postburn periods some of the changes which were described looked as if they could have been due to the postburn volume effects. Has Dr. Jelenko redescribed well-known oxygen consumption changes that occur with and following resuscitation or injury?

Dr. Carl Jelenko, III (closing). I do not know how long the surface coating remains. It takes only 400 μg per square centimeter of tissue to realize the effect, and we are putting on considerably more than this. Both in vivo and in vitro, we have measured the effect in terms of evaporative water loss, and not in terms of the generation of epoxides, hydroperoxides, and other materials. We are currently looking at that, but there are some data out of the food industry that indicate that the breakdown rate is temperature-, water-, pH-dependent, and also is a function of the contact of the material with protein, which would be the situation in the excised wound. The thing that is particularly disturbing is that the material appears to penetrate intact skin.

There really should not be any difference between the burned rabbits in the control and in the treated group. They were all burned by the same technique, using the same time to burn, by the same technician, and the subjects chosen for treatment at the various times, or for control, were selected at random, so that we should have obviated a problem with depth of burn or with the sorts of effects that Dr. Pruitt suggests.

With regard to postburn volume effects, none of the animals were resuscitated. None were given anything but the one dose of topical lipid and put back in their cages. All were allowed to eat and drink ad libitum. The amount of food and water taken in by all was approximately the same. There was no statistical difference.

I agree with Dr. Hunt. I hope we can clean up the toxicity problem. There are some clues, also coming out of the food industry, that such materials as histidine, vitamin E, pH buffered at 7, relative humidity maintained at about 35 percent, cobalt, all will protect this particular lipid from being broken down in air and markedly increase the induction time for the formation of the hydroperoxides.

With regard to the mechanism whereby healing occurs, I hope that the problem is as simple as he describes. If the healing were related to tissue oxygen, saving metabolic energy, then the animals treated immediately postburn should also show the same metabolic effect—which they do.

We have previously reported some work that demonstrated the full eschar had the capability of actively transporting sodium and potassium for at least a day. Histologically, in the depths of this wound, there seemed to be some cells that may be alive. Perhaps this lipid has something to do with maintaining the viability of these cells, very much as the topical antibacterial agents now have created a situation in which we cannot determine what is a full-thickness and a partial-thickness burn until after it is healed, or not, as the case may be.

Total body potassium in surgical patients

Harry M. Shizgal, M.D.,* Robert S. Kurtz, M.D., *and* **C. Douglas Wood, M.D.,**
Montreal, Quebec, Canada

The efficacy of parenteral nutrition was evaluated by quantitating the body cell mass and its supporting extracellular environment by measuring total exchangeable sodium (Na_e), total body water (TBW), and total exchangeable potassium (K_e). The TBW and Na_e were measured by isotope dilution by using tritiated water and sodium-22, respectively. Total exchangeable potassium was determined indirectly using the formula: $K_e = R \times (TBW) - Na_e$, where R is the ratio of the sum of sodium plus potassium content to the water content in a whole blood sample. The indirect measurement of K_e was validated by simultaneously determining K_e indirectly and directly, by K-42 dilution, in 15 normal, five uremic, and 14 dogs rendered hypo-osmolar by intramuscular Pitressin and a water load. The correlation between the two measurements of K_e was excellent with a correlation coefficient of 0.98. Similarly, the simultaneous determination of K_e both indirectly and by K-42 dilution in 20 patients with a variety of illnesses resulted in a mean difference of −0.7 percent and a correlation coefficient of 0.99. The experimental data thus validates the indirect measurement of K_e. TBW, Na_e, and K_e were simultaneously determined in four groups of surgical patients; 13 normal patients, eight with longstanding sepsis, five with starvation, and six with chronic sepsis who, in addition, received intravenous hyperalimentation. K_e expressed as a function of TBW was reduced in the patients with sepsis and starvation, but normal in similar patients receiving parenteral hyperalimentation. The reverse was observed in the Na_e, expressed as a function of TBW, which was elevated in the septic and starved patients, but normal in patients receiving intravenous hyperalimentation.

From the Department of Surgery, Royal Victoria Hospital and McGill University, Montreal, Quebec, Canada.

INTRAVENOUS hyperalimentation is administered to the chronically stressed surgical patient in order to preserve the body cell mass. Moore and co-workers[7] defined the body cell mass as that component of body composition which is rich in potassium, exchanging energy, and performing work. It is the protein-containing cellular component of body composition as opposed to the extracellular supporting component and the triglyceride stores in adipose tissue. Thus, measuring the body cell mass would be an ideal method of assessing the efficacy of parenteral nutrition. Unfortunately, it is impossible to quantitate this variable directly. Instead, nitrogen balance has been employed as an indirect measurement of either the destruction or preservation of the body cell mass. Another approach has been

Supported by a grant from the Medical Research Council of Canada.

Presented at the Thirty-fifth Annual Meeting of the Society of University Surgeons, St. Louis, Mo., Feb. 14-16, 1974.

*Medical Research Council of Canada Scholar.

the measurement of total exchangeable potassium.[1, 7] A linear relationship between exchangeable potassium and body cell mass has been postulated because of the constancy of intracellular potassium concentration.[6] The validity of this postulate was recently confirmed by the demonstration of a linear correlation between total body potassium and total body nitrogen.[5] The measurement of total body potassium, however, poses many problems.

The measurement of total exchangeable potassium by isotope dilution, in the clinical setting, is both expensive and inconvenient because of the short half-life of the potassium radioisotopes that are available. The half-life of potassium-42 is 12.4 hours and that of potassium-43 is 22 hours. Total body potassium has also been determined using a total body counter to quantitate the naturally occurring radioactive potassium-40.[2, 10] However, this approach requires an expensive installation. In addition, the calibration of the total body counter remains a serious problem.[2]

In the present study, a new method for the measurement of total exchangeable potassium is described. In addition, the experimental validation of this technique, and its application to test the efficacy of parenteral nutrition is presented.

METHODS AND MATERIALS

Total exchangeable potassium is determined indirectly by a technique which is based on the hypothesis that the ratio (R) of sodium content (Na) plus potassium content (K) divided by the water content (H_2O)

$$R = \frac{Na + K}{H_2O} \qquad (1)$$

is constant for all of the soft tissues within each individual. If this ratio is indeed the same for all the tissues, it would thus also hold for the sum of the tissues within the individual,

$$R = \frac{Na_e + K_e}{TBW} \qquad (2)$$

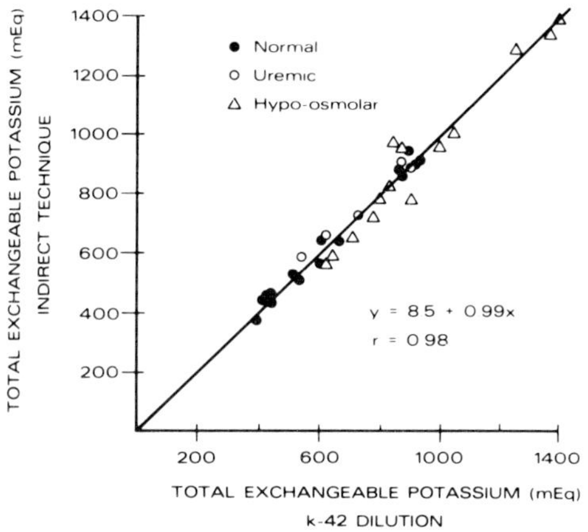

Fig. 1. Total exchangeable potassium was simultaneously determined indirectly and directly, by K-42 dilution, in 15 normal, 5 uremic, and 14 dogs in a hypo-osmolar state. The regression between the two sets of measurements is given by the equation $Y = 8.5 + 0.99x$ with a correlation coefficient of 0.98.

where Na_e = total exchangeable sodium, K_e = total exchangeable potassium, and TBW = total body water which can be rearranged such that

$$K_e = R \times TBW - Na_e \qquad (3)$$

In these studies, total exchangeable potassium was calculated by determining the constant R from a whole blood sample while the total body water and total exchangeable sodium were determined by isotope dilution. The total body water was determined by injecting a known mass of tritiated water intravenously and measuring the equilibrated plasma tritium concentration at 24 hours. The latter was determined in a protein-free filtrate of plasma using standard liquid scintillation counting techniques. Exchangeable sodium was simultaneously determined by injecting a known mass of sodium-22 intravenously, and measuring the plasma sodium-22 concentration at 24 hours in a deep-well scintillation counter and the plasma sodium concentration by flame photometry. In addition, the sodium-22 excreted during the 24 hour equilibration period was measured. Exchangeable sodium was calculated as described by Moore and co-workers.[7]

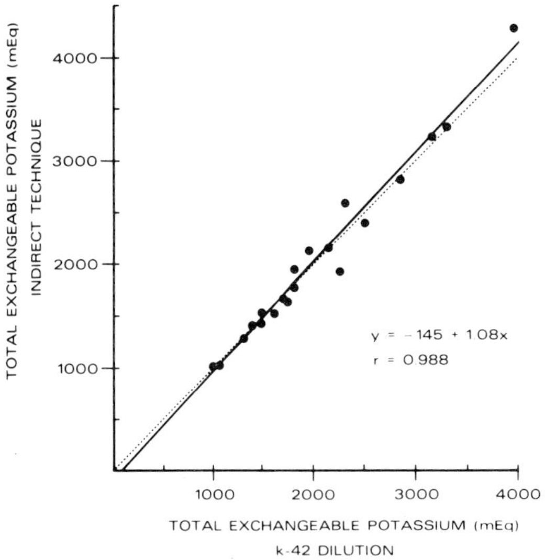

Fig. 2. Total exchangeable potassium was simultaneously determined both indirectly and directly by K-42 dilution in 20 patients with a variety of illnesses. The broken line is the line of identity. The regression between the two sets of measurements is given by the solid line and the equation Y = – 145 + 1.08x. The correlation coefficient is 0.988.

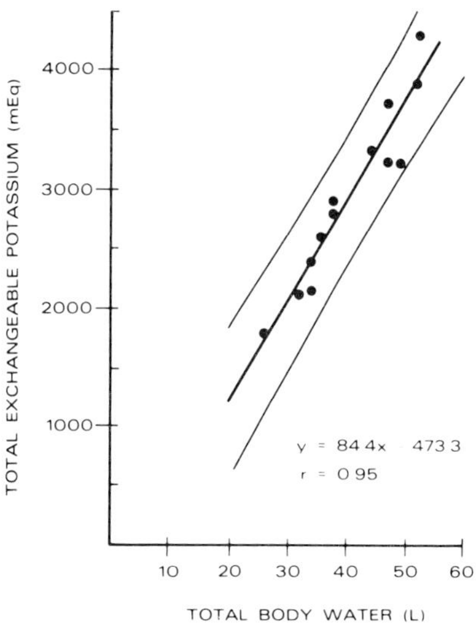

Fig. 3. The total exchangeable potassium is plotted as a function of total body water in 13 normal patients, resulting in a correlation coefficient of 0.95. The regression is given by the equation 84.4x – 473.3. In addition, the 95 percent confidence limits are denoted.

The constant R was determined in each case by directly measuring the sodium and potassium content in a whole blood sample, by flame photometry, while the water content was determined by desiccating to a constant weight. The exchangeable potassium was subsequently calculated using Equation 3.

To validate this indirect technique, exchangeable potassium was determined indirectly, as described above, and directly by isotope dilution using potassium-42.[7] Measurements were carried out in 15 normal dogs, 5 dogs rendered uremic by bilateral ureteral ligation, and 14 dogs which received 2 L. of 5 percent glucose in water intravenously and intramuscular Pitressin to create a hypo-osmolar state. The indirectly determined exchangeable potassium was compared to the measurement obtained by potassium-42 dilution in a heterogeneous group of 20 patients many of whom were in a terminal state with extensive neoplastic disease. The experimental data validating this indirect technique has been described in detail elsewhere.[8, 11]

Following its experimental validation, the above technique was employed in studying four groups of surgical patients.

Group 1. Thirteen normal patients who were in hospital for either investigation or elective surgery. Their nutritional status appeared normal.

Group 2. Eight patients with severe longstanding sepsis. The majority of these patients required prolonged stays in the intensive-care unit. These patients did not receive a significant amount of parenteral calories or nitrogen.

Group 3. Five patients who were admitted to hospital in a state of chronic malnutrition secondary to either a stenosing esophageal lesion or simply due to decreased oral intake.

Group 4. Six patients with long-standing sepsis who were similar to the patients in Group two, except that they received intravenous hyperalimentation as described by Dudrick and co-workers.[3]

RESULTS

In both the normal dogs and in those with either uremia or hypo-osmolarity due to a water load, there was an excellent correla-

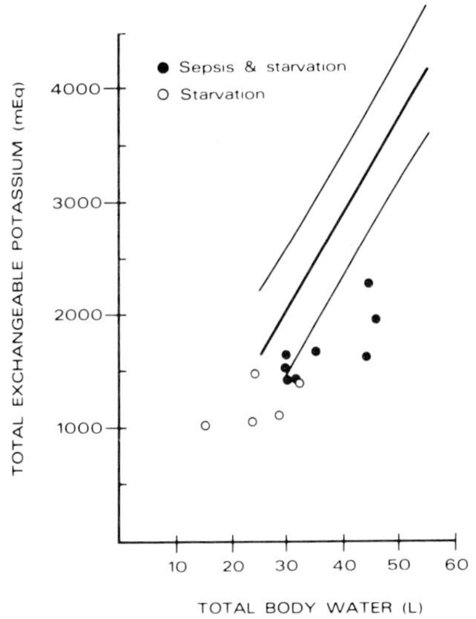

Fig. 4. Total exchangeable potassium is plotted as a function of total body water in eight patients with long-standing sepsis and five patients with chronic starvation. The regression and 95 percent confidence limits for the 13 normal patients plotted in **Fig. 3** are also included.

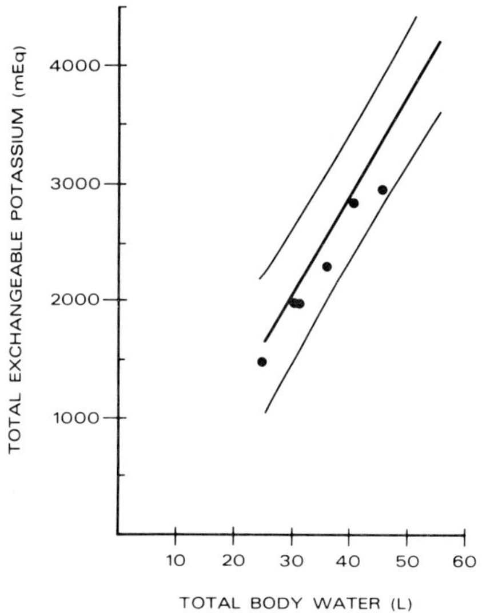

Fig. 5. Total exchangeable potassium is plotted as a function of total body water in the six patients with long-standing sepsis and intravenous hyperalimentation. Included are the regression line and the 95 percent confidence limits for the 13 normal patients plotted in Fig. 3.

tion between the indirect and direct measurement of exchangeable potassium (Fig. 1). The resultant regression was almost identical to the line of identity with an intercept of 8.5 and a slope of 0.99. The correlation coefficient was 0.98. Similarly, there was a close correlation between the two measurements of exchangeable potassium in the 20 patients studied (Fig. 2). The exchangeable potassium in these patients ranged from 1,020 to 4,303 mEq. Nevertheless, the correlation coefficient was 0.988 and the mean percentage difference between the two sets of measurements were –0.7 percent.

In Fig. 3, the exchangeable potassium is plotted as a function of the total body water for the 13 normal patients studied. Included is the regression and the 95 percent confidence limits; within which are 95 percent of the population represented by this sample of 13 normal patients. The exchangeable potassium is plotted as a function of total body water for both the septic and starved patients (Fig. 4), and the septic patients who received hyperalimentation (Fig. 5). The regression and 95 percent confidence limits for the normal patients are included in both figures. It is apparent from Fig. 4 that, in the majority of the septic and starved patients, the exchangeable potassium was significantly less than the range defined by the normal group. On the other hand, in the septic patients receiving intravenous nutrition, the exchangeable potassium was within the normal range.

In a similar fashion, the exchangeable sodium is plotted as a function of total body water for the septic and starved patients (Fig. 6) and the septic patients with parenteral nutrition (Fig. 7). Included in both figures, is the regression line and 95 percent confidence limits as defined by the 13 normal patients. In contrast to exchangeable potassium, the exchangeable sodium increased with sepsis and starvation (Fig. 6) and returned toward normal with hyperalimentation.

The data for the four groups studied is summarized in Table I.

DISCUSSION AND CONCLUSIONS

Edelman and co-workers[4] demonstrated, in a large group of heterogeneous patients, a close correlation between the serum sodium

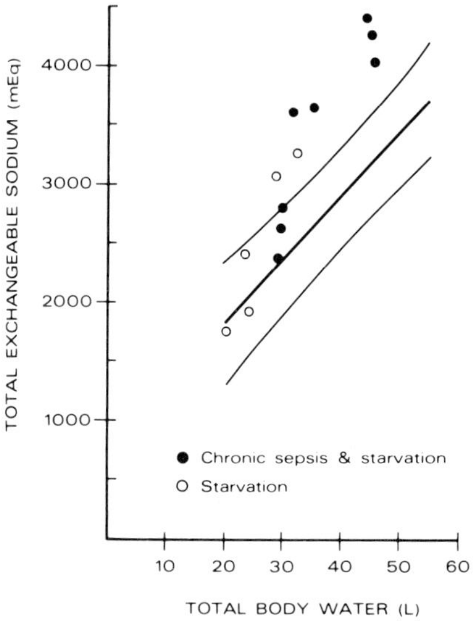

Fig. 6. Total exchangeable sodium is plotted as a function of total body water for the eight patients with long-standing sepsis and five patients with chronic starvation. Included are the regression line and the 95 percent confidence limits for the 13 normal patients.

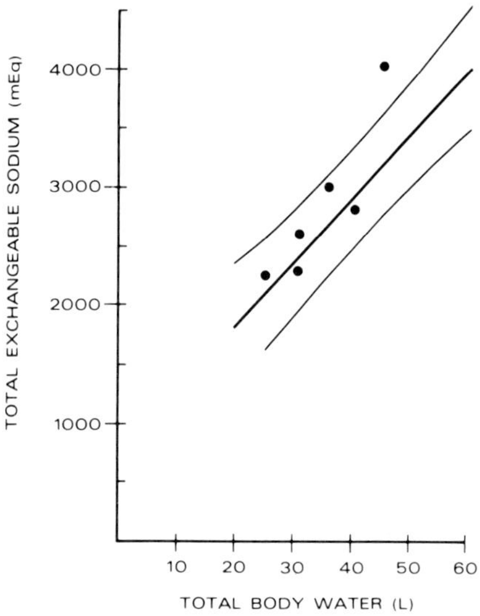

Fig. 7. Total exchangeable sodium is plotted as a function of total body water for the six patients with long-standing sepsis who received parenteral hyperalimentation. Included are the regression line and 95 percent confidence limit for the 13 normal patients studied.

concentration and the sum of exchangeable sodium plus exchangeable potassium divided by the total body water.[4] This relationship implied that an osmotic gradient did not exist between the intracellular and extracellular compartments, and that the electrolytes, of which sodium and potassium are the principal cations, are the major source of the osmotic activity in body water. The same is implied by the hypothesis upon which the indirect measurement of total exchangeable potassium is based. The validity of this hypothesis is supported by the experimental data which demonstrated a close correlation between the direct and indirect measurement of total exchangeable potassium in both the experimental animal and in a group of patients. Many of these patients were seriously ill with abnormally low total exchangeable potassium. Nevertheless, the accuracy of the indirect total exchangeable potassium measurement was unaffected.

The validity of this indirect measurement of total exchangeable potassium is thus supported by the experimental data. The measurement is simple to perform and requires neither expensive installations nor costly isotopes. Its major disadvantage is that it is an indirect technique. Although we have experimentally demonstrated its validity in both normal animals and patients and in those with a variety of pathologic conditions, the possibility exists that under certain unique situations this technique may not be valid. Another disadvantage is that the experimental error in the exchangeable potassium measurement is the sum of the experimental error in the measurement of the ratio R, total body water, and total exchangeable sodium. The necessity to measure exchangeable sodium and body water is not a disadvantage because the techniques employed are simple and the body composition parameters measured are important.

Total exchangeable potassium has been used by numerous investigators as a measure of the body cell mass.[1, 7] The relationship between total exchangeable potassium and the body cell mass is based on the constancy of the intracellular potassium concentration. Potassium is the principal intracellular cation with less than 2 percent of the total body potassium in the extracellular compartment. In addition, cellular tissue has a constant

Table I

	No. of patients	K_e/TBW (mEq./L.)	Na_e/TBW (mEq./L.)	Na_e/K_e
Normal	13	70.8 ± 1.7	73.4 ± 1.5	1.03 ± 0.14
Chronic sepsis	8	46.2 ± 1.8	99.6 ± 3.6	2.21 ± 0.15
Starvation	5	48.6 ± 4.2	96.4 ± 4.9	2.09 ± 0.26
Chronic sepsis and intravenous nutrition	6	64.7 ± 1.6	85.2 ± 2.6	1.32 ± 0.05

potassium-to-nitrogen ratio of approximately 3 mEq per gram.[6] Recently, a direct correlation has been demonstrated between the total body nitrogen as determined by neutron activation analysis, and total body potassium measured with a whole-body counter.[5] Furthermore, changes in the total body nitrogen, which occurred with uremia or following abdominal surgery, were accompanied by parallel changes in the total body potassium.

In the present study, total exchangeable potassium was employed as a measure of body cell mass to assess parenteral nutrition. In the patients with long-standing sepsis and starvation, the total exchangeable potassium was decreased while the total exchangeable sodium was increased when compared to normal patients. In addition, there was a significant increase in the ratio of exchangeable sodium to exchangeable potassium. These findings are similar to those observed by Moore and co-workers and are indicative of a contraction of the body cell mass, while the extracellular supporting component of body composition appears to expand. The administration of intravenous hyperalimentation to a similar group of patients restored the relationship between total exchangeable potassium and total body water to normal. Similarly, total exchangeable sodium, expressed as a function of total body water, and the ratio of exchangeable sodium to exchangeable potassium returned toward normal. A possible explanation of these body composition changes in the patients receiving intravenous hyperalimentation, is that the total exchangeable potassium increased while the total exchangeable sodium and the total body remained unchanged. If the total body water is unchanged, a significant increase in body cell mass would occur without any change in body weight. Furthermore, it would indicate that intravenous hyperalimentation preserved the body cell mass in these patients. Preliminary data from current investigations in our laboratory indicates that this is indeed the case. Unfortunately, the data in the present report involved discreet measurements in four different groups of patients, and not measurements before and after a period of intravenous hyperalimentation. Thus, our data do not rule out the possibility that there was a decrease in both the exchangeable sodium and total body water without any change in the total exchangeable potassium. The latter would also result in a normal relationship between total exchangeable potassium and total body water, as was seen in Fig. 5, and between total exchangeable sodium and total body water as was observed in Fig. 7. Further studies to distinguish these possibilities are in progress.

The marked difference recorded between the various groups of patients studied would support the use of the technique described in this report to evaluate a patient's nutritional status. Thus, in addition to using this approach to quantitate the efficacy of parenteral nutrition, as in the present report, this technique can also be employed to determine a patient's status prior to a major surgical procedure. This would determine whether a preoperative period of nutritional support was warranted. In addition, this approach can be utilized to determine if parenteral hyperalimentation should be instituted.

REFERENCES

1. Bernard, R. W., and Stahl, W. M.: Total body potassium measurements as a guide to

intravenous alimentation, Ann. Surg. **178:** 559, 1973.
2. Cohn, S. H., and Denbrowski, C. S.: Absolute measurement of whole body potassium by gamma-ray spectrometry, J. Nucl. Med. **11:** 239, 1970.
3. Dudrick, S. J., Wilmore, P. W., Vars, H. M., and Rhoads, J. E.: Long-term total parenteral nutrition with growth development and positive nitrogen balance, SURGERY **64:** 134, 1968.
4. Edelman, I. S., Leibman, J., O'Meara, M. P., and Birkenfeld, L. W.: Interrelations between serum sodium concentration, serum osmolarity and total exchangeable sodium, total exchangeable potassium, and total body water, J. Clin. Invest. **37:** 1236, 1958.
5. Harvey, T. C., Jain, S., Dykes, P. W., James, H., Chen, N. S., Chettle, D. R., Ettinger, K. V., Fremlin, J. H., and Thomas, B. J.: Measurement of whole body nitrogen by neutron-activation analysis, Lancet **2:** 395, 1973.
6. Moore, F. D., and Boyden, C. M.: Body cell mass and limits of hydration of the fat free body: their relation to estimated skeletal weight, Ann. N. Y. Acad. Sci. **110:** 62, 1963.
7. Moore, F. D., Olsen, K. H., McMurrey, J. D., Parker, H. V., Ball, M. R., and Boyden, C. M.: The body cell mass and its supporting environment, Philadelphia, 1963, W. B. Saunders Co.
8. Shizgal, H. M., and Wood, C. D.: A simplified technique for measuring total exchangeable potassium. In preparation.
9. Snedecor, G. W.: Statistical methods, Ames, Iowa, 1956, The Iowa State College Press.
10. Tyson, I., Sebastian, G., James, R. L., Bikerman, V., and Burrows, B. A.: Body potassium measurements with a total body counter, J. Nucl. Med. **11:** 255, 1970.
11. Wood, C. D., and Shizgal, H. M.: The indirect measurement of total body potassium, Clin. Res. **21:** 1080, 1973.

DISCUSSION

Dr. Paul Richard Schloerb (Kansas City, Kan.). Certainly, we all try to extract all the information we can from serum concentrations, and are well aware of the fact that these often do not match up very well with body composition. Over ten years ago, this interrelationship was first documented by Edelman, and later by Bowling.

This is a slide taken from Bowling, and the dotted line, as you can see, which goes almost through zero, represents Edelman's data. The solid line is another series of about 100 patients, representing Bowling's data. On the ordinate we have total body water—or total body water on the abscissa, and on the ordinate we have the sum of total body sodium plus total exchangeable body potassium, divided by their respective serum concentrations. This is unique, because it probably represents, if you assume all the measurement errors are random errors, a perfect correlation, something unique in biology and medicine—particularly remarkable because these jaundiced patients represent all forms of fluid electrolyte derangement, and a wide variety of diseases.

What this says is that a low serum sodium may reflect a low body potassium, and for any given volume of body water, as Dr. Shizgal has said, this expression must remain constant. It also provides the basis for calculation of total body sodium or total body potassium, provided one knows total body water and either body sodium or body potassium.

The next slide shows Bowling's computation, where exchangeable body potassium is 0.9 times this expression of +321, with a very, very high correlation.

Now, recognizing that this 0.9 is less than 1, and this factor of 321 over at the right tends to correct—they actually tend to cancel out; so that this, then, becomes not unlike Dr. Shizgal's formula, where R is in his study, sodium and potassium in blood, and here we have serum sodium plus serum potassium, which serves equally well as an expression R, as shown by Bowling over ten years ago.

I think this is useful information, but the problem is that Dr. Shizgal, in Montreal, has used sodium-22. We have used sodium-22 in the past, as have others, but the Food and Drug Administration has zeroed in on sodium-22, with its two and one-half-year half-life and its bone-seeking characteristics. Sodium-22 is no longer available in this country.

Dr. Robert M. Zollinger, Jr. (Cleveland, Ohio). I think there are two points worthy of discussion. The factor R appears to be strongly dependent upon the hematocrit; I wonder whether or not whole blood with this potassium concentration in red cells, which is not really representative of tissue cells—whether this is a fair representation of what is going on in the body as a whole.

Second, I would like to point out that the isotope dilution method is not yet dead. This is potassium-43 equilibrium in a man going out about five days, and the upper line represents the fall in specific activity in serum and plasma—or, rather, saliva—whereas the lower dots coming up represent that within the red cell itself; it is approximately forty hours before a stable specific activity is obtained.

This, of course, is one of the disadvantages of the isotope method for exchangeable potassium, that a forty-hour period is really needed. But I think the slide also shows that the red cell does not immediately equilibrate its potassium with that in the serum. Therefore, this makes me worry more about the R factor in the patients with sepsis, or perhaps someone that has had a recent transfusion, as to whether this factor will hold up to be truly representative of the patient as a whole.

Dr. Hastings Kemper Wright (New Haven, Conn.). We have heard one immediate clinical application already; this is prevention of protein depletion in patients with sepsis. There is a second major application, I think, and that is in identifying patients who are protein depleted, who present for elective surgery; e.g., the cirrhotic patient—and in allowing some measure for a rate of repletion in patients.

I would like to ask the authors whether they have identified such patients that common-sense clinical observation would not show to be protein depleted, used hyperalimentation, and then operated on those patients. If so, how long did it take to replete these patients?

Dr. Harry M. Shizgal (closing). This is the equation which Dr. Edelman published and which relates the serum sodium concentration to this ratio. You can easily say: Well, why not just measure the serum sodium concentration, measure the exchangeable sodium, which we can do quite easily, measure total body water, and calculate K_e? And the reason was that we have to assume that this contant is the same for all patients.

So, to get around it, what we do in effect is to calculate these constants by determining our R ratio. What we are really saying is that we calculate the ratio R by using a representative soft tissue, and the soft tissue we use is whole blood which makes it slightly different from just applying this equation.

Now, if you think about it, the implication of Edelman's equation, and the slide that Dr. Schloerb showed states that there is no significant osmotic gradient between the extracellular and the intracellular compartment. And, therefore, if that is true, you can calculate the ratio R from whole blood—from any tissue in the body. We have done this in a large series of rats where we measured the R from seven or eight different tissues in about twenty rats, and the ratio came out about the same.

We have also used plasma and serum to calculate R. By measuring the sodium content, not concentration, potassium content, and water content, we find that R is the same whether we are using whole blood, plasma, or serum.

The reason we keep on using whole blood is that it is an indirect technique, and we are always worried that we may run into some situation where this may not hold, where there may be a difference between the cellular constituents of osmotic pressure and the intracellular constituents, even though the osmotic pressure is the same, and that we may not have such a great error if we are using a cellular component.

We are looking at the problem of trying to assess the nutritional status of patients, and we have had a bit of experience with several older patients who presented looking as if they had come out of a concentration camp and have found that they fall within a normal range. On the other hand, we have had the experience of a patient in the intensive-care unit with severe pancreatitis who was grossly obese, and the fellows were having trouble hyperalimenting her. Since everyone said, "Well, she's obese, and she can afford to lose all that weight," they did not hyperaliment her, and she is on one of those slides which shows the chronic septic patient. In effect, although she did not lose a lot of weight, she did destroy her body cell mass; her potassium fell precipitously; and she died obese.

Are there educational advantages to a surgical clerkship in a university hospital?

Sidney Levitsky, M.D.,* Rene L. Nerenberg, M.A., C. Thomas Bombeck, M.D., *and* **Lloyd M. Nyhus, M.D.,** *Chicago, Ill.*

The participation of five community hospitals in the surgical education program for undergraduate students has allowed us to study the differences in the quality of the clerkship between university-type hospitals staffed by a full-time faculty and community hospitals staffed by a voluntary part-time faculty. In a clerkship evaluation, certain characteristics such as motivation, attitude, and behavioral identification with professorial models are difficult to define and measure objectively. Other factors such as cognitive knowledge and problem-solving can be more readily evaluated and were measured in 357 students in 1972 and 1973 by comparing student total and surgical scores on the University Clinical Comprehensive Examination and the National Board of Medical Examiners test (Part II). Although students were initially distributed at random between hospitals, numbers of students who planned academic careers usually managed to switch to a university clerkship, thus apparently giving bias to the university group. Nevertheless, analysis of variance between groups revealed no differences in either year. Thus, the surgery clerkship setting appeared to bear no relationship to student achievement as measured by these examinations. Perhaps a better index of the worthiness of an educational environment may be an evaluation of how it motivates the student to sustain a high degree of scholarship and achievement after the completion of the clerkship.

From the Department of Surgery and the Center for Educational Development of the Abraham Lincoln School of Medicine of the University of Illinois College of Medicine, Chicago, Ill.

In January of 1970, the University of Illinois College of Medicine embarked on a major reorganization program; among its goals was an expansion of the medical school class. For a variety of reasons, including a commitment to extend health science teaching into the community throughout the state, building additional university hospitals to accommodate this expansion was felt to be undesirable, and, therefore, the assistance of several community hospitals in metropolitan Chicago was sought. The participation of three of these five community hospitals in the surgical undergraduate education program and the large number of students in the class seemed to provide a unique opportunity for us to study the differences in the quality of the clerkship between university-type hospitals staffed by a full-time faculty and community hospitals staffed by voluntary part-time faculty. The initiation of this study was based on a preconceived bias on the part of the authors (S. L. and

Presented at the Thirty-fifth Annual Meeting of the Society of University Surgeons, St. Louis, Mo., Feb. 14-16, 1974.

Reprint requests: Sidney Levitsky, M.D., Department of Surgery, Abraham Lincoln School of Medicine of the University of Illinois, College of Medicine, P. O. Box 6998, Chicago, Ill. 60680.

*Established Investigator, American Heart Association.

L. M. N.) that the surgical clerkship in a classical university hospital setting should provide the medical student with a higher degree of scholarship than found in the community hospital.

In order to determine whether the setting of a student's clerkship affects the degree of scholarship attained, one considers such aspects as cognitive knowledge, problem-solving skill, and additional factors such as motivation, attitude, and behavioral identification with professorial models. Since the latter variables are difficult to define and to measure objectively, this study concentrated on the former—those variables which relate most directly to classical conceptions of academic achievement.[6, 9, 11, 12] These skills were measured in 357 students in 1972 and 1973 by employing student total and surgical scores on the University of Illinois Clinical Comprehensive Examination and National Board of Medical Examiners test (Part II). Additional data were obtained by surveying other Departments of Surgery.

METHODS

Students. Although the students at the University of Illinois College of Medicine entered medical school as a homogeneous group, varying experiences and faculty exposures during the basic science years may have resulted in the development of specific prejudices in regard to the type of hospitals they preferred for clinical training. Although students were initially distributed at random between hospitals, an undetermined number of students who planned academic or specialty careers usually managed to switch to a university clerkship, thus apparently giving bias to the university group. Scores of this group on the total and the surgery subset of both the National Board and Comprehensive examinations were compared with scores of the group trained in the community hospitals.

Complete examination data were available for 188 of 204 (92 percent) students in the Class of 1972 and for 169 of 192 (88 percent) students in the Class of 1973. Students in special situations such as those involved in the independent study program who might not take the formal clerkship in surgery or students who took the National Board examination at a time other than that of the regular members of the class were not included.

Hospitals. The university hospital experience encompassed three institutions that fulfilled the following criteria: (1) Attending staff is full-time with no outside private practice. (2) Entire attending staff is engaged in laboratory or clinical research. (3) Majority of operative procedures are performed by the resident staff under the supervision of the attending staff. (4) Majority of patients are indigent or rely entirely on third-party payees for entire medical care costs. (5) Majority of intern and resident staff are United States medical school graduates.

The university-type hospitals include a state-supported university hospital, a Veterans Administration hospital, and a large county hospital. These hospitals were involved in surgical teaching for 67 and 65 percent of the class for the years 1972 and 1973, respectively (Table I). The University hospitals, within a one-block radius of each other, have 773 surgical beds, a bed-student ratio of 6.5, and a student-faculty ratio of 8.8.

The surgical program at the metropolitan community hospitals involved three of the five hospitals associated with the College of Medicine and another Veterans Administration hospital with a part-time staff. These hospitals were characterized by: (1) Part-time voluntary staff, all of whom were involved in the private practice of surgery; (2) few members of the staff were engaged in clinical research; (3) majority of operative procedures were performed by the private surgical practitioner; (4) majority of patients relied on third party payees supplemented by personal funds to meet medical costs; and (5) majority of house officers were foreign medical graduates. These hospitals have 959 surgical beds with a bed-student ratio of 16 and are dispersed throughout the City of Chicago.

Educational programs. The general curricular objectives were the same in all institutions. The students were assigned three to

Table I. *Comparison of surgery and total scores on National Boards Part II and University of Illinois Clinical Comprehensive by university and community hospital clerkships*

	University			*Community*			
	No. of students	*Mean*	*Standard deviation*	*No. of students*	*Mean*	*Standard deviation*	*F-ratio**
Class of 1972	127			61			
National Board Part II							
Surgery		467	±93		474	±102	0.24
Total		489	±90		498	±94	0.39
Clinical Comprehensive							
Surgery		69	±10		70	±9	0.58
Total		67	±5		68	±4	0.48
Class of 1973	110			59			
National Board Part II							
Surgery		478	±101		503	±107	2.43
Total		502	±98		515	±96	0.69
Clinical Comprehensive							
Surgery		57	±10		57	±10	0.03
Total		61	±6		61	±5	0.75

*None of the F ratios are significant.

five patients per week, obtained a history from the patient, performed a physical examination, and participated in the preoperative work-up, the intraoperative procedure (scrub), and the postoperative care. At the university hospitals, formal teaching exercises consisted of service attending and specialty rounds at least three times weekly, surgical pathology conferences, daily clinical seminars, Professor's Rounds, weekly mortality and morbidity conferences, and daily rounds with the house staff. Similarly, the community hospitals had attending rounds (limited for the most part to the private patients of the attending surgeon), clinical seminars, monthly staff-mortality conferences, and daily rounds with the house staff. There were weekly "grand rounds" and surgical-radiology conferences for all students held at the University hospital but were rarely attended by the students assigned to the community hospitals. On reviewing critiques submitted by students and faculty advisory teams from both types of hospitals, it was noted that the students felt that they received the major amount of teaching in both educational settings from the house staff. Major sources of dissatisfaction at the university hospitals involved the students devoting large blocks of time to non-educational "scut" activities, i.e., finding x-ray films, obtaining laboratory data, etc. On the other hand, students at the community hospitals felt that they were isolated from the mainstream of group educational activities, i.e., visiting professors, research seminars, etc., and had limited contact with subspecialty consultants.

Examinations. National Board Part II is an examination consisting of approximately 850 to 900 multiple-choice items sampling a broad range of clinically relevant information; the surgery subtest includes 140 to 150 items. The University of Illinois Clinical Comprehensive examination measures cognitive knowledge in more depth by use of branching patient management problems. The problems are constructed to involve the student in a series of exercises involving sequential analysis designed to simulate the clinical situation as colsely as possible. In addition, the Clinical Comprehensive examination includes approximately 180 multiple-choice items which test complex intellectual processes such as interpretation of data and

Table II. *Survey of Departments of Surgery, 1972-73, compared with data from the University of Illinois*

	1972	*1973*	*Total*	*Univ. of Ill.* *1972*	*Univ. of Ill.* *1973*
No. questionnaires sent			104		
No. questionnaires returned			48		
No. questionnaires used			24		
Average No. students per medical school class	89	101		188	169
Average No. students taking surgery at university hospital	72	82		127	110
Average No. full-time surgery faculty	21.3	22.2		14	13
Average student-surgical faculty ratio at university hospital	5.4	5.1		9.1	8.5
Average % students at university hosiptal	82	83		68	65

problem-solving. Thus, in the two examinations, the students are assessed both on cognitive knowledge and on their ability to use their knowledge to make interpretations and to solve problems.

For both examinations, a total score and a discipline subtest score are derived. However, the methods of obtaining the total score and of reporting all scores differ in the two examinations. All National Board scores are reported in standard score units with a mean of 500 and a standard deviation of 100, standardized on the total national group of examinees. The total score and the subtest scores are based on the total number of items answered correctly. Unacceptable performance on the examination is defined as a score more than 2.1 standard deviations below the mean. There is no minimum passing level for the subtests. Scores on the University of Illinois Clinical Comprehensive examination are reported in terms of percent of maximum possible points. The total score is a weighted sum of all subtest scores; unacceptable performance is defined in advance on the basis of required competencies and is independent of the actual performance of a group. The comprehensive is a certifying examination administered to all University of Illinois students in their senior year.

Means and standard deviations for the two samples (Class of 1972 and Class of 1973) were computed and analysis of variance was used to compare means of the two groups and total scores for the two examinations described above. With analysis of variance, if an experimental condition (clerkship training) has been influential, then it should be reflected in differences between the mean scores of the groups beyond any differences between these groups likely to arise by chance alone.[4]

Medical school survey. To obtain additional data regarding the importance of a full-time faculty for medical student surgical teaching, a request for information was sent to the Department of Surgery Chairmen of 104 medical schools for the years 1972 and 1973. The data requested included: (1) total and surgery test scores on the National Board examination (Part II); (2) percentage of the class receiving surgical training at the University hospital; and (3) the number of full- and part-time surgical faculty at the university hospital. In order to preserve anonymity, a stamped addressed envelope was enclosed and the survey form did not contain any information about institutional identification.

RESULTS

Examinations. Table I reports the mean scores and standard deviations for the two groups of students on the total test and the surgical subtest for both the University of Illinois Clinical Comprehensive examination and the National Board (Part II) examination for 1972 and 1973, respectively. An analysis of variance between groups revealed no significant differences on any measure in either year.

Table III. *Correlations between surgery National Board scores and other variables (Data obtained from survey of Departments of Surgery, 1972-1973)*

*Correlations**	*1972*	*1973*	*No.*†
$r_{1,2}$	−0.153	−0.167	24
$r_{1,3}$	−0.125	−0.193	24
$r_{1,2\cdot3}$‡	−0.090	+0.015	24
$r_{2,3}$	+0.857	+0.900	24
$r_{2,4}$	−0.091	+0.072	18

*r_1 = ratio of students in a University Hospital to full-time surgical faculty; r_2 = surgery scores on National Board Part II; r_3 = total scores on National Board Part II; r_4 = ratio of students at University Hospital to total number of students in class.

†Number of completed surveys.

‡Partial r between 1 and 2 controlling for the effect of 3.

Medical school surgical survey. One hundred and four chairmen of departments of surgery were surveyed and asked to complete the data form previously outlined. Of the 48 chairmen who replied, the data were incomplete or unusable in 24 cases (Table II). Of the remaining 24, only 18 reported numbers of students per class resulting in a total of 2,127 and 2,378 students, respectively, for each of the years studied. Because of the anonymity of the replies, it was impossible to determine bias by either the returnees or by those who failed to return the questionnaire. It was hypothesized that lower student-faculty-ratios and higher percent of students in university hospitals would be associated with higher mean scores on National Board examinations. However, as noted in Table III, there was no significant correlation between these variables. Similarly, there was no significant correlation between the surgery score and the percentage of students in either class taking their surgical clerkship at a university hospital. Thus, schools having a majority of students training at university hospitals did not score higher than schools having a major percentage of students training at community hospitals. A significantly positive correlation ($p < 0.01$) between total and surgical National Board scores was found, suggesting the commonality between disciplines and its strong relationship to surgical scores.

There was great difficulty in evaluating the data for the part-time faculty at university hospitals, with the number varying from none to 387. Several comments indicated that the majority of part-time faculty positions were honorary rather than actual teaching positions.

DISCUSSION

The results of this study, namely, that the educational setting appears to be immaterial in determining medical student examination performance in surgery, may have far-reaching governmental and economic ramifications. Over the past decade, societal needs translated into political pressures have resulted in a rapid increase of medical students and schools. However, the financing of medical school activities has not kept up with these accelerating needs, so that expanding or new schools have been forced to seek alternative educational settings for their students rather than relying solely on the traditional university-type hospitals. In addition, recent changes in the financing of medical care, views that medical care is a right of all citizens, and the maldistribution of physicians have caused a shift of emphasis away from traditional university hospitals to community hospitals. Thus, new community-based medical schools have arisen and older medical schools have formed educational partnerships with community hospitals to meet the joint needs of producing new physicians and providing additional health care to local communities.[3, 13, 14] Concomitant with this rapid increase has been a concern regarding the quality of the educational process. It is to this question that the present study is addressed.

The problem of evaluating clinical competence following a surgical clerkship has been the subject of numerous studies. The major criticism of the examinations used in this study may be that they are not sufficiently sensitive to reflect the subtle differences between clerkships based in different settings. The University of Illinois Clinical Comprehensive examination consisting of multiple-choice type questions and patient management problems has been internally validated as to consistency and construction. These studies indicate that there are significant differences between groups taking the same examination at different levels of training.[7, 10] Questions have been raised as to how well grades achieved on the National Board examination correlate with medical school grades.[1] Problems in interpreting these data arise when some schools or departments use the National Board scores to determine wholly or partially the school grade. In interpreting National Board data for the survey, it is important to consider the proportion of students in each senior class who took the examination, when they took it, and the motivation involved (whether or not it was a graduation requirement). Since we were unable to control for these factors in the survey, the results with regard to National Board scores may not be decisive.

While these examinations reveal similarities in cognitive knowledge between the different types of hospitals, they do not measure surgical clinical competency. The latter may be defined as a bedside "real-life" demonstration of the application of knowledge, skills, and attitudes. Schwartz and Gonnella[12] have found low correlation between examination (cognitive knowledge) scores and clinical performance scores, a finding which suggests that each of these entities may measure different aspects of clerkship competence. However, unless a systematic approach is made to define operationally the level of clinical performance required of a student at a particular stage of training, the grade may reflect the unstructured, informal, personal encounters that usually transpire between faculty and students in any large hospital. Moreover, direct observation as a means of evaluating clinical skills requires an inordinate amount of faculty time and examiner training to achieve a high degree of interrater agreement.[5] Cowles[2] has suggested that quantification of "critical comments" may be a more valid measure of clinical performance. However, this methodology also requires a large expenditure of faculty time.

While there may be some scholarship differences between the hospitals, all of the students were registered at the same medical school and shared a "commonality of experiences" outside the surgical clerkship. These shared experiences may very well have diluted the advantages of one clerkship over another. By submitting surgical students to pre- and postclerkship testing, McCarthy and King[8] were able to show a progressive increase in pretest scores as students progressed through a greater variety of clerkships, again illustrating the importance of common experience.

If the results of these data from cognitive examinations are to be accepted then one might assume that the learning environment is immaterial and that learning at the clerkship level is purely self-motivated. Thus, while a university environment may add enrichment for the medical student, it may not be absolutely necessary. In addition, our data also reveals that students and schools with high total examination scores consistently perform at a higher level on surgical tests, irrespective of the student-faculty ratio. Nevertheless, it is difficult to reject totally the hypothesis that the presence of a full-time staff, frequent conferences, rounds, and a research-oriented faculty, reflecting the totality of commitment of scholarship common to a university environment, does not result in measurable superiority. Perhaps a better index of the worthiness of an educational setting may be an evaluation of how it motivates the student to sustain a high degree of scholarship and achievement after the completion of the clerkship.

The authors wish to express their appreciation to Ms. Christine H. McGuire and Mr. Thomas Bligh of the Center for Educational Development for criticism and statistical advice and to Ms. Patricia Kuhar for secretarial assistance.

REFERENCES

1. Carol, B., and Pigman, W.: The correlation between medical school grades and National Board examination scores, J. Med. Educ. **41:** 477, 1966.
2. Cowles, J. T.: A critical-comments approach to the rating of medical students' clinical performance, J. Med. Educ. **40:** 188, 1965.

3. Evans, R. L., Pittman, J. G., and Perers, R. C.: The community-based medical school—Reactions at the interface between medical education and medical care, N. Engl. J. Med., **288:** 713, 1973.
4. Hays, W. L.: Statistics for the social sciences, ed. 2, New York, New York, 1973, Holt, Rinehart and Winston, pp. 457-523.
5. Hinz, C. F., Jr.: Direct observation as a means of teaching and evaluating clinical skills, J. Med. Educ. **41:** 150, 1966.
6. Hubbard, J. P., Levit, E. J., Schumacher, C. F., and Schnabel, T. G.: An objective evaluation of clinical competence: New technics used by the National Board of Medical Examiners, N. Engl. J. Med. **272:** 1321, 1963.
7. Joorabchi, B., Olson, C. J., and Page, G. G.: Relationship between type of pediatric clerkship and performance on pediatric examination, J. Med. Educ. **48:** 356, 1973.
8. McCarthy, W. H., and King, T. C.: Evaluating patterns of surgical clerkship programs, J. Med. Educ. **43:** 367, 1968.
9. McGuire, C. H.: A process approach to the construction and analysis of medical examinations, J. Med. Educ. **38:** 556, 1963.
10. McGuire, C. H., and Babbott, D.: Simulation technique in the measurement of problem-solving skills, J. Educ. Meas. **4:** 1, 1967.
11. Sanazaro, P. J., and King, T. C.: An exploratory study of undergraduate programs in surgery, J. Med. Educ. **42:** 289, 1967.
12. Schwartz, G. F., and Gonnella, J. S.: The surgical clerkship: Assessment of clinical competence, J. Surg. Res. **14:** 373, 1973.
13. Willard, W. R.: New medical schools: Some preliminary considerations, J. Med. Educ. **35:** 93, 1960.
14. Willard, W. R.: The development of the medical school as a community resource, J. Public Health **54:** 1041, 1964.

Objectives and methods in undergraduate surgical education

Ralph G. DePalma, M.D., Robert J. Izant, M.D., Alf Jordan, M.D., William D. Holden, M.D., *Cleveland, Ohio and* **T. Joseph Sheehan, Ph.D.,*** *Hartford Conn.*

During a recent curriculum reorganization, we defined two distinct, but related, processes in surgical clerkship: (1) introductory goals—to teach skills needed by all physicians, and (2) core goals—to teach skills unique to surgery. Three years ago, third-year students were assigned to the surgical service as their first clinical experience, Introductory Clerkship (IC). Objectives of IC were: (1) development of skills in history-taking, physical examination, use of medical records, and application of laboratory procedures; (2) development of skills in synthesis of data and problem-solving; and (3) orientation to the clinical setting and integration into a professional team. Objectives unique to surgery were attained in Core Surgical Clerkship (CSC). During CSC the students were assigned to specialty areas or to senior faculty members with more broadly defined objectives: (1) recognition of surgically treated disease; (2) understanding metabolic and physiologic effects of trauma; (3) correlation of disordered physiology and surgical pathology; (4) development of appropriate affective responses to urgent problems; (5) recognition of the effects of surgery on psychological, economic, and social aspects of patients and family; and (6) acquisition of common psychomotor techniques. Definition of objectives resulted in better teaching methods and better evaluation of student performance. Formal involvement of residents in undergraduate education and initial exposure of students to surgery created a more favorable education environment.

From the Department of Surgery, Case Western Reserve University and University Hospitals of Cleveland

IN RECENT YEARS, as the practice of medicine has increased in complexity,[1, 3] clinical disciplines first responded by altering and expanding graduate residency training through specialization. These alterations in graduate education occurred more rapidly and independently than changes in undergraduate education. There was discontinuity between undergraduate and graduate education, and goals for undergraduate medical education became indistinct.[4, 7, 14] Although performance could be defined on completion of a specific surgical residency, no general agreement existed about the goals of undergraduate surgical education.[6]

We describe objectives and methods for undergraduate core surgical education stressing the use of a surgical service for teaching clinical skills common to all physicians. This report, describing goals and attitudes of students and faculty, cannot be presented

Presented at the Thirty-fifth Annual Meeting of the Society of University Surgeons, St. Louis, Mo., Feb. 14-16, 1974.

*Present address: Head, Research in Health Education, University of Connecticut Health Center, Hartford, Conn.

as scientific data. We emphasize the need for a clear definition of objectives to integrate undergraduate and graduate surgical programs, provide data for evolution of performance, appraise educational methods, and ensure accuracy of faculty communication.

EVOLUTION OF CHANGE

Changes in undergraduate surgical education span a period of over twenty years beginning with innovative recommendations made by the Committee of Medical Education (CME) in 1960. These included teaching by subject committee and introduction of three phases: Phase 1, Normal Biology of Man; Phase 2, Pathologic Physiology and Principles of Medicine; Phase 3, Clinical Medicine and Patient Care. A progress report for the period of 1946 to 1962 has been presented by Ham.[8] The Division of Research in Medical Education (DORIME) was formed in 1958 to guide curricular changes in coordination with the faculty.

The Committee on Clinical Teaching, chaired by Dr. W. D. Holden in 1964, reported to CME on the status of undergraduate education. Based on these recommendations, CME then proposed a series of changes in the undergraduate curriculum affecting the third and fourth years. Important changes were completion of basic clinical experience by the end of the third year and the proposed use of surgical patients and faculty for introductory clerkship. In addition, the fourth year was to be an optional program with electives in advanced clinical science and increased patient responsibility.

In 1967, the Phase 3 Committee, chaired by Dr. John Murphy of the Department of Medicine and composed of clerkship directors in the various clinical disciplines described specific educational goals for introductory and core experiences. Goals were developed with the assistance of Dr. Joseph Sheehan of DORIME, Mager's publications,[12, 13] and the *Taxonomy of Education Objectives/Handbooks I and II*.[2, 11]

Objectives were divided within three domains: (1) the *cognitive domain,* performances varying from simple recall to highly original ways of synthesizing new material; (2) the *affective domain,* performances emphasizing feelings—emotions varying from simple interest in and attention to phenomena to complex but internally consistent qualities of character and conscience; (3) *psychomotor domain,* performances emphasizing skills requiring neuromuscular coordination.

In 1968, the proposal for the third year of clinical experience was accepted by the general faculty and objectives were applied to existing clerkships. The revised program, including introductory clerkships in surgery, began in 1970. To integrate further undergraduate and graduate education, a Committee on Surgical Education became a function of the Department of Surgery; its first charge has been to develop goals of basic surgical education for the first two graduate years.

INTRODUCTORY CLERKSHIP

Introductory Clerkship (IC) is a period of five weeks at the beginning of the third year. Its purpose is to develop skills needed by all physicians and prepare the student for core clerkships. Students initially assigned to medicine, surgery, or pediatrics perform their first Core Clerkship on that service. The introductory period seeks to advance skills partially learned in Phases 1 and 2, Clinical Science. Common objectives for introductory clerkship were more readily formulated than core objectives. These goals, and student activities directed toward their achievement, are:

1. To advance his skills and knowledge of collecting medically related information through interview or medical history, physical examination, medical records, and laboratory procedures to the extent that he can completely and efficiently work up patients.
   a. The student examines two preoperative patients weekly.
   b. Abnormal physical findings or disordered physiology is observed at operation.
   c. Work-ups by students are presented at daily conferences of their peers and surgical fellows.

d. After appraisal by faculty, student work-ups are expected to be of such quality that they become part of the hospital record.

2. To organize and synthesize medical information and begin to apply this information in a problem-solving manner in the case method with the goal of resolving the patient's medical problem.
   a. The student recognizes hypovolemia, shock due to other causes, hypoxemia, sepsis, and major organ failure.
   b. Using a problem-oriented approach, the student lists anatomic and physiologic derangements and formulates a plan of therapy.
3. To become sufficiently familiar with the hospital in order to be able to function as a member of the "professional team." This includes activities or functions of the hospital as well as organization of the hospital.
   a. Students are initially assigned geographically, not to services; they continue core clerkship in the same area, but on a specific service.

Objectives for history and physical examination are complex and performances not easily classified. Interviewing patients requires skills in both cognitive and affective domains; physical examination also involves psychomotor skills as does performance of basic laboratory analyses (blood counts and urinalyses). For the purpose of evaluation, introductory objectives have been further subdivided (Table I). These same performances are evaluated at the end of introductory clerkship and on all subsequent core clerkships.

Table I. *Introductory performance objectives*

Performance	*Type of objective*
Initial data collection (history, physical, laboratory)	Cognitive, affective, psychomotor
Follow-up data collection	Affective, cognitive, psychomotor (student must take the initiative in obtaining follow-up data)
Organization of data	Cognitive
Synthesis/problem-solving	Cognitive
Content/application of basic science knowledge	Cognitive
Participation in patient care	Affective, cognitive, psychomotor
Relationships with patients, staff and peers	Affective

CORE SURGICAL CLERKSHIP

The core surgical clerkship is a two-month period. Goals of core clerkship have been classified for increasingly complex performance. The goals and objectives of core clerkship are:

Cognitive goals

1. *The student becomes familiar with diseases amenable to surgical correction or attenuation.* He is able to recognize surgical diseases and methods of diagnosis, and techniques or procedures employed in their treatment. He differentiates common surgical and non-surgical diseases with the use of history and physical findings, and is able to select appropriate laboratory and x-ray studies.
2. *The student comprehends the effect of trauma, shock, sepsis, and surgical intervention.* He is able to enumerate the common disorders of metabolism and physiology associated with trauma. He is able to contrast similar effects in varying types of injury. Using these principles, he is able to participate in resuscitation, correct hypovolemia, and maintain cardiopulmonary function.
3. *The student correlates disordered physiology observed preoperatively and pre- and postoperative physical findings with the pathology seen at operation.* He is able to determine the anatomic and physiologic consequences of surgical intervention along with the range of therapeutic choices for specific cases he has studied. The ability to extrapolate for his own cases is the most complex attainment expected.

Affective goals

4. *The student performs as a member of a surgical team in an environment which requires prompt decisions and*

Table II. *Content of undergraduate seminars**

Subject	*Content*	*No. of hours*
Surgical biology	Body compartments	1
	Fluid balance	1
	Wound healing, collagen dynamics	1
	Bone growth, repair	1
	Immunology, neoplasms, and chemotherapy	1
	Transplantation	1
	Bleeding and clotting	1
	Energy metabolism; shock	1
	Oxygen transport	1
	Surgical infections	1
	Lipid dynamics	1
	Total	11
Approach to surgical problems	Life support systems	1
	Triage, multiple trauma	1
	Responses to trauma and surgery	2
	ENT emergencies	1
	Ophthalmologic emergencies	1
	"Minor" injuries	1
	Total	7
Common entities	The acute abdomen	1
	Gastrointestinal bleeding	1
	Portal hypertension	1
	Hematologic disorders	1
	Shock: clinical correlates	1
	Thermal injuries	2
	Total	7
Disease of organ systems	Endocrines	3
	Breast	1
	Esophagus and stomach	1
	Small bowel	1
	Biliary system	2
	Appendicitis	1
	Colon/rectum	1
	Hernias	1
	Peripheral vascular disease	2
	Heart, congenital and acquired	2
	Lungs	1
	Total	16

*Total of 41 hours obtained at weekday seminars with faculty during a two-month period.

responses. He is able to respond to rapid adjustment demanded by surgical illnesses. He is expected to accept responsibility for night and emergeny work but not to develop completely the life-style demanded of the surgical milieu.

5. *The student understands the emotional effects of surgical intervention and comprehends the effects of surgery on the social and economic status of the patient and his family.* He behaves in a consistent and stable manner when faced with the need for surgical intervention. He values the dignity of the patient and allays the fears of the patient and family; at the same time, he is able to understand and accept the risks of surgical intervention.

Psychomotor goals

6. *The student acquires common manual techniques and procedures used for diagnosis and therapy.* The student regards this as an important goal; however, the surgical faculty emphasizes that psychomotor skills are not critical at the core level. These skills best develop under careful supervision: (1) aseptic technique and wound dressing; (2) suture of simple laceration under local anesthesia; (3) poise in the operating room and the ability to function as a second assistant; (4) intestinal intubation, thoracentesis, and paracentesis; (5) endotracheal intubation; (8) use of splints and other methods of fracture immobilization.

The objectives are outlined on beginning the clerkship. Students become familiar with the contents of a standard textbook of surgery. Familiarity on a recognition level is their objective. Distinctions between recognition of disease entities, determining implications, predicting consequences, and selecting surgical intervention are explained. It is made clear at the onset that in two months they will not see every surgical illness.

The importance of affective objectives is explained; the relationship between affective and cognitive achievement is illustrated. The student is not to abruptly change his values to those of the more advanced in surgery or to become a house officer. Some attempt this at the expense of achieving cognitive objectives.

The students are then assigned for one

month with rotations through general surgery, emergency room, and anesthesia. Objectives and achievements are again discussed. In the second month, the student selects two surgical services as electives.

The operating room experience is valuable provided its problems are recognized and controlled. Appropriate participation implies that the student is (1) able to see and feel pathologic lesions; (2) able to ask questions of the attending surgeon; (3) prepared with basic knowledge of anatomy and pathology; (4) not expected to hold retractors for extended periods.

All students are excused from other duties to participate daily in a one-hour seminar with a senior faculty member. To prepare for these discusions, students are given a syllabus outlining content (Table II). Specialty conferences for students are also held on a weekly basis or during their rotations (Table III). The faculty emphasizes active learning, independence, critical thinking, and understanding the relationships between scientific conclusions and clinical practice.[5, 10] Basic science is related to the approach to the surgical patient. Entities caused by a variety of diseases, such as gastrointestinal bleeding, are discussed as units. Finally, organ systems are discussed by faculty from various specialties.

Each student is assigned to a faculty preceptor, but is responsible for establishing the depth and this relationship. Experience with preceptors confirms the observation of Sanazaro and King[15] that there are marked differences in educational philosophy among faculty. These can limit the benefit of this experience unless preceptors are selected who have actively participated in formulating objectives.

Table III. *Content of specialty conferences**

Specialty	*Subject*	*No. of hours*
Neurosurgery	Craniocerebral trauma Pressure cone phenomena CNS neoplasms Neural pathways Pain ablative procedure Hydrocephalus: mechanisms and therapy	8
Pediatric Surgery	Neonatal physiology Infant and child as surgical patient Fluid balance Neoplasms in childhood/hemangiomata Intersex problems Congenital malformations: GI tract, abdominal wall, and cloacal area Hernias in childhood	8
Urology	Urinary retention Diagnosis and surgical methods Tumors, bladder and kidney Prostatic disease Stone formation and treatment Urinary diversion	8
Orthopedics	Common fractures Arthritis: role of surgery Scoliosis Congenital malformations	6
Plastic Surgery	Head and neck tumors Maxillofacial trauma Cleft lip and palate Hand	4
	Total:	34

*Saturday and late afternoon conferences.

TEACHING FELLOWS

Surgical residents from the second, third, and fourth postgraduate years were selected as teaching fellows responsible for assisting the students in attaining introductory objectives. The teaching residents conducted rounds with students, selected patients for work-up, held daily conferences to present those work-ups, and supervised the numbers and kinds of patients that students were to examine.

The residents were enthusiastic about this assignment and reported that the advantages important to their own development were (1) improved teaching abilities; (2) a different quality of contact with senior faculty; (3) exposure to basic teaching techniques; and (4) an opportunity for a comprehensive basic science and clinical review.

The residents regarded the independence and responsibility they were permitted in planning students' activities as an important asset of the program. The formal recognition of the teaching role of residents in undergraduate medical education has been long overdue.[16] These residents influenced the other house staff in helping meet the goals required for students because of their understanding of student objectives. This created a more favorable environment for undergraduate education.

EVALUATION

The surgical faculty evaluated the subsequent performance of students receiving their introductory clinical experience on surgery at University Hospitals. The records of 25 students of the classes of 1972, 1973, and 1974 were examined to determine: (1) achievement of skills common to all physicians evaluated by the faculty in other disciplines; (2) surgical and other discipline evaluation of over-all performance by comparison; and (3) possible bias or influence toward surgery and a surgical career choice.

Although the grading system here does not permit class ranking of students who perform satisfactory work, the evaluation procedure used for all clerkships is uniform. Students are rated Excellent, Good, Satisfactory, Poor, and Unsatisfactory for each of the introductory performances (Table I). All students with introductory experiences on surgery performed satisfactorily on subsequent clerkships in the other disciplines. Detailed narrative descriptions of attitudes and recommendations for improvement are also made. Each student is permitted to read evaluations of his performance.

Honors performance on core clerkships is based on ratings of Excellent for introductory skills, basic science knowledge, and achievement of objectives unique to each clerkship. Of three students who received Honors by surgical faculty for introductory and core experience, two were subsequently rated Honors on other core clerkships.

Four of 25 students receiving introductory clerkships over three years applied for straight surgical internships. An increasing proportion of the whole class applied for surgical training in recent years; however, no undue influence has been created by the surgical introductory experience. The core and option experiences appear more important in influencing career choice than introductory exposure.

On completing core clerkship, student performance is evaluated by both senior faculty and responsible residents. No formal examinations are given; cognitive achievement is assayed by performance in seminars (Table II), which approximate the content of the clerkship. Attitudinal and psychomotor performances are often more effectively reported by house officers than by attending faculty. The written appraisals of six to ten individuals comprise the final measure of each student's performance.

Students are asked to evaluate their own achievements and to suggest revisions of the clerkship in two meetings with the clerkship directors, once during and once at the end of the clerkship. The feedback from these sessions is used to modify the clerkship; the faculty functions in this capacity not only as teacher but as manager of the learning system.[17] An important observation made by students has been that identical clinical exposure cannot be provided since uniform rotations make assignments too brief. With the exception of the emergency service and anesthesia, two-week rotations are now minimum clinical assignments.

DISCUSSION

This experience demonstrates that surgical patients provide an excellent base for teaching skills needed by all physicians. Especially effective education results when the pathology is exposed at operation and disordered physiology understood. Diagnoses become obvious; therapeutic success or failure is dramatically demonstrated. As shown, introductory exposure on a surgical service does not influence career choice, but the result of the total program, including core and option experience, is reflected in an increase in the proportion of the class applying for straight surgical internships: nine percent of the class in 1964 increasing progressively to 18 percent in 1974. Negative attitudes expressed by students about surgeons as physicians are now notably absent. The fact that many students now have their first major clinical experience on a surgical service probably relates to more positive student attitudes.

Developing objectives for undergraduate

surgical education is the first step toward more effective planning of a basic surgical education. It is obvious that simply listing objectives does not ensure their achievement; the active participation of the faculty in formulating objectives is critical. Surgical education is continually evolving; future changes in its structure should be made by surgical faculties which are self-critical, aware of changing requirements of medical education, and familiar with educational techniques.

Responsible educators may question the value of classifying objectives. Arbitrary division may oversimplify human performance. Critics state that it is not possible to think or perform complex psychomotor tasks in the absence of knowledge or positive attitudes toward those tasks, or to think without emotion. Valid points of disagreement exist, especially in defining affective objectives. The immeasurable influence of past experience makes it impossible to predict specific behavior resulting from a particular attitude. Thus, differing individual attitudes result in similar behavior while like attitudes may produce variable responses. In spite of these limitations, education must begin with a clear idea of desired performance when the experience is completed and surgery is not an exception. The surgical faculty recognized that achievement of affective objectives was critical in surgical performance. In adopting affective objectives, the faculty assumed responsibility for guiding emotional responses and attitudes.

With attainment of affective objectives, attention can be directed toward developing comprehensive congnitive and psychomotor goals for surgeons, especially in their early education. This must be done to ensure a broad education in basic surgery before specialty residency training. Recently, the interface between medical school and the graduate years has become blurred.[9] Relationships between the last two years of undergraduate and the first two years of graduate surgical education have yet to be integrated. In effect, granting an M.D. degree after three years, incorporating internship into residency programs, and the fluidity of an optional fourth year contribute to a difficult period in the education of young surgeons. At the present time, planning of this entire period must be individualized. To appraise the wisdom of changes in this early and critical period, surgical educators must first agree upon goals for core surgical education and basic graduate education.

The authors wish to thank Miss Sharon Lillevig for assistance in editing and preparation of the manuscript.

REFERENCES

1. Austen, W. G., and Kinney, T. D.: The content of undergraduate medical education: In the future of medical education, Durham, N. C., 1973, Duke University Press, pp. 71-86.
2. Bloom, B. S., editor: Handbook I: Cognitive domain, *in* Taxonomy of educational objectives: The classification of educational goals (series), New York, 1956, David McKay, Inc.
3. Child, C. G., III, and Wedgewood, R. J.: *In* O. Cope, editor: Our primary purpose in man, mind and medicine, Philadelphia, 1968, J. B. Lippincott Co., pp. 120-122.
4. Comroe, J. H., Jr.: Objectives of medical education, J. Med. Educ. **37:** 17, 1962.
5. Coppola, E. D., and Gonnella, J. S.: A nondirective approach to clinical instruction in medical school, J. A. M. A. **205:** 487, 1968.
6. Egdahl, R. H.: A survey of some attitudes and practices in surgical education, J. Med. Educ. **44:** 1024, 1969.
7. Elrick, H.: The clinical education of the medical student, J. Med. Educ. **42:** 453, 1967.
8. Ham, T. H.: Medical education at Western Reserve University, N. Engl. J. Med. **267:** 868, 916, 1962.
9. Holden, W. D.: The interface between undergraduate and graduate medical education, Surgery **70:** 498, 1971.
10. King, T. C., Maxwell, J. G., Richard, R. C., Stevens, L. E., and Reemtsma, K.: Research in undergraduate surgical education: Innovation and evaluation, J. Med. Educ. **43:** 373, 1968.
11. Krathwohl, D. R., Bloom, B. S., and Massia, B. B., editors: Handbook II: Affective domain, *in* Taxonomy of educational objectives: The classification of educational goals (series), New York, 1956, David McKay, Inc.
12. Mager, R. F.: Preparing instructional objectives, Palo Alto, 1962, Fearon Publishers.
13. Mager, R. F.: Goal analysis, Belmont, Calif., 1972, Fearon Publishers.

14. Reichman, F., Browning, F. E., and Hinshaw, J. R.: Observation of undergraduate teaching in action, J. Med. Educ. **39:** 147, 1964.
15. Sanazaro, P. J., and King, T. C.: An exploratory study of undergraduate programs in surgery, J. Med. Educ. **42:** 289, 1967.
16. Sedlacek, W. E.: Attitudes of residents toward their complex role in medical education, J. Med. Educ. **43:** 344, 1968.
17. Stritter, F. T., and Bowles, L. T.: The teacher as manger: A strategy for medical education, J. Med. Educ. **47:** 93, 1972.

DISCUSSION

Dr. Erle E. Peacock, Jr. (Tucson, Ariz.). From the vantage point of one getting ready to leave the Test Committee of the National Board of Medical Examiners for the Surgery Test Committee, I would like to make a few highly prejudiced comments involving what I believe to be a mistake in utilizing the National Boards in the study of the first paper presented. There are three points.

The first point is that a third control which could have been used was omitted, and that is the control of people who had had no clerkship in surgery. There are considerable data available on this now, because many students are taking the National Board in the spring of the junior year, before they have had any surgery, or who have elective courses in their medical schools and have taken no surgery. Although these data have not been subjected to the same thoughtful and critical analysis to which Dr. Levitsky and his group submitted their data, my general impression from looking at the raw data is that there is less than five points' difference in the scores on the National Boards, strongly suggesting that a third control would have fit in beautifully with the other two experimental controls.

The second point is that I do not share the authors' confidence that the National Board test in surgery measures problem-solving ability, particularly in the almost anti-intellectual frame into which many educators are pushing the importance of problem-solving at this time.

As an example, University of Arizona scores were included here, and for the two years one would note that the first year the University of Arizona students scored seventy-seventh out of 79—two from the bottom—in their performance.

Although many other things happened in the second year of this study, such as adding more faculty, and so forth, two very important things happened. These students were told that, even though the University had a pass-fail system, the Department of Surgery intended to deal with scores and grades and that a passing grade of 70 on a National Board exam would be needed to complete the course. You will see in that second year, our scores ranked just above the norm—an enormous jump when this incentive was applied.

I recall once at North Carolina that Dick Peters and I were literally infuriated when nine students who had performed beautifully under ward clerkships failed the National Boards. We found out that not one of the nine owned a textbook of surgery. They were given ten days to buy a textbook and to take a repeat examination of a previous National Board exam. Every one of the nine scored in the eighth and ninth percentile ten days later, strongly suggesting that what the National Board of Medical Examiners' exam really measures, or only correlates with, is one's association with a standard textbook of surgery.

The third point is that the National Board of Medical Examiners' examination is a very difficult examination. It is so difficult that in many years only half of the questions are answered correctly. When you realize that the elevator operator can score 20 percent correctly by simply marking *(a)* all the way down, and that the junior AOA student from a land-grant college in the East will score no better than 50 percent, you recognize then that there are only 30 percent of those questions in there which measure the entire spectrum of premedical and medical education.

To select one tiny little thing, like the difference in a clerkship, and try on the basis of only 30 percent of those questions to make a selective difference, I believe, was not warranted.

Dr. Frank Gordon Moody (Salt Lake City, Utah).

Dr. Levitsky has certainly confirmed an impression we have had in Salt Lake, because we have used the community hospitals rather extensively in our educational programs, and one might challenge his criteria and methods for testing, but certainly our impressions would go along with what he has shown us here today.

It sounds a little bit pre-Flexnerian that you can just send the students out to the community hospital where fellows are involved in a very active practice and come out with an educational experience that they think is positive. I think one of the variables here that has not been discussed is the type of individuals who are practicing in these community hospitals. I would conclude that there probably is an educational director at these hospitals, that he has a group of individuals who are interested in at least having the students around in order to make it a positive educational and motivational experience.

Dr. John Ervin Jesseph (Indianapolis, Ind.). We have had a long experience at Indiana with the farm system; anticipating, for the same historical reasons, some years ago the things that people have commented on this morning. Our farm system began with the first two years of school, and now that we have the largest medical school in the country in terms of enrollment, our 1974 class will be 315 entering freshmen.

We have to use hospitals in our center and one large private hospital in the city. The same question that Dr. Levitsky posed to us—is there a bias in the educational experience—has come to us from a different source. We have not answered it as a matter of introspection, but, rather, it has come to us through the grumbly student who flunks something. He then has the impression that he has been disfavored by being sent to one of the hospitals other than in the center.

We have come to the same conclusion,. that it does not really matter. We have simply proved to ourselves again that a good student will do well pretty near any place, and a poor student will be a poor student.

Generalities are not safe. Each of us functions in a system, and the set of hospitals is quite different from each of the others. Perhaps Dr. DePalma gives us one clue, at least, as to how we might regulate this whole business, and that is that a clearly stated, succinct, and workable set of objectives, agreed to by our faculty and having at least spiritual agreement among all of the faculty, is important to learn certain basic things. It matters little whether there is an optional clerkship, whether the clerkship is two months or three in length. We have to agree about what we want the students to learn and see to it that they have the opportunity.

Dr. Lucian L. Leape (Boston, Mass.). I was also a bit depressed to have reaffirmed something that many of us observe, that is, that the teachers really often do not have much influence over what the students learn. Nonetheless, we can take a great step forward in surgical education if we take the game-playing out of it and let the student know the basis upon which he is being judged.

Certainly, in grading sessions I have sat in on, the effective performance is usually based on whether the student shows a lot of interest and is around, rather than his particular acquisition of particular attitudes and certain skills, and therefore we all respond to the interested student.

I would like to ask Dr. Levitsky if he has, in effect, done that. Do your sudents at the various places receive an indication of what is expected of them, and, in effect, are you clearly stating to both groups what the objectives of your courses are? And, I think, if you do do that, they will achieve them regardless of the setting.

Dr. James C. Thompson (Galveston, Texas). We must be careful about extrapolating Dr. Levitsky's data, as he suggested, to the formation of new medical schools. What he is measuring is the teaching ability of faculties that are selected in a community that has had a long-standing and relatively good history of medical education by a full-time faculty, well established in a medical school. Presumably the faculty exerted careful selection of those hospitals that their students were going to be sent to.

I think I understood Dr. Levitsky to say that one of the problems was whether it was legitimate for new medical schools to start out with community hospital arrangements. That is a vastly different problem, which is starting in a small, semirural town in Middle America a brand new medical school which consists of a small basic science building and five community hospitals which are widely scattered. Without this history, without this entire past experience in teaching, I think it would be vastly different, and I do not think that the data are extrapolatable.

Dr. John A. Waldhausen (Hershey, Pa.). Did these students who had a clerkship in surgery, either at a community or a university hospital, have comparable clerkships in other fields? In other words, were the ones at a community hospital always at a community hospital for medicine, pediatrics, etc., or did they have at times a university exposure? I would think that if you had a clerkship in medicine at the university, and then went to the community hospital for your surgical experience, there would be some carry-over of some disciplines that the university hospital gave you.

Dr. Jeremiah George Turcotte (Ann Arbor, Mich.). At Michigan the junior year consists of four major clerkships. All the students do take the National Board; it is required for passing into the next year; so they are well motivated. They used to take it in the spring, and it was found that there was a significantly lower grade on the National Board in that discipline which the students had not yet had the opportunity to take in the form of a clerkship. In other words, if surgery was in the spring, they were taking their National Board prior to taking the surgery clerkship, whereas three quarters of the class would have had their surgery clerkship.

The difference is statistically significant, and has resulted in a change in our policy, that they will all take the National Boards now in the fall, so that they have all had the opportunity to take clerkships in all major areas.

Dr. Lawrence W. Way (San Francisco, Calif.). One of the inevitable consequences of embarking upon the business of writing explicit objectives is almost always the construction of a highly structured clerkship. At times, it may eventually turn out to be a trap, because inevitably more and more conferences are generated to sort of cover the area of these highly complex objectives, and the student's learning of the material becomes divorced from the clinical setting.

I would like to ask if there is any objective measurements of the value of the great increase in structure and the listing of these objectives, as far as student learning is concerned.

Dr. Sidney Levitsky (closing). When we initiated this study and looked at the first results, we were concerned that we might become pariahs or "traitors to our class" in that we presumably had data that were contrary to our previous visceral reactions.

In reply to Dr. Peacock, the National Board examination measures cognitive knowledge but does not measure surgical performance at the bedside. It has been shown by our group at the University of Illinois as far as the comprehensive examinations are concerned that motivation is a very strong factor in determining how the student will perform. In addition, many of these examinations are measuring minimal competence. They are not measuring the entire spectrum of scholarship that we are trying to evaluate. So I think we have a problem in that the inadequacy of the examination makes hard, solid conclusions difficult to accept.

Initially when the students were spread throughout the different community hospitals, there was a mad scramble to get to the university hospitals. They knew, if they wanted to get a surgical internship in a high-quality place, the professor of surgery had to know them. Perhaps this study may alleviate some of these students' fears.

In reply to Dr. Moody, the enthusiasm expressed by the part-time faculty at the community hospitals has been and remains excellent. This was the first time they had had students, and they were very excited and receptive. Many times there were more one-on-one encounters than might have occurred at the university hospital. In addition, it has been shown by other investigators that the much greater part of the student teaching is not done by the faculty, but really is done by the house staff, and perhaps this factor might have been an equalizer.

We agree with Dr. Jesseph that in our survey the good student does well any place; the poor student does poorly in whatever environment you put him.

One of the reasons why we found some of the data from other institutions could not be included in our study was that there was such a great variation in the organization of different medical schools as to the number of full-time faculty in some of the community hospitals—some had none, some had a few—and the entire distribution was quite variable. So we arbitrarily picked certain schools that fitted our criteria and used those in the study.

Dr. Leape, as far as objectives are concerned, when these initial students were being trained, they were not given objectives. At the present time, with our new curriculum, they are given a list of objectives.

Dr. Waldhausen, some of the students did take medicine and pediatrics at the community hospital, as well as surgery. Some received all of their training at the university hospital except for surgery. This distribution was quite variable, and we have no hard data numbers to support one group or the other. But the commonality of experience between different fields is a real one. It has been shown, in the past by Dr. King, that a student will perform differently on the same surgical exam whether that examination is given in September, when all the students are starting with zero knowledge, as opposed to the student starting on a surgical clerkship in May or June, when he has had other clerkships.

Dr. Ralph G. DePalma (closing). In answer to the question about the explicit objectives, the existence of explicit objectives does not imply a highly structured, highly rigid program. The objectives are given to the student at the beginning of the clerkship. They are reviewed with the student in the middle of the clerkship, and they are again reviewed at the end of the clerkship.

Now, there is an inherent danger in formulating behavioral objectives that educators have recently recognized. You can see that it would be easy to produce a stereotypic type of individual. We must allow for individuality and recognize that similar behavior may result from widely varying attitudes, or the reverse.

So I would like to emphasize that the inclusion of these congnitive objectives in our clerkship involves about 43 hours of senior faculty time per month. However, the experience for the student, including the cognitive and affective objectives, can be quite different for individual students.

Microcrystalline collagen as a topical hemostatic agent for vascular surgery

William M. Abbott, M.D., *and* **W. Gerald Austen, M.D.,** *Boston, Mass.*

Microcrystalline collagen (MCC) is a recently developed material that possesses promise as a topical hemostatic agent. The potential for using MCC in vascular surgery was studied in canine iliac artery anastomoses, and four basic requirements were evaluated: hemostatic effectiveness; hemodynamic effects; gross anatomic change; and effects on vessel wall structure. The results with MCC were compared to gauze pressure alone (control) and treatment with oxidized cellulose (OXY). All four requirements were satisfied by MCC. MCC was subjectively superior in controlling suture-line hemorrhage and 50 percent more effective as judged by the incidence for additional sutures to accomplish hemostasis. There were no adverse hemodynamic effects after four weeks or four months. Angiography showed satisfactory intraluminal anatomy after four months in all instances and was similar to controls in frequency and degree of angiographic abnormalities. Histologic appearance was also similar to controls. Stress-strain curves, although showing some loss of distensibility as compared to normal, were identical to dissected but untreated vessels. OXY seemed less satisfactory in meeting these requirements. On the basis of these studies it seems logical to use MCC in vascular surgery when a topical hemostatic agent is needed.

From the Department of Surgery, Massachusetts General Hospital, and Harvard Medical School, Boston, Mass.

THE AVAILABILITY of a safe, effective topical hemostatic agent would be extremely helpful in vascular surgery to control hemorrhage from arterial suture lines as well as from dissected surrounding tissues. Such bleeding may be particularly vexing because of the local and systemic use of heparin. In small diseased vessels additional sutures used to control anastomotic bleeding may compromise the lumen as well as worsen the bleeding because of tearing of tenuous tissue structures. Thus, topical hemostatic agents may often be tried before sutures are used.

Presented at the Thirty-fifth Annual Meeting of the Society of University Surgeons St. Louis, Mo., Feb. 14-16, 1974.

The most popular topical agents are oxidized cellulose cloth and gelatin sponge. Recently a new topical hemostatic agent, microcrystalline collagen, has become available for investigation. This material is a water-insoluble hydrochloric acid salt of bovine hide collagen considered to be in the form of microcrystals of submicron size.[3, 5, 6] The product is a fluffy, off-white flourlike powder, but it can also be rendered into a clothlike web. Several studies have indicated that this is an effective topical hemostatic agent in controlling hemorrhage from wounds in solid organs.[7, 8, 13] The purpose of this study was to investigate its potential for use in vascular surgery to aid in hemostasis around arterial anastomoses.

METHODS

Twenty-three mongrel dogs weighing between 20 and 25 kilograms were used in the study. The abdominal aorta and common iliac vessels were bilaterally exposed. The anastomotic site selected was the common iliac vessel because the size of this vessel (5 to 6 mm.O.D.) was large enough to facilitate reproducible anastomoses, but small enough to be susceptible to technical and other problems such as postoperative scarring. The common iliac vessel was transected and an end-to-end anastomosis carried out with the use of a running No. 6-0 non-absorbable suture. The dogs were then divided into two groups. In 12 dogs, anastomotic bleeding on the right was controlled by simple gauze pressure and subsequent additional sutures as required. On the left side, the anastomoses were immediately packed with microcrystalline collagen* (MCC) plus gentle pressure with gauze. A hemostatic protocol was followed for all anastomoses. After three minutes, the anastomosis was inspected and if hemostasis had not been accomplished, the hemostatic maneuver was repeated. If after three attempts hemostasis was still incomplete, additional sutures were used to arrest the suture-line bleeding. Following hemostasis, whether or not sutures were required, anastomoses on the left again had MCC packed around them. On the right, they were not treated further and served as controls.

In 11 additional dogs, the left iliac anastomosis was treated with MCC as just described. On the right side, the anastomoses were treated with oxidized cellulose cloth (OXY), also according to the hemostatic protocol. These anastomoses were also left with the OXY wrapped around them whether or not sutures were required, and, therefore, served as a "positive" control with a currently used hemostatic agent. Following the procedure all animals were restudied at four weeks and four months.

In the testing of any topical hemostatic agent it seems necessary to satisfy four basic requirements: (1) It must be effective as a hemostatic agent. (2) There must be no adverse hemodynamic effects at the anastomosis. (3) There must be no adverse gross anatomic effects. (4) There must be no adverse effects on vessel wall structure.

Hemostatic effectiveness. All anastomoses were constructed by one investigator in such a way as to allow some anastomotic hemorrhage. Each anastomosis was judged as to the amount of time required to accomplish hemostasis by the three methods utilized. In addition, the frequency which additional sutures were needed to control the bleeding, and the number of sutures required were recorded.

Adverse hemodynamic effects. Arterial flow was measured directly in the distal iliac arteries by square wave electromagnetic flow monitoring equipment (Statham SP-2202). Pressure gradients were searched for by measurement of proximal arterial pressure in the aorta and distal pressure in the profunda femoris artery. All pressures were monitored by Hewlett-Packard 267AD pressure transducers. Pressure and flow data were simultaneously recorded on a multiple-channel recorder (Sanborn 7700, Hewlett-Packard) prior to and after the iliac vascular anastomoses. Pressures and flows were again recorded at the time of definitive study either after four weeks or four months.

Adverse gross anatomic effects. The presence of local scarring, infection, and adhesions to surrounding tissues was estimated at the time of definitive study. Aortoiliac angiograms were performed in all animals at four weeks and after four months in those animals which had not been killed earlier. Angiograms were accomplished by transbrachial retrograde catheterization of the abdominal aorta. Identical technique was used for serial angiograms to minimize variations caused by radiologic projections. Angiograms were independently analyzed; any deviation from a completely normal appearance was recorded as an abnormality. Degree of abnormality was estimated as percent narrowing using calipers to compare the anastomoses with the diameters of the proximal and distal vessels.

*Kindly provided by Dr. John H. Tenery, Avicon, Inc., Ft. Worth, Texas.

Adverse effects on structure. At the time of sacrifice, the anastomoses and surrounding proximal and distal vessel were removed for histologic study by conventional techniques. Structural properties of the vessels were also studied by analyzing stress-strain curves with the use of a method developed in this laboratory for other experiments.[9] Early in the studies it was found that stress-strain data generated from the iliac arteries used for the anastomoses was unreliable because of varying exposure to the hemostatic agents. For the remaining studies, the effects of operative dissection and the presence of either MCC or OXY around dissected arteries and veins was studied at four weeks and four months in carotid arteries and external jugular veins without anastomoses.

Stress-strain analysis was conducted by placing small segments of test vessel into a hydraulic chamber with pressure or stress then generated by a constant volume infusion. The pressure-volume response curves derived were then transcribed to tension versus strain curves where strain was measured geometrically as two-dimensional elongation. The curves were statistically analyzed by paired, two tail T tests at tension levels of 5, 10, 40, 100, and 200 dynes/cm.$^2 \times 10^4$.

RESULTS

In the 23 dogs there were 46 anastomoses available for evaluation; 12 control or untreated, 23 treated with MCC, and 11 treated with OXY.

Hemostatic effectiveness. Hemostatic effectiveness was difficult to quantitate since it was not possible to consistently make anastomoses that would bleed similarly from experiment to experiment. Nevertheless, all anastomoses bled to some extent and all required additional maneuvers to control it. Subjectively, the MCC possessed a high degree of hemostatic effectiveness and was clearly superior to pressure or OXY in accomplishing hemostasis. MCC-treated anastomoses also seemed to be associated with less blood loss. The time required to accomplish hemostasis was highly variable and was obscured because of the frequent requirement for additional sutures. However, the trend was definitely in favor of a shortened time to hemostasis for MCC-treated anastomoses.

Table I. *Blood flow through iliac artery anastomoses: Mean flow (ml./min.)*

*Time of study**	*Untreated*	*MCC treated*	*OXY treated*
Preanastomosis	133 ± 17	141 ± 18	136 ± 16
Postanastomosis	142 ± 18	150 ± 21	142 ± 15
4 wk. later	127 ± 21	136 ± 14	133 ± 19
4 mo. later	129 ± 16	139 ± 17	101 ± 14

*No significant differences noted.

There were also differences in the frequency in which additional sutures were required to ultimately control bleeding. Of 12 control anastomoses, six required one or more additional sutures or a frequency of 50 percent. Of the 11 OXY-treated anastomoses, five, or 45 percent, required additional sutures. In contrast, only six of the 23 MCC-treated anastomoses required additional sutures. This is a frequency of only 26 percent, which is almost 50 percent less than control. Although not statistically significant, the frequency difference verifies the subjective conclusion that MCC was hemostatically effective for anastomotic bleeding and at least partially satisfied the requirement.

Hemodynamic effects. Pressure and flow determinations were carried out prior to and immediately after all anastomoses, and again at the time of death either at four weeks or four months. Mean flow was quite similar in all groups as seen in Table I. Preanastomosis flow averaged about 135 ml. per minute and proximal and distal pressures were equal at about 140/120 mm. Hg. No pressure gradient was found in any experiment. Immediately after the anastomosis, flow was slightly higher, probably as a result of post-occlusion hyperemia. At the time of death in both the four-week and four-month interval groups, the flows were quite close to preanastomosis flow in all instances except that of the four-month group treated with OXY. In this group, the mean flow seemed distinctly lower at 101 ml. per minute. Although not statistically significant, this slight diminution of mean flow suggests potential problems

Table II. *Frequency of angiographic abnormalities*

	Un-treated (%)	*MCC treated (%)*	*OXY treated (%)*
Abnormal at 4 wk.	22	16	22
Abnormal at 4 mo.	34	25	42
Percent increase	55	56	91
Percent progressive	50	40	67

Table III. *Degree of angiographic abnormalities*

	Un-treated (%)	*MCC treated (%)*	*OXY treated (%)*
Percent narrowing at 4 wk.	8	4	12
Percent narrowing at 4 mo.	14	13	25

in this group; this finding was supported by the angiographic studies to be described later. However, since there were no detectable hemodynamic differences in vessels treated with MCC compared with controls, MCC satisfied the hemodynamic requirement, at least for the period of four months.

Gross anatomic effects. At the time of definitive study, the degree of local scarring, the presence of infection, and the amount of adhesion formation to the anastomotic area was assessed. There was little difference between control and MCC-treated anastomoses at either time period. Although moderate adhesion formation and soft scar was present on both sides at four weeks, there was little further change at four months. There was only scant MCC remaining at four weeks, and after four months, no grossly identifiable MCC was found at the operative sites. There were no signs of infection at any anastomosis. Around the OXY-treated anastomoses there was rather dense scarring, often with obliteration of the local anatomic relationships. Adhesion formation, however, was similar to that of control and MCC-treated anastomoses.

The angiographic studies were quite revealing. Angiograms were available in nine of 12 control, 16 of 23 MCC-treated, and seven of 11 OXY-treated anastomoses. With the very critical interpretation employed, angiographic abnormalities were found with considerable frequency in all groups. Table II shows the frequency with which these occurred. At four weeks, 22 percent of the control anastomoses had abnormalities as compared to 16 percent of MCC-treated anastomoses. At four months, abnormalities were found in 34 percent of the controls and 25 percent of the MCC-treated anastomoses. These are each about a 55 percent increase in frequency from the early to the later time interval. At four months, 42 percent of OXY-treated anastomoses were abnormal as compared to 22 percent at four weeks, which represents a 91 percent increase. This suggests a greater progression of narrowing with time in those vessels treated with OXY. In the smaller number of angiograms performed serially there was progression of the abnormality in 50 percent of control anastomoses, 40 percent of MCC-treated anastomoses, and 67 percent of OXY-treated anastomoses. The latter result further suggests a more extremely progressive nature of the narrowing in OXY-treated vessels.

The degree of angiographic abnormality is illustrated in Table III. Although the frequency with which abnormalities occurred was fairly high, in the untreated and MCC-treated vessels the abnormality was only of a relatively minor degree, being at 14 percent and 13 percent narrowing, respectively, at four months. The OXY-treated anastomoses, however, had a greater degree of narrowing compared to controls at both time intervals with a 25 percent narrowing seen in four-month studies. Since there was little difference between untreated and MCC-treated vessels in the frequency or degree of angiographic abnormality as well as in local scarring and adhesions, the requirement regarding adverse anatomic effects does seem satisfied by MCC. That this requirement cannot be satisfied by OXY is also suggested from the data.

Structural effects. Careful analysis of

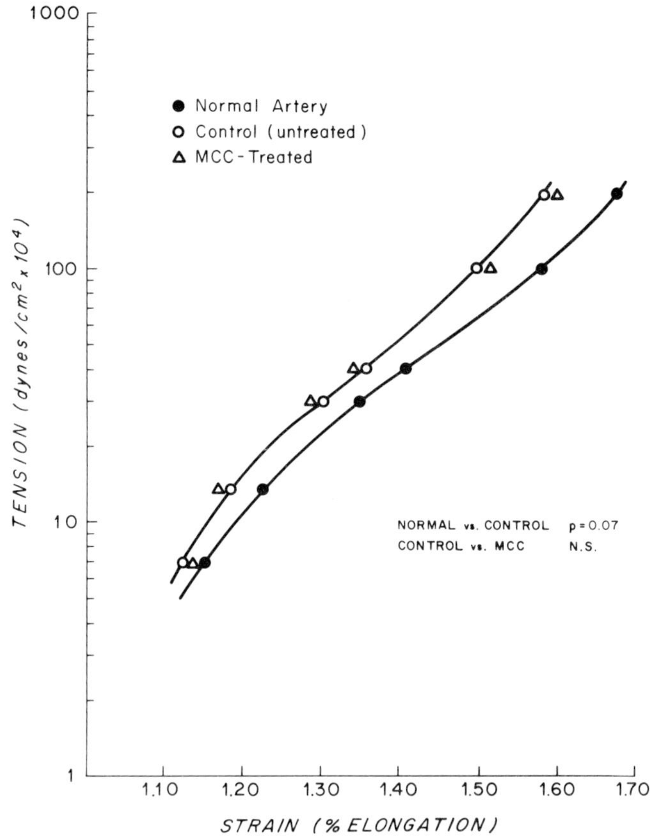

Fig. 1. Stress-strain relationships in arteries (four-month studies). Stress-strain curves for normal carotid artery compared to carotid artery dissected but untreated and dissected and treated with MCC. Compared to normal, stiffening or loss of distensibility is seen after dissection and MCC treatment but no difference between them is observed.

microscopic sections was carried out with the histologist not knowing how the vessel had been treated. No consistent differences between control and MCC-treated vessels were observed, except for the presence of residual MCC in those vessels so treated. In vessels sectioned after four months, however, even microscopically there was very little identifiable MCC remaining. Fibrosis and inflammatory reaction surrounded all vessels but did not distinguish between those not treated or treated with MCC. The changes which did occur were confined to the peri-adventitial region and there was no recognizable change in any vessel in the medial or intimal layers. Although difficult to quantitate, there was seemingly a slightly greater periadventitial inflammatory response and fibrous tissue reaction in those vessels treated with OXY, noted especially in the four-week group.

The results of the in vitro stress-strain analysis testing correlated with the histologic findings. Fig. 1 shows stress-strain curves for normal carotid arteries and arteries four months after dissection alone and dissection plus packing with MCC. There is a shift to the left of the latter two curves which denotes stiffening. Paired t tests on comparable data points reveal that although there is no statistical difference between normal artery and dissected artery that the trend toward stiffening of the vessel wall is probably real ($P = 0.07$). Comparison of dissected with MCC-treated vessels revealed no statistical difference. The data for OXY-treated arteries (not shown) was similar.

Fig. 2 shows stress-strain curves for normal,

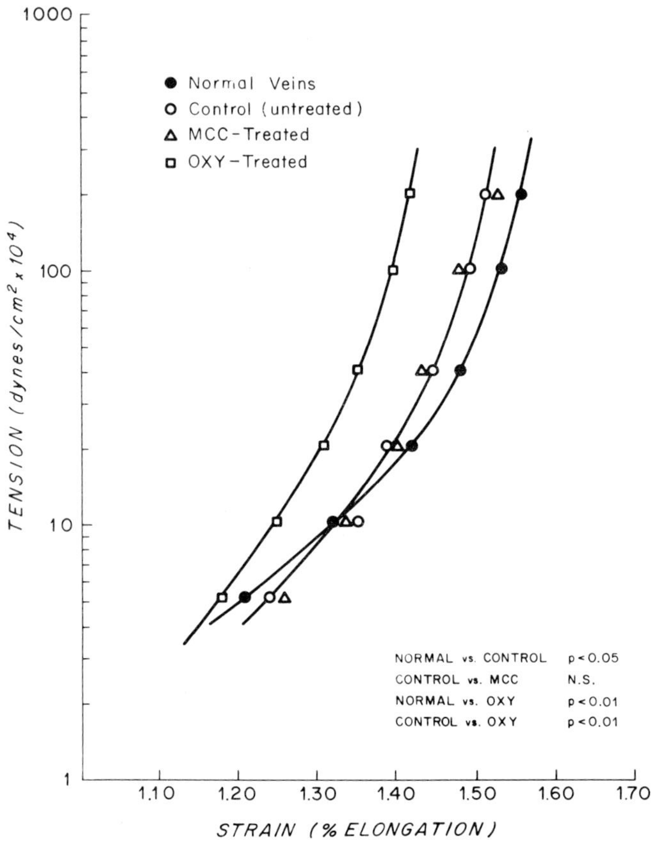

Fig. 2. Stress-strain relationships in veins (four-month studies). Stress-strain curves for normal jugular vein compared to vein dissected but untreated and dissected and treated with MCC or OXY. Compared to normal, stiffening or loss of distensibility is seen in all operated vessels. No differences are seen between untreated and MCC-treated vessels, whereas OXY-treated vessels show greater stiffening than the others.

dissected, MCC-treated, and OXY-treated jugular vein. Dissection and MCC treatment resulted in changes from normal again manifested by stiffening, significant at the $P < 0.05$ level. There was no statistical difference between dissected and MCC-treated vessels. There was greater stiffening in the OXY-treated veins which was significantly different ($P < 0.01$) from both normal and dissected veins.

Stiffening in this setting is probably secondary to the inflammatory response. The scarring due to dissection is real, but since the presence of MCC did not enhance the inflammatory response over that due to dissection as denoted either histologically or as increased stiffening, the fourth, or structural effect requirement also seems satisfied by MCC. Again, OXY seems to be less satisfactory in meeting this requirement.

DISCUSSION

Microcrystalline collagen, derived from bovine corium, has been demonstrated in both animal and human studies to be minimally antigenic, and safe for potential use as a topical hemostatic agent without dangers of sensitization, anaphylactic reaction, or other toxicity.[12] Its method of action in accomplishing hemostasis has not been completely clarified, but it is now thought to be primarily mediated by platelets.[11] Platelets have a known affinity for collagen, and collagen is also capable of initiating both platelet aggregation and the platelet release reaction.[4] Collagen and platelets together form a tenacious adhesive mass which then probably forms a hemostatic plug directly at the bleeding site. In addition, to its interaction with platelets, microcrystalline collagen has now been shown to shorten the reaction time of the intrinsic clotting system by about 60 percent.[11] The hemostatic plug which results from the direct interaction of collagen and blood leading to coagulation may be responsible for the greater effectiveness of microcrystalline collagen as compared to other topical agents such as oxidized cellulose. Oxidized cellulose in contact with blood swells and transforms from a white gauzelike cloth to an almost black, adhesive substance. This probably does not actually initiate coagulation but merely sticks to the bleeding surface and causes hemostasis by pressure.

The relative importance of the two possible mechanisms of action of MCC remains to be elucidated, but MCC has been shown in dogs to be effective in the presence of clotting factor deficiencies such as Factors VIII and IX.[11] In the presence of depressed platelet counts, it has seemingly been less effective. From the clinical standpoint, however, it has been observed to be effective in the presence of systemic heparinization[1] and, therefore, may be potentially useful during cardiovascular reconstructive surgery.

On the basis of studies reported herein, it appears that microcrystalline collagen is an effective and safe topical hemostatic agent for use in vascular surgery to control anastomotic hemorrhage. Four distinct requirements for such an agent were evaluated and in each instance they were partially or completely satisfied by microcrystalline collagen.

The evaluation of hemostatic effectiveness, although somewhat subjective, demonstrated that MCC was superior to pressure or oxidized cellulose in controlling hemorrhage from arterial end-to-end anastomoses. The results are supported by other studies showing hemostatic effectiveness recorded as a shortened time to hemostasis accomplished by topical MCC in experimental wounds of the brain, pancreas, kidney, liver, and spleen.[7, 8] An even better demonstration of such effectiveness comes from the work of Wilkinson and associates,[13] who showed with statistical significance, less blood loss from skin graft donor sites in man after treatment with microcrystalline collagen. Although statistical significance could not be demonstrated in the experiments with vascular anastomoses, hemostasis was more readily accomplished in those treated with MCC. The fact that fewer MCC-treated anastomoses required additional sutures and fewer were associated with angiographic abnormalities is probably important as illustrating the potential danger of additional suturing in small vessel anastomoses.

The remaining requirements regarding the absence of adverse effects on hemodynamics, gross anatomy, and vessel wall structure all reveal little difference between control and MCC-packed anastomoses at any time period. The information from the angiographic studies, however, requires further comment. Critically interpreted angiograms showed a fairly high incidence of abnormalities in both the control of MCC-treated groups, but no differences between these or the degrees of abnormality. There was also a seemingly greater incidence of abnormalities in the four-month groups as compared to the four-week groups, the reason for which is not completely clear. Four months is a relatively short time in the course of a vascular anastomosis which must be measured in years. Although progression was similar in both MCC-treated and untreated vessels, the fact that any progression was observed demands longer-term information to absolutely ensure safety. Studies to determine this are in progress. Further, in these studies MCC was left packed around the anastomosis which in actuality is not necessary since after hemostasis is secure, MCC may be grossly totally removed without creating rebleeding. This even further lessens the likelihood of significant problems with MCC over that from natural events alone.

Data from the stress-strain studies suggest that at least some of the angiographic changes may be due to varying degrees of scar tissue formation. Parallel shifts of stress-strain curves to the left have been shown in previous studies to be secondary to stiffening or loss of distinsibility caused by periadventitial fibrous tissue reaction rather than actual change in the vessel wall itself.[2] The more extreme angiographic and histologic change in OXY-treated vessels correlated well with the maximum stiffening seen in stress-strain curves which is consistent with this interpretation. The long-term significance of such loss of distinsibility is not known. It has been shown, however, that loss of distensibility is associated with aging and gradual dilatation and may be associated with aneurysm formation.[10] More important, however, progressive fibrous tissue reaction can also possibly lead to stenotic lesions of hemodynamic significance and peripheral circulatory ischemia in the watershed. Hence, the less the stiffening, the better.

Some changes from normal distensibility was seen in vessels subjected only to simple operative dissection. This loss of distensibility was more pronounced in veins than in arteries which means that venoarterial anastomoses such as in bypass grafts may be more susceptible to agents which enhance the inflammatory response. It is therefore important that in both arteries and veins, the presence of MCC did not at all enhance the inflammatory response and hence the stiffening.

It has been suggested that treatment with oxidized cellulose may be harmful, at least as utilized during these studies where the material was wrapped and left around the anastomosis. In fact, the manufacturer specifically recommends against this practice because of the risk of enhancing foreign body reaction with stricture formation. These risks are probably real, based upon the data from these experiments. There was a question of diminution of flow in four-month experiments, a greater incidence and degree of angiographic abnormality, a slightly greater inflammatory reaction seen histologically, and finally, increased stiffness in OXY-wrapped vessels. These facts lead to the conclusion that OXY should definitely not be used in the way it was in these experiments. When a topical agent is necessary during vascular procedures, in view of the hemostatic superiority of MCC, it would seem that this agent may be a more logical choice as soon as it becomes available.

The authors gratefully acknowledge the help of Dr. James Caulfield, Department of Pathology, for the preparation and evaluation of the histologic material, and Dr. Chris Athanasoulis, Department of Radiology, for the performance and interpretation of angiograms, and the technical assistance of Messrs. Peter Mione and Steven Wieland.

REFERENCES

1. Abbott, W. M.: Unpublished observations.
2. Abbott, W. M., Mundth, E. D., and Austen, W. G.: Autogenous vein grafts: Effects of simple storage on structural properties, Surg. Forum **24:** 260, 1973.
3. Battista, O. A., Erdi, N. Z., Ferraro, C. F., and Karasinski, F. J.: Novel microcrystals of polymers, part II, J. Appl. Polymer Sci. **11:** 481, 1967.
4. Deykin, D.: Emerging concepts of platelet function, N. Engl. J. Med. **290:** 144, 1974.
5. Hait, M. R.: Microcrystalline collagen: A new hemostatic agent, Am. J. Surg. **120:** 330, 1970.
6. Hait, M. R., Battista, O. A., Stark, R. B., and McCord, C. W.: Microcrystalline collagen as a biologic dressing, vascular prosthesis, and hemostatic agent, Surg. Forum **20:** 51, 1969.
7. Hait, M. R., Robb, C. A., Borgmann, A. R., and Tippett, L. O.: Comparative evaluation of Avitene microcrystalline collagen hemostat in experimental animal wounds, Am. J. Surg. **125:** 284, 1973.
8. Morgenstern, L.: Use of microcrystalline collagen for splenic hemostasis in experimental splenic injury, presented at the Southern California Chapter of the American College of Surgeons, Palm Springs, Calif., Jan. 18, 1973.
9. Mundth, E. D., Wright, J. E. C., and Austen, W. G.: Development of a method for stress/strain analysis of cardiac valvular tissue, Curr. Top. Surg. Res. **3:** 67, 1971.
10. Roach, M. R., and Burton, A. C.: The effect of age on the elasticity of human arteries, Can. J. Biochem. Physiol. **164:** 330, 1961.
11. Tenery, J. H.: Personal communication.
12. Tenery, J. H., and Clemmons, R. H.: Technical report, Code No. 072-3310-005, Oct. 9, 1972, Alcon Laboratories, Inc.
13. Wilkinson, T. S., Tenery, J. H., and Jufi, D.: The skin graft donor site as a model for

evaluation of hemostatic agents, Plast. Reconstr. Surg. **51:** 541, 1973.

DISCUSSION

Dr. Erle E. Peacock, Jr. (Tucson, Ariz.). Some years ago Dr. H. F. Siegler, now at Duke, and I published in the *Annals of Surgery* some data showing the results of using acid-swollen ficin-digested bovine skin collagen as a hemostatic agent in a very brutal fatal hemorrhage in dogs and in people. The hypothesis for the experiment was that in addition to hemostatic possibilities, the advantages of a sponge over a gel would be very effective —a sponge with open interstices would allow cells to come in, and it would form the structure for a new Glisson's capsule, or a new Gerota's fascia, or a new pleura after a decortication procedure. The mortality rate in the gel-foam or other-treated animals was 75 percent; with the use of the bovine collagen, it was 15 percent.

In addition, four patients were treated at the North Carolina Memorial Hospital with what we classified as potentially fatal hemorrhage in the portal area or caudate lobe, which could not be resected. The survival rate was 100 percent.

In summary, this reached the stage of management that Ethicon, who helped us develop this sponge, figured that it would cost them $35 apiece to prepare these and deliver them to your operating room. They felt the expense was so high and the need was so small that they overruled it, and it never appeared.

I think, in view of the beautiful data you have just seen, and those experiments which did show that a sponge could be compressible, so that you would not get necrosis of cellular tissue behind it, and that a sponge with open interstices provide the framework for cells to line up and synthesize a new connective tissue capsule—is such that maybe we can now get those big, blanket sponges made for the pelvis, the lung, the surface of the liver, the kidney, and so forth.

Dr. Julius H. Jacobson, II (New York, N. Y.). I simply rise to say that we have been using this material clinically and have come to the old conclusion that there is still no substitute for a well-placed suture. We have not found that it has been particularly effective or more effective than the gloved finger. I am always a little suspicious when one has to do very accurate measurements to determine a difference between two substances.

Have you used this clinically? We may not be applying it right. We just simply pat it over the surface with our fingers. I imagine there might be some trick that you have learned that has made it more effective.

Dr. Graeme L. Hammond (New Haven, Conn.). I agree fully with Dr. Jacobson's remarks. However, one place where this conceivably could be very helpful could be in coronary anastomoses on heparinized patients. I would like to know if there is any work with the heparinized animal.

Dr. Thomas Knight Hunt (San Francisco, Calif.). I would like to present another interesting fact that my colleague, Dr. Michaley has worked out in our laboratory. Of course, the rationale for the use of collagen is really to aggregate platelets and initiate the coagulation from that point, but it turns out that the platelet attaches to collagen in a very limited area of its molecular structure; it is possible to use synthetic peptides for the same purpose. This may open up a new class of hemostatic agents which can be delivered in a variety of forms—on a blanket, as Erle has suggested, or, for that matter, in a fluid medium, or impregnated on another medium that might present it to the surgical bleeding surface in a more preferable manner.

Dr. Peacock. That field is called solid state pharmacology, and it is going to be very important to us.

Dr. William M. Abbott (closing). The matter of cost is going to be a very real concern, and I have absolutely no information about that at this particular time. There is going to be a cost-benefit ratio type of situation that is going to play a definite role in the ultimate utilization of this material.

There are some instances in which we are somewhat reluctant to use additional sutures, and I think that the correlation in our data between an increase in angiographic abnormality and an increase in the utilization of sutures probably verifies that point; additional sutures do run the additional risk of slight narrowing or stenotic effects in anastomoses, especially if it is a relatively small one.

We have applied this pretty much as the people who have developed it have told us. It comes as a fairly fluffy powder. In order to put it onto a bleeding surface, it is best compressed as much as it possibly can be, and then put on and pinched, actually, on the anastomosis, or bleeding surface, and held there with gentle pressure for several minutes. If bleeding continues, it can then be teased and flushed away, and a second or third application can be made.

In cardiovascular surgery, heparin is very frequently used; microcrystalline collagen does seem to be effective in this setting. We have done no experiments with this up to this point, but I think that the mode of action does come via the platelet situation, and there must be platelets present in order for it to initiate coagulation and result in hemostasis. It has been also found to be effective in intrinsic clotting factor deficiencies, whereas in patients or in animals with depressed platelet counts it has not worked as well.

Emerging concepts in the control of surgical infections

J. Wesley Alexander, M.D., Sc.D., *Cincinnati, Ohio*

From the Department of Surgery, University of Cincinnati Medical Center, Cincinnati, Ohio

THE EXPLOSION of scientific knowledge has provided the opportunity to explore new methods of therapy which have changed and improved surgical practice remarkably during the past few decades. However, surgical infection continues to be a major unsolved problem, partly because of these advances. Attention on new therapeutic approaches has arisen because of a growing concern with nosocomial infections and the realization that antimicrobial drugs have both limited usefulness and definite liabilities.

This presentation will provide a personal and admittedly biased view of the progress and direction of current research as it may apply to the management of surgical infections. Emphasis will be placed on the development of new and emerging concepts. There are four broad areas in which new developments might influence the control of surgical infections. These are related to environmental and technical factors, the bacteria themselves, antimicrobial agents, and immune defense mechanisms of the patient.

THE ENVIRONMENT AND SURGICAL TECHNIQUE

The principles of antisepsis and asepsis were well established by the early 1900's. Numerous modifications and improvements have been developed, but as Wangensteen and associates[16] so aptly stated in a recent historical review of surgical infection, "since the beginning of the 20th century, there have been essentially no original surgical innovations to protect the patient during operation."

THE MICROBES

Man lives in contact with a myriad of microorganisms on every epithelial surface exposed to the outside environment. It is indeed remarkable that so few infections actually occur, reflecting the extraordinary efficiency of the epithelial barriers and primary lines of immune defense. Whenever surgical or traumatic wounds penetrate the epithelial barriers, there is a direct correlation between the number of contaminating organisms and the incidence and degree of infection developing in the wound. However, the number of bacteria necessary to initiate an infection, often designated as the critical inoculum, varies remarkably with the local microenvironment.

Competitive colonization by "non-pathogenic" bacteria has been tried in certain highly susceptible populations of patients such as newborns. However, there is growing awareness that any bacterium can become pathogenic, and the practice has not gained much favor. On another potential front, genetic manipulation of the microbial environment has not been successful in achieving a therapeutic advantage. Thus, there have been no major advances in the

Supported in part by United States Public Health Service Grant No. 5-POI-GM15428-06.

Presented at the Thirty-fifth Annual Meeting of the Society of University Surgeons, St. Louis, Mo., Feb. 14-16, 1974.

study of microbes themselves which have been beneficial to the control of surgical infections.

THE ANTIMICROBIAL DRUGS

New therapeutic agents with antimicrobial activity are being developed continually. While highly beneficial in selected instances, their use may be frankly deleterious and has made the problem of nosocomial infections even more complex. Surface and contaminating flora are readily suppressed by effective antimicrobial agents, but the "parade of pathogens" and the changing nature of infections since the introduction of antibiotic agents have served to emphasize adaptability within the microbial world. We have learned, often by sad experience, that a therapeutically induced ecological vacuum in a host's microbial environment will soon be filled, often with opportunistic pathogens of impressive virulence and antibiotic resistance. Unfortunately, antibiotic agents have provided only a partial solution to the changing problem of surgical infections, and no new therapeutic concepts seem to be emerging in the area of antimicrobial drugs.

DEFENSES OF THE HOST

With the frustration that has developed from pursuing other strategies of attack and with the rapid expansion of knowledge in the field of immunology, it has been a natural consequence to re-examine immune defense mechanisms in surgical infections. Host defenses against infection represent a complex interplay of cellular and humoral components which have been and are being dissected with difficulty. While highly interdependent, these can be separated into three categories which can be discussed independently: the phagocytic cells, the opsonins, and the vascular response.

PHAGOCYTIC CELLS

Neutrophils. The use of potent chemotherapeutic agents, especially in the management of malignant disease, has led to an increasing frequency of severe neutropenia and prolonged periods of bone marrow depression which are often associated with septic complications. Transfusion of leukocytes from another individual to provide protection during these periods has been of significant, albeit very brief, benefit in selected patients,[8] and the practical application of leukocyte transfusion has been possible only recently with the development of appropriate technology for leukophoresis. The value of the techniques could be increased significantly if large numbers of functionally active neutrophils could be stored for long periods of time to allow development of cell banks. Typing of leukocyte antigens and matching of donor-recipient combinations to increase survival and decrease immunological reactions against these antigens would then be possible. Methods of leukocyte storage for ultimate transfusion-replacement therapy are currently being investigated under contracts from the Blood Resources Branch of the National Institutes of Health.

Table I. *Selected diseases in which an impairment of the antibacterial function of neutrophils has been associated with an increased susceptibility to infection*

Hereditary diseases	*Acquired diseases*
Chronic granulomatous disease of childhood (CGD)	Severe burn injury
Variants of CGD	Advanced malignancy
Myeloperoxidase deficiency	Kwashiorkor
Severe G6PD deficiency	Severe trauma
Chediak-Higashi syndrome	Newborn infants
	Iron deficiency anemia
	Diabetes mellitus
	Sepsis
	Drug therapy

Discovery of chronic granulomous disease of childhood focused worldwide attention on abnormalities of the antibacterial function of neutrophils as a factor in the genesis of bacterial infections. Since then, functional abnormalities have been found to be associated with the development of infection in a variety of hereditary and acquired diseases (Table I). Important among these have been several surgical disorders including burn injury, severe trauma, and immunosuppression for transplantation. In burn patients,

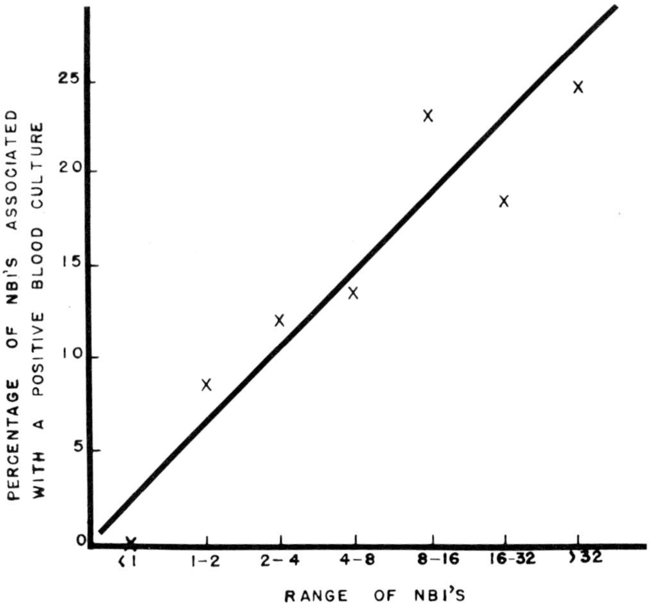

Fig. 1. Association of abnormalities of neutrophil function with positive blood cultures in burn patients. The ability of neutrophils to kill ingested bacteria decreases as the neutrophil bactericidal index (NBI) increases. (From Alexander, J. W., and Meakins, J. L.: A physiological basis for development of opportunistic infections, Ann. Surg. 176: 273, 1972.)

Table II. *Relationship of hyperalimentation, sepsis, and neutrophil function in seriously burned patients**

Type of hyper-alimenta-tion	*Size burn (T/3°)*	*Average NBI*	*No. of septic death/total No. patients studied*
None	61.5/50.2	11.6	4/6
IV	54.2/42.5	10.6	2/13
Oral	60.7/47.7	2.1	1/8

*The neutrophil bactericidal index (NBI) was measured using *S. aureus* as the test organism. Higher values reflect poorer function.

it has been possible to establish a direct relationship between the degree of functional abnormality of circulating neutrophils and the development of life-threatening infections[2] (Fig. 1). Also of importance has been the demonstration of a naturally occurring cyclic variation in the antibacterial function of circulating neutrophils, in both man (Fig. 2) and experimental animals.[3] In our studies of burn patients, septic episodes have occurred primarily at intervals of relatively impaired function. Despite this association, the pattern of cyclic variation of antibacterial function of neutrophils has been found to vary with different types of organisms, suggesting that there are related but specific enzymatic pathways of intracellular killing.[2] We have postulated that the cyclic variation in neutrophil function partially explains unexpected periods of both resistance and susceptibility to the development of infection in surgical and traumatic wounds (Fig. 3). The regulatory mechanism for the variation of cyclic variation in neutrophil function has not yet been elucidated, but it does not appear to be under endocrinologic control.[3]

Perhaps of greatest importance among more recent studies has been the observation that nutritional supplementation can prevent acquired abnormalities of neutrophil function.[10] In a recent study of burn patients at the Cincinnati Shriners Burns Institute, a dramatic improvement in neutrophil function in seriously burned patients was found when compared to earlier patients. Associated with this improvement was an increased resistance to infection as evidenced by a lowered incidence of sepsis and death from in-

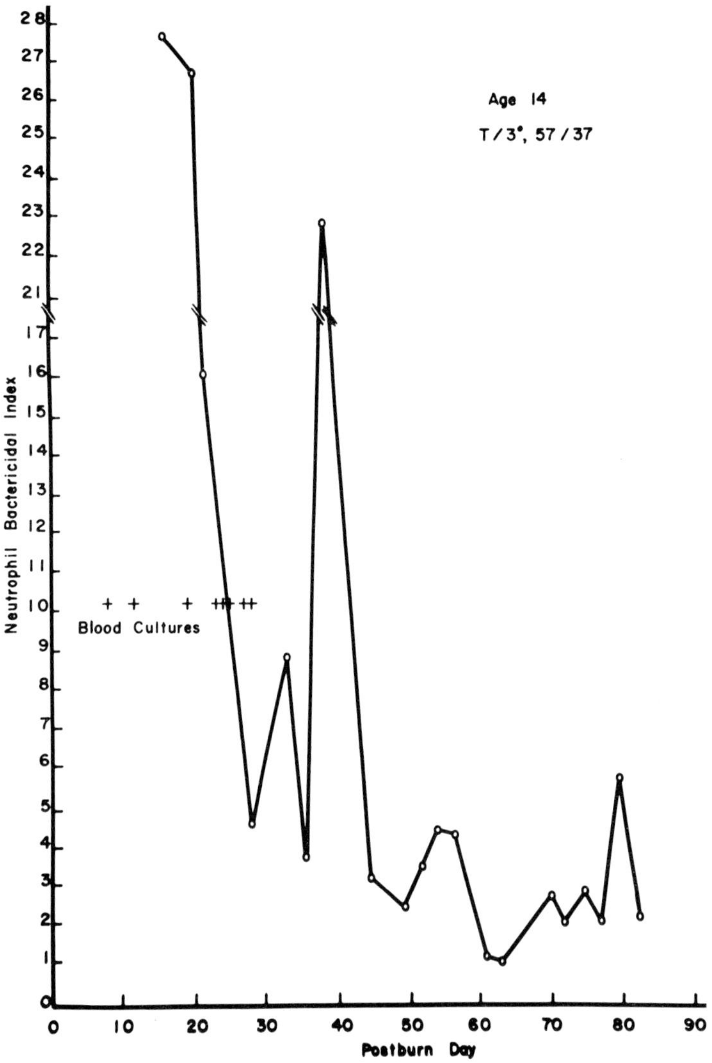

Fig. 2. Serial measurements of the neutrophil bactericidal index in a seriously burned patient. A cyclic variation of the antibacterial function of the patient's neutrophils occurred during the period of observation. Note that the development of positive blood cultures was associated with portions of the cycle where neutrophil function was relatively worse. (From Alexander, J. W., and Meakins, J. L.: A physiological basis for development of opportunistic infections. Ann. Surg. 176: 273, 1972.)

fection (Table II). This improvement appeared to be related to an increased intake of minerals and trace elements during nutritional supplementation by oral hyperalimentation. However, this suggestion awaits laboratory confirmation.

Mononuclear phagocytes. The reticuloendothelial system (RES) has been actively investigated for several decades, but its precise role in the genesis of surgical infections is not yet defined. Recent laboratory data suggest that the activity of this important system can be expanded by both specific and nonspecific stimuli,[11, 12] and activation of macrophages serves to increase resistance in laboratory animals to a number of microbial pathogens which are of increasing importance in immunodepressed patients. It is entirely conceivable that this type of stimulation could lead to increased resistance

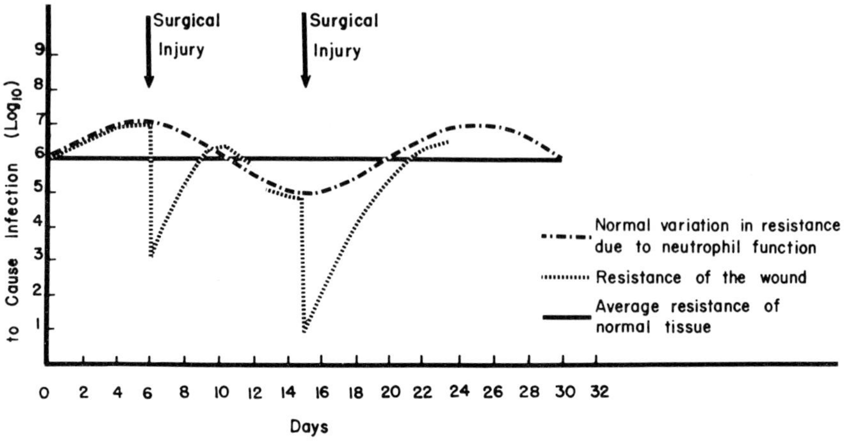

Fig. 3. The resistance of tissue to infection can be expressed as the number of bacteria necessary to cause infection. In normal tissues this number is approximately 10^6 for *Staphylococcus aureus*, but it may vary considerably for different organisms. The resistance of normal tissue to infection is markedly reduced by a factor of approximately 10,000 in a surgical wound closed by silk sutures. Resistance gradually recovers with the development of increased vascularity of the wound and exceeds normal tissues by the fifth or sixth day. The resistance of normal tissue to infection is probably modified in most people by the normally occurring cyclic variation in antibacterial function of their circulating neutrophils. Thus, the degree of susceptibility of injured tissue may vary with the temporal relationship of injury to the phase of this cycle. (From Alexander, J. W.: Nosocomial infections, *in* Current Problems in Surgery, Chicago, 1973, Year Book Medical Publishers, Inc.)

in certain patients such as those with burn injury or severe trauma where there is a clear depression of reticuloendothelial system activity.

Lymphocyte mediators. Transfer factor is another emerging therapeutic agent which has potential value in the treatment of surgical infections.[7] The dialyzable fraction from extracts of sensitized human lymphocytes contains this factor which can be passively transferred to recipients in small quantities to expand immunological reactivity against certain infectious agents. It has already been shown to be of value in a few conditions such as mucocutaneous candidiasis and leprosy. Its potential value in other conditions where thymic-dependent lymphocyte (T cell) function is impaired (such as in burns, during chemotherapy, and following radiation injury) has not been quantitated. It is probable that it will be of value in conditions associated with a high incidence of opportunistic infections including fungal and viral agents. The role of other lymphocyte mediators or lymphokines is being actively investigated.[6, 11]

THE OPSONINS

In man, the efficiency of phagocytic cells is often highly dependent upon the complex system of serum proteins loosely classified as "opsonins." This term refers to antibodies, components of the complement system, and perhaps other less clearly defined serum proteins. Opsonins interact with particulate matter and foreign antigens to increase cellular recognition and removal by phagocytosis.

Specific antibody. Antibody has been known to play a protective role in infection since the turn of the century. However, until recently, its therapeutic application in surgical infections was limited largely to the control of tetanus and infection with other organisms which produce exotoxin. The rising problem of septic death in burn patients caused by *Pseudomonas aeruginosa* prompted the development and trial of a new polyvalent vaccine, and the results of the initial five-year study of active immunization with this vaccine were recently analyzed.[1] This study included 322 vaccinated patients with burn injuries involving 20 percent or more

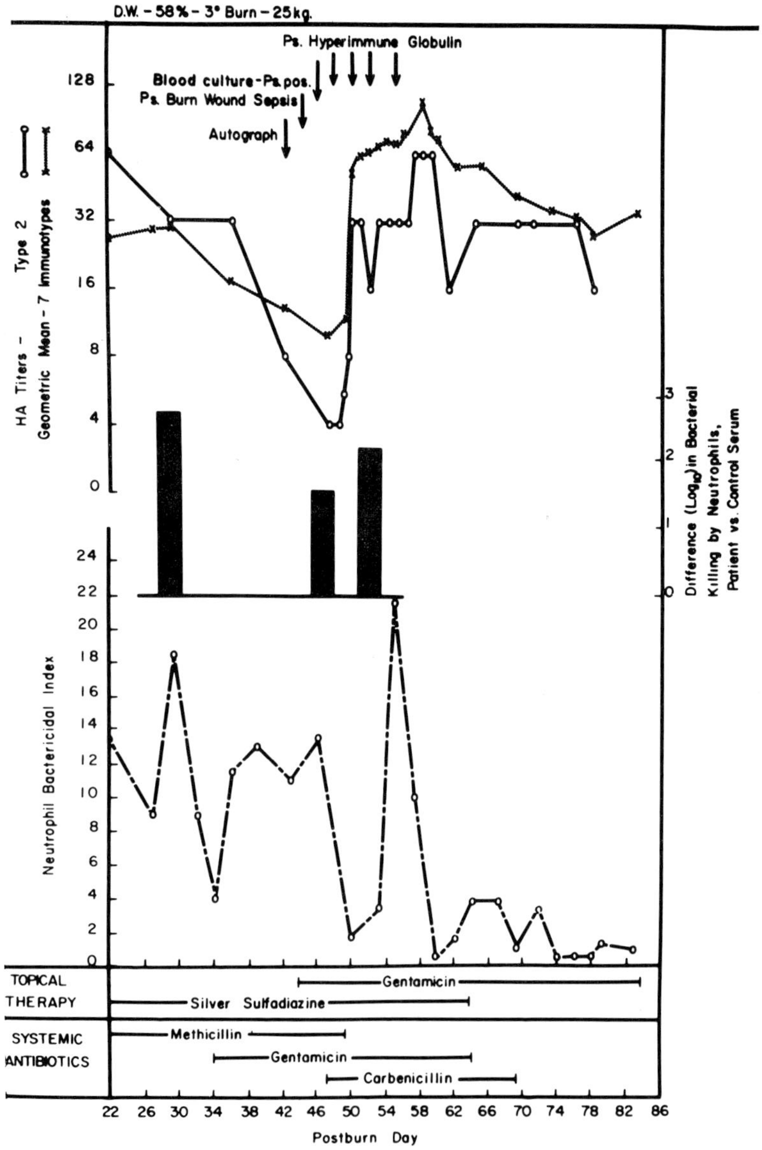

Fig. 4. Serial measurements of antibody titers and neutrophil function in a patient with a severe burn who was heavily colonized with type 2 *P. aeruginosa*. Initially high antibody titers were protective in this patient despite abnormal neutrophil function. However, infection of the burn wound was associated with a preferential consumption of type 2 antibody from the serum and a fall in opsonic activity against the corresponding bacterium. Associated with this fall and the presence of abnormal neutrophil function, the patient became septic. However, passive administration of immune antibody resulted in improvement of opsonic activity of the serum, elevation of serum antibody levels, and survival of the patient. (From Jones, C. E., Alexander, J. W., and Fisher, M. W.: A clinical evaluation of Pseudomonas hyperimmune globulin, J. Surg. Res. 14: 87, 1973.)

of their total body surface area who survived for five days after admission without evidence of Pseudomonas septicemia. In a consecutive group of 75 similar but non-vaccinated patients treated immediately before the onset of the study, death from Pseudomonas sepsis occurred in 14.7 percent, and Pseudomonas bacteremia occurred in 18.7 percent. With increasing effectiveness of vaccine regimens, the incidence of Pseudom-

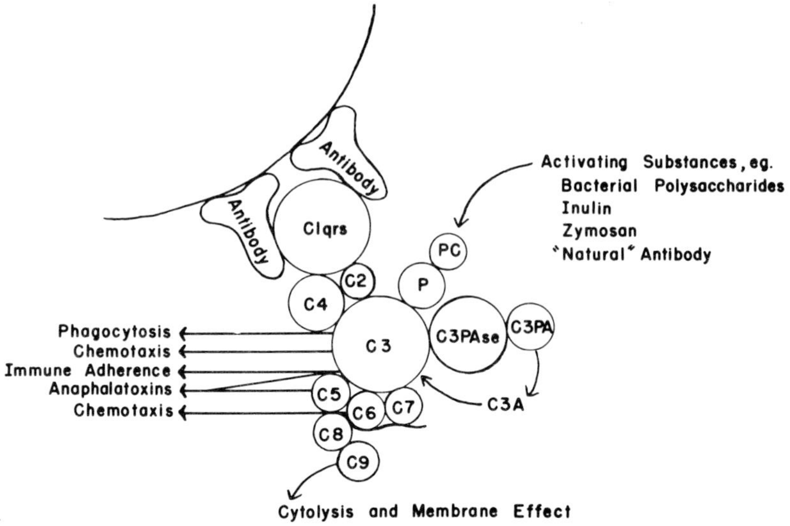

Fig. 5. Schematic representation of the current concept of the complement system. C1 through C9 are the components of the classical pathway. The other components are part of the alternate pathway: PC = properdin convertase, P = properdin, C3PAse = C3 proactivator convertase, C3PA = C3 proactivator, and C3A = C3 activator.

onas bacteremia fell to 6 percent. In the initial patients with maximal dose vaccination alone, death from Pseudomonas occurred in 3.1 percent. However, with the availability of a hyperimmune anti-Pseudomonas gamma globulin to treat vaccine failures with bacteremia, death from Pseudomonas infection did not occur in the last 186 vaccinated patients. The effectiveness of both active vaccination and the passive administration of hyperimmune globulin has been supported by statistically valid studies in other burn centers.[13]

Immunological studies performed during this time showed that the IgM class of antibody was far less important than the IgG class in immune resistance to *P. aeruginosa*. Additional studies showed that immune IgG antibody was extremely effective, both in prevention of *P. aeruginosa* infection and in its therapeutic management. This observation may be related to the ability of immune antibodies to opsonize bacteria in the absence of complement.[5] The presence of immune antibody generated either by active vaccination or by passive administration has also been shown to increase resistance to the corresponding organism in the presence of deficiencies in other components of host defense such as abnormal neutrophil function. Another important observation was that immune antibody to a specific strain of Pseudomonas could be preferentially consumed during the course of infection with that strain (Fig. 4). This observation helps to explain the sudden emergence of septicemia during heavy colonization with a single type of organism.

Complement, the amplification system. Although specific antibody provides a high degree of selectivity for immune reactions, the effects of complement activation produce most of the important biological responses, thus acting as an amplification system in immune reactions (Fig. 5). The classical pathway consists of eleven serum proteins. This cascade of protein interaction is initiated by certain antigen-antibody complexes which bind the C1 trimolecular complex thereby activating Cls. The remainder of the components, C4, C2, and C3 through C9, are activated sequentially to cause the full expression of complement system activity which includes phagocytosis, chemotaxis, immune adherence, cytolysis of susceptible membranes, and release of anaphylotoxins and vasoactive substances.

Several years ago, it was noted that sera

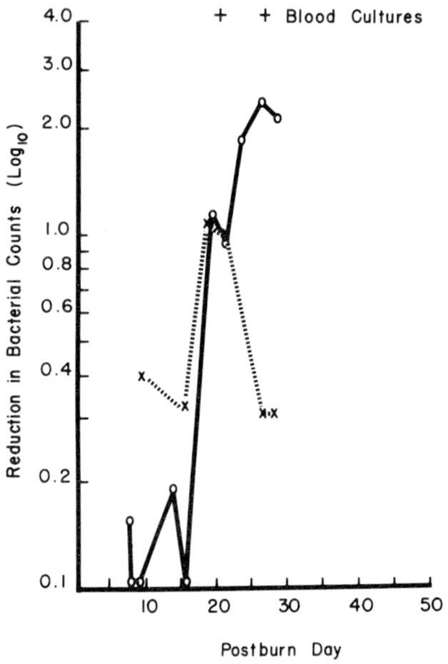

Fig. 6. Tests of opsonic activity on the serum from a 47-year-old man with a severe burn injury (68 percent total/56 percent, third degree burn (Patient 4). The temporal sequence of opsonic activity of the burn sera for *Pseudomonas aeruginosa* is shown as a solid line whereas the dotted line represents opsonic activity for *E. coli.* Values of activity for normal human serum were 2.23 ± 0.36 for *P. aeruginosa* and 3.00 ± 0.20 for *E. coli.* Opsonic activity for both *P. aeruginosa* and *E. coli* was decreased during the first 15 days with opsonic activity for *P. aeruginosa* returning to normal values, presumably because of the induction of immune antibodies by vaccination. Opsonic activity for *E. coli* was improved temporarily, but with the development of septicemia, this activity fell sharply, indicating a consumption of critical components of the opsonic system. See text. (Adapted from Bjornson, A. B., and Alexander, J. W.: Alterations of serum opsonins in patients with severe thermal injury, J. Lab. Clin. Med. To be published.)

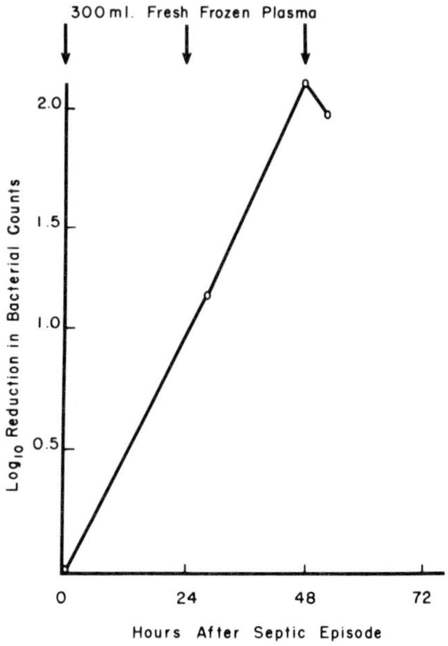

Fig. 7. Opsonic activity for *E. coli* in serum taken from a 61-year-old recipient of a cadaveric kidney transplant. At the time of the initial sample, the patient had severe pneumonia caused by *H. influenzae* which became clinically apparent three days before. The administration of 900 ml. of fresh frozen plasma over the next 48 hours restored opsonic activity with associated clinical improvement. Samples were drawn before administration of each unit of plasma.

which was markedly deficient in C2 could support opsonic activity normally but not hemolysis, but C3-deficient sera could not support either type of activity. The probability arose that there was another mechanism to activate the terminal components of the complement system by bacterial cell walls which did not involve the earlier components to a significant degree. This mechanism is now called the alternate pathway or bypass mechanism and is known to be related to the properdin system described originally by Pillemer and co-workers.[14] In some biological systems "natural" antibody, interacting with bacterial cell walls or certain polysaccharide substances, appears to participate in the complement system by this bypass mechanism.[5] Recently, it has been shown that the activating substances interact with properdin to activate C3.[9] This step may require an enzyme which activates properdin which has been designated properdin convertase.[14] One of the cleaved portions of the C3 molecule then activates C3 proactivator convertase, in turn acting on C3 proactivator (C3PA) to form C3 activator (C3A) which again cleaves C3. By continuation of the circuit, there is a powerful amplification system in which only small amounts of polysaccharide and antibody are necessary to trigger the reaction. This recently discovered alternate pathway now appears to be responsible for many of the deficiencies of host resistance

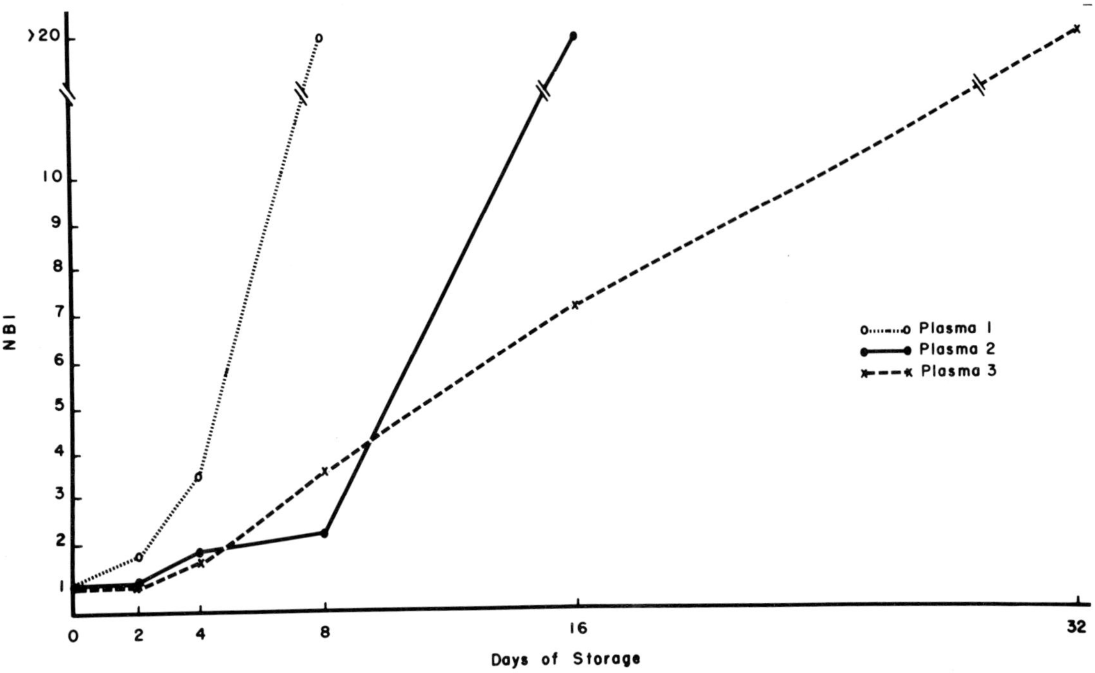

Fig. 8. Opsonic activity of plasma, samples from three donors, taken from ACD blood stored under standard conditions at 4° C. Samples were taken shortly after the time of the drawing and at 2 4, 8, 16, and 32 days. Each plasma sample was converted to serum by the addition of calcium ion and frozen. Final testing of all samples was done at a single time using normal human neutrophils and 2 percent concentration of each sample. In contrast to previous figures, the NBI was expressed as the ratio of the remaining viable bacteria after incubation of neutrophils and bacteria with later samples compared to the initial sample. The only variable in the test was the length of storage of the sample. Opsonic activity began to diminish within four days with marked loss between the eighth and thirty-second day.

which were previously not understood. Several types of abnormalities involving the alternate pathway have been shown to be related to acute or recurrent infections. While some of these are still not completely understood, others are clearly correctable with our present state of knowledge.

An investigation of the opsonic activity of serum obtained from patients with burns involving 36 to 85 percent of their total body surface area showed reduced opsonic activity for *Pseudomonas* and *E. coli* for 4 to 28 days postburn[4] (Fig. 6). These opsonic alterations both preceded and followed the onset of septic episodes, suggesting that they not only contributed to the pathogenesis of sepsis but could also occur as a consequence of sepsis. Further studies have shown that the C3 molecule was altered in patients with large burns in such a way that it could not be activated by C3 activator, suggesting the presence of an inhibitor. The relationship of this inhibitor to burn toxins has not been determined.

The data from Fig. 6 indicate that there was consumption of opsonic factors from the serum of the patient at the time of infection. This patient had been actively immunized with a Pseudomonas vaccine which elicited the synthesis of heat-stable immune antibody to Pseudomonas which did not require participation of the alternate pathway. Therefore, once this antibody appeared, the patient's serum supported opsonization of Pseudomonas to a normal degree. However, opsonins supporting phagocytosis of *E. coli* were consumed during infection with *E. coli.* Since the infection was caused by

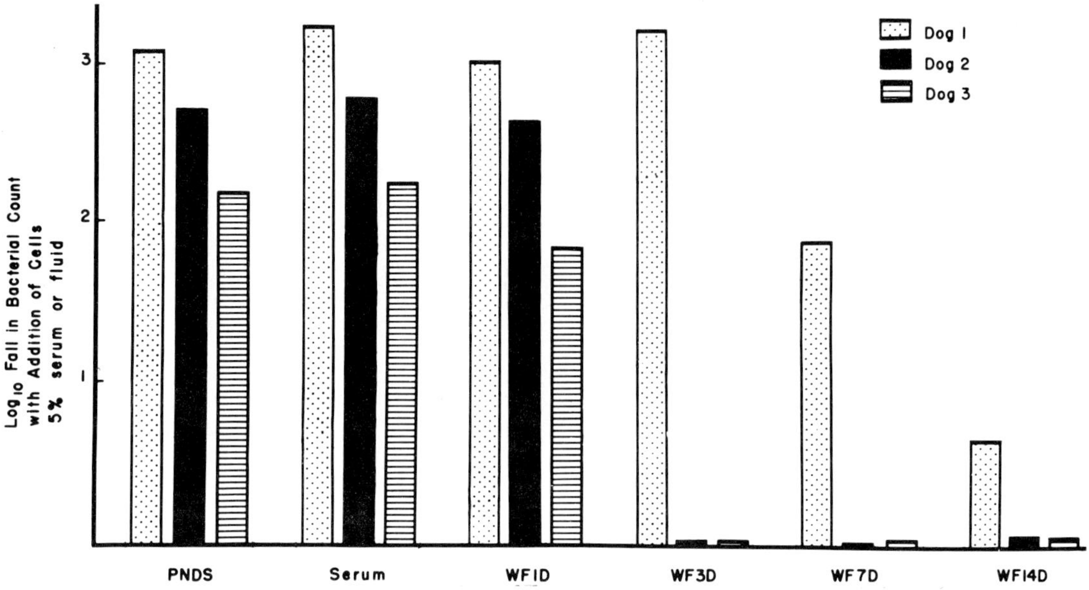

Fig. 9. Opsonic activity of serum and samples of wound fluid (WF) aspirated from stainless steel cylinders at 1, 3, 7, and 14 days after implantation into the subcutaneous tissues of dogs. All tests were performed using a five percent concentration of the serum or wound fluid. The bars measure the difference in the killing of *E. coli* in the presence of this fluid with and without the addition of normal neutrophils. A slight decrease in opsonic activity was detected in fluids taken from the cylinders on the first postoperative day with a marked decrease in activity subsequently.

E. coli, reduction of opsonic activity could have occurred from consumption of either specific antibody or components of the alternate pathway. Opsonic consumption is also suggested by the data collected on the patient shown in Fig. 7. Serum from this patient had no opsonic activity for *E. coli* during an episode of pneumonia caused by *H. influenzae,* indicating a severe deficiency of components of the alternate pathway. However, the administration of frozen plasma corrected the defect, returning opsonic activity to normal levels, and the patient recovered from the infective episode. These and similar findings from other patients provide strong support to the hypothesis that consumption of important opsonic proteins, especially those involving the alternate pathway of complement, can occur during active infection. I have named this condition "consumptive opsoninopathy," and its real importance is that it can be corrected, at least in certain instances, by the passive administration of plasma or blood containing a full component of normal serum proteins.

Recent interest in this problem has stimulated us to examine the loss of opsonic activity in whole blood stored under standard banking conditions at 4° C. The opsonic activity of plasma converted to serum by the addition of Ca^{++} is shown in Fig. 8 for three donors. Significant activity was lost during prolonged storage. However, both fresh frozen plasma and plasma from which the cryoprecipitate had been removed retained full opsonic activity in other experiments. Attempts to fractionate the important components of the opsonic system from plasma are being conducted in several laboratories including our own, and it appears that selected components may soon be available to correct precise deficiencies. These would have the advantage of not carrying the risk of transmitting infectious hepatitis or other diseases associated with transfusion therapy.

Table III. *Data collected from a 62-year-old man with a history of recurrent wound infections between 1967 and 1974**

	Patient values	*Normal values*
E. coli opsonic activity (%)	54.5	99
Pseudomonas opsonic activity (%)	91	99
C3B (U./ml.)	10.25	24
C3 breakdown with inulin (%)	0	54
C3PA (mg. %)	13.75	14.75
C3PA breakdown with inulin (%)	0	19

*He had a normal childhood and no episodes of septicemia.

Increasing numbers of patients with deficiencies of opsonic proteins are currently being recognized. Partial data from one such patient is shown in Table III. The antibacterial function of this patient's neutrophils was normal, but his serum failed to support normal opsonization of *E. coli* and *P. aeruginosa*. There was a reduced amount of native C3 in his serum, and the addition of inulin to his serum failed to activate the alternate pathway of complement. Final analysis of the problem may lead to correction of the defect and the performance of surgical procedures without associated infection.

Since some of the opsonic proteins undergo degradation during in vitro storage at 4° and 20° C., it seemed probable that collection of serum in wounds or body cavities would also lose opsonic activity. This question was studied both in man and experimental animals and found to be true. Fluid collected from sterile surgical wounds had a progressive decrease in the ability to opsonize *E. coli* (Fig. 9), with changes being evident as early as the first postoperative day. This loss might help to explain the development of wound infections which became apparent for the first time several days after a surgical procedure. It also provides additional laboratory support for the use of closed sterile suction devices for the drainage of potential dead spaces to prevent the accumulation of fluid and encourage the apposition of viable tissues.

THE VASCULAR RESPONSE

Diminished perfusion with blood has a markedly adverse effect on cellular function. During severe infections, especially those associated with septic shock, numerous vasoactive substances are released from anoxic or dead cells and from bacteria. These activate multiple complex systems including the kallekrein, complement, clotting, and autonomic nervous system to release mediators which effect altered nutrient flow, thus compounding the problem. As information accumulates concerning mediators and their regulation, we come closer to useful therapeutic management of septic conditions. This goal has only begun to be achieved and will become of increasing importance in the future.

CONCLUSIONS

Many changes and improvements have occurred in surgical care which have allowed successful management of numerous patients who would not have been salvageable only a few years ago. Surgery of patients at the extremes of age, severe trauma, the transplantation of organs, operations of longer and greater complexity, and the administration of chemotherapeutic agents, are a few among many factors that have contributed to an increased complexity of the problem of surgical infections. It is appropriate that we should continue a vigorous attempt to limit infection as a complication and to search for new methods to accomplish this end.

Observation of established principles of asepsis and antisepsis is obviously our most important ally, but it is unfortunate that no new concepts involving environmental control or surgical techniques have arisen in this century which aid in the control of surgical infection. It is also unfortunate that antimicrobial drugs have not been effective in controlling the rising problem, nor are they likely to do so.

Most of the conditions associated with an increased incidence of infection have accompanying abnormalities of normal host defense mechanisms as a basis for the susceptibility. Immune mechanisms which defend against microbial invasion are complex but becoming increasingly understood.

Prominent among the acquired abnormalities which have been defined are neutropenia, defects of the antibacterial function of neutrophils, and depression of the reticuloendothelial system. There is compelling evidence that these abnormalities, once defined, can be improved. Transfusion of neutrophils can be accomplished with therapeutic benefit in leukopenic patients, and the feasibility of long-term storage of leukocytes for transfusion is being investigated. The acquired abnormality of neutrophil function following burn injury can be prevented by nutritional supplementation, and analysis of current data suggests that trace elements may be involved. Expansion of RES activity is being accomplished by using both specific and non-specific stimuli. Also of potential benefit, is the use of exogenous transfer factor to increase specific thymus dependent immunity to certain infections.

The opsonic system acts in concert with the cellular defenses, and an increasingly important role in natural immunity is being attributed to activity of the alternate pathway of complement. It is now being appreciated that reduction in serum opsonins from any cause can lead to an increased susceptibility to infection, and many conditions may be associated with lowered opsonins. Severe burn injury, for example, can be associated with the presence of an inhibitor of the complement system which reduces opsonic activity. Active infection can result in the consumption of opsonic proteins, a condition we now call consumptive opsoninopathy. Such a depletion can potentially be corrected since both cryoextracted plasma and fresh frozen plasma contain all of the components necessary for opsonization. Single components may soon be available for replacement therapy, thus avoiding the risk of hepatitis and other transmissible diseases. More classically, studies conducted during the last decade have shown that active immunization of seriously burned patients can protect against invasive Pseudomonas infection. Hopefully, this trial can serve as a prototype for the development of vaccines against other problem pathogens. At the present time, the passive administration of immune anti-Pseudomonas antibody has been a valuable aid in the treatment of established, life-threatening infections.

Obviously, the future can not be predicted accurately, but the current direction and progress of clinical and basic research in surgical infections suggest that the emphasis on immunological mechanisms is appropriate.

REFERENCES

1. Alexander, J. W., and Fisher, M. W.: Pseudomonas immunization in burn disease, Proceedings of Conference on Endotoxin, Vienna, 1973. To be published.
2. Alexander, J. W., and Meakins, J. L.: A physiological basis for the development of opportunistic infections, Ann. Surg. **176:** 273, 1972.
3. Alexander, J. W., Meakins, J. L., Randall, M., and Mitchell, M.: Lack of pituitary, adrenal, thyroid, gonadal, and pineal endocrine control of cyclic changes in the antibacterial function of neutrophils, J. Res. **14:** 266, 1973.
4. Bjornson, A. B., and Alexander, J. W.: Alterations of serum opsonins in patients with severe thermal injury, J. Lab. Clin. Med. **83:** 372, 1974.
5. Bjornson, A. B., and Michael, J. G.: Factors in normal human serum that promote bacterial phagocytosis, presented at the International Endotoxin Conference, 1972, J. Infect. Dis. **128:** S182, 1973.
6. David, J. R.: Mediators produced by sensitized lymphocytes, Fed. Proc. **30:** 1730, 1971.
7. Fundenberg, H. H., Levin, A. S., Spitler, L. E., Wybran, J., and Byers, V.: The therapeutic uses of transfer factor, Hosp. Prac. **9:** 95, 1974.
8. Graw, R. G., Jr., Herzig, G., Perry, S., and Henderson, E. S.: Normal granulocyte transfusion therapy. Treatment of septicemia due to gram-negative bacteria, New Eng. J. Med. **287:** 367, 1972.
9. Götze, O., and Muller-Eberhard, H. J.: The role of properdin in the alternate pathway of complement activation, J. Exp. Med. **139:** 44, 1973.
10. Lennard, E. S., Alexander, J. W., Craycraft, T. K., and MacMillan, B. G.: Association of

improved antibacterial defense with oral hyperalimentation in burn patients. Submitted for publication.
11. Mackaness, G. B.: Resistance to intracellular infection, J. Infect. Dis. **123:** 439, 1971.
12. McGregor, D. D., and Koster, F. T.: The mediator of cellular immunity. IV. Cooperation between lymphocytes and mononuclear phagocytes, Cell. Immunol. **2:** 317, 1971.
13. Parke-Davis and Company. Data in research files.
14. Pillemer, L., Blum, L., Lepow, I. H., Ross, O. A., Todd, E. W., and Wardlaw, A. C.: The properdin system and immunity: I. Demonstration and isolation of a new serum protein, properdin, and its role in immune phenomena, Science **120:** 279, 1954.
15. Stitzel, A. E., and Spitzer, R. E.: The utilization of properdin in the alternate pathway of complement activation: Isolation of properdin convertase, J. Immunol. **112:** 56, 1974.
16. Wangensteen, O. H., Wangensteen, S. D., and Klinger, C. F.: Surgical cleanliness, hospital salubrity, and surgical statistics, historically considered, SURGERY **71:** 477, 1972.

Index to volume 75

AUTHOR INDEX*

A

ABBOTT, WILLIAM M., AND AUSTEN, W. GERALD. Microcrystalline collagen as a topical hemostatic agent for vascular surgery, 925

ABOUNA, GEORGE M., VEAZEY, PHILIP R., AND TERRY, DANIEL B., JR. Intravenous infusion of hydrochloric acid for treatment of severe metabolic alkalosis, 194

ABRAMSKY, O., AND GOLDSCHMIDT, Z.: Treatment and prevention of acute hepatic encephalopathy by intravenous levodopa, 188

ABSOLON, KAREL B. (*See* Agostini et al.), 213

ACKERMAN, NORMAN B. The blood supply of experimental liver metastases. IV. Changes in vascularity with increasing tumor growth, 589

ACLAND, R. D. Microvascular anastomosis: a device for holding stay sutures and a new vascular clamp, 185

ADROUNY, GEORGE A. (*See* Hewitt et al.), 1

AGOSTINI, JUAN C., RAMIREZ, RUBEN G., ALBERT, SOLOMON N., GOLDBAUM, LEO R., AND ABSOLON, KAREL B. Successful reversal of lethal carbon monoxide intoxication by total body asanguineous hypothermic perfusion, 213

AKIYAMA, HIROSHI, AND HIYAMA, MAMORU. A simple esophageal bypass operation by the high gastric division, 674

ALBERT, SOLOMON N. (*See* Agostini et al.), 213

ALEXANDER, J. WESLEY. Emerging concepts in the control of surgical infections, 934

ALEXANDER-WILLIAMS, JOHN. How to be an adequate vagotomist, 308

ALMEIDA CHAVEZ LUIS, ALBANO. (*See* Marchesini, Almeida Chavez Luis, and Cravo), 621

ALPERS, DAVID A. (*See* Binnington et al.), 805

ALTMAN, R. PETER. (*See* Lilly, Weintraub, and Altman), 664

ANDERSON, ANN P. (*See* Jelenko et al.), 892

ANDERSSON, A., HOFER, P.-A., HOLMLUND, D. E. W., AND WENDEL, H. Pinhole colonic perforation in breech-born infants, 617

ANDROULAKIS, JOHN A. (*See* Skandalakis et al.), 233

ANTOINE, JOHN E. (*See* Doberneck and Antoine), 87

ARIMA, EITOKU, FONKALSRUD, ERIC W., AND NEERHOUT, ROBERT C. Experiences in the management of surgically correctable biliary atresia, 228

ARMSTRONG, RAYMOND G. (*See* Haff and Armstrong), 715

*January, pp. 1-154; February, pp. 155-318; March, pp. 319-476; April, pp. 477-630; May, pp. 631-804; June, pp. 805-966.

AUSTEN, W. GERALD. (*See* Abbott and Austen), 925

AUSTIN, GEORGE, LAFFIN, DAVID, AND HAYWARD, WILLIAM. Physiologic factors in the selection of patients for superficial temporal artery to middle cerebral artery anastomosis, 861

B

BAEZ, A. (*See* Haimov et al.), 447

BALDERSON, GLENDA. (*See* Hardie et al.), 651

BAN, ICHIRO. (*See* Shionoya et al.), 695

BASOLI, ANTONIO. (*See* Stefanini et al.), 597

BAUE, ARTHUR E. (*See* Chaudry, Sayeed, and Baue), 220

BECKER, HORST D., REEDER, DAVID D., AND THOMPSON, JAMES C. Direct measurement of vagal release of gastrin, 101

—, —, AND —. Effect of atropine on basal and food-stimulated serum gastrin levels in man, 701

BEIL, ARTHUR R., JR. (*See* Frantz et al.), 471

BELZER, FOLKERT O. The role of paramedical personnel in organ procurement (editorial), 315

—, SALVATIERRA, OSCAR, PERLOFF, DOROTHEE, AND GRAUSZ, HENRY. Surgical correction of advanced fibromuscular dysplasia of the renal arteries, 31

BENFIELD, JOHN R. (*See* Schick et al.), 348

BERGAN, JOHN J. (*See* Kornmesser and Bergan), 80

BERGER, MICHAEL, SCHUESSLER, JOHN S., CARVAJAL, HUGO F., LORENTZ, WILLIAM B., JR., TRAVIS, LUTHER B., AND TYSON, KENNETH R. T. Obturator intestinal obstruction following renal allotransplantation: relief with hyperosmolar enemas, 746

BERNE, THOMAS V. (*See* Moore, Berne, and English), 357

BERNSTEIN, EUGENE F. (*See* Crissey and Bernstein), 543

BERR, F. (*See* Grundmann et al.), 178

BINNINGTON, H. BRADLEY, SUMNER, HATTON, LESKER, PEGGY, ALPERS, DAVID A., AND TERNBERG, JESSIE L. Functional characteristics of surgically induced jejunal neomucosa, 805

BISMUTH, H. (*See* Lecompte et al.), 161

BJORKEN, CHRISTER. (*See* Groth et al.), 725

BLUMENBERG, ROBERT M., AND GELFAND, MICHAEL L. A simple and inexpensive tunneler for use in peripheral vascular surgery, 305

BOGGAN, M. D. (*See* Friesen et al.), 517

BOLINGER, R. E. (*See* Friesen et al.), 517

BOMBECK, C. THOMAS. (*See* Levitsky et al.), 908

BONNET-EYMARD, JACQUES. (*See* Hanson et al.), 557

BORODY, CYRIL, AND MOUZAS, GEORGE L. The protection of the skin of fracture patients immobilized in plaster of Paris, 638

BOWEN, JOHN C., FLEMING, WILLIAM H., AND THOMPSON, JAMES C. Increased gastrin release following penetrating central nervous system injury, 720
BRADLEY, E. L., III. Measurement of hepatic blood flow in man, 783
—. Pulse contour vs. dye-dilution methods (letter to editors), 317
BRAZIER, JOHN, COOPER, NORMAN, MALONEY, JAMES V., JR., AND BUCKBERG, GERALD. The adequacy of myocardial oxygen delivery in acute normovolemic anemia, 508
BRODMAN, RICHARD F., HACKETT, RAYMOND L., FINLAYSON, BIRDWELL, AND PFAFF, WILLIAM W. Microangiography of the renal vasculature following total renal artery occlusion, 734
—, PFAFF, WILLIAM W., FINLAYSON, BIRDWELL, AND HACKETT, RAYMOND L. Venous drainage of the ischemic kidney, 584
BROELL, J. (*See* Halmagyi et al.), 763
BROWN, ROBERT S. (*See* Drucker et al.), 487
—. (*See* Pindyck et al.), 11
BUCHWALD, HENRY, COYLE, JOHN J., AND VARCO, RICHARD L. Effect of small bowel bypass on gastric fuction: postintestinal exclusion hypersecretion, a phenomenon in search of a syndrome, 821
—, GEBHARD, ROGER L., AND VARCO, RICHARD L. Relative secretion of cholesterol-4-^{14}C in the bile fistula rabbit, 266
BUCKBERG, GERALD. (*See* Brazier et al.), 508
BURROWS, L. (*See* Haimov et al.), 447

C

CALLAWAY, DIANNE. (*See* Jelenko et al.), 892
CAMERON, JOHN L. (*See* Sterioff, Orringer, and Cameron), 56
CARBONI, MANLIO. (*See* Stefanini et al.), 597
CARLSON, PAUL A. Length of residency (letter to editors), 318
CARRINGTON, CHARLES B. (*See* Sachatello, Hahn, and Carrington), 107
CARVAJAL, HUGO F. (*See* Berger et al.), 746
CERNY, JOSEPH C. (*See* Lindenauer, Cerny, and Morley), 705
CHAUDRY, IRSHAD H., SAYEED, MOHAMMED M., AND BAUE, ARTHUR E. Effect of adenosine triphosphate–magnesium chloride administration in shock, 220
CHIARILLO, LUIGI. (*See* Reul et al.), 682
CHO, SANG IN, DERHAGOPIAN, ROBERT P., KRANE, ROBERT S., AND NABSETH, DONALD C. Regional organ preservation program in the New England area, 528
CHRISTIANSEN, CHRISTINE. (*See* Wells and Christiansen), 49
CHRISTOUDIAS, GEORGE (*See* LeVeen et al.), 299
CLUNIE, G. J. A. (*See* Hardie et al.), 651
COLLINS, JOHN A. Problems associated with the massive transfusion of stored blood, 271
COOKE, PAUL A., AND EHRENFELD, WILLIAM K. Successful management of mycotic aortic aneurysm: report of a case, 132
COOLEY, DENTON A. (*See* Reul et al.), 682
COOPER, NORMAN. (*See* Brazier et al.), 508
COYLE, JOHN J. (*See* Buchwald, Coyle, and Varco), 821
CRABO, BO G. (*See* Rebelo et al.), 319
CRAIG, C. C. (*See* Friesen et al.), 517
CRAVO, MARCO AURELIO. (*See* Marchesini, Almeida Chavez Luis, and Cravo), 621
CRISSEY, MICHAEL M., AND BERNSTEIN, EUGENE F. Delayed presentation of carotid intimal tear following blunt craniocervical trauma, 543
CROSBY, I. (*See* Friesen et al.), 517
CUDNIK, D. B. (*See* Friesen et al.), 517
CUMMINGS, MICHAEL C. (*See* Dodsworth et al.), 811
CUSSEN, L. J. (*See* MacMahon et al.), 660

D

DARDIK, HERBERT. The young surgeon's dilemma (letter to editor), 630
—, DARDIK, IRVING, AND VEITH, FRANK J. Exposure of the tibial-peroneal arteries by a single lateral approach, 377
DARDIK, IRVING. (*See* Dardik, Dardik, and Veith), 377
DEBAKEY, LOIS. Reply: Honesty in authorship (letter to editor), 802
—. Rewriting and the byline: is the author the writer? 38
DELANEY, JOHN P., AND SCARPINO, JON. Reply to letter to editors by Rhodes, Lopez-Majano, and Wagner, 154
DEPALMA, RALPH G., IZANT, ROBERT J., JORDAN, ALF, HOLDEN, WILLIAM D., AND SHEEHAN, JOSEPH T. Objectives and methods in undergraduate surgical education, 915
DERHAGOPIAN, ROBERT P. (*See* Cho et al.), 528
DIAZ, CARLOS. (*See* LeVeen et al.), 299
DIETZMAN, RONALD H. (*See* Rebelo et al.), 319
DI LUZIO, N. R. (*See* Olcay et al.), 64
DOBERNECK, RAYMOND C., AND ANTOINE, JOHN E. Deglutition after resection of oral, laryngeal, and pharyngeal cancers, 87
DODSWORTH, JOHN, JAMES, J. HOWARD, CUMMINGS, MICHAEL C., AND FISCHER, JOSEF E. Depletion of brain norepinephrine in acute hepatic coma, 811
DON, HILLARY F. (*See* Hanson et al.), 557
DORIGHI, JOHN A., KAMINSKI, DONALD L., AND WILLMAN, VALLEE L. The effect of endogenous secretin and cholecystokinin on pentagastrin-stimulated innervated and denervated gastric mucosa, 755
DRAPANAS, THEODORE. (*See* Hewitt et al.), 1
—. (*See* Olcay et al.), 64
DREWS, JOHN A. Reply (letter to editor), 630
DRINKER, PHILIP A. (*See* Hanson et al.), 557
DRUCKER, MICHAEL R., PINDYCK, FRANK, BROWN, ROBERT S., ELWYN, DAVID H., AND SHOEMAKER, WILLIAM C. The interaction of glucagon and glucose on cardiorespiratory variables in the critically ill patient, 487
—. (*See* Pindyck et al.), 11
DUNPHY, J. ENGLEBERT. Surgery in the twenty-first century, 332

E

ECKERT, CHARLES. (*See* Wu, Jordan, and Eckert), 790
EDMUNDS, L. HENRY, JR. (*See* Wagner, Edmunds, and Heilbron), 91
EGDAHL, RICHARD H. Hypertonic glucose and improved critical organ performance (editorial), 145
EHRENFELD, WILLIAM K. (*See* Cooke and Ehrenfeld), 132
EIDEMILLER, LARRY R. (*See* Snider, Porter and Eidemiller), 613

EISENBERG, H. (*See* Zimmerman et al.), 550
ELWYN, DAVID H. (*See* Drucker et al.), 487
ENGLISH, THOMAS S. (*See* Moore, Berne, and English), 357
ESPERANZA-GARCÍA, CARLOS (*See* Hernández-Jáuregui, Esperanza-García, and González-Angulo), 631

F

FERACI, ROBERT P., AND SCHOUR, LIONEL. Parabiotic inhibition of murine sarcoma growth, 430
FIALLOS, E. (*See* Friesen et al.), 517
FINLAYSON, BIRDWELL. (*See* Brodman et al.), 584, 734
FISCHER, JOSEF E. (*See* Dodsworth et al.), 811
FISCHER, RONALD P. (*See* Fulton and Fischer), 881
FLEMING, WILLIAM H. (*See* Bowen, Fleming, and Thompson), 720
FONKALSRUD, ERIC W. (*See* Arima, Fonkalsrud, and Neerhout), 228
FORBES, GLENN S., GLENN, W. W. L., AND LANGE, R. C. Xenon-133 radiospirometry in electrophrenic respiration: diaphragm pacing, 398
FOX, CHARLES L., AND STANFORD, JOHN W. Comparative efficacy of hypo-, iso-, and hypertonic sodium solutions in experimental burn shock, 71
FRANCO, D. (*See* Lecompte et al.), 161
FRANTZ, STEPHEN L., KAPLITT, MARTIN J., BEIL, ARTHUR R., JR., AND STEIN, HARRY L. Ascending aorta–bilateral femoral artery bypass for the totally occluded infrarenal abdominal aorta, 471
FRIESEN, R. H. (*See* Friesen et al.), 517
FRIESEN, S. R., CROSBY, I., BOGGAN, M. D., FIALLOS, E., LEES, J. M., CUDNIK, D. B., UNDERWOOD, J., III, PECKLER, M. S., CRAIG, C. C., FRIESEN, R. H., BOLINGER, R. E., AND MCGUIGAN, J. E. An experimental study of the antral gastrin mechanism, 517
FRONEK, ARNOST, AND WITZEL, THOMAS. Hemodynamics of the terminal vascular bed in canine hemorrhagic shock, 408
FUCHS, RICHARD. (*See* Heppenstall et al.), 874
FULTON, ROBERT L., AND FISCHER, RONALD P. Pulmonary changes due to hemorrhagic shock: resuscitation with isotonic and hypertonic saline, 881

G

GEBHARD, ROGER L. (*See* Buchwald, Gebhard, and Varco), 266
GEELHOED, GLENN W., MILLAR, ROGER C., AND KETCHAM, ALFRED S. Hernia presentation of cancer in the groin, 436
GEIS, W. PETER. (See Groth et al.), 725
GELFAND, MICHAEL L. (*See* Blumenberg and Gelfand), 305
GERVIN, ALFRED S., MASON, KENNETH, LIMBIRD, TOM, AND SILVER, DONALD. Ultrapore filter–induced thrombocytopenia, 566
GILES, G. R. (*See* Keighley et al.), 578
GLENN, WILLIAM W. L. Magnification and coronary artery surgery (editorial), 629
—. (*See* Forbes, Glenn, and Lange), 398
GLOTZER, DONALD J. (*See* Silen and Glotzer, 535
GLOVER, JOHN L. (*See* Yaw et al.), 140
GOLDBAUM, LEO R. (*See* Agostini et al.), 213
GOLDSCHMIDT, Z. (*See* Abramsky and Goldschmidt) 188
GONDOS, BERNARD. (*See* Schick et al.), 348
GONZÁLEZ-ANGULO, AMADOR. (See Hernández-Jáuregui, Esperanza-García, and González-Angulo), 631
GRAHAM, EDMUND F. (*See* Rebelo et al.), 319
GRASSI, G., AND ORECCHIA, C. A comparison of intraoperative tests of completeness of vagal section, 155
GRAUSZ, HENRY. (*See* Belzer et al.), 31
GRAY, STEPHEN W., SKANDALAKIS, JOHN E., SORIA, RAUL E., AND ROWE, JOSEPH S., JR. Strangulated obturator hernia, 20
—. (*See* Skandalakis, Rowe and Gray), 148
—. (*See* Skandalakis et al.), 233
GRISELL, T. W. (*See* Yaw et al.), 140
GROTH, CARL G., HATHAWAY, WILLIAM E., GUSTAFSON, AKE, GEIS, W. PETER, PUTNAM, CHARLES W., BJORKEN, CHRISTER, PORTER, K. A., AND STARZL, THOMAS E. Correction of coagulation in the hemophilic dog by transplantation of lymphatic tissue, 725
GRUNDMANN, R., PITSCHI, H., BERR, F., AND PICHLMAIER, H. Nonpulsatile vs. pulsatile canine kidney perfusion, 178
GUMP, F. E. (*See* Halmagyi et al.), 763
GUSTAFSON, AKE. (See Groth et al.), 725

H

HACKETT, RAYMOND L. (*See* Brodman et al.), 584, 734
HAFF, RODERICK C., AND ARMSTRONG, RAYMOND G. Trends in the current management of primary hyperparathyroidism, 715
HAHN, IL SONG. (*See* Sachatello, Hahn, and Carrington), 107
HAIMOV, M. The crossover femoropopliteal bypass, 610
—, BURROWS, L., BAEZ, A., NEFF, M., AND SLIFKIN, R. Alternatives for vascular access for hemodialysis: experience with autogenous saphenous vein autografts and bovine heterografts, 447
HALFORD, PETER. (*See* Shim and Halfor), 416
HALLMAN, GRADY L. (*See* Reul et al.), 682
HALMAGYI, D. F. J., BROELL, J., GUMP, F. E., AND KINNEY, J. M. Hypermetabolism in sepsis: correlation with fever and tachycardia, 763
HANSON, E. LAWRENCE, DRINKER, PHILIP A., DON, HILLARY F., VAN DEVANTER, STEPHEN H., BONNET-EYMARD, JACQUES, AND MOORE, FRANCIS D. Venoarterial bypass with a membrane oxygenator: successful respiratory support in a woman following pulmonary hemorrhage secondary to renal failure, 557
HARDIE, I. R., CLUNIE, G. J. A., BALDERSON, GLENDA, LEDITSCHKE, J. F., AND LESLIE, I. J. A simplified kidney preservation system: further development and results of extended perfusion, 651
HARDY, MARK A. (*See* Stamford and Hardy), 496
HATHAWAY, WILLIAM E. (*See* Groth et al.), 725
HAYAKAWA, BETTY. (*See* Schick et al.), 348
HAYWARD, WILLIAM. (*See* Austin, Laffin, and Hayward), 861
HEILBRON, DAVID C. (*See* Wagner, Edmunds, and Heilbron), 91
HEPPENSTALL, R., BRUCE, LITTOOY, FRED N., FUCHS, RICHARD, SHELDON, GEORGE F., AND HUNT, THOMAS K. Gas tensions in healing tissues of traumatized patients, 874

Hernández-Jáuregui, Pablo, Esperanza-García, and González-Angulo, Amador. Morphology of the connective tissue grown in response to implanted silicone rubber: a light and electron microscopic study, 631
Hewitt, Robert L., Lolley, David M., Adrouny, George A., and Drapanas, Theodore. Protective effect of glycogen and glucose on the anoxic arrested heart, 1
Hewitt, William F. Scientists and medical writing (letter to editor), 802
Hirai, Masafumi. (*See* Shionoya et al.), 695
Hiyama, Mamoru. (*See* Akiyama and Hiyama), 674
Hobson, Robert W. (*See* Wright and Hobson), 453
Hofer, P.-A. (*See* Andersson et al.), 617
Hoff, J. (*See* Richards and Hoff), 253
Holden, William D. (*See* DePalma et al.), 915
Holmlund, D. E. W. (*See* Andersson et al.), 617
Hornung, Mario A., and Krementz, Edward T. Specific tissue and tumor responses of chimpanzees following immunization against human melanoma, 477
Hughes, Edward F. X. Halsted and American surgery, 169
Humphrey, Edward W. (*See* Schwartz et al.), 750
Hunt, Thomas K. (*See* Heppenstall et al.), 874

I

Inahara, Toshio, and Pineda, Jose D. Extraperitoneal endarterectomy for unilateral iliofemoral occlusive disease, 771
Izant, Robert J. (*See* DePalma et al.), 915

J

Jacobs, S. I. (*See* Keighley et al.), 578
James, B. E. (*See* MacMahon et al.), 660
James, J. Howard. (*See* Dodsworth et al.), 811
Jelenko, Carl, III, Wheeler, Mogan L., Anderson, Ann P., Callaway, Dianne, and Scott, Robert A., Jr. Topical lipid protection of burned subjects and their wounds, 892
Jordan, Alf. (*See* DePalma et al.), 915
Jordan, Francis R. (*See* Wu, Jordan, and Eckert), 790

K

Kaminski, Donald L. (*See* Dorighi, Kaminski, and Willman), 755
Kaplitt, Martin J. (*See* Frantz et al.), 471
Karmody, Allastair M., and Lempert, Neil. "Smooth loop" arteriovenous fistulas for hemodialysis, 238
Kartchner, Mark M., and Bogosian, A. J. Routine venography in placement of the Mobin-Uddin vena cava filter: dual filter placement in a patient with an accessory vena filter (cardinal vein), 137
Kawai, Seiichi. (*See* Shionoya et al.), 695
Keighley, M. R. B., Lister, D. M., Jacobs, S. I., and Giles, G. R. Hazards of surgical treatment due to microorganisms in the bile, 578
Keramidas, Dimitris C. Congenital incomplete prepyloric diaphragm in infants and children, 690
Ketcham, Alfred S. (*See* Geelhoed, Millar, and Ketcham), 436
King, Terry D., and Mills, Noel L. Nonoperative closure of atrial septal defects, 383
King, William, III. (*See* Tompkins and King), 243
Kinley, C. E., Paasche, P. E., MacDonald, A. S., and Marble, A. E. Stress vascular anastomosis in relation to host artery: synthetic graft diameter, 28
Kinney, J. M. (*See* Halmagyi et al.), 763
Kitahama, Akio. (*See* Olcay et al.), 64
Kormesser, Thomas W., and Bergan, John J. Anatomic control of vertebral arteriovenous fistulas, 80
Krane, Robert S. (See Cho et al.), 528
Krementz, Edward T. (See Hornung and Krementz), 477
Kurtz, Robert S. (*See* Shizgall, Kurtz, and Wood), 898

L

Laffin, David. (*See* Austin, Laffin, and Hayward), 861
Lagergren, H., Olsson, P., and Swedenborg, J. Inhibited platelet adhesion: a nonthrombogenic characteristic of a heparin-coated surface, 643
Lange, R. C. (*See* Forbes, Glenn, and Lange), 398
Lecompte, Y., Franco, D., Martin, E. D., and Bismuth, H. Liver arterialization with portacaval shunt in the cirrhotic rat, 161
Leditschke, J. F. (*See* Hardie et al.), 651
Lees, J. M. (*See* Friesen et al.), 517
Lemmi, Carlos A. E. (*See* Moore, Sinclair, and Lemmi), 203
Lempert, Neil. (*See* Karmody and Lempert), 238
Lesker, Peggy. (*See* Binnington et al.), 805
Leslie, I. J. (*See* Hardie et al.), 651
LeVeen, Harry H., Piccone, Vincent A., Jr., Diaz, Carlos, Christoudias, George, Slade, Walter, and Norstrand, Iris. A simplified correction of subclavian steal syndrome, 299
Levitsky, Sidney, Nerenberg, Rene L., Bombeck, C. Thomas, and Nyhus, Lloyd M. Are there educational advantages to a surgical clerkship in a university hospital?
Lillehei, Richard C. (*See* Rebelo et al.), 319
Lilly, John R., Weintraub, William H., and Altman, R. Peter. Spontaneous perforation of the extrahepatic bile ducts and bile peritonitis in infancy, 664
Limbird, Tom. (*See* Gervin et al.), 566
Lindenauer, S. Martin, Cerny, Joseph C., and Morley, George W. Ureterosigmoid conduit urinary diversion, 705
Lister, D. M. (*See* Keighley et al.), 578
Littooy, Fred N. (*See* Heppenstall et al.), 874
Lockwood, Dean H. (*See* White et al.), 829
Lolley, David M. (*See* Hewitt et al.), 1
Lopez-Majano, Vincent. (*See* Rhodes, Lopez-Majano, and Wagner), 153
Lorentz, William B., Jr. (*See* Berger et al.), 746

M

McDermott, F. T. (*See* MacMahon et al.), 660
MacDonald, A. S. (*See* Kinley et al.), 28
McGuigan, J. E. (*See* Friesen et al.), 517
MacMahon, R. A., Cussen, L. J., McDermott, F. T., and James, B. E. Thymidine incorporation in esophageal wounds of zinc-deficient rats, 660
Maloney, James V., Jr. (*See* Brazier et al.), 508
Marble, A. E. (*See* Kinley et al.), 28

MARCHESINI, JOÃO BATISTA, ALMEIDA CHAVES LUIS, ALBANO DE, AND CRAVO, MARCO AURELIO. Amyloidoma (a solitary nodule of the lung), 621
MARCHIORO, THOMAS L., AND TREMANN, JAMES A. A simplified method of ureteroileotomy in renal homotransplantation 129
MARTIN, E. D. (*See* Lecompte et al.), 161
MASON, EDWARD E. (*See* Thomas and Mason), 461
MASON, KENNETH. (*See* Gervin et al.), 566
MATSUBARA, JUNICHI. (*See* Shionoya et al.), 695
MAZZARIELLO, RODOLFO M. Transcholecystic extraction of residual calculi in common bile duct, 338
MILLAR, ROGER C. (*See* Geelhoed, Millar, and Ketcham), 436
MILLER, ROBERT H. (*See* Olcay et al.), 64
MILLS, LAWRENCE J. (*See* Warshaw and Mills), 296
MILLS, NOEL L. (*See* King and Mills), 383
MOODY, FRANK G. (*See* Rikkers and Moody), 421
MOORE, FRANCIS D. (*See* Hanson et al.), 557
MOORE, THOMAS C., BERNE, THOMAS V., AND ENGLISH, THOMAS S. Accelerated rejection of 36 immediate posttransplant functioning machine-preserved human cadaveric kidneys, 357
—. SINCLAIR, MICHAEL C., AND LEMMI, CARLOS A. E. Elevation in host splenic and in allograft parenchymal and capsular histidine decarboxylase activity and weights following renal allografting in rats, 203
MORLEY, GEORGE W. (See Lindenauer, Cerny, and Morley), 705
MOSES, ARNOLD M. (*See* Neumann and Moses), 869
MOUZAS, GEORGE L. (*See* Borody and Mouzas), 638
MOXLEY, RICHARD T., III. (*See* White et al.), 829
MURPHY, WILLIAM R. C. (*See* Schwartz et al.), 750
MYERS, M. BERT. Reply to letter by Ravitch (letter to editors), 476

N

NABSETH, DONALD C. (*See* Cho et al.), 528
NAJARIAN, JOHN S. (*See* Toledo-Pereyra, Simmons, and Najarian), 368
NAKATA, YUKIFUMI. (*See* Shionoya et al.), 695
NEERHOUT, ROBERT C. (*See* Arima, Fonkalsrud, and Neerhout), 228
NEFF, M. (*See* Haimov et al.), 447
NERENBERG, RENE L. (*See* Levitsky et al.), 908
NEUMANN, PATRICIA J., AND MOSES, ARNOLD M. Altered action of parathyroid hormone by chlorpropamide, 869
NICKEL, W. O. (*See* Sarin and Nickel), 442
NICOLOFF, DEMETRE M. (*See* Schwartz et al.), 750
NORSTRAND, IRIS. (*See* LeVeen et al.), 299
NYHUS, LLOYD M. (*See* Levitsky et al.), 908

O

OLCAY, ISIK, KITAHAMA, AKIO, MILLER, ROBERT H., DRAPANAS, THEODORE, TREJO, RAFAEL A., AND DI LUZIO, N. R. Reticuloendothelial dysfunction and endotoxemia following portal vein occlusion, 64
OLSSON, P. (*See* Lagergren, Olsson, and Swedenborg), 643
ORECCHIA, C. (*See* Grassi and Orecchia), 155
ORRINGER, MARK B. (*See* Sterioff, Orringer, and Cameron), 56

P

PAASCHE, P. E. (*See* Kinley et al.), 28
PATRASSI, NERI. (*See* Stefanini et al.), 597
PECKLER, M. S. (*See* Friesen et al.), 517
PERLOFF, DOROTHEE. (*See* Belzer et al.), 31
PETER, MICHAEL. (*See* Schick et al.), 348
PFAFF, WILLIAM W. (*See* Brodman et al.), 584, 734
PHILPOTT, GORDON W. Undergraduate medical education in Great Britain (editorial), 150
PICCONE, VINCENT A., JR. (*See* LeVeen et al.), 299
PICHLMAIER, H. (*See* Grundmann et al.), 178
PINDYCK, FRANK, DRUCKER, MICHAEL R., BROWN, ROBERT S., AND SHOEMAKER WILLIAM C. Cardiorespiratory effects of hypertonic glucose in the critically ill patient, 11
—. (*See* Drucker et al.), 487
PINEDA, JOSE D. (*See* Inahara and Pineda), 771
PITSCHI, H. (*See* Grundmann et al.), 178
POLK, HIRAM C., JR. Diminished surgical infection by systemic antibiotic administration in potentially contaminated operations (editorial), 312
—. (*See* Robertson and Polk), 123
PORTER, JOHN M. (*See* Snider, Porter, and Eidemiller), 613
PORTER, K. A. (*See* Groth et al.), 725
POZEFSKY, THOMAS. (*See* White et al.), 829
PRESSMAN, PETER I. Interscapulothoracic amputation for the complications of breast cancer: a new approach, 796
PUTNAM, CHARLES W. (*See* Groth et al.), 725

R

RAM, M. D. (See Watanatittan and Ram), 740
RAMIREZ, RUBEN G. (*See* Agostini et al.), 213
RAVITCH, MARK M. No need for autoclavable information (letter to editors), 471
REBELO, A. EIRA, GRAHAM, EDMUND F., CRABO, BO G., LILLEHEI, RICHARD C., AND DIETZMAN, RONALD H. Surgical preparation, perfusion techniques, and cryoprotectants used in successful freezing of the kidney, 319
REEDER, DAVID D. (*See* Becker, Reeder, and Thompson), 101, 701
REUL, GEORGE J., JR., WUKASCH, DON C., SANDIFORD, FRANK M., CHIARILLO, LUIGI, HALLMAN, GRADY L., AND COOLEY, DENTON A. Surgical treatment of abdominal angina: review of 25 patients, 682
RHODES BUCK A., LOPEZ-MAJANO, VINCENT, AND WAGNER, HENRY N., JR. Arteriovenous shunting after sympathectomy (letter to editors), 153
RICHARDS, T., AND HOFF, J. Factors affecting survival from acute subdural hematoma, 253
RIKKERS, LAYTON F., AND MOODY, FRANK G. Estimation of functional reserve of normal and regenerating dog livers, 421
RIOS, ANGELYN, AND SIMMONS, RICHARD L. Experimental cancer immunotherapy using a neuraminidase-treated non-viable frozen tumor vaccine, 503
RITCHIE, W. P. Influence of vasopressin and topical bile salts on the gastric mucosal barrier of the subhuman primate, 853
ROBERTSON, HOWARD D., AND POLK, HIRAM C., JR. The mechanism of infection in patients with diabetes mellitus: a review of leukocyte malfunction, 123
ROSOFF, C. B. (See Zimmerman et al.), 550

ROWE, JOSEPH S., JR. (*See* Gray et al.), 20
—. (*See* Skandalakis Rowe, and Gray), 148
—. (*See* Skandalakis et al.), 233
RUTHERFORD, ROBERT B. The academic surgeon and the emergency department, 259

S

SACHATELLO, CHARLES R., HAHN, IL SONG, AND CARRINGTON, CHARLES B. Juvenile gastrointestinal polyposis in a female infant: report of a case and review of the literature of a recently recognized syndrome, 107
SALTHOUSE, T. N. Nomarski differential-interference contrast microscopy: application in dermal wound healing studies, 59
SALVATIERRA, OSCAR. (*See* Belzer et al.), 31
SANDIFORD, FRANK M. (See Reul et al.), 682
SARIN, C. L., AND MICKEL, W. O. Hemodynamics of coronary circulation during ventricular fibrillation, 442
SAYEED, MOHAMMED M. (*See* Chaudry, Sayeed, and Baue), 220
SCHICK, PETER, BENFIELD, JOHN R., GONDOS, BERNARD, HAYAKAWA, BETTY, SHORS, EDWIN, SHIMADA, KOICHIRO, AND PETER, MICHAEL. Experimental lobar pneumonia in canine lung grafts, 348
SCHORS, EDWIN. (*See* Schick et al.), 348
SCHOUR, LIONEL. (*See* Feraci and Schour), 430
SCOTT, ROBERT A., JR. (*See* Jelenko et al.), 892
SCHUESSLER, JOHN S. (See Berger et al.), 746
SCHWARTZ, MICHAEL L., MURPHY, WILLIAM R. C., NICOLOFF, DEMETRE M., AND HUMPHREY, EDWARD W. Factors altering pulmonary capillary perfusion, 750
SHEEHAN, T. JOSEPH. (*See* DePalma et al.), 915
SHELDON, GEORGE F. (*See* Heppenstall et al.), 874
SHIM, WALTON T. K., AND HALFORD, PETER. Method for maintaining the neonate's intraoperative core temperature, 416
SHIMADA, KOICHIRO. (*See* Schick et al.), 348
SHINJO, KENZO. (*See* Shionoya et al.), 695
SHIONOYA, SHIGEHIKO, BAN, ICHIRO, NAKATA, YUKIFUMI, MATSUBARA, JUNICHI, SHINJO, KENZO, HIRAI, MASAFUMI, KAWAI, SEIICHI, SUZUKI, SHOICHI, AND TSAI, WEN HSIUNG. Diagnosis, pathology, and treatment of Buerger's disease, 695
SHIZGAL, HARRY M., KURTZ, ROBERT S., AND WOOD, C. DOUGLAS. Total body potassium in surgical patients, 898
SHOEMAKER, WILLIAM C. (*See* Drucker et al.), 487
—. (*See* Pindyck et al.), 11
SHUMACKER, H. B. (*See* Yaw et al), 140
SILBER, SHERMAN JAY. Chronic salt-loading of donor and recipient in renal transplantation, 573
SILEN, WILLIAM, AND GLOTZER, DONALD J. The prevention and treatment of the persistent perineal sinus, 535
SILVER, DONALD. (*See* Gervin et al.), 566
SIMMONS, RICHARD L. (*See* Rios and Simmons), 503
—. (*See* Toledo-Pereyra, Simmons, and Najarian), 368
SINCLAIR, MICHAEL C. (*See* Moore, Sinclair, and Lemmi), 203
SKANDALAKIS, JOHN E. (*See* Gray et al.), 20
—, ROWE, JOSEPH S., JR., AND GRAY, STEPHEN W. Surgical anatomy (editorial), 148
—, —, —, AND ANDROULAKIS, JOHN A. Identification of vagal structures at the esophageal hiatus, 233
SKILLMAN, JOHN JOAKIM. Postoperative deep vein thrombosis and pulmonary embolism: a selective review and personal viewpoint, 114
SLADE, WALTER. (*See* LeVeen et al.), 299
SLIFKIN, R. (*See* Haimov et al.), 447
SNIDER, RICHARD L., PORTER, JOHN M., AND EIDEMILLER, LARRY R. Inferior vena caval obstruction caused by expansion of an abdominal aortic aneurysm: report of a case and review of the literature, 613
SORIA, RAUL E. (*See* Gray et al.), 20
SPARK, R. (*See* Zimmerman et al.), 550
STAMFORD, WILLIAM P., AND HARDY, MARK A. Fatty acid absorption in jejunal autograft and allograft, 496
STANFORD, JOHN W. (*See* Fox and Stanford), 71
STARZL, THOMAS E. (*See* Groth et al.), 725
STEFANINI, PARIDE, CARBONI, MANLIO, PATRASSI, NERI, AND BASOLI, ANTONIO. Beta-islet cell tumors of the pancreas: results of a study on 1,067 cases, 597
STEIN, HARRY L. (*See* Frantz et al.), 471
STERIOFF, SYLVESTER, ORRINGER, MARK B., AND CAMERON, JOHN L. Colon perforation associated with steroid therapy, 56
STREMPLE, JOHN F., AND WATSON, CHARLES G. Serum calcium, serum gastrin, and gastric acid secretion before and after parathyroidectomy for hyperparathyroidism, 841
SUMNER, HATTON. (*See* Binnington et al.), 805
SUZUKI, SHOICHI. (*See* Shionoya et al.), 695
SWEDENBORG, J. (*See* Lagergren, Olsson, and Swedenborg), 643

T

TERNBERG, JESSIE L. (*See* Binnington et al.), 805
TERRY, DANIEL B., JR. (*See* Abouna, Veazey, and Terry), 194
THOMAS, JOHN W., AND MASON, EDWARD E. The effects of gastric exclusion operations on pancreatic exocrine secretion, 461
THOMPSON, JAMES C. (*See* Becker, Reeder, and Thompson), 101, 701
—. (*See* Bowen, Fleming, and Thompson), 720
TILNEY, NICHOLAS L. A broadening of vision: observation on the practice of surgery in a university hospital in Great Britain, 776
TOLEDO-PEREYRA, LUIS H., SIMMONS, RICHARD L., AND NAJARIAN, JOHN S. Prolonged survival of canine orthotopic small intestinal allografts preserved for 24 hours by hypothermic bloodless perfusion, 368
TOMPKINS, RONALD K., AND KING, WILLIAM, III. Investigations of the enterobiliary metabolism of lecithin, 243
TOSATTI, BIANCA. Transplantation and reimplantation in the arts, 389
TRAVIS, LUTHER B. (*See* Berger et al.), 746
TREJO, RAFAEL A. (*See* Olcay et al.), 64
TREMANN, JAMES A. (*See* Marchioro and Tremann), 129
TSAI, WEN HSIUNG. (*See* Shionoya et al.), 695
TYSON, KENNETH R. T. (*See* Berger et al.), 746

U

UNDERWOOD, J., III. (*See* Friesen et al.), 517

V

VAN DEVANTER, STEPHEN H. (*See* Hanson et al.), 557
VARCO, RICHARD L. (*See* Buchwald, Coyle, and Varco), 821
—. (*See* Buchwald, Gebhard, and Varco), 266
VEAZEY, PHILIP R. (*See* Abouna, Veazey, and Terry), 194
VEITH, FRANK J. (*See* Dardik, Dardik, and Veith), 377

W

WAGNER, OTTO A., EDMUNDS, L. HENRY, JR., AND HEILBRON, DAVID C. Vascular pressure-flow relationships in denervated and reimplanted lungs, 91
WAHLE, W. M. (*See* Yaw et al.), 140
WARSHAW, ANDREW L., AND MILLS, LAWRENCE J. Starch pleuritis: a postthoracotomy syndrome possibly caused by surgical glove powder, 296
WATANATITTAN, SUKAWAT, AND RAM, M. D. Nonsimultaneous bilateral breast carcinoma, 740
WATSON, CHARLES G. (*See* Stremple and Watson), 841
WEINTRAUB, WILLIAM H. (*See* Lilly, Weintraub, and Altman), 664
WELLS, SAMUEL A., JR., AND CHRISTIANSEN, CHRISTINE. The transplanted parathyroid gland: evaluation of cryopreservation and other environmental factors which affect its function, 49
WENDEL, H. (*See* Andersson et al.), 617
WHEELER, MOGAN L. (*See* Jelenko et al.), 892
WHITE, JOHN J., MOXLEY, RICHARD T., III, POZEFSKY, THOMAS, AND LOCKWOOD, DEAN H. Transient kwashiorkor: a cause of fatty liver following small bowel bypass, 829
WILLMAN VALLEE L. (*See* Dorighi, Kaminski, and Willman), 755
WITZEL, THOMAS. (*See* Fronek and Witzel), 408
WOOD, C. DOUGLAS. (*See* Shizgal, Kurtz, and Wood), 898
WRIGHT, CREIGHTON B., AND HOBSON, ROBERT W. Hemodynamic effects of femoral venous occlusion in the subhuman primate, 453
WU, KWANG-TZEN, JORDAN, FRANCIS R., AND ECKERT, CHARLES. Lipoma, a cause of paralysis of deep radial (posterior interosseous) nerve: report of a case and review of the literature, 790
WUKASCH, DON C. (*See* Reul et al.), 682

Y

YAW, PETER B., GRISELL, T. W., WAHLE, W. M., SHUMACKER, H. B, AND GLOVER, JOHN L. Fate of a nylon vascular prosthesis for aortic replacement: 14 year follow-up study, 140

Z

ZIMMERMAN, C. E., EISENBERG, H., SPARK, R., AND ROSOFF, C. B. Transvenous adrenal destruction: clinical trials in patients with metastatic malignancy, 550
ZUIDEMA, GEORGE. A single step (editorial), 626

SUBJECT INDEX*

A

Abdominal angina, surgical treatment of: review of 25 patients (Reul et al.), 682
aorta, infrarenal, totally occluded, ascending aorta–bilateral femoral artery bypass for (Frantz et al.), 471
aneurysm, inferior vena caval obstruction caused by expansion of: report of case and review of literature (Snider, Porter, and Eidemiller), 613
Academic surgeon and emergency department (Rutherford), 259
Acid absorption, fatty, in jejunal autograft and allograft (Stamford and Hardy), 496
gastric, serum calcium, and serum gastrin secretion before and after parathyroidectomy for hyperparathyroidism (Stremple and Watson), 841
hydrochloric, for treatment of severe metabolic alkalosis, intravenous infusion of (Abouna et al.), 194
Adenosine triphosphate–magnesium chloride administration in shock, effect of (Chaudry et al.), 213
Adhesion, platelet, inhibited: non-thrombogenic characteristic of heparin-coated surface (Lagergren, Olsson, and Swedenborg), 643
Adrenal destruction, transvenous: clinical trials in patients with metastatic malignancy (Zimmerman et al.), 550
Alkalosis, metabolic, severe, intravenous infusion of hydrochloric acid for treatment of (Abouna et al.), 194
Allograft and autograft, jejunal, fatty acid absorption in (Stamford and Hardy), 496
and host splenic parenchymal and capsular histidine decarboxylase activity and weights following renal allografting in rats, elevation in (Moore et al.), 203
renal, in rats, elevation in host splenic and in allograft parenchymal and capsular histidine decarboxylase activity and weights following (Moore et al.), 203
small intestinal, orthotopic, canine, preserved for 24 hours by hypothermic bloodless perfusion, prolonged survival of (Toledo-Pereyra et al.), 368
Allotransplantation, renal, obturator intestinal obstruction following: relief with hyperosmolar enemas (Berger et al.), 746
American surgery and Halsted (Hughes), 169
Amputation, interscapulothoracic for complications of breast cancer: new approach (Pressman), 796
Amyloidoma (solitary nodule of lung) (Marchesini, Almeida Chaves Luis, and Cravo), 621
Anastomosis, microvascular: device for holding stay sutures and new vascular clamp (Acland), 185
superficial temporal artery–to–middle cerebral artery, physiologic factors in selection of patients for (Austin, Laffin, and Hayward), 861

*January, pp. 1-154; February, pp. 155-318; March, pp. 319-476; April, pp. 477-630; May, pp. 631-804; June, pp. 805-966.

Anastomosis—Cont'd
vascular, in relation to host artery, stress at: synthetic graft diameter (Kinley et al.), 28
Anatomic control of vertebral arteriovenous fistulas (Kornmesser and Bergan), 80
Anatomy, surgical (Skandalakis et al.) (editorial), 148
Anemia, normovolemic, acute, adequacy of myocardial oxygen delivery in (Brazier et al.), 508
Aneurysm, aortic, abdominal, inferior vena caval obstruction caused by expansion of: report of case and review of literature (Snider, Porter, and Eidemiller), 613
mycotic, successful management of: report of case (Cooke and Ehrenfeld), 132
Angina, abdominal, surgical treatment of: review of 25 patients (Reul et al.), 682
Anoxic arrested heart, protective effect of glycogen and glucose on (Hewitt et al.), 1
Antibiotic administration, systemic, in potentially contaminated operations, diminished surgical infection by (Polk) (editorial), 312
Antral gastrin mechanism, experimental study of (Friesen et al.), 517
Aorta, ascending–bilateral femoral artery bypass for totally occluded infrarenal abdominal aorta (Frantz et al.), 471
Aortic aneurysm, abdominal, inferior vena caval obstruction caused by expansion of: report of case and review of literature (Snider, Porter, and Eidemiller), 613
mycotic, successful management of: report of case (Cooke and Ehrenfeld), 132
replacement, fate of nylon vascular prosthesis for: 14 year follow-up study (Yaw et al.), 140
Arterialization, liver, with portacaval shunt in cirrhotic rat (Lecompte et al.), 161
Arteriovenous fistulas, "smooth loop," for hemodialysis (Karmody and Lempert), 238
vertebral, anatomic control of (Kornmesser and Bergan), 80
shunting after sympathectomy (Rhodes et al.) (letter to editors), 153; reply (Delaney and Scarpino), 154
Artery(ies), coronary, surgery and magnification (Glenn) (editorial), 629
femoral, bilateral–ascending aorta bypass for totally occluded infrarenal abdominal aorta (Frantz et al.), 471
host, stress at vascular anastomosis in relation to: synthetic graft diameter (Kinley et al.), 28
occlusion, renal, total, microangiography of renal vasculature following (Brodman et al.), 734
renal, surgical correction of advanced fibromuscular dysplasia of (Belzer et al.), 31
superficial temporal, –to–middle cerebral artery anastomosis, physiologic factors in selection of patients for (Austin, Laffin, and Hayward), 861
tibial-peroneal, by single lateral approach, exposure of (Dardik et al.), 377
Arts, transportation and reimplantation in (Tosatti), 389

Atresia, biliary, surgically correctable, experiences in the management of (Arima et al.), 228
Atrial septal defects, nonoperative closure of (King and Mills), 383
Atropine on basal and food-stimulated serum gastrin levels in man, effect of (Becker, Reeder, and Thompson), 701
Author the writer, is: Rewriting and by-line (DeBakey), 38
Authorship, honesty in (DeBakey) (letter to editors; reply to letter by Hewitt), 802
Autoclavable information, no need for (Ravitch) (letter to editor), 476; reply (Myers), 476
Autograft(s) and allograft, jejunal, fatty acid absorption in (Stamford and Hardy), 496
vein, saphenous, autogenous, and bovine heterografts, experience with: alternatives for vascular access for hemodialysis (Haimov et al.), 447

B

Beta-islet cell tumors of pancreas: results of study on 1,067 cases (Stefanini et al.), 597
Bilateral breast carcinoma, non-simultaneous (Watanatittan and Ram), 740
Bile duct, common, transcholecystic extraction of residual calculi in (Mazzariello), 338
extrahepatic, and bile peritonitis in infancy, spontaneous perforation of (Lilly, Weintraub, and Altman), 664
hazards of surgical treatment due to microorganisms in (Keighley et al.), 578
salts, topical, and vasopressin on gastric mucosal barrier of subhuman primate, influence of (Ritchie), 853
and upper and lower small intestinal washings of bile fistula rabbit, relative secretion of cholesterol-4-^{14}C in (Buchwald et al.), 266
Biliary atresia, surgically correctable, experiences in management of (Arima et al.), 228
Blood flow, hepatic, in man, measurement of (Bradley), 783
stored, problems associated with massive transfusion of (Collins), 271
supply of experimental liver metastases: changes in vascularity with increasing tumor growth (Ackerman), 589
Bloodless perfusion, hypothermic, prolonged survival of canine orthotopic small intestinal allografts preserved for 24 hours by (Toledo-Pereyra et al.), 368
Body asanguineous hypothermic perfusion, total, successful reversal of lethal carbon monoxide intoxication by (Agostini et al.), 213
Bowel, small, bypass, cause of fatty liver following: transient kwashiorkor (White et al.), 829
on gastric secretory function, effect of: postintestinal exclusion hypersecretion, phenomenon in search of syndrome (Buchwald, Coyle, and Varco), 821
secretory function: postintestinal exclusion hypersecretion, phenomenon in search of syndrome (Buchwald, Coyle, and Varco), 821
Brain norepinephrine in acute hepatic coma, depletion of (Dodsworth et al.), 811
Breast cancer, interscapulothoracic amputation for complications of: new approach (Pressman), 796
carcinoma, bilateral, non-simultaneous (Watanatittan and Ram), 740
Breech-born infants, pinhole colonic perforation in (Andersson et al.), 617
Buerger's disease, diagnosis, pathology, and treatment (Shionoya et al.), 695
Burn shock, experimental, comparative efficacy of hypo-, iso-, and hypertonic sodium solutions in (Fox and Stanford), 71
subjects and their wounds, topical lipid protection of (Jelenko et al.), 892
By-line and rewriting: is author the writer? (DeBakey), 38
Bypass, ascending aorta–bilateral femoral artery, for totally occluded infrarenal abdominal aorta (Frantz et al.), 471
esophageal, operation, simple, by high gastric division (Akiyama and Hiyama), 674
femoropopliteal, crossover (Haimov), 610
small bowel, cause of fatty liver following: transient kwashiorkor (White et al.), 829
on gastric secretory function, effect of: postintestinal exclusion hypersecretion, phenomenon in search of syndrome (Buchwald, Coyle, and Varco), 821
venoarterial, with membrane oxygenator: successful respiratory support in woman following pulmonary hemorrhage secondary to renal failure (Hanson et al.), 557

C

Calcium, serum, gastric acid secretion, and serum gastrin before and after parathyroidectomy for hyperparathyroidism (Stremple and Watson), 841
Calculi, residual, in common bile duct, transcholecystic extraction of (Mazzariello), 338
Cancer, breast, interscapulothoracic amputation for complications of: new approach (Pressman), 796
in groin, hernia presentation of (Geelhoed et al.), 436
immunotherapy, experimental, using a neuraminidase-treated non-viable frozen tumor vaccine (Rios and Simmons), 503
oral, laryngeal, and pharyngeal, deglutition after resection of (Doberneck and Antoine), 87
Capillary perfusion, pulmonary, factors altering (Schwartz et al.), 750
Capsular and parenchymal histidine decarboxylase activity and weights, host splenic and allograft, following renal allografting in rats, elevation in (Moore et al.), 203
Carbon monoxide intoxication, lethal, by total body asanguineous hypothermic perfusion, successful reversal of (Agostini et al.), 213
Carcinoma, breast, bilateral, non-simultaneous (Watanatittan and Ram), 740
Cardiorespiratory effects of hypertonic glucose in critically ill patient (Pindyk et al.), 11
variables in critically ill patient, interaction of glucagon and glucose (Drucker et al.), 487

Carotid intimal tear following blunt craniocervical trauma (Crissey and Bernstein), 543
Cava, vena, filter, Mobin-Uddin, routine venography in placement of: dual filter placement in patient with accessory vena filter (cardinal vein) (Kartchner and Bogosian), 137
Cerebral artery, middle, –to–superficial temporal artery anastomosis, physiologic factors in selection of patients for (Austin, Laffin, and Hayward), 861
Chlorpropamide, altered action of parathyroid hormone by (Neumann and Moses), 869
Cholecystokinin and secretin, endogenous, on pentagastrin-stimulated innervated and denervated gastric mucosa, effect of (Dorighi, Kaminski, and Willman), 755
Cholesterol-4-^{14}C in bile and upper and lower small intestinal washings of bile fistula rabbit, relative secretion of (Buchwald et al.), 266
Cirrhotic rat, liver arterialization with portacaval shunt (Lecompte et al.), 161
Clamp, vascular, new, and device for holding stay sutures: microvascular anastomosis (Acland), 185
Clerkship, surgical, in university hospital, are there educational advantages to? (Levitsky et al.), 898
Coagulation in hemophilic dog by transplantation of lymphatic tissue, correction of (Groth et al.), 725
Collagen, microcrystalline, as topical hemostatic agent for vascular surgery (Abbott and Austen), 915
Colon perforation associated with steroid therapy (Sterioff et al.), 56
  pinhole, in breech-born infants (Andersson et al.), 617
Coma, hepatic, acute, depletion of brain norepinephrine in (Dodsworth et al.), 811
Congenital incomplete prepyloric diaphragm in infants and children (Keramidas), 690
Core temperature, intraoperative, neonate's, method for maintaining (Shim and Halford), 416
Coronary artery surgery and magnification (Glenn) (editorial), 629
Craniocervical trauma, blunt, delayed presentation of carotid intimal tear following (Crissey and Bernstein), 543
Cryopreservation and other factors which affect its function, evaluation of: transplanted parathyroid gland (Wells and Christiansen), 49
Cryoprotectants, perfusion techniques, and surgical preparation used in successful freezing of kidney (Rebelo et al.), 319

D

Decarboxylase, histidine, activity and weights, host splenic and allograft parenchymal and capsular, following renal allografting in rats, elevation in (Moore et al.), 203
Deglutition after resection of oral, laryngeal, and pharyngeal cancers (Doberneck and Antoine), 87
Department, emergency, and academic surgeon (Rutherford), 259
Dermal wound healing studies, application in: Nomarski differential-interference contrast microscopy (Salthouse), 59
Diabetes mellitus, mechanism of infection in patients with: review of leukocyte malfunction (Robertson and Polk), 123
Diaphragm pacing: xenon-133 radiospirometry in electrophrenic respiration (Forbes et al.), 398
Dilemma, young surgeon's (Dardik) (letter to editors), 630
Disease, Buerger's, diagnosis, pathology, and treatment (Shionoya et al.), 695
  occlusive, iliofemoral, unilateral, extraperitoneal endarterectomy for (Inahara and Pineda), 771
Division, gastric, high, simple esophageal bypass operation by (Akiyama and Hiyama), 674
Drainage, venous, of ischemic kidney (Brodman et al.), 584
Duct, bile, common, transcholecystic extraction of residual calculi in (Mazzariello), 338
  extrahepatic, and bile peritonitis in infancy, spontaneous perforation of (Lilly, Weintraub, and Altman), 664
Dye-dilution vs. pulse contour methods (Bradley) (letter to editors), 317
Dysplasia, fibromuscular, advanced, of renal arteries, surgical correction of (Belzer et al.), 31

E

Education, surgical, undergraduate, objectives and methods in (DePalma et al.), 915
Educational advantages to surgical clerkship in university hospital, are there? (Levitsky et al.), 898
Electrophrenic respiration, xenon-133 radiospirometry in: diaphragm pacing (Forbes et al.), 398
Embolism, pulmonary, and postoperative deep vein thrombosis: selective review and personal viewpoint (Skillman), 114
Emergency department and academic surgeon (Rutherford), 259
Encephalopathy, hepatic, acute, by intravenous levodopa, treatment and prevention (Abramsky and Goldschmidt), 188
Endarterectomy, extraperitoneal, for unilateral iliofemoral occlusive disease (Inahara and Pineda), 771
Endotoxemia and reticuloendothelial dysfunction following portal vein occlusion (Olcay et al.), 64
Enemas, hyperosmolar, relief with: obturator intestinal obstruction following renal allotransplantation (Berger et al.), 746
Enterobiliary metabolism of lecithin, investigations of (Tompkins and King), 243
Esophageal bypass, operation, simple, by high gastric division (Akiyama and Hiyama), 674
  hiatus, identification of vagal structures at (Skandalakis et al.), 233
  wounds of zinc-deficient rats, thymidine incorporation in (MacMahon et al.), 660
Exclusion, gastric, operations on pancreatic exocrine secretion, effects of (Thomas and Mason), 461
Exocrine secretion, pancreatic, effects of gastric exclusion operations of (Thomas and Mason), 461

Extraction, transcholecystic, of residual calculi in common bile duct (Mazzariello), 338
Extraperitoneal endarterectomy for unilateral iliofemoral occlusive disease (Inahara and Pineda), 771

F

Factors altering pulmonary capillary perfusion (Schwartz et al.), 750
Fatty acid absorption in jejunal autograft and allograft (Stamford and Hardy), 496
Femoral artery, bilateral–ascending aorta bypass for totally occluded infrarenal abdominal aorta (Frantz et al.), 471
venous occlusion in subhuman primate, hemodynamic effects of (Wright and Hobson), 453
Femoropopliteal, bypass, crossover (Haimov), 610
Fever and tachycardia, correlation with: hypermetabolism in sepsis (Halmagyi et al.), 763
Fibromuscular dysplasia, advanced, of renal arteries, surgical correction of (Belzer et al.), 31
Filter, ultrapore–induced thrombocytopenia (Gervin et al.), 566
vena cava, Mobin-Uddin, routine venography in placement of: dual filter placement in patient with accessory vena filter (cardinal vein) (Kartchner and Bogosian), 137
Fistulas, arteriovenous "smooth loop," for hemodialysis (Karmody and Lempert), 238
vertebral, anatomic control of (Kornmesser and Bergan), 80
bile, rabbit, relative secretion of cholesterol-4-^{14}C in bile and upper and lower small intestinal washings of (Buchwald et al.), 266
Flow, blood, hepatic, in man, measurement of (Bradley), 783
Flow-pressure relationships, vascular, in denervated and reimplanted lungs of dogs (Wagner et al.), 91
Fracture patients immobilized in plaster of Paris, protection of skin of (Boroda and Mouzas), 638
Freezing, successful, of kidney, surgical preparation, perfusion techniques, and cryoprotectants used in (Rebelo et al.), 319

G

Gas tensions in healing tissues of traumatized patients (Heppenstall et al.), 874
Gastric acid, serum calcium, and serum gastrin secretion before and after parathyroidectomy for hyperparathyroidism (Stremple and Watson), 841
division, high, simple esophageal bypass operation by (Akiyama and Hiyama), 674
exclusion operations on pancreatic exocrine secretion, effects of (Thomas and Mason), 461
mucosa, innervated and denervated, pentagastrin-stimulated, effect of endogenous secretin and cholecystokinin on (Dorighi, Kaminski, and Willman), 755
mucosal barrier of subhuman primate, influence of vasopressin and topical bile salts (Ritchie), 853
Gastric—Cont'd
secretory function, effect of small bowel bypass on: postintestinal exclusion hypersecretion, phenomenon in search of syndrome (Buchwald, Coyle, and Varco), 821
Gastrin, antral, mechanism, experimental study of (Friesen et al.), 517
direct measurement of vagal release of (Becker et al.), 101
release, increased, following penetrating central nervous system injury (Bowen, Fleming, and Thompson), 720
serum, basal and food-stimulated, levels in man, effect of atropine on (Becker, Reeder, and Thompson), 701
gastric acid secretion, and serum calcium before and after parathyroidectomy for hyperparathyroidism (Stremple and Watson), 841
Gastrointestinal polyposis, juvenile, in female infant: report of case and review of literature of recently recognized syndrome (Sachatello et al.), 107
Gland, parathyroid, transplanted: evaluation of cryopreservation and other environmental factors which affect its function (Wells and Christiansen), 49
Glove powder, surgical, postthoracotomy syndrome possibly caused by: starch pleuritis (Warshaw and Mills), 296
Glucagon and glucose on cardiorespiratory variables in critically ill patients, interaction of (Drucker et al.), 487
Glucose and glucagon on cardiorespiratory variables in critically ill patient, interaction of (Drucker et al.), 487
and glycogen on anoxic arrested heart, protective effect of (Hewitt et al.), 1
hypertonic, in critically ill patients, cardiorespiratory effects of (Pindyck et al.), 11
and improved critical organ performance (Egdahl) editorial), 145
Glycogen and glucose on anoxic arrested heart, protective effect of (Hewitt et al.), 1
Grafts, lung, canine, experimental lobar pneumonia in (Schick et al.), 348
synthetic, diameter: stress at vascular anastomosis in relation to host artery (Kinley et al.), 28
Great Britain, observation on practice of surgery in university hospital: broadening of vision (Tilney), 776
undergraduate medical education in (Philpott) (editorial), 150
Groin, hernia presentation of cancer in (Geelhoed et al.), 436

H

Halsted and American surgery (Hughes), 169
Healing, wound, studies, dermal, application in: Nomarski differential-interference contrast microscopy (Salthouse), 59
Heart, arrested, anoxic, protective effect of glycogen and glucose on (Hewitt et al.), 1
Hematoma, subdural, acute, factors affecting survival from (Richards and Hoff), 253
Hemodialysis, alternatives for vascular access: experience with autogenous saphenous vein autographs and bovine heterografts (Haimov et al.), 447

Hemodialysis—Cont'd
"smooth loop" arteriovenous fistula for (Karmody and Lempert), 238
Hemodynamic(s) effects of femoral venous occlusion in subhuman primate (Wright and Hobson), 453
of terminal vascular bed in canine hemorrhagic shock (Fronek and Witzel), 408
Hemophilic dog by transplantation of lymphatic tissue, correction of coagulation in (Groth et al.), 725
Hemorrhage, pulmonary, secondary to renal failure, successful respiratory support in woman following: venoarterial bypass with membrane oxygenator (Hanson et al.), 557
Hemorrhagic shock, canine, hemodynamics of terminal vascular bed in (Fronek and Witzel), 408
pulmonary changes due to: resuscitation with isotonic and hypertonic saline (Fulton and Fischer), 881
Hemostatic agent, topical, for vascular surgery, microcrystalline collagen as (Abbott and Austen), 915
Heparin-coated surface, non-thrombogenic characteristic of: inhibited platelet adhesion (Lagergren, Olsson, and Swedenborg), 643
Hepatic blood flow in man, measurement of (Bradley), 783
coma, acute, depletion of brain norepinephrine in (Dodsworth et al.), 811
encephalopathy, acute, by intravenous levodopa, treatment and prevention of (Abramsky and Goldschmidt), 188
Hernia, obturator, strangulated (Gray et al.), 20
presentation of cancer in groin (Geelhoed et al.), 436
Heterografts, bovine, and autogenous saphenous vein autografts, experience with: alternatives for vascular access for hemodialysis (Haimov et al.), 447
Hiatus, esophageal, identification of vagal structures at (Skandalakis et al.), 233
Histidine decarboxylase activity and weights, host splenic and allograft parenchymal and capsular, following renal allografting in rats, elevation in (Moore et al.), 203
Homotransplantation, renal, simplified method of ureteroileotomy in (Marchioro and Tremann), 129
Honesty in authorship (DeBakey) letter to editors; (reply to letter by Hewitt), 802
Hormone, parathyroid, by chlorpropamide, altered action of (Neumann and Moses), 869
Hospital, university, are there educational advantages to surgical clerkship in? (Levitsky et al.), 908
in Great Britain, observation on practice of surgery in: broadening of vision (Tilney), 776
Hydrochloric acid for treatment of severe metabolic alkalosis, intravenous infusion of (Abouna et al.), 194
Hypermetabolism in sepsis: correlation with fever and tachycardia (Halmagyi et al.), 763
Hyperosmolar enemas, relief with: obturator intestinal obstruction following renal allotransplanation (Berger et al.), 746
Hyperparathyroidism, primary, trends in current management of (Haff and Armstrong), 715
Hypersecretion, exclusion, postintestinal, phenomenon in search of syndrome: effect of small bowel bypass on gastric secretory function (Buchwald, Coyle, and Varco), 821
Hypertonic glucose in critically ill patient, cardiorespiratory effects of (Pindyck et al.), 11
and isotonic saline, resuscitation with: pulmonary changes due to hemorrhagic shock (Fulton and Fischer), 881
Hypothermic bloodless perfusion, prolonged survival of canine orthotopic small intestinal allografts preserved for 24 hours by (Toledo-Pereyra et al.), 368
perfusion, asanguineous, total body, successful reversal of lethal carbon monoxide intoxication by (Agostini et al.), 213

I

Iliofemoral occlusive disease, unilateral, extraperitoneal endarterectomy for (Inahara and Pineda), 771
Immunization against human melanoma, specific tissue and tumor responses of chimpanzees following (Hornung and Krementz), 477
Immunotherapy, cancer, experimental, using a neuraminidase-treated non-viable frozen tumor vaccine (Rios and Simmons), 496
Infection in patients with diabetes mellitus, mechanism of: review of leukocyte malfunction (Robertson and Polk), 123
surgical, diminished, by systemic antibiotic administration in potentially contaminated operations (Polk) (editorial), 312
emerging concepts in control of (Alexander), 934
Infrarenal abdominal aorta, totally occluded ascending aorta–bilateral femoral artery bypass for (Frantz et al.), 471
Infusion, intravenous, of hydrochloric acid for treatment of severe metabolic alkalosis (Abouna et al.), 194
Injury, central nervous system, penetrating, increased gastrin release following (Bowen, Fleming, and Thompson), 720
Interscapulothoracic amputation for complications of breast cancer: new approach (Pressman), 796
Intestinal obstruction, obturator, following renal allotransplantation: relief with hyperosmolar enemas (Berger et al.), 746
post-, exclusion hypersecretion, phenomenon in search of syndrome: effect of small bowel bypass on gastric secretory function (Buchwald, Coyle, and Varco), 821
small, allografts preserved for 24 hours by hypothermic bloodless perfusion, prolonged survival of (Toledo-Pereyra et al.), 368
upper and lower, washings and bile of bile fistula rabbit, relative secretion of cholesterol-4-^{14}C in (Buchwald et al.), 266

Intimal tear, carotid, following blunt craniocervical trauma, delayed presentation of (Crissey and Bernstein), 543
Intoxication, carbon monoxide, lethal, by total body asanguineous hypothermic perfusion, successful reversal of (Agostini et al.), 213
Ischemic kidney, venous drainage of (Brodman et al.), 584
Isotonic and hypertonic saline, resuscitation with: pulmonary changes due to hemorrhagic shock (Fulton and Fischer), 881

J

Jejunal autograft and allograft, fatty acid absorption in (Stamford and Hardy), 496
  neomucosa, functional characteristics of surgically induced (Binnington et al.), 805
Juvenile gastrointestinal polyposis in female infant: report of case and review of literature of recently recognized syndrome (Sachatello et al.), 107

K

Kidneys, cadaveric, human, machine-preserved, functioning, immediate posttransplant, accelerated rejection of 36 (Moore et al.), 357
  ischemic, venous drainage of (Brodman et al.), 584
  perfusion, canine, nonpulsatile vs. pulsatile (Grundmann et al.), 178
  preservation system, simplified: further development and results of extended perfusion (Hardie et al.), 651
  surgical preparation, perfusion techniques, and cryoprotectants used in successful freezing of (Rebelo et al.), 319
Kwashiorkor, transient: cause of fatty liver following a small bowel bypass (White et al.), 829

L

Laryngeal, pharyngeal, and oral cancers, deglutition after resection of (Doberneck and Antoine), 87
Lecithin, investigations of enterobiliary metabolism of (Tompkins and King), 243
Leukocyte malfunction, review of: mechanism of infection in patients with diabetes mellitus (Robertson and Polk), 123
Levodopa, intravenous, treatment and prevention of acute hepatic encephalopathy by (Abramsky and Goldschmidt), 188
Lipid protection, topical, of burned subjects and their wounds (Jelenko et al.), 892
Lipoma, cause of paralysis of deep radial (posterior interosseous) nerve: report of case and review of literature (Wu, Jordan, and Eckert), 790
Liver arterialization with portacaval shunt in cirrhotic rat (Lecompte et al.), 161
  dog, normal and regenerating, estimation of functional reserve of (Rikkers and Moody), 421
  fatty, following small bowel bypass, cause of: transient kwashiorkor (White et al.), 829
  metastases, experimental, blood supply of: changes in vascularity with increasing tumor growth (Ackerman), 589

"Loop, smooth," arteriovenous fistulas for hemodialysis (Karmody and Lempert), 238
Lung(s), denervated and reimplanted, of dogs, vascular pressure-flow relationships in (Wagner et al.), 91
  grafts, canine, experimental lobar pneumonia in (Schick et al.), 348
  solitary nodule of (amyloidoma) (Marchesini, Almeida Chavez Luis, and Cravo), 621
Lymphatic tissue, correction of coagulation in hemophilic dog by transplantation of (Groth et al.), 725

M

Machine-preserved human cadaveric kidneys, functioning, immediate posttransplant, accelerated rejection of 36 (Moore et al.), 357
Magnesium chloride-adenosine triphosphate administration in shock, effect of (Chaudry et al.), 213
Magnification and coronary artery surgery (Glenn) (editorial), 629
Malignancy, metastatic, clinical trials in patients with: transvenous adrenal destruction (Zimmerman et al.), 550
Management, current, of primary hyperparathyroidism, trends in (Haff and Armstrong), 715
Medical education, undergraduate, in Great Britain (Philpott) (editorial), 150
  writing, scientists and (Hewitt) (letter to editors), 802; reply (DeBakey), 802
Melanoma, human, specific tissue and tumor responses of chimpanzees following immunization against (Hornung and Krementz), 477
Membrane oxygenator, venoarterial bypass with: successful respiratory support in woman following pulmonary hemorrhage secondary to renal failure (Hanson et al.), 550
Metabolic alkalosis, severe, intravenous infusion of hydrochloric acid for treatment of (Abouna et al.), 194
Metabolism, enterobiliary, of lecithin, investigations of (Tompkins and King), 243
Metastases, liver, experimental, blood supply of: changes in vascularity with increasing tumor growth, 589
Metastatic malignancy, clinical trials in patients with: transvenous adrenal destruction (Zimmerman et al.), 550
Methods, pulse contour vs. dye-dilution (Bradley) (letter to editors), 317
Microangiography of renal vasculature following total renal artery occlusion (Brodman et al.), 734
Microcrystalline collagen as topical hemostatic agent for vascular surgery (Abbott and Austen), 915
Microorganisms in bile, hazards of surgical treatment due to (Keighley et al.), 578
Microscopic study, electron and light: morphology of connective tissue grown in response to implanted silicone rubber (Hernández-Jáuregui, Esperanza-García, and González-Angulo), 631
Microscopy, contrast, differential-interference, Nomarski: application in dermal wound healing studies (Salthouse), 59

Microvascular anastomosis: device for holding stay sutures and new vascular clamp (Acland), 185
Mobin-Uddin vena cava filter, routine venography in placement of: dual filter placement in patient with accessory vena filter (cardinal vein) Kartchner and Bogosian), 137
Mucosa, gastric, innervated and denervated, pentagastrin-stimulated, effect of endogenous secretin and cholecystokinin on (Dorighi, Kaminski, and Willman), 755
Mucosal barrier, gastric, of subhuman primate, influence of vasopressin and topical bile salts on (Ritchie), 853
Myocardial oxygen delivery in acute normovolemic anemia, adequacy of (Brazier et al.), 508

N

Neomucosa, jejunal, surgically induced, functional characteristics of (Binnington et al.), 805
Neonate's intraoperative core temperature, method for maintaining (Shim and Halford), 416
Nerve, radial (posterior interosseous), deep, lipoma, cause of paralysis of: report of case and review of literature (Wu, Jordan, and Eckert), 790
Neuraminidase-treated nonviable frozen tumor vaccine, experimental cancer immunotherapy using (Rios and Simmons), 503
New England area, regional organ preservation program in (Cho et al.), 528
Nodule, solitary, of lung (amyloidoma) (Marchesini, Almeida Chavez Luis, and Cravo), 621
Nomarski differential-interference contrast microscopy: application in dermal wound healing studies (Salthouse), 59
Norepinephrine, brain, in acute hepatic coma, depletion of (Dodsworth et al.), 811

O

Obturator hernia, strangulated (Gray et al.), 20
  intestinal obstruction following renal allotransplantation: relief with hyperosmolar enemas (Berger et al.), 746
Occlusion, artery, renal, total, microangiography of renal vasculature following (Brodman et al.), 734
  vein, portal, reticuloendothelial dysfunction and endotoxemia following (Olcay et al.), 64
Occlusive disease, iliofemoral, unilateral, extraperitoneal endarterectomy for (Inahara and Pineda), 771
Operations, exclusion, gastric, on pancreatic exocrine secretion, effects of (Thomas and Mason), 461
  potentially contaminated, diminished surgical infection by systemic antibiotic administration in (Polk) (editorial), 312
Oral, laryngeal, and pharyngeal cancers, deglutition after resection of (Doberneck and Antoine), 87
Organ, critical, performance, hypertonic glucose and (Egdahl) (editorial), 145
  preservation program, regional, in New England area (Cho et al.), 528
  procurement, role of paramedical personnel in (Belzer) (editorial), 315
Oxygen, myocardial, delivery in acute normovolemic anemia, adequacy of (Brazier et al.), 508
Oxygenator, membrane, venoarterial bypass with successful respiratory support in woman following pulmonary hemorrhage secondary to renal failure (Hanson et al.), 550

P

Pacing, diaphragm: xenon-133 radiospirometry in electrophrenic respiration (Forbes et al.), 398
Pancreas, beta-islet cell tumors of: results of study on 1,067 cases (Stefanini et al.), 597
Pancreatic exocrine secretion, effects of gastric exclusion operations on (Thomas and Mason), 461
Parabiotic inhibition of murine sarcoma growth (Feraci and Schour), 430
Paralysis of deep radial (posterior interosseous) nerve, lipoma, cause of: report of case and review of literature (Wu, Jordan, and Eckert), 790
Paramedical personnel, in organ procurement, role of (Belzer) (editorial), 315
Parathyroid gland, transplanted: evaluation of cryopreservation and other environmental factors which affect its function (Wells and Christiansen), 49
  hormone by chlorpropamide, altered action of (Neumann and Moses), 869
Parenchymal and capsular histidine decarboxylase activity and weights, host splenic and allograft, following renal allografting in rats, elevation in (Moore et al.), 203
Patient, critically ill, cardiorespiratory effects of hypertonic glucose in (Pindyck et al.), 11
Pentagastrin-stimulated innervated and denervated gastric mucosa, effect of endogenous secretin and cholecystokinin on (Dorighi, Kaminski, and Willman), 755
Perforation, spontaneous, of extrahepatic bile ducts and bile peritonitis in infancy (Lilly, Weintraub, and Altman), 664
Perfusion, bloodless, hypothermic, prolonged survival of canine orthotopic small intestinal allografts preserved for 24 hours by (Toledo-Pereyra et al.), 368
  capillary, pulmonary, factors altering (Schwartz et al.), 750
  extended, further development and results of: simplified kidney preservation system (Hardie et al.), 651
  hypothermic, asanguineous, total body, successful reversal of lethal carbon monoxide intoxication by (Agostini et al.), 213
  kidney, canine, nonpulsatile vs. pulsatile (Grundmann et al.), 178
  techniques, surgical preparation, and cryoprotectants used in successful freezing of kidney (Rebelo et al.), 319
Perineal sinus, persistent, prevention and treatment of (Silen and Glotzer), 535
Peripheral vascular surgery, simple and inexpensive tunneler for use in (Blumenberg and Gelfand), 305
Peritonitis, bile, in infancy, spontaneous perforation of extrahepatic bile ducts and (Lilly, Weintraub, and Altman), 664

Peroneal-tibial arteries by a single lateral approach, exposure of (Dardik et al.), 377
Personnel, paramedical, in organ procurement, role of (Belzer) (editorial), 315
Pharyngeal, laryngeal, and oral cancer, deglutition after resection of (Doberneck and Antoine), 87
Plaster of Paris, protection of skin of fracture patients immobilized in (Boroda and Mouzas), 638
Platelet adhesion, inhibited: non-thrombogenic characteristic of heparin-coated surface (Lagergren, Olsson, and Swedenborg), 643
Pleuritis, starch: postthoracotomy syndrome possibly caused by surgical glove powder (Warshaw and Mills), 296
Pneumonia, lobar, experimental, in canine lung grafts (Schick et al.), 348
Polyposis, gastrointestinal, juvenile, in female infant: report of case and review of literature of recently recognized syndrome (Sachatello et al.), 107
Portacaval shunt in cirrhotic rat, liver arterialization with (Lecompte et al.), 161
Portal vein occlusion, reticuloendothelial dysfunction and endotoxemia following (Olcay et al.), 64
Potassium, body, total, in surgical patients (Shizgal, Kurtz, and Wood), 898
Powder, glove, surgical, postthoractomy syndrome possibly caused by: starch pleuritis (Warshaw and Mills), 296
Prepyloric digaphragm, congenital incomplete, in infants and children (Keramidas), 690
Preservation, organ, program, regional, in New England area (Cho et al.), 528
  system, kidney, simplified: further development and results of extended perfusion (Hardie et al.), 651
Pressure-flow relationships, vascular, in denervated reimplanted lungs of dogs (Wagner et al.), 91
Primate, subhuman, hemodynamic effects of femoral venous occlusion in (Wright and Hobson), 453
  influence of vasopressin and topical bile salts on gastric mucosal barrier of (Ritchie), 853
Procurement, organ, role of paramedical personnel in (Belzer) (editorial), 315
Program, regional, organ preservation, in New England area (Cho et al.), 528
Prosthesis, vascular, nylon, for aortic replacement, fate of: 14 year follow-up study (Yaw et al.), 140
Pulmonary capillary perfusion, factors altering (Schwartz et al.), 750
  changes due to hemorrhagic shock: resuscitation with isotonic and hypertonic saline (Fulton and Fischer), 881
  embolism and deep vein thrombosis, postoperative: selective review and personal viewpoint (Skillman), 114
  hemorrhage secondary to renal failure: successful respiratory support in woman following: venoarterial bypass with membrane oxygenator (Hanson et al.), 557
Pulsatile vs. nonpulsatile canine kidney perfusion (Grundmann et al.), 178
Pulse contour vs. dye-dilution methods (Bradley) (letter to editors), 317

R

Radial (posterior interosseous) nerve, deep, lipoma, cause of paralysis of: report of case and review of literature (Wu, Jordan, and Eckert), 790
Radiospirometry, xenon-133, in electrophrenic respiration: diaphragm pacing (Forbes et al.) 398
Reimplantation and transplantation in the arts (Tosatti), 389
Rejection, accelerated, of 36 immediate posttransplant functioning machine-preserved human cadaveric kidneys (Moore et al.), 357
Renal allografting in rats, elevation in host splenic and in allograft parenchymal and capsular histidine decarboxylase activity and weights following (Moore et al.), 203
  allotransplantation, obturator intestinal obstruction following: relief with hyperosmolar enemas (Berger et al.), 746
  arteries, surgical correction of advanced fibromuscular dysplasia of (Belzer et al.), 31
  failure, successful respiratory support in woman following pulmonary hemorrhage secondary to: venoarterial bypass with membrane oxygenator (Hanson et al.), 557
  homotransplantation, simplified method of ureteroileotomy in (Marchioro and Tremann), 129
  transplantation, chronic salt-loading of donor and recipient in (Silber), 573
  vasculature following total renal artery occlusion, microangiography of (Brodman et al.), 734
Reply to letter to editor by Dardik (Drews), 630
Residency, length of (Carlson) (letter to editors), 318
Respiration, electrophrenic, xenon-138 radiospirometry in: diaphragm pacing (Forbes et al.), 398
Respiratory support, successful, in woman following pulmonary hemorrhage secondary to renal failure: venoarterial bypass with a membrane oxygenator (Hanson et al.), 557
Reticuloendothelial dysfunction and endotoxemia following portal vein occlusion (Olcay et al.), 64
Rewriting and by-line: is author the writer? (DeBakey), 38

S

Saline, isotonic and hypertonic, resuscitation with: pulmonary changes due to hemorrhagic shock (Fulton and Fischer), 881
Salt-loading, chronic, of donor and recipient in renal transplantation (Silber), 573
Salt, bile, topical, and vasopressin on gastric mucosal barrier of subhuman primate, influence of (Ritchie), 853
Saphenous vein autografts, autogenous, and bovine heterografts, experience with: alternatives for vascular access for hemodialysis (Haimov et al.), 447
Sarcoma, murine, growth, parabiotic inhibition of (Feraci and Schour), 430
Scientists and medical writing (Hewitt) (letter to editors), 802; reply (DeBakey), 802

Secretin and cholecystokinin, endogenous, on pentagastrin-stimulated innervated and denervated gastric mucosa, effect of (Dorighi, Kaminski, and Willman), 755
Secretion, exocrine, pancreatic, effects of gastric exclusion operations of (Thomas and Mason), 461
Secretory function, gastric, effect of small bowel bypass on: postintestinal exclusion hypersecretion, phenomenon in search of syndrome (Buchwald, Coyle, and Varco), 821
Section, vagal, comparison of intraoperative tests of completeness of (Grassi and Orecchia), 155
Sepsis, hypermetabolism in: correlation with fever and tachycardia (Halmagyi et al.), 763
Septal defects, atrial, nonoperative closure of (King and Mills), 383
Serum calcium, serum gastrin, and gastric acid secretion before and after parthyroidectomy for hyperparathyroidism (Stremple and Watson), 841
  gastrin, basal and food-stimulated, levels in man, effect of atropine on (Becker, Reeder, and Thompson), 701
Shock, burn, experimental, comparative efficacy of hypo-, iso-, and hypertonic sodium solutions in (Fox and Stanford), 71
  effect of adenosine triphosphate–magnesium chloride administration in (Chaudry et al.), 213
  hemorrhagic, canine, hemodynamics of terminal vascular bed in (Fronek and Witzel), 408
  hemorrhagic, pulmonary changes due to: resuscitation with isotonic and hypertonic saline (Fulton and Fischer), 881
Shunt, portacaval, in cirrhotic rat, liver arterialization with (Lecompte et al.), 161
Shunting, arteriovenous, after sympathectomy (Rhodes et al.) (letter to editors), 153; reply (Delaney and Scarpino), 154
Silicone rubber, implanted, morphology of connective tissue grown in response to: light and electron microscopic study (Hernández- Jáuregui, Esperanza-García, and González-Angulo), 631
Sinus, perineal, persistent, prevention and treatment of (Silen and Glotzer), 535
Skin of fracture patients immobilized in plaster of Paris, protection of (Boroda and Mouzas), 638
Sodium solutions, hypo-, iso-, and hypertonic, in experimental burn shock, comparative efficacy of (Fox and Stanford), 71
Splenic, host, and allograft parenchymal and capsular histidine decarboxylase activity and weights following renal allografting in rats, elevation in (Moore et al.), 203
Starch pleuritis: postthoracotomy syndrome possibly caused by surgical glove powder (Warshaw and Mills), 296
Steal, subclavian, syndrome, simplified correction of (LeVeen et al.), 299
Step, a single (Zuidema) (editorial), 626
Steroid therapy, colon perforation associated with (Sterioff et al.), 56
Stress at vascular anastomosis in relation to host artery: synthetic grafts diameter (Kinley et al.), 28
Subclavian steal syndrome, simplified correction of (LeVeen et al.), 299
Subdural hematoma, acute, factors affecting survival from (Richards and Hoff), 253
Subhuman primate, influence of vasopressin and topical bile salts on gastric mucosal barrier to (Ritchie), 853
Successful management of mycotic aortic aneurysm: report of case (Cooke and Ehrenfeld, 132
Surgeon, academic, and emergency department (Rutherford), 259
  young, dilemma (Dardik) (letter to editors), 630
Surgery, American, and Halsted (Hughes), 169
  coronary artery, and magnification (Glenn) (editorial), 629
  in twenty-first century (Dunphy), 332
  in university hospital in Great Britain, observation on practice of: broadening of vision (Tilney), 776
  vascular, peripheral, simple and inexpensive tunneler for use in (Blumenberg and (Gelfand), 305
Surgical anatomy (Skandalakis et al.) (editorial), 148
  clerkship in university hospital, are there educational advantages to? (Levitsky et al.), 908
  correction of advanced fibromuscular dysplasia of renal arteries (Belzer et al.), 31
  education, undergraduate, objectives and methods in (DePalma et al.), 915
  glove powder, postthoracotomy syndrome possibly caused by: starch pleuritis (Warshaw and Mills), 296
  infection, diminished, by systemic antibiotic administration in potentially contaminated operations (Polk) (editorial), 312
    emerging concepts in control of (Alexander), 934
  patients, total body potassium in (Shizgal, Kurtz, and Wood), 898
  preparation, perfusion techniques, and cryoprotectants used in successful freezing of kidney (Rebelo et al.), 319
  treatment of abdominal angina: review of 25 patients (Reul et al.), 682
  treatment due to microorganisms in bile, hazards of (Keighley et al.), 578
  vascular, microscrystalline collagen as topical hemostatic agent for (Abbott and Austen), 925
Sutures, stay, device for holding, and new vascular clamp: microvascular anastomosis (Acland), 185
Sympathectomy, arteriovenous shunting after (Rhodes et al.) (letter to editors), 153; reply (Delaney and Scarpino), 154
Syndrome, postintestinal exclusion hypersecretion, phenomenon in search of: effect of small bowel bypass on gastric secretory function (Buchwald, Coyle, and Varco), 821
  postthoracotomy, possibly caused by surgical glove powder: starch pleuritis (Warshaw and Mills), 296

Syndrome—Cont'd
recently recognized, juvenile gastrointestinal polyposis in female infant: report of case and review of literature of (Sachatello et al.), 107
subclavian steal, simplified correction of (LeVeen et al.), 299
Systemic antibiotic administration in potentially contaminated operations, diminished surgical infection by (Polk) (editorial), 312

T

Tachycardia and fever, correlation with: hypermetabolism in sepsis (Halmagyi et al.), 763
Techniques, perfusion, surgical preparation, and cryoprotectants used in successful freezing of kidney (Rebelo et al.), 319
Temperature, core, intraoperative, neonate's, method for maintaining (Shim and Halford), 416
Temporal artery, superficial, –to–middle cerebral artery anastomosis, physiologic factors in selection of patients for (Austin, Laffin, and Hayward), 861
Thrombocytopenia, ultrapore filter–induced (Gervin et al.), 566
Thrombogenic, non-, characteristic of heparin-coated surface: inhibited platelet adhesion (Lagergren, Olsson, and Swedenborg), 643
Thrombosis, vein, deep, postoperative, and pulmonary embolism: selective review and personal viewpoint (Skillman), 114
Thymidine incorporation in esophageal wounds of zinc-deficient rats (MacMahon et al.), 660
Tibial-peroneal arteries by a single lateral approach, exposure of (Dardik et al.), 377
Tissue, connective, grown in response to implanted silicone rubber, morphology of: light and electron microscopic study (Hernández-Jáuregui, Esperanza-García, and González-Angulo), 631
healing, of traumatized patients, gas tensions in (Heppenstall et al.), 874
lymphatic, correction of coagulation in hemophilic dog by transplantation of (Groth et al.), 725
and tumor responses, specific, of chimpanzees following immunization against human melanoma (Hornung and Krementz), 477
Transcholecystic extraction of residual calculi in common bile duct (Mazzariello), 338
Transfusion, massive, of stored blood, problems associated with (Collins), 271
Transplantation of lymphatic tissue, correction of coagulation in hemophilic dog by (Groth et al.), 725
and reimplantation in the arts (Tosatti), 389
renal, chronic salt-loading of donor and recipient in (Silber), 573
Transplanted parathyroid gland: evaluation of cryopreservation and other environmental factors which affect its function (Wells and Christiansen), 49
Trauma, craniocervical, blunt, delayed presentation of carotid intimal tear following (Crissey and Bernstein), 543
Traumatized patients, gas tensions in healing tissues of (Heppenstall et al.), 874
Treatment and prevention of acute hepatic encephalopathy by intravenous levodopa (Abramsky and Goldschmidt), 188
of severe metabolic alkalosis, intravenous infusion of hydrochloric acid for (Abouna et al.), 194
Tumor(s), beta-islet cell, of pancreas: results of study on 1,067 cases (Stefanini et al.), 597
growth, increasing, changes in vascularity with: blood supply of experimental liver metastases (Ackerman), 589
and tissue responses, specific, of chimpanzees following immunization against human melanoma (Hornung and Krementz), 477
vaccine, frozen, non-viable, neuraminidase-treated experimental cancer immunotherapy using (Rios and Simmons), 503
Tunneler, simple and inexpensive, for use in peripheral vascular surgery (Blumenberg and Gelfand), 305

U

Ultrapore filter–induced thrombocytopenia (Gervin et al.), 566
Undergraduate medical education in Great Britain (Philpott) (editorial), 150
surgical education, objectives and methods in (DePalma et al.), 915
University hospital, are there educational advantages to a surgical clerkship in? (Levitsky et al.), 908
in Great Britain, observation on practice of surgery in: broadening of vision (Tilney), 776
Ureteroileotomy in renal homotransplantation, simplified method of (Marchioro and Tremann), 129
Ureterosigmoid conduit urinary diversion (Lindenauer, Cerny, and Morley), 705
Urinary diversion, conduit, ureterosigmioid (Lindenauer, Cerny, and Morley), 705

V

Vaccine, tumor, frozen, non-viable, neuraminidase-treated, experimental cancer immunotherapy using (Rios and Simmons), 503
Vagal release of gastrin, direct measurement of (Becker et al.), 101
section, comparison of intraoperative tests of completeness of (Grassi and Orecchia), 155
structures at esophageal hiatus, identification of (Skandalakis et al.), 233
Vagotomist, adequate, how to be (Alexander-Williams) (editorial), 308
Vascular access for hemodialysis, alternatives for: experience with autogenous saphenous vein autografts and bovine heterografts (Haimov et al.), 447
anastomosis in relation to host artery, stress at: synthetic graft diameter (Kinley et al.), 28
bed, terminal, in canine hemorrhagic shock, hemodynamics of (Fronek and Witzel), 408
clamp, new, and device for holding stay sutures: microvascular anastomosis (Acland), 185

Vascular—Cont'd
pressure-flow relationships in denervated and reimplanted lungs of dogs (Wagner et al.), 91
prosthesis, nylon, for aortic replacement, fate of: 14 year follow-up study (Yaw et al.), 140
surgery, microcrystalline collagen as topical hemostatic agent for (Abbott and Austen), 925
peripheral, simple and inexpensive tunneler for use in (Blumenberg and Gelfand), 305
Vascularity with increasing tumor growth, changes in: blood supply of experimental liver metastases (Ackerman), 589
Vasculature, renal, following total renal artery occlusion, micoroangiography of (Brodman et al.), 734
Vasopressin and topical bile salts on gastric mucosal barrier of subhuman primate, influence of (Ritchie), 853
Vein occlusion, portal, reticuloendothelial dysfunction and endotoxemia following (Olcay et al.), 64
saphenous, autografts, autogenous, and bovine heterografts, experience with: alternatives for avascular access for hemodialysis (Haimov et al.), 447
thrombosis, deep, postoperative, and pulmonary embolism: selective review and personal viewpoint (Skillman), 114
Vena cava filter, Mobin-Uddin, routine venography in placement of: dual filter placement in patient with accessory vena filter (cardinal vein) (Kartchner and Bogosian), 137
Vena caval obstruction, inferior, caused by expansion of abdominal aortic aneurysm: report of case and review of literature (Snider, Porter, and Eidemiller), 613
Venoarterial bypass with membrane oxygenator: successful respiratory support in woman following pulmonary hemorrhage secondary to renal failure (Hanson et al.), 557
Venography, routine, in placement of Mobin-Uddin vena cava filter: dual filter placement in patient with accessory vena filter (cardinal vein) (Kartchner and Bogosian), 140
Venous drainage of ischemic kidney (Brodman et al.), 584
occlusion, femoral, in subhuman primate, hemodynamic effects of (Wright and Hobson), 453

W

Wounds, espophageal, of zinc-deficient rats, thymidine incorporation in (MacMahon et al.), 660
healing, dermal, studies, application in: Nomarski differential-interference contrast microscopy (Salthouse), 59
topical lipid protection of burned subjects and their (Jelenko et al.), 892
Writing, medical, and scientists (Hewitt) (letter to editors), 802; reply (DeBakey), 802

X

Xenon-133 radiospirometry in electrophrenic respiration: diaphragm pacing (Forbes et al.), 398

Z

Zinc-deficient rats, thymidine incorporation in esophageal wounds of (MacMahon et al.), 660